INFERTILITY COUNSELING

Infertility Counseling: A Comprehensive Handbook for Clinicians, Second Edition, is a comprehensive, multidisciplinary textbook for all health professionals providing care for individuals facing reproductive health issues. It is the most thorough and extensive book currently available for clinicians in the field of infertility counseling, providing an exhaustive and comprehensive review of topics. It addresses both the medical and psychological aspects of infertility, reviewing assessment approaches, treatment strategies, medical counseling issues, third-party reproduction, alternative family building, and postinfertility counseling issues. Each chapter follows the same format: introduction, historical overview, literature review, theoretical framework, identification of clinical issues, suggestions for therapeutic interventions, and future implication. This edition also includes extensive appendixes of psychological and legal tools useful to all clinicians, including an Internet database of resources and an extensive glossary of terminology.

Sharon N. Covington is an Assistant Clinical Professor in the Department of Obstetrics and Gynecology at the Georgetown University School of Medicine in Washington, DC. She is also currently the Director of Psychological Support Services at Shady Grove Fertility Reproductive Science Center in Rockville, Maryland. A clinical social worker and psychotherapist for more than thirty years, she practices individual, couple, and group psychotherapy as well as the highly specialized area of infertility counseling.

Linda Hammer Burns is an Assistant Professor in the Department of Obstetrics, Gynecology, and Women's Health at the University of Minnesota Medical School and the Director of Counseling Services at the Reproductive Medicine Center in Minneapolis, Minnesota. She has been a psychologist for more than twenty years, providing individual and couple counseling in women's health psychology, with a special focus on reproductive health psychology.

Infertility Counseling

A COMPREHENSIVE HANDBOOK FOR CLINICIANS

SECOND EDITION

Edited by

SHARON N. COVINGTON

Assistant Clinical Professor
Department of Obstetrics and Gynecology
Georgetown University School of Medicine
Washington, DC

LINDA HAMMER BURNS

Assistant Professor
University of Minnesota Medical School
Department of Obstetrics, Gynecology, and
Women's Health
Minneapolis, MN

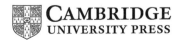
CAMBRIDGE
UNIVERSITY PRESS

CAMBRIDGE UNIVERSITY PRESS
Cambridge, New York, Melbourne, Madrid, Cape Town, Singapore, São Paulo

Cambridge University Press
32 Avenue of the Americas, New York, NY 10013-2473, USA

www.cambridge.org
Information on this title: www.cambridge.org/9780521853637

Second edition first published 2006

Printed in the United States of America

A catalog record for this publication is available from the British Library.

Library of Congress Cataloging in Publication Data

Infertility counseling : a comprehensive handbook for clinicians / edited by Sharon N.
Covington, Linda Hammer Burns. – 2nd ed.
  p. ; cm.
Includes bibliographical references and index.
ISBN-13: 978-0-521-85363-7 (hardback)
ISBN-10: 0-521-85363-X (hardback)
ISBN-13: 978-0-521-61949-3 (pbk.)
ISBN-10: 0-521-61949-1 (pbk.)
1. Infertility – Patients – Counseling of – Handbooks, manuals, etc.   I. Covington,
Sharon N.   II. Burns, Linda Hammer.
[DNLM: 1. Infertility – psychology.   2. Counseling.   3. Psychotherapy.
4. Reproductive Techniques, Assisted – psychology.   WP 570 I4363   2006]
RC889.I5615   2006
616.6'92–dc22   2006008215

ISBN-13   978-0-521-85363-7 hardback
ISBN-10   0-521-85363-X hardback

ISBN-13   978-0-521-61949-3 paperback
ISBN-10   0-521-61949-1 paperback

For our husbands,

Barry Truitt Covington and Sheldon Robert Burns,

and our growing families,

Brendan Truitt Covington, Laura Stratford Covington,

Michelle Covington Harmon, Scott Newcomer Harmon;

and Sean Covington Harmon;

Evan Robert Burns, Alicen Burns Spaulding,

and Stephen Alan Parlin Spaulding.

You will always be the wind beneath our wings.

Contents

List of Contributors

Sharon N. Covington, MSW
Assistant Clinical Professor
Department of Obstetrics and Gynecology
Georgetown University School of Medicine
Washington, DC USA

Director of Psychological Support Services
Shady Grove Fertility Reproductive Science Center
Rockville, MD USA

Linda Hammer Burns, PhD
Assistant Professor
University of Minnesota Medical School
Department of Obstetrics, Gynecology, and Women's
  Health
Minneapolis, MN USA

Director of Counseling Services
Reproductive Medicine Center
Minneapolis, MN USA

Linda D. Applegarth, EdD
Associate Professor of Psychology
Departments of Obstetrics & Gynecology,
  Reproductive Medicine, and Psychiatry
Weill Medical College of Cornell University
New York, NY USA

Director of Psychological Services
Institute for Reproductive Medicine
Weill Medical College of Cornell University
The New York Presbyterian Hospital
New York, NY USA

Eric Blyth, PhD
Professor of Social Work
University of Huddersfield
Huddersfield, England, UK

Jacky Boivin, PhD
Senior Lecturer and Associate Professor
Cardiff University

School of Psychology
Cardiff, Wales, UK

Dorothy A. Greenfeld, MSW
Associate Clinical Professor
Department of Obstetrics and Gynecology
Yale University School of Medicine
New Haven, CT USA

Director of Psychological Services
Yale Fertility Center
New Haven, CT USA

Jacqueline N. Gutmann, MD
Clinical Associate Professor
Associate Director, Division of Reproductive
  Endocrinology
Thomas Jefferson University
Philadelphia, PA USA

Jean M. Haase, MSW
Social Worker
Reproductive Endocrinology and Infertility
  Program
University Hospital
London Health Sciences Centre
London, ON Canada

Hilary Hanafin, PhD
Director of Counseling Services
Center for Surrogate Parenting
Beverly Hills, CA USA

Michaela Hynie, PhD
Associate Professor
Department of Psychology
York University
Toronto, ON Canada

Nancy Stowe Kader, RN, PhD
Director, Health Policy and Bioethics

Pal-Tech, Inc.
Arlington, VA USA

Roger D. Kempers
Professor of Obstetrics and Gynecology
Emeritus, Mayo Clinic School of Medicine
Rochester, MN USA

Immediate Past President IFFS
Past Medical Director
American Society for Reproductive Medicine
Editor Emeritus
Fertility and Sterility

William R. Keye, Jr., MD
Clinical Associate Professor
Department of Obstetrics and Gynecology
University of Michigan
Ann Arbor, MI USA

Director of the Division of Reproductive
   Endocrinology and Infertility
Department of Obstetrics and Gynecology
William Beaumont Hospital
Royal Oak, MI USA

Sheryl A. Kingsberg, PhD
Associate Professor
Departments of Reproductive Biology and Psychiatry
Case Western Reserve University School of Medicine
Cleveland, OH USA

Chief, Division of Behavioral Medicine
Department of Obstetrics and Gynecology
University Hospitals of Cleveland
Cleveland, OH USA

Susan Caruso Klock, PhD
Associate Professor
Departments of Clinical Obstetrics & Gynecology and
   Psychiatry
Northwestern University Medical School
Chicago, IL USA

Psychologist
Northwestern Medical Faculty Foundation
Reproductive Endocrinology and Infertility Program
Chicago, IL USA

Donald B. Maier, MD
Associate Professor
Division of Reproductive Endocrinology and
   Infertility
Department of Obstetrics and Gynecology
University of Connecticut Health Center
Farmington, CT USA

Director, Division of Reproductive Endocrinology
   and Infertility
St. Francis Hospital and Medical Center
Hartford, CT USA

Louise U. Maier, PhD
Psychologist
Private Practice
Avon, CT USA

Christopher R. Newton, PhD
Assistant Professor
Departments of Obstetrics & Gynecology and
   Psychology
University of Western Ontario
London, ON Canada

Psychologist
University Hospital, London Health Sciences
   Centre
London, ON Canada

William D. Petok, PhD
Assistant Clinical Professor
Department of Obstetrics and Gynecology
University of Colorado Health Sciences
   Center
Denver, CO USA

Psychologist
Private Practice
Baltimore, MD USA

Krista Redlinger-Grosse, ScM
Instructor
Genetic Counseling Graduate Program
University of Minnesota
Minneapolis, MN USA

Genetic Counselor
Fairview-University Maternal Fetal Medicine
   Center
Minneapolis, MN USA

Patricia L. Sachs, MSW
Social Worker
Shady Grove Fertility Reproductive Science
   Center
Rockville, MD USA

Covington & Hafkin and Associates
Rockville, MD USA

Linda P. Salzer, MSS
Social Worker
Private Practice
Englewood, NJ USA

Gretchen Sewall, RN, LICSW
Health Promotion and Counseling Service
Seattle Reproductive Medicine
Seattle, WA USA

President
Donor Secure
Edmonds, WA USA

Cheri Schoonveld, MS
Assistant Professor
Genetic Counseling Graduate Program
University of Minnesota
Minneapolis, MN USA

Genetic Counselor
Fairview-University Maternal Fetal Medicine Center
Minneapolis, MN USA

Margaret E. Swain, RN, JD
Attorney
Private Practice
Baltimore, MD USA

Janet E. Takefman, PhD
Assistant Professor
Department of Obstetrics & Gynecology
McGill University
Montreal, QC Canada

Director of Psychological Services
McGill Reproductive Centre
Montreal, QC Canada

Petra Thorn, PhD
Psychologist
Private Practice
Moerfelden, Germany

Affiliated Lecturer
Protestant University of Applied
  Sciences
Darmstadt, Germany

Christianne Verhaak, PhD
Psychologist
Department of Medical Psychology and
  Obstetrics & Gynecology
Radboud University Medical Center
Nijmegen, The Netherlands

Katherine E. Williams, MD
Clinical Instructor, Associate Director
Department of Psychiatry & Behavioral
  Sciences
Behavioral Neuroendocrinology Program
Women's Wellness Center
Stanford University School of Medicine
Stanford, CA USA

Laurel N. Zappert, MS
Clinical Research Associate
Stanford University
Department of Psychiatry & Behavioral
  Sciences
Stanford, CA USA

Foreword

It is remarkable to see how much the specialty of infertility counselinghas matured and established itself since the publication, just six years ago, of the first edition of this important book. I was privileged then, as I am again now, to write the Foreword for this textbook, which has become the standard of reference for the profession. As noted by the editors in their preface, the continuing enthusiasm that has welcomed this text both nationally and internationally has created the demand to bring all critical chapters up to today's leading edge of knowledge, as well as to add several relevant and important new ones in this second edition.

Today, with the continued rapid advances in the assisted reproductive technologies, there is a much clearer recognition of the psychosocial issues that may arise over the course of treatment for infertile patients as well as the critical role played in their management by mental health professionals. Infertility counseling has become an indispensable adjunct to the practice of reproductive medicine, particularly in those countries at the forefront of new developments in the field. It is gratifying to see that over recent years, infertility counseling has gained appropriate recognition on an even broader international level, which is addressed in depth in Chapter 31, Global Perspectives on Infertility Counseling. Of note has been the collegial networking internationally among national counseling organizations and mental health professionals that ultimately led to the formation of an international association, the International Infertility Counseling Organization (IICO). IICO continues to grow and evolve, and currently it is made up of national organizations from ten countries. IICO has a liaison with the International Federation of Fertility Societies (IFFS) and also meets regularly in conjunction with the annual meetings of other major infertility organizations, such as the American Society for Reproductive Medicine (ASRM) and the European Society of Human Reproduction and Embryology (ESHRE). Within its educational mission, IICO provides postgraduate courses with national and international congresses as well as symposia, workshops, and social gatherings. These efforts generate informative dialogue among both medical and mental health professionals concerning critical legislation and regulations in other countries, practice guidelines, credentialing of mental health professionals, research on the psychosocial aspects of infertility and medical treatment outcomes, and creating standards of practice in infertility counseling worldwide.

All infertility professionals are indebted to coeditors Sharon N. Covington, MSW, and Linda Hammer Burns, PhD, as well as their distinguished contributing authors for making this textbook as complete and comprehensive as it is, covering the breadth and scope of the field. This new second edition will, ultimately, make it possible to provide superior clinical care for all patients worldwide. Not only have the editors provided an invaluable service to their discipline by fostering this important text, but they both continue to provide strong leadership in medical organizations at both the national and international levels. Linda Hammer Burns has played an indispensable role in organizing IICO and is currently its chair. Sharon Covington has been equally active as a founding member of the Mental Health Professional Group (MHPG) of ASRM, serving on many ASRM committees, including the Society of Asssisted Reproductive Technologies (SART) Executive committee and as chair, along with Linda Hammer Burns, of the MHPG of the ASRM. Both have contributed their expertise through contributions to other professional texts and as reviewers for respected journals in the field, in addition to their mentoring of mental health professionals and clinicians new to the field of reproductive health counseling.

I have known and admired them both for many years, going back to the time when I was editor-in-chief of *Fertility and Sterility* and it was my pleasure to be able to publish a number of Sharon Covington's important juried scientific contributions, as well as calling on both as reviewers. Through their tireless efforts and devotion to excellence, both have distinguished themselves in advancing their field and helping to establish infertility counseling as an indispensable discipline in the integrated care of infertility patients.

This book will benefit all who read it. As I wrote in my previous Foreword, it is designed for serious students and practitioners of infertility counseling. It will be a valuable resource text for medical libraries and will grace the personal libraries of mental health professionals, students of reproductive medicine, clinicians, and educators alike.

Roger D. Kempers
February, 2006

Preface

When we wrote (edited) the first edition of this book, our motivation was simple and straightforward: to provide a definitive textbook on infertility counseling. We had worked in the field for a number of years, nurtured its growth and development as a professional specialty, and mentored many entering the field, yet there was no single, scholarly text for professionals. So, with this simple idea the original text was born. Little did we realize the impact it would have on the profession of infertility counseling, the field of reproductive medicine, or on us, both professionally and personally. We are still amazed when we hear (as we have many times) people around the world refer to it as 'the purple bible.' This text is not an updated version of the original book, as is often the case, but a new book entirely that offers updated versions of each chapter as well as several new topics. This is not to say we did not think all of the topics from the original book were not important or relevant, but only that limits of space necessitated a reshuffling. As such, the original text will remain relevant and the new one of equal and parallel importance.

Since the first edition was published, the profession of infertility counseling has evolved and so have our own professional perspectives. One of the most significant changes has been the development of an international perspective on infertility counseling. This has been triggered by our own travel instincts (and Linda's predilection for visiting infertility clinics wherever she travels) but also interest in our textbook that has brought us contacts, questions, and requests for consultations from around the world. Recognizing this, Linda spearheaded the formation of the International Infertility Counseling Organization (IICO) – with the support and helpful guidance of Sharon who was a founding member of the Mental Health Professional Group of the American Society of Reproductive Medicine. Although IICO continues to experience (as all new organizations) growing pains, it has been successful in bringing together professionals from around the world, providing educational opportunities and a mechanism for professional collaboration, and fostering the development of new infertility counseling societies. Dr. Roger Kempers, who was so very helpful during his tenure at ASRM and supportive of our first book, has been equally, if not more, helpful in the development of IICO in his position as chair of the International Federation of Fertility Societies (IFFS). We owe him a special debt of gratitude not only for his professional and personal support, but for his unyielding validation of the professional development of infertility counseling and a collaborative approach to treatment of infertile patients in acknowledging the importance of psychosocial aspects of infertility.

It was not particularly surprising, as such, when our ever loyal editor, Nat Russo, approached us with his usual enthusiasm and insistence about updating the original text but with a more international perspective. Although we willingly embraced the idea, little did we realize then how this new approach would exponentially complicate the project, creating new and unique challenges for us – as well as our contributors.

To our contributors who met these challenges with varying degrees of dread and/or excitement, we owe a very special thank you. All are respected (and busy) professionals in their own right and their efforts here are exceptional. We appreciate each of them for their professional expertise, effort, and time. A special thanks to those who provided extra doses of personal encouragement and kindness – especially when our own spirits or stamina waned. Many of the contributors have played significant roles in the professional development of infertility counseling worldwide and continue to do so through an array of professional activities. While many contributors were authors in the first edition, some are new to this volume and, as such, faced unanticipated hurdles and problems. Despite the distinct trials and travails of this edition, we wish to express our appreciation for each author's willingness to contribute their expertise and knowledge and for their patience and tolerance of our suggestions, critiques, and 'improvements' of their work. Although we realize we have become rather notoriously exacting editors (applying the same exacting standards to our own work), we hope (and think) that despite our often rigorous demands, we have kept their friendships and they are well aware of our very deep appreciation.

As before, we must also thank our respective practices and colleagues. Over the years, Sharon has seen her practice expand at Shady Grove Fertility Reproductive Science Center from one office, one doctor, and five staff members, to one of the largest practices in the United States with eight offices, eighteen physicians, and more than 250 employees . . . and still growing. The list of all the important people at Shady Grove who have helped and supported me along the way is too extensive to include, yet a few (though not exclusively) stand out: Dr. Robert Stillman, Dr. Michael Levy, Dr. Eric Widra, and Dr. Arthur Sagoskin for helping me define the collaborative reproductive healthcare model through their respect and belief in psychological services (and me); and nurses Karen Moore, Kathy Bugge, and Michele Purcell for their exceptional skill, compassion, and encouragement in our work together over the years. Just as important are the extraordinary group of clinical social workers who have joined me in my practice – Patricia Sachs, Carol Toll, Ellen Eule, Erica Hanson, Michelle Hester, and Carol Miller. They have been patient with me throughout this revision, picked up extra work without complaint, always kept their good nature despite my distraction, and continued to remind me of the importance of this project. I would also like to thank Dr. Larry Nelson at the National Institutes of Health for giving me the opportunity to work on his research team, and for his commitment to the psychological needs of women struggling with premature ovarian failure. Special appreciation goes to Nancy Hafkin, PhD, my friend of more than forty years and cotherapist for more than twenty, for helping (and putting up with) me throughout this process with patience, humor, and when needed, clinical interpretation. Thanks, also, to Linda Applegarth, EdD, who was a personal friend before we began to share the journey in our professional careers of infertility counseling and whose understanding and support have been so important to me along the way. I feel so blessed to have had the opportunity to do work that I love with people that I love working with.

Linda has remained at the University of Minnesota Medical School, Department of Obstetrics, Gynecology, and Women's Health, and the Reproductive Medicine Center. Although he is retired now, special thanks will always be owed to Dr. George Tagatz, who decades ago offered me a job and allowed me to design and implement an infertility counseling program that became an integral part of patient care and the model and impetus for this book. Dr. Theodore (Ted) Nagel was there that day when Dr. Tagatz asked (on behalf of both of them), "Linda, how would you like to work here?" And despite the vicissitudes of our respective careers, we are both still here – in large part due to Dr. Nagel's determined refusal to allow either of us to retire – even when it seemed like a good idea. Over the years, I have come to appreciate not only his professional mentoring but his quick wit, extraordinary intelligence, and personal kindness. He has, more than any other colleague, tolerated my big ideas (even when skeptical) and supported my various other commitments and interests without complaint – and more often than not, offered his own ideas and insights. In addition, there are other professionals including physicians, nurses, and secretarial staff who have, over the decades, provided rewarding and edifying professional as well as personal relationships. These include, but, of course, are not limited to, Dr. Mark Damario; Bonnie Le Roy, MS; Mary Ahrens, MS; Selina Blatz, NP; Mary Danich, NP; Rosie Drechnik, NP; Deb Pearo, RN; Neda Tasson, RN; Rachel Radman; and Kim Hockett. In addition, I owe a very special debt of gratitude to colleague, mentor, and friend Sue V. Petzel, PhD. She has been there from the very beginning as an exceptionally talented mentor and colleague who I not only appreciate but respect immensely. Now, after years of astutely avoiding the field of infertility counseling, she too has become intrigued with the field and the fascinating patients we assist. A simple thank you is really inadequate and, as such, it is my hope that she is well aware of how grateful I am for her professional guidance and personal friendship. Finally, I feel especially privileged and blessed to have had a career that has been so intellectually stimulating and professionally rewarding and has allowed me to work with colleagues who not only gave me respect and support, but an enjoyable camaraderie.

As we continue to practice as infertility counselors, we realize that it is our patients who have provided us with the clinical experience and expertise to enable us to contribute to this field through professional development and writing. As such, we owe a special debt of gratitude to our patients, both past and present. In their suffering and resilience they taught us, and from their pain and transcendence we learned. We feel honored and privileged to have been included in their journeys through infertility, pregnancy loss, childlessness, and for many, eventual parenthood. We are who we are today and who we have become (personally and professionally) because of these special clients, and this project (as with the previous book) would have been impossible without them.

It goes without saying that we are grateful to our families to whom we are not simply indebted – we are probably overdrawn! Through the journey of this book, we have seen the birth of Sharon's first grandchild and the marriage of Linda's daughter – in the same month! Throughout the usual family transitions, personal and family crises, professional challenges, and daily hassles, our families have helped us keep our equilibrium (sometimes tenuously) with their steadfast love and support. Once again, our children offered generous assistance – even though they are now young adults with lives of their own and live (most of them) at some distance. Again, our children were our computer experts (not only for us but for our contributors), research assistants, secretarial staff, and general *aides-de-camp*. We wrote through wedding plans, baby preparations, babysitting, computer crashes, cross-country relocations, and natural disasters with our single-minded determination, creating only slight (albeit justified) grumbles. Our husbands, despite their own crises and challenges, have never wavered in their support of our work and this project, providing limitless encouragement and comfort. More than anyone else, they have borne the brunt of the stressful challenges of this book, tolerating our self-imposed work schedules, including working during vacations, filling in on a myriad of responsibilities that

we were forced to relinquish, and yet still they always supplied us with kindness, love, and a sense of humor – particularly when our spirits lagged or our nerves were frayed. Once again, this book is dedicated to our very special husbands and families including our newest members, because it could never have happened without their blessing, love, and hard work, in addition to our own.

Finally, we must thank each other. It was Sharon who noted that twice in her life she had "married someone I hardly knew" – once personally and once professionally – and both times it has led to exceptional, long-lasting 'marriages.' Our collaboration and collaborative abilities continue to mystify even us. Although we often felt at the end of our tethers and overwhelmed by the work, we never felt that way with each other. We have never disagreed or had a different vision of what this book could or should be. Somehow, despite both positive and negative stressors in our personal and professional lives, we were able to remain focused and working – usually due to large doses of humor and Sharon's ever present reminder to 'just breathe.' The qualities that helped us through the first book (communication, intelligence, good humor, and work ethic) have also made this book possible. And as before, we not only learned to appreciate each other more, but we also learned a great deal about ourselves. For its own unique reasons, this book *was* more challenging than the last, yet also more rewarding. In the end, we are not only appreciative and proud of the work we have produced here, but of the friendship and collaboration that enabled it.

Sharon N. Covington
Linda Hammer Burns

1 Psychology of Infertility

LINDA HAMMER BURNS AND SHARON N. COVINGTON

A child within my mind. I see
The eye, the hands. I see you also there.
I see you waiting with an honest care,
Within my mind, within my body....

– Elizabeth Jennings

Yearning for children and the heartbreak of barrenness have been a part of life since the beginning of mankind, chronicled throughout history by religious accounts, myths, legends, art, and literature. Whether driven by biological drive, social necessity, or psychological longing, the pursuit of a child or children has compelled men and women to seek a variety of remedies, sometimes even extreme measures. In fact, in all cultures involuntary childlessness is recognized as a crisis that has the potential to threaten the stability of individuals, relationships, and communities. Every society has culturally approved solutions to infertility involving, either alone or together, alterations of social relationships (e.g., divorce or adoption), spiritual intercession (e.g., prayer or pilgrimage to spiritually powerful site), or medical interventions (e.g., taking of herbs or consultation with 'medicine man').[1] While spiritual and medical remedies for infertility are common and often used early on by infertile couples, social solutions demanding the alteration of relationships have been shown to be the last alternative individuals or couples usually consider.[1] Typically, infertile couples are reluctant to jeopardize or disturb close relationships (perhaps because social changes are usually permanent) because they hope or believe infertility will be a temporary problem. By the same token, reluctance to consider solutions may be due to the hope and promise often attributed to medical and/or spiritual interventions. Nonetheless, infertile couples use all three measures – social, spiritual, and medical – as remedies for their involuntary childlessness; numerous examples of these remedies exist throughout history and across all cultures.[1] One of the most renowned social solutions to involuntary childlessness is King Henry VIII of England, who changed the religion and laws of a country to accommodate the need for a child (albeit a male child).

Divorce, polygamy, and extramarital affairs remain, as they have long been, social solutions to infertility, as do various forms of adoption and fostering. Examples of other social solutions include the continuing practice in some cultures of multiple wives in response to infertility (or lack of a son) or the custom in some cultures requiring a sibling (usually an eldest son) to provide one of his children to a younger, childless sibling. Community involvement in the realignment of social relationships is exemplified by the native peoples of two small islands off the coast of South America in which infertility was addressed by raiding the neighboring island to steal small children for childless women. Demonstrable in each of these examples is the social and emotional distress and expense of solutions involving the alteration of social relationships, thus explaining, in part, the reluctance of individuals to pursue these alternatives until other remedies have been exhausted.

Since antiquity, the appeal of religious faith and the power of belief in spirits and gods as a remedy for infertility can be found in all cultures. Fertility symbols, special gods, and fertility rites and customs are apparent from the highly erotic art of India, to the Celtic goddess of fertility carved into stoned walls of ancient Irish castles, to specially shaped and painted Navajo pottery. In ancient Greece, a common offering to the gods was terracotta votives in the shape of the affected organ (e.g., vagina, uterus, or penis).[2] In addition, the special spiritual power of certain places to enhance fertility can be seen in a phallic-shaped rock on the island of Maui in Hawaii; as well as in the pilgrimages made by infertile women of the Carib tribe in Mexico to Isla de las Mujeres (Island of Women) and by many infertile Roman Catholic women to Medjugorje in Bosnia-Herzegovina. Nevertheless, the importance of faith either as a means of solving infertility or as a source of comfort cannot be minimized, and religious faith remains a powerful resource (or painful burden) for many infertile individuals around the world, even today.

Infertility affects between 80 million and 168 million people in the world today. Approximately one in ten couples experience primary and/or secondary infertility.[3,4] The majority of men and women live in the developing world, are infertile due to sexually transmitted diseases or underlying, untreated health conditions (e.g., malnuitrition) while in the developing world increasing age in women is a major causal factor in infertility.[5] Global rates of infertility vary dramatically – from prevalence rates of about 5% in some developed countries to as high as more than 30% in sub-Saharan Africa.[6] Rates of primary infertility worldwide are generally 1 to 8% with rates of secondary infertility reaching as high as 35%. The rates of infertility are the highest in the world in what has been termed the 'infertility belt,' stretching across central and southern Africa.[7]

Although infertility is a global issue impacting individual and social well-being, the wide variance in incidence rates contributes to significant and unique psychosocial consequences as a result of *where* an individual experiences involuntary childlessness. This 'stratification of infertility' refers to the ways in which the infertility experience is affected by economic, social welfare, and public health issues. These issues include the preponderance of poverty, malnutrition, obesity, smoking, sexually transmitted diseases, or other conditions that impact general health and/or fertility; ignorance of reproduction, sexual health, and/or fertility preservation; lack of availability or access to high-quality medical treatments; and/or the inability to access medical treatments for cultural, religious, or legislative reasons. Any and all of these factors can and do contribute to infertile individuals traveling across national or international borders in pursuit of medical treatments to facilitate reproduction and/or parenthood – a phenomenon often termed 'reproductive tourism.' In short, as a global condition, infertility is not only a medical condition but also a social and emotional condition, in which a shift in emphasis has occurred from coping with childlessness through social means (e.g., participating in rearing the children of others) to a dependence on medical interventions – even when accessing them can be challenging.[8] This process has been referred to as the 'medicalization of infertility' – the phenomenon in which healthy, yet childless, individuals become patients, undergoing an array of medical treatments and assuming the passive patient role in patient–physician interactions – all in pursuit of parenthood.[9]

Infertility counseling, as an emergent specialty within the mental health professions, has gained recognition and respect for its professional contributions through patient care, research, and education as well as for the identification of the need for expert care and treatment of this unique population in conjunction with complex medical treatment. In this book the term *infertility counselor* refers to any mental health professional (e.g., social worker, family therapist, psychiatrist, or psychologist) who has special training in reproductive medicine. In fact, a major goal and purpose of this book is to define the standard of care and practice, professional competency, and legal responsibilities for infertility counselors worldwide by providing a knowledge base on which to provide optimum clinical care with evidence-based therapeutic interventions.

As a clinical textbook, this book provides a comprehensive overview of the array of clinical issues and therapeutic interventions useful for the practicing infertility counselor as well as for the mental health professional who encounters a few patients with reproductive issues (current or past) requiring a clinical understanding of the relevant issues. This textbook (like its predecessor) has eight sections that reflect the breadth of the experience and issues confronted by individuals and couples experiencing infertility: assessment; treatment modalities; medical counseling issues; third-party reproduction and other means of alternative family building; postinfertility issues; and infertility counseling practice issues. Each chapter follows the same format regardless of the topic addressed in the chapter: an introduction to the topic, historical overview, review of the literature, clinical issues, therapeutic interventions, and future implications. This format is designed to provide both students and professionals with a consistent and predictable treatment of each topic and a basis for comparison across topics, thereby enabling optimum and professionally competent clinical care using evidence-based practice principles. This chapter outlines the scope and depth of issues involved in infertility counseling including:

■ A historical overview of medical approaches to infertility and the emergence of infertility counseling in collaborative patient care;

■ A review of advances in the scientific study of psychological responses to infertility;

■ A discussion of the importance of theoretical frameworks as a basis for developing clinical interventions, including relevant infertility-specific psychological theories; and

■ A summary of clinical issues and therapeutic interventions, which will provide a context for the chapters in this text.

HISTORICAL OVERVIEW

The Trobrian Islanders attributed pregnancy to spirits, not sexual intercourse. Chukchi female shamans said they made children via their sacred stones, not through sexual intercourse or any contribution from men. Australian Ingarda peoples thought women became pregnant by eating special foods or by embracing a sacred tree hung with umbilical cords from previous births. The Batak peoples believed no woman could become pregnant unless umbilical cords and placentas were buried under her house.[10] Ancient Hindus believed that conception was facilitated by the worship of the *lingam* (erect penis) and *yoni* (female genitalia) and that a hole in a rock or cloven tree symbolized the female birth passage. Therefore, a woman could improve her fertility by passing through a hole in trees or rocks – a ritual that continues to be practiced in some parts of the world even today.[11]

Women in ancient Africa were encouraged to eat the eye of a hyena with licorice and dill to aid conception that was guaranteed to occur within three days while Siberian women were encouraged to eat spiders to facilitate conception.[11] According to African custom, to ensure pregnancy men applied a special powder made from the crushed roots of nine trees to the penis to enable sexual intercourse three times a night, while African women used vaginal pessaries made of wool dipped in peanut oil and wrapped in two cloves of garlic.[12] In ancient Arabia, amulets and/or fertility symbols were commonly worn as pendants to encourage conception, particularly by Egyptian women. Additionally, many cultures used fertility fetishes and symbols such as statuettes of pregnant females or of males with large phalluses to maximize fertility.[11] Even today, amulets, herbal remedies, and traditional rituals continue to be used by many infertile men and women, often in conjunction with conventional medical treatment, in hopes of achieving the longed-for pregnancy (child).

In antiquity, menstruation and fertility were believed to be influenced by the waxing and waning of the moon. As a result, astrology and numerology were considered important fertility treatments by providing correct numbers and/or days of the month for maximizing fertility and achieving pregnancy. It is generally accepted that ancient peoples had little understanding of human reproduction and as such sterility. With little understanding of the equal contributions of male and female reproductive cells or the role of sexual intercourse in fertilization, reproduction was thought to be a singularly female phenomenon and the role of the male was considered unnecessary and/or ceremonial. This ignorance probably contributed to valuing women for their reproductive abilities but also to blaming women when conception and pregnancy failed. Throughout history and across cultures, there are countless examples of social, religious, and cultural glorification, even idealization of motherhood, and the vilification and maltreatment of infertile or 'barren' women. Infertile women were (and still may be) accused of witchcraft; socially isolated and ostracized; physically abused; divorced, abandoned, or forced to accept their husband's additional wives; or murdered (often by their husband or their husband's family). In Japanese, the word for infertile women is *umazume*, which is literally translated as 'stone woman.' The characters used spell 'no-life woman' or 'nonbirthing woman.' *Umazume* is considered one of the worst words in the entire Japanese language and it is rarely used because, according to traditional custom, the presence of a stone woman could make a whole village wither.[13] In various African, Asian, and Pacific cultures men fear(ed) female vaginal blood, which is not only viewed as polluting but also thought to weaken any man touched by it.[14]

Science altered our understanding of reproduction and fertility when, in 1677, Dutch scientist Anton Leeuwenhoek became the first to identify spermatozoa with the newly invented microscope. In 1765, through experiments with dogs, Italian priest and physiologist Lazzaro Spallanzani became the first to discover that mammalian reproduction required both the male sperm and female oocyte, that is, that the embryo was the "product of male seed, nurtured in the soil of the female."[15] However, it was not until the nineteenth century that human reproduction (and infertility) became more clearly illuminated. In 1826, German biologist Karl von Baer discovered the mammalian oocyte and identified mammalian embryonic development of animals. Together with Heinz Christian Pander and based on the work by Caspar Friedrich Wolff, he described the germ-layer theory of embryological development and the principles that became the foundation for comparative embryology.[16] The next year, Swiss physiologist and histologist Albert von Kolliker identified the function of spermatozoa and that sperm originated from the testes. In 1839, Augustus Gendrin suggested that ovulation controlled menstruation, thereby dispelling the long-standing belief that menstruation was controlled by the moon and lunar phases.

By the early twentieth century, the pieces of the reproductive puzzle were beginning to fall into place. Still, it was only in the middle of the twentieth century and later that physicians medically addressed infertility as a couples issue in which both partners were medically evaluated rather than viewed as a woman's medical problem (defect).[17] Nevertheless, infertility treatment continued to maintain a paradigmatic example of a medical situation in which throughout much of its history physicians were men, patients were women, and the focus of medical treatment was on the sexual organs.[8] Despite evidence that men were and are infertile as often as women, throughout history and across cultures, women have disproportionately borne the medical, social, and cultural burden of a couple's failure to conceive. This is a situation that has become even more prominent with the advent of assisted reproductive technologies in which the female partner undergoes disproportionately more treatment, regardless of the etiology of the infertility diagnosis.[8] This paradigm did not dramatically shift despite the advent of assisted reproductive technology (ART), which began with the birth of Louise Brown in Great Britain in 1978. Her conception via in vitro fertilization (IVF) was the result of the groundbreaking work of British physicians Patrick Steptoe and Robert Edwards which began the modern era of human reproduction in which reproduction did not require sexual intercourse, used an array of assisted reproductive technologies, and could be facilitated by various forms of donated gametes, embryos, and surrogacy.

Infertility counseling, as a profession, emerged almost in tandem with the major medical advancements in the field of reproductive medicine, particularly assisted and third-party reproduction. Although the psychological impact of infertility was addressed in the literature beginning in the 1930s, infertility counseling has emerged as a recognized profession and mental health specialty only within the past thirty years.[18] Historically, the role of the mental health professional in the treatment of infertility was to cure the infertile patient's neurosis thereby curing their infertility. This approach fell into disfavor in the 1970s as mental health professionals working in infertility clinics began providing psychological support, crisis intervention, and education to ameliorate the stress of infertility and enhance the patient's quality of life.[19] Today, the role of the infertility counselor has expanded to meet the psychosocial challenges of assisted reproduction and includes assessment, support, treatment, education, research, and consultation.[18,20,21]

Throughout history and across cultures, medical solutions to infertility have been diverse and varied such as relics, charms, incantations, eating special foods, vaginal treatments, treatments to enhance male sexual potency, and special potions and/or poultices. Whether 'primitive' medical treatments or the more sophisticated assisted reproductive technologies of today, medical treatments for infertility have always been actively pursued and held particular power and influence for infertile couples. It may be argued that medical solutions to involuntary childlessness became even more powerful and appealing to the infertile by the end of the twentieth century with the advent of assisted reproductive technologies and advanced third-party reproduction.

REVIEW OF LITERATURE

Original investigations into the psychological aspects of infertility focused on individual psychopathology (particularly in women), sexual dysfunction, and infertility-specific distress. Furthermore, early research was largely based on theoretical speculations or anecdotal information rather than scientifically rigorous investigations. Much of the research focused on psychological distress, was exploratory, relied on researcher-designed instruments rather than standardized measures, lacked control or comparison groups, and was plagued by small numbers. While research on the medical aspects of infertility has expanded exponentially, research on the psychosocial aspects of infertility continues to lag behind by comparison. Nevertheless, the overall quality and quantity of studies have dramatically improved in recent decades with an increasing number of infertility counselors acting as researchers investigating a wider array of issues such as the impact of stress on infertility; gender differences in response to infertility; cross-cultural issues; and complicating medical conditions.

Recently, the focus of research on the psychological aspects of infertility has shifted from individual psychopathology to more holistic/interactive views of infertility and to the impact of advancing assisted reproductive technologies. Consequently, there has been a shift from a singular focus on the individual to assessments and interventions aimed at groups, such as couples and families. In addition, while research and clinical experience continue to indicate that the vast majority of infertile men and women do not experience significant levels of psychological trauma or psychopathology, the use of advanced medical technology and/or third-party reproduction involving a plethora of additional stressors may increase psychological distress during specific periods of the treatment cycle. As such, investigations into responses to assisted reproduction have involved the interactive aspects of medical technology and individual and couple response, as well as medical outcome. In addition, the focus of both medical and psychosocial research has become more 'evidence-based': how research findings can provide direction for the identification of clinical issues and therapeutic interventions that are most beneficial and effective.

Van Balen and Inhorn contend that research on the psychosocial aspects of infertility has historically been hampered because infertility was: (1) considered a medical condition rather than a social problem worthy of social analysis (particularly in Western societies); (2) a taboo subject not easily talked about even in 'neutral' research settings; (3) an issue emerging in Western societies at a time of changing social beliefs about parenthood, women's roles, and the importance of children in the lives of men and women; and (4) research-focused on psychosocial responses to assisted reproductive technologies and less on the experience of involuntary childlessness or 'disrupted reproduction' and its impact on the lives of individuals and couples.[22]

In recent decades, however, infertility has gained increasing attention from various social and behavioral scientists who have brought a wider variety of investigative approaches and research methods, in contrast to traditional psychologically oriented qualitative and quantitative methods. Examples of new research methodologies include the ethnographic model typically used in anthropology,[23] in which data are collected on the basis of reproductive life histories and/or narratives in individual studies;[24–27] grounded-theory methodology; discourse analysis (e.g., the analysis of newspaper accounts);[28] and ethnographic, qualitative case studies.[29] These are but a few examples of the different research approaches that provide different perspectives, exciting insights, and important findings that help provide a greater understanding of the psychosocial impact of infertility, thereby facilitating the work of infertility counselors by identifying significant clinical issues and/or beneficial therapeutic interventions.

While the scientific rigor of psychosocial investigations has dramatically improved, some significant gaps in the research remain, particularly regarding the psychosocial needs of the underserved (reproductive stratification) as well as the counseling needs of culturally diverse patients and reproductive tourists. A continuing and significant problem regarding research on the psychosocial issues of involuntary childlessness is that the preponderance of research to date has focused predominantly on white, heterosexual women living in developed countries and who, generally, are better educated and have higher socioeconomic status. Far less research has focused on culturally diverse men and women with limited financial or education resources, from developing countries, and/or who have limited access to treatment or specifically assisted reproduction.[30] The World Health Organization (WHO) has recognized the importance of sterility as a health issue of global concern, particularly in developing countries. WHO has acknowledged the challenges of lack of heterogeneity in the developing world particularly regarding assisted reproductive technologies, inconsistent access to or availability of quality infertility services in the developing world, as well as the lack of consistent standards regarding the quality of infertility services.[3] By contrast, little attention has focused on the psychosocial needs and/or the provision of mental health services in the developing world. Similar challenges exist regarding the wide variation of attitudes regarding counseling and mental heath services and the lack of consistent standards regarding the quality of available infertility counseling services. As such, underserved, culturally diverse, infertile couples seeking infertility treatment either in their home country or across international borders remain an area that not only received minimal research attention, but, as a result, also failed to benefit from clearly identified clinical and therapeutic interventions based on research evidence.

Psychosocial Interventions for Infertility

For several decades the provision of psychosocial support and/or counseling services have been requested by patients, suggested by professionals, legislated, and/or recommended on the basis of evidence-based research. Infertile patients have requested psychological services in conjunction with or as an adjunct to medical treatment for infertility[31–33] or through consumer advocacy organizations (e.g., ISSUE, ICSI, CHILD, Resolve). Recommendations for infertility counseling have also been mandated by legislation and/or regulatory bodies.[34–39] At the same time, infertility counseling services have been recommended and/or mandated by medical professional organizations, most often in conjunction with specific medical treatments.[40–43] Mental health professionals have also made recommendations for the provision of psychological counseling services.[20,21,44–46]

In a review of current research, Boivin addressed the effectiveness of psychosocial interventions for infertility in terms of the following questions: 1) Do psychosocial interventions improve well-being?, 2) Do psychosocial interventions increase pregnancy rates?, and 3) Are some interventions more effective than others?[47] The review involved a systematic search of all published and unpublished papers in any language and any source that (1) described a psychosocial intervention and (2) evaluated its effect on at least one outcome measure in an infertile population. A total of 380 studies met the criteria but only 7% were independent evaluation studies. Analysis of these studies showed that psychosocial interventions were more effective in reducing negative affect than in changing interpersonal functioning (e.g., marital and social functioning). Pregnancy rates were unlikely to be affected by psychosocial interventions. It was also found that group interventions that had emphasized education and skills training (e.g., relaxation training) were significantly more effective in producing positive change across a range of outcomes than counseling interventions that emphasized emotional expression and support and/or discussion about thoughts and feelings related to infertility. Men and women were found to benefit equally from psychosocial interventions. This review highlighted the lack of well-controlled, scientifically rigorous studies based on classic experimental methods. This review examined thirty years of research, yet produced only twenty-five independent studies evaluating psychosocial interventions for infertile individuals of which only eight met minimum requirements for good quality studies. By contrast, during the same period almost 400 papers were published in which psychosocial interventions for infertility were strongly recommended. In short, there remains a significant, even urgent need for high quality studies to unequivocally address the effectiveness of psychosocial interventions. Boivin suggests that future research should address (1) who benefits from psychological interventions, (2) which types of interventions are most beneficial to which patients, and (3) when is the optimum time to provide psychological interventions. In summary, by not simply recommending, but by providing evidence-based research through controlled investigative methodology, infertility counselors can provide more effective psychological interventions with greater confidence.

THEORETICAL FRAMEWORK

In both psychology and medicine, theories or theoretical frameworks are the basis for the academic scientific method. Theories (as a collection of interrelated ideas and facts) are developed to describe, explain, predict, and/or change (manage) behavior or mental processes. The purpose of theories is to better understand previous conditions that led to a thought, behavior, interaction, or phenomenon. As such, the scientific method involves (1) stating the problem, (2) forming a theory, (3) developing a hypothesis, (4) testing the hypothesis through a variety of research methods, and (5) replicating the results of the tested hypothesis. As such, theories or theoretical frameworks are a fundamental component of the research process, while at the same time facilitating and enhancing patient care by identifying relevant clinical issues and therapeutic interventions most beneficial and effective in curing or ameliorating sympatology,

improving well-being, and/or enhancing the outcome of treatment.

While the focus of the academic approach in medicine and counseling is research, the focus of the applied or clinical approach to medicine and counseling is implementation of knowledge gained from research for the immediate and practical benefit of individuals, couples, and families. In fact, clinicians and researchers do not have mutually exclusive roles and many infertility counselors are involved in both research and clinical work (i.e., application of research findings) to some extent over the course of their careers. The basic premise of applied psychology is the use of psychological principles and theories to overcome practical problems (e.g., reproductive medicine or health psychology). Infertility counseling is a specialty area with specific theoretical frameworks, clinical issues, and therapeutic interventions based on the scientific model of evidence-based medicine or treatment.

Theoretical approaches to infertility and, as such, infertility counseling have historically been based on a specific theoretical perspective or specific principles of theories adapted and applied to infertility. Recently, interest in developing infertility-specific theoretical frameworks, that contribute to a greater understanding of the psychosocial impact of infertility, has been growing. Infertility-specific theoretical frameworks aid infertility counselors as both researchers and clinicians by identifying the psychosocial phenomena of infertility, relevant issues, treatment modalities, and beneficial interventions to minimize psychosocial distress and trauma.

Evolution of Infertility-Specific Theoretical Frameworks

Over the years, infertility-specific theoretical frameworks have evolved from what have been termed *psychogenic infertility theories* or *psychosomatic medicine* approaches, in which demonstrable psychopathology was thought to play an etiological role in infertility.[48] The foundation of *psychogenic infertility theories* was Freudian psychoanalytic approaches in which psychological (and medical) disorders were thought to be due to an individual's unresolved conflicts and/or an unconscious defense mechanisms that caused or contributed to sterility.[49] The psychogenic infertility model (also sometimes referred to as the *psychosomatic medicine approach*) was introduced in the 1930s and reached its height of popularity during the pronatalist period of the 1950s and 1960s, particularly in the United States. At a time when up to 50% of infertility problems could not be accurately medically diagnosed or treated, psychological explanations of potential causes or treatment modalities were considered helpful and reasonable. However, the vast majority of these theories focused on psychological (and subconscious) disturbances in women, contending that neurotic conflicted feelings about motherhood or their own mothers prevented conception and the assumption of adult roles. Fischer described two personality styles in women contributing to infertility: the weak, emotionally immature, overprotected type, and the ambitious, masculine, aggressive, and dominating career-type.[50] The 'weak' woman was thought to be unable to separate or differentiate from her mother or express her anger in a direct fashion, or she had an abnormal fear of sex, motherhood, pregnancy, and labor that inhibited reproductive ability. 'Ambitious' women were infertile because "becoming pregnant meant accepting sexual feelings, being comfortable in competing with a stronger maternal figure, giving up the fantasy of remaining a child, and not having to compete with an unborn child."[51] Typically, 'psychogenically infertile' men were thought to have domineering mothers who over controlled their sons by threatening withdrawal of love, expecting conformity to their rigid moral codes, or creating anxiety within their sons as a result of their own sexual inhibitions.[52] Men, too, were thought to have conflicted feelings about parenthood or masculinity causing infertility.[53] This theory was recycled during the sexual revolution of the 1960s in descriptions of the 'new impotence' – men experiencing impotence as a result of performance pressure from 'liberated' women who expected sexual encounters to be mutually rewarding.[54]

Psychogenic infertility theories fell into disfavor partly as a result of the increased ability of reproductive medicine to diagnose and treat infertility problems. During the past thirty years, infertility of unknown etiology has been significantly reduced in large portions of the world, eliminating the necessity and/or feasibility of psychological causes of reproductive failure. More importantly, several reviewers of the psychogenic infertility literature concluded that the preponderance of studies revealed no consistent or striking evidence of psychological causes of infertility.[55–58]

Subsequently, *psychological sequelae* or *psychological consequences theories* emerged during the late 1970s in the United States and a worldwide consumer movement emphasizing that experience of infertility and treatment for it are emotionally difficult and all-encompassing, impacting all aspects of an individual and couple's life. Hence, infertility was the *consequence* and not the *cause* of involuntary childlessness.[30,59] Menning was one of the first to suggest a *psychological sequelae* or

psychological consequences approach that included the recommendation of psychological support services in conjunction with or as an adjunct to infertility treatment.[59] This model was initially presented using a combination of theoretical frameworks including developmental models, crisis theory, bereavement models, and a predictable pattern to develop a stage theory of infertility. Accordingly, the inability to procreate impaired the completion of adult tasks of intimacy and generativity creating a period of emotional disequilibrium, with the potential for either maladjustment or positive growth facilitating resolution and homeostasis for individuals or couples. Furthermore, infertility evoked typical feelings and psychological responses to infertility that followed a predictable pattern based on the stages of bereavement; involved recognition of the loss; gave meaning to the experience and attained effective resolution through personal growth; and overcame the losses of infertility.[59]

In general, the *psychological sequelae* approach provided a broad view of the interrelationships of individual, couple, family, society, and reproductive medicine; integrated different theoretical frameworks; conceptualized infertility as a major life crisis involving stress and grief; and provided a framework for the provision of counseling services. As such, the *psychological sequelae model* was valuable in stimulating the development of consumer advocacy and support organizations; increasing awareness among mental health and medical professionals of the importance of the psychosocial aspects of infertility; and legitimizing adjustment to infertility as a problem worthy of empirical study.[60] Still, the *psychological sequelae* approach was not without flaws and criticism in that it continued to apply a medical model to the complex psychosocial experience of infertility and failed to consider the social and cultural factors influencing the experience of involuntary childlessness and treatment for it.[30]

Subsequently, several different approaches have been suggested including the *psychological cyclical model*,[61] the *psychological outcome approach*,[30] and the *psychosocial context approach*. According to the *psychological cyclical model*, involuntary childlessness increases stress levels causing physiological changes that influence treatment outcome. As such, the *cyclical model* suggests that the psychological distress of infertility can and does have biological consequences that can (and may) influence conception whether or not medical treatment is used.[62] However, the *cyclical model* historically failed to address stress levels in the male partner and/or identify what levels of stress were significant (and counterproductive) for specific individuals under particular circumstances or situations.

The *psychological outcome approach* is, to some extent, an elaboration on the *psychological cyclical model* in that it involves an integrated mind–body, family system, and biopsychosocial perspective to research and clinical practice and recognizes the influence of psychobiological factors (e.g., stress) on conception and treatment outcome. The focus of the *psychological outcome approach* is the psychosocial response to infertility treatment of individuals, couples, and subsequent families as well as psychotherapeutic interventions that impact treatment outcomes. An example is the Heidelberg Model,[46] in which solution-focused counseling was found to be helpful for infertile couples, particularly couples who were highly stressed and who experienced deterioration of mood and sexual problems over the course of treatment.

The *psychosocial context approach* addresses how infertility is an experience that occurs within a social structure (e.g., marriage, family, community, and culture) and context (e.g., culture or religion). Although infertility can be a painful psychological trauma and life-altering phenomenon that is isolating and stigmatizing, it is not simply an individual psychological experience but a social experience that occurs within the context of the individual's or couple's life and social milieu. As such, infertility is better understood as a 'process' rather than a single event or series of isolated events. The *psychosocial context approach* is also a less individualistic model that takes a more holistic, global approach to understanding the psychosocial phenomena of infertility and the provision of treatment. It addresses cultural, religious, and environmental factors (e.g., natural or manmade disasters such as hurricanes or terrorist attacks) that can and do intensify or somehow influence the infertility experience for individuals and couples. Furthermore, the *psychosocial context approach* addresses the issues of stratification of medical and mental health services for infertility (e.g., uneven availability of infertility treatment services); reproductive tourism (e.g., culture clashes when patients travel across borders for reproductive treatment); and, finally, the influence of culture and/or religion on psychosocial response to infertility as well as the acceptability of medical treatments, mental health care, and/or family-building options.

Ultimately, both the *psychological outcome* and *psychosocial context* approaches provide perspectives by increasing our understanding of individual, couple and cultural differences, providing greater knowledge of clinical issues and effective therapeutic interventions to improve patient well-being and response to treatment. Ultimately, theory development in infertility should expand even further to include the integration of empir-ical research, clinical practice, psychotherapeutic interventions, and social policy issues acknowledging the universal and global context in which infertility is experienced and in which treatment is provided both medically and psychologically.[30] As noted throughout this book, how theoretical frameworks have been developed and/or applied in infertility vary according to the issue or topic being addressed. As such, the *psychosocial context approach* to theoretical frameworks in infertility may be more relevant as it acknowledges that the theoretical framework of individual identity may be highly applicable to individual psychotherapy or psychopathology but less useful within the context of cross-cultural counseling, while stress and coping theories or bereavement theories may have more universal application.

Infertility-Specific Theoretical Frameworks

Grief and Bereavement Approaches

Infertility involves grief and loss whether it is a profound distinct loss at the onset of treatment or a gradual accumulation of losses over time. The losses of infertility may involve the loss of individual and/or couple's health, physical and psychological well-being, life goals, status, prestige, self-confidence, and assumption of fertility, loss of privacy and control of one's body, and anticipatory grief at the possibility of being childless.[63,64] Grieving may also involve mourning relationships altered by infertility whether allowed to slip away or actually lost or forever changed. As with any grief response, the level of attachment (the desire for parenthood, child, or baby) is directly proportionate to the level of grief an individual or couple experiences. As such, infertility may typically involve grief responses such as shock, disbelief, anger, blame, shame, and guilt, while over time, feelings of loss of control, diminished self-esteem, chronic bereavement, anxiety, and depression may persist.

Building on bereavement approaches to infertility, Burns and Covington suggested the *keening syndrome of infertility-specific grieving*.[21] Within this context *keening* refers to the traditional Irish custom of grieving in which women weep and wail while preparing the deceased for burial, while men watched in somber silence (often sharing alcoholic beverages which typically lead to the cultural phenomenon known as the 'Irish Wake'). The keening syndrome of infertility refers to the way in which many couples grieve the losses of infertility: Women weep and men watch – with men often emotionally distancing themselves from the couple's shared loss. This phenomenon can result in husbands becoming the 'forgotten mourners' because the husband is less verbal and expressive with his grief or unable to express it in the same open manner as his wife. Ultimately, failure to acknowledge and appropriately grieve the losses of infertility has an impact on a couple's long-term adjustment to infertility, as well as prospective decisions regarding treatment and family-building alternatives. In many ways, this approach highlights not only gender differences in grief and mourning but also how women often assume the role of primary mourner, bearing an unequal share of the emotional burden of a couple's grief. Some have suggested that this is because women are proportionately more distressed than men, while others argue that it represents a common marital or cultural pattern in which women assume greater responsibility for the couple's emotional well-being and expressiveness. It may also reflect how infertility treatment is disproportionately geared toward women.

By contrast, Unruh and McGrath objected to the application of traditional grief and loss theory to infertility because it failed to address the ongoing, chronic nature of infertility.[65] They identified infertility as a *chronic sorrow* for the infertile, typically involving numerous losses over an extended period of time. In fact, infertility-specific grief may never be completely mourned, transcended, or fully integrated. According to the *chronic infertility-specific grief model*, even after parenthood has been achieved or childlessness accepted, infertility can, and often does, periodically reemerge only to be remourned from a different perspective or vantage point in the couple's or individual's life.

It has been suggested that infertility is a *disenfranchised grief* in that infertility is a loss that can lead to intense grief, although others may not recognize it or perceive it as minor.[66] Disenfranchised grief has three categories, all of which are to some extent often experienced by infertile couples. It is a grief in which (1) the lost relationship loss has no legitimacy, is socially unrecognized, or unacknowledged (e.g., yearned-for child, miscarriage); (2) the loss itself is not recognized as significant to others in the couple's social network or culture (e.g., failed treatment cycle or chemical pregnancy); and (3) the griever is not recognized as having suffered a loss and justified in grieving. Disenfranchised grief is recognized as a more complicated bereavement because the usual supports that facilitate grieving and the healing process are absent. Furthermore, there are some situations around which losses are so socially stigmatizing that individuals are reluctant to acknowledge their loss. Infertility may be so socially unacceptable that the shame of the diagnosis, treatments for it, and/or family-building alternatives may be lead the infertile individual to keep his or her losses hidden to minimize social stigma.

Individual Identity Theories

Infertility as an experience that alters an individual's identity and sense of a self was suggested as *integration of infertility into sense of self* model by Olshansky, who contended that the internalization of the infertility experience is instrumental in managing the narcissistic wounds of infertility.[27] According to this theoretical approach, infertility alters an individual's sense of self by creating or exacerbating feelings of deficiency, hopelessness, and shame. Both infertile men and women experience altered self-concept and self-image as a result of infertility, although they may experience it differently. Women often feel inadequate and deficient for failing to fulfill personal and societal roles, while men often feel inferior, ashamed, and angry. In short, whether infertility involves an actual pregnancy loss or the loss of the couple's wished-for child, it is a loss that is experienced as a narcissistic injury as well as a symbolic loss of self.[67] A core concept of this theory is that individuals experiencing infertility must integrate and incorporate infertility into their individual identity, sense of self, or self-definition. In so doing, the individual is then able to move beyond a personal identity of oneself as 'infertile' and transcend the experience through overcoming, circumventing, or reconciling the identity of self as infertile.[27]

In considering the impact of infertility on women, Unruh and McGrath suggest that infertile women have (1) the right to have control over their bodies, particularly their reproductive capabilities, and to actively participate in their healthcare; (2) been commonly blamed for the conditions that have caused them personal distress; (3) been socialized to value themselves primarily for their childbearing roles; and (4) more in common with each other than their differences in fertility.[65] Another theoretical approach that addresses identity issues in infertile women is Kikendall's application of self-*discrepancy theory*. According to this theoretical approach, infertility is a personal identity crisis in which a woman experiences a conflict between her ideal sense of self as mother or woman and her real sense of self as infertile.[68]

Stress and Coping Theories

Taymor and Bresnick were the first to refer to infertility as a *stressor* and *crisis* involving interaction among physical conditions predisposing to infertility, medical interventions addressing infertility, reactions of others, and individual psychological characteristics.[69] Stanton and Dunkel-Schetter applied stress and coping theory to infertility, noting that infertility is characterized by the dimensions of what individuals find stressful: unpredictability, negativity, uncontrollability, and ambiguity.[60] Furthermore, infertile couples typically perceive infertility as carrying the potential for both harm (e.g., loss of a central role) and benefit (e.g., strengthening of the marital relationship). Additionally, infertility is a stressor that is both controllable (e.g., deciding whether or not to pursue medical treatment or a specific treatment) and uncontrollable (e.g., attaining conception).[70]

Within the context of the infertility, individuals may experience a single acute stressor (i.e., crisis) such as diagnosis of a genetic disorder or cancer as the cause of infertility and, as such, is a discrete, time-limited crisis involving specific coping strategies to adapt to the crisis. However, for the majority of couples, infertility is more likely to be experienced as a chronic stressor in that emotional distress and demanding treatments and events accumulate over an extended period of time requiring different coping strategies to successfully adjust, adapt, and maintain emotional and marital equilibrium regardless of the ultimate outcome. Whether acute or chronic, infertility is a life crisis typically perceived or experienced as an insolvable problem threatening important life goals, taxing personal resources, and potentially arousing unresolved problems from the past. The application of stress and coping theory to infertility provides a greater understanding of (1) the conditions under which infertility is likely to be perceived as stressful; (2) factors most likely to facilitate or impede adjustment in infertile couples or individuals (i.e., identifying optimum coping strategies); (3) guidance in defining what constitutes successful psychological adjustment to infertility; and (4) what therapeutic interventions may be most beneficial for enhancing treatment outcome and/or reducing stress.

Social Construction and Stigma Theories

Infertility is experienced within the context of ever changing interpersonal relationships, predominantly family relationships. The individual develops a sense of self within the context of social interactions, family systems, religion, personal values, culture, and language often based on narratives that contribute to the construction of a sense of self and one's life. The concept of *stigma* in infertile men and women contains a self-perception of loss, role failure, and diminished esteem.[71] This theoretical framework is the foundation for understanding infertility as a cultural, religious, and existential experience.

Stigma involves the failure to fulfill cultural norms and extends to the social identity of the whole person, polluting his or her other accomplishments.[72] Stigma has been identified as theoretical framework applicable to both gender-specific infertility and infertility-specific individual distress within cultural contexts.[73,74] Infertile men and women typically experience feelings of defectiveness, inadequacy, inferiority, worthlessness, shame, and guilt – feelings that have been found to be culturally universal responses. Although men and women do not appear to differ in feelings of stigma regarding infertility, men with male-factor infertility seem to be more stigmatized than men without male-factor infertility, and women seem more stigmatized by infertility regardless of the diagnosis.[75] In short, infertility, as an externally invisible 'defect,' increases feelings of inferiority, differentness, and spoiled identity.[76,77]

Stigma has been found to be a significant theoretical framework across cultures in that different facets of infertility cause social isolation in specific cultures or social circumstances. Accordingly, Gonzalez noted that social stigma was experienced as failure to fulfill a prescribed societal norm as well as an assault on personal identity. However, infertility could also be a *transformational process* in which an individual has mourned the loss of reproductive function and parenting roles and struggled to make restitution for the perceived stigma and powerlessness associated with nonfulfillment of a prescribed societal norms, exclusion from cherished societal rituals, and deprivation of familial ties of descent.[78]

Family Systems Theory

Infertility thwarts a couple's movement forward into the next stage of marriage and family life (i.e., 'family expansion') for the couple as well as the members of their extended families. As such, infertility is an *intergenerational family developmental crisis* preventing parents and siblings from proceeding through life cycle stages (e.g., not yet grandparents, inability to share parenthood with siblings). It is a crisis of family developmental genealogy in which infertility jeopardizes and compromises the family's generative potential. Family system theory has been applied to infertility in a variety of contexts (e.g., cultural factors, diagnosis of genetic disorders, family-building alternatives, and the impact of family 'secrets,' particularly regarding third-party reproduction). Furthermore, family systems theory and therapeutic interventions have been integrated into infertility counseling diagnosis and treatment, as exemplified by the identification of resiliency as an individual and family strength potentially facilitating adjustment to infertility not only for the infertile couple, but also their extended family.[79]

Matthews and Matthews, using the family life stage model, suggested that the identity confusion and role adjustment of infertility precipitates family stress and crisis.[76] Accordingly, infertility as a 'transition to non-parenthood' represents the infertile couple's inability to make the anticipated transition to parenthood, resulting in confused life tasks, uncertain roles, and blurred boundaries in their own relationship as well as their relationship with their families of origin. Furthermore, the distinction between 'the biological condition of infertility' and 'the social condition of involuntary childlessness' is an important determinant in how individuals and family systems experience infertility and involuntary childlessness.

Family boundary ambiguity refers to ambiguity in family relationships and roles that impact and even impair marital and family functioning. The longed-for child is experienced by the infertile couple as 'psychologically present but physically absent,' blurring the boundaries and thereby creating ambiguity in the couple's marital system, as well as their extended families.[80] The ambiguous boundaries of infertile couples are emotionally painful and can have long-lasting effects for couples because over time, the longed-for child becomes an idealized child, who represents idealized portions of each spouse. Or the failure of the child to arrive may be perceived as caused by the negative characteristics (faults) of themselves or their partner. In response to infertility, some couples create rigid boundaries around the issue of infertility, protecting themselves against invasions of privacy but potentially contributing to isolation and alienation from friends and family. Other couples create boundaries that are too permeable, sharing too much information with others or disregarding their partner's personal boundaries.

Another application of family system theory is *complex adoption*, which refers to the cultural and social influences, historical circumstance, and scientific developments that have facilitated the creation of families via various forms of adoption and assisted reproduction.[81] Complex adoption includes various forms of adoption including adoption of older children through foster placement or institutional care; open adoptions in which birth parents have an ongoing relationship with the adoptive family; international or intercountry adoptions; transracial adoptions; as well as the wide array of medically assisted third-party reproduction (e.g., donated gametes, embryos, and gestational carrier facilitated parenthood). Although these forms of adoption present new avenues of parenthood, they also present new challenges to the process of family formation, family dynamics, and the psychosocial needs of both parents and children in these families.

Phase or Stage Theory

Read has suggested an *infertility counseling model* based, in large part, on the needs and recommendations of the Human Fertilization and Embryology Authority.[82] The model incorporates the grief counseling models of Kubler-Ross (denial, anger, bargaining, depression, and acceptance) and Worden (accept the reality of the loss; work through the pain of grief; adjustment in the environment that acknowledges the lost loved one; and emotionally relocate and move on with life) as well as the helping model of Egan (exploration, new understanding, and action). Read's infertility counseling model involves fives stages: (1) diagnosis, (2) managing feelings, (3) planning action, (4) understanding medical treatment, (5) and awaiting treatment outcomes. According to Read, the stages of this model may be repeated as the individual and/or couple adapts to the loss.

Blenner's stage theory of infertility described the experience of moving from the prediagnosis to post-treatment as *passages* based on three concepts: (1) engagement, (2) immersion, and (3) disengagement. The stages within these concepts were: (1) experiencing a dawning of awareness, (2) facing a new reality, (3) having hope and determination, (4) intensifying treatment, (5) spiraling down and letting go, (6) quitting and moving out, and (7) shifting the focus.[83]

Diamond and colleagues described five distinct phases of infertility. They are: *Dawning, Mobilization, Immersion, Resolution,* and *Legacy*.[84] During the *Dawning* phase, couples become increasingly aware that they are having a problem conceiving and eventually seek medical assistance. *Mobilization* marks the first step into the medical arena during which the couple begins diagnostic testing. If a definitive diagnosis is made, it can cause shock, disbelief, and denial, particularly if it is secondary infertility. Problems may emerge in the relationship as the couple faces the first of what will probably be many losses. *Immersion* is the most complex and demanding phase, as the couple undergoes more and more testing and treatment. This stage is marked by feelings of being in 'limbo' or 'not yet parents' because they cannot move ahead to the next stage of the life cycle: parenting. Late in the *Immersion* phase, couples may face family-building alternatives they never thought they would have to consider: decisions about donor gametes, donor embryos, or adoption. The *Resolution* phase consists of three overlapping subphases: (1) ending medical treatment, (2) acknowledging and mourning the loss of not having a genetically shared (or related) child, and (3) refocusing on other possibilities such as prenatal adoption, traditional adoption, or childlessness. The *Legacy* phase encompasses the aftermath of the infertility experience including the marital, sexual, and parenting problems that may emerge as a consequence of infertility, particularly when partners have not adequately handled the significant losses of it.

Deveraux and Hammerman suggested a model of infertility counseling that involves integrating infertility into identity; empowering infertile individuals; managing infertility; and recognizing loss and grief as inherent aspects of infertility.[85] The primary objective of this model is facilitating the integration of infertility into the individual's sense of self and away from identification of himself or herself as solely individual. Accordingly, the stages of this model involve (1) integration of infertility into the individual's definition of self, (2) acknowledging that the infertile individual is the 'expert,' (3) promoting acceptance of infertility, (4) acknowledging the losses of infertility, (5) facilitating grief and bereavement, (6) assigning homework, (7) fostering and encouraging individual empowerment, (8) facilitating transcendence of the infertility experience through acceptance (rather than resolution), (9) promoting responsibility (versus control), and (10) encouraging self-advocacy. This model encourages a variety of therapeutic interventions including the use of cognitive restructuring, journaling, development of rituals, the use of metaphors and analogies, pragmatic problem-solving and creative decision making, and techniques that facilitate bereavement, integration of the infertility experience, and problem-solving. It provides a model for planning therapeutic sessions.

Cooper-Hilbert applied a variety of family system couple's developmental stages and tasks to the counseling of infertile couples.[86] These developmental stages focused on the expansion of the couple dyad; establishing a nuclear family relationship; fulfilling parental roles as individuals and couples; and redefining relationships with one's family-of-origin. According to this model, the primary goal of the initial stage of psychotherapy is normalization of the couple's infertility experiences. In the second stage, the goal is assessment and treatment of any serious individual psychological disorder; encouragement of the expression and acknowledgment of the partner's feelings about infertility; and continued normalization of feelings regarding infertility. Additionally, the therapist provides assistance with separating their sexuality, self-image, and self-esteem from the issue of childbearing. During the final stage of psychotherapy, the goal is accepting infertility and moving on from it. Integral to this stage is facilitating planful coping, goal setting, decision making, stress management, and giving meaning to the infertility experience.

CLINICAL ISSUES

Infertility is recognized around the world as a distressing experience with the potential for threatening individual, marital, family, and social stability. There is some evidence that certain circumstances enhance infertility-specific distress including preexisting medical or mental health problems, cultural or religious issues, and gender-specific infertility diagnosis. Distress may be the result of the experience of involuntary childless or disrupted reproduction, the infertility diagnosis itself, or the demands of the medical treatment regimes to treat infertility. *Gender-specific diagnosis* addresses the unique way in which men and women experience infertility differently, and the consequences of being the 'identified patient.'

With the globalization of infertility care, the importance of providing *culturally-sensitive infertility counseling* is even more paramount. The psychology of infertility for diverse populations and circumstances (as distinct from white, middle-class, heterosexual, young, first-married couples) involves the recognition of disparate responses and unique social circumstances, typically influencing therapeutic approaches and counseling interventions. Knowledge of cross-cultural factors in infertility can assist the therapist's provision of appropriate support, direction, and intervention, as well as improving establishment of the therapeutic alliance. Infertility is experienced within a context that has an impact on the infertile couple's experience of infertility as well as their perspective, approach to treatment or family-building options, and psychological adjustment. Providing culturally-sensitive infertility counseling not only improves patient care and satisfaction, but cultural competency from the infertility counselor is also fundamental to professional standards of care, particularly in terms of the global nature of infertility and the issue of reproductive tourism.

Medical Counseling Issues

Although an understanding of the psychology of infertility is fundamental to infertility counseling, it is also paramount that the infertility counselor be knowledgeable of reproductive medicine, including medical diagnosis and current treatment options for infertility. As a basis for this understanding, an overview of the *medical aspects of infertility* is provided, as well as a review of medical conditions or circumstances of particular relevance to infertility and its treatment. This includes not only knowledge of the basic infertility work-up and treatment options but also the various forms of assisted reproduction including third-party reproduction. Additionally, medical factors impacting fertility such as preexisting genetic disorders or genetic conditions causing infertility are also important. In short, it is important that infertility counselors have a comprehensive understanding of reproductive medicine and that their knowledge base always remain current, as reproductive medicine is a dynamic and ever evolving field. As such, the medically knowledgeable infertility counselor is better able to provide accurate patient education and guidance; collaborate with other professionals on the reproductive medicine team; and assess patient response to treatment.

Medical conditions affecting fertility include conditions causing infertility (e.g., cancer treatment or genetic disorders), resulting in infertility (e.g., premature ovarian failure), or affecting infertility treatment (e.g., endometriosis). *Medically complicating conditions* or special medical circumstances often involve a variety of psychological issues with the potential for precipitating emotional crisis and understandably impacting emotional well-being as well as reproductive treatment decisions. Diagnosis of a disease or genetic disorder (whether related or unrelated to infertility) during the course of infertility evaluation or treatment can result in a dual crisis of health and fertility in which the patient must deal with illness (even mortality) that amplifies the typical reactions to infertility of loss, defectiveness, and abnormality. Finally, it has become increasingly common for infertile patients, as well as gamete donors, to undergo *genetic counseling* and/or genetic screening for reasons of parental age, reproductive or medical history of genetic disorders, or diagnosis of the reproductive problem. Understandably, the process of genetic counseling and/or the diagnosis of a genetic problem can cause significant emotional distress and complicate adjustment to infertility.

For couples who may have spent years of anticipation, time, energy, and money to conceive a much desired pregnancy, pregnancy loss or the death of a newborn is especially bitter and cruel. *Pregnancy loss* (whether spontaneous or planned) can be an emotionally traumatic experience involving varying degrees of grief, diminished self-esteem, and marital distress. Spontaneous losses – ectopic pregnancy, miscarriage, stillbirth, or infant death – can potentially trigger acute grief responses, clinical depression, and/or the reemergence of unresolved past losses. Planned terminations (e.g., for reasons of multifetal reduction or

genetic defects) are often grieved and mourned in the same manner as spontaneous losses, although social stigma associated with abortion may increase isolation and guilt about the 'chosen' loss of a longed-for child.

Infertility Counseling Practice Issues

Infertility counseling is an amalgam of medicine and mental health and, while a relatively new, still evolving field, has taken on a *global perspective* in which mental health professionals worldwide (i.e., social workers, psychologists, psychiatrists, psychiatric nurses, and family therapists) have become increasingly important professionals in reproductive medicine, genetics, and perinatalogy. Infertility counselors are mental healthcare providers, researchers, reproductive medical team collaborators, and educators, as well as a supportive resource to colleagues. The practice of infertility counseling has required not only additional clinical skills but also increasing adaptability by including more culturally diverse counseling skills (e.g., reproductive tourists), legal and ethical knowledge, and the growing use of telecommunication for education, information access, and communication with colleagues and patients. A major goal of infertility counseling is improving the quality of infertile patients' lives during and after treatment, ameliorating the impact of infertility, facilitating patient transcendence of the infertility experience so as to minimize long-term harm or distress, and ensuring the healthy adjustment of all participants, particularly in families created via complex (third-party) reproduction or adoption and for children with a legacy of parental infertility.

To achieve this goal, the practice of infertility counseling has evolved into a model of collaborative reproductive healthcare. Infertility counselors, whether independent or employees of a reproductive clinic, need to be versatile and adaptable to work with a variety of relationships – patients, treatment team, colleagues, advocacy and community organizations, and more. They also need to develop practice management skills that further the collaborative reproductive healthcare model, which may seem in contrast, at times, with traditional mental health practices. Furthermore, infertility counseling is not practiced in a vacuum but rather in a global environment, with increasing ethical and legal challenges. Infertility counselors often are confronted with *ethical issues* generated by rapidly changing and advancing technology and social topography. Just as variable are the *legal issues* faced by infertility counselors regarding practice standards, competency, laws and regulations, as well as matters occurring from third-party reproduction.

Infertility counselors must abide by the professional standards of their particular profession (e.g., social work and psychology) while at the same time maintaining the highest professional standards regarding infertility counseling. Professional competency in infertility counseling involves maintaining an awareness of current standards of ethical practice (locally and globally), legal responsibilities, appropriate record keeping, and collaboration with other professionals (e.g., medical, mental health, and legal professionals) working in reproductive medicine. To further these objectives, practitioners in an increasing number of countries have formed professional infertility counseling organizations, often under the umbrella of reproductive medical societies. Recently, these groups have joined together to form the International Infertility Counseling Organization (IICO), further reflecting the global perspective of this profession.

THERAPEUTIC INTERVENTIONS

The clinical issues of reproductive medicine, psychosocial components of impaired fertility, and professional competency provide the knowledge base upon which infertility counselors approach a variety of therapeutic interventions. These areas include:

■ assessment;
■ treatment modalities;
■ third-party reproduction and other means of alternative family-building;
■ postinfertility issues.

Assessment

Infertility counseling or the psychological care of the infertile individual or couple including assessment and treatment, can take place within a wide array of contexts and circumstances, such as self-referral for psychotherapy or mandatory preparation and educational counseling prior to medical treatment. Infertility counselors may provide psychological assessment, screening, and psychotherapy; diagnosis and treatment of disorders; and psychometric testing and/or administration measures of infertility-specific distress. *Psychosocial assessment* generally involves gathering information in a structured manner about the individual/couple's personal history, psychiatric history, and current level of functioning, as well as a review of the infertility experience in terms of its impact on marriage, psychiatric health, relationships, reproductive history, and sexual history. The clinical interview provides the framework

for assessment. When combined with psychological testing, information from the clinical interview is used to facilitate assessment, so as to develop and implement a treatment plan. Like other forms of psychological treatment, infertility counseling involves interventions based on careful psychosocial assessment of the patient or couple; and may identify disturbance, psychopathology, and/or possibly the need for psychotropic medication.

While there is no evidence of increased incidence of psychiatric problems in infertile patients, individuals may develop psychological distress in response to the stresses of medical treatment or experience the reemergence of preexisting psychopathology (e.g., depression and eating disorders) over the course of infertility treatment. Whether newly emergent or preexisting, emotional distress can impair quality of life, have an impact on medical treatment, and pose challenging management problems for medical staff. As such, psychological care involves a variety of treatment modalities including *psychiatric or psychopharmacological treatment*. Whether psychiatric care is adjunctive or primary care, the practitioner must be aware of the unique treatment demands and challenges of patients undergoing infertility treatment, while also requiring psychiatric care. As a result, the infertility counselor and treatment team must be cognizant of the treatment needs of both medical and mental health diagnosis.

Finally, competent and optimum infertility counseling involves the provision of care based on sound theoretical, clinical, and therapeutic principles, which need to be supported by evidence found in grounded research. However, despite overwhelming recommendations in the literature in the past forty years for psychosocial intervention, there is poor integration of research into infertility counseling practice. An *evidence-based treatment approach* uses empirically supported assessment strategies and techniques, emphasizing diverse methods in addition to the clinical interview and assessment measures. Infertility counselors increasingly will be called upon to support the effectiveness of their psychosocial interventions based upon empirical evidence, especially in regard to financial reimbursement from third-party payers (i.e., insurance companies) and, thus, will need to develop practice-based research skills.

Treatment Modalities

Infertility counselors use a variety of treatment modalities, rarely endorsing a single approach, as noted throughout this text. It is generally recognized that various treatment modalities (individual, couple/family, support and therapy groups) are used in infertility counseling, based upon theoretical and therapeutic approaches such as psychodynamic therapy, cognitive-behavioral treatment, marriage and family therapy, strategic/solution-focused brief therapy, sex therapy, crisis intervention, grief counseling, and implications/decision-making counseling. *Individual counseling* is useful for addressing personal distress and dysfunction, whether caused or exacerbated by infertility. It provides a safe and trusting relationship with the therapist, allowing growth and healing from the pain of infertility or past psychological injury or illness. *Couple counseling* is useful in addressing relationship or marital problems, particularly those involving communication, decision making, and conflict resolution. It is a particularly appropriate approach as infertility is usually a 'couple problem,' involving the grieving of shared losses for both partners, interrupted sexual practices, and considerable couple stressors (e.g., financial strain and extended medical treatment). *Group counseling* is helpful to couples and individuals needing validation or personal perspective in promoting psychological growth. Group members aid in normalizing and sharing the infertility experience, as well as ameliorating feelings of isolation and stigma. Additionally, there is some evidence that some forms of group interventions may improve medical treatment outcomes.

Within the context of these three methods of therapy delivery, different counseling approaches may be used. *Behavioral medicine* as a therapeutic approach to infertility is helpful in that it integrates cognitive-behavioral therapy and health psychology, emphasizing the patient's role in medical care. It offers stress management and coping interventions, such as cognitive restructuring, guided imagery, and relaxation techniques. An area of increasing interest to patients and reproductive healthcare providers are *complementary and alternative medical (CAM) approaches* to infertility. While some of these methods have been used to treat infertility for thousands of years, it has been only recently that these treatments have been pursued and investigated as an adjunct to traditional Western medical interventions treatment of infertility. A variety of CAM methods are being used by infertility patients, including acupuncture, homeopathy, vitamins, herbs, mind–body techniques, body manipulation and energy techniques, although the efficiency of most remain questionable. Another area of importance is *sexual counseling*, which is often both necessary and beneficial for infertile couples who typically encounter problems related to sexual health either as a result of medical treatment or in response to the infertility diagnosis. Whether the infertility counselor provides these counseling services or refers to another professional for adjunctive care, it is evident that diverse treatment modalities are beneficial in assisting infertile patients.

Third-Party Reproduction and Other Means of Alternative Family-Building

For some infertile couples, medical treatments will not be successful and they must reconsider previous decisions about parenthood; decide whether to maintain their family as it is (e.g., couple or single-child family); or pursue other family-building alternatives, such as adoption or third-party reproduction. All of these alternatives involve the conscious decision to relinquish the family they had planned to have; redefine the meaning of family (or their family); and grieve the experience of pregnancy, birth, and/or a genetically-shared, biological child. For some couples, childlessness may be redefined as *child-free*, and their decision not to continue medical treatment may involve enhancing the benefits of couplehood; redefining the meaning of family; or the pursuit of other life goals. For other couples, remaining childless means significant social stigma and social isolation, particularly for the wife, who may be divorced, maltreated, or abandoned by her husband, his family, and/or even her own.

Adoption or foster care is a family-building alternative preferred by other couples for whom medical treatment has failed or who decide for a variety of reasons to discontinue infertility treatment. Adoption involves the same rewards (and travails) of parenthood as well as the opportunity to share lives with a child needing parents. Finally, the pursuit of parenthood through the various forms of *third-party reproduction* (donated sperm, oocytes, or embryos, surrogacy, and gestational carrier) is another means of family-building, although it may challenge traditional beliefs, moral views, or customs, especially when it involves lesbian and gay couples, unmarried individvals, and/or older women.

While considerations of adoption and childlessness seem fairly straightforward to most infertile individuals, third-party reproduction can be daunting in its complexity and implementation. To a large extent, current practices in third-party reproduction are based on traditions associated with *sperm donation*, used therapeutically for more than 100 years and historically involving donor anonymity and secrecy. However, the development of assisted reproduction technologies (e.g., IVF) over the past thirty years now enables couples to build their family through the use of *donated oocytes and embryos* and to use the services of surrogates and gestational carriers. The psychological complexities of these forms of family-building have precipitated considerations and recommendations for the care of all participants – recipients and donors – involving assessment, preparation, education, and support.

Couples considering the use of donated sperm, oocytes, or embryos must first address the emotional consequences of reproductive failure as individuals and as couples. Having decided to build their family through the use of donated gametes or embryos, they, as the *recipient couple*, must grieve the biological, genetically-shared child they had hoped for. In addition, they must mutually agree that their best alternative to genetic parenthood is assisted reproduction and the use of donated sperm, oocytes, or embryo. Furthermore, they must decide on the form of donation with which they are comfortable and to which they have access – anonymous donor or known donor (e.g., family member) – and on their level of openness about the child's conception. Additional considerations include access and/or availability of their desired form of donation and legislative, regulatory, or professional guidelines regarding the gamete/embryo donation. Gamete/embryo donation is not a universally available family-building alternative and is typically governed by legislation or regulations, which couples may or may not perceive as beneficial. As a result, there has been an increase in 'reproductive tourism' – infertile couples traveling across national or international borders in pursuit of the family-building option that best suits them. However, the legal and cultural context in which treatment is undertaken as well as where the family will eventually reside are important considerations for the couple as well as the infertility counselor.

The other patient participants in third-party reproduction are the *donors, surrogates*, and *gestational carriers* who facilitate parenthood for infertile couples. Preparation of gamete donors varies. Anonymous *sperm donor* preparation has primarily been restricted to medical screening while *oocyte donors* have received more extensive psychological assessment and preparation because the donation process is medically intrusive and demanding. *Embryo donors* are usually infertile couples who have completed their families and wish to donate their 'unused' cryopreserved embryos or extra embryos from a current IVF cycle that they do not plan to use themselves. Preparation of embryo donors has involved assessment of couple agreement as well as helping them understand the implications of their donation, socially, legally, and psychologically. Preparation of *surrogates and gestational carriers* has typically involved psychological assessment, education, definition of the reproductive relationship parameters, and ongoing support, sometimes even after the pregnancy and relinquish-

ment of the child as the 'ultimate gift.' However, just as patients are traveling across borders in pursuit of treatments, potential donors and carriers also can be reproductive tourists perhaps to help a family member or for financial gain. As such, the requirements of culturally-sensitive infertility counselors is all the more important and relevant.

Postinfertility Counseling Issues

Despite technological advances that have pushed back the biological clock, the medical treatment process for infertility eventually must come to an end, either by an active or passive decision or with a pregnancy. *Ending treatment*, just as beginning it, can be a difficult and complex process, replete with emotions. 'When is enough, enough?' is a question patients and caregivers struggle with, and the infertility counselor has the opportunity to play a special role in making a 'good-enough' ending for both parties through exit counseling strategies. The *pregnancy after infertility* is a precious one, yet often it is fraught with anxiety and worry. Psychological adjustment to this unique pregnancy typically presents a myriad of new issues, including possible multiple gestation, potential serious maternal/fetal health risks, decisions regarding multifetal reduction, complications requiring high-tech intervention and prolonged bed rest, or adjustment to a pregnancy that is not genetically linked to or carried by the 'contracting' mother. In short, previously infertile pregnant women and their spouses, expecting a blissful experience, are often surprised by an exceedingly challenging experience of pregnancy, which understandably, can diminish their happiness and expectations while increasing their distress.

Family adjustment after infertility entails all the normal developmental tasks of parenthood and family life, but often with unique demands. Special issues for *parenting after infertility* may involve older parenthood, parenting multiples, parenting an only child after secondary infertility, or the complex dilemmas of parenting after third-party reproduction. Parenthood against a backdrop of reproductive loss and highly technical medical conception requires special psychological preparation, education, and adjustment to its special joys and challenges. Similarly, the *impact on children* created through assisted reproductive technology has become an increasing focus of attention for infertility counselors. A key aspect to helping families adjust concerns assisting parents in developing and discussing a plan regarding disclosure of the circumstances of their child(ren)'s conception and/or birth. In short, just as technology has grown, so too has the role of the infertility counselor in the long-term adjustment of individuals, couples, and families affected by impaired fertility.

FUTURE IMPLICATIONS

As a new and emerging mental health profession, infertility counseling applies mental health treatment to the fields of reproductive medicine, genetic medicine, and perinatology. Over the past thirty years, it has seen dynamic growth in terms of the number of professionals working in the field, the amount of scientific research, professional development, and increasing presence in a wide variety of infertility clinics and medical treatment facilities. As such, it is safe to say that infertility counseling is a new, as well as a dynamically growing, field of mental health marked by a group of multidisciplinary professionals working together with a wide variety of medical professionals to provide comprehensive patient care; increase consumer awareness and education; and improve patient response to medical treatment. Future developments in this field involve its continuing definition as a mental health profession; professional qualifications and standards of practice for caregivers; and education and training for professionals wishing to enter the field. It also means being prepared and adapting to future medical developments (e.g., gonadal tissue cryopreservation, in vitro oocyte maturation and embryonic stem cell culture, and cloning) that can and will impact infertility counseling, clinical issues, and therapeutic interventions as well as the families created by these technologies. Worldwide, mental health professionals working in the field of infertility counseling have provided comprehensive patient care while establishing programs, standards of professional education, practice guidelines, and, recently, professional qualifications and quality assurance for consumers.

As with all new fields, infertility counseling has had its growing pains, and there will no doubt be more. In the past, the most important challenge facing infertility counseling was recognition of the importance of the field and the role of the infertility counselor as an important member of the treatment team. In the future, the most significant challenge is credentialing in infertility counseling: the establishment of a credentialing process that defines the field and criteria for credentialing for infertility counselors internationally. In the future, credentialing in infertility counseling will have to address: What are the competencies that an infertility counselor should possess? Are these competencies the same for all areas of practice within the profession?

How can these competencies be assessed? The answers to these questions will need to be addressed on a national and international level, and will help in defining the future of the infertility counseling profession.

SUMMARY

■ Although infertility has existed since the beginning of time, the social and historical context of reproductive choice has changed dramatically in the last century and become significantly more complex for couples medically, socially, culturally, and psychologically.

■ While research and clinical experience continue to indicate that the vast majority of infertile men and women do not experience significant levels of psychological trauma, the use of advanced medical technology and/or third-party reproduction may increase psychological distress during specific periods of treatment.

■ There has been an evolution in the psychological theoretical view of infertility over the years. Infertility-specific theoretical frameworks aid infertility counselors, as both researchers and clinicians, by identifying the psychosocial phenomena of infertility, relevant issues, treatment modalities, and beneficial interventions to minimize psychosocial distress and trauma.

■ Clinical intervention combines an understanding of the medical and psychological aspects of infertility. Intervention is based on careful assessment, use of appropriate treatment modalities, and an understanding of the complex issues and circumstances involved in infertility counseling practice.

REFERENCES

1. Rosenblatt PC, Peterson P, Portner J, et al. A cross-cultural study of responses to childlessness. *Behav Sci Notes* 1973; 8:221–31.
2. Lyons AS, Petrocelli RJ. *Medicine: An Illustrated History*. New York: Abradale Press, 1987.
3. Vayena E, Rowe P, Peterson H. Assisted reproductive technologies in developing countries: Why should we care. *Fertil Steril* 2002; 78:13–5.
4. Butler P. Assisted reproduction in developing countries – facing up to the issues. *Progress in Reproductive Health* 2003; 63:1–8.
5. Fidler A, Bernstein J. Infertility: From a personal to a public health problem. *Public Health Rep* 1999; 114:494–511.
6. Daar A, Merali Z. Infertility and social suffering: The case of ART in developing countries. In: E Vayena, P Rowe, D Griffin, eds. *Report of a Meeting on Medical, Ethical, and Social Aspects of Assisted Reproduction*. 2001, Sept. 17–21, Geneva, Switzerland: WHO; 2001; 16–21.

7. Datta B, Okonofua F. What about us? Bringing infertility into reproductive care. *Quality/Calidad/Qualite* 2002; 13:1–31.

8. Marsh M, Ronner W. *The Empty Cradle: Infertility in America from Colonial Times to the Present.* Baltimore: Johns Hopkins University Press, 1996.

9. Greil AL. Infertile bodies: Medicalization, metaphor, and agency. In: MC Inhorn, F Van Balen, eds. *Infertility Around the Globe: New Thinking on Childlessness, Gender, and Reproductive Technologies.* Los Angeles, CA: University of California Press, 2002; 101–18.

10. Walker BG. *The Woman's Encyclopedia of Myths and Secrets.* New York: Harper & Collins, 1983.

11. Johnston DR. The history of human infertility. *Fertil Steril* 1963; 14:261–9.

12. Sha JL. *Mothers of Thyme: Customs and Rituals of Infertility and Miscarriage.* Ann Arbor, MI: Lida Rose Press, 1990.

13. Kittredge C. *Womansword: What Japanese Words Say About Women.* Tokyo: Kodansha International, 1987.

14. Gillison G. Images of nature in Gimi thought. In: C MacCormack, M Strathern, eds. *Nature, Culture, and Gender.* Cambridge: Cambridge University Press, 1980; 143–73.

15. Foote RH. The history of artificial insemination: selected notes and notables. *J Anim Sci* 2002; 80 (E-Suppl. 2): 1–10.

16. Wood C, Trounson A. *Clinical In Vitro Fertilization.* Berlin: Springer-Verlag, 1984.

17. Laborie F. Social alternatives to infertility. In: P Stephenson, M Wagner, eds. *Tough Choices: In Vitro Fertilization and the Reproductive Technologies.* Philadelphia: Temple University Press, 1993; 37–52.

18. Covington SN. The role of the mental health professional in reproductive medicine. *Fertil Steril* 1995; 64:895–7.

19. Bresnick E, Taymor ML. The role of counseling in infertility. *Fertil Steril* 1979; 32:154–6.

20. Boivin J, Kentenich H, eds. Guidelines for Counselling in Infertility. *ESHRE Monographs.* London: Oxford University Press, 2002.

21. Burns LH, Covington SN. eds. *Infertility Counseling: A Comprehensive Handbook for Clinicians.* New York: Parthenon, 1999.

22. Van Balen F, Inhorn MC. Interpreting infertility: A view from the social sciences. In: MC Inhorn, F Van Balen, eds. *Infertility Around the Globe: New Thinking on Childlessness, Gender, and Reproductive Technologies.* Los Angeles, CA: University of California Press, 2002; 3–32.

23. Inhorn MC. The 'local' confronts the 'global': Infertile bodies and the new reproductive technologies in Egypt. In: MC Inhorn, F Van Balen, eds. *Infertility Around the Globe: New Thinking on Childlessness, Gender, and Reproductive Technologies.* Los Angeles, CA: University of California Press, 2002; 263–82.

24. Kirkman M. Thinking of something to say: Public and private narratives of infertility. *Health Care for Women Int.* 2001; 22:523–35.

25. Pashigan MJ. Conceiving the happy family: infertility and marital politics in northern Viet Nam. In: MC Inhorn, F Van Balen, eds. *Infertility Around the Globe: New Thinking on Childlessness, Gender, and Reproductive Technologies.* Los Angeles, CA: University of California Press, 2002; 134–51.

26. Riessman CK. Positioning gender identity in narratives of infertility: south Indian women's lives in context. In: MC Inhorn, F Van Balen, eds. *Infertility Around the Globe: New Thinking on Childlessness, Gender, and Reproductive Technologies.* Los Angeles, CA: University of California Press, 2002; 152–70.

27. Olshansky EF. Identity of self as infertile: An example of theory-generating research. *Adv Nurs Sci* 1987; 9:54–63.

28. Gannon K, Glover L, Abel P. Masculinity, infertility, stigma and media reports. *Soc Sci Med* 2004; 59:1169–75.

29. Sundby J. Infertility and health care in countries with less resources: case studies from sub-Saharan Africa. In: MC Inhorn, F Van Balen, eds. *Infertility Around the Globe: New Thinking on Childlessness, Gender, and Reproductive Technologies.* Los Angeles, CA: University of California Press, 2002; 247–59.

30. Greil A. Infertility and psychological distress: A critical review of the literature. *Social Science Medicine* 1997; 45:1679–784.

31. Royal Commission on New Reproductive Technologies (Canada). *Proceed with Care* (No. Volumes 1 and 2): Minister of Government Services, 1993.

32. Warnock M. The Warnock Report. *Brit Med J* 1985; 29:187–9.

33. The New York State Task Force on Life and the Law. *Assisted Reproductive Technologies: Analysis and Recommendations for Public Policy.* Albany, NY, 1998.

34. Human Fertilisation and Embryology Authority. *Revised HFEA Code of Practice* (No. 6th edition). London, 2004.

35. Ministerial Committee on Assisted Reproductive Technology. *Assisted Human Reproduction: Navigating our Future*: Department of Justice, New Zealand Government, 1994.

36. King's Fund Centre Counselling Committee. *Counselling for Regulated Infertility Treatments* (report): Kings Fund Centre, 1991.

37. Herbert M, Chenier NM, Norris S. Bill C-6: Assisted Human Reproduction Act. Statues of Canada. Library of Parliament, 2004.

38. Infertility Treatment Authority. Donor Treatment Procedure Information Register. Australia, 1998.

39. Szoke H. Regulation of assisted human reproductive technology: The state of play in Australia. In I Freckleton, K Petersen, eds. *Controversies in Health Law.* Leichhardt, NSW: The Federation Press, 1999.

40. American Society for Reproductive Medicine. Guidelines for gamete and embryo donation: A practice committee report. *Fertil Steril* 2002; 77:Suppl 5.

41. American Society for Reproductive Medicine. Guidelines for psychological assessment donors and recipients. *Fertil Steril* 2002; 77:Suppl 5.

42. ESHRE task force on ethics and law. Gamete and embryo donation. *Human Reprod* 2002; 17:1407–8.

43. Bruhat MA. Recommendations of obstetricians and gynecologists of the diagnosis, treatment, cost and results of the treatment of infertility health services. *Human Reprod* 1992; 7:1335–7.

44. Sundby J, Olsen A, Schei B. Quality of care for infertility patients: An evaluation of a plan for hospital investigation. *Scandinavian J Social Medicine* 1994; 22:139–44.

45. Klock SC, Maier D. Guidelines for the provision of psychological services at the University of Connecticut Health Center. *Fertil Steril* 1991; 56:680–5.

46. Wischmann T, Stammer H, Gerhard I, et al. Couple counseling and therapy for the unfulfilled desire for a child:

The two-step approach of the 'Heidelberg infertility consultation.' In: B Strauss, ed. *Involuntary Childlessness: Psychological Assessment, Counseling, and Psychotherapy*. Seattle: Hogrefe & Huber Publishers, 2002; 127–50.

47. Boivin J. A review of psychosocial interventions in infertility. *Social Science Medicine* 2003; 57:2325–41.

48. Berg BJ, Wilson JF, Weingartner PJ. Psychological sequelae of infertility treatment: The role of gender and sex-role identification. *Soc Sci Med* 1991; 33:1071–80.

49. Benedek T. Infertility as a psychosomatic defense. *Fertil Steril* 1952; 3:527–41.

50. Fischer IC. Psychogenic aspects of infertility. *Fertil Steril* 1953; 4:466–71.

51. Rothman D, Kaplan AH, Nettles E. Psychosomatic infertility. *Am J Obstet Gynecol* 1962; 83:373–81.

52. Belonoschkin B. Psychosomatic factors and matrimonial infertility. *Int J Fertil* 1962; 7:29–36.

53. Rubenstein BB. An emotional factor in infertility: A psychosomatic approach. *Fertil Steril* 1951; 2:80–6.

54. de Watteville H. Psychologic factors in the treatment of sterility. *Fertil Steril* 1957; 8:12–24.

55. Walker HE. Psychiatric aspects of infertility. *Urol Clin North Am* 1978; 5:481–8.

56. Denber HCB. Psychiatric aspects of infertility. *J Reprod Med* 1978; 20:23–9.

57. Edelmann RJ, Connolly KJ. Psychological aspects of infertility. *Br J Med Psychol* 1986; 59:209–19.

58. Noyes RW, Chapnick EM. Literature on psychology and infertility: A critical analysis. *Fertil Steril* 1964; 15:543–58.

59. Menning BE. The emotional needs of infertile couples. *Fertil Steril* 1980; 34:313–19.

60. Stanton AL, Dunkel-Schetter C. Psychological adjustment to infertility. In: AL Stanton, C Dunkel-Schetter, eds. *Infertility: Perspectives from Stress and Coping Research*. New York: Plenum Press, 1991; 3–16.

61. van Balen F. The psychologization of infertility. In: MC Inhorn, F Van Balen, eds. *Infertility Around the Globe: New Thinking on Childlessness, Gender, and Reproductive Technologies*. Los Angeles, CA: University of California Press, 2002; 79–98.

62. Wischmann TH. Psychogenic infertility: Myths and facts. *J Asst Reprod Genetics* 2003; 20:485–94.

63. Lukse MP, Vacc NA. Grief, depression, and coping in women undergoing infertility treatment. *Obstet Gynecol*, 1999; 93:245–51.

64. Kuchenhoff J. Unfulfilled desire for children – what is the grief for men? *Ther Umsch* 1999; 56:260–4.

65. Unruh AM, McGrath PJ. The psychology of female infertility: Toward a new perspective. *Health Care Women Int* 1985; 6:369–81.

66. Harvey JH. *Disenfranchised Grief: New Directions, Challenges, and Strategies for Practice*. Champaign, IL: Research Press, 2002.

67. Leon I. *When a Baby Dies: Psychotherapy for Pregnancy and Newborn Loss*. New Haven: Yale Press, 1990.

68. Kikendall KA. Self-discrepancy as an important factor in addressing women's emotional reactions to infertil-

ity. *Professional Psychology Research Practice* 1994; 25: 214–20.

69. Taymor ML, Bresnick E. Emotional stress and infertility. *Infertility* 1979; 2:39–47.

70. Stanton AL. Cognitive appraisals, coping processes, and adjustment to infertility. In: AL Stanton, C Dunkel-Schetter, eds. *Infertility: Perspectives from Stress and Coping Research*. New York: Plenum Press, 1991; 87–108.

71. Singer D, Hunter M, eds. *Assisted Human Reproduction: Psychological and Ethical Dilemmas*. London Whurr Publishers, 2003.

72. Goffman E. *Stigma: Notes on the Management of Spoiled Identity*. Englewood Cliffs, NJ: Prentice Hall, 1963.

73. Niederberger C. Middle Eastern masculinities in the age of new reproductive technologies: Male infertility and stigma in Egypt and Lebanon. *J Urol* 2005; 174:1368–9.

74. Sandelowski M, de Lacey S. The uses of a 'disease': Infertility as rhetorical vehicle. In: MC Inhorn, F Van Balen, eds. *Infertility Around the Globe: New Thinking on Childlessness, Gender, and Reproductive Technologies*. Los Angeles, CA: University of California Press, 2002; 33–51.

75. Nachtigall RD, Quiroga SS, Tschann JM, et al. Stigma, disclosure, and family functioning among parents with children conceived through donor insemination. *Fertil Steril* 1997; 68:1–7.

76. Matthews R, Matthews AM. Infertility and involuntary childlessness: The transition to nonparenthood. *J Marriage Fam* 1986; 48:641–9.

77. Miall CE. Perceptions of informal sanctioning and the stigma of involuntary childlessness. *Deviant Behav* 1985; 6:383–403.

78. Gonzalez LO. Infertility as a transformational process: A framework for psychotherapeutic support of infertile women. *Issues Ment Health Nurs* 2000; 21:619–33.

79. Daly, Kerry J. Crisis of genealogy: Facing the challenges of infertility. In: HI McCubbin, EA Thompson, et al., eds: *Resiliency in Families*. Sage Publications, Inc, 1999; 1–39.

80. Burns LH. Infertility as boundary ambiguity: One theoretical perspective. *Fam Process* 1987; 26:359–72.

81. Shapiro VB, Shapiro JR, Paret IH. *Complex Adoption and Assisted Reproductive Technology: A Developmental Approach to Clinical Practice*. New York: Guildford Press, 2001.

82. Read J. *Counselling for Fertility Problems*. London: Sage Publications Ltd, 1995.

83. Blenner JL. Passage through infertility treatment: A stage theory. *IMAGE: Journal of Nursing Scholarship* 1990; 22:153–8.

84. Diamond R, Kezur D, Meyers M, et al. *Couple Therapy for Infertility*. New York: Guildford Press, 1999.

85. Deveraux LL, Hammerman AJ. *Infertility and Identity: New Strategies for Treatment*. San Francisco: Jossey-Bass Publishers, 1998.

86. Cooper-Hilbert B. *Infertility and Involuntary Childlessness: Helping Couples Cope*. New York: WW Norton, 1998.

2 Medical Aspects of Infertility for the Counselor

WILLIAM R. KEYE, JR.

Fortunately when religion was strong and science weak, men mistook magic for medicine; now, when science is strong and religion weak, men mistake medicine for magic.

– Thomas Szasz

The term *infertility* is commonly used to describe a condition or disease characterized by the inability to conceive during one year of sexual intercourse without contraception.[1] This time interval is chosen because of the observation that approximately 25% of young couples will conceive within the first month, 60% within six months, and 80% within twelve months of unprotected sexual intercourse.[2] However, many couples consider themselves to be infertile if they conceive but, due to a miscarriage, are unable to deliver a living child. *Primary infertility* is defined as the failure to conceive by a couple who has never conceived, while *secondary infertility* refers to the failure to conceive by a couple who had previously conceived. In general, the evaluation and treatment of couples with primary or secondary infertility, as well as the causes, are similar.

While the prevalence of infertility is difficult to ascertain in developing countries, it is estimated that approximately 14% of married couples in the United States, Canada, Denmark, Scotland, and Sweden report that they are infertile. In rural Nigeria, the prevalence of primary and secondary infertility has been reported to be 12.9% and 54.1%, respectively.[3] While there is an impression that infertility has become more prevalent, recent data suggest this is not true in the developed world. In the United States, the proportion of couples experiencing infertility has apparently not changed since 1965.[4] What is increasing is the demand for medical services for infertility, and the publicity and public awareness of infertility, and its new high-tech treatments such as in vitro fertilization (IVF). The causes of infertility may be categorized as seen in Table 2.1.[5] The major causes of infertility include (1) failure to ovulate, (2) failure to deliver adequate numbers of healthy sperm to the fallopian tubes, (3) structural or functional abnormalities of the fallop-

ian tubes, (4) endometriosis or adhesions in the pelvis of the woman that interfere with capture of the egg by the fallopian tube, (5) poor timing or technique of intercourse, (6) infections of the reproductive tract, (7) immunological barriers to fertilization or implantation, and (8) an abnormal uterine lining that may interfere with implantation of the embryo. The infertility work-up is designed to evaluate each of these potential causes and to screen for the presence of underlying conditions or diseases. It is also important to note that an individual couple may have more than one reason for their infertility. Therefore, one should not assume that once an abnormality is found that there are no other contributing factors and should evaluate both partners even if a disorder is diagnosed in one partner.

This chapter

- identifies the etiology of infertility;
- reviews diagnostic testing in evaluation of male and female infertility;
- discusses current treatment options.

HISTORICAL OVERVIEW

The first written reference to infertility dates back to the Egyptians and the Kahoun papyrus (2200–1950 BC).[6] The Egyptians described procedures to diagnose infertility (e.g., a failure to detect on the breath the odor of garlic after it had been placed in the vagina) and therapeutic measures (e.g., douching with garlic or wine). Hippocrates (460–370 BC) was the first Greek author to discuss infertility and believed that pregnancy was not likely to occur unless the penis actually entered the uterine cavity and the semen of the male mixed with a 'semen concentrate' produced by the female. The Roman author Soranus, who lived in the second

TABLE 2.1. Causes of infertility[5]

Disorders of ovulation	30%
Abnormality of semen	22%
Abnormal fallopian tubes	17%
Unexplained	14%
Other disorders: cervical and uterine disorders, immunological problems, infection, sexual dysfunction	12%
Endometriosis	5%

century AD and who is considered by some to be the father of gynecology, believed that infertility was the result of the improper timing of intercourse and that the most fertile time of the menstrual cycle was just after the end of menstrual flow. He also believed that hot baths reduced fertility. It was not until the sixteenth century that our understanding of fertility and infertility became more scientifically based when Vesalius (1514–1564) described the female reproductive tract and Spellanzani described the process of fertilization. In the 1800s, infertility was thought to be primarily a mechanical problem caused by disorders of the cervix or malposition of the uterus. As a result, the treatment of infertility focused on the female and was, for the most part, surgical with an emphasis on dilatation of the cervix, removal of pelvic adhesions, and surgical repositioning of the uterus.

Modern practice in infertility is based almost entirely on observations and insights gained during the 1900s (Figure 2.1). For example, the relationship between body temperature and the phases of the menstrual cycle was first described in 1904. The recording of the basal body temperature (BBT) became the most commonly used and the most cost-effective method of detecting ovulation. Additional tests to document ovulation were introduced late in the twentieth century, and today commonly measure progesterone in the blood, look at the histological pattern of the lining of the uterus to determine if ovulation has occurred, or use ultrasound to assess follicular activity. Another example of the instrumental work of the early years of the twentieth century is the understanding of the interaction of sperm and cervical mucus. Although this interaction had been observed and described by J. Marion Sims[7] in 1888, its importance in achieving pregnancy was recognized by Huhner[8] in 1913.

Tests used to evaluate the fallopian tubes have changed very little in the past sixty years. In 1920, Isidor Rubin[9] described an office-based test in which oxygen was introduced through the cervix into the uterus and the resistance to flow measured. It was assumed that the fallopian tubes were open when there was little resistance and obstructed when there was a great deal of resistance. This test was later proven to be of little predictive value and has been replaced by the hysterosalpingogram (HSG), which was first described by Rindfleisch[10] in 1910. Hysterosalpingography involves the introduction of an x-ray contrast material into the cervix and uterus and gives a permanent radiological image of the shape and size of the uterine cavity and the fallopian tubes.

Evaluation of the fallopian tubes was limited to the HSG until the 1940s when Palmer,[11] working in Paris, began to use laparoscopy to evaluate the pelvic organs. While this technique was soon popular in Europe and Great Britain, physicians in North America did not adopt laparoscopy in the evaluation of female infertility until the 1960s. During the 1970s and 1980s, not only was the laparoscope used to evaluate the pelvis and diagnose pelvic adhesions and endometriosis, but it also became an important therapeutic tool as gynecologists learned to operate in the pelvis with it.

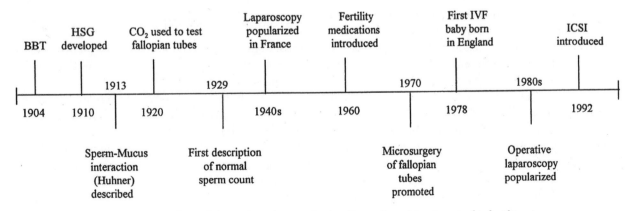

Figure 2.1. A timeline of the major advances in the diagnosis and treatment of infertility since 1900.

Evaluation of male infertility began with the microscopic observation of sperm by van Leeuwenhoek in the seventeenth century. However, the modern approach to the analysis of sperm can be traced to the description of what was thought to be a normal sperm count by Macomber and Sanders[12] in 1929. Much later in the twentieth century, the World Health Organization published a manual that standardized the techniques of semen analysis, as well as the normal range of sperm and semen parameters such as sperm density (count), motility, and morphology.[13] Perhaps the most significant advance in the treatment of infertility occurred in 1978 in England, when Robert Edwards and Patrick Steptoe announced the birth of the first baby conceived outside the human body. After almost a century of research on the process of fertilization, this announcement changed forever the evaluation and treatment of infertile couples. Now, almost thirty years later, tens of thousands of babies are born each year around the world via IVF. The process of IVF has quickly progressed from a medical curiosity to a cornerstone of infertility treatment.

Since 1990, several major developments have occurred. The first is a technique known as intracytoplasmic sperm injection (ICSI), in which a single sperm is injected into a single oocyte to create a fertilized oocyte. This technique has been the most significant advance in the treatment of male-factor infertility because it has made it possible for men who produce only a few or dysfunctional sperm to father a child. To complement this development, urologists developed relatively simple outpatient procedures to obtain sperm directly from the epididymis, microsurgical epididymal sperm aspiration (MESA), and testicle, testicular sperm extraction (TESE). The second major advancement has been the recent discovery of a means to freeze oocytes. Although not fully developed to date, this advance has the potential for dramatically changing the treatment of infertility in women with age-related factors and ovarian failure. The third major development has been preimplantation genetic diagnosis, which has made it possible to determine if an embryo is likely or not to produce a child with a genetic predisposition to one of many inheritable diseases. The fourth development has occurred in the field of medical economics, with an increasing interest and emphasis on cost-effective tests and treatments. While a greater appreciation of the cost-effectiveness of infertility care may streamline the evaluation of infertile couples, it also runs the risk that economic considerations will become the only factors considered in the choice among several therapeutic options. As a result, some couples may be forced by economic concerns to choose a therapy with which they may feel psychologically or ethically uncomfortable. In addition to economic factors, barriers to the access to care for fertility problems include lack of information among patients and their care providers and cultural bias against infertility treatment.[14] Finally, the fifth major development in the 1990s has been the focus on the psychosocial, regulatory, legal, and ethical aspects of reproduction. As we have become technologically more sophisticated and capable of manipulating genes (as well as oocytes, sperm, and embryos), society has become more interested in both the planning and oversight of artificial and third-party reproduction[15] while professionals have been more interested in establishing professional standards of care, whether medical or psychological care of the infertile.

REVIEW OF LITERATURE

Only recently has there been an emphasis on well-designed basic research studies of infertility. During most of recorded history, reports and studies of fertility and infertility treatments have consisted largely of anecdotes, uncontrolled trials, and descriptive studies. This is rapidly changing, however, and now "evidence from clinical trials is fundamental to ethical medical practice"[16] and is an important adjunct to clinical experience, patient preferences, and unique circumstances.

Clearly, the attempt to form a scientific basis for the clinical care of the infertile couple has begun to pay off, as those tests (e.g., postcoital tests) that were found to have little predictive value have been largely discarded, as have treatments that have been shown to be largely ineffective (e.g., empiric thyroid hormone therapy).

Current areas of research include the following:

■ Using medications in unconventional ways, such as the treatment of irregular menstruation with drugs typically used to treat breast cancer[17] or the use of antidepressant medications to improve fertility in women[18]
■ Identifying abnormalities of the lining of the uterus that may cause infertility[19]
■ Freezing human ovaries or ovarian tissue to preserve fertility in women about to undergo cancer chemotherapy or pelvic radiation[20]
■ Transplanting ovarian tissue or ovaries[21]
■ Using preimplantation diagnosis (PGD) to provide information to assist older patients in deciding whether it is worthwhile to continue to continue treatment[22]
■ Using nontraditional, alternative therapies such as acupuncture, phytoestrogens, or hyperbaric oxygen in the treatment of infertility.[23] The results of these

research efforts may change the content and style of infertility care in the future.

CLINICAL ISSUES

When Couples Should Seek Care

Based on the statistics presented earlier, couples should consider seeking medical care if they have not conceived during twelve months of unprotected sexual intercourse. However, some couples may benefit from earlier medical intervention.[24] For example, those who may be experiencing difficulty with sexual intercourse, have a known genetic disorder, or have a history of infertility in a previous relationship should consider medical evaluation earlier. In addition, women should consider obtaining a medical consultation or evaluation either before the first attempts are made to conceive or after six months of unsuccessful attempts if they do not have regular menstrual periods, have had or are suspected of having endometriosis, pelvic surgery or pelvic infections, have a history of cancer, or are attempting to conceive after age thirty-five. Finally, men who have problems with ejaculation, history of cancer treatment, or are known to have a history of infertility, infections, surgery, injuries, or developmental abnormalities of the male reproductive tract should seek care prior to or soon after deciding to attempt conception. This recommendation to obtain medical care for infertility is based not only on the assumption that medical treatments may enhance a couple's chances of conceiving, but also because infertility may be the presenting symptom of numerous underlying medical conditions. Individuals may be infertile because of diseases such as pituitary tumors, thyroid problems, endometriosis, or cancer or as a result of congenital or heritable conditions such as Klinefelter's syndrome or Rokitansky-Küster-Hauser syndrome. The early detection of underlying diseases and/or disorders may simplify infertility therapy and may improve not only chances of conception, but also the quality of an individual's life. In rare instances, it can also be life-saving. Thus, the treatment of infertility should not be seen as a purely elective process, because it clearly has potential health benefits.

Infertility Team

The care of the infertile man or woman should be provided by a team of professionals. While a family physician or internist can obtain an appropriate history and perform an adequate examination in a young man or woman with an uncomplicated history,

the care of most infertile women is best provided by a general obstetrician–gynecologist or a specialist in female infertility known as a reproductive endocrinologist. A reproductive endocrinologist is an obstetrician–gynecologist who has taken an additional two- or three-year fellowship and passed written and oral examinations. The American Board of Obstetrics and Gynecology offers a certificate of special competence in the field of reproductive endocrinology to those who complete the fellowship and pass the examinations. The specialist should be involved early in the care of the following groups of infertile women: older than thirty-five years who have had previous infertility; pelvic surgery, infection, or pelvic pain; cancer; congenital abnormalities of the reproductive tract; infertility for greater than two to three years, endometriosis, polycystic ovary syndrome or diseases of the fallopian tubes, and couples considering in vitro fertilization (IVF).[25] The reproductive endocrinologist usually has a nursing staff with special expertise in reproductive disorders. While the physician establishes the treatment plan, supervises the care of the patient, and performs surgery and IVF, nurses provide much of the day-to-day care by answering questions, instructing and educating patients with respect to tests and treatments, and performing simple office procedures. They also see and absorb much of the emotional reactions experienced by infertile couples. As a result, nurses must be knowledgeable about the impact of infertility, its tests, and treatments on emotions and relationships so that they can provide supportive care in an empathic and nonjudgmental manner or make appropriate referrals to a qualified infertility counselor. Many infertility practices also have a part- or full-time mental health professional such as a social worker or psychologist, who provides an array of services ranging from evaluation of couples' psychological and social background, to providing education and support in preparation for assisted reproductive technologies, to counseling couples about how to better cope with the stress of the infertility work-up and treatment.

The infertile male usually is initially seen by the gynecologist who is providing care for his wife or female partner. The gynecologist usually orders the initial semen analysis and, if it is abnormal, refers the man to a urologist. There are no formal fellowships for urologists wishing to specialize in the treatment of male-factor infertility. Urologists with special interest in male infertility often have additional training beyond their residency in general urology. They may have sophisticated semen or hormone laboratories in their office, may conduct research into male infertility, and may be part of an IVF team, working side by side with the other team members listed above. A urologist who has had additional training in infertility may be a better choice than a general urologist when there are severe abnormalities of semen quality or quantity that may require MESA or TESE. Even when there is a significant semen or sperm problem, the reproductive endocrinologist usually coordinates most of the care because the eventual treatment often involves female-focused treatments such as intrauterine insemination, in vitro fertilization, or intracytoplasmic sperm injection. Most sophisticated infertility teams also have an embryologist on staff. The embryologist is usually a laboratory scientist with a masters or doctorate degree who is responsible for the fertilization of the eggs and the growth of the embryos in conjunction with IVF, as well as the laboratory evaluation of the male and preparation of the sperm for intrauterine insemination. The proper use and collaboration of all of these professionals is essential to efficient and effective therapy and treatment success. Because of the rapid expansion of new and highly technical options for therapy, designing the best strategy for each couple is not easy. In addition, there usually is more than one reasonable treatment plan for any infertile person or couple. Just as there is no single best treatment plan for each infertile person, there is no ideal team either.

Initial Appointment

The initial visit is perhaps more important than any other visit that may follow because it establishes the foundation for all future visits. Ideally, it should involve both partners (if there is a partner) and focus on reviewing not only the medical but also the psychological, religious, and social or cultural aspects of the individual or couple's infertility problem. The goal should be to develop a plan or outline for future care that will meet both the individual's and the couple's goals and needs. It is common practice to have infertile individuals or couples complete and return a detailed infertility questionnaire before their first visit with the reproductive endocrinologist. Such a questionnaire is available for a small charge from the American Society for Reproductive Medicine (see www.asrm.org). In addition, it is recommended that all relevant previous records including x-ray examinations and/or surgical videos be available for review at the initial visit. During the initial interview, it is helpful to have a few minutes alone with each member of the couple, as well as interviewing them together. An individual may be more willing to share information about previous pregnancies, elective terminations, extramarital relationships, and/or sexually transmitted diseases if their partner is not present.

Because of the expanding number of treatment options, it is becoming more common for couples to seek advice from several specialists before embarking on a program of evaluation or treatment. Infertile couples are commonly as interested in interviewing the infertility physician and team as the physician or team is in interviewing the couple.

The content of the initial interview should consist of a discussion of the following topics:

■ Duration of infertility and results of any previous evaluation and treatment

■ Menstrual, gynecological, and obstetric history in the female

■ Urological history in the male including the results of all previous sperm assays including allergies to medications, current use of medications, herbs or alternative therapies, current illnesses or system diseases, surgeries of the reproductive tract, urological infections, exposure to sexually transmitted diseases, vasectomy, and/or pregnancy with a different partner

■ Medical history including a history in the woman should include allergies to medications, current use of medications, herbs or alternative therapies, previous illnesses or current systemic diseases, previous pregnancies, contraceptive techniques, surgeries, systemic disease, pelvic infections, abnormal pap smears, exposure to sexually transmitted diseases, abortions, or sterilization.

■ Family history of genetic disorders, birth defects, mental retardation, multiple miscarriages, or infertility in one or both partners including report from genetic counselor, in event couple has been counseled

■ Previous relationships in which infertility may have been an issue

■ Lifestyle, including diet; exercise; use of alcohol, tobacco, or recreational drugs; exposure to environmental toxins; or occupational factors including any cultural, religious, or legal factors that may influence their treatment

■ Sexual practices and the frequency and timing of intercourse, as well as the presence of pain with intercourse, erectile dysfunction, or retrograde ejaculation

■ Reasons why the individual or couple may be seeking medical care at the present time

■ Goals and expectations, including the motives for seeking infertility care

■ Beliefs about why they have not conceived and about the process of conception itself

■ The unique psychosocial and cultural environment in which the couple is trying to conceive, including pressure exerted by a partner, extended family, community, religion, or other stresses

■ The individual's psychosocial and cultural responses to his or her infertility and the possible need for referral for appropriate counseling or other special accommodations (e.g., translator, special condoms for sperm collection)
■ The acceptability of tests and treatments such as donor insemination, IVF, selective reduction, and preimplantation genetic diagnoses
■ Financial and other resources or limitations or constrictions (e.g., reproductive tourists with time-limited visas)

Following this detailed history, a physical examination will be performed, either at the initial visit or a subsequent visit before extensive testing or treatment begins. In addition, in some practices the infertile couple may meet with a mental health professional (infertility counselor) or health educator to discuss issues of concern, as well as strategies for coping with the stress associated with infertility and its evaluation and treatment.

Once these issues have been addressed, the physician may outline a plan for evaluation and/or treatment and provide a decision-tree and timeline for the couple. Most couples will find the medical evaluation and treatments less stressful if they know in advance how the information gained from tests will be used and how long it will take to complete the evaluation or course of therapy. This approach establishes a partnership between the infertility team and the infertile couple or individual and may reduce the tension that is an inevitable part of the process. It is only after all these issues have been discussed that an appropriate plan can be developed. However, it should be noted that caregivers must be prepared to adapt this approach given the cultural background of the patients. In some cultures, a collaborative partnership in terms of treatment is less acceptable than in most Western cultures and patients prefer the physician to take a more paternalistic/authoritative approach to their care.

One of the initial visits will include a physical examination of the female. The examination should include height, weight, a general physical assessment, blood pressure, hair distribution, breast development and an attempt to elicit breast secretions, and abdominal and pelvic examinations. If the male's history or semen analysis suggests a problem, he is usually referred to a urologist for a physical examination, evaluation, and treatment.

If the individual or couple has decided to follow through with the infertility team, the visit should conclude with the discussion of a strategy so that the individual or couple may return home to think about, discuss, and commit to additional care. It is advisable that

the physician write down the important points that have been discussed, so the couple can review them later. The plan should consist of an outline of tests and treatments, together with brief descriptions of their costs and odds of success. Some practices may also include a discussion about healthcare insurance/coverage/benefits and financial aspects of infertility care. Finally, a list of local resources, bibliography, or patient education brochures (available from patient support groups, professional orgnizations, and some pharmaceutical companies) may be of value to the infertile individual or couple.

Most infertile individuals are concerned that their diet, exercise program, or other aspects of their lifestyle may be the cause of their infertility. As such, it may be helpful to address these concerns during their initial visit, using it as an opportunity to provide patient education and treatment if needed. There is now significant evidence that the use of tobacco, alcohol, and marijuana negatively impact both male and female fertility. Present data indicate that approximately 13% of both male and female infertility can be linked to cigarette smoking. Because of these data and the detrimental effects of smoking on nonreproductive organs, the healthcare provider should discourage smoking in all patients, but especially in those who are trying to conceive or plan to conceive in the future.[26] Additionally, obesity is another factor impacting fertility in men and women. Excessive exercise (leading to little body fat) may impact fertility in women, while certain forms of exercise may be detrimental to male reproduction (e.g., bicycling). For men, exposure to toxic agents and heat as well as excessive masturbation near the time of ovulation may decrease fertility. All too often, patients are undereducated about how their own health efficacy behaviors can improve their fertility and may, instead, turn to 'alternative or adjunctive' treatments (e.g., acupuncture) when altering their own behaviors may be just as effective, or more so.

Infertility Evaluation

The diagnostic evaluation of infertility is designed to identify the cause or causes of infertility and determine the most effective and cost-efficient approach to therapy. In general, the least invasive, least expensive, and least painful diagnostic tests are done first. Before proceeding with the diagnostic evaluation, the clinician and individual or couple should agree on the extent of testing and establish a timeline for testing. Finally, many couples appreciate receiving a decision-tree that outlines how the diagnostic work-up and treatment plan will be influenced by the results of the diagnostic tests.

As shown in Table 2.2, an infertility evaluation consists of some or all of the following tests: determination of ovulation, evaluation of the production and delivery

---

TABLE 2.2. Evaluation of the infertile couple

Detection of ovulation
  Menstrual history
  Basal body temperature
  Serum progesterone
  Endometrial biopsy
  Serial ultrasound examinations

Evaluation of production and delivery of sperm
  Semen analysis

Evaluation of fallopian tubes
  Hysterosalpingogram
  Infusion of dye into the tubes at laparoscopy

Evaluation of the uterine cavity
  Hysterosalpingogram
  Hysteroscopy
  Sonohysterogram

Evaluation of pelvic cavity (adhesions, endometriosis)
  Laparoscopy

Evaluation of transportation of sperm in female
  Postcoital examination

---

of sperm, determination of patency of the fallopian tubes and size and shape of the uterine cavity, evaluation of the pelvic cavity with a search for endometriosis or adhesions, and evaluation of sperm transport within the female reproductive tract.

Detecting Ovulation

Detection of ovulation is extremely important because the treatment of infertility resulting from a failure to ovulate is among the most successful of all infertility treatments. The menstrual history is often by itself a reliable indicator of the presence or absence of ovulation. A history of regular, cyclic, predictable, and painful menstrual periods usually indicates that ovulation is occurring. However, the patient who is not ovulating may still have menstrual periods, although they usually occur less frequently than every thirty-five days, at unpredictable intervals, and without menstrual cramps. An inexpensive, convenient, and noninvasive approach to the documentation of ovulation is to chart the basal body temperature (BBT) each day through one or two menstrual cycles. A woman who is ovulating will usually have an early morning temperature that is less than 98°F (36.6°C) during the first half of the menstrual cycle and higher than 98°F (36.6°C) during the second half of the menstrual cycle. However, the BBT does not give specific enough information to determine the day of ovulation, and it is not a good method for predicting which day ovulation actually occurs. However, because

some women find it impractical and stressful to take their BBT, the detection of progesterone within the blood can also be used to determine if ovulation has occurred. About the time of the ovulation, the ovary begins to produce progesterone, and once the level of progesterone exceeds three nanograms per milliliter of serum, the temperature rises and one can be reasonably certain that ovulation has occurred.[27] The progesterone value is most reliable when testing occurs approximately one week after the assumed day of ovulation or approximately one week before the anticipated onset of the next menstrual period. Some physicians obtain a biopsy of the endometrium (uterine lining). The histological appearance of the endometrium under a microscope change, after ovulation and in response to the secretion of progesterone. However, the endometrial biopsy is typically expensive and often uncomfortable for women. Serial ultrasound examinations of the ovaries is another way of assessing ovulation that may provide presumptive evidence of ovulation. However, because this approach is not always accurate and can be expensive, it is not recommended.

If it is determined that a woman is not ovulating, a search for specific causes of the ovulation disorder should be performed. Over-the-counter ovulation predictor kits are often helpful in determining the day of ovulation in women with regular monthly periods. However, they are not a substitute for a BBT or blood progesterone test in women with irregular periods because they may occasionally produce false-positive or false-negative results and do not provide proof of ovulation. Also, they are an additional expense and may give patients a false sense of confidence about the accuracy of ovulation prediction.

From the moment of birth, the number and quality of a woman's oocytes decreases until she reaches menopause at about age fifty. Many years prior to the menopause, there is a significant decline in fertility due to the spontaneous and gradual death of the oocytes in her ovaries. The extent to which her oocytes have decreased and the impact of this decrease on her fertility can be estimated by measuring a hormone, that is, follicle-stimulating hormone (FSH), in her blood. As the number of oocytes decrease, the FSH value increases. While the test is not perfectly accurate, it is used by most fertility specialists, along with other fertility tests results, to predict the likelihood of achieving a pregnancy with any of the fertility treatments.

In rare situations, this normal process of ovarian aging is accelerated in young women (eighteen to thirty-five years) who will experience symptoms similar to menopause, a condition called premature ovarian failure (POF). Fortunately, women who experience premature ovarian failure are not always menopausal and may still have a 5–10% chance of conceiving. However, the resumption of ovulation and return of fertility is unpredictable and intermittent so it is impossible to predict the best time to have intercourse in order to conceive. A common sense approach would be to recommend the woman have coitus two to three times a week so sperm will be present in her reproductive tract when and if ovulation occurs.[28]

Unfortunately, the loss of oocytes with age is an irreversible process. While there are effective treatments for almost any other cause of female-factor fertility, there is no effective therapy that can restore fertility once most of the normal, healthy oocytes have disappeared. As a result, most women, no matter the age, become very sad when they are informed that their FSH blood test value is high, their chances of conceiving are low, and there is no way to replace their oocytes or restore their fertility. They often express disbelief or anger and may seek a second opinion, hoping to receive a better prognosis. For most of these women, their only options are using donated oocytes, adoption, or childlessness. For obvious reasons, these women should be offered professional counseling in addition to medical care.

Evaluation of the Production and Delivery of Sperm

It has been estimated that 40–60% of all couples with infertility have an identifiable cause that may be attributed to the male partner.[29] The initial evaluation should include a reproductive history that includes questions regarding coital frequency, timing, and sexual functioning, duration of infertility, childhood illnesses, systemic adult illnesses, prior surgery, sexually transmitted diseases, and exposure to toxic substances. Their reproductive history should include questions about any pregnancies, births, or pregnancy losses with other partners and use of birth control including vasectomy. The standard test of male fertility is semen analysis, which should be performed early in the course of the infertile couple's evaluation. A minimum of two analyses should be performed several weeks apart to properly assess male fertility. It is important that clinicians use a laboratory capable of performing an appropriate semen analysis. Laboratories usually perform a semen analysis and report the results according to the recommendations of the WHO.[13] The parameters and normal values recommended by the WHO are seen in Table 2.3. Often, small hospital laboratories or independent laboratories may not use these standards, and consequently confidence in the results may be lacking – misleading patients about their actual reproductive capabilities or problems. If a semen analysis report does not give the normal range of values and all of the parameters as outlined by the WHO, another semen sample should be obtained and evaluated in a more sophisticated laboratory. In addition, the laboratory should have a quality control program and proper certification. The semen analysis should be obtained through masturbation, after at least one day, but no more than ten days, of abstinence[30] into a clean container that does not contain soap residue or other substances or residues that may be harmful to the sperm. For those men who have personal, cultural, or religious objections to the collection of a sample in this way, special condoms can and should be provided that facilitate collection of the sample during intercourse. Standard, over-the-counter condoms used for contraception and prevention of disease transmission are not recommended because they are toxic to the sperm.

If there is a consistent abnormality in the quality or numbers of sperm seen on two or more occasions, an evaluation of the male by a urologist is indicated. The urologist takes a general medical, surgical, reproductive, and sexual history, as well as a history of possible exposure to toxic substances, including medications, tobacco, alcohol, and recreational drugs.[31] Various medications may interfere with normal sperm production by inhibiting the production of hormones by the pituitary or the testicles, by directly affecting the testicle itself, or by interfering with ejaculation. In addition, the use of tobacco, alcohol, and marijuana is associated with an abnormal sperm count, morphology, or function and, as such, diminished fertility.

Physical examination of the male may detect systemic diseases, endocrine disorders, infections, or developmental abnormalities of the male reproductive system, including congenital absence of the vas deferens. Because congenital bilateral absence of the vas deferens (CBAVD) occurs more often in men who carry a gene for cystic fibrosis, known as the cystic fibrosis transmembrane conductance regulator (CFTR), those in whom this abnormality is found should undergo genetic testing and counseling (and testing of their partner) and a CFTR mutation analysis performed before the couple starts any fertility treatments. These men should also have an evaluation of their kidneys and ureters to look for congenital abnormalities of the urogenital system. In addition, abnormalities of the

TABLE 2.3. Normal semen analysis parameters from the World Health Organization[13]

Volume	≥2.0 mL
PH	≥7.2–8.0
Count	≥20 million/mL
Motility	≥50%
Progressive motility	≥25%
Morphology	30% normal forms

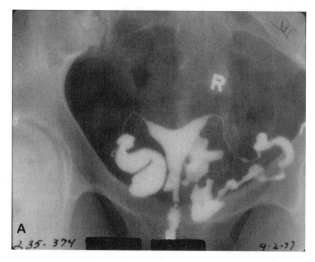
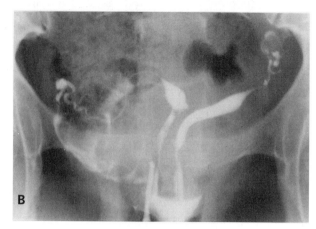

Figure 2.2. **A.** A normal hysterosalpingogram that shows swelling of the right fallopian tube because of obstruction of its distal end. The left tube is normal caliber and opens into the peritoneal cavity. **B.** A hysterosalpingogram of a double uterus and normal fallopian tubes.

urethra may lead to the deposition of sperm outside the vagina during intercourse. Finally, infertile men may also have a collection of varicose veins within the scrotum known as a varicocele. Large varicoceles may interfere with both the number and quality of sperm. Surgical correction of a varicocele may occasionally have a dramatic impact on the number and quality of sperm thereby improving fertility.

Blood tests to detect hormonal causes of male infertility should be performed if there is (1) an abnormal semen analysis with a sperm concentration of less than 10 million/ml, (2) impotence or difficulty ejaculating, or (3) historical or physical findings consistent with specific hormone disorders. The minimal hormone evaluation should include the measurement of serum testosterone and follicle-stimulating hormone (FSH) concentrations.[29] Other tests such as an evaluation of urine for sperm, an ultrasound examination of the scrotum, cultures of semen for bacteria, antisperm antibodies, and sperm viability tests may be indicated by other abnormalities of the semen analysis.

Finally, as many as 18% of men with a decreased number of sperm that cannot otherwise be accounted for, have a missing fragment of their Y chromosome (microdeletions).[32] Genetic testing should be recommended to men who have few or no sperm and no evidence of an obstruction of their vas deferns or epididymis and to men with CBAVD.

Unfortunately, men with azoospermia and/or testicular failure to produce sperm, regardless of age, are understandably alarmed and saddened to learn that there are no effective treatments or therapies to restore fertility. Both the man and/or his partner may have difficulty grasping the reality of their situation – perhaps seeking a second opinion, hoping to receive a

better prognosis. However, the reality is that for these couples their only alternatives are dramatically altered with their only alternatives being the use of donor sperm, adoption, or childlessness. As such, these couples should be offered professional counseling in addition to medical care.

Evaluation of the Fallopian Tubes

A potentially correctable cause of female infertility is obstruction or blockage of the fallopian tubes. While this may occasionally be congenital, it more often follows a pelvic infection or pelvic surgery. It has been estimated that approximately 15% of women who have a single episode of a pelvic infection caused by chlamydia or neisseria gonorrhoeae will have obstruction of the fallopian tubes.[33] As noted earlier, detection of an obstruction of the fallopian tubes is usually accomplished by hysterosalpingography (HSG). In this procedure, a colorless liquid, known as x-ray contrast material, is injected into the opening of the cervix, and its flow through the uterus and the fallopian tubes is observed via an x-ray machine. A series of pictures are taken, and the location and type of obstruction may be detected. This procedure usually takes only fifteen minutes to perform and is usually associated with mild-to-moderate menstrual-like cramps. If an abnormality of the fallopian tubes is detected, a laparoscopy can identify the specific nature and extent of disease of the fallopian tube. An HSG showing obstruction of the fallopian tubes with the presence of hydrosalpinges is seen in Figure 2.2A, and a double uterus with normal fallopian tubes is seen in Figure 2.2B.

Abnormalities of the cavity of the uterus are uncommon, but often very treatable causes of infertility. Pedunculated submucosal fibroids, endometrial polyps,

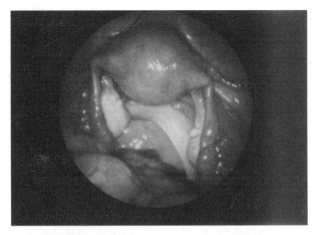

Figure 2.3. The appearance of normal pelvic organs as seen through a laparoscope.

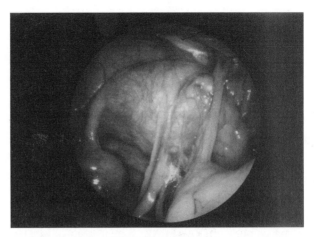

Figure 2.4. The laparoscopic appearance of pelvic adhesions.

and uterine septae are the most common abnormalities of the cavity and are all easily treated. Other less common abnormalities such as a bicornuate uterus or diethylstilbestrol (DES) exposure are not generally remediable nor do they necessarily need treatment. The hysterosalpingogram, used to detect abnormalities of the fallopian tubes, is also used by most reproductive endocrinologists to detect abnormalities of the uterus. Once an abnormality has been detected, the exact nature and extent of the abnormality may be determined by performing an ultrasound exam after the infusion of saline into the cavity, a sonohysterogram, or by viewing the cavity through a thin telescope, a procedure known as hysteroscopy.

Evaluating the Cervix

The postcoital examination of the cervix has long been a standard part of the infertility evaluation of a couple. It is designed to evaluate the transport of sperm within the female reproductive tract. However, there is a great deal of controversy regarding its validity, because the interpretation of the test results is extremely subjective and the results have not been found to predict future fertility.[34] During the test, which is usually performed on the day of or within two days prior to ovulation, a couple is instructed to have intercourse without the use of vaginal lubricants. The woman then comes into the office several hours later, and the nurse or physician obtains a sample of mucus from the cervix. The quality of the mucus is then evaluated, and the sample is viewed through a microscope in the office. The sperm are counted and their motility determined. Because of its poor predictive value and because in vitro fertilization or the direct insemination of sperm into the uterus bypasses the cervix, the postcoital test is rarely performed today. Furthermore, many patients found the testing stressful and distasteful.

Evaluation of the Pelvic Cavity

Laparoscopy is an outpatient surgical procedure during which a telescope is placed through a small incision in the umbilicus or navel. The pelvic cavity is then visualized, and the various pelvic structures viewed. Figure 2.3 shows the appearance of a normal pelvis as seen through the laparoscope. Figure 2.4 shows adhesions within the pelvis. Laparoscopy is clearly indicated in women with infertility and either moderate-to-severe pain with their periods or pain with intercourse. In addition, women who have a history of pelvic surgery or pelvic infections may have pelvic scar tissue and often benefit from laparoscopy. Women who have had an abnormal HSG indicating blockage of the fallopian tubes are also candidates for laparoscopy unless they choose to use IVF. Finally, many women with otherwise unexplained infertility are candidates for laparoscopy. However, laparoscopy is the most expensive of the diagnostic procedures, and many physicians now delay or omit laparoscopy in women who have no significant pain and no history of pelvic infections or surgery, if the HSG and pelvic ultrasound are normal. The role of laparoscopy in the evaluation of infertile woman is evolving, and indications for its use are changing. Once an evaluation has or has not, been completed and the information obtained from the laparoscopy has been evaluated, a course of therapy can be laid out for the patient. The course of therapy will usually be dictated or determined by the results of the diagnostic tests. However, there are often several different treatment options.

THERAPEUTIC INTERVENTIONS

Using the tests described above, a possible reason for a couple's infertility will be found in approximately 85% of cases.[5] No explanation or reason will be found for the other 15%. Once an explanation has, or has not, been found, a treatment program can be presented to the infertile individual or couple.

Induction of Ovulation

Women who do not have monthly menstrual periods will almost always respond to ovulation-inducing drugs (so-called 'fertility drugs'), unless they have experienced ovarian failure (e.g., menopause). There are two commonly used classes of drugs to induce ovulation. The first are termed antiestrogens and consist of either clomiphene citrate or tamoxifen citrate. While clomiphene citrate is approved by the U.S. Food and Drug Administration (FDA) for ovulation induction, tamoxifen is not. Clomiphene and tamoxifen are available in tablet form and are taken for five or more days during the early part of the menstrual cycle. Approximately one week after the last tablet is taken, ovulation usually occurs, and the couple should have intercourse several times around this time. These drugs may cause hot flashes but are usually free of other side effects, except for a multiple pregnancy rate of approximately 6–8%. If ovulation does not occur after use of these drugs, the course of medication is usually repeated at a higher dosage. Approximately 60–70% of women will ovulate on clomiphene or tamoxifen, and 30–40% will conceive within six months of therapy. Because most women who conceive on clomiphene will do so in the first four months, the extended use of clomiphene for more than four to six months is considered inappropriate or questionable. Recently, researchers have reported that another class of antiandrogens, known as aromatase inhibitors, are also effective in inducing ovulation in some women. However, experience with these drugs is limited and they are not approved by the FDA for this indication.

The other class of ovulation induction medications are known as gonadotropins. These drugs are similar to the human hormones produced by the pituitary gland, and are either extracted and purified from human urine, or produced from Chinese hamster ovaries using recombinant technology. They are given by intramuscular or subcutaneous injection and tend to stimulate several follicles to grow and for several oocytes to ovulate. Of those who conceive on these medications, 15–20% will have a multiple pregnancy. Because of the potential for multiple follicular development and a condition called hyperstimulation syndrome, close monitoring in the form of blood hormone tests and pelvic ultrasound examinations is commonly performed. In its most mild form, hyperstimulation syndrome is characterized by multiple ovarian cysts; while in its most severe form it is marked by the production of a large amount of free fluid in the abdominal cavity and around the lungs. It may cause abdominal pain, marked weight gain, difficulty breathing, and, rarely, death due to blood clots that may cause a stroke or other catastrophic events. The syndrome is usually more severe if a woman conceives in the month in which she receives the gonadotropin. These medications are much more expensive, more potent than the antiestrogens, and administered via injections.

Fallopian Tube Surgery

When the infertility investigation detects scar tissue or adhesions within the fallopian tubes, surgery may restore fertility to normal. The scar tissue may be limited to one small segment of the tube, and the rest of the tube may be remarkably normal. If the scar tissue is located near the junction of the tube and the uterus, the small segment of the tube containing the scar tissue can be removed and the healthy ends sewn back together. Another procedure, transcervical balloon tuboplasty, uses small probes or catheters passed from within the uterus and out into the tubes to open the blocked area, if the obstruction at the junction of the tube and ovary is due to delicate scar tissue or a plug of mucus wedged into the tube. Pregnancy rates following these procedures may approach 50% if the rest of the tube is normal and there are no other infertility factors.

In the case of a previous tubal ligation, surgery known as microsurgical tubal reanastomosis may restore fertility. The surgery requires magnification, very small sutures, and special training in gynecological microsurgery. If the previous tubal ligation has not removed or damaged the majority of the length of the fallopian tube and there are no other possible causes of infertility, an experienced microsurgeon can reanastomose the fallopian tubes and restore fertility in nearly 75% of women.

If scar tissue is blocking the distal end of the fallopian tube adjacent to the ovary, surgery may also be successful. This surgery is often performed through the laparoscope and may restore fertility in as few as 10% or as many as 60–70% of women, depending on the extent of scar tissue. Unfortunately, there is an increased risk of an ectopic or tubal pregnancy after restorative tubal surgery. The greatest advantage of tubal surgery is that the woman may have more than one pregnancy after a single successful tubal surgery.

Treatment of a Poorly Developed Lining of the Uterus

A successful intrauterine pregnancy requires a receptive and healthy uterine lining. Several therapies have been shown to improve the condition of the uterine lining. For some women who are extremely thin or engaged in extremely strenuous exercise, weight gain and restoration of normal eating habits along with a reduction in exercise may restore the lining of the uterus to normal by increasing the production of estrogen and progesterone by the ovaries. For others, ovulation induction medications may be necessary to stimulate greater production of estrogen or progesterone by the ovaries, which will, in turn, improve the lining of the uterus. Finally, the administration of progesterone by intramuscular injection or vaginal suppository or gel may restore fertility to normal in women with a thin uterine lining. However, our understanding of the role of the uterine lining in conception is incomplete and the validity of some of these therapies has yet to be established.

Treatment of Abnormal Sperm Transportation

If the number of sperm reaching the fallopian tubes after intercourse is inadequate because of low sperm count, the inability to deposit adequate numbers of sperm into the vagina during intercourse or an abnormal interaction between the sperm and the cervical mucus, placement of sperm directly into the uterus may lead to a successful pregnancy. The success of intrauterine insemination (IUI) requires processing of the sperm in the laboratory. Approximately two hours before the insemination is to be done, a semen sample is obtained through masturbation, and the sperm are separated from the semen by the use of a sperm 'washing' technique or the passage of the semen sample through a column of material that allows the sperm to swim out of the semen. Once prepared, the sperm are then placed into the uterine cavity using a thin catheter placed through the cervix during a pelvic speculum examination at ovulation. This process takes only thirty to sixty seconds and is usually painless. The woman then leaves the office and goes about her usual daily activities. The other important factor in successful IUI is the appropriate timing. IUI may be performed approximately fourteen days before the next anticipated menstrual period, within eighteen to thirty-six hours of a positive ovulation detection test, or approximately thirty-six hours after the administration of human chorionic gonadotropin (hCG) given to trigger ovulation. Some physicians advocate two or more inseminations each month. Success rates vary according to the quality and number of sperm, the presence of other female reproductive disorders, and age of the woman. For a woman under the age of thirty-five using normal sperm with a cervical factor, the monthly chances of achieving a pregnancy with IUI are approximately 10–15%. If poor

transportation of sperm in the female reproductive tract is the result of an infection of the cervix, a course of antibiotic therapy may be successful.

Treatment of Endometriosis

Endometriosis is a common condition characterized by the presence of uterine lining tissue in locations outside the uterus. It is commonly found in and around the ovaries and fallopian tubes and may cause pelvic pain and infertility. While it is present in only 3–10% of all women of reproductive age, it is found in 30–35% of women with infertility. Exactly how endometriosis contributes to infertility is unknown, although it often causes infertility by stimulating the formation of ovarian cysts and forming scar tissue. Fortunately, not all women with endometriosis will be infertile.

In cases of endometriosis, surgery and drug therapy have been used to improve pregnancy rates. Several medications are commonly used in the treatment of endometriosis, including birth control pills, progesterone, danazol, and gonadotropin-releasing hormone (Gn-RH) agonists. These medications are most useful in treating the pain of endometriosis and, perhaps, preventing its recurrence, but less useful in treating infertility. By themselves, they have not been shown to improve fertility. They may, however, be useful in reducing the volume of disease before surgery or reducing the likelihood of adhesion formation or recurrence of endometriosis after surgery. While most women will tolerate and respond well to one or more of these medications, each medication has its own set of side effects which many women find distressing and, as a result, limit its usefulness. Typical side effects include hot flashes, headaches, mood changes, vaginal dryness, acne, facial hair growth, and weight gain.

The most successful approach to the treatment of endometriosis appears to be surgery. The surgical removal of mild endometriosis may not only improve fertility but can also be useful in reducing pelvic pain. Surgical removal of extensive endometriosis and restoration of the normal anatomical relationships between the ovaries and the fallopian tubes may dramatically improve fertility so that as many as 50–60% of women will conceive after surgery. While most surgery for endometriosis can be performed on an outpatient basis through a laparoscope, occasionally a laparotomy and postoperative hospitalization are required.

Treatment of Uterine Abnormalities

Abnormalities of the uterine cavity may either prevent pregnancy or increase the chance of miscarriage. The most common abnormalities are fibroids, adhesions, polyps, and congenital abnormalities, such as a septum dividing the cavity into halves. Another abnormality of the uterine cavity occurs in women who were exposed to DES during the first three months of their mother's pregnancy. The inside of the uterus in women with this abnormality has the appearance of the letter *T* instead of an inverted triangle. Women with a T-shaped uterus caused by DES exposure may have more difficulty conceiving and carrying a pregnancy to term. In the past, adhesions or polyps were treated by performing a dilatation and curettage (D&C), and fibroids and congenital abnormalities were treated by performing a laparotomy and using a scissors to cut out the abnormal tissue. Today, however, almost all uterine surgery for these conditions is performed through a hysteroscope, a small telescope placed through the cervix.

Treatment of Male Infertility

A few infertile men may have a congenital or acquired deficiency in the secretion of the pituitary hormones, luteinizing hormone (LH) and follicle-stimulating hormone (FSH). In these cases, there is inadequate stimulation of the testes and poor or no sperm production. Normal production of sperm and testosterone may be induced by administration of LH and FSH (by intramuscular injection using a preparation of human menopausal gonadotropins), of a Gn-RH agonist to stimulate pituitary production of LH and FSH, or of hCG, which mimics the action of LH. One or more of these therapies are usually effective if the testes are normal.

There are numerous other hormonal therapies that have been studied and used in men who have a normal pituitary gland but produce sperm in reduced numbers. They include clomiphene, tamoxifen, low-dose testosterone, human menopausal gonadotropins, thyroid hormone, vitamins A, C, and E, and zinc. Unfortunately, while these treatments may benefit an occasional individual, none has been proven consistently successful in the treatment of low-sperm production.

The surgical treatment of a varicocele eliminates more than 90% of varicoceles and has been shown to improve semen quality in the majority of men. However, it is not currently possible to state that varicocele repair improves fertility due to methodologic limitations of the scientific studies published.[35] Microsurgical procedures, such as MESA and TESE, may restore fertility in men who have had a previous vasectomy or have accidental transection of the vasa during pelvic surgery or a previous hernia repair. Surgery may also be helpful when there is obstruction or other abnormalities of the ejaculatory duct. Unfortunately, fertility is not always restored after surgery due to either scar tissue formation in the vas deferens or antisperm antibodies in the testes. However, up to 75% of men may father children after surgical repair of a previous vasectomy.

Finally, men who cannot deliver sperm or ejaculate usually have sperm in their testes. A biopsy of their testes or aspiration of fluid from their epididymus may yield sufficient sperm that can be injected into eggs to produce embryos at IVF. These procedures are preferred to surgery when the female partner is near forty years old, when she has a cause of infertility that requires IVF, when surgery is too expensive for the couple, or when the odds of successful surgery are low.[36]

Assisted Reproduction

While IVF was originally designed to overcome irreversible disorders of the fallopian tubes, it has become an appropriate treatment for virtually all forms of infertility in men and women. In addition, when coupled with the donation of oocytes from younger women, it has been highly successful in helping women older than forty conceive.

IVF consists of several steps. The first step is the stimulation of the ovaries to produce multiple oocytes or follicles. In response to clomiphene, human menopausal gonadotropins, or FSH, most women will produce at least four to six and as many as twenty to thirty mature oocytes. The goal is not to obtain the greatest number of oocytes but to obtain several good-quality oocytes, capable of being fertilized. During ovulation stimulation with medications, blood tests are obtained and pelvic ultrasound examinations are performed to monitor the response of the ovaries.

Once the oocytes have reached an appropriate maturity, they are collected using a needle introduced into the pelvis through the vagina and guided by ultrasound. The oocytes, once collected, are sent to an embryology laboratory, where they are mixed with large numbers of sperm in a small laboratory dish. Alternatively, a single sperm may be injected into a single oocyte to achieve fertilization. This procedure is called intracytoplasmic sperm injection or ICSI. Within twenty-four hours, evidence of fertilization can be observed through a microscope. The fertilized oocytes are allowed to divide into two-, then four-, then six- to eight-celled embryos over the next forty-eight to seventy-two hours. The embryos are graded according to their quality. Those embryos that divide rapidly and consist of individual cells that are round and equally sized are considered high quality and have a greater chance of implanting. At the time of embryo transfer, the couple is consulted and a final decision is made regarding how many embryos will be transferred into the uterus. Of course, an initial discussion of the number of embryos to transfer should take place early in the discussion of IVF. In some countries, the maximum number of embryos that can be transferred is federally regulated, while in other countries there are voluntary guidelines. The transfer of a larger number of embryos may result in an unacceptable risk of multiple pregnancy without a significant improvement in singleton pregnancy rate. As a result, some countries have strict limitations on the number of embryos transferred and do not allow for individualization after consideration of each patient's unique circumstances.

The transfer of embryos occurs during a pelvic examination using a thin, soft catheter. The embryos are loaded into the end of the catheter, and the catheter is passed painlessly through the cervix into the uterine cavity. During the weeks following the transfer of the embryos, most women receive progesterone by intramuscular injection, vaginal suppository, or gel. Approximately two weeks later, blood pregnancy tests are done. Blood pregnancy tests are preferred to home pregnancy tests because of their reliability, sensitivity, and ability to quantify the pregnancy hormone hCG.

The success of IVF has recently improved, so that approximately one in every three IVF cycles will result in the birth of a baby. However, some programs have recently reported success rates of 40–50% or even higher, per attempt.

Two additional procedures are sometimes used to improve pregnancy rates:

Assisted hatching. Under some conditions, there is an impaired ability of embryos to implant in the uterine lining because the outer membrane of the embryo, the zona pellucida, is too thick or too hard. Assisted hatching may improve implantation by making a small opening in the zona pellucida that surrounds the oocyte. This procedure takes place just minutes before the embryos are transferred to the uterus and allows them to make better contact with the lining of the uterus, increasing implantation and therefore pregnancy rates. This is usually performed when the woman is older than thirty-seven or has failed to conceive in two previous IVF attempts. However, the benefit of assisted hatching has not been established.

Blastocyst transfer. While most embryos are transferred after seventy-two hours of growth, some are transferred after approximately 120 hours of growth, when they contain approximately 100 cells and are blastocysts. The benefits of transferring one or two blastocysts are a high pregnancy rate and a low-high-order multiple pregnancy rate.

Third-Party Reproduction

Many persons who cannot produce their own sperm or oocytes wish to have children. While adoption is one alternative, some couples may choose to use sperm or oocytes from a known or anonymous donor. In the case of a woman without a fertile male partner, sperm from a donor can be inseminated into her cervix or uterus with a reasonable chance of success. There are many commercial sperm banks throughout the world that provide sperm collected from donors who have been screened for genetic diseases, infections, and other undesirable traits. The sperm is frozen and quarantined for six months and then thawed for insemination at the time of ovulation each month. If the infertile woman has diseased or absent fallopian tubes, donated sperm can also be used during an IVF cycle to fertilize her oocytes in the laboratory.

In the case of a woman who does not produce oocytes or have a normal uterus, traditional surrogacy is an option. The traditional surrogate is a gestational carrier and oocyte donor. The traditional surrogate is inseminated with the sperm of the infertile woman's husband. This procedure is relatively uncomplicated medically and much simpler than the other option, oocyte donation, for the woman who does not produce oocytes. However, traditional surrogacy has greater psychological risks as the woman is relinquishing at birth a child to whom she is genetically related. Following the pregnancy and birth, the surrogate relinquishes the child to the intended parents and is adopted by the rearing mother. The traditional surrogate is both the genetic and birthmother and, as a result, her legal 'rights' to the offspring have led to this practice being a less popular reproductive choice for surrogates and intended parents. Today most couples prefer to use a donated oocyte with a gestational carrier. Surrogacy remains an uncommon or illegal form of reproduction in a majority of countries worldwide.

In oocyte donation, a woman, referred to as an egg or oocyte donor, volunteers to receive fertility drugs and undergo the retrieval of her oocytes just as though she were undergoing IVF. Her oocytes are then fertilized with sperm from the infertile woman's partner or donated sperm. The fertilized oocytes are then transferred into the uterus of the infertile woman so that she may carry and deliver the baby.

Finally, in the case of a woman who does not have a normal uterus but has functioning ovaries, gestational carrier is an option. In gestational carrier pregnancies, the infertile woman receives fertility drugs and undergoes oocyte retrieval as though she were undergoing IVF. Her oocytes are fertilized by her partner's sperm or donated sperm, but the resulting embryos are transferred into the uterus of another woman, called a gestational carrier. After delivery of the baby, the infertile woman or couple become the legal parents of the baby via adoption by the genetically related parents. This procedure is obviously more complicated than insemination of a traditional surrogate, but it does make it possible for the infertile woman or couple to have a genetically-shared child. Thus, women without a normal uterus or functioning ovaries or men without sperm can still participate actively in overcoming their childlessness, using the new reproductive technologies and/or a third party. However, as stated earlier, these forms of third-party reproduction involve complex psychosocial issues warranting counseling of all parties involved.

FUTURE IMPLICATIONS

The past twenty years have been dominated by advances in medical technology. However, the next twenty years will not only see technological advances but also a much greater involvement by the nonmedical community in the economics and ethics of these new advanced reproductive technologies.

As we gain greater understanding of the role of the uterine lining in implantation and learn how to identify embryos with the greatest potential for implantation, we will be able to achieve higher success rates in IVF without a high rate of multiple pregnancies. In addition, not only will we be able to evaluate the genetic constitution of each embryo, but we will also be able to correct some genetic abnormalities and prevent some types of birth defects. And while these technologies may provide more opportunities for reproductive parenthood, they also present greater ethical challenges for couples and clinicians as the potential for designer children becomes technologically possible.

Recent advances in the manipulation and preservation of eggs will also have important implications for infertile women. The treatment of female-factor infertility due to advanced maternal age or ovarian incompetence may be dramatically changed by oocyte freezing. In the future, it may be possible for women to select oocytes from a commercial oocyte bank or even to cryopreserve their own oocytes for use later in their lives. In addition, women who must undergo chemotherapy

for the treatment of cancer may have their ovaries biopsied or removed and frozen. After recovery from the chemotherapy and cancer, the ovaries may be thawed and the unstimulated oocytes stimulated and matured in the laboratory. Finally, in the future women with polycystic ovary syndrome who are unable to produce mature oocytes for IVF may have unstimulated oocytes retrieved from their ovaries and matured in the laboratory before insemination.

None of these technological developments will take place in a social vacuum, however. Society is becoming increasingly involved through legislation, regulation, and the rationing of financial resources for artificial reproduction. Hopefully, regulation of reproduction will be a positive force that will lead to a common agreement regarding the limits of artificial reproduction, as well as to an increased level of confidence and trust in the clinicians and scientists who provide such care worldwide.

Unfortunately, rationing of healthcare may pose a serious threat to the treatment of infertility services in the future. To the fertile population, to adults past their reproductive years, and to medical practitioners in most medical specialties, using limited financial resources for the treatment of infertility is not a priority. While the potential will exist for overcoming infertility for virtually every infertile individual, only time will tell how, when, and for whom these exciting technologies will be provided.

SUMMARY

■ Infertility is defined as the inability to conceive during twelve months of sexual intercourse without contraception.

■ Approximately 8–14% of couples will experience infertility.

■ Causes of infertility include:

Failure to ovulate

Failure to produce or deliver adequate numbers of healthy sperm to the fallopian tubes

Obstruction of the fallopian tubes

Endometriosis or adhesions involving the ovaries or fallopian tubes

Poor timing of technique of intercourse

Possible infections of the reproductive tract

Immunological barriers to fertilization or implantation

An unreceptive lining of the uterus

Genetic factors.

■ Efficient and effective delivery of care involves a multidisciplinary team consisting of physicians, nurses, mental health professionals, urologists, andrologists, and embryologists.

■ The medical work-up of the infertile couple consists of:

Determination of ovulation and the number of competent oocytes in the ovaries

Evaluation of the semen through a semen analysis and sperm function tests

Evaluation of the uterus and fallopian tubes by hysterosalpingogram

Evaluation of the pelvic organs by laparoscopy.

■ Treatment options include:

Fertility drugs to induce ovulation or enhance hormone production

Surgery of the uterus or fallopian tubes

Drug or hormone therapy to improve sperm production

Surgery of the male reproductive tract to improve delivery of adequate numbers of sperm

Insemination of sperm

Assisted reproduction: IVF, ICSI, assisted hatching, and blastocyst transfer.

■ Using third-party reproduction, women and men now 'have a baby' via donor sperm, donor oocytes, donor embryos, traditional surrogacy, and/or gestational carrier.

■ Preimplantation genetic diagnosis makes it possible for women and men with some genetic disorders to have children who will not develop the disease.

■ In the future, the new reproductive technologies may include cloning, oocyte freezing, and cryopreservation of ovaries. The limitations and barriers to these technologies are likely to be more social and ethical than medical or technological.

REFERENCES

1. American Society for Reproductive Medicine. 1993 Committee Opinion on Definition of "infertility."

2. Olsen J. Subfecundity according to the age of the mother and father. *Dan Med Bull* 1990; 37:281–2.

3. Strickler RC. Factors influencing fertility. In: WR Keye Jr, RJ Chang, RW Rebar, R Soules, eds. *Infertility: Evaluation and Treatment*. Philadelphia: Saunders, 1995; 8–9.

4. Mosher WD. Infertility: Why business is booming. *Am Demogr* 1987; 9:42–3.

5. Taylor PJ, Collins JA. Overview of the prevalence of unexplained infertility and the investigations necessary to make the diagnosis. In: PJ Taylor, JA Collins, eds. *Unexplained Infertility*. Oxford: Oxford University Press, 1992; chapter 2.

6. Shamma FN, DeCherney AH. Infertility: A historical perspective. In: WR Keye, RJ Chang, RW Rebar, MR Soules, eds. *Infertility: Evaluation and Treatment*. Philadelphia: Saunders, 1995; 3–7.

7. Sims JM. Sterility and the value of the microscope in diagnosis and treatment. *Trans Am Gynecol Soc* 1888; 77:886.

8. Huhner M. *Sterility in the Female and Its Treatment*. New York: Robman Co, 1913.

9. Rubin IC. Non-operative determination of fallopian tubes in infertility: Intrauterine inflation with oxygen and production of a subphrenic pneumoperitoneum, a preliminary report. *JAMA* 1920; 75:661.

10. Rindfleisch W. Darstellung des Cavum Utere. *Berl Klin Wochenschr* 1910; 17:780.

11. Palmer R. Instrumentation et technique de la coelioscopie gynécologique, *Gynecol Obstet* 1947; 46:420–31.

12. Macomber D, Sanders MR. The spermatozoa count. *N Engl J Med* 1929; 200:981–4.

13. World Health Organization. *WHO Laboratory Manual for the Examination of Human Semen and Sperm-Cervical Mucus Interaction*. 3rd ed. Cambridge: Press Syndicate of the University of Cambridge, 1992.

14. Jain T, Hornstein MD. Disparities in access to infertility services in a state with mandated insurance coverage *Fertil Steril* 2005; 84:221–3.

15. The President's Council on Bioethics. Reproduction and Responsibility: The Regulation of New Biotechnologies. www.bioethics.gov.2004.

16. Practice Committee of the American Society for Reproductive Medicine. Interpretation of clinical trial results. *Fertil Steril* 2004; 82:S-55–S-61.

17. Garcia-Velasco JA, Moreno L, Pacheco A, et al. The aromatase inhibitor letrozole increases the concentration of intraovarian androgens and improves the in vitro fertilization outcome in low responder patients: A pilot study. *Fertil Steril* 2005; 84: 82–7.

18. Meller W, Burns LH, Crow S, et al. Major depression in unexplained infertility. *J Psychosom Obstet Gynaecol* 2002; 23:27–30.

19. Palomino WA, Fuentes A, Gonzalez RR, et al. Differential expression of endometrial integrins and progesterone receptors during the window of implantation in normo-ovulatory women treated with clomiphene citrate *Fertil Steril* 2005; 83: 587–93.

20. Oktay K, Sonmezer M. Ovarian tissue banking for cancer patients: Fertility preservation, not just ovarian cryopreservation. *Hum Repro* 2004; 19:477–80.

21. Donnez J, Dolmans MM, Demylle D, et al. Livebirth after orthotopic transplantation of cryopreserved ovarian tissue. *Lancet* 2004; 364:1405–10.

22. Platteau P, Staessen C, Michiels A, et al. Preimplantation genetic diagnosis for aneuploidy screening in women older than 37 years. *Fertil Steril* 2005; 84:319–24.

23. Paulus WE, Zhang M, Strehler E, et al. Influence of acupuncture on the pregnancy rate in patients who undergo assisted reproductive therapy. *Fertil Steril* 2002; 77:721–4.

24. Keye WR Jr. Initial approach to the infertile couple. In: WR Keye Jr, RJ Chang, RW Rebar, R Soules, eds. *Infertility: Evaluation and Treatment*. Philadelphia: Saunders, 1995; 76–81.

25. Practice Committee of the American Society for Reproductive Medicine Committee Opinion. Optimal Evaluation of the Infertile Female. *Fertil Steril* 2004; 82, S169–S172.

26. The Practice Committee of the American Society for Reproductive Medicine. Smoking and infertility. *Fertil Steril* 2004; 81:1181–6.

27. Cedars M. Prediction, detection and evaluation of ovulation. In: WR Keye Jr, RJ Chang, RW Rebar, MR Soules, eds. *Infertility: Evaluation and Treatment*. Philadelphia: Saunders, 1995; 107–14.

28. Nelson LM, Covington SN, Rebar R. An update: Spontaneous premature ovarian failure is not an early menopause. *Fertil Steril* 2005; 83:1327–32.

29. American Urologic Association and American Society for Reproductive Medicine. Joint report on optimal evaluation of the infertile male. *Fertil Steril* 2004; 82, S123–S130.

30. The Practice Committee of the American Society for Reproductive Medicine. Smoking and infertility. *Fertil Steril* 2004; 81:1181–6.

31. Carter MD, Hollander MB, Lipschultz LI. Drug clues to male infertility. *Contemp Obstet Gynecol* 1994; 27:30–44.

32. Najmabadi H, Huang V, Yen P, et al. Substantial prevalence of microdeletions of the Y-chromosome in infertile men with idiopathic azoospermia and oligospermia detected using a sequence-tagged site-based mapping strategy. *J Clin Endocrinol Metab* 1996; 81:1347–52.

33. Westrom L. Influence of sexually transmitted diseases on sterility and ectopic pregnancy. *Acta Eur Fertil* 1985; 16: 21–4.

34. Griffith CS, Grimes DA. The validity of the postcoital test. *Am J Obstet Gynecol* 1990; 162:615–20.

35. American Urological Association and American Society for Reproductive Medicine. Report on Varicocele and Infertility. *Fertil Steril* 2004; 82, 5142–5.

36. American Urological Association and American Society for Reproductive Medicine. Report on management of obstructive azoospermia. *Fertil Steril* 2004; 82, S137–S141.

3 The Psychology of Gender-Specific Infertility Diagnoses

WILLIAM D. PETOK

Women are not men's equals in anything except responsibility. We are not their inferiors, either, or even their superiors. We are quite simply different races.

– Phyllis McGinley, 1959

Infertility affects men and women in approximately equal proportions, although there may be some regional variations.[1,2] For example, over half the cases of infertility reported in sub-Saharan Africa are male factor.[3] Worldwide, it is generally accepted that the breakdown of organic causes of infertility is: 35% male factor, 50% female factor, 5% other, and 10% unexplained with combined male- and female-factor infertility accounting for 20% of all infertility.[4]

While women have historically been the focus of infertility treatment due to medical necessity, myths, cultural beliefs and traditions, it is now clear that male-factor infertility plays a significant role in a couple's efforts to achieve a pregnancy. Accumulating knowledge of male factors contributing or causing infertility, from advances in diagnostic techniques and treatments, has helped to equalize both the medical and psychological understanding of the impact of infertility. At the same time, this has helped to promote a better understanding of the emotional impact of male and female infertility on men and women as individuals and make the experiences of infertility a shared one.

This chapter

■ describes factors determining gender-specific diagnoses of infertility;

■ explains treatments for gender-specific diagnoses and their psychological implications;

■ explores the psychological and emotional meaning to a man or woman of a gender-specific diagnosis;

■ examines some of the differences between men and women in their reactions to infertility.

HISTORICAL OVERVIEW

Biblical references to infertility abound, but the psychological reactions to infertility seem limited to the women in these ancient stories. In Genesis, Abraham and Sarah had such difficulty conceiving that Abraham, with Sarah's blessing, took Hagar as his concubine and produced a male heir (Ishmael) with Hagar, commonly known today as a surrogate. However, the Bible provides very little insight into Abraham's feelings about his wife's infertility or Sarah's feelings about her childlessness, although it notes that Sarah laughed incredulously when God eventually promises her a child. Perhaps the laughter was out of anger, shock, or relief. Later, we get a glimpse of her jealous feelings about her surrogate son, Ishmael, when she asks her husband to drive Ishmael and his mother from their camp.

In the book of Samuel, we are introduced to Hannah, the second of Elkanah's two wives. She had no children, but her counterpart had two sons by their mutual husband. While Elkanah appears not to understand his wife's feelings about her infertility, the wife's feelings are abundantly clear. When she appears depressed, weeping and refusing to eat, her husband asks, "... Why are you brokenhearted? Am I not better to you than ten children?" (I Samuel 1:8). However, as with all good stories and perhaps as part of ancient wisdom for a glimmer of hope for the childless, the outcome is positive and Hannah conceives and bears a child.

Popular culture also frequently portrays women's psychological reactions to infertility. In Jane Smiley's *A Thousand Acres* the heroine has had five miscarriages. Carlos Fuentes uses infertility as a motivational theme in *Aura*. And there is no doubt about the emotion Sylvia Plath portrays in her poem, *Barren Woman*. The artwork of Freda Kahlo also employs images of infertility, as does the play, *Tally's Folly*, by Lansford Wilson. In a rare glimpse into male reactions to infertility, Michael Chabon's *Son of the Wolfman* does look at a man's emotional response to a couple's inability to conceive.

With progress in the medical aspects of the field, reporting on the psychosocial aspects of infertility has also grown in complexity. It is not unusual to see articles on assisted reproductive technology in newspapers, popular periodical publications, and television news – or celebrity biographies or accounts of royal infertility tribulations. While the focus of these accounts is often on the scientific techniques available to help achieve pregnancy and a child, a sidebar or accompanying story will highlight the emotional issues at stake for the couple or individuals using these medical advances.

REVIEW OF LITERATURE

Hardy and Makuch,[5] in an international review of gender, infertility and assisted reproductive technology (ART), note that, across cultures, women are more likely to define the term 'mother' as a function of both biology and the interaction between a woman and child. Motherhood is the result of pregnancy and childbirth and later nurturing. Men seem to define their relationship to a child as a function of their role in conception. Fatherhood is more related to ownership of children. This traditional view, they note, is changing in many societies as fathers become increasingly involved in child upbringing. Nevertheless, the conceptual notion elaborated by their work highlights a difference between men and women of great significance and with profoundly different meanings for each gender. Infertility denies a woman the important function of mothering over many years. At the same time, the loss for a man becomes a failure to create a commodity that will carry on his name and genetic line.

Research on female and male reactions to infertility has focused on the psychological response of men to male-factor infertility, general studies about women's reactions to infertility, Polycystic Ovarian Syndrome (PCOS), premature ovarian failure (POF) and their psychological sequelae, and various treatments and comparison studies of gender differences in reaction to infertility. Genetic causes of both female and male infertility men have been identified, but little specific research exists on the psychological outcomes. Cancers that effect the reproductive systems of men and women, either directly or through radiation or chemotherapeutic treatments, are similarly recognized in the literature. A number of methodological problems have hampered research in the field including the use of convenience samples that compromise generalizability and a failure to analyze the influence of variables such as diagnosis and treatment length.[6] Infertile men have been studied with less frequency than infertile women. Because many of the treatments are aimed at women, a fre-

quent criticism of the existing research is that the needs of infertile men have not been identified and therefore remain unmet.[7,8]

Unfortunately, there is a limited body of literature that examines specific gender-related diagnoses and the resulting psychological reactions of the diagnosed. Regardless, a substantial body of literature supports the notion that being the partner with the identified source of the fertility problem is one of several factors that yields a more negative response. It is important to note that in some cultures, women receive all the treatment focus because a diagnosis of male-factor infertility is socially unacceptable.[3] Men experience more distress when male-factor infertility is diagnosed than do women when female-factor is found.[9,10] At the same time, women report stronger overall negative reactions to infertility. The stronger responses of women to their infertility than those of men is probably due to multiple factors: the more invasive nature of medical work-ups for infertile women and the different social contexts in which men and women are raised, and therefore must negotiate the experience of being unable to produce a child. For example, considering individuals in treatment via in vitro fertilization (IVF), women report significantly higher levels of depression, and state and trait anxiety than their partners. Men report more suppression of their anxiety and anger than women.[11] Finally, many of the medical treatments for infertility that use hormonal medications are provided to women. These medications have known side effects that can produce psychological symptoms as mild as minor mood swings and as profound as full-blown psychotic reactions. Men do not typically receive similarly powerful medications for their treatment.[12]

Psychological Response in Men to Male-Factor Infertility

Male-factor infertility can be the result of problems in delivery of sperm such as an absent vas deferens or other obstructive azoospermia conditions, chromosomal conditions such as Klinefelter's syndrome, hormonal problems such as acquired or congenital deficiency in the secretion of pituitary hormones, ejaculatory problems such as retrograde ejaculation, testicular damage from infections such as mumps, cancer treatment, prior vasectomy, or injury. Previously thought to be a contributor to male-factor infertility, the significance of varicocele has come under recent scrutiny and, as such, is considered a less significant causal factor in male-factor infertility.[13] This is also the case for sperm-antibodies once thought to be a major factor and now primarily relevant in postvasectomy reversal situations. Although seen less frequently today than in the past, men (and women) may experience reproductive tract malformations as a result of exposure to diethylstilbestrol (DES) in utero – ironically a medication used to prevent miscarriage. Age, unlike in women, is not typically seen as a factor in male infertility. At the same time, increased age can affect a man's level of sexual desire and capacity. Consequently, older men who are attempting to start families may experience difficulty due to erectile problems or other age-related health issues that compromise sexual capacity.

While there is no doubt that a diagnosis of male factor is stressful, the great majority of men appear to manage it well.[14] Most of the research regarding men's reactions to infertility looks at aggregate groups and does not separate out specific diagnoses. The majority of authors have noted that men typically adopt coping styles that incorporate denial, distancing, or avoidance.[12] In addition, most research has indicated that general male response to infertility is less negative than their female counterparts, with the exception of a male-factor diagnosis.

In an early study specifically addressing a diagnosis of azoospermia,[15] ten of the sixteen men in the sample experienced some form of temporary 'impotence' subsequent to diagnosis. While the author does not specify, one suspects he is referring to the more contemporary diagnosis of erectile dysfunction. Interviews collected from the men suggest that their inability to achieve erection was directly related to an emotional reaction to their diagnosis. Feuer[16] found that men diagnosed with oligospermia felt the negative psychological impact to a greater extent than other men with different diagnoses in the study. The supposition is that the uncertain nature of the diagnosis led to the increased depression and social isolation experienced as well as reduced self-esteem and marital satisfaction. A review of the literature on vasectomy indicates that, in general, adverse psychological events are the least common in men who made the decision for vasectomy jointly with their wives. Potential predictors of psychosexual problems for men who obtained vasectomies include preexisting emotional instability, excessive concerns about masculinity, and confusion of the procedure with castration.[17]

Mason[18] conducted in-depth interviews with men, primarily from Great Britain, all diagnosed with male-factor infertility. The twenty-two men in her research primarily responded to articles in self-help publications about her work. These men discussed their pain and how they learned to cope with the fact that they would not produce their own biological children. Guilt, shame, anger, isolation, loss, and a sense of personal failure were common themes in these interviews.

Of unique interest is the research of Gannon and colleagues,[19] which notes that media reports in Great Britain have described a crisis in male fertility based on newspaper accounts of declining sperm counts. The authors reviewed newspaper accounts of male fertility between 1992 and 1998. They conclude that infertile men are being stigmatized because they are perceived as being deficient of a critical component that defines masculinity.

However, others[20] see the stigma as a result of having broken the group norm of producing children. Regardless, these men also describe feelings of guilt, despair, loneliness, isolation, and stress. This constellation of emotional responses can leave the infertile man feeling less than a man, diminished and powerless in his masculinity.[21] When men and women with no fertility problems were interviewed about their views of infertile men and women, male infertility was associated with higher levels of stigma than female infertility. In addition, when the cause of the infertility was attributed to male factor, it was viewed as the result of sexual dysfunction. Those interviewed felt that the infertile men would see themselves as having tarnished egos or failed sexual prowess.[22]

Other research has looked at groups of men with varying diagnoses. One study[23] found that infertile men suffered more psychological distress and greater somatic symptoms than their fertile counterparts. Stigmatization, loss of potency, role failure, and reduced self-esteem were reactions of the men described in the work of Natchtigall[24] and his associates. The impact of the diagnosis on marital relationships and a decrement in self-esteem is a common finding in similar studies.[21] Feelings of personal and sexual inadequacy, sexual dysfunction, depression, hostility, and guilt have been reported.[25] Dhillon[26] and associates used psychometric measures to study equal-sized groups of fertile men, men with unexplained infertility, and men with abnormal semen analyses based on World Health Organization criteria. Both groups of infertile men underwent treatment with intra uterine insemination (IUI). No differences were found on the psychometric measures between the groups. The authors offered a variety of explanations for their results including research that suggested men may be more willing than women to find comfort in roles other than parenting, and that a man's true feelings are best derived from interview rather than psychometric data.

Boivin[27] and colleagues compared Swedish men with male-factor diagnoses undergoing intracytoplasmic sperm injection (ICSI) and IVF. They hypothesized that male ICSI patients would experience more distress than their IVF counterparts due to the higher level of male-factor diagnoses compared to IVF patients. In addition, they hypothesized that the greatest difference in distress scores would take place during the active stages of these procedures, that is, when men were required to produce a sperm sample and find out if the oocytes had been fertilized. Daily data on emotional, physical, and social reactions to infertility were obtained and the emotional subscale data were divided into distress and optimism variables. Interestingly, no significant differences were found between the two groups of men with the exception of the ICSI patients reporting more distress during the two days prior to the active stages of treatment. The researchers concluded that men undergoing ICSI experienced more anticipatory anxiety than those in the IVF group. Furthermore, the researchers noted that the availability of the ICSI procedures may help reduce feelings of loss and hopelessness because ICSI offers an alternative to donor insemination and a possible solution to their infertility that enables them to have the desired genetically shared child with their partner. Other researchers had determined that providing a sperm sample could increase anxiety about being able to perform during this crucial stage of treatment.[28] While not dealing with specific male-factor diagnosis infertility, Pook and colleagues[29–31] have demonstrated that distress due to infertility has a predictive value for changes in sperm concentration and motility.

It has long been noted that men with infertility diagnoses have a tendency to somaticize. Because male infertility implies a lack of masculinity and is, therefore, stigmatizing, many men keep their diagnosis a secret. This secrecy can increase stress levels. Conrad and colleagues[32] investigated whether or not men tended to suppress their emotions and have a higher degree of alexithymia, which is difficulty in identifying and communicating feelings. They pointed to earlier research establishing links between nonexpression of emotions and somatic complaints as explanatory for the symptom of somatization found in infertile men. The research of Conrad and colleagues confirmed that, in the sample of German men they studied, higher levels of alexithymia occurred than in healthy controls. However, the infertile men were lower in alexithymia when compared with a group of psychosomatic outpatients known to have a high rate of alexithymia. It appears that infertile men were inclined to repress their feelings about infertility. Furthermore, it seems that difficulty in identifying and expressing feelings was common in this sample of men.

Issues of masculinity related to infertility appear to be global in nature. Tarlatzis and colleagues[33] found that infertile Greek men had a greater tendency to repress feelings of anxiety and had a greater probability for psychosomatic illness than their infertile wives. In addition, a high rate of sexual dysfunction was found in this sample. Chinese men were found to have higher self-esteem as well as more marital and sexual satisfaction than their wives in another study. Fifty-nine married infertile couples from medical centers in Taipei, Taiwan, completed psychometric questionnaires. Overall, the men had significantly less distress than their wives.[34] The authors suggested that because in Chinese society in-laws play a significant role, particularly in marital satisfaction, a difference exists from patterns typically found in the West. The role that sons play in their parents' old age was presumed to be an important factor because childlessness is one of three ways a son can dishonor his parents according to Chinese proverbs. Furthermore, a son can take another wife if his first wife fails to produce a child, presumably reducing the stress that he feels if no pregnancy occurs.

In some African cultures, infertility is seen as solely a woman's problem, and thus the diagnosis of male-factor infertility is unacceptable. Consequently if male-factor infertility is the problem, there is typically significant denial by all parties (husband, wives, and even caregivers) and a lack of treatment. This cultural norm is presumably to protect the male ego and the 'superior' role of the male in the society and family.[35,36] In one qualitative study of racially and educationally diverse men seeking treatment for infertility in Cape Town, South Africa,[37] the majority of the men noted emotional reactions brought on by their childlessness. Guilt, sadness, pain and emptiness, feelings of being left out, and inadequacy were identified. Being defined as a man because of one's children was also a significant theme. In Egypt, male-factor infertility is a crisis of masculinity, with the ultimate social price usually paid by the wife because her husband can divorce her and take a new wife despite her lack of 'blame.'[38] Nevertheless, for men in many Middle Eastern countries the emasculation that infertility brings is compounded by the newer treatments, such as ICSI, which create more stigma and secrecy due to complicated restrictions that Islam has on third-party donation of gametes.[39] An Iranian study of infertile couples showed that some men and women in Islamic countries had psychological reactions similar to their Western counterparts. Men whose partners eventually conceived reported significantly less stress than those whose partners did not conceive.[40]

In general, male-factor infertility research dealing with the psychological sequelae finds that while men do suffer emotional insults in more Western cultures, they tend to be protected from similar outcomes in others. This is particularly so in cultures that are less egalitarian with regard to gender roles.

Psychological Response in Women to Female-Factor Infertility

Female-factor infertility can be the result of hormonal abnormalities that prohibit ovulation or do not properly prepare the endometrium to receive a fertilized ovum, compromised cervical mucous, obstruction or damage to the fallopian tubes and the adjacent structures of the pelvic peritoneum from disease, surgery or endometriosis, and uterine factors such as congenital defects, fibroids or polyps. Medical conditions, typically hormonally related, including PCOS, POF, and endometriosis can also be a cause of female-factor infertility. Because ovulation is an age-related function, aging can and does have an impact on female fertility. Female circumcision, a practice common in twenty-six African countries, can also lead to infection and infertility.[41,42]

Infertility has a variety of psychological impacts on a woman. Grief and depression, anger, guilt, shock and denial, and anxiety are the most commonly mentioned emotional themes in descriptive reports.[43] Competence and self-esteem are compromised because women typically feel incapable of accomplishing what other women seem to do with apparent ease.[44] Failure is another descriptor often used with regard to sexual and reproductive functions (further reinforced by medical diagnostic terms, such as premature ovarian 'failure' or 'incompetent' cervix), as well as failure as a woman. A variety of factors have been identified with higher levels of distress in women experiencing infertility. Poor self-esteem and a primary investment in the motherhood role with regard to identity and self-image top the list. Lengthier treatment also seems to increase marital and sexual distress for women. Unresolved diagnostic status appears to be another factor that produces acute distress in women. One study found that 32% of women in the early stages of infertility treatment might be at risk for developing clinically relevant mental health problems[45] as measured by the Twelve Item General Health Questionnaire and three multiitem scales from the Short Form Health Survey Questionnaire.

In evaluating research with control groups prior to 1988, Dunkel-Schetter and Lobel[43] highlighted the variability of results obtained. In two well-designed studies[46,47] that used both control groups and standardized measures, no significant differences were found between infertile women and control subjects on a variety of psychological measures. Other studies have reported differences in satisfaction with some aspects of

life and higher anxiety levels in infertile women versus controls. Dunkel-Schetter and Lobel's summary indicates that the dominant pattern across studies was that on most dimensions, there are no differences with the exception of anxiety and emotional distress. When significant differences did exist, the studies were generally weaker in design.

In discussing major experiences in the reproductive lives of women, Stanton[48] and colleagues note that infertility is not experienced as a discrete event. Instead, it is a sequence that can cover many years having an impact on many aspects of a woman's life. With respect to normative groups, the researchers noted that women experiencing infertility are a variable group. Some display equal adjustment to their noninfertile counterparts, while others evidence less positive psychological outcomes. Nevertheless, 49% of women interviewed reported that infertility was the most upsetting event of their lives and women are more likely than men to experience stress specific to infertility.[14] Because diagnostic and treatment procedures for women are typically more invasive than for men, this is not surprising. As a result, infertility can be a more significant loss for women.[49] It is also possible that women generally appraise negative events as more stressful than men.[50]

Unfortunately, as with male-factor infertility research, there is a limited body of literature on specific types of female-factor infertility and women's psychological reactions to them, PCOS and POF being exceptions. Hardy and Makuch,[5] in a recent literature review, highlight the difference in the way men and women view childbearing, with women more likely to experience depression and anxiety than men. For example, Domar and colleagues[51] demonstrated that infertile women were twice as likely to be depressed as their fertile counterparts. Women with identified causes for their infertility had significantly higher depression scores than those with unexplained or undiagnosed infertility.

International findings regarding female reactions to their infertility cover wide ground. A Chinese study that employed control groups and standardized measures[52] found that infertile women in China suffered moderate to severe levels of mental pressure, and more depression symptoms and self-isolation than control group subjects. A study, lacking in controls, found anxiety and depression in infertile Japanese women correlated with a lack of support from their husbands.[53] In a study of Western European women by Oddens and colleagues[54] the researchers using a control group and standardized measures found that only 28% of the subjects had female-factor infertility diagnoses. In the aggregate of all subjects, negative feelings were higher in the patient group with the largest differences seen for shock, embarrassment, anger, feeling hurt and depressed. In a Kuwaiti study, conducted in 2004, that assessed the effect of infertility on Arab women, the researchers used an age-matched sample of pregnant women as controls. The infertile women evidenced higher levels of tension, hostility, anxiety, depression, self-blame, and suicidal ideation than the control group women. The researchers noted that childlessness typically causes significant social stigmatization for Arabic women that puts them at risk for serious social and emotional consequences.[55] Infertile Greek women report depression, high rates of defensive anxiety, and numerous psychosomatic symptoms.[33] A 2005 Israeli study of 242 women in treatment at a regional infertility center asked women to respond to a list of difficulties that included items such as anticipation of treatment results, negative feelings aroused by the patient's fertility problem, and disruption of the patient's functioning at work. In addition, the women were asked to complete a questionnaire about infertility-specific distress and well-being. The researchers found that while there was great variability in women's responses, women who reported high levels of difficulty from their infertility also reported higher levels of emotional distress.[56]

Sub-Saharan Africa, with its extremely high rate of infertility, has also been the subject of research.[37,41] Women in many African cultures have low status and gain value from their capacity to reproduce and/or provide sexual satisfaction to the male partner. Consequently, blame for infertility, regardless of its origin, is affixed to the female member of a couple.[57] Infertility in African women frequently causes marital disharmony, leading to divorce. Women are often blamed for the infertility and men engage in polygamy in an attempt to have children.[58] Divorce because of infertility is common among infertile Nigerian women.[59] The women in the study by Orji et al. noted that divorce was the result of abuse by the husband's family, their husband taking a second or third wife, and accusations of being a witch. Abuse can take place because children are considered a connection between ancestors and future generations and a barren woman provides no such connection for her husband's family.

In one of the diagnosis-specific studies of women with PCOS, Austrian women were compared with Moslem immigrants to Austria. Cultural issues put Moslem women under greater pressure to reproduce and when they are unable, they suffer more in their marriages and social group than do Austrian women.[60] Another PCOS study, which looked at five quality-of-life variables, found that emotions and infertility were the second and third lowest in order of concern for women with PCOS. Weight gain was the most important factor for these women.[61]

In an interesting comparison of women with infertility due to endometriosis or tubal sterility, those with endometriosis were found to experience higher levels of anxiety. The authors had hypothesized that gender role conflicts would be found in women with endometriosis. Results of the interviews and questionnaire data confirmed the original hypothesis. The conflict seemed to be characterized by a negative experience of menarche and puberty, early gynecological problems, and negative sexual experiences.[62]

Kitzinger and Willmott[63] evaluated women with PCOS. Infertility was one of the symptoms of their condition that left them feeling less feminine than their fertile counterparts. These women used words such as 'freakish,' 'abnormal,' and not 'proper' in describing themselves. They viewed themselves as decidedly different from other women and therefore less feminine. This stigmatization was a 'theft of womanhood.'

POF affects between 1 and 5% of women below forty,[64] and involves the cessation of ovulatory and endocrine ovarian function in women younger than forty.[65] Possible causes of POF include genetic factors such as Turner's syndrome and Fragile X syndrome, enzyme deficiencies, ovarian damage from medical interventions such as radiation and chemotherapy for cancer, and autoimmune factors. A small percentage of women with the disorder have idiopathic POF. Because residual follicles and oocytes may have episodic function, some research indicates that 20% of women with POF will have sporadic ovulation and as many as 8% have reported pregnancies.[66] Pregnancies in women with POF have been reported after bouts of amenorrhea lasting several years.[65]

Orshan and colleagues,[64] in a phenomenological study of six women with idiopathic POF, reported that a common experience was a perceived lack of support from healthcare providers regarding the symptoms that subsequently led to the diagnosis. The women in this study felt that healthcare providers did not understand the ramifications and emotional consequences of the diagnosis. Some women in the study described the diagnosis as a death, complete with loss, grief, depression, and the emptiness frequently experienced in mourning. In addition, women in this study had feelings of premature aging associated with medical regimens used for women going through an age-appropriate menopause.

The theme of feeling unsupported by healthcare providers was reiterated in an observational study of 100 women with POF.[67] Women reported feeling confusion, depression, anxiety, emptiness, loss, shock, anger, denial, relief (to know what was wrong), and curiosity when first hearing their diagnosis. Many of the women felt that their physicians lacked knowledge, sensitivity, and helpful suggestions for dealing with POF. When women felt that they had been given thorough and accurate information about the disorder, they felt better emotionally. The results of the study indicated that women find receiving a diagnosis of POF emotionally traumatic. Negative body image, characterized by feeling old, unfeminine, less healthy, empty, and worthless were described. The authors suggest that the word *failure* in the diagnosis contributes to a sense of defectiveness in women and that it may be more helpful to use *ovarian insufficiency* when describing the disorder.

THEORETICAL FRAMEWORK

No single theoretical framework applies universally to male or female factor infertility. However, theoretical frameworks that have been or may be applicable include Freudian theory, Goffman's stigma theory, Kohut's self-psychology theory, and grief and loss theory. In addition, family systems theory and Mahlstedt's description of specific losses related to grief and loss theory can be used to understand the issues extant for both men and women.

Specific gender-based theories do suggest issues related to infertility. Families have long relied on women to provide nurturance, both emotional and physical, to husbands, children, and aging parents.[68] Consequently, mothering is an essential role for a woman. Without the opportunity to do so, she is deprived of an important aspect of womanhood. At the same time, Barnett and Baruch[69] contend that a woman's psychological health is not dependent on fulfilling the role of mother and wife. They suggest that women who are mothers may benefit from that role depending on their other roles and the assistance they receive in fulfilling their family and workplace obligations.

Levinson[70] notes that in all societies a man is expected to marry and assume certain familial responsibilities. Producing offspring connects a man to other components of life including his original family, ethnicity and occupation, and places him within the larger world. Starting a family is, from Levinson's perspective, an important developmental task. Fatherhood gives men a sense of importance and gratification, particularly when things go well. By extension, these connections are missing for a man who does not create a family.

McGrath and colleagues[71] cite infertility as one of the unique female-specific reproductive events hypoth-

esized for placing women at risk for depression. They highlight research on women's roles as caretakers and marital confidants as contributory factors. While relationships tend to bring greater satisfaction to women, strains in those relationships produce a greater risk factor for depression than similar strains or problems in other areas of life. So, caretaking can have a detrimental side to it. And husbands more often than wives report being understood and affirmed by their spouses. Consequently, a married woman undergoing the emotional stress of infertility is less likely to be understood and have her feelings validated, leaving her at risk for depression.

Freudian Theory

Male Factor
Competition with one's father is a familiar theme in Freudian theory. Male-factor infertility, which can lead to the use of donor sperm, can be viewed as an emotional disturbance from this theoretical point of view. Gerstel[72] believed that a male-factor infertility diagnosis if compounded with a revived oedipal conflict, would necessarily lead to severe psychopathology in a couple using donor sperm as well as in the resulting child. While some psychoanalytic literature continues to be published in this area, most of current psychoanalytic thinking approaches family-of-origin issues and the manner in which men are parented as determinants in how they manage the crisis of infertility. If, for example, a man has not had a close relationship with his father, masculinity can be measured by his ability to impregnate his wife. Virility and fertility can become confused, leading to the belief that failure to reproduce is the loss of total sexual function and therefore manhood. Men who are emasculated by their infertility may reject third-party reproduction techniques because it would signify a further loss of their manhood.[21]

Female Factor
Karen Horney wrote about women from a psychoanalytic perspective. A woman's goal of independence and/or career success was not important because motherhood or dedication to a male partner were critical.[21] Her psychology of self included the actual self, the real self, and the idealized self. Loss of fertility therefore involves losses in all three domains. Infertility represents a deep narcissistic wound to the idealized self.

Olshansky[73] has proposed that Relational Cultural Theory (RCT) is a useful way of understanding why infertile women might be vulnerable to depression. RCT is a theory of psychological development that frames healthy interpersonal relationships as the key to healthy psychological growth. Based on the work of Miller[74] and others, it incorporates relational aspects of psychological growth to understand psychological development in women. Work is also being done to understand how this model applies to both men and women.[75]

RCT differs from classic psychodynamic beliefs that autonomy and individuation are the key components of a psychologically healthy person. The newer model does not preempt individuation but moderates it with connectedness. Growth into relationships is the key. A healthy and strong sense of self is developed within the context of mutually healthy interpersonal relationships. Growth in relationships enhances growth in self. Connectedness, an important component of RCT, recognizes that people do not live in isolation from one another. Healthy relationships require a sense of being part of another person either via sharing ideas and values or feelings. Additional key components of RCT include empathy, mutuality, reciprocity, and authenticity. From the RCT perspective, infertility presents repeated and sustained interference with significant relationships and can lead to depression in infertile women. Olshansky[73] suggests that to manage the narcissistic wounds of infertility, internalization of the experience is necessary. To refocus their lives from infertility as the definition of self to a more integrated perception, some infertile women must incorporate infertility as a portion of identity so that it is one of many defining experiences as opposed to *the* defining experience.

Stigma Theory

According to Goffman[76] (p. 3), stigma is an attribute that extensively discredits an individual, reducing him or her "from a whole and usual person to a tainted, discounted one." The assumption is that people who are stigmatized have (or are believed to have) an attribute that sets them apart as different and therefore devalued in the eyes of others. Goffman[76] suggests that stigmatized individuals acquire ambivalence about themselves. Stigma arises through physical deformities, individual character deformities, or through deviation from the group identity. Miall[77] suggests that infertility is most closely associated with Goffman's physical deformity type.

The concepts of shame and blame have received considerable attention in psychotherapy with infertile individuals. In general, for shame to be present, something reasonably good must have been taking place and was subsequently made worse.[78] Infertility diagnoses that are gender-specific fit this description quite well because they attack an individual's sense of well-being. In pronatalist societies, the validation of social identity

is formed by the cultural construction of gender roles linked to reproduction.[79] Therefore, the concept of being the 'other' and culturally rejected, forced into isolation and denied the social expression of grief and sympathy, which infertile women can hold, is caused by a perceived deviation from the group norm.[20] Miall[80] discussed how infertility could stigmatize women in two ways. When a woman has female-factor infertility, she has a social role disability. All the respondents in her research described their infertility as a type of failure or an inability to work normally. They also felt that a public awareness of their fertility problems would cause others to view them in a new and damaging light. When women are married to a man with male-factor infertility, they acquire a 'courtesy stigma.' That is, they share the stigma attached to their male partner's infertility or a type of guilt by association with someone who has a stigmatizing attribute.

Nathanson[78,81] described the cognitive phase of the shame experience as a search of memory for similar experiences followed by layered associations to:

■ matters of personal size, strength, ability, or skill ("I am weak, incompetent, stupid");
■ dependence/independence (Sense of helplessness);
■ competition ("I am a loser");
■ sense of self ("I am defective");
■ personal attractiveness ("I am ugly or deformed");
■ sexuality ("There is something wrong with me sexually");
■ issues of seeing and being seen (The urge to escape from the eyes before which we have been exposed);
■ wishes and fears about closeness (The sense of being shorn of all humanity. A feeling that I am unlovable. The wish to be left alone).

The great majority of these cognitions can be present when an individual is diagnosed with infertility. According to Nathanson, the intensity of the shame experience is directly proportional to the gulf between the idealized self and the actual experience. Because most individuals approach their fertility in an idealized fashion, this gap can be wide. That is, most individuals rarely consider the possibility that conceiving will be difficult. When it is difficult, the resulting emotional experience can be shame-laden based on the cognitions listed above.

Self-Psychology Theory

Kohut's expansion of psychoanalytic theory into a psychology of self views happiness and well-being as dependent on a stable sense of self.[82] Infertility can produce an altered self-concept and self-image, predictable factors that affect both men and women, although often for different reasons. Men typically feel angry, ashamed, and inferior to their fertile peers. Women feel inadequate and deficient because they have failed to fulfill societal and personal roles.

Grief and Loss Theory

Grief and loss models have been applied to the psychological responses of men and women to infertility. Grief associated with infertility is similar to that sustained with the death of a child.[83] Losses of adulthood can be triggers for depression.[84] Infertility poses losses that are potentially multiple and any one of them can trigger an adverse reaction. In addition to the psychological losses described below, physical losses can include the loss of potency and/or a loss of interest in intercourse. Stages of grief and loss are described elsewhere.[82] A significant problem for individuals and couples is that contemporary North American society presently provides no mourning rituals for couples who deal with miscarriage or other failures in conception. This complicates the normal grieving that takes place in other situations of loss.[84]

CLINICAL ISSUES

It is well established that women view the role of mother as an important determinant of their femininity and that men, to a somewhat lesser extent, see their ability to father a child as one important representation of their masculinity. Consequently, a gender-related factor that prevents conception is an insult to that portion of the psyche that represents gender, sex role identification, and ego definition or sense of self. Significantly, motherhood is seen as the defining role for women in the vast majority of cultures – whether this is a cultural bias or simply a reality of nature and a continuation of the species. Consequently, anything that disrupts this role has the potential for yielding negative assessments such as being considered selfish or unfulfilled, cold or unnurturing. Women are susceptible to this in far greater degree than men because fatherhood is typically seen as secondary to career and economic pursuits and a more parallel role in conjunction with these pursuits than the primary and sole role of motherhood is for women. Therefore, men are typically subject to less social pressure to parent – although they may be subject to equal amounts of social pressure to father a child. Social support networks can be more disrupted for infertile women than men. When an infertile woman's friends become parents, the space given to friendship activities can be consumed with caretaking, domestic and sometimes occupational pursuits, leaving her without a significant source of emotional support. Her losses are compounded by her infertility. Men, on the other hand, seem to undergo relatively few changes in their friendships with other men when their peers become fathers and they do not.[11] Infertility makes one feel 'out of sync' with one's peers. This phenomenon seems to be felt more by men when it is male-factor and they are 'holding up' their wives. A man's distress may be more indirect in that he does not feel badly for himself as much as responsible and guilty for distress that causes his wife, who is ready to be a mother, to feel badly.

Although significant numbers of men and women attending infertility clinics indicate that they would seek counseling if offered, a surprisingly low percent actually accept it.[85] Counseling interventions for infertility have frequently been based on a bereavement model with the aim of helping couples mourn their losses associated with failure to achieve pregnancy. While this may be appropriate for women, this model does not appear to fit the experience of infertile men. Consequently, the best counseling interventions for women may alienate men.[7] To address these various concerns, Pook and colleagues[86] examined why infertile men engaged in counseling services. Their data suggest that a man's knowledge of his number of impaired sperm parameters and his anxiety and depression scores affected whether or not he was willing to use counseling. Counseling users had higher depression and anxiety scores as well as greater numbers of impaired sperm parameters. In summary, although some research has indicated that the majority of men and women attending infertility clinics do not avail themselves of counseling services, counseling seems to be an important resource for a segment of patients. Furthermore, when offered and undertaken, infertility counseling may be most useful when it is tailored to the needs of the patient (e.g., identifying and treating emotional problems, or providing support and education) rather than using a bereavement model of 'one size fits all.' This may be even more relevant with gender-specific infertility diagnosis.

Clinical components of a gender-specific diagnosis can determine the scope that therapeutic interventions will encompass for the infertility counselor. For women with PCOS, the concomitant constellation of hirsutism, weight problems, and menstrual irregularity as well as infertility requires the clinician and patient to be knowledgeable about the medical problems underlying the infertility. Quality-of-life issues, increased stress, and body image problems compound the losses of the associated infertility and comprehensive counseling must deal with these as well. Similarly, women with POF or endometriosis underlying their infertility will likely have experienced gynecological problems and negative sexual experiences in addition to the problem of infertility. Successful interventions will take these factors into account. Endometriosis, POF, and PCOS patients may derive benefit from individual and group interventions. At the same time, all may be well served by couple's counseling that provides educational information about the underlying medical problems as well as dealing with the specific clinical issues inherent in infertility. Often, male partners of women with endometriosis are frustrated on multiple levels: They have been thwarted in efforts to help achieve a pregnancy and sexual interaction is greatly diminished because intercourse can be painful for their partner. Both members of the couple can feel inadequate, incompetent, and guilty. Consequently, both members of the couple can benefit from education about the nature of the disease to dispel any notions they have about personal responsibility for the disorder. In addition, they can benefit from therapy that encourages nonintercourse sexual activity. The woman may feel unattractive and undesirable. Interventions that encourage attention to self, such as taking time for self-pampering activities, can be useful. Journaling is another clinical intervention that can address some of the negative feelings that a woman with PCOS or other female-factor infertility related disorders can develop.[87,88]

Gender-specific diagnoses can frequently influence core beliefs that a person holds about his or her ability to fulfill a societal sex role. Men with male-factor diagnoses can feel 'less than' and sexually inadequate, creating feelings of inadequacy that become generalized to other arenas of their lives. As a result, counseling efforts must address not only issues of generativity in terms of carrying on a family line, but also the sexual component of manhood. Knowledge about potential sexual problems and their treatment necessarily comes into play. While it may be easier and appropriate to refer a man who has developed erectile dysfunction subsequent to a male-factor infertility diagnosis to a sex therapist, this is a risky approach. In so doing, the infertility counselor (or medical caregiver) may be facilitating emotional compartmentalization for him and his partner. As such, an important treatment goal for the infertility counselor is viewing the couple and each partner as complete persons who have been affected in multiple areas of their lives by one diagnosis. This consideration requires a breadth of skill and understanding of the myriad of implications of infertility as well as wide array of effective treatment interventions including individual therapy, marriage and family counseling, sex therapy, and so on.

The issue of responsibility or blame for some misfortune is common. Individuals like to have something on which to blame hard luck. It is not unusual for an individual to attach personal blame when a gender-specific infertility diagnosis is rendered. Blaming oneself for prior improper acts such as sexual promiscuity, illicit drug use, or other risky behavior are common reactions to a diagnosis. And self-blame appears to affect men and women similarly, although women are seemingly more susceptible.[89] Some cultures do tend to place all blame for infertility on women,[57] regardless of diagnosis. Of course, when other marital issues are extant, it is possible for one member to blame the other for the infertility diagnosis. For example, a wife who was a virgin at the time of their marriage could easily blame a husband with a greater premarital sexual history for his male-factor diagnosis.

Shame and stigma are clinical issues for both male-factor and female-factor infertility. Zolbrod[90] describes the shame that artificial insemination patients felt because medical personnel were present during a 'sex act.' Their shame was related to a sense of loss of control over their bodies and their lives. It would not be surprising to find that feelings of personal exposure also contributed to their shame. Shame related to the perceived defect of infertility or feeling of lack of personal competence can also be present. Similarly, shame can be present when female-factor infertility is present. Feelings of being a sexual failure, or otherwise defective, influence feelings of shame. Stigmatization from a reproductive system failure and subsequent loss of either the ability to conceive or carry a child to term can have clinical ramifications. In both male- and female-factor infertility, the individual is at risk for feeling helpless or deformed in some way.

THERAPEUTIC INTERVENTIONS

In general, it has been established that benefits accrue to infertile individuals who receive psychosocial interventions.[91] Therapeutic implications of male-factor and female-factor infertility can be explored from both medical and emotional variables. In addition, increasing mobility has made it possible for individuals from one culture to easily transplant themselves into another, subsequently seeking medical care for infertility. Awareness of different cultural values becomes imperative for the infertility counselor in these situations.

Exploring the Implications of Male-Factor Infertility

To explore the implications for male-factor infertility, the infertility counselor should inquire about the man's understanding of his infertility diagnosis and his feelings related to it as well as his partner's understanding of the diagnosis and her feelings. Initial interventions can be made with the man alone, later adding his partner in, so as not to embarrass him if he finds the discussion difficult. In addition, some men may be less willing to talk with their partner present, preferring to allow her to speak for him. Once the clinician feels that the man has a good grasp of the situation, adding his partner in, as a potential source of support and emphasizing the teammate nature of their relationship, can be useful. Despite the common notion that men are less likely to discuss their feelings, clinical experience indicates that many men want to explore their emotions regarding their diagnosis. They may lack a sufficient vocabulary to do this and clinicians are in a position to help them develop the language to describe their experience.

Implications of Medical Conditions

The most frequent causes of male-factor infertility are difficulties with sperm production, sperm transport, and fertilization. Genetic disorders, illness, injury or ingestion or exposure to toxic materials, mumps, orchitis and testicular cancer all can obliterate the ability to produce sperm. Male-factor infertility can also be the result of inherited or genetic disorders such as congenital bilateral absence of the vas deferens (CBAVD) or Klinefelter's syndrome. Toxic agents, reactive oxygen stress, tobacco smoke, alcohol abuse, and recreational drugs have all been implicated in male-factor infertility. Overheating of the testicles from hot tubs or laptop computer use has also been implicated. Previous advice regarding underwear for men was to avoid briefs in favor of boxer shorts because briefs could cause overheating and impair sperm production. Recent research has questioned this advice.[92] Finally, a vasectomy performed at an earlier stage of life is a distinct barrier to reproduction.

It is important that the infertility counselor be knowledgeable about the medical aspects of male-factor infertility, and is able to communicate and educate this information to patients. All too often, one of the consequences of stigma and shame related to male-factor infertility is that patients have not felt comfortable enough or educated enough to ask caregivers about their diagnosis. This can cause not only undue emotional distress, but may also result in treatment decisions based on inaccurate information or misunderstandings. Furthermore, health behavioral changes that the patient could or should make to maximize his fertility (e.g., stopping alcohol or tobacco usage) may not have been encouraged or facilitated by caregivers. Masculinity, virility, fertility, and male roles can all have

cultural determinants that influence a man's emotional response to infertility. An exploration of fundamental beliefs and cultural values of the man and his partner are important, especially when they may differ but not be obvious.[21]

Although the counselor might assume that a man, or woman for that matter, has been asked questions about alcohol, tobacco, or recreational drug use by medical personnel, it is useful to repeat these questions in a counseling session. Clinical experience indicates that an individual will more readily disclose this information in a therapy setting in which issues of confidentiality are usually well discussed. If, for example, an individual is using marijuana to reduce the stress he feels going through treatment for male-factor infertility, information about the potential detrimental effect on sperm count will be helpful to him.

Age seems not to play the same role in fertility for men as it does with women. There is evidence that with increasing age in men, there is associated delayed conception, although a direct correlation between age and fecundity has not been strongly established. Other confounding factors, such as decreases in coital frequency with age, age-related medical conditions (e.g., Type 2 diabetes), or side effects of medications to treat age-related illnesses (e.g., osteoarthritis), may occur.[93]

For some time, it was thought that most male-factor infertility was the result of idiosyncratic problems that could not be treated. Few treatment options existed, especially for azoospermia. The most common intervention was insemination with the husband's sperm after it was diluted with a medium and centrifuged. Failure of this procedure usually led to consideration of donor insemination (DI) or therapeutic donor insemination, not a treatment for infertility but, rather, a family-building alternative. Furthermore, DI involves some measure of stigma as well as the equally vexing problem of disclosure. When, as is often the case, male-factor infertility is unexplained with no apparent etiology or identifiable causative factor, the man and his partner often find adjustment much more challenging because it is an emotionally ambiguous situation in which resolution and closure typically feel elusive.[94]

Recently, a significant number of male-factor infertility problems are diagnosable and treatable with sophisticated and effective procedures, albeit with their own set of psychosocial issues. The advent of microsurgery techniques in 1977 now provide reproductive opportunity to a large number of men affected by male-factor infertility. These new techniques include ICSI, microsurgical epididymal sperm aspiration (MESA), and testicular sperm extraction (TESE). MESA and TESE provide solutions to sperm-transport problems and ICSI is a solution for problems of sperm penetration of the oocyte and sperm mobility and morphology (the embryologist can choose a specific healthy sperm to use for ICSI). And while these procedures provide new hope and opportunity for men with male-factor infertility to have the genetically linked offspring they want, the procedures still require that his female partner undergo a significant series of interventions. She will have ovulation induced, and IVF is used to maximize conception probabilities even if her own fertility is not impaired. This necessarily requires ovum retrieval and transfer of the embryo, both invasive procedures. In short, even though male-factor infertility can be treated today with a wide array of medical interventions, the medical treatments still require major medical treatment of the female partner. This 'imbalance' of medical treatment can result in its own fair share of emotional and marital consequences and should be consequences the infertility counselor and clinician is always on the alert for and prepared to address.

Genetic advances have improved the understanding of several forms of male-factor infertility. It now appears that azoospermia and oligospermia may be due to genetic disorders that involve CBAVD, microdeletions on the Y chromosome, and/or subtle abnormalities in other genes that are not apparent from gross karyotyping.[95] Consequently, it is clear that men with CBAVD may be at increased risk for cystic fibrosis even though they are frequently asymptomatic. When their infertility is uncovered, the presence of the genetic problem and possible life-threatening or life-altering medical problem comes to light (see Chapter 14).

Testicular cancer and Hodgkin's disease are cancers that frequently occur in younger men and subsequently impact their fertility either as a disease in and of itself or as a consequence of treatment for cancer. If testicular cancer is diagnosed early enough, fertility may not already be impaired. Similarly, sperm quality may be satisfactory at the time of diagnosis for Hodgkin's. When sperm abnormalities do not exist prior to treatment of these cancers, cryopreservation of sperm is useful[96] because chemotherapy for these cancers can impair fertility. Although this has not always been the case, an increasing number of cancer specialists now offer pretreatment cryopreservation of sperm to young men diagnosed with cancer, with an eye to future fatherhood in adulthood. This increased practice gained further momentum from consumer awareness programs to preserve fertility in cancer patients. Counseling for testicular cancer patients is strongly advised because the integrity of self-esteem, sexuality, fertility, and masculinity is so closely associated with this particular reproductive organ.[97,98]

Since the mid-1970s, microsurgery has permitted vasectomy reversal for men whose life circumstances change and who now wish to father children. Approximately 6% of the 500,000 men who annually have vasectomies in the United States seek reversal of the procedure.[99] Vasovasostomy (VVS), a surgical procedure that restores continuity and repairs blockage of the vas deferens, is used to reverse the effects of vasectomy. In some cases, a vasoepididymostomy (VE), which bypasses blockages in the epididymis, is performed. If VVS or VE are unsuccessful, percutaneous epididymal sperm aspiration (PESA) or percutaneous vasal sperm aspiration (PVSA) along with IUI have been used with success.[100] A significant number of men who seek VVS or VE are in second marriages and want to establish a family with a new spouse.[101] But men may be ambivalent about starting new families, particularly if a first marriage has already produced children who are now older. Despite the sophistication of the surgery for vasectomy reversal, men may be reluctant to undergo invasive and potentially expensive procedures. Furthermore, having already experienced a failed marriage, a man may have legitimate concern about his ability to have a successful second marriage. Consequently, it can be useful for counselors to explore the man's feelings about his new marriage and his desire to have children in it.

These new technologies do create reproductive choices for men, not all of which are without potential adverse consequences. ICSI provides a method for men with severe defects in spermatogenesis to reproduce. At the same time, MESA and TESE make it possible for genetic mutations to be transmitted. As a result, the Health Council of The Netherlands has banned MESA and TESE. In short, these new technologies provide parenthood with the possibility of transmitting a genetic disorder to offspring, and additional counseling for couples considering the use of ICSI, MESA, and TESE is recommended.[21] This may be educational, implications, supportive counseling, psychotherapy, and/or genetic counseling (see Chapter 15).

The availability of a genetically shared pregnancy makes ICSI, MESA, and TESE desirable for couples where male-factor infertility is at issue. At the same time, there are significant additional factors for consideration by these couples. These procedures have been used as medical treatment options or a diagnostic tool for male-factor infertility. Infertility counselors and medical caregivers share a concern about the option of 'donor backup' often offered along with the more advanced technologies in the event of fertilization failure. Donor backup, unlike ICSI, MESA, and TESE, does not allow a genetically-shared pregnancy and is not a treatment for male-factor infertility but, rather, a family-building alternative. However, this distinction is not always clear to couples in their anxious, determined, and even myopic drive to conceive. Under these circumstances, treatment decisions are more complicated due to the potential for transmitting genetic anomalies, having children with chromosomal disorders, achieving a pregnancy via donor sperm, and/or having a multiple pregnancy with different genetic fathers. Consequently, couples considering ICSI, MESA, and TESE should be informed about the possibilities and the risks associated with their use. While the medical technology is quite miraculous, the psychosocial and ethical complexities are significant making the necessity for proper counseling all the more imperative. Pretreatment counseling should help couples make informed decisions by helping them consider all potential treatment outcomes and understand the distinction between medical procedures that facilitate reproduction and provide opportunity for family-building.[21]

Implications of the Emotional Response

The idea of psychologically integrating medical information about themselves into their sense of self is difficult and aversive for some men. If they refuse to accept the reality of male-factor infertility diagnosis and its associated implications, some men resort to inappropriate methods for handling their feelings. They may act out sexually by having affairs or using prostitutes, compulsive masturbation, or internet sexual activity (e.g., pornography or dating) to validate their masculinity. Bullying, controlling, or attaching blame to a wife or medical caregiver is another inappropriate mechanism for coping. Escape via alcohol, drugs, gambling, or internet addiction have also been observed. For men with these types of impulse control problems, support groups that focus specifically on the problem, such as Alcoholics Anonymous or Gamblers Anonymous, can be adjuncts to more traditional counseling strategies. An important intervention goal is to increase the man's sense of competence and ability to soothe himself in healthy rather than destructive ways. Consequently, insight into the function of the inappropriate behavior coupled with strategies for change become therapeutic components that complement each other.

Male-factor infertility can also trigger changes to a man's body image or sexual functioning that are intrusive and distressing to the man as well as his partner. He may experience flashbacks of prior sexual vulnerability residual to adolescence or spontaneous and negative visual imagery of a body defect have been reported.[102] For men who have a history of sexual abuse or trauma, the experience of infertility can trig-

ger reemergence of posttraumatic symptoms or other psychological symptoms.[103] Counseling that focuses on these issues in ways that do not retraumatize the man are best. For example, methods that draw distinctions between past traumatic events and the relative safety of his current situation can help heal traumatic wounds. In addition, helping the man to see his competencies and survival capacity is also useful.

A variety of factors can make it difficult for a man to maintain positive self-esteem and self-image. These include preexisting shame about his body, heightened guilt feelings, or misperceptions about previous behavior that might have caused his infertility. There is clinical evidence that men who are more devastated and have significant problems with a male-factor diagnosis will be those who (1) were emotionally close to their fathers while growing up, and/or have positive internalized images of fatherhood; (2) highly value their genetic heredity or bloodlines; (3) have preexisting narcissistic wounds regarding body image and masculinity; and (4) have preexisting sexual problems.[104] To ensure that a man does not become overwhelmed with feelings of defectiveness or depression, several clinical treatment approaches can be considered. Infertility counselors can help men process feelings so that they do not view a future child, conceived via donor sperm, as a reminder of an impairment or what they perceive as personal deficits or defects. Because men are often socialized to see themselves as responsible for the well-being of their families and spouses, they may be reluctant to share their distress with partner or caregivers. As a result, they may agree to medical interventions, such as donor insemination (DI), to please a wife or avoid confrontation rather than address their own feelings and make a positive and collaborative decision to use DI for family-building with their partner. Overall it is important that a man be clear that his choice is one that he owns and not one that he will regret or for which he will hold his partner responsible at some point in the future.

Most importantly, men with male-factor infertility must integrate the diagnosis into their ego and lives enabling them to make reproductive choices that are their own: providing them with ownership of their choices, lives, and the children they parent, however those children are created. Working through emotional reservations reduces the hazards to a positive father–child bond. Cognitive-behavioral therapy (CBT) approaches that reduce thoughts of helplessness and other depressive symptoms are also useful and successful tools.[105,106]

When family-building decisions lead to donor insemination, some men may resist the idea of donor gametes because they feel they will not be a 'real' father to a resulting child. Helping the man understand that parenthood is more than genetic in nature is another essential component of intervention. Conveying the message that the social context in which a child is raised may have a far greater impact than the child's genetic origins, can be useful. Assisting men to see their role as father as an ongoing process rather than a finite event is essential. Questioning a man about the qualities that he values in his own father can help him accomplish this, as he begins to understand the dynamic nature of fatherhood.

While the specific emotional reactions of a man with male-factor infertility are important, recognition of the dyadic nature of most infertility is equally significant. The great majority of male-factor infertility takes place in the context of heterosexual marriages. Therefore, husbands must be able to acknowledge and accept their wives' feelings of loss without simultaneously feeling responsible, blamed, or shamed. His losses are primary but his wife's are also important, not only to her but also to the relationship as a whole. Acceptance and validation of her feelings can enhance the strength and closeness in a marital relationship, allowing each to recognize, confirm, and share their pain and loss as a result of his infertility. By communicating, acknowledging, and validating each of their perspectives, couples can make infertility a shared experience with a shared meaning. With a shared definition of the experience, couples are more likely to move on from the trauma and disappointments of infertility in a positive and healthy fashion. Interventions that encourage dialogue and incorporate couples and family therapy approaches have been used to accomplish these goals.[107,108]

Exploring the Implications of Female-Factor Infertility

Similar to men, to explore the implications for female-factor infertility, inquiries into a woman's understanding of her infertility diagnosis and her feelings about it must be made. However, female fertility is finite, unlike male fertility that has the ability to maintain itself into old age because testicular function does not experience a complete age-related decline as ovarian function does with menopause.[109,110] This significant difference does have both medical and emotional consequences for women and must be taken into account by those who counsel them.

Implications of Medical Conditions

Like male-factor infertility, female-factor infertility may be the result of either infertility-specific disorders or medical conditions/disorders impacting reproduction. Age-related factors such as diminished ovarian reserve, declining quality of oocytes, menstrual abnormalities/irregularities, and elevated levels of follicular-stimulating hormone (FSH) levels as well as reduced uterine receptivity can compromise fertility. Increased maternal age also increases the risk of miscarriage and offspring with chromosomal abnormalities and/or age-related birth defects (e.g., Down syndrome). Congenital anomalies including Turner's syndrome and Rokitansky-Küster-Hauser syndrome as well as chromosomal abnormalities that subvert either reproductive system development or later functioning are also causes of female-factor infertility. Hysterectomy or oophorectomy due to cancer, other diseases, or treatments related to cancer/disease treatment such as radiation or chemotherapy may reduce fertility or cause permanent sterility. Medical conditions such as endometriosis, POF, or PCOS impair female fertility through hormonal imbalance, disease process impacting the reproductive cycle, and/or the reproductive tract. Uterine anomalies including fibroids or scarring due to the use of certain forms of intrauterine devices used as birth control are also potential causes of female infertility. Women may experience infertility due to blocked fallopian tubes due to sexually transmitted disease(s), genital mutilation, surgical scarring, abdominal injury, and/or infection such as pelvic inflammatory disease (PID). Finally, although less prevalent than in the past, women (and men) may experience infertility due to reproductive tract malformations as a result of exposure to DES in utero.

Age-related female-factor infertility can have a set of highly emotional factors attached to it. Not the least of these is the fact that, at least in Western cultures, women are waiting until later in life to have children. Couples marry later and therefore delay childbearing. Women's career priorities, advanced education, control over fertility, and financial concerns are other contributing factors to this trend. In the United States, women have their children later than they did twenty years ago, with mothers over the age of thirty accounting for one in three births in 1992.[111] In Spain, the average age of women at the time of the birth of their first child was twenty-eight years of age in 1975, yet by 1995, that age was thirty.[112] Similarly, in The Netherlands average maternal age for a first child was 24.6 years in 1970 and 29.1 years in 1999.[113] Age-related steadily declining fertility rates in women take a sharp drop at thirty-five. An estimated one-third of women who delay a first pregnancy until age thirty-five or older will have problems with conception. And if a woman waits until age forty to attempt conception, she faces a 50% chance of difficulty achieving a pregnancy and carrying the fetus to term without fetal abnormality. Oocytes decline in quality as a woman ages. This can result in increased follicular atresia, chromosomal abnormalities, menstrual abnormalities, and elevated FSH levels resulting in declining fertility. Finally, problems with uterine receptivity to pregnancy maintenance increase with age.[111]

Reasons for waiting to have children can be numerous and compelling. Completing educational goals, building a career, taking care of aging parents, inability to find a suitable partner, changing life circumstances or perspective in oneself or partner may be reasons why a woman waits (intentionally or unintentionally) until older to begin her childbearing. With the 'biological clock ticking,' the realization of a lost opportunity to bear, nurture, and raise children often increases the desire to experience pregnancy and have children. Women observing friends and colleagues becoming pregnant and opting for a different lifestyle can trigger this desire. Family, religious, or cultural pressure can be instrumental as well: It is not unusual for a childless woman to be questioned, frequently in well-meaning ways, about why she has no children. Aging or terminally ill parents provide another impetus to create a family that may not have existed earlier in life. Producing a grandchild can provide evidence of 'true' adulthood, and in some cultures, the birth of a child signifies another rite of passage. Consequently, there may be familial pressure to have a child. And remarriage in middle age can instigate a reevaluation of a decision to remain childless or perhaps the desire to have additional children with a new spouse who may or may not already have children. All or any of these factors can influence a woman who previously had no children to seek them later in life. Age can provide a certain perspective on life. At the same time, attempting to have children later in life can introduce a new set of stresses rendering perspective at best, less effective or, at worst, lost.

Reproductive endocrinologists routinely recommend an increasing intensity of treatment regimens for women with age-related infertility. Typically, initial treatment focuses on ovulation induction (medically or with superovulation) with or without IUI (intrauterine inseminations). Should these treatments fail, IVF is typically the next treatment step. However, as age increases, even with superovulation inducing medications, fewer oocytes are produced, retrieved, and/or fertilized leaving fewer embryos to be transferred, resulting in lower implantation and pregnancy rates and increased miscarriage rates due to age. If these treatments are unsuccessful due to ovarian failure or poor oocyte quality, the next line of treatment is donated oocytes. Donor oocyte offers women with ovarian failure a better chance of pregnancy and parenthood.[114,115] It is generally accepted that patients considering the use of donated gametes have counseling to explore issues related not only to the inherent losses of infertility, but also expectations regarding donors, privacy, and disclosure matters as well as a variety of other pertinent factors (see Chapters 17 and 18). In the event that the woman has fully functioning ovaries but no uterus (i.e., due to Rokitansky syndrome or loss of uterus to cancer), she may undergo ovulation stimulation with her retrieved oocytes fertilized with her spouse's sperm. These embryos are then transferred to a gestational carrier who carries the pregnancy for her. In the worst of all possible cases when a woman has lost both ovarian function and uterine function, a traditional surrogate or gestational carrier with donated oocytes may be her only pathways to reproductive parenthood in which a child has a genetic connection to her partner but not to her.

Solutions for genetic disorders that disrupt fertility for women rely on some form of third-party reproduction assistance. Women born with Turner's syndrome, a chromosomal anomaly characterized by only one X chromosome instead of two, have early loss of all oocytes and nonfunctional ovaries at birth. Other aspects of their reproductive system, fallopian tubes, uterus, cervix, and vagina are intact in these women and they are able to carry a pregnancy generated with donor oocytes. Although they have no genetic connection to the resultant child, they do have the opportunity to experience pregnancy and childbirth. However, there is a significant risk of death from rupture or dissection of the aorta and prescreening of these women with echocardiography to rule out risks is strongly recommended;[116] the use of a surrogate may be indicated. Women with Rokitansky-Küster-Hauser syndrome have functioning ovaries but congenital absence of the vagina and/or uterus. This is a congenital defect (not a genetic disorder that can be transmitted to her offspring) and, as such, many women with this disorder can achieve parenthood of a genetically-shared offspring through the use of gestational carriers. These pregnancies are achieved through ovarian stimulation and oocyte retrieval followed by IVF with the husband's sperm and embryo transfer to the gestational carrier.[117] Both disorders, with their concomitant infertility and medical problems, can trigger an array of emotional issues that may have been dormant prior to attempts at conception. Losses of body image, sexual function, and female identity issues can be significant. In addition, stigma associated with a body defect can be present. Therapeutic interventions that address grieving will be important. In addition, interventions that enhance other aspects of the woman's femininity can be useful. Cognitive-behavioral therapy to address negative thoughts can play a role. Discussions about the significance of the nurturing component of motherhood are also useful.

Endometriosis, the presence of uterine lining tissue outside the uterus, can be a painful chronic medical condition that causes chronic pain or pain during intercourse and during ovulation. It is found in 30–35% of women with infertility.[118] However, a clear causal relationship between endometriosis and infertility has yet to be established and the mechanism by which endometriosis contributes to infertility is speculative at best. With early-stage disease, it appears that surgical treatment (removal) can increase pregnancy rates as well as reduce pelvic pain associated with the disease. Medication regimens for endometriosis to reduce pain and/or prevent recurrence have not been shown to improve fertility rates. Furthermore, side-effects from these medications can be significant including mood changes, vaginal dryness, headaches, hirsutism, and hot flashes. IVF is one treatment option particularly if endometriosis has caused tubal blockage, although evidence is inconclusive as to its effectiveness.[118] Counseling infertile women with endometriosis should explore probabilities of success with various treatments as well as potential avenues to childbearing should they be unsuccessful in achieving a pregnancy. Mind–body approaches have been used to reduce stress that can contribute to the pain associated with endometriosis.[104] These techniques allow a woman to reduce potential sources of stress. Relaxation techniques such as focused breathing, imagery, and progressive muscle relaxation can be helpful as can journaling.

Abnormally high levels of androgens, irregularity or absence of the menstrual cycle, and ovarian cysts characterize PCOS, the most common hormonal reproductive problem in women of childbearing age. In addition to affecting fertility, it can impact a woman's insulin production, heart, and blood vessels. Altered appearance due to increased acne and hirsutism are also complications of the condition. Weight loss, because it can reverse insulin resistance with its attendant anovulation, is a first-line therapy.[119]

Medical treatments designed to increase fertility and decrease other symptoms of PCOS have included clomiphene citrate, used for ovulation induction, low-dose recombinant FSH,[120] gonadotropin-releasing hormone (GnRH) therapy,[121] tamoxifen citrate, a nonsteroidal selective estrogen receptor modulator[122] and metformin, a medication used to treat diabetes mellitus and found helpful in restoring insulin sensitivity in women with PCOS.[123] Surgical treatment with laparoscopic ovarian drilling (LOD)[124,125] has been used with women who are resistant to clomiphene citrate therapy or those who failed ovulation induction with gonadotropins. LOD treatment is physically invasive and involves general anesthesia, surgical incision, and the destruction of portions of the ovary via electrocautery or laser. The psychological components of PCOS are related to stigmatizing factors associated with the physical characteristics of the disorder, stress, and the potentially depressing thoughts that can occur with chronic medical conditions. Weight loss, a difficult thing for many to accomplish, is an area of intervention in which counselors can make a contribution. Work with patients to establish and monitor reasonable and achievable goals can enhance a woman's sense of control and reduce shame and stigma. Moderate levels of exercise are another component of weight loss programs for PCOS patients. Directing patients to support networks for this purpose is useful. Stress reduction techniques that can be used include focused breathing, relaxation techniques, and visual imagery. Helping patients to establish a more positive outlook can enhance their self-esteem and feelings of self-worth.

Premature ovarian failure (POF) is the spontaneous cessation of normal ovarian function prior to age forty. The literature on POF establishes a connection between the disorder and psychological distress.[67] Clearly, a diagnosis of POF can be life changing not only in the recognition of significant problems with fertility but also with additional underlying medical conditions. Groff et al.[67] offer specific guidelines for clinicians to present the diagnosis most effectively and with the least traumatic outcome. These include face-to-face delivery of the diagnosis with enough time available to provide thorough information on the disorder, offering information on support groups, and referral for psychological counseling and/or spiritual support. Noting that most women want guidance on how to cope with the emotional components of POF, Nelson and associates[126] recommend that clinicians lead patients in this direction. Statements that attest to the difficulty that many patients have emotionally accepting a POF diagnosis can provide entrée to a discussion. They further recommend helping patients identify individuals with whom they will feel comfortable discussing the emotional aspects of the diagnosis.

Tubal blockages are a significant physical cause of female-factor infertility. Some tubal blockages are the result of tubal sterilization, a form of birth control intended to be permanent, which can be reversed. A small number of women who have tubal sterilization have regrets and seek reversal. A strong correlation exists between regrets and youthful age and to changes in marital situation.[128] Research indicates that women who reported substantial conflict with their husbands or partners before tubal sterilization were more than three times as likely to regret their decision and more than five times as likely to request a reversal than women who did not report such conflict. Few women undergo this procedure, known as tubal reanastomosis. In addition to skill of the surgeon, the success of sterilization reversal depends on the age of the woman and the length of fallopian tube remaining after the initial sterilization procedure.[129] IVF is often used in place of sterilization reversal, but no randomized controlled studies exist comparing the two procedures.[129] The psychological issues that these patients present can be addressed with therapies that seek to identify the reason for a tubal sterilization and to normalize the woman's response to a stressful interpersonal situation. Guilt associated with having made a 'bad decision' and feeling penalized is possible. Cognitive strategies to reduce guilt and reverse irrational thinking are useful.[130]

Tubal disease is responsible for 25–35% of female infertility, with pelvic inflammatory disease (PID) the most frequent cause. An increase in infertility rates is noted with repeated infection episodes. Tubal occlusions can be either proximal or distal. A variety of approaches to the diagnosis of tubal infertility, including laparoscopy with chromopertubation, hysterosalpingography, onohysterosalpingography, and salpingoscopy, involve invasive procedures. Chlamydial serology is a noninvasive technique used to assess the presence of previous infection with Chlamydia trachomatis. Therapeutic approaches for proximal tubal occlusion include transcervical tubal cannulation and tubocornual anastomosis. Salpingostomy and fimbrioplasty are available for the treatment of distal tubal occlusion. Finally, IVF is a commonly used strategy for the treatment of all types of tubal dysfunction.[129] While no randomized controlled trials exist comparing IVF and tubal surgery for infertility, younger women with adequate ovarian reserve and mild to moderate tubal disease do better than older women with severe tubal disease in achieving subsequent pregnancies. All the invasive procedures for both diagnosis and treatment of tubal blockage can have psychological effects. Women treated for tubal blockages or other surgeries of the reproductive tract can experience deterioration of their sexual life.[130,131] Fear and anxiety prior to surgery and postoperative depression have also been observed. Behavioral interventions to improve coping skills for the medical treatments are useful. In addition,

stress reduction techniques serve these patients well because many of the medical procedures are stress inducing, not to mention the obvious stress of failure to achieve a pregnancy. Men can have a difficult time appreciating the psychological issues that their partners face with tubal disease. Therefore, it is also useful to hold sessions with the woman and her partner to improve emotional support between the two.

Cancer of the female reproductive organs can include cervical, uterine, and ovarian forms. Of these, reproductive-aged women are most frequently affected by cervical cancer. Surgery has replaced radiation therapy for women with early-stage cervical cancer and can spare the ovaries. Women who require hysterectomy for their cervical cancer can become mothers if oocytes are retrieved, fertilized via IVF, and the resultant embryo(s) are transferred to a gestational carrier.[96] Young women with ovarian tumors of low malignant potential can receive conservative surgery because of the excellent prognosis of these tumors. Patients wishing to conceive after diagnosis occasionally require ovulation induction. Cancer presents a set of emotional issues for any patient, and reproductive cancers have the additional issue of fertility loss. In addition, women who elect to use sophisticated ART procedures to preserve their fertility are faced with additional stress from the procedures themselves and the uncertainty of a child resulting from them. The loss of femininity associated with reproductive cancers can be profound. Counseling interventions that address not only these losses but also teach coping strategies are important. Some women will be receptive to bibliotherapy interventions. Books such as Harold Kushner's *When Bad Things Happen to Good People* or Norman Cousins' *Anatomy of an Illness as Perceived by the Patient* provide insight from spiritual and mind–body approaches to healing. When oophorectomy is necessary, use of embryos derived from the patient's oocytes retrieved prior to surgery is possible. However, they must normally be cryopreserved until her system is free from the deleterious effects of any postoperative chemotherapy. In addition, she must have an intact, healthy uterus. Cryopreservation of oocytes is not yet assumed to be safe. Furthermore, cryopreservation and subsequent transplantation of ovarian tissue is currently under investigation with some reported limited success.[132] If this technology is successful and the ethical issues inherent in such procedures are adequately addressed, it offers a promising solution for women whose cancers require surgical removal of their ovaries.[132] (See Chapter 14.)

Similar issues may exist for women with breast cancers where chemotherapy can result in permanent ovarian failure.[96] Women with cancers for which treatment can impair future reproductive capacity face the dual dilemma of life-threatening disease and infertility. The resulting psychological sequelae can include not only anxiety about recurrent cancer but also lost fertility and, perhaps, shortened life expectancy. Counseling with these women, and men with cancers as well, must take both facts into account. Depression and anxiety are commonly seen in individuals with cancer diagnoses. Research on reducing these psychological sequelae indicates that a variety of factors can reduce anxiety and depression including the following: preparing the patient for a possible diagnosis of cancer; providing the patient as much information about the diagnosis as desired; providing written information; presenting the information clearly; discussing the patient's questions the same day; talking about the patient's feelings and being reassuring; using the word *cancer*; discussing the severity of the situation, life expectancy, and how the cancer might affect other aspects of life; and encouraging the patient to be involved in treatment decisions.[133] Counselors are in a position to help both physicians and patients with these recommendations. In addition, counselors can help patients make decisions with their partners about reproduction options. For example, when it is clear that a patient's cancer is terminal, is posthumous reproduction something that is desired by the diagnosed individual? Clearly, this is more easily accomplished when a man is the patient because semen can be obtained and frozen for later use. The use of frozen embryos from a woman with terminal cancer raises additional issues regarding a surrogate carrier after the patient's demise.

Implications of the Emotional Response

Stress as a consequence of and perhaps a contributor to female-factor infertility is a well-established finding.[56] Furthermore, it appears that infertile women experience greater levels of distress than do infertile men. When infertile partners are evaluated, women experience more psychosocial distress than men with respect to anxiety, cognitive disturbance, depression, and hostility.[134] While anxiety and depression scores for infertile women are lower than women with other medical conditions, they are statistically similar to those obtained by women with serious medical conditions.[135] Stress for women can be associated with not only the diagnosis but also the treatment procedures, many of which are either physically or pharmacologically invasive. Intrusive thoughts and avoidant ideation along with anxiety and depression are characteristic of the normal response to traumatic stressors. Infertility and its treatment have been described as traumatic

for women. Intrusive ideation has been demonstrated to be predictive of infertility-specific distress and dysfunction.[136] Psychosocial distress and other psychological factors have also been implicated in dropout rates for infertility treatment.[137,138] And because psychological factors, such as stress, can be improved by intervention, and demographic and other factors are immune to treatment, patient counseling for these variables has been advised for women.[139]

The literature on stress and women involved in infertility treatment has led to the development of treatment programs aimed at reducing stress. Many of these treatments adopt a mind–body approach.[142] Group and individualized interventions have been used and significant positive results in reducing anxiety, depression and other psychological components of stress have been achieved[141–143], and some reports indicate an improvement in pregnancy rates with these types of interventions as well.[144]

Shame associated with failure to reproduce and feelings of inadequacy are found in women with female-factor infertility. Therapeutic techniques such as cognitive-behavioral interventions, eye movement desensitization and reprocessing (EMDR), hypnosis, and insight therapies can all be used with shame issues. The stigmatizing effect of female-factor infertility includes the exclusion of the woman from societal rituals and the deprivation of ties of descent. Therapeutic interventions can include insight-oriented therapies and cognitive behavioral interventions designed to alter irrational thoughts.

Older individuals may benefit from understanding their motivations for seeking children. Typically, three separate yet overlapping goals exist for these women: (1) the desire to have a genetic child, (2) the desire to experience pregnancy, and (3) the desire to become a parent. An evaluation of these goals and determination of which takes personal precedence can help a woman decide which treatment option to pursue. For example, an older woman whose primary goal is to experience a pregnancy will do best if she seeks donor oocytes. If a genetic child is primary, then IVF with or without a GC is indicated if physiologically possible. If parenting is the primary goal, other alternative family-building techniques such as adoption or foster parenting can be considered.[111]

Insight-oriented approaches for female-factor patients have been recommended to help process the loss and subsequent grief, if fertility treatment fails. And loss and grief, components of the emotional response to an inability to have a genetic child, pregnancy, or parent, are normal and can be framed that way by counselors. This seems to provide relief

TABLE 3.1. Factors to consider when treating infertile men and women

	Women	Men
Stresses felt	Higher levels Interpersonal health	Lower levels Occupational
Significant reported effects of infertility	Biological clock Jealous of others with children	Lost power to reproduce Worry about partner's reactions
Coping styles employed	Escape/avoidance Positive reframing Seek social support	Instrumental Problem-focused

to women.[56] Patients who can approach their losses in this way will be more able to accept alternative solutions for parenting should they be necessary.

Clearly, gender differences exist in the way men and women cope with infertility. Coping strategies that appear to work better for women than men include escape and avoidance, positive reframing of the situation, and seeking social support.[145] It may be that women use escape and avoidance because certain social situations remind them of their infertility. Avoiding those interactions is protective. At the same time, women appear to find it easier to discuss their infertility (thereby venting their feelings) with others outside the marriage than do men.[146] Data also suggest that infertile women who receive unsupportive social interactions develop more depressive symptoms and overall psychological distress.[147] Fortunately, significant opportunities for social support currently exist in patient support groups that have sprung up throughout the world, as well as online support groups (see Resources). Counselors are in a unique position to provide referral to these organizations. Individuals who are reluctant to engage in face-to-face meetings can be encouraged to peruse websites of support organizations as a way of desensitizing themselves to the idea of discussing their infertility with someone else. Counselors can also hold discussions regarding material that patients have obtained through these sources, helping patients sort out which information is useful to them.

Women with infertility related to endometriosis, POF, PCOS, or PID could experience difficulty with the sexual aspects of their relationships. Endometriosis can cause significant pain on intercourse and therefore produce an avoidance of sexual interaction. While women with PCOS appear to engage in intercourse at a similar rate to control subjects,[148] they tend to find themselves less sexually attractive. PID, with its chronic pelvic pain, can lead to low sexual desire. Similarly, women whose infertility is cancer-related will likely experience distur-

bances in their sexual images. Counseling efforts for these patients that takes into account their sexual relationships is important.

IVF as a treatment for a variety of infertility problems affecting women has achieved respected status in the medical community. Nevertheless, live birth rates, depending on age of the woman, can be as low as 25%.[149] Success rates as low as one in four can therefore be a significant factor in psychological outcomes for women undergoing IVF. Hynes et al.[150] determined that women were more depressed and had lower levels of self-esteem after a failed cycle than they did before. As noted by others, cognitive coping strategies were useful for these women and practitioners are advised to use them with comparable patients.

Table 3.1 provides a brief summary of factors to consider when providing psychosocial counseling to infertile men and women.

FUTURE IMPLICATIONS

Advances in the science of infertility diagnosis and treatment have played a role in our understanding of gender-specific infertility. As knowledge accumulates in the medical realm, knowledge related to the psychological components of infertility has experienced rapid growth. It is likely that future medical advances will propel psychological knowledge further. Certainly there is already room for more descriptive research on various gender-specific diagnoses of infertility, which will lead to more appropriate psychological interventions.

At a minimum, more research is necessary in how men react to a diagnosis of male-factor infertility. If and how men with differing diagnoses react is another direction for the future. And there is more room for research on how men react to female-factor diagnoses in their partners and vice versa. Investigations into why more men do not seek counseling and what counselor attributes work best with male-factor patients are called for. Finally, research that goes beyond descriptive and investigates the effectiveness of various interventions with men is called for.

Similarly, research with female-factor infertility patients must go beyond the descriptive and aggregate studies that have provided the bulk of information to date. Research on psychosocial interventions with women appears ready to go forward. Now longitudinal and experimental research regarding various techniques and their effectiveness is needed. Advances in cryopreservation of gametes and other reproductive tissue, genetic testing, and other reproductive technologies will provide the next generation of assisted reproductive technology with new options for childbearing. Similarly, research with stem cell lines may open doors to remediation of conditions that currently cause a variety of gender-specific infertility.

SUMMARY

■ Developments in medical research have clarified that male- and female-factor diagnoses account for approximately equivalent amounts of infertility.
■ Limited research exists on the effects of male-factor diagnoses relative to that available for female-factor diagnoses.
■ Typically, the diagnosed individual within a couple has a more negative response.
■ Stress seems to be a larger clinical issue for infertile women than infertile men.
■ Research into effective psychotherapeutic strategies for both infertile men and women is necessary to improve outcomes for both genders.
■ Despite the gender-specific diagnosis, therapeutic interventions need to focus on the couple while acknowledging the effect on the individual.

REFERENCES

1. Thonneau P, Marchand S, Tallec A, et al. Incidence and main causes of infertility in a resident population (1,850,000) of three French regions (1988–1989). *Hum Reprod* 1991; 6:811–16.
2. Henning K, Strauss B. Psychological and psychosomatic aspects of involuntary childlessness: State of research at the end of the 1990s. In: B Strauss, ed. *Involuntary Childlessness: Psychological Assessment, Counseling and Psychotherapy*. Seattle, WA: Hogrefe and Huber; 2002; 3–18.
3. Inhorn MC. Global infertility and the globalization of new reproductive technologies: Illustrations from Egypt. *Soc Sci Med* 2003; 56:1837–51.
4. Leiblum SR. *Infertility: Psychological Issues and Counseling Strategies*. New York: John Wiley & Sons, 1997.
5. Hardy E, Makuch MY. Gender, infertility and ART. In: E Vayena, PJ Rowe, PD Griffin, eds. *Current Practices and Controversies in Assisted Reproduction*. Geneva: World Health Organization, 2002; 272–80.
6. Berg BJ. A researcher's guide to investigating the psychological sequelae of infertility: Methodological considerations. *J Pyschosom Obstet Gynaecol* 1994; 15:147–56.
7. Glover L, Abel PD, Gannon K. Male subfertility: Is pregnancy the only issue? Psychological responses matter too – and are different in men. *BMJ* 1998; 316:405–6.
8. Berg BJ, Wilson JF, Weingartner PJ. Psychological sequelae of infertility treatment: The role of gender and sex-role identification. *Soc Sci Med* 1991; 33:1071–80.
9. Connolly KJ, Edelmann RJ, Cooke ID. Distress and marital problems associated with infertility. *Jour Reprod & Infant Psych* 1987; 5:49–57.
10. Mikulincer M, Horesh N, Levy-Shiff R, et al. The contribution of adult attachment style to the adjustment to infertility. *Br J Med Psychol* 1998; 71:265–80.
11. Beaurepaire J, Jones M, Thiering P, et al. Psychosocial adjustment to infertility and its treatment: Male and female responses at different stages of IVF/ET treatment. *J Psychosom Res* 1994; 38:229–40.
12. Daniluk JC. Gender and infertility. In: SR Leiblum, ed. *Infertility: Psychological Issues and Counseling Strategies*. New York: John Wiley & Sons, 1997:103–25.
13. Silber SJ. The varicocele dilemma. *Hum Reprod Update* 2001; 7:70–7.
14. Freeman EW, Boxer AS, Rickels K, et al. Psychological evaluation and support in a program of in vitro fertilization and embryo transfer. *Fertil Steril* 1985; 43:48–53.
15. Berger DM. Impotence following the discovery of azoospermia. *Fertil Steril* 1980; 34:154–6.
16. Feuer GS. The psychological impact of infertility on the lives of men. *Dissertation Abstracts International* 44(3-A), 1983; 706–7.
17. Rogstad KE. The psychological effects of vasectomy. *Sex Marital Ther* 1996; 11:265–72.
18. Mason MC. *Male Infertility—Men Talking*. London: Routledge, 1993.
19. Gannon K, Glover L, Abel P. Masculinity, infertility, stigma and media reports. *Soc Sci Med* 2004; 59:1169–75.
20. Whiteford LM, Gonzalez L. Stigma: The hidden burden of infertility. *Soc Sci Med* 1993; 40:27–36.
21. Zolbrod AP, Covington SN. Recipient counseling for donor insemination. In: LH Burns, SN Covington, eds. *Infertility Counseling: A Comprehensive Handbook for Clinicians*. New York: Parthenon, 1999; 325–44.
22. Miall CE. Community constructs of involuntary childlessness: Sympathy, stigma, and social support. *Canadian Rev Soc Anthro* 1994; 31:392–421.
23. Kedem P, Mulciner M, Nathanson Y, et al. Psychological aspects of male infertility. *Br J Med Psychol* 1990; 63:73–80.
24. Nachtigall R, Becker G, Wozny M. The effects of gender specific diagnosis on men's and women's response to infertility. *Fertil Steril* 1992; 57:113–21.
25. Irvine SCE. Male infertility and its effect on male sexuality. *Sex Marital Ther* 1996; 11:273–80.
26. Dhillon R, Cumming CE, Cumming DC. Psychological well-being and coping patterns in infertile men. *Fertil Steril* 2000; 74:702–6.
27. Boivin J, Shoog-Svanberg A, Andersson L, et al. Distress level in men undergoing intracytoplasmic sperm

injection versus in-vitro fertilization. *Hum Reprod* 1998; 13:1403–6.

28. McGrade JJ, Tolor A. The reaction to infertility and infertility investigation: A comparison of the response of men and women. *Infertility* 1981; 4:7–27.

29. Pook M, Tuschen-Caffier B, Krause W. Is infertility a risk factor for impaired male fertility? *Hum Reprod* 2004; 19:954–9.

30. Pook M, Krause W, Rohrle B. Coping with infertility: Distress and changes in sperm quality. *Hum Reprod* 1999; 14:1487–92.

31. Pook M, Rohrle B, Krause W. Individual prognosis for changes in sperm quality on the basis of perceived stress. *Psychother Psychosom* 1999; 68:95–101.

32. Conrad R, Schilling G, Langenbuch M, et al. Alexithymia in male infertility. *Hum Reprod* 2001; 16:587–92.

33. Tarlatzis I, Tarlatzis BC, Diakgiannis I, et al. Psychosocial impacts of infertility on Greek couples. *Hum Reprod* 1993; 8:396–401.

34. Lee TY, Sun GH. Psychosocial response of Chinese infertile husbands and wives. *Arch Androl* 2000; 45:143–8.

35. Inhorn MC. Sexuality, masculinity, and infertility in Egypt: Potent troubles in the marital and medical encounters. *Jour Men's Stud* 2002; 10:343–59.

36. Mabasa LF. The sociocultural aspects of infertility in a black South African community. *Jour of Psychol Africa; South of the Sahara, the Caribbean, & Afro-Latin America* 2002; 12:65–79.

37. Dyer SJ, Abrahams N, Mokoena NE, van der Spuy ZM. 'You are a man because you have children': Experiences, reproductive health knowledge and treatment-seeking behaviour among men suffering from couple infertility in South Africa. *Hum Reprod* 2004; 19:960–7.

38. Inhorn MC. "The worms are weak": Male infertility and patriarchal paradoxes in Egypt. *Men and Masculinities* 2003; 5:236–56.

39. Inhorn MC. Middle Eastern masculinities in the age of new reproductive technologies: Male infertility and stigma in Egypt and Lebanon. *Med Anthropol Q* 2004; 18:162–82.

40. Nasseri M. Cultural similarities in psychological reactions to infertility. *Psych Rep* 2000; 86:375–8.

41. Toubia N. Female circumcision as a public health issue. *NEJM* 1994; 331:712–16.

42. Inhorn MC, Buss KA. Infertility, infection and iatrogenesis in Egypt: An anthropological epidemiology of blocked tubes. *Med Anthropol* 1993; 15:217–44.

43. Dunkel-Schetter C, Lobel M. Psychological reactions to infertility. In: AL Stanton, C Dunkel-Schetter, eds. *Infertility: Perspectives From Stress and Coping Research.* New York: Plenum, 1991; 29–57.

44. Daniluk JC. *Women's Sexuality Across the Lifespan.* New York: Guilford Press, 1998.

45. Souter VL, Hopton JL, Penney GC, et al. Survey of psychological health in women with infertility. *J Pschosom Obstet Gynaecol* 2002; 23:41–9.

46. Paulson JD, Haarmann BS, Salerno RL, et al. An investigation of the relationship between emotional maladjustment and infertility. *Fert Steril* 1988; 49:258–62.

47. Freeman EW, Garcia CR, Rickels K. Behavioral and emotional factors: Comparisons of anovulatory infertile women with fertile and other infertile women. *Fert Steril* 1983; 40:195–201.

48. Stanton AL, Lobel M, Sears S, et al. Psychological aspects of selected issues in women's reproductive health: Current status and future directions. *J Con Clin Psych* 2002; 70:751–70.

49. Abbey A, Andrews FM, Halman LJ. Gender's role in response to infertility. *Psych of Women Q* 1991; 15:295–316.

50. Miller SM, Kirsch N. Sex differences in cognitive coping with stress. In: RC Barnett, L Biener, GK Baruch, eds. *Gender and Stress.* New York: Free Press, 1987; 278–307.

51. Domar AD, Broome A, Zuttermeister, PC, et al. The prevalence and predictability of depression in infertile women. *Fertil Steril* 1992; 58:1158–63.

52. Lu Y, Yang L, Lu G, Sun Q. Mental status and coping style of infertile women. *Chin Ment Health J* 1996; 10:169–70.

53. Matsubayashi H, Hosaka T, Izumi S, et al. Increased depression and anxiety in infertile Japanese women resulting from lack of husband's support and feelings of stress. *Gen Hosp Psychiatry* 2004; 26:398–404.

54. Oddens BJ, den Tonkelaar I, Nieuwenhuyse H. Psychosocial experiences in women facing fertility problems – a comparative survey. *Hum Reprod* 1999; 14:255–61.

55. Fido A, Zahid MA. Coping with infertility among Kuwati women: Cultural perspectives. *Int J Soc Psychiatry* 2004; 50:294–300.

56. Benyamini Y, Gozlan M, Kokia E. Variability in the difficulties experienced by women undergoing infertility treatments. *Fertil Steril* 2005; 83:275–83.

57. Savage OMN. Artificial donor insemination in Yaounde: Some sociocultural considerations. *Soc Sci Med* 1992; 35:907–13.

58. Araoye MO. Epidemiology of infertility: Social problems of the infertile couples. *West Afr J Med* 2003; 22:190–6.

59. Orji EO, Kuti O, Fasuba OB. Impact of infertility on marital life in Nigeria. *Int J Gynaecol Obstet* 2002; 79:61–2.

60. Schmid J, Kirchengast S, Vytiska-Binstorger E, et al. Psychosocial and sociocultural aspects of infertility – a comparison between Austrian and immigrant women. *Anthropol Anz* 2004; 62:301–9.

61. McCook JG, Reame NE, Thatcher SS. Health-related quality of life issues in women with polycystic ovary syndrome. *J Obstet Gyn Neon Nurs* 2005; 34:12–20.

62. Strauss B, Didzus A, Speidel H. A study of the psychosomatic aspects of endometriosis. *Psychother Psychosom Med Psychol* 1992; 42:242–52.

63. Kitzinger C, Willmott J. 'The thief of womanhood': Women's experience with polycystic ovarian syndrome. *Soc Sci Med* 2002; 54:349–61.

64. Orshan, SA, Furniss KK, Forst C, et al. The lived experience of premature ovarian failure. *J Obstet Gynecol Neonatal Nurs* 2001; 30:202–8.

65. Pal L, Santoro N. Premature ovarian failure (POF): Discordance between somatic and reproductive aging. *Ageing Res Rev* 2002; 1:413–23.

66. Rebar RW, Connolly HV. Clinical features of young women with hypergonadotrophic amenorrhoea. *Fertil Steril* 1990; 53:804–10.

67. Groff AA, Covington SN, Halverson LR, et al. Assessing the emotional needs of women with spontaneous premature ovarian failure. *Fertil Steril* 2005; 83:1734–41.

68. Brannon L. *Gender: Psychological Perspectives*. Needham Heights, MA: Allyn & Bacon, 1996.

69. Barnett RC, Baruch GK. Social roles, gender and psychological distress. In: RC Barnett, L Biener, GK Baruch, eds. *Gender and Stress*. New York: Free Press, 1987; 122–43.

70. Levinson DJ, *The Seasons of a Man's Life*. New York: Alfred A. Knopf, 1978.

71. McGrath E, Keita GP, Strickland BR, et al., eds. *Women and Depression: Risk Factors and Treatment Issues*. Washington, DC: American Psychological Association, 1990.

72. Gerstel G. A psychoanalytic view of artificial donor insemination. *Am J Psychother* 1963; 17:64–77.

73. Olshansky E. Identity of self as infertile: An example of theory-generating research. *Adv Nurs Sci* 1997; 9:54–63.

74. Miller JB. *Toward a New Psychology of Women*. Boston MA: Beacon, 1986.

75. Bergman S. Men's psychological development: A relational perspective. *Stone Center Working Paper Series, paper #48*. Wellesley, MA: The Stone Center. 1991.

76. Goffman E. *Stigma: Notes on the Management of Spoiled Identity*. Englewood Cliffs, NJ: Prentice-Hall, 1963.

77. Miall CE. Perceptions of informal sanctioning and the stigma of involuntary childlessness. *Deviant Beh* 1985; 6:383.

78. Nathanson DL. About emotion. *Psych. Annals* 1993; 23:543–55.

79. Martin E. *The Woman in the Body: A Cultural Analysis of Reproduction*. Boston, MA: Beacon Press, 1987.

80. Miall CE. The stigma of involuntary childlessness. *Soc Prob* 1986; 33:268–82.

81. Nathanson DL. Shame transactions. *Transactional Anal Jour* 1994; 24:121–9.

82. Burns LH, Covington SN. Psychology of infertility. In: LH Burns, SN Covington, eds. *Infertility Counseling: A Comprehensive Handbook for Clinicians*. New York: Parthenon, 1999; 3–25.

83. Mahlstedt PP. Psychological issues of infertility and assisted reproductive technology. *Urol Clin North Am* 1994 Aug; 21; 557–66.

84. White R, David H, Cantrell W. Pyschodynamics of depression: Implications for treatment. In: B Usdin, ed. *Depression: Clinical, Biological, and Psychological Perspectives*. New York: Brunner/Mazel, 1977; 308.

85. Boivin J. Is there too much emphasis on psychosocial counseling for infertile patients? *J Assist Reprod Genet* 1997; 14:184–6.

86. Pook M, Rohrle B, Tuschen-Caffier B, Krause W. Why do infertile males use psychological couple counselling? *Patient Educ Couns* 2001; 42:239–45.

87. Pennebaker JW. Putting stress into words: Health, linguistic, and therapeutic implications. *Beh Res Ther* 1993; 31:539–48.

88. Domar AD, Dreher H. *Healing Mind, Healthy Woman*. New York: Henry Holt and Co., 1996.

89. Anderson KM, Sharpe M, Rattray A, et al. Distress and concerns in couples referred to a specialist infertility clinic. *Jour Psychosom Res* 2003; 54:353–5.

90. Zolbrod AP. The emotional distress of the artificial insemination patient. *Med Psychother* 1988; 1:161–72.

91. Boivin J. A review of psychosocial interventions in infertility. *Soc Sci Med* 2003; 57:2325–41.

92. Munkelwitz R, Gilbert BR. Are boxer shorts really better? A critical analysis of the role of underwear type in male subfertility. *J Urol* 1998; 160:1329–33.

93. Ford WC, North K, Taylor H, et al. Increasing paternal age is associated with delayed conception in a large population of fertile couples: Evidence for declining fecundity in older men. The ALSPAC Study Team (Avon Longitudinal Study of Pregnancy and Childhood). *Hum Reprod* 2000; 15:1703–8.

94. Nachtigall RD, Tschann JM, Quiroga SS, et al. Stigma, disclosure, and family functioning among parents of children conceived through donor insemination. *Fertil Steril* 1997; 68:83–9.

95. Reijo R. Diverse spermatogenic defects in humans caused by Y chromosome deletions encompassing a novel RNA-binding protein gene. *Nature Genet* 1995; 10: 383.

96. Maier DB, Maier LU. Patients with medically complicating conditions. In: LH Burns, SN Covington, eds. *Infertility Counseling: A Comprehensive Handbook for Clinicians*. New York: Parthenon, 1999; 179–97.

97. Rieker PP. How should a man with testicular cancer be counseled and what information is available to him? *Semin Urol Oncol* 1996; 14:17–23.

98. Green D, Galvin H, Horne B. The psycho-social impact of infertility on young male cancer survivors: A qualitative investigation. *Psychooncology* 2003; 12:141–52.

99. Parekattil SJ, Kuang W, Agarwal A, et al. Model to predict if a vasoepididymostomy will be required for vasectomy reversal. *J Urol* 2005; 173:1681–4.

100. Qiu Y, Yang DT, Wang SM. Restoration of fertility in vasectomized men using percutaneous vasal or epididymal sperm aspiration. *Contraception* 2004; 69: 497–500.

101. Sperling H, Lummen G, Otto T, et al. The need for further reproductive medical advice after vasectomy reversal. *World J Urol* 1999; 17:301–4.

102. Zolbrod AP. *Getting Around the Boulder in the Road: Using Imagery to Cope with Fertility Problems*. Lexington, MA: The Center for Reproductive Problems, 1990.

103. Burns LH. Psychological changes in infertility patients. In: A Rosen, ed. *Frozen Dreams: Psychodynamic Dimensions of Infertility and Assisted Reproduction*. Hillsdale, NJ: Analytic Press, Inc., 2005; 3–29.

104. Zolbrod AP. *Men, Women and Infertility: Intervention and Treatment Strategies*. New York: Lexington Books, 1993.

105. Tuschen-Caffier B, Florin I, Krause W, et al. Cognitive-behavioral therapy for idiopathic infertile couples. *Psychother Psychosom* 1999; 8:5–21.

106. Hunt J, Monach JH. Beyond the bereavement model: The significance of depression for infertility counseling. *Hum Reprod* 1997 Nov; 12:188–94.

107. Stammer H, Wischmann T, Verres R. Counseling and couple therapy for infertile couples. *Fam Proc* 2002; 41:111–22.

108. Diamond R, Kezur D, Meyers M, et al. *Couple Therapy for Infertility*. New York: Guilford Press, 1999.

109. Ng KK, Donat R, Chan L, et al. Sperm output of older men. *Hum Reprod* 2004; 19:1811–15.

110. Hermann M, Untergasser G, Rumpold H, et al. Aging of the male reproductive system. *Exp Gerontol* 2000; 35:1267–79.

111. Rosenthal MB, Kingsberg SA. The older infertile patient. In: LH Burns, SN Covington, eds. *Infertility Counseling: A Comprehensive Handbook for Clinicians*. New York: Parthenon, 1999; 283–95.

112. Bosch X. Investigating the reasons for Spain's falling birth rate. *Lancet* 1998; 12:887.

113. te Velde ER, Pearson PL. The variability of female reproductive ageing. *Hum Reprod Update* 2002; 8:141–54.

114. Sauer MV, Paulson RJ, Lobo RA. Reversing the natural decline in human fertility: An extended trial of oocyte donation to women of advanced reproductive age. *JAMA* 1992; 268:1270–5.

115. Paulson RJ, Boostanfar R, Saadat P, et al. Pregnancy in the sixth decade of life: Obstetric outcomes in women of advanced reproductive age. *JAMA* 2002; 288:2320–3.

116. Beski S, Gorgy A, Venkat G, Craft IL, et al. Gestational surrogacy: A feasible option for patients with Rokitansky syndrome. *Hum Reprod* 2000; 15:2326–8.

117. Keye WR. Medical aspects of infertility of the counselor. In: LH Burns, SN Covington, eds. *Infertility Counseling: A Comprehensive Handbook for Clinicians*. New York: Parthenon, 1999; 27–46.

118. Pritts EA, Taylor RN. An evidence-based evaluation of endometriosis-associated infertility. *Endocrinol Metab Clin North Am* 2003; 32:653–67.

119. Homburg R. The management of infertility associated with polycystic ovary syndrome. *Reprod Biol Endocrinol* 2003; 14(1):109.

120. Lopez E, Gunby J, Daya S, et al. Ovulation induction in women with polycystic ovary syndrome: Randomized trial of clomiphene citrate versus low-dose recombinant FSH as first line therapy. *Reprod Biomed Online* 2004; 9:382–90.

121. Cardone VS. GnRH antagonists for treatment of polycystic ovarian syndrome. *Fertil Steril* 2003; 80(Suppl 1): S25–31.

122. Nardo LG. Management of anovulatory infertility associated with polycystic ovary syndrome: Tamoxifen citrate an effective alternative compound to clomiphene citrate. *Gynecol Endocrinol* 2004; 19:235–8.

123. Fedorcsak P, Dale PO, Storeng R, et al. The effect of metformin on ovarian stimulation and in vitro fertilization in insulin-resistant women with polycystic ovary syndrome: An open-label randomized cross-over trial. *Gynecol Endocrinol* 2003; 17: 207–14.

124. Cleemann L, Lauszus FF, Trolle B. Laparoscopic ovarian drilling as first line of treatment in infertile women with polycystic ovary syndrome. *Gynecol Endocrinol* 2004; 18:138–43.

125. Amer SA, Li TC, Ledger WL. Ovulation induction using laparoscopic ovarian drilling in women with polycystic ovary syndrome: Predictors of success. *Hum Reprod* 2004; 19:1719–24.

126. Nelson LM, Covington SN, Rebar RR. An update: Spontaneous premature ovarian failure is not an early menopause. *Fertil Steril* 2005; 83:1327–32.

127. Platz-Christensen JJ, Tronstad SE, Johansson O, et al. Evaluation of regret after tubal sterilization. *Int J Gynaecol Obstet* 1992; 38:223–6.

128. Jamieson DJ, Kaufman SC, Costello C, et al. US Collaborative Review of Sterilization Working Group. A comparison of women's regret after vasectomy versus tubal sterilization. *Obstet Gynecol* 2002; 99:1073–9.

129. Kodaman PH, Arici A, Seli E. Evidence-based diagnosis and management of tubal factor infertility. *Curr Opin Obstet Gynecol* 2004; 16:221–9.

130. Lalos A, Lalos O, Jacobsson L, et al. The psychosocial impact of infertility two years after completed surgical treatment. *Acta Obstet Gynecol Scand* 1985; 64:599–604.

131. Lalos A, Lalos O, Jacobsson L, et al. Psychological reactions to the medical investigation and surgical treatment of infertility. *Gynecol Obstet Invest* 1985; 20:209–17.

132. Beerendonk CC, Braat DD. Present and future options for the preservation of fertility in female adolescents with cancer. *Endocr Dev* 2005; 8:166–75.

133. Schofield PE, Butow PN, Thompson JF, et al. Psychological responses of patients receiving a diagnosis of cancer. *Ann Oncol* 2003; 14:48–56.

134. Wright J, Duchesne C, Sabourin S, et al. Psychosocial distress and infertility: Men and women respond differently. *Fertil Steril* 1991; 55:100–8.

135. Domar AD, Zuttermeister PC, Friedman R. The psychological impact of infertility: A comparison with other medical conditions. *J Psychosom Obstet Gynaecol* 1993; 14 Suppl: 45–52.

136. Miller SM, Mischel W, Schoreder CM, et al. Intrusive and avoidant ideation among females pursuing infertility treatment. *Psychology and Health* 1998; 13:847–58.

137. Domar AD. Impact of psychological factors on dropout rates in insured infertility patients. *Fertil Steril* 2004; 81:271–3.

138. Smeenk JM, Verhaak CM, Stolwijk AM, et al. Reasons for dropout in an in vitro fertilization/intracytoplasmic sperm injection program. *Fertil Steril* 2004; 81:262–8.

139. Smeenk JM, Verhaak CM, Eugster A, et al. The effect of anxiety and depression on the outcome of in-vitro fertilization. *Hum Reprod* 2001; 16:1420–3.

140. Domar AD, Seibel MM, Benson H. The mind/body program for infertility: A new behavioral treatment approach for women with infertility. *Fertil Steril* 1990; 53: 246–9.

141. Domar AD, Zuttermeister PC, Seibel MM, et al. Psychological improvement in infertile women after behavioral treatment: A replication. *Fertil Steril* 1992; 58: 144–7.

142. Domar AD, Friedman R, Zuttermeister PC. Distress and conception in infertile women: A complementary approach. *J Am Med Womens Assoc* 1999; 54:196–8.

143. Domar AD, Clapp D, Slawsby E, et al. The impact of group psychological interventions on distress in infertile women. *Health Psychol* 2000; 19:568–75.

144. Domar AD, Clapp D, Slawsby EA, et al. Impact of group psychological interventions on pregnancy rates in infertile women. *Fertil Steril* 2000; 73:805–11.

145. Jordan C, Revenson TA. Gender differeneces in coping with infertility: A meta-analysis. *Jour Behav Med* 1999; 22:341–58.

146. Brand HJ. The influence of sex differences on the acceptance of infertility. *J Reprod Infant Psychol* 1989; 7:129–31.

147. Mindes EJ, Ingram KM, Kliewer W, et al. Longitudinal analyses of the relationship between unsupportive social interactions and psychological adjustment among women with fertility problems. *Soc Sci Med* 2003; 56:2165–80.

148. Elsenbruch S, Hahn S, Kowalsky D, et al. Quality of life, psychosocial well-being, and sexual satisfaction in women with polycystic ovary syndrome. *J Clin Endocrinol Metab* 2003; 88:5801–7.

149. Lalwani S, Timmreck L, Friedman R, et al. Variations in individual physician success rates within an in vitro fertilization program might be due to patient demographics. *Fertil Steril* 2004; 81: 944–6.

150. Hynes GJ, Callan VJ, Terry DJ, et al. The psychological well-being of infertile women after a failed IVF attempt: The effects of coping. *Br J Med Psychol* 1992; 65: 269–78.

4 Cross-Cultural Issues in Infertility Counseling

MICHAELA HYNIE AND LINDA HAMMER BURNS

> *The life history of the individual is first and foremost an accommodation to the patterns and standards traditionally handed down in his community.*
>
> – Ruth Benedict, 1934

Involuntary childlessness is a universally stigmatizing condition that threatens the stability and well-being of individuals, couples, and the larger society. Children provide many benefits to the couple and the community. They stabilize or cement marital relationships; enlarge and strengthen kinship ties; validate individual roles; offer spiritual comfort or religious redemption; provide financial benefits; ensure immortality; afford a legacy for property or values; and afford a unique interpersonal relationship. Infertility can thus trigger a myriad of psychosocial consequences with cultural, religious, and social ramifications for both men and women.

Although the value and importance of children may be universal, the meaning of children, and thus childlessness, may vary across cultures. Culture, religion, kinship/family values, beliefs about health and illness, and gender roles all influence how individuals and cultural groups experience and interpret infertility. These influential factors are typically all considered under the umbrella of 'culture.' The term 'culture' usually refers to the distinctive customs, manners, values, religious behavior, and other social and intellectual aspects of a society. Culture has also been defined more broadly, however, to include differences on the basis of age and gender, sexual orientation, disability, education, and/or economic status.[1] These other dimensions also have a strong influence on reactions to and consequences of infertility, and thus an awareness of diversity along all of these social and demographic dimensions is essential in counseling. However, these dimensions each require a detailed specific treatment, and go beyond the scope of what can be covered here. This chapter therefore focuses on the narrower definition of culture, one informed primarily by the history of cross-cultural research.

The American Psychological Association (APA) guidelines propose that 'culture' is the learned "belief sys-tems and value orientations that influence customs, norms, practices and social institutions including psychological practices . . . and organizations."[2] Although this definition of culture is narrower in scope than some, it still casts a broad net. Culture, conceptualized in this manner, determines and reflects the meaning of our thoughts, language, and behavior.[1] Even similar words spoken by people of different cultural backgrounds may carry very different meanings, especially when discussing issues of relationships, emotions, and well-being. It is impossible to understand a person, or communicate effectively with them, without understanding their cultural context. Cultural sensitivity is therefore essential for successful multicultural and cross-cultural counseling, and cultural context may be especially important when considering issues of infertility.

The Need for Cultural Awareness

Medical and mental health professionals working in the field of reproductive medicine are under growing pressure to adapt medical diagnoses and treatments to work with individuals from various cultural, ethnic, and/or religious backgrounds. Indeed, the need for mental health professionals to be sensitive to their clients' cultural context has never been greater. Medical and mental health caregivers are more and more likely to work with clients who come from a cultural background and worldview that differs from their own.[3]

Although awareness of the need for cultural sensitivity is a relatively new issue, cultural diversity is not a new phenomenon, nor is it limited to a subset of nations. The populations of most countries consist of a number of ethnic groups of varying sizes that have existed side by side with the majority culture for generations, although not all countries actively acknowledge the existence or importance of minority groups. In the United States, for example, where culture is typically defined by race, mainstream culture is often represented as white or of European descent. The 2000 U.S. Census, however, showed that two thirds of the population described themselves as white[4] with the remainder being primarily of African American, Hispanic/Latino or Asian descent, but with many other ethnicities represented as well in smaller numbers. Likewise, most countries in Africa, Asia, Latin America, and Europe also tend to be represented as culturally homogenous, but are often comprised of multiple ethnic communities, with these communities differing widely in socioeconomic status, language, religion, and worldviews from the majority. Even those countries most often represented as culturally homogenous (e.g., Japan and Iceland) are in reality multicultural, if not in theory. In essence, all countries and communities must address diversity issues in one form or another. Today people are citizens of the world as much as they are citizens of a particular nation or cultural group, but even countries that appear (or maintain a self-perception of) culturally homogenous must address diversity issues in one form or another (e.g., immigration, cross-cultural marriage, and international adoption).

Not only are most countries characterized by the presence of multiple long-standing communities, each with their own ethnic and religious heritage, worldviews and beliefs, but many nations are also the destination of a large number of immigrants. In the years 1995–2000, the United States had the highest net immigration in the world, with an average of 760,000 immigrants per year. This is almost double the net immigration of the next highest country, the Russian Federation with 394,000.[5] Likewise, according to survey on ethnic diversity conducted by Statistics Canada in 2002, about 23% of non-Aboriginal Canadians over the age of fifteen were born in a country other than Canada. Another 17% of Canadians were born in Canada but had at least one parent who was born elsewhere. In other words, approximately 40% of the current Canadian population are either first- or second-generation immigrants to Canada.

Residents of Canada, the United States, and Australia are accustomed to thinking of their countries as destinations for immigration, but immigration rates are high in Europe as well. In 2001, more than 175,000 non-European immigrants acquired citizenship in Germany, more than 88,000 acquired citizenship in the United Kingdom, and almost 45,000 acquired citizenship in The Netherlands.[6] Likewise, there are large movements of people across Africa, Latin America, and Asia. Rwanda, for example, was among the top five countries in terms of the number of immigrants arriving between 1995 and 2000.[5] Furthermore, these numbers actually underestimate the movement of peoples. In addition to immigrant communities, many nations are also the destination for migrant workers, some of whom are long-term residents (with or without legal documents).

Immigration creates somewhat different concerns in terms of cultural diversity. There is an assumption that immigrants arrive with the values, norms, and beliefs of their heritage culture but that these values change to match those of the host culture, as immigrants learn about, adapt to, and interact with the new culture. In reality, though, immigrants do not completely abandon their former cultural beliefs and replace them with new ones.[7] Rather, some values of the new culture are acquired over time but some of the values of their heritage culture are retained, often over several generations.[8,9] Moreover, the values that are most likely passed from generation to generation are those that pertain to family-related norms, values, and domestic life.[10] This would, understandably, include beliefs about childbearing and fertility. Thus, descendents of immigrant parents or grandparents may appear to be fully assimilated to their host culture, but may have fundamental assumptions and beliefs about family relationships that are more similar to those of their parents and grandparents than of the mainstream culture in which they currently reside.

The Need for Awareness of Spirituality and Religion

There has also been an increasing awareness among medical and mental health caregivers that spiritual well-being is an important dimension to physical and emotional health, and that there is a generally positive relationship between religious involvement and health outcomes, including mental health.[11] Historically and globally, the majority of individuals have been found to have explicit religious beliefs and practices. Although religion may no longer play as large a role in social life in Western nations as it once did, many people around the world still regard their spiritual faith to be of central importance in their lives.

The majority of individuals in a given nation often practice the same religion, yet the norm is for there to be multiple religious groups within each country, each with their own belief system, worldview, and guidelines for behavior. There are five major monotheistic religions (i.e., Judaism, Christianity, Islam, Zoroastrianism, and Sikhism) and six major polytheistic spiritual traditions (i.e., Hinduism, Buddhism, Janism, Shintoism, Confucianism, and Taoism). According to

TABLE 4.1. Major World Religions by Population[12]

1. **Christianity** 2.1 billion
   - **Roman Catholicism**: 1.1 billion
   - **Protestantism**: 350 million
   - **Eastern Orthodoxy**: 240 million
   - **Anglican**: 84 million
   - **Oriental Orthodoxy, Assyrians, and other Christians**: 350 million
2. **Islam** 1.3 billion
   - **Sunnism**: 940 million
   - **Shi'ism**: 170 million
3. **Secular/Irreligious/Agnostic/Atheist** 1.1 billion
4. **Hinduism** 900 million
5. **Chinese traditional religion** 394 million
6. **Buddhism** 376 million
   - **Mahayana**: 185 million
   - **Theravada**: 124 million
7. **Primal indigenous** 300 million; **African traditional and diasporic** 100 million; and **Spiritism** 15 million
8. **Sikhism** 23 million
9. **Judaism** 14 million

2003 statistics on world religions, more than half of the world's population is monotheistic (Christian 33%, Muslim 20%, Sikh 0.39%, and Judaism 0.23%).[12] The polytheistic religion with the largest number of adherents are Hindu (13%) and Buddhism (6%). Thirteen percent of people in the world adhere to spiritual beliefs and traditions of indigenous cultures, although they often do so in tandem with a formal theistic religion. Only 2% of the world's population is atheist while 12% are nonreligious, although it is interesting to note that half of the nonreligious acknowledge theistic beliefs but do adhere or align with a specific formal religion (see Table 4.1).

Although there is a great diversity between and within these religious traditions regarding beliefs and practices, they agree that human beings can and should transcend hedonistic and selfish tendencies to grow spiritually and to promote the welfare of others.[13] There is also general agreement among the world religions about what moral principles and values promote spiritual enlightenment and personal and social harmony.[14] Also common to all world religions are prayer, spiritual enlightenment, a consideration of others above one's self, and a belief that moral values should be taught and transmitted from one generation to the next.[15,16]

Through these rituals, practices, and beliefs, religion can thus be a source of meaning and strength for a couple or individual as they cope with infertility. However, religious beliefs may also provide limits on the acceptability of various treatment options. In providing a culturally-sensitive approach, infertility counselors must consider religion as a potential asset as well as a potential liability for infertile men and women. Religious faith, spiritual leaders, and the community of their faith may provide individuals and couples with comfort and sanctuary in the maelstrom of infertility. Conversely, these factors might make the experience of infertility that much more painful, stigmatizing, onerous, and isolating. It is therefore paramount that the infertility counselor be aware of the impact of faith and religion on the infertile couple and how religion is, for them, either a benefit or burden.

The Need for Awareness of Reproductive Stratification and Reproductive Tourism

Finally, and of particular relevance for infertility counselors, are couples and individuals who travel to access medical and reproductive services. Many countries have only limited access to reproductive technologies in terms of the overall number of clinics; the variety of services available; and which individuals are permitted access to these services. Various forms of third-party reproduction are restricted in many countries for legal, ethical, or religious reasons. Additionally, the conditions under which certain treatments are available may be unacceptable to some infertile couples (e.g., identified gamete donation and oocyte-sharing). National differences in the limitations placed on assisted reproduction have led to steadily increasing rates of reproductive tourism.[17] Couples and individuals who can afford to do so are increasingly likely to travel to seek assisted reproductive technology (ART) services that, for whatever reason, are not available to them in their home country or are less expensive in a different country.

Reproductive tourists create special challenges in infertility counseling. These individuals are not residents in the country to which they have traveled for treatment and are therefore not likely to be aware of or familiar with the host country's cultural values or the dominant language. The consequence of this is that infertility counselors are faced with even greater disparities between their own cultural worldviews and those of their clients. Communication can be extremely difficult, further aggravated by the need to have knowledge of (or translator knowledge of) specific, complicated medical terms. Furthermore, caregivers and/or patients may be less motivated to overcome these challenges because of the temporary nature of the couple's (or individual's) residence in the country. The difficulties of successful multicultural counseling under these circumstances may be magnified, but the solutions to these challenges are similar. An effective multicultural counselor needs to learn about their client's particular cultural worldview and be sensitive to how it may differ from their own. They must be prepared to afford appropriate translating services and adapt patient education, assessment, and preparation services to meet the unique needs of these patients.

In short, the growing awareness of the reality of multiculturalism is forcing medical and mental health professionals to establish a working knowledge of the cultural and religious perspectives of the psychosocial meanings and implications of infertility, as well as psychological diagnosis and treatment of infertile men and women. Cultural and religious groups differ in the acceptability of various remedies to infertility, involuntary childlessness, or disrupted reproduction. In providing assistance to all infertile couples, it is therefore important for caregivers to be cognizant of the couple's religious and cultural background and how these factors may influence their experience of infertility, treatment options, and acceptable remedies for their childlessness within their culture or religion.

This chapter focuses on cultural and religious factors influencing the experience and treatment of infertility and the impact these issues have on infertility counseling. It is beyond the scope of this chapter to address every experience of infertility, involuntary childlessness, or interrupted reproduction in terms of every culture or religion. Instead, it will provide the infertility counselor with a basis for approaching and assessing cultural, religious, and ethnic issues influencing care and treatment as well as the standards of practice in multicultural infertility counseling.

This chapter addresses:

- sensitivity to one's own cultural characteristics;
- awareness of specific cultural and religious concerns pertaining to infertility treatment, counseling, and solutions to involuntary childlessness;
- recognition of some major dimensions along which cultures vary, and their consequences for infertility counseling;
- familiarity with current professional standards on multicultural counseling and the integration of spirituality in infertility counseling.

HISTORICAL OVERVIEW

The first step in acquiring cultural sensitivity is to recognize the influence of one's own culture on one's worldview. The importance of recognizing one's own worldview as a cultural bias cannot be overstated, but the difficulty in achieving this awareness should not be underestimated. One is more likely to recognize the influence of culture when considering other people's belief systems than when considering one's own. There

is a tendency to apply the term *culture* to other people's beliefs and worldviews but to see one's own values as natural and obviously true.[18,19] This is especially the case for members of a society's majority group. The majority worldview, by definition, predominates in the media, the health system and mainstream educational institutions, thereby reinforcing a sense that the majority (and thus one's own) cultural assumptions are simply truisms.

Insight into the influence of one's own culture on one's beliefs, assumptions, values, and worldviews may be particularly relevant for those who counsel infertile couples. Although having children is both desired and expected in all cultures, the meanings attached to children and parenthood, perceptions of infertility, sexuality, and medicine, and the nature of communication about these issues vary widely from culture to culture.[7,20] For example, while modern Western medical practices and beliefs exist in virtually all cultures, most non-Western cultures have their own history of medical beliefs and practices that coexist alongside the Western medical model[21] and these beliefs often differ fundamentally from it. Western medical practices focus on diseases and on the individual, while most non-Western models of health are holistic, with an emphasis on the balance between various elements in the physical, social, and spiritual environment. Thus, the person is seen as just one part of a larger environmental, social, and spiritual system. Moreover, the social roles of healer and patient are often defined differently across cultures, resulting in widely varying expectations of what should occur in a therapeutic relationship and with whom this relationship should be sought.[22]

Achieving cultural awareness can be particularly difficult for mental health professionals because most of what is known and taught in both psychology and counseling is derived from work on and by, middle- and upper-class North Americans and Western Europeans.[18,23,24] As a result, most assumptions, goals, and therapeutic techniques are particular to a Western, and most often North American, mainstream worldview. However, these assumptions, goals, and techniques are almost always taught and applied as if they are culturally neutral and universal.

As such, until fairly recently, diversity was not considered an issue professionally or therapeutically. This worldview began changing in the 1950s and 1960s with the civil rights movement in the United States. This period was marked by political and social shifts that first sensitized some mental health professionals to the failure of mental health services to address the needs of minority populations. Perceptions that psychoanalysis and psychotherapy were failing visible minorities, and even oppressing them by labeling diversity or cultural phenomena as illness, coincided with calls for change in the education and training of mental health professionals. It took another twenty years, however, for the publication of the first position paper suggesting that counseling ethnically diverse clients required specific competencies beyond that of traditional counseling.

In 1980, the first position paper on multicultural counseling was developed by the Counseling Division of the American Psychological Association Education and Training Committee.[25] The paper described a model in which three dimensions of multicultural competencies were identified as fundamental to multicultural counseling. These three dimensions were: (1) beliefs/attitudes toward multicultural counseling; (2) knowledge of multicultural counseling; and (3) skills to practice multicultural counseling. The aforementioned paper was not formally accepted by the division, but was subsequently published by Sue and colleagues, in 1982, and continues to be the dominant model in multicultural counseling.[26]

Shortly thereafter, the American Psychological Association and the American Counseling Association both published statements regarding the importance of including cultural diversity and multiculturalism in counseling education and training.[27] This was the beginning of a rapid growth in the recognition of diverse needs in diverse populations. Most mental health professions and medical organizations have since affirmed the importance of acknowledging and addressing cultural and ethnic diversity. The Diagnostic and Statistical Manual of Mental Disorders, Forth Edition (DSM-IV) and International Classification of Diseases, Ninth Edition (ICD-9) were prepared with a culturally diverse population in mind,[28] the U.S. Surgeon General recently prepared a report specifically addressing the importance of providing adequate mental healthcare for members of ethnic and cultural minorities[29], and, since the 1990s, numerous counseling textbooks have been published with guidelines for how to become a culturally-sensitive counselor.

Despite the widespread endorsement of multicultural awareness, however, real change has been slow to come. Some of the first proponents of the multicultural counseling movement recently reported their frustration at how little change has actually occurred in how counseling is taught and practiced.[26] Research in the United States, where the call for multicultural counseling has perhaps been the loudest and longest, suggests that minority clients are still less likely to use outpatient mental health services than clients of the majority culture, and that they are far more likely to terminate counseling after only one contact with their counselor.[30] The number of research articles in the leading clinical psychology journals that specifically address ethnic minority populations has remained around 5% for the last twenty years[28], and very little research has addressed how multicultural competencies actually work in therapy[31] or how they are accepted or received by different consumers of counseling.[24]

Thus, despite twenty-five years of affirming and promoting the need to address cultural diversity, it seems that there is still a belief that therapeutic theories and approaches to counseling are universal and apply to all people of all cultural backgrounds. It is clear that there continues to be a need to actively promote research, teaching, and education about culture as a fundamental component of counseling, rather than as an afterthought to the traditional program. This lack may be particularly apparent in the context of infertility counseling. Although there is a substantial body of research addressing cultural differences and issues in infertility and infertility treatments, there is very little if any to be found that evaluates approaches to infertility counseling with multicultural populations. Sue and colleagues suggest that resistance to multicultural counseling can be traced back to a fundamental 'ethnocentric monoculturalism.'[26] Individually and professionally, mental health professionals remain hampered by an inability to recognize that their own worldview is not natural and true, but a product of their own particular culture. Thus, the need to elevate awareness of one's own cultural biases remains an essential first step.

Religion and Spirituality in Therapy and Counseling

The cultural bias described above may also extend to the relative blindness Western counselors have historically exhibited with respect to the role of religion and spirituality in counseling and therapy. Religion, spirituality, and the role of faith have always been recognized as significant components of culture, although the interface of spirituality and religion with mental health and psychology is a fairly recent development. In fact, religion may be viewed as much as a culture in and of itself, as it is a system of beliefs. Despite evidence of the clear benefits of religious activities (e.g., prayer, confession, and seeking strength and comfort from faith or a religious community), Western psychology and psychotherapy have been slow in recognizing religion as a resource and asset.[32] In fact, religion was, for some time, viewed as a psychological liability, a reinforced learned behavior (according to Skinner), or wish-fulfillment (according to Freud).

Nonetheless, religious beliefs have had a place in the development of psychological practice. Modern existential psychotherapy is an example of a therapy that is clearly based on a traditional religious framework, encouraging the transcendence of suffering by finding meaning in suffering.[33] Moreover, elements of religious practice have increasingly found their way into medical and mental health practices. For example, mindfulness and meditation, which are derived primarily from traditional Hinduism and Buddhism, encourage the cultivation of a sense of inner calm, harmony, and transcendence to achieve spiritual growth. Applied in Western medicine and counseling, 'mindfulness meditation' (i.e., focusing on the present moment) has been found to be useful as a physiological relaxation technique; a means of changing neurological functioning; a type of positive addiction; a form of cognitive restructuring; and a means of promoting spiritual and existential growth.[34] Importantly, it has also been applied successfully to coping with the experience of infertility.[32,35] Moreover, as will be seen below, spiritual leaders also typically play a central role in counseling infertile couple in cultures that have a more holistic traditional healthcare system.

A formalized movement to "meld the wisdom of the world's spiritual traditions with the learning of modern psychology"[36] has also developed, beginning with the diversity movement in psychology in the United States. The specialty disciplines of the psychology of religion and pastoral psychology/counseling emerged in the late 1990s.[37] Pastoral psychology is a distinct branch of psychology/psychiatry associated with religion, with the objective of offering relief through spiritual investigation or practices. Pastoral psychology arose out of a growing acknowledgment by the medical, psychological, and counseling professions of the importance that religion and spiritual beliefs play in people's psychological well-being. Pastoral psychology may be provided by mental health professionals or by clergy using psychotherapeutic principles and techniques with parishioners. As such, it combines spirituality and religious teachings with counseling practice.

In sum, an individual's spiritual perspective and religious beliefs may be highly relevant to understanding his or her problems, worldview, culture, and experience, particularly as it relates to the experience of infertility, childlessness, medical treatment, and family-building alternatives. The contribution of religious beliefs and practices to well-being has only recently been incorporated into counseling and psychotherapy in Western medicine, and even then, only a subset of religious practices and beliefs have been identified and accepted by mental health professionals. Religion and spirituality have always been a core component of counseling in other medical systems, however, and need to be recognized by counselors working with clients from these cultures. The recognition that religion and spirituality are relevant to coping, meaning, and well-being, but that religious beliefs vary widely within any given culture, highlights the need for infertility counselors to identify and understand the specific religious beliefs of their clients, regardless of their clients' cultural background.

REVIEW OF LITERATURE

Cross-Cultural Experience of Childlessness

Few studies have explicitly compared cultures in their reactions to infertility. One exception is a study of involuntary childlessness in which seventy-eight societies were examined. Despite the randomness of geographic distribution, geography was not found to be a significant factor in reactions to infertility. Although many cultures did not have specific solutions to childlessness, people did not accept childlessness passively. Within cultures in which there were remedies, solutions to childlessness fell into one of three categories: (1) medical interventions; (2) prayer or spiritual interventions; and (3) realignment of social relationships (e.g., divorce, polygamy, and adoption). Across the majority of cultures, medical and spiritual solutions were typically the first choices while realignment of social relationships was the last or *least* acceptable solution to childlessness (particularly polygamy). The researchers found that "...it is 'human' to be concerned about childlessness.... People pray, or take drugs, or cast spells...before they try to change social relationships by adding a spouse, ending a marital relationship, or quaisimarital relationship, or adopting or fostering." An additional finding of this study was that women were significantly more likely to be blamed for childlessness than men – a fact attributed to the ubiquity of women's low social status across cultures. Men were blamed in only one culture (Bemba). Either both sexes were equally blamed or no one was blamed in six cultures (Chukchee, Gon, Ifugao, Kikuyu, Basseri, and Papago).[38]

Cross-Cultural Sensitivity among Infertility Treatment Providers

Blenner conducted in-depth interviews of twenty-eight health providers in a major American city to examine how healthcare providers approach treatment of culturally diverse infertile patients.[39] The findings revealed three types of healthcare providers: (1) culturally unaware; (2) culturally nontolerant; and (3) culturally sensitive. *Culturally unaware providers* failed to recognize cultural diversity and treated all clients the same (in other words, they displayed rigidity). These caregivers perceived culturally different patients as noncompliant and lacking in motivation and labeled them as difficult, uncooperative, and uncommitted. Understandably, culturally different patients were more likely to terminate treatment with a culturally insensitive provider. *Culturally intolerant providers* recognized cultural differences but were unwilling to tolerate cultural conflicts or to change or adapt treatment protocols. As a result, these providers terminated treatment or made referrals to more culturally tolerant providers. *Culturally sensitive providers* were aware of cultural differences; acquired information about the patient's cultural beliefs; worked within patient limitations; and adapted tests and treatment protocols to meet clients' needs to make them more culturally compatible with the clients' belief systems. Blenner concluded that culturally diverse infertile patients particularly need providers who are tolerant and sensitive to cultural differences as they are more likely to suffer significant levels of stigma and social isolation and to find little empathy within their communities regarding their involuntary childlessness.

Impact of Religion on Infertility Treatment

Religion is an intrinsically important aspect of all cultures. It has a profound impact on individual and societal beliefs and practices regarding childlessness, reproduction, and assisted reproduction. However, although much has been written about the acceptability of specific treatments according to various religious beliefs, little research has examined the influence (positive/negative) of religiosity on overall the experience of infertility and/or patient decisions regarding treatment for it.

Although general religiosity and religion as a demographic descriptive have been included in research on the psychosocial impact of infertility, only recently has the impact of spirituality on the psychological impact of potential resource been included in or been the focus of research. In one study of nearly 200 infertile women, high levels of religiosity and spirituality were significantly correlated with low levels of psychological distress.[40] These findings were replicated in a recent study on the role of spirituality in the psychosocial well-being of 138 women with premature ovarian failure (POF). The researchers found that women with POF who had higher spiritual well-being were significantly more likely to report higher overall functional well-being.[41]

Religious beliefs were found to play a central role in decisions around infertility treatments in Asia and Persian Gulf countries in one study.[42] This survey found that ARTs was practiced in twenty Asian countries with half the treatments centers (>600) located in Japan. Taiwan was the only country that had specific legislation regarding treatment, with six other countries having some kind of ministerial regulations. Although the majority of Asian countries did not have legal regulations regarding ARTs, therapeutic decisions in Asia were found to be influenced by religious beliefs and prevailing cultural norms.

Fertility status may interact with religious beliefs to influence treatment decisions and may even override cultural and religious norms. For example, despite the importance of religious beliefs in determining attitudes regarding ARTs in Japan, infertile couples were found to have a very favorable attitude toward ARTs while laypersons' attitudes were less affirmative. In this study, the main reason for disapproving of new reproductive technologies was that "it conflicts with the way of nature," but the main reason for approving was that "it is a treatment for infertility." Thus, fertility status seemed to change the manner in which people evaluated reproductive technologies.[43]

Similar results were obtained in a study comparing attitudes toward gamete donation in Iranian and British women. The survey study involved fifty fertile and fifty infertile Iranian women and fifty fertile and twenty-five infertile British women.[44] The researchers noted that in Islamic Iran, any form of gamete donation is forbidden by religion and society and, as such, Iranian respondents were expected to be influenced by religion to a greater extent than the more secular and/or Christian women from Great Britain. The researchers therefore compared the extent to which the women regarded God's will as responsible for their infertility as well as evaluating the women's beliefs about the acceptability of assisted reproduction. Iranian women were more likely to endorse the role of God's will in infertility than were British women regardless of fertility/infertility status. The researchers speculated that Iranian women's greater attachment to faith might be a factor that *helps* them, in that Iranian women, in contrast to Western women, were not been found to be emotionally distressed following failed IVF cycles. Interestingly, however, fertile women from both countries were more in agreement with each other than with their infertile counterparts regarding the acceptability of gamete donation, while nationality had no significant effect. Both British and Iranian fertile women were more likely to endorse oocyte and sperm donation as acceptable remedies to childlessness than were their infertile counterparts.

By contrast, in a study that assessed the impact of religious beliefs on assisted reproduction in Turkey, researchers found that despite Islam being the predominant religion, most individuals found assisted reproduction acceptable. Questionnaires were used to assess the opinions of 400 individuals (232 women, 168 men) in a major Turkish city. The majority (67%) of the respondents considered themselves religious; 65% were married; 5% divorced; 64% had children; and 4% were infertile. Although 66% had graduated from high school or university, less than one-third actually knew what oocyte donation was. Fifteen percent completely objected to oocyte donation although men were more likely to favor it than women.[45]

THEORETICAL FRAMEWORK

Perspectives on Multiculturalism

There are a number of different approaches to research and education about multiculturalism, which differ in terms of their fundamental assumptions about the nature of cultural differences.[46] *Etic* approaches assume that there are universal psychological processes and that it is only the contents of these processes that differ from culture to culture. This perspective allows one to compare cultures on various dimensions and to apply similar therapeutic processes with clients of different cultural backgrounds. *Emic* approaches assume that every culture is unique and can only be understood from the perspective of that culture's unique psychology. From this perspective, universal approaches in research and counseling are neither possible nor fruitful.[1,18,47]

The etic/emic distinction refers to two end points along a dimension of universalism and relativism. Where one stands with respect to these positions reflects an underlying philosophical orientation about human nature. Regardless of one's position on this distinction, however, there is an agreement that cultural sensitivity requires cultural awareness. To some extent, both of these approaches have informed the present discussion of cultural differences. An etic perspective is presented in the discussion of cross-cultural comparisons that are believed to result from overarching cultural differences on universal dimensions or traits. Specific issues in infertility are also presented from an emic within-culture position to expose infertility counselors to a range of beliefs and norms around infertility and, thus, assist them in asking relevant questions about beliefs, norms, and expectations of clients from different cultural backgrounds.

With respect to the discussion of cultural differences, it is also important to remember that individuals within cultures vary. Once again, this is obvious with respect to individuals within one's own culture. We are aware that not everyone from our own culture shares the exact values or beliefs and perceive and expect to encounter a wide range of individual differences. However, there is a powerful and well-documented tendency to perceive members of other social groups, *them* as opposed to *us*, as being highly similar to one another in terms of values, personality traits, and even physical characteristics, which can then lead to stereotyping.[48] The following descriptions of cultural differences should, therefore, be relied upon primarily for an analysis of one's own cultural biases and as a guide to information seeking when working with clients whose cultural background differs from one's own. One cannot assume that a cultural norm is descriptive of every member of a given population. Rather, one must be willing to learn from and ask questions of the client and allow the client to describe their cultural and religious perspective and define their own personal experience.

Individualism and Collectivism across Cultures

One way of gaining understanding into the influence of culture on one's worldview, in general, and reactions to infertility, in particular, is from the perspective of *individualism* and *collectivism*. Individualism and collectivism are the most studied dimensions in cross-cultural psychology.[49,50] Individualism and collectivism refer to culture-level differences in self-definitions, goal priorities, relationships and the relative importance of social norms and personal attitudes.[51] *Individualist cultures* are those in which the goals of individuals take priority over the goals of the in-group and where personal attitudes, rather than social norms, are expected to play the primary role in determining people's behavior. Individualism is associated with highly industrialized wealthy nations, such as the United States, Canada, Australia, Britain, and the countries in Northern Europe.

In contrast, *collectivist cultures* are those in which members of the community place the needs and goals of their important groups, most notably their family or kinship group, ahead of their own individual needs. In general, collectivism is associated with agricultural societies where people are highly dependent on one another for survival. These cultures are typically characterized by large extended families that may have strict hierarchical roles, whether patriarchal or matriarchal. Social norms are typically clearly defined in these cultures, and play an important role in determining behavior.[52]

The psychological characteristics associated with these constructs have been measured in more than fifty different countries and are thought to be among the most significant dimensions on which cultures differ. They are also believed to act as organizing principles for many of the differences observed between cultures, and have special relevance to issues of parenthood and the family. The individual-level psychological characteristics associated with individualism and collectivism have been referred to as *independence* and *interdependence*, or as *idiocentrism* and *allocentricism*. *Independence*, or *idiocentrism*, is characterized by an independent sense of self. This is a sense of the self as a separate, unique, fixed entity, with an emphasis on individual traits and abilities, and an ease in moving from group to group. In individualist cultures there is a strong emphasis on personal freedom and personal fulfillment as well as personal control. Maintaining personal consistency across situations is seen as both important and healthy. Thus, people from individualist cultures typically go to great lengths to feel and appear consistent in different social situations and feel very uncomfortable if inconsistency between their behavior and their attitudes is brought to their attention. The need to maintain consistency results in a greater focus on themselves and their inner states than on their environment.[52,53] There is also less differentiation between members of the in-group (i.e., family or kinship group) and out-group members than one sees in other cultures.[54]

At a psychological level, people from collectivist cultures are said to be *interdependent*, or *allocentric*. Members of these cultures are believed to develop an interrelated, or interdependent, sense of self. They are interdependent in that their bonds with their in-group (e.g., family) define who they are and how they experience their self-concept. As a result, these bonds cannot easily be broken. Moreover, because interdependent people see themselves in terms of their roles and memberships in the groups they belong to, they experience themselves differently in different social situations.[55]

An interdependent sense of self has several important psychological, social, and interpersonal consequences. Because interdependent people from collectivist cultures define themselves in terms of their group memberships, being a good group member is their primary goal. As a result, interdependent people place a strong emphasis on working to maintain the well-being of their families as a whole, rather than emphasizing their own personal well-being. Furthermore, they value fitting in with their social groups and fulfilling their roles and obligations to their important social groups. From an early age, children in collectivist cultures are trained to focus their attention on others' responses and behaviors, which in adulthood results in greater awareness of and attention to one's social environment than to one's inner states.[52,53] Thus, the pursuit of harmony includes conforming to the expectations of the people with whom they are interacting and avoiding behaviors that would disrupt close relationships. However, this desire for harmony and awareness of others does not typically extend beyond the members of the in-group[54] (e.g., family or kinship circle). It is therefore primarily family members who play a central role in important decisions, especially decisions that will influence the well-being of the family, including, for example, decisions about whom and when to marry[55–58] and when to have children.

Individualism and collectivism were originally thought to be two end points of a single continuum,[59] and when speaking of these characteristics at the level of a given culture, the tendency is still to distinguish between collectivist and individualist cultures.[52] Now, however, the psychological constructs associated with this cultural difference are considered to be two orthogonal dimensions and thus the psychological topography is more complex than originally believed. People can be high on one, both, or neither of these characteristics. Moreover, individuals in a given culture will vary in the extent to which they personally endorse the culture-level orientation on these dimensions. It should also be noted that there may be many types of individualism and collectivism that are defined by different characteristics in different cultures. One must therefore be very careful to avoid assuming that all individuals from collectivist cultures share the same traits and characteristics. Nonetheless, there are some distinct patterns that have been observed. Individualism and collectivism can have a profound impact on personality, coping, communication, and well-being and, thus, have important consequences for counseling, and therapy generally, and infertility counseling, in particular. Furthermore, these cultural differences can, and do, impact willingness and receptiveness to pretreatment educational counseling and/or infertility-specific psychotherapy.

The United States stands out as a clear outlier in terms of individualism. Members of the white middle class of the United States are notably higher in terms of individualism than members of all other cultures, including those from ethnic subcultures within the United States. Canada, Britain, and Australia are somewhat lower on individualism but are still among the highest in the world on this measure.[53] Northern Europeans are also relatively high on individualism, whereas Southern Europeans tend to be somewhat higher on interdependence.

Those cultures that score the highest on collectivism are China and India, but other East and South Asian countries are also very high on this characteristic, followed by African, South American, and Middle Eastern countries, which are somewhat lower but overall still highly collectivist.[49] As noted above, individuals in some cultures, such as Japan[50] and Turkey,[60] tend to be high on both dimensions. Thus, one cannot assume that individuals from highly collectivist cultures are *necessarily* low on individualism, although this may often be the case.

The cultural distribution of collectivism and individualism is an important point for infertility counselors to recognize. Counseling theory and practice was largely developed by and in the United States, a culture that is more extreme in terms of individualism and collectivism than virtually every other culture in the world. Counseling theory and practice have therefore historically emphasized a highly individualist sense of self and focused on the individual alone, rather than considering a person's social context.[1,61] Thus, the natural inclination of Western-trained mental health professionals is to emphasize personal fulfillment and self-determination, an inclination that is born out of their own individualism, further augmented by highly individualist counseling theories and training. This approach, however, may be highly inappropriate for clients from more collectivist backgrounds. It is therefore imperative that infertility counselors recognize these influences.

CLINICAL ISSUES

Culture and Family Roles

There is no question that infertility has been found to be stressful for individuals and couples in all cultures. Couples and individuals who have been identified as infertile consistently report experiencing high levels of anxiety and depression, lower self-esteem, and generalized stress and emotional distress. This holds true whether they live in China[62] or Japan;[63,64] India[65] or Bangladesh;[66] Iran[67] or Kuwait;[68] Nigeria[69] or South Africa;[70] or Brazil.[71] Comparable levels of distress have been observed between Western and non-Western cultures.

For people from individualist cultures, well-being derives from attaining one's personal goals[50] and life satisfaction is determined more by one's own inner states and feelings.[71] Motives for having children are thus more closely linked to personal joy and pleasure.[72] Indeed, personal joy and pleasure is often listed as a primary reason for wanting children.[73] Individuals in individualistic cultures are less influenced by social role expectations and are less likely to feel pressured to become parents by members of their extended family or social community. Parenthood is seen as an entirely personal decision for the couple, and

infertility is thus likely to be seen as a private and personal loss. Of lesser importance is how infertility may harm others beyond the couple.

By contrast, for individuals and couples in collectivist cultures, group membership is central to the self concept and thus well-being is dependent upon being able to carry out social roles and obligations.[52] Social norms determine the definition of a satisfactory life, and life satisfaction is strongly influenced by one's ability to meet these normative expectations.[71] A sense that one has failed in one's roles is extremely distressing in collectivist cultures and great efforts are made to avoid this. Fulfillment of roles is particularly important within families. Families are the most important social unit in these cultures, with relationships and obligation to parents often taking clear precedence over spousal relationships. Adults, and especially women, are expected to marry and have children and are often socially isolated and even actively derogated if they do not do so. The social role of an adult demands parenthood, particularly motherhood.[74–78] Not surprisingly, then, infertility may be extremely stressful in collectivist cultures because, above and beyond one's personal desire for children, infertility signifies a failure to fulfill one's social role and obligations, potentially threatening important in-group relationships.

An example of infertility-specific distress in collectivist versus individualistic cultures is a study that compared infertile Chinese couples with infertile couples in Europe, Canada, and the United States. For infertile Chinese couples only, the in-laws' response (particularly the husband's parents) played an important role in the couple's ability to cope with infertility (particularly the wife's) and negatively impacted the couple's marital satisfaction.[62] Similarly, in Vietnam, childbearing provides women the opportunity for stronger sentimental ties with her husband and his family through generational links between the worlds of the living and deceased (i.e., ancestor worship and descent). As such, children are required to improve individual happiness, family harmony, and marital satisfaction. Thus, infertility has serious social consequences for Vietnamese women because it impedes her integration into her marital family through conventional and traditional means, that is, childbearing.[79]

The stress of role loss for infertile women, in particular, has been observed in other, non-Asian cultures as well. In Egypt, infertility had significant negative consequences for women, often enhanced by the woman's social status as a result of the monogenetic, male procreation belief system that is the basis for Egyptian patriarchy, evidenced by the patrilineal kinship patterns and family life. For illiterate, poor, urban Egyptian women, motherhood is a mandatory role and, as such, infertility magnified other forms of oppression they experienced in their lives. Involuntary childlessness or 'missing motherhood' was the major source of suffering for many infertile Egyptian women – marring identities, testing faith in God, and enveloping their lives in sadness.[80]

Because marriage in collectivist cultures is embarked upon, in large part, for continuation of the family, the marriages of childless couples are under even greater strain than they would be in individualist cultures. Illustrative of this strain, a retrospective study of newly married couples in Shanghai found that infertile couples were twice as likely to divorce as fertile couples.[74,81] Similarly, 45% of first marriages that ended in divorce in Ethiopia were primarily due to infertility.[82] Likewise, in Nigeria and other parts of sub-Saharan Africa, infertility was found to cause marital disharmony leading to divorce because women were typically blamed for the infertility and men responded by engaging in polygamy in an attempt to have children.[83] Although polygamy is a long-standing cultural remedy for infertility, it is not without significant consequences, particularly for infertile women. For example, 30% of Nigerian women were found to have diagnosable psychopathology, which was attributed to infertility and the consequences of polygamy.[69]

In short, the social and cultural aspects of infertility in patrilineal African societies including Botswana,[84] Egypt,[80,85,86] Gambia,[87,88] Nigeria,[89–92] and South Africa[70] have significant negative personal, marital, familial, and social consequences particularly for women who described their lives without children as meaningless, fruitless, miserable, shameful, or desolate. It is the norm for childless women in these cultures to be blamed for the couple's infertility, leading to maltreatment of her by her husband and/or his family (e.g., physical or emotional abuse, divorce, abandonment, polygamy, or murder). If she does remain in the family system, her role and status as wife is typically diminished significantly (e.g., family servant). Divorced, infertile women may be cast out of their community and excluded from inheriting property or from participating in family life. Moreover because male-factor infertility is a significant social stigma, it is often the wife who bears the brunt of this stigma, frequently through blame, denigration or social ostracization, which is justified by religious beliefs or indigenous spiritual beliefs or traditions. Involuntary childlessness may therefore be particularly traumatic for women in developing countries who have limited alternative roles to motherhood and may suffer significant negative social consequences in addition to the personal loss of motherhood.

Infertility for women in matrilineal societies is also socially complex and associated with significant psychosocial trauma. In a matrilineal kinship system, the children born to a woman belong to her descent group, and her husband, considered a 'stranger' in his wife's kinship group, has no right over his wife's children. Children have a great value to the woman's family. An example is the matrilineal culture of Macua in northern Mozambique in which an infertile woman may divorce her husband as a solution to her childlessness, while her husband is generally blamed for the woman's childlessness. These women (with the support of their family) put greater emphasis on conception than on marriage. As a result, most of the women had had several sexual partners, a fertility-seeking strategy that was condoned by their families but had the potential of actually causing infertility through sexually transmitted infections. And although these women may have been supported in their fertility-seeking strategies, childless women in the Macua culture were stigmatized and excluded from social events and ceremonies because childless women had no alternative roles to motherhood; experienced significant emotional distress; and received little social support for these feelings.[93]

In summary, although infertility-specific distress seems to be similar and experienced at the same level in both men and women in both individualistic and collectivistic cultures, differences arise around *what* is experienced as stressful within the context of individualistic and collectivist cultures. In collectivist cultures, social pressure resulting in strained marital, social, and/or social relationships is the predominant stressor. In individualist cultures, stressors that involve personal loss (e.g., sense of self) are more significant and profound.

Culture, Causes of Infertility, and Treatment Preferences

People from individualist and collectivist cultures also differ in terms of how malleable they see themselves and the world. Compared to those from individualist cultures, people from collectivist cultures see themselves as having less control over their environment and are more inclined to put their energy into adapting themselves to their environment than vice versa.[53] Those from individualist cultures see the self as constant and fixed and are therefore more inclined to seek to change their situation and current environment to fit their needs. Consistent with these differences in perceived control. Tweed and his colleagues found that individuals of Chinese and Japanese ethnicity (i.e., individuals from more collectivist cultures) coped differently in response to stress than those of European ethnicity.[94] Compared to those of European heritage, individuals with an East Asian background were more likely to use coping strategies that emphasized controlling or managing the self rather than the environment. Examples of this internal control included distancing themselves from the event; accepting the event; and waiting things out.

These general differences in perceived control may be reflected in how couples of different cultural backgrounds cope with their infertility. Couples from collectivist cultures may be more fatalistic and less aggressive about seeking medical treatment in response to their infertility than those from individualist cultures. Indeed, Islam teaches that infertility is God's will and thus is to be accepted. Research suggests that women from various Muslim countries are indeed more likely to attribute their childlessness to God's will (e.g., Baruch).

However, the importance many cultures place on biological children as a link to ancestors, and the stigma associated with childlessness, may be so great in collectivist cultures that their members may be more willing to try a greater number of solutions to overcome their childlessness than couples from more individualist cultures. For example, researchers compared infertile couples of Turkish origin living in Germany with infertile German couples and immigrant Turkish mothers.[95] The women of Turkish origin experienced a greater intensity in their desire to have children; were younger at the start of infertility treatment; and were more likely to experience emotional distress due to infertility. Furthermore, Turkish couples were more motivated to have a biological child and more willing to pursue invasive forms of medical treatments in pursuit of this goal. Interestingly, Turkish mothers in this study had more social contact outside the family than their infertile counterparts and were more likely to see themselves as having two identities than did the infertile women of either Turkish or German heritage. Researchers noted that a comparison between the two migrant groups of Turkish women indicated that the infertile women were less acculturated; less likely to want to remain in Germany; had been married longer; and were more likely to have had an arranged marriage. The researchers concluded that all of these factors contributed to an openness to consider reproductive medicine, with a high degree of willingness to pursue invasive medical treatments without question or evaluation.

Similarly, in her study of Vietnamese women, Pashigian found that because the most negative consequence for infertile Vietnamese women was divorce, childlessness was considered a more significant social problem than having too many children.[79] As a result of the severity of the possible consequences of infertility, the women in this study felt compelled to undergo med-

ical treatment for infertility even if it meant intermittent treatment over years, with treatment undertaken whenever funds were available and the women could afford time away from work.

Ironically, the desire and social pressure to have children may be so great that many couples are willing to violate religious and social beliefs to seek treatment. In an investigation comparing the impact of assisted reproductive technologies on male-factor infertility and stigma in Egypt and Lebanon, more than 70% of the study participants underwent IVF/ICSI for the treatment of long-standing male-factor infertility, because gamete donation is seen as adulterous in Islam, and may, therefore, have significant social and religious consequences.[86]

Israel, another pronatalist country in the Middle East, has some of the most liberal reproductive laws in the world – the Public Health (In Vitro Fertilization) Regulation 1987 and the Public Health (Semen Banks) Regulations 1979.[96] As a result, surrogacy legislation in Israel allows couples with serious infertility problems to pursue ARTs even though to do so does not comply with Jewish *religious* law.[97] In a study of stigma and coping, infertile Israeli women were found to have fully internalized the pronatalist culture (or motherhood imperative) in which they lived and actively avoided exposure of their 'hidden disability.'[98] As a result, these women were willing to go to any lengths to have a child, including explicitly violating religious laws regarding third-party reproduction.

The cultural difference in perspectives on control can also extend to yielding more control to those with authority. Thus, one may also see a greater reliance on medical professionals as well as on traditional healers or community/religious leaders to take the initiative regarding interventions to address childlessness. A willingness to place more trust in authority figures is suggested by the study comparing Turkish and German citizens of Turkey, described above, where the infertile women of Turkish descent were willing to accept invasive treatment without question.[99]

A slightly different perspective on treatment was noted in research by Paxson, who investigated the impact of infertility and assisted reproductive technologies in Greece.[100] Paxson noted that according to Greek tradition, motherhood completes a woman by effectively demonstrating her proficiency at being a *good* woman, fulfilling her kinship roles and social contracts. Modern urban Greek women are expected to be both self-actualizing (i.e., independent, a feministic approach) and self-sacrificing (i.e., collectivist, a traditional approach to womanhood). In contrast to the Euro-American approach, assisted conception is seen as 'giving nature a helping hand' or as a typical and natural use of technology. Women in urban Greece view ARTs as a technology of motherhood that is consistent with both choice and individual well-being, enabling a woman to fulfill both goals. In contrast, women in rural Greece view ARTs as a technology that facilitates motherhood and allows her to fulfill traditional definitions of motherhood and womanhood. As such, it is consistent with a traditional ethic of service rooted in village life in which it is morally appropriate to keep hidden anything that would draw public attention to family matters (e.g., sexual matters).[101] This study highlights beliefs about infertility and ARTs across cultures (e.g., Greek versus European and American beliefs) but also illustrates differences in beliefs within a culture (urban versus rural Greeks). This is just one example of how cultures can differ within national boundaries (i.e., urban versus rural residency) as well as across national boundaries. As such, these intracountry differences can become yet another significant factor influencing cross-cultural counseling.

In sum, a substantial body of research suggests that cultures differ in terms of how individuals in them relate to others and the priority they place on family integrity. These differences have far-reaching consequences on many aspects of behavior, attention, expression, and personality. Perhaps what is most important for Western-trained mental health professionals to recognize is that Western culture is, in fact, the anomaly in this regard and that the history of counseling and mental healthcare has been strongly influenced by this bias. Most clients from non-Western cultures will express a stronger investment in interdependence, and thus their relationships to others, than in their own individual goals. A first step in cultural awareness is therefore recognition of how the mental health professional's own assumptions about mental health and well-being, communication, and family relationships may be influenced by these pervasive factors in their own cultural background and professional training.

Religion and Infertility

Like psychology, most of the world's major religions offer a framework for understanding human experience; guidelines for personal development; the maintenance of social relationships; and a method for addressing human suffering. Religion offers a unique focus on the sacred as well as the opportunity for transformation or transcendence. The literatures of the major religions share concerns regarding existential issues. The Tao Te Ching, Dhammapada, Qu'an, Talmud, Torah, and New Testament Bible repeatedly address these issues including: (1) the awareness of the presence of good and evil; (2) the inevitability

of suffering, disease, old age, and death; and (3) the struggle to make meaning out of chaos.[102] They therefore embody a well-developed meaning-making system for understanding illness and misfortunes, such as unwanted childlessness. However, approaches to assisted reproduction vary across the major religions.[103]

Judaism allows the practice of all techniques of assisted reproduction when the oocyte and sperm originate from the wife and husband, respectively. Jewish religious authorities continue to debate the acceptability of the use of donated gametes. Originally, Jewish law prohibited the use of donated gametes for a variety of reasons including incest, lack of genealogy, and the problem of inheritance. The Jewish religion does not forbid the practice of surrogate motherhood in the case of full surrogacy. The dilemma regarding the use of oocyte donation revolves around who should be considered the mother, the oocyte donor or the gestating mother. Jewish law states that the child is related to the woman who finished its formation, the one who gave birth. From the religious point of view, the child will belong to the father who gave the sperm and to the woman who gave birth.[104]

By contrast, the attitude toward reproductive practice differs among the various branches of Christianity. Roman Catholicism does not accept the practice of any form of assisted reproduction; however, the majority of Protestant denominations and Anglicans permit it. Christian tradition views the embryo as a human being from conception, and therefore abortion and/or the destruction of embryos is strictly forbidden by some conservative forms of Christianity. In Latin America, the majority of the population claims to be Roman Catholic, a fact that dramatically influences medical practice and legislation regarding treatment for infertility. However, in a survey study involving members of the Latin American Network of Assisted Reproduction, it was found that despite the specific instructions of the Roman Catholic Church regarding assisted reproduction, couples' reproductive decisions were guided primarily by social interactions and their own conscience – often in conflict with religious law.[105]

Similarly, in a study that examined the psychological responses of Chilean women who had become mothers via oocyte donation, the majority of whom were Roman Catholic, significant distress was found among the Roman Catholic women due to the "dissociation between progeniture and motherhood." This was based on the Roman Catholic belief that gamete donation is an intromission of a third party into the privacy of the marriage. As a result, many women felt isolated and burdened – an outcome for which they felt ill-prepared. Furthermore, 59% of women expressed the need for more active psychological counseling to address the cognitive dissonance precipitated by creating a family in a way that was incongruent with their personal values and/or religious traditions.[106]

According to Islam, assisted reproduction is acceptable only if it involves the husband and the wife. Thus, in almost all Muslim countries of the Middle East, third-party reproduction (sperm, oocyte, embryo donation, or surrogacy) as well as traditional adoption are forbidden or viewed as less acceptable because they are perceived to be adulterous or to be violations against legal inheritance.[96,99,107] Islam encourages medical treatment for infertility, such as intrauterine insemination (IUI), IVF, and frozen embryo transfer (FET) which are deemed appropriate interventions as long as they do not involve gamete donation.[108] At the same time, Islamic law encourages acceptance by the couple that the marriage will remain childless, although this may leave the marriage and/or the position of the wife vulnerable to divorce, polygamy, and/or maltreatment. Thus, Islam provides support for a variety of options for childless couples, encouraging limited forms of medical treatment (use of their own gametes), but also explicitly speaking to childlessness as a possible outcome.

Beyond the major religions and spiritual traditions described in the introduction, there are also traditions indigenous to particular cultures that share spiritual assumptions, while not being an organized religion per se.[32] Many indigenous belief systems portray life as sacred and individuals in these cultures perceive themselves as interrelated through spiritual dimensions; respect and communing with nature; and understand human development as a spiritual journey. Witchcraft, belief in evil spirits, voodoo, magic, and mythologies, as well as the performance of culture-based rituals and traditions, are often practiced in tandem with an organized religion or the religion of the majority group. It may therefore be necessary to ask clients about specific spiritual beliefs above and beyond those affiliated with their professed religious affiliations.

A preference for faith healers and traditional medicine is typically linked to a belief that infertility is part of an imbalance or problem in the larger social, spiritual, or physical environment. Among the Macau of Mozambique, for example, researchers found that a variety of fertility rites during a girl's childhood are designed to enhance her fertility in adulthood or prevent infertility.[93] In this matrilineal society, "incompatibility of the blood between spouses" was one legitimate cause of infertility. When infertility did occur, couples turned to traditional healers: herbal, spiritual, and/or Islamic healers.

In fact, the use of traditional healers and traditional medicine is widespread in most non-Western cultures, although with education, there is a greater tendency to rely on Western medicine alone.[68] For example, in a study of Kuwaiti women, those women who were illiterate were more likely to attribute the cause of their infertility to supernatural causes such as evil spirits, witchcraft, and God's retribution, while educated women blamed nutritional, marital, and psychosexual factors for their infertility. Faith healers and traditional healers were considered as the first treatment choice among illiterate women, while educated women opted for infertility treatment at a medical clinic.[68]

Similarly, a study of the consequences of infertility in a predominantly Muslim population in the slums of Bangladesh found traditional beliefs existing side by side with Western medical ones.[66] Researchers interviewed sixty randomly chosen men and women and infertile women. In both groups of respondents, the leading causes of infertility were perceived to be evil spirits; physiological defects in women; psychosexual problems; and/or physiological defects in men. Herbalists and traditional healers were considered the leading treatment option for women, while for men it was remarriage, followed by herbalists and traditional healers.

Although religious beliefs can be a source of strength and solace for individuals facing involuntary childlessness, these beliefs may also contribute to their feelings of distress. In a study in South Africa that examined case studies of infertile individuals and religious leaders representing the faiths of the infertile individuals, remarkable differences were found between Indian and African worldviews compared with those of 'coloureds' and whites. However, the impact of religion on the handling of infertility was found to be similar across the different religions. The individuals' level of involvement with religion; their personal conception of God; and their sense of self in relation to God appeared to be important factors influencing the impact of religion on the experience of infertility. The most pervasive theme that emerged was that of infertility being seen as punishment for wrongdoing.[109]

What seems clear from research on religion and infertility is that the pursuit of guidance from spiritual healers often occurs in parallel with seeking medical treatment and advice and can provide a great deal of support during the process. Various tenets and practices of religion and spirituality include mindfulness and mediation, prayer, values, acceptance, forgiveness, evoking hope, serenity, and behavioral approaches to enhancing spirituality including practicing particular rituals (e.g., sacraments, holy days, and dances),

CROSS-CULTURAL ISSUES IN INFERTILITY COUNSELING

compassionate sacrificial service, fasting, or pilgrimages, all of which may be of benefit to individuals struggling with infertility. However, religious beliefs and practices may also result in guilt and self-blame in response to infertility and may influence clients' comfort with various treatment options. It is therefore essential to explore religious and spiritual beliefs from all of these different perspectives, as well as recognize and support these practices as coping mechanisms.

Cultural Resistance to Infertility Counseling

Reproductive medicine and infertility counseling are fairly new fields in medicine and, as a result, many infertile men and women are unaware of the practical applications of infertility counseling or its importance in comprehensive patient care in reproductive medicine. Research has shown that the majority of infertile men and women do *not* voluntarily seek counseling regarding involuntary childlessness, reproductive losses, infertility treatment, or family-building alternatives – even when counseling is legally mandated or encouraged.[110] Reasons for reluctance to seek counseling are numerous and varied: cultural stigma regarding mental health diagnosis; resistance to use of mental health professionals (particularly if the professional is from a different culture/race); financial expense of counseling; ignorance of advantages and/or benefits of infertility counseling; confusion about how to access and/or use available mental healthcare systems or services; and/or lack of confidence in counseling in general or a specific counselor's capabilities/qualifications. However, many individuals have negative feelings about counseling which they may view as a superfluous 'luxury' for self-involved, self-indulgent, weak-minded individuals unable to manage their problems on their own. All or some of these factors can contribute to significant client resistance before the counseling session has even begun.

As a result, many infertile men and women arrive at their appointment with the infertility counselor ill-informed, unprepared, apprehensive, and, basically, resistant. Sometimes resistance involves common topic-specific issues such as conflict (e.g., coercion, abuse, or violence) or sexuality (e.g., dysfunction or female circumcision), while sometimes resistance involves infertility-specific issues such as third-party reproduction (e.g., use of donor gametes, embryos, and gestational carrier); gender-specific infertility diagnosis; and/or adoption. Resistance may be covert rather than overt, with the individual and couple presenting as pleasant and cooperative but affectively flat, unforthcoming, and detached from the counseling pro-

cess. Or resistance may be overt hostility and refusal to participate in counseling. Consequently, neutralizing resistance and engaging the infertile patient(s) must be the primary goal of the initial session and the greatest challenge. As such, at the outset of the initial session the infertility counselor should state the purpose of the interview and outline the psychotherapy or preparation and educational counseling process (e.g., use of the interpreter, purpose of the interview, history-taking process, and review of educational materials). In fact, the infertility counselor may need to use all of his or her very best skills to engage the culturally resistant, most importantly by 'joining' through the use of phrases from their language; display a willingness to learn about their culture and their personal perspective through open-ended questions; allowing the client to describe their perspective of infertility in terms of their culture and religion; using humor whenever possible; exhibiting a sense of curiosity about their culture and religion; using positive body language; and culture-specific gestures (e.g., bowing head). Still, the infertility counselor must be prepared for the possibility that, at the end of the interview, they have little or no understanding of their clients, their history, or their infertility experience, and little confidence that the clients have gained anything useful from the interview.

THERAPEUTIC INTERVENTIONS

Becoming a More Culturally-Sensitive Infertility Counselor

Infertility counseling is a relatively new field that has grown up, as it were, alongside the field of reproductive medicine. While professionals in the field have worked to define the roles and responsibilities in patient care, there has been a consistent awareness of the need to be culturally sensitive and present. This seems to be an even more pressing need as an increasing number of patients find their way to infertility clinics across national or international boundaries. As such, providing appropriate patient care means providing care that is knowledgeable about the medical treatments *and* the cultural issues. Culturally adaptive infertility counseling involves being aware of the multiple layers of problems, meanings, and cultural differences in any given situation.

In 2003, the American Psychological Association published *Guidelines on Multicultural Education, Training, Research, Practice, and Organizational Change for Psychologists.* The goal of the guidelines was to provide: (1) the rationale and needs for addressing multiculturalism and diversity; (2) basic information, relevant terminology, and current empirical research that support and underscore the importance of the guidelines; (3) references to enhance the goals of the guidelines; and (4) paradigms that broaden the purview of psychology as a profession. While these guidelines are directed to psychologists, the message applies to all mental health professionals to expand their view of their own cultural heritage; identify and define their own sense of cultural identity; integrate their cultural identity into their other various social identities; and develop their knowledge of other cultures.

Sue and Sue have suggested that, in working toward becoming a more culturally aware clinician, the counselor should accomplish (or work toward) the following:[30]

■ moving from being culturally unaware to being aware and sensitive to his or her own cultural heritage and to valuing and respecting cultural differences;
■ being comfortable with the differences existing between themselves and clients in terms of culture, race, religious beliefs, and even cultural biases regarding gender;
■ being fluent in other languages (including ability to use medical terms), knowing how to work appropriately with a translator, and/or being able to problem solve translation challenges. Many major medical centers offer translators on staff, but this is more of a challenge for smaller private clinics. With an informal translator (e.g., spouse or family member) the patient may have difficulty discussing private matters; confidentiality is easily broken; or there is a danger of information being skewed to agree with the translator's perspective or agenda.
■ being sensitive to circumstances (personal biases, degree of ethnic identity, sociopolitical influences) that may dictate referral of a minority client to a counselor of his or her own race/culture or a more culturally sensitive counselor;
■ attempting to achieve a cultural 'match' with the client to facilitate therapeutic alliance;
■ becoming familiar with the cultural issues unique to infertility as well as their particular community;
■ enhancing cultural awareness through self-education, for example, volunteering in community minority organizations, travel, literature, university coursework, attending different religious services, and studying different language(s);
■ acknowledging and being aware of his or her own racist attitudes, beliefs, and feelings.

More infertility-specific guidelines are suggested by Gacinski and colleagues.[99] These authors suggest that the infertility counselor working with infertile couples from a different culture consider asking clients some key questions as a starting point for helping them adjust to infertility treatment and counseling:

■ *Do you discuss the fertility problem with others in your social circle? Who can you confide in?* All too often, the issue of childlessness is so stigmatizing that the couple or one partner is unable to talk about it with anyone, resulting in further isolation.
■ *Do you feel pressure from relatives?* If children are highly valued in a culture, the couple's childlessness may be a stigma for the family as well as the couple.
■ *What do you do in your spare time?* If the woman is not working (perhaps as an émigré she is unable to get a work permit), the state of quasi-waiting for parenthood can increase her stress. Alternatively, she may not pursue career interests or goals in hopes of parenthood.
■ *In male sterility: Is it accepted by your partner and/or his family?* Male infertility is highly stigmatizing across many cultures and many myths about it continue to exist. It is important to determine not only his feelings about the diagnosis but also what the partner's feelings are and those of their families.
■ *Have you visited a doctor or caregiver in your home country, for example, during your holiday?* Some couples continue complementary treatments (e.g., herbal or spiritual therapies) while being treated with ARTs.
■ *Have you considered spiritual treatments customary to your culture or talked to a spiritual leader (e.g., priest)?* Some couples are combining 'traditional' and Western medicine although they often do not disclose this out of fear of a negative response from the caregiver. However, some traditional treatments have been found to interact negatively with infertility treatments so patients should be carefully and tactfully educated.
■ *Can you imagine a time when you would like to end treatment?* Many couples expect that treatment will be quickly successful and the thought of abandoning treatment or putting a limit on it is unfathomable. Helping them consider this prospect is an important part of counseling. In addition, the infertility counselor should help them become active participants in the treatment process, considering their right and responsibility to choose the treatments that are best for them.
■ *Are there alternatives to a biologically-linked child for you?* Even with couples (and cultures) in which a child genetically-linked to each partner is the primary focus; infertility counselors should help the couple investigate and consider alternatives. This is especially important for couples with poor prognosis and for whom parenthood is highly valued or for whom the stigma of childlessness is significant.

Using a Cultural Genogram

One tool that may be particularly useful for working with culturally diverse clients is the cultural genogram. The genogram is a tool used in both family therapy and genetic counseling to take a family history, gather information, and diagram family patterns and dynamics in a time-efficient manner while creating an easily read diagram. It has been suggested that this is also a useful tool for developing a 'cultural history' for a couple/family, thereby increasing cultural competence as an infertility counselor.[111, 113]

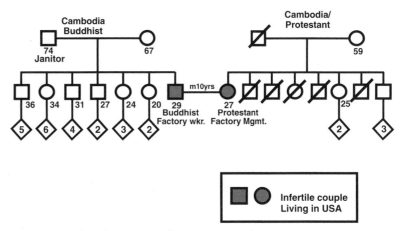

Figure 4.1. Cultural genogram of immigrant couple.

A cultural genogram provides a quick and efficient method of gathering information about a couple's marital and family history as well as cultural dynamics such as religion; ethnic background; emigration history/status; cultural values (collectivism vs. individualism); emotional expressiveness; communication patterns; patterns of closeness; and conflict.[114–117] Figure 4.1 demonstrates the intergenerational nature of infertility as well as the myriad of factors influencing a couple's experience of infertility including religion, culture, emotional expressiveness and closeness, and the dilemmas of collectivism versus individualism. In this genogram, an immigrant couple is from the same country, but the wife emigrated as a small child under traumatic circumstances in which most of her family died and the husband emigrated as a late adolescent. They are affected by uneven acculturation, demonstrated by the wife's greater command of the language and willingness to pursue Western medical treatments and the husband's limited understanding of the language and a strong desire for his wife to use traditional herbal and spiritual remedies.

Using a genogram in infertility counseling enables the infertility counselor to take a cultural history as well as assess family values and dynamics; other stressors; and family history of reproductive issues (e.g., family history of cystic fibrosis and miscarriage). By using a genogram to diagram the infertile couple's familial milieu, information can be efficiently gathered and shared with other professionals as well as the couple themselves. It can be used as an effective therapeutic tool through soliciting the patient's participation in diagramming their marriage and family. In addition, through examination of the completed genogram, individuals and couples are often better able to identify cultural, emotional, and/or physical factors impacting their experience of infertility. As such, the genogram

provides a framework for including and addressing the culturally-sensitive questions suggested by Gacinski, Yuksel, and Kentenich.[99] It also gives the infertility counselor an opportunity to provide culturally-sensitive treatment in an efficient and expeditious manner.

Individualism–Collectivism and the Therapeutic Interview

The guidelines above offer specific approaches to working with clients from diverse cultural backgrounds. However, there are also more general issues that arise from differences in individualism and collectivism that may influence the success of the guidelines described earlier. These factors relate to basic and overarching aspects of communication and therapeutic process. For example, it has frequently been reported that since most non-Western collectivist cultures have a tradition of advice being given by elders or healers to those in distress, clients from these cultures may expect and feel more comfortable with more directive forms of counseling.[24] A therapist who is unwilling to give advice may be seen as lacking knowledge and/or expertise; unwilling to provide comfort and support; or failing to understand the clients' problems. Keeping this in mind, the mental health professional assisting a couple in managing the crisis of infertility should consider adapting these directive approaches to include coping strategies that are congruent with a collectivist culture, should the couple indicate a preference for a more directive approach.

Individualism–collectivism can also have a significant impact on emotional expression. Although there may be shared universal patterns across cultures that distinguish how basic emotions are expressed, there are also subtle and important cultural differences regarding which expressions are controlled and with whom.[118]

Collectivist cultures emphasize the importance of maintaining harmony with others. As a result, they value restraint in emotional expression. In particular, these cultures emphasize the importance of limiting the expression of emotions like anger and contempt that might disrupt close relationships.[54] Thus, a couple in counseling may be extremely reluctant to express any anger they feel toward each other and especially medical caregivers. In these cases, other means of discussing their experience of infertility may need to be explored.

In contrast, people in individualist cultures value open emotional expression, and pay more attention to their emotional states.[50,53] In individualist cultures, emotional states are taken as important information in evaluating one's environment and one's self.[71] This is not the case in collectivist cultures. As a consequence, clients from collectivist cultures may not focus on their emotional state to the same extent as those from individualist cultures and may report fewer emotions overall. For people from more collectivist cultures, it can be more appropriate and common to express distress in psychosomatic ways rather than in terms of directly expressed emotion.[8,119] A successful multicultural counselor must therefore be willing to consider the variety of ways in which distress may be expressed and recognize that it may not always be in terms of explicit emotions.

Addressing Religion as an Infertility Counselor

A competent multicultural infertility counselor needs to consider not only issues of culture, but also of religion. Thus, beyond appropriate initial and continuing professional education, the infertility counselor also needs a set of culturally sensitive proficiencies regarding religion and spirituality:

■ A nonjudgmental, accepting, and empathic relationship with the client that allows for discussion of religious and/or spiritual concerns, particularly those relating to the individual's and/or couple's experience of infertility, treatment, and viable remedies for childlessness;
■ An openness and willingness to take time to understand the individual's and/or couple's spirituality as it may relate to infertility and other health concerns;
■ Some familiarity with culturally related values, beliefs, and practices that are common among the patient population likely to be served;
■ Comfort in asking and talking about spiritual issues with patients;

■ A willingness to seek information from appropriate professionals and coordinate care concerning patients' spiritual traditions;[11]
■ A willingness to think more globally and openly about spirituality and religion as factors in the lives of individuals and couples, and differentiating this from participation in religious institutions;
■ A willingness to offer religion and spirituality (e.g., hope, acceptance, forgiveness, mindfulness and meditation, values, serenity, and community) as potential resources for coping with infertility;
■ A recognition of how religion may be an asset and/or liability in the experience of infertility, treatment, and/or family-building endeavors for infertile individuals and couples.

Addressing religion and spirituality with infertile couples can be challenging as religion may be both a resource and a burden, a source of comfort or a source of pain. Faced with existential dilemmas, psychological distress, and social stigma, many infertile men and women experience a 'crisis of faith' or find comfort in their faith that helps them meet the challenges of infertility. For some couples, religion may provide opportunities to maintain hope and give meaning to their experiences of suffering and loss inherent in the infertility experience. They may find comfort by venting their anger at God(s) or at religious ceremonies that involve children. In contrast, they may find peace, meaning, and comfort in their religious community and/or its rituals. The infertility counselors should therefore be aware of the couple's religion (and their interpretation of it); be open to discussing the couple's spiritual or religious dilemmas and needs; and have available religious resources, including religious leaders, within their community to whom they can refer couples for spiritual assistance and support. As such, it is important too that both partners be helped to identify and articulate their spiritual perspective and struggles. Is one partner waiting for a miracle while the other is experiencing infertility as a punishment? Is one partner feeling disillusioned with his/her faith while the other is finding strength and hope through his or her religious beliefs?[120] By facilitating open discussions, the infertility counselor can provide a safe environment for discussion of sensitive and potentially volatile issues.

FUTURE IMPLICATIONS

The role of the infertility counselor has become an increasingly integral part of the treatment of infertility and on the treatment team. At the same time more patients are crossing geographic, cultural, religious, and personal boundaries to pursue medical treatments for involuntary childlessness and/or infertility in cities and countries far from home.[121] As such, the importance of providing culturally-sensitive infertility counseling is increasingly essential and necessary. Professional development, collaboration, and an awareness of cultural diversity are integral elements for the culturally-sensitive infertility counselor, as is an appreciation of the importance of culture as an essential healing resource for ourselves and for our patients.

SUMMARY

■ The growing number of patients crossing geographic, cultural, religious, and personal boundaries to pursue medical treatments for infertility, emphasizes the importance and necessity of providing culturally-sensitive infertility counseling.

■ Culture, religion, kinship/family values, beliefs about health and illness, and gender roles all influence how individuals and cultural groups experience and interpret infertility.

■ Religion and spirituality are fundamental parts of culture but can be challenging as they may be experienced as a resource (comfort) or a burden (punishment).

■ Individualism and collectivism refer to cultural differences. In individualist cultures, the goals of individuals take priority over the goals of the in-group. In contrast, in collectivist cultures the needs of the family or kinship group take precedence over individual needs. Cultural levels of collectivism and individualism can and do influence how individuals and couples experience infertility.

■ Even countries that appear culturally homogenous are multicultural to some degree, requiring an awareness of diversity issues and the impact of culture on the provision of infertility treatment and infertility counseling.

■ One cannot assume that a cultural norm is descriptive of every member of a given population. Rather, one must be willing to learn from and ask questions of the client; allow the client to describe their cultural and religious perspective; and define their own personal experience.

■ There are specific skills and techniques the infertility counselor can and should learn to become more culturally-sensitive and specific questions and approaches that have been found to be useful when dealing with culturally different infertile patients.

Acknowledgment

The authors would like to thank Azzi Momen for her editorial assistance in the preparation of this chapter.

REFERENCES

1. Pederson PB. Cross-cultural counseling: Developing culture-centered interactions. In: G Bernal, JE Trimble, AK Burlew, FTL Leong, eds. *Handbook of Racial and Ethnic Minority Psychology*. Thousand Oaks, CA: Sage, 2003; 487–503.
2. American Psychological Association. *Guidelines on Multicultural Education, Training, Research, Practice, and Organizational Change for Psychologists*. Washington, DC: American Psychological Association, 2002.
3. Leong FTL, Santiago-Rivera AL. Climbing the multiculturalism summit: Challenges and pitfalls. In: P Pederson, ed. *Multiculturalism as a Fourth Force*. Brunner/Mazel, 1999; 61–72.
4. US Census Bureau. http://factfinder.census.gov.; c2000 [cited 2005 Apr 1].
5. Dovidio JF, Esses VM. Immigrants and immigration: Advancing the psychological perspective. *J Soc Issues* 2001; 34:375–87.
6. Eurostat. http://europa.eu.int/comm/eurostat/. 2005 [cited 2005 Apr 1].
7. Berry JW. Immigration, acculturation, and adaptation. *J Appl Psychol* 1997; 46:5–68.
8. Marin G, Balls Organista P, Chun KM. Acculturation research: Current issues and findings. In: G Bernal, JE Trimble, AK Burlew, FTL Leong, eds. *Handbook of Racial and Ethnic Minority Psychology*. Thousand Oaks, CA: Sage, 2003; 208–19.
9. Phinney JS. Ethnic identity in adolescents and adults: Review of research. *Psychol Bull* 1990; 108:499–514.
10. Hynie, M. From conflict to compromise: Immigrant families and the processes of acculturation. In: DM Taylor, ed. *Diversity with Justice and Harmony: A Social Psychological Analysis*. Ottawa, Canada: Department of Citizenship and Immigration, 1996; 97–123.
11. Miller WR, Thoreson CE. Spirituality, religion, and health: An emerging research field. *American Psychologist* 2003; 58:24–35.
12. http://www.cia.gov/cia/publications/factbook/geos/xx.html. August 30, 2005.
13. Richards PS, Bergin AE. *A Spiritual Strategy for Counseling and Psychotherapy*. Washington, DC: American Psychological Association, 1997.
14. Richards PS, Rector JM, Tjeltveit AC. Values, spirituality, and psychotherapy. In: WR Miller, ed. *Integrating Spirituality into Treatment: Resources for Practitioners*. Washington, DC: American Psychological Association Press, 1999; 133–60.
15. Smith H. *The World's Religions: Our Great Wisdom Traditions*. San Francisco, CA: Harper Collins, 1991.
16. Smith H. *Forgotten Truth: The Common Vision of the World's Religions*. San Francisco. Harper Collins, 1992.
17. Fathalla MF. Current challenges in assisted reproduction. In: E Vayena, PJ Rowe, PD Griffin, eds. *Current*

Practices and Controversies in Assisted Reproduction. Geneva: World Health Organization, 2005; 3–13.

18. Kim U, Berry JW. Introduction. In: U Kim, JW Berry, eds. *Indigenous Psychologies: Research and Experience in Cultural Context.* Newbury Park, CA: Sage, 1993; 1–29.

19. Maio GR, Olson JM. Values as truisms: Evidence and implications. *J Pers Soc Psychol* 1998; 74:294–311.

20. Molock, SD. Racial, cultural, and religious issues in infertility counseling. In: LH Burns, SN Covington, eds. *Infertility Counseling: A Comprehensive Handbook for Clinicians.* New York: The Parthenon Publishing Group, 1999; 249–65.

21. Mulatu, MS, Berry JW. Health care practice in a multicultural context: Western and non-Western assumptions. In: SS Kazarian, DR Evans, eds. *Handbook of Cultural Health Psychology.* San Diego, CA: Academic Press, 2001; 45–61.

22. Huff RM, Kline MV. Health promotion in the context of culture. In: RM Huff, MV Kline, eds. *Promoting Health in Multicultural Populations.* Thousand Oaks, CA: Sage Press, 1999; 3–21.

23. McFadden J. Historical approaches to transcultural counseling. In: J McFadden, ed. *Transcultural Counseling* Alexandria, VA: American Counseling Association, 1999; 3–21.

24. Rawson D, Whitehead, G, Luthra M. The challenge of counseling in a multicultural society. In: S Palmer, P Laungani, eds. *Counseling in a Multicultural Society.* London: Sage; 1999; 6–34.

25. Fraga ED, Atkinson DR, Wampold BE. Ethnic group preferences for multicultural counseling competencies. *Cult Divers Ethnic Minor Psychol.* 2004; 10:53–65.

26. Sue DW, Carter RT, Casas JM, et al. *Multicultural Counseling Competencies: Individual and Organizational Development.* Thousand Oaks, CA: Sage; 1998.

27. D'Andrea M, Daniels J. Promoting multiculturalism and organizational change in the counseling profession: A case study. In: JG Ponterotto, JM Casas, LA Suzuki, CM Alexander, eds. *Handbook of Multicultural Counseling.* Thousand Oaks, CA: Sage; 1995; 17–33.

28. Johannes CK, Erwin PG. Developing multicultural competence: Perspectives on theory and practice. *Couns Psychol Q.* 2004; 17:329–38.

29. Iwamasa GY, Sorocco KH, Koonce DA. Ethnicity and clinical psychology: A content analysis of the literature. *Clin Psychol Rev.* 2002; 8:931–44.

30. Sue DW, Sue D. *Counseling the Culturally Different: Theory & Practice.* 3rd ed. New York: John Wiley & Sons; 1999.

31. Fuertes JN, Brobst K. Clients' ratings of counselor multicultural competency. *Cult Divers Ethnic Minor Psychol.* 2002; 8:214–23.

32. Hays, PA. *Addressing Cultural Complexities in Practice: A Framework for Clinicians and Counselors.* Washington, DC: American Psychological Association, 2001.

33. Yalom I. *Existential Psychotherapy.* New York: Basic Books, 1980.

34. Marlatt GA, Kristeller JL. Mindfulness and meditation. In WR Miller, ed. *Integrating Spirituality into Treatment: Resources for Practitioners.* Washington, DC: American Psychological Press, 1999; 67–84.

35. Domar AD, Clapp D, Slawsby E, et al. The impact of group psychological interventions on distress in infertile women. *Health Psychology* 2000; 19:568–75.

36. Cortigight B. *Psychotherapy and Spirit.* Albany, NY: State University of New York Press, 1997.

37. Miller W, ed. *Integrating Spirituality into Treatment. Resources for Practitioners.* Washington, DC: American Psychological Association, 1999; 15.

38. Rosenblatt PC, Peterson P, Portner J, et al. A cross-cultural study of responses to childlessness. *Beh Science Notes* 1973; 8:221–31.

39. Blenner JL. Healthcare providers' treatment approaches to culturally diverse infertile clients. *J Transcult Nurs* 1991; 2:24–31.

40. Domar AD, Penzias A, Dusek JA, et al. The stress and distress of infertility: Does religion help women cope? *Sexuality, Reproduction and Menopause* 2005; 10:45–51.

41. Covington, SN, Fitzgerald OR, Calis KA, et al. Spiritual well-being is significantly associated with functional well-being in women with spontaneous premature ovarian failure. *Fertil Steri* 2005; 84:S232.

42. Schenker JG, Shushan A. Ethical and legal aspects of assisted reproduction practice in Asia. *Hum Reprod* 1996; 11:908–11.

43. Shirai Y. Japanese Attitudes toward assisted procreation. *J Law Med Ethics* 1993; 21:43–53.

44. Baluch B, Fallone A, Anderson R, et al. Women's attitude to egg donation and sperm donation: A cross-cultural study. *J Hum Behav* 1994; 31:5–8.

45. Isikoglu M, Senol Y, Berkkanoglu M, et al. Public opinion regarding oocyte donation in Turkey: First data from a secular population among the Islamic world. *Hum Reprod* 2006; 21:318–23.

46. Carter RT, Quresh A. A typology of philosophical assumptions in multicultural counseling and training. In: JG Ponterotto, JM Casas, LA Suzuki, CM Alexander, eds. *Handbook of Multicultural Counseling.* Thousand Oaks, CA: Sage; 1995; 239–62.

47. Church AT. Culture and personality: Toward an integrated cultural trait psychology. *J Pers* 2000; 68:651–703.

48. Taylor SE. A categorization approach to stereotyping. In: DL Hamilton, ed. *Cognitive Processes in Stereotyping and Intergroup Behavior.* Hillsdale, NJ: Erlbaum; 1981; 365–76.

49. Church, AT Lonner WJ. The cross-cultural perspective in the study of personality: Rationale and current research. *J Cross Cult Psych* 1998; 29:32–62.

50. Oyserman, D, Coon HM, Kemmelmeier M. Rethinking individualism and collectivism: Evaluation of theoretical assumptions and meta-analyses. *Psychol Bull* 2002; 128:3–72.

51. Triandis HC. *Individualism and Collectivism.* Boulder, CO: Westview Press; 1995.

52. Triandis HC. Individualism-collectivism and personality. *J Pers.* 2001; 69:907–24.

53. Heine SJ. Self as cultural product: An examination of East Asian and North American selves. *J Pers.* 2001; 69:881–906.

54. Matsumoto D, Takeuchi S, Andayani S, Kouznetsova N, Krupp D. The contribution of individualism vs. collectivism to cross-national differences in display rules. *Asian J of Soc Psychol.* 1998; 1:147–65.

55. Markus H, Kitayama S. Culture and self: Implications for cognition, emotion and motivation. *Psychol Rev*. 1998; 98:224–53.

56. Dion KK, Dion KL. Cultural perspectives on romantic love. *Pers Relatsh*. 1994; 1:5–17.

57. Doherty RW, Hatfield E, Thompson K, Choo P. Cultural and ethnic influences on love and attachment. *Pers Relatsh*. 1994; 1:391.

58. Lalonde RN, Hynie M, Pannu M, et al. The role of culture in interpersonal relationships: Do second generation South Asian Canadians want a traditional partner? *J Cross Cult Psych*. 1994; 35:503–24.

59. Hofestede C. *Culture's Consequences: International Differences in Work Related Values*. Beverly Hills, CA: Sage; 1980.

60. Uskul, AK, Hynie, M, Lalonde, RN. Interdependence as a mediator between culture and interpersonal closeness for Euro-Canadians and Turks. *J Cross Cult Psych*. 2004; 35:174–91.

61. Jackson ML. Multicultural counseling: Historical perspectives. In: JG Ponterotto, JM Casas, LA Suzuki, CM Alexander, eds. *Handbook of Multicultural Counseling*. Thousand Oaks, CA: Sage; 1995; 3–16.

62. Lee TY, Sun GH. Psychosocial response of Chinese infertile husbands and wives. *Arch Androl*. 2000; 45:143–8.

63. Matsubayashi H, Hosaka T, Izumi S, et al. Increased depression and anxiety in infertile Japanese women resulting from lack of husband's support and feelings of stress. *Gen Hosp Psychiatry*. 2004; 26:398–404.

64. Matsubayashi H, Hosaka T, Izumi S, et al. Emotional response of infertile women in Japan. *Hum Reprod*. 2001; 16:966–9.

65. Dhaliwal LK, Gupta KR, Gopalan S, et al. Psychological aspects of infertility due to various causes – prospective studies. *Int J Fertil Womens Med*. 2004; 49:44–8.

66. Papreen N, Sharma A, Sabin K, et al. Living with infertility: Experiences among urban slum populations in Bangladesh. *Reprod Health Matters*. 2000; 8:33–44.

67. Nasseri M. Cultural similarities in psychological reactions to infertility. *Psychol Rep*. 2000; 86:375–8.

68. Fido A, Zahid MA. Coping with infertility among Kuwaiti women: Cultural perspectives. *Int J Soc Psychiatry*. 2004; 50:294–300.

69. Aghanwa HS, Dare FO, Ogunniyi SO. Sociodemographic factors in mental disorders associated with infertility in Nigeria. *J Psychosom Res*. 1999; 46:117–23.

70. Dyer SJ, Abrahams N, Hoffman M, et al. 'Men leave me as I cannot have children': Women's experiences with involuntary childlessness. *Hum Reprod*. 2002; 17: 1663–8.

71. Suh E, Diener E, Oishi S, Triandis HC. The shifting basis of life satisfaction judgments across cultures: Emotions versus norms. *J Pers Soc Psychol*. 1998; 74:482–93.

72. Meade RD, Singh L. Motives for child-bearing in America and India. *J Cross-Cult Psychol*. 1973; 4:89–110.

73. Hoffman LW. The value of children to parents and child-drearing patterns. *Soc Behav*. 1987; 2:123–41.

74. Lee TY, Chu TY. The Chinese experience of male infertility. *West J Nurs Res*. 2001; 23:714–25.

75. Mabasa LF. Sociocultural aspects of infertility in a black South African community. *J of Psychology in Africa*. 2002; 12:65–79.

76. Remennick L. Childless in the land of imperative motherhood: Stigma and coping among infertile Israeli women. *Sex Roles*. 2000; 43:821–41.

77. Riessman CK. Stigma and everyday resistance practices: Childless women in South India. *Gend Soc*. 2000; 14:111–35.

78. Runganga AO, Sundby J, Aggleton P. Culture, identity and reproductive failure in Zimbabwe. *Sexualities*. 2001; 4:315–32.

79. Pashigian MJ. Conceiving the happy family: Infertility and marital politics in northern Vietnam. In: MC Inhorn, F van Balen, eds. *Infertility Around the Globe: New Thinking on Childlessness, Gender, and Reproductive Technologies*. Los Angeles, CA: University of California Press; 2002; 134–49.

80. Inhorn M. *Infertility and Patriarchy: The Cultural Politics of Gender and Family Life in Egypt*. Philadelphia: University of Pennsylvania Press; 1996.

81. Che Y, Cleland J. Infertility in Shanghai: Prevalence, treatment seeking, and impact. *J Ob Gyn*. 2002; 22: 643–8.

82. Tilson D, Larsen U. Divorce in Ethiopia: The impact of early marriage and childlessness. *J Biosoc Sci*. 2000; 32:355–72.

83. Araove MO. Epidemiology of infertility: Social problems of the infertile couples. *West Afr J Med*. 2003; 22:190–6.

84. Upton RL. 'Infertility makes you invisible': Gender health and the negotiation of fertility in northern Botswana. *J South Af Stud*. 2001; 27:349–62.

85. Inhorn M, Buss K. Ethnography, epidemiology and infertility in Egypt. *Soc Sci Med*. 1994; 39:671–86.

86. Inhorn MC. Privacy, privatization, and the politics of patronage: Ethnographic challenges to penetrating the secret world of Middle Eastern, hospital-based in vitro fertilization. *Soc Sci Med*. 2004; 59:2095–108.

87. Sundby J. Infertility in the Gambia: Transitional and modern health care. *Patient Educ Couns*. 1997; 31:29–37.

88. Sundby J. Infertility and health care in countries with less resources: case studies from sub-Sahara Africa. In: MC Inhorn, F van Balen, eds. *Infertility Around the Globe: New Thinking on Childlessness, Gender, and Reproductive Technologies*. Los Angeles, CA: University of California Press; 2002; 247–59.

89. Koster-Okekan W. Olorun a shi e ni inu. God will open your womb: Causes, treatment and consequences of infertility among Yoruba women in Nigeria. *Medische Antropologie*. 1998; 10:43–58.

90. Okonofua FE, Harris D, Odebiyi A. The social meaning of infertility in southwest Nigeria. *Health Transition Rev*. 1997; 7:205–20.

91. Onah N. The sociocultural perception and implications of childlessness in Anambra State. In: MN Kisekka, ed. *Women's Health Issues in Nigeria*. Nigeria: Tamaza Publishing; 1992; 183–90.

92. Ikechebelu JI, Adinma JIB, Orie EF, et al. High prevalence of male infertility in southeastern Nigeria. *J Ob Gyn*. 2003; 23:657–9.

93. Gerrits, T. Social and cultural aspects of infertility in Mozambique. *Patient Educ Couns*. 1997; 31:39–48.

94. Tweed RG, White K, Lehman DR. Culture, stress, and coping: Internally- and externally-targeted control strategies of European Canadians, East Asian Canadians, and Japanese. *J Cross Cult Psych*. 2004; 35:652–68.

95. David M, Yuksel E., Kentenich H. The desire to have children and migration: On the psychosocial situation of infertile Turkish couples in Germany. *Geburtshilfe Frauenheilkd*. 2002; 62:33–44.

96. Lee RG, Morgan D. *Human Fertilisation & Embryology: Regulating the Reproductive Revolution*. London: Blackstone Press Ltd, 2001.

97. Honig D, Nave O, Adam R. Israeli surrogacy law in practice. *Isr J Psychiatry Relat Sci*. 2000; 37:115–23.

98. Remennick L. Childless in the land of imperative motherhood: Stigma and coping infertile Israeli women. *Sex Roles*. 2001; 43:821–41.

99. Gacinski L, Yuksel E, Kentenich H. The unfulfilled desire for a child of oriental couples – Infertility counseling and treatment of Turkish immigrants in Germany. In: B Strauss, ed. *Involuntary Childlessness: Psychological Assessment, Counseling, and Psychotherapy*. Seattle: Hogrefe & Huber Publishers; 2002; 51–60.

100. Paxson H. *Making Modern Mothers: Ethics and Family Planning in Urban Greece*. Los Angeles: University of California Press; 2004.

101. Tarlatzis I, Tarlatzis BC, Diakogiannis I, et al. Psychosocial imports of infertility on Greek couples. *Hum Reprod*. 1993; 8:396–401.

102. Sanderson C. Linehan M. Acceptance and forgiveness. In W. Miller, ed., *Integrating Spirituality into Treatment. Resources for Practitioners*. Washington, DC: American Psychological Association, 1999; 199–216.

103. Schenker JG. Women's reproductive health: Monotheistic religious perspectives. *Int J Gynacol Obstet*. 2000; 70:77–86.

104. Schenker JG. Infertility evaluation and treatment according to Jewish law. *Eur J Obstet Gynecol Reprod Biol*. 1997; 71:113–21.

105. Zegers-Hochschild F. Attitudes towards reproduction in Latin America. Teachings from the use of modern reproductive technologies. *Hum Reprod Update*. 1999; 5:21–5.

106. Zegers-Hochschild F, Pachero IM, Fabres C, et al. Psychological characteristics of Chilean women participating in an in vitro fertilization program (IVF/ET) with donated oocytes (OD). *Fertil Steril*. 1998. Abstract 0-076.S29.

107. Baluch B, Manyande, A, Aghassa MM, et al. Failing to conceive with in vitro fertilization: The Middle Eastern experience. *Psychol Rep*. 1993; 3:1107–10.

108. Craft I, al-Shawaf T. IVF versus GIFT. *J Assist Reprod Genet*. 1992; 9:424–7.

109. Sewpaul V. Culture, religion, and infertility: A South African perspective. *Brit J Soc Work*. 1999; 29: 742–54.

110. Boivin J, Scanlan LC, Walker SM. Why are infertile patients not using psychosocial counseling? *Hum Reprod*. 1999; 14:1384–91.

111. Hardy KV, Laszoloffy TA. The cultural genogram: Key to training culturally competent family therapists. *J Marital Fam Ther*. 1995; 21:227–37.

112. Odell M, Shelling G, Young KS, et al. The skills of the marriage and family therapist in straddling multicultural issues. *Am J Fam Ther*. 1994; 22:145–55.

113. Sodowsky GR, Taffe RC, Gatkin TB, et al. Development of the Multicultural Counseling Inventory: A self-report measure of multicultural competencies. *J Couns Psychol*. 1994; 41:127–48.

114. Friedman H, Krakaue S. Learning to draw and interpret standard and time-line genograms: An experimental comparison. *J Fam Psychol*. 1994; 41:127–48.

115. Keiley MK, Dolbin M, Hil J, et al. The cultural genogram: Experiences from within a marriage and family therapy training program. *J Marital Fam Ther*. 2002; 28:165–78.

116. McGoldrick M, Giodana J, Pearce J. *Ethnicity and Family Therapy*. 2nd ed. New York: Guilford; 1996.

117. McGill DW. The cultural story in multicultural family therapy. *Fam Soc*. 1992; 73:339–49.

118. Scherer KR, Wallbott HG. Evidence for universality and cultural variation of differential emotion response patterning. *J Pers Soc Psychol*. 1994; 66:310–28.

119. Mesquita B, Karasawa M. Different emotional lives. *Cognition & Emotion*. 2002; 16:127–41.

120. Kolata G. Infertile foreigners see opportunity in U.S. *New York Times*. 1-4-1998.

121. Hart VA. Infertility and the role of psychotherapy. *Issues Ment Health Nurs*. 2002; 23:31–41.

5 Psychosocial Evaluation of the Infertile Patient

SUSAN CARUSO KLOCK

Fear cannot be banished, but it can be calm and without panic; and it can be mitigated by reason and evaluation.
— Vannevar Bush

INTRODUCTION

The role of the mental health professional in evaluating infertility patients has evolved over the past two decades. While some mental health professionals may not believe in the 'assessment' portion of their work with infertility patients, many believe it is an integral part of their role in trying to understand what each couple needs as they approach treatment. Most programs now have a mental health provider as part of their treatment team, either on-site or as a designated consultant. This chapter describes the role of the mental health professional in providing psychosocial evaluation to the infertile couple.

The chapter

■ reviews the basic and specific areas that need to be addressed in the evaluation of an infertile couple;
■ addresses the use of psychological testing in the context of the evaluation.

HISTORICAL OVERVIEW

The role of the mental health professional in the evaluation and screening of infertility patients is relatively new, having evolved over the past twenty to twenty-five years. The use of a mental health professional either as a treatment team member or as a consultant is the norm in most academically based and large private practices in the industrialized world. However, there are still some physicians who do not use a mental health professional to work with their patients. They generally believe that they are able to counsel their own patients about the psychosocial aspects of infertility treatment and feel that an additional psychological referral is: (1) an added stress, (2) an unnecessary expense, and/or, (3) insulting to their patients. Nevertheless, mental health professionals continually work to demonstrate

their value in the reproductive medicine clinical setting. As this role continues to grow and develop, so too, hopefully, will outcome studies demonstrating the clinical utility of their role with infertility patients and the benefit to patients. Kentenich (in Boivin et al.) listed how infertility treatment differs from other types of medical consultation, and therefore, justifies the inclusion of a mental health professional in the provision of infertility care. He stated, "the focus of the treatment is: (1) the unfulfilled wish for a child (as opposed to the specific identification of a diagnosis or disease process); (2) the creation of a third person; (3) often unsuccessful; and (4) has an impact on the sexual and marital functioning of two partners, that fertility clinics should address the psychosocial needs of their patients."[1]

REVIEW OF LITERATURE

The goals of infertility treatment are to "accomplish a thorough investigation, to treat any abnormalities that are uncovered, to educate the couple to the workings of the reproductive system, to give the couple some estimate of their fertility potential, to counsel for adoption when appropriate, and to provide emotional support."[2] And while all team members contribute to patient care, it is the primary role of the mental health professional to address the psychosocial issues that emerge as the couple confronts infertility. The mental health professional evaluates, diagnoses, and treats psychological disorders. In addition, the infertility counselor provides patient education, an arena for facilitating decision making, a forum for discussing ethical and cultural issues related to treatment, and emotional follow-up when the treatment results in a pregnancy and especially, when it does not.

Typically, the initial psychosocial evaluation or consultation with the infertile couple is the first contact that the mental health professional has with the couple; therefore, providing knowledgeable, compassionate care is imperative. It is well known that infertility and its treatment are psychologically stressful, with virtually hundreds of articles published on the psychological concomitants of infertility treatment.[3] The stressfulness of infertility can be related to numerous issues,[4] including the blocking or postponement of an important life goal (having a child), marital discord related to infertility, the cyclical nature of treatment, the side effects of fertility medications, and the disappointment when treatment success rates do not match patient expectations. While it has been known for some time that infertility is stressful, it has been only recently that clinicians have acknowledged the need for psychosocial consultation as an integral part of infertility treatment.[5] To quote Christie,[6] "the physician needs to acquire a holistic perspective on infertility, so that he can assess somatic, psychological and social factors in each diagnostic work-up. Only then will he be in a position to evaluate and manage the complex human problems that can emerge during the diagnosis and treatment of a couple's infertility."

Although the majority of patients do not develop overt psychiatric disorders in response to involuntary childlessness, investigators have documented the occurrence of anxiety and depressive symptoms,[7–9] marital difficulties,[9,10] and changes in sexual functioning[9,11] during or after infertility treatment. The results from several studies indicate that women report greater infertility-related psychological stress than men.[12,13] In addition, occasionally an infertile patient may present with a significant preexisting psychiatric disorder; in which case, pregnancy may be contraindicated, based on concerns for both the patient and the potential child. If parenthood/pregnancy is not contraindicated, for the patient with a preexisting psychiatric disorder, special pretreatment preparation and care are warranted. For these reasons, many authors have recommended the routine provision of psychological services, both evaluation and treatment, to individuals and couples presenting for infertility treatment, especially those undergoing assisted reproductive technologies. Despite the expressed need for psychological services for infertile patients, there has been a paucity of information regarding the content of an initial psychosocial consultation and the identification of patient groups for whom a psychosocial consultation may be recommended or required. For example, some clinics may recommend a psychosocial consultation for all new patients, regardless of how much treatment they have previously received. Other clinics may recommend psychosocial consultations for subgroups of patients, depending on the type of treatment they are receiving, including in vitro fertilization (IVF), donor insemination (DI), oocyte donation (OD), and embryo donation (ED). Due to the nature of the treatment, there are several issues that need to be addressed with infertile patients that are not routinely covered in a typical first-visit psychological consultation.

THEORETICAL FRAMEWORK

The purpose of a psychological assessment is to gather information about an individual that describes their personal history and current level of functioning. The assessment can gather pieces of information in two ways: (1) a clinical interview and (2) psychological testing. In the clinical interview, specific questions are asked to obtain information about patients' history (family, education, occupation, and social history) and to ascertain their perception of the current event(s) leading to the psychological consultation. The clinical interview is also essential for assessing mental status and general interpersonal style via direct experience with the interviewer. Psychological interviews are not standardized and are subject to the biases of the interviewer and the interviewee. Psychological tests, on the other hand, are used when one wants to gather information about patients in a standardized manner and compare their responses to a preestablished norm. The role of psychological testing in the evaluation of infertile patients is discussed later in the chapter.

CLINICAL ISSUES

For the majority of men and women, having a child is an essential developmental milestone that cements their entry into adult social status. Most couples assume that they will be able to conceive effortlessly when they want to. When they try to conceive and are unsuccessful, many face, for the first time in their lives, the inability to meet a highly desired goal. This in turn begins to erode their previously held belief that they can do whatever they set their mind to, as long as they work hard enough. The couple then begins treatment and is exposed to a new world of medical technology, an invasion into their sexual and reproductive life, cyclical treatment demands, financial pressure, work absences, and relatively low per-cycle success rates. All of these factors over time can erode self-esteem, stress a previously solid marriage, and generally wreak havoc in a couple's life. For those less able to cope, these stresses can lead to the development of depression, anxiety disorders, obsessive-compulsive disorders, or sexual dysfunction.

For those more able to cope, their life is still turned upside down, and they are forced to question previously held beliefs about their life, their role in life, and their belief in a predictable, just world. The primary need for a psychological consultation is to aid in coping with the enormous psychological consequences of infertility and its treatment. A secondary reason that supports the use of a psychological consultation for infertility patients is patient satisfaction. It is the opinion and observation of many that patients are more satisfied when they believe that their psychological, as well as physical, health is being attended to by their physician. While some doctors continue to hold to the belief that they will insult their patients if they recommend a psychological consultation, today it is widely accepted and acknowledged worldwide that the majority of patients welcome the opportunity and feel more satisfied with their overall care when psychosocial support is available and offered.

Who Should Be Seen?

The question of who should have a psychosocial evaluation can be answered relatively easily. A psychological consultation with every infertile couple during the diagnostic work-up would be the ideal. While it may be impossible to see every infertile couple, the stakes become higher when patients begin to undergo an assisted reproductive technology procedure and/or make use of third-party reproduction options, such as DI, OD, ED, or gestational surrogacy. In these situations, it is widely believed that a psychological evaluation of all parties should be mandated due to the extraordinary circumstances around the possible conception of a child.[5,14] In addition, Dennerstein and Morse[15] reported that any patient who is perceived by the physician to be psychiatrically-at-risk should be referred. "These include patients with psychosomatic symptoms or current psychiatric disorder; past psychiatric treatment; where there is concern about motivation; stability of the marriage and capacity of parenthood; and those with unrealistic expectations of treatment." Ningel and Strauss[16] have stated that, in principle, psychological counseling should be available to all infertility patients. Availability to all patients would maximize the identification of at-risk individuals or couples and provide easy segue way to psychotherapy if it were needed. If psychosocial consultations remain on an 'as needed' basis, patients who are referred may feel stigmatized, which could result in increased attempts to mask or deny their difficulties. When operating on a routine basis, the role of the mental health professional is normalized, and the mental

health professional (infertility counselor) is viewed as just another member of the treatment team whose goal it is to aid the patient.

Some countries (United Kingdom, Canada, and Switzerland, for example) are required to offer psychological counseling to infertility patients or require that patients participate in counseling before proceeding with their treatment plan. The Human Fertilization and Embryo Authority[17] (HFEA) delineates three types of counseling to be offered depending on the couple and treatment context and provides a thorough outline for the provision of counseling to infertility patients. Canada passed legislation mandating counseling in licensed fertility treatment centers. Boivin and colleagues from several European nations in 2001 published infertility counseling guidelines[1] under the auspices of the European Society of Human Reproduction and Embryology (ESHRE). These guidelines describe the purpose and objectives for providing psychosocial care and counseling to infertility patients in both general and specific (e.g., high distress, end of treatment, and third-party reproduction) situations. This comprehensive outline is particularly useful in that it describes the purpose and objectives of counseling. It does not, however, specify exclusion criteria for couples who may not be deemed appropriate for treatment or explicate qualifications for persons who provide infertility counseling.

The Ethics Committee of the American Society for Reproductive Medicine (ASRM) recently published a report on "Child-rearing ability and the provision of fertility services."[18] This report describes the nature of the competing interests of the parties involved, that is, the infertility program that provides treatment, couples seeking treatment, and the potential child. The report presents the following conclusions: (1) fertility programs may withhold treatment to couples or individuals who may be unable to provide adequate childrearing for offspring; (2) fertility programs may treat persons who medically qualify (except in clear cases of significant harm to offspring); (3) fertility programs should develop written policies and procedures for making determinations to withhold services on the basis of concerns about the childrearing capacities; (4) a program's assessment of a patient's childrearing capacity should be made jointly among members of the program; and (5) persons with disabilities should not be denied fertility services except in rare cases where well-substantiated concerns exist.[18] Specific criteria are not provided in this report for withholding treatment but concerns regarding psychiatric illness, substance abuse or domestic abuse as they relate to the ability to provide adequate childrearing are provided as examples of when a program may withhold infertility treatment. Finally, the report states that, "the well-being of offspring is an overriding ethical concern that should be taken into account in determining whether to provide infertility services."[18, p. S209]

Psychological consultation for infertility patients should be available to any individual or couple who is self-referred. For those patients undergoing IVF, DI, OD, or ED, a routine psychological consultation should take place at least two weeks prior to the start of treatment. This allows the couple time to consider the many psychological, social, religious, and legal issues brought up during the psychological consultation. It may be indicative of a potential problem if patients want to rush through the evaluation process (both medical and psychological). They may be trying to push an unwilling partner through the treatment ("If I don't do it now, my husband won't do it"), deny their ambivalence ("I'd better do it now, or I'll lose my nerve"), or mask underlying pathology ("Let's get this over with"). When the medical and psychosocial evaluation happens over time, it tends to let the treatment team get to know the couple better, and issues or problems can emerge and be dealt with without the urgency and panic that might occur if a shortened timetable is used.

A research focus on the need for and utilization of infertility counseling has emerged over the past several years.[19] One recent prospective, randomized study of pre-IVF counseling indicated that, although the levels of depression and anxiety remained in the normal range for participants, routine pre-IVF counseling was judged acceptable by 80% of participants. Of those queried, 65% expected that counseling would be helpful. Among the 20% of participants in the study who refused counseling, reasons such as lack of time and knowledge of who could provide counseling were noted as obstacles.[20]

Who Should Do the Evaluation?

There are many different types of mental health practitioners, including psychiatrists, psychologists, social workers, psychiatric nurses, and a variety of therapists who have postgraduate training in a social science. Mental health professionals doing infertility-related work should also meet the fundamental requirements described by the Mental Health Professional Group (MHPG) of the ASRM and the ESHRE Guidelines. These guidelines provide the minimum training and experiential requirements for mental health practitioners in this area.

Globally, there is no consensus (and some controversy) regarding requirements or specialty licensure for infertility counselors. In the United States, the MHPG of the ASRM has begun exploring the various benefits and obstacles to credentialing and certification of infertility counselors. In other countries, Boivin et al. have noted that an agreed set of criteria for who should counsel has not been developed but that individuals providing counseling must be trained mental health professionals and have a working knowledge of the medical aspects of reproduction.[1]

An extremely important component of these guidelines is the recommendation that the infertility-related mental health professionals have a thorough working knowledge of the medical aspects of the infertility workup and treatment. Familiarity with procedures, medications, and various treatment protocols is a necessary foundation enabling the mental health clinician to work effectively with medical team professionals and communicate with patients. Patients seen by counselors without this background complain, with good reason, that they have to educate such counselors about the medical aspects of treatment, which is another hassle and expense for them. The interested reader should refer to Chapter 2 on Medical Aspects of Infertility in this book. Other excellent reviews include Rein and Schiff[21] and Hardy and Fox[22] regarding the evaluation and treatment, respectively, of the infertile couple. For a more thorough understanding of reproductive endocrinology, the reader should review Speroff and colleagues'[2] *Clinical Gynecologic Endocrinology and Infertility*. Last, clinicians can always update their fund of knowledge by attending one of the postgraduate courses at the annual meetings of professional societies such as ASRM, ESHRE, Canadian Fertility and Andrology Society, FLASEF [See Resources]. These courses provide up-to-the-minute information on the rapidly developing infertility treatment techniques and their psychological consequences.

What Is Being Assessed?

What is the mental health professional assessing during the psychological consultation with infertility patients? First, they are assessing all the usual content areas addressed in a psychological intake interview, such as the presenting problem, psychological history, social history (including current relationship and sexual functioning), medical history, family history, and current mental status. In addition to these topics, the infertility assessment includes a review of the treatment about to be undertaken, the implications of the treatment, a discussion of the perceived stress of the treatment, social support for the treatment, legal and ethical issues, expectations of treatment success, and the treatment plan. These are typically covered in the first hour, with additional time scheduled as needed.

The goal of the psychosocial evaluation is to:

- prepare patients for the treatment that they are about to undergo;
- raise issues that they may not have considered thus far, so that these can be discussed prior to treatment;
- screen for individuals who may benefit from psychological treatment either before or during infertility treatment;
- evaluate patents for any preexisting psychopathology or social dysfunction that would preclude or impact infertility treatment.

THERAPEUTIC INTERVENTIONS

Psychosocial Evaluation

Preparing for the Interview

Some logistics to consider prior to the interview include: (1) boundaries of confidentiality, (2) clarification of the mental health professional's role, and (3) documentation of the consultation. Health Insurance Portability and Accountability Act (HIPAA) regulations in the United States and other information-sharing regulations require that the patient understand what information is being collected and how the information is being used. The patient should be made aware of the nature of the information exchange between the psychologist and the treatment team. For example, if the mental health professional is part of the treatment team, he or she may be expected to provide relevant psychological information to the attending reproductive endocrinologist or other staff members. The nature of the consultation and consent to participate in the consultation should be discussed with the patient before the interview. According to the American Psychological Association (APA), "Informed consent includes an explanation of the nature and purpose of the assessment, fees, involvement of third parties, and limits of confidentiality and sufficient opportunity for the patient to ask questions and receive answers."[23, p. 13, section 9.03a] For example, if a single woman is being seen for a routine consultation regarding DI use and the consultation is geared toward determining if she is psychologically appropriate to receive the treatment, then that purpose must be clearly explicated to the patient before the interview; additionally, the patient would need to understand what portions of the assessment information would be shared (if any) with the treatment team, fees for the assessment, and whether she can ask any questions about the process. If a patient understands that information would be shared with others or be used to make a treatment decision, it may prompt the patient to be less than forthcoming with sensitive information during the interview. Disclosure about the purpose of the assessment is necessary to fully inform the patient. Additionally, the physicians and nurses who may describe the psychological consultation to the patient should be clear about the nature of the consultation as well. In the informed consent process, the patient needs to understand the implications of the assessment and/or therapy and actively agree to participate in it. The informed consent process is based on the ethical principle of respect for persons and the individual's autonomy to participate or not in the requested activity. The consent may be a written document the patient and therapist sign, or a structured discussion that is documented in the patient's chart. Regardless of the form it takes, obtaining informed consent is a process by which the therapist and patient communicate the goals, method, and conditions of the consultation or therapy. This can clarify the expectations of both parties and decrease misunderstandings and miscommunications. In the case of psychotherapy in the context of infertility, many mental health professionals now also obtain consent to engage in a psychotherapeutic relationship.

Consent from the patient is needed for exchange of information to other health professionals and should be documented in the patient's chart after it has been obtained. The mental health professional must also be careful to maintain privacy boundaries for information that patients do not wish to be shared. A common example of information that a patient may not want her physician to know is previous sexual or reproductive trauma. As with any other type of consultation, the mental health professional's first obligation is to maintain patient confidentiality, but it is also to encourage patients to share any medically relevant information with their physician. In addition, the mental health professional should be aware of the laws governing the creation and storage of psychiatric records. For example, in some states, psychiatric and psychological reports and records are kept in a separate medical record to protect patient privacy. If this is the case, then only documentation of basic information (date, purpose, and time of interview; recommendation(s); and plan) in a couple's medical chart is appropriate, and the major portion of the confidential information should be kept in a separate location. Some infertility counselors maintain this practice even if it is not legally mandated in their locale.

Preparation of a couple for the interview can be done by the physician or nurse on the team. In many practices, a couple is informed that the psychological consultation is a routine part of the diagnostic work-up; therefore, the couple learns early on that this is an expected part of the treatment process, just like an ultrasound examination or other procedure. In addition, the couple's primary nurse or treatment coordinator is responsible for helping schedule the psychological consultation appointment. Often, it is helpful for a couple to briefly meet and say hello to the mental health professional prior to the interview, so that their anxiety about the interview is minimized.

A couple can be told briefly about the purpose of the interview, which is to learn more psychosocial information about them that may impact their infertility treatment, to ease their psychological adjustment to the infertility diagnosis and treatment, and to act as a resource, should they need one. In addition, the consultation provides a couple with the opportunity to discuss the ethical, religious, and moral issues related to treatment, to review treatment success rates, to ask questions about the informed-consent process, and to seek assistance in decisions about ending treatment and obtaining counseling regarding adoption or child-free living. In some cases, health education may also be part of the interview in that it may be the infertility counselor's responsibility to address issues related to smoking cessation, chemical abuse/addiction, and/or obesity. It is often useful to encourage patients to come prepared with their own questions or concerns to make the best use of the interview. It is helpful to provide written information for patients that they receive prior to the appointment, explaining the purpose/goals of the interview, what to expect, preparations, and cost.

Content of the Evaluation Interview

The foundation for the clinical interview for infertility patients is the same as a general psychological interview with elaboration and greater detail in obtaining information in areas related to reproductive history, marital history, sexual functioning, and cultural and religious issues. Given the nature of infertility (i.e., the majority of patients are married or in a committed relationship), the identified patient is most often a couple, not an individual woman alone. Therefore, the husband or partner's presence at the psychological evaluation is imperative. Not only does this give the clinician another source of information about the couple's history, but more importantly, it can also provide a snapshot of how the couple works (or does not work) together in conceptualizing and coping with infertility. The absence of the husband or partner on repeated occasions can indicate significant marital discord or ambivalence about treatment and/or parenthood on his part.

A useful model for the structured clinical interview is the Comprehensive Psychosocial History for Infertility[24] (CPHI, see Appendix 3). The CPHI provides clinicians with the structure for an interview that covers the needed content areas specific to infertile populations. As the authors note, the CPHI can be used by a variety of health professionals. It covers the spectrum of issues relevant to the emotional status of infertile patients, as well as issues relevant to a couple's functioning, and it can help identify 'red flag' issues that may be indicators that a couple is at risk for a poor adjustment to infertility treatment or that, in more serious cases, infertility treatment may need to be postponed or denied.

The content areas in the CPHI are self-explanatory. As a clinician goes through each section, information can be elicited from one or both partners about each area. It may be a good idea to begin by addressing the infertility history question to the woman because (1) she is usually the primary recipient of diagnostic and treatment interventions; (2) it is often easier for the woman to break the ice in the initial part of the interview; and (3) she can provide a role model for her husband or partner about how to talk about the emotionally sensitive issues related to infertility.

Gathering information. The first thing a clinician needs to determine is whether patients are accurate and reliable informants. Because of the high socioeconomic status of the majority of infertility patients, this is generally not a problem, but in some instances individuals may not be able to give reliable information or may be purposefully deceptive. A second fundamental cognitive prerequisite is that individuals fully understand the medical procedure(s) that are about to be performed and are cognitively able to provide informed consent. Patients must be able to understand a procedure's risks, benefits, and chances for success. Occasionally, a patient with little education will come for treatment, or may speak another language, and may not comprehend the nature of the treatment and its risks and benefits. When language is an issue, it is important for the infertility counselor to have an impartial translator available to interpret.

In discussion of a couple's reproductive history, it is important to spend some time asking the infertile partner (if one has been identified) how he or she feels about being the 'one with the problem.' If the infertile partner has been identified, he or she may feel isolated, embarrassed, ashamed, and sad about the diagnosis but may be unable to talk to his or her partner about it. The infertile person often feels a huge sense of responsibility for being the one preventing a pregnancy and typically has fears that the fertile partner will leave or feel resentment. In the context of the consultation, it is useful to have both partners talk about their reaction to the infertility diagnosis and its impact on their self-esteem and marital equilibrium (see Chapter 3).

Marital or relationship history and the impact of the infertility are other topics to be addressed in the consultation interview. The circumstances surrounding courtship, marriage, and current marital situation can provide information about many aspects of the marriage, including how a couple handles relationship discord, emotional support of one another, division of labor, decision making, and expression of emotional needs. During this discussion, the motivation of each partner to pursue infertility treatment and become a parent also emerges.

An unfortunate, but somewhat common, scenario is the couple seeking infertility treatment as a way to mend a faltering relationship or guarantee the continuation of a relationship. For example, an older woman in a relationship with a younger man may feel pressured to pursue infertility treatment to prove to her partner that she is still able to provide children or to ensure that he will not abandon her for a younger, fertile woman. Contingencies for the continuation of the relationship may rest on the outcome of the infertility treatment. In this situation, both partners will perceive an inordinate amount of pressure on the outcome of the treatment and want to begin treatment as soon as possible. However, it is advisable to slow the couple down and try to address this situation prior to beginning treatment.

In addition to the social support supplied within the marriage, a clinician will also want to assess the availability and quality of the social support from family and friends, as well as the cultural context in which they live. This is taken into consideration along with the tendency of a couple to be open or private regarding their infertility diagnosis and treatment. It is also important to determine if there are any cultural or religious factors influencing their response to infertility and treatment options. Often men and women differ in regard to how open they are with family and friends regarding their infertility. Problems can arise when one partner tells too many people too much about the infertility diagnosis and treatment or refuses to respect the other's need for privacy or support. This can cause a rift in the relationship and/or prompt unwanted intrusions or questions from family and friends. Therefore, initial discussion about a plan for the type and amount of disclosure is often helpful.[25]

Obtaining an accurate psychiatric history for both partners is essential. Due to the demographics of infertility patients, in general, partners are usually high-functioning, but this does not preclude the existence of a past or current psychiatric illness. The psychiatric history is important because it may impact the adjustment to pregnancy and the patient's ability to parent. For example, if a woman has major depression, discontinuation of antidepressants during infertility treatment and the possible reemergence of depression during pregnancy and the postpartum period need to be carefully considered. A psychiatric illness does not rule out the possibility of infertility treatment, but it needs to be assessed in order to make arrangements for the maintenance of psychiatric stability during treatment, pregnancy, and the transition to parenthood.

Although it is not included in the CPHI, it is a good idea to discuss a couple's legal history. It is extremely rare that a patient will have a legal history relevant to the infertility treatment, but legal history is relevant if it relates to instances of child neglect, endangerment, or abuse. Also relevant are legal entanglements indicating current alcoholism or drug addiction (e.g., 'Driving Under the Influence' arrest), particularly in women. If such a history is found, then further information regarding the specific charges, reparation, or rehabilitation should be obtained. An additional legal issue pertains to 'reproductive tourists,' patients who travel to another country to obtain treatment that is unavailable or expensive in their own country. Visa restrictions may have an impact on treatment timelines and patient motivation. In one country, couples may receive treatment that is banned in another.

During the course of the structured interview, the individual's and couple's style of coping will become evident. Most infertility patients tend to use problem-focused coping, which may be a reason why they choose to seek infertility treatment. This style of coping is generally helpful, but couples need to understand that treatment outcome is not related to the amount of planning, medical compliance, and behavioral change that they undergo. This may be the first time that a couple experiences a situation in which the attainment of a highly desired goal is not related to the effort that they expend toward meeting that goal. This irony is one of the key components of the stressfulness of infertility treatment to otherwise highly effective and successful people.

Managing expectations. Infertility treatment is a less-than-perfect art. The per-cycle pregnancy and take-home-baby rates generally vary from clinic to clinic and procedure to procedure, depending on a couple's diagnosis. Therefore, it is important for mental health professionals to be aware of the success rates for their clinic in order to talk candidly about a couple's expectations for treatment success. More often than not, a couple is not able to absorb all the information given to them during the medical consultation, including success-rate information.[26] Moreover, they may hear the statistics and inflate them, based on information specific to the couple. For example, a thirty-year-old couple may have been told that they have a 35% chance of getting pregnant with use of gonadotropin medications and intrauterine insemination. They may tell themselves that because they are relatively young, have been in treatment a short time, and are 'good people,' their own chances for success are higher. This increasing optimism sets up an inaccurate expectancy that can lead to a dysphoric or even depressive reaction in the event that the cycle is unsuccessful. In the course of the psychological consultation, it is important for mental health professionals to ask a couple about their perception of the chances for treatment success and help them maintain a cautiously optimistic attitude.

In the past twenty-five years since the advent of IVF, mental health professionals have had to talk to couples about their thoughts and feelings about extracorporeal creation of embryos, freezing and thawing of embryos, and disposition of unused embryos. Usually, within the context of this discussion, a couple also is made aware of the likelihood of a multiple pregnancy and the option of selective reduction. All of these issues are jarring to the couple who 'just wants to have a baby.' Couples, out of necessity, are forced to discuss and make decisions about things they never thought possible. In the psychosocial evaluation, mental health professionals can discuss each of these issues and elicit any religious, cultural, or moral differences between the partners as well as acceptability of the options for patients. Some individuals may object to the cryopreservation of embryos; others may disagree with one another regarding the disposition of unused embryos. The mental health professional can play a pivotal role in helping couples discuss their differences and come to a consensus regarding these important decisions. The decision can then be conveyed to the treatment team to allow greater clarity in clinical care and fewer last-minute decisions and/or misunderstandings, and additionally avoiding iatrogenetic distress.

Issues regarding multiple pregnancy and selective reduction are increasingly common. During the consultation, a couple may, for the first time, have the time to think about the implications of a multiple pregnancy and the possibility of parenting twins, triplets, or more. Couples often resist discussions of multiple pregnancy during the psychological consultation because they are solely focused on the goal of getting pregnant. They may dismiss these discussions by stating that they would be delighted with a 'family' instead of just one child

TABLE 5.1. Psychosocial contraindications to infertility treatment
Treatment or pregnancy may significantly worsen an active psychiatric illness
Active substance dependence with concomitant chaotic lifestyle
One partner is coercing the other to proceed with treatment
One or both partners are unable or unwilling to provide consent for the treatment
A legal history related to child endangerment is discovered
Infertility treatment is used to compensate for a sexual dysfunction
Decisions about privacy and disclosure in third-party reproduction cannot be resolved
Use of a family member gamete donor would cause significant familial discord
Custody arrangements for the potential child of a known gamete donor have not been agreed to by all parties
Serious marital discord

and may minimize concerns about the welfare of the mother and infants in multiple pregnancies. It may take some redirection to help them understand the importance of preemptive discussion to aid in possible decision making later on. It is a difficult clinical situation, if there is a multiple pregnancy and the partners disagree with one another about their course of action. Again, as with the issue of cryopreservation of embryos, multiple pregnancy rates should be discussed with patients by their physician; while mental health professionals should focus on the partners' emotional and moral reaction to the possibility and aid in decision making if a difference is identified.

Communicating recommendations. After completion of the interview, clinicians can begin summarizing the information and coming up with impressions and recommendations. Most couples are high-functioning and psychologically aware. Therefore, mental health professionals may only need to remind the couple about adaptive coping skills, provide them with information or educational materials regarding the treatment, and offer further follow-up as needed. Unfortunately, treatment may be contraindicated in a minority of cases. In general, infertility treatment is contraindicated and may be denied or postponed under certain circumstances. The contraindications for infertility treatment are listed in Table 5.1. When a clinic denies or postpones treatment to an individual or couple, the decision can be conveyed verbally to the patient and then reiterated in a follow-up letter. It is helpful if the letter recapitulates the reasons that were discussed with the patient and also includes appropriate referral information, if necessary. The letter can be cosigned by the attending physician, the mental health professional, and the medical director to decrease the focus on the mental health professional and to limit the amount of manipulation that may take place from the patient.

When one of these situations occurs, the evaluating clinician has to carefully review his or her boundaries prior to making treatment recommendations. If further infertility treatment is contingent on the solution of a problem that requires psychotherapy, and the evaluating clinician is an employee of the infertility program, it is advisable for the evaluating clinician to refer the couple to a different treating clinician. In cases when a problem is identified, but it is not serious enough to preclude treatment, then the conflict of interest between the evaluating and treating clinicians is not as great. If the evaluating clinician feels that there is a conflict of interest between themselves, the couple, and the program, it is wise to refer to a colleague not affiliated with the infertility program and then obtain consent from the couple that the evaluating clinician receive information about their treatment progress when infertility treatment is desired in the future. This is often a time-consuming and difficult boundary to maintain, but for all concerned, it is the best option for keeping couples' needs in the forefront and to reduce the likelihood of biased treatment.

Related to this issue is the communication of the results of the psychosocial evaluation to the team and the sharing of information obtained in the interview. Clinicians may want to write a note in the medical record indicating:

▮ date and time of the interview;
▮ general content of the interview ("Reviewed couple's history and discussed the emotional concomitants of the treatment.");
▮ impression regarding the couple's preparedness for treatment ("The couple appear to be appropriate candidates for this treatment." or "Further clarification and treatment of marital difficulties need to be completed before initiation of treatment.");
▮ plan ("routine social support follow-up offered") or referral (e.g., for marital therapy); and
▮ indication of full intake summary report and its location ("Full intake note dictated on . . . , filed in separate psychological record.").

It is a good idea to inform couples that the recommendation will be shared with the team and that in the event of postponement or refusal of treatment the information will be shared with the attending physician. In keeping within the boundaries of confidentiality among mental health professionals, it is important for patients to know that specific information obtained in the history is not shared with the treatment team. This applies to all information but is especially important in cases in which there have been previous pregnancy terminations, sexual abuse, or legal problems.

The final purpose of the psychosocial evaluation is to provide couples with the feeling that they have an open door to a person with expertise in reproductive psychology who can be a resource to them in the future. Clinicians should leave time at the end of the interview for questions and long-term treatment planning. After the initial consultation, many couples find it useful to come in for a consultation when considering ending treatment and/or moving to adoption. Also, in cases of a pre-IVF oocyte donor or sperm donor evaluation, it is a good idea to call after the completion of the first treatment cycle to check in with patients and see how they are feeling. This is usually a welcome opportunity to talk about their emotional reaction to treatment.

Psychological Testing

Role in the Evaluation of Infertility Patients

In general practice, the interview provides the majority of information gathered during the routine psychological evaluation of an infertile couple. This information is easy to obtain and is usually reliable. There may be cases in which the clinician wants a second source of information to provide confirmation of refutation of the interview material. In these cases, the use of psychological testing may be helpful.

Psychological cognitive tests were developed around the turn of the century as a way of assessing the skills and competencies of a large group of people on a uniform set of tasks. Personality tests were developed to get the unique response of an individual to standardized testing material in a controlled situation. The test results received from one individual can then be compared with the test's established norms for the representative sample to which the individual belongs. Testing is a useful source of additional information, but it is not a substitute for a clinical interview. Before discussion of the use of psychological tests with infertility patients, some basic background on the characteristics of psychological tests may be helpful.

Characteristics of Psychological Tests

Psychological tests can be either projective, such as the Rorschach inkblot test, in which a person's response to ambiguous stimuli is interpreted, or objective, such as the Minnesota Multiphasic Personality Inventory (MMPI), in which a person's answers to direct questions with a true or false response are scored via empirically derived scoring criteria. In both cases, responses are compared to preestablished norms. The difference between projective and objective tests is the degree to which the test administrator interprets the results: Projective tests are subject to greater interpretation than objective tests. Psychological tests can assess multidimensional characteristics, such as personality or intelligence, or a single psychological construct or attribute, such as anxiety or depression. The utility of either type of test is dependent on how well it answers the question that a clinician wants answered. For example, within the context of infertility, if it were known that a woman who had high levels of anxiety needed more anesthesia and nursing support during a laparoscopy, then pretreatment anxiety testing would be useful in determining which patients were more anxious to plan for greater anesthesia and nursing coverage. In this example, an anxiety test would be useful in helping plan the allocation of clinical resources. But before a test can be used to predict behavior, two important characteristics about the test must be established: validity and reliability.

Validity and reliability are two key concepts in the theory of test construction.[27] In their simplest form, validity refers to how well a test measures what it purports to measure, and reliability refers to how consistently the measure assesses what it purports to measure. A test is essentially useless if it does not have moderate to high levels of validity and reliability. How do you know if a test is valid and/or reliable? There are several types of validity. One is called *content* validity, referring to the extent to which the items on a test assess the construct that it is trying to assess. For example, a test assessing depression should include items known to be symptoms of depression. A second type of validity is called *criterion-related* validity, referring to the process of checking to see whether a score on a test is correlated with an actual behavior hypothesized to be measured by the test. For example, scores on a depression test would be correlated with clinicians' ratings of depression. The extent to which the scores on the test and the clinicians' ratings corresponded would be the degree to which the test had criterion-related validity. A third type of validity is *construct* validity, referring to how well a test correlates with other measures of the same con-

struct. For example, we would expect that a new measure of depression would be highly correlated with an older measure of depression. The test constructors usually investigate all these types of validity before a test becomes widely used. Prior to using a test, it is important for clinicians to understand the degree of validity the measure has to know its strengths and limitations in a given situation.

Reliability refers to the consistency of a test. There are two types of reliability, internal consistency and test–retest reliability. *Internal consistency* refers to the intercorrelation of items on a test and the extent to which they measure the same construct. For example, on a measure of depression, all the items should be related to the construct of depression and should correlate with one another. *Test–retest reliability* refers to the correlation of test scores over time. It reflects the extent to which the score on a test given at time one will be similar to the score obtained on the same test at time two. A final word about reliability: Reliability is not necessarily correlated with validity. A test may be very reliable to the extent that it consistently yields the same result time after time, but it may not be valid to the extent that it does not measure the construct of interest.

Literature Review on Psychological Testing

In addition to the clinical interview, some clinicians working with infertile patients routinely use psychological tests, usually personality tests, to obtain further information. While numerous measures, including the MMPI, MMPI-2, Symptom Checklist 90 (SCL-90) Speilberger's State-Trait Anxiety Inventory (STAI), and the Beck Depression Inventory (BDI), have been used to evaluate infertile patients in clinical research, their utility in the clinical context for predictive purposes has not been demonstrated.

Several researchers have used psychological tests with infertility patients. They have generally addressed one of the following points: (1) identification of psychopathology among idiopathic infertile women; (2) assessment of personality and other psychological constructs among IVF participants; and (3) assessment of depression, anxiety, locus of control, and/or coping among pregnant and nonpregnant infertility patients to determine if psychological variables correlate with pregnancy outcome. There have been no studies addressing the clinical utility of psychological tests in predicting psychological outcome among general infertility patients.

IVF participants seem to be the most studied group of infertility patients[8,28,29]. During the mid- to late

1980s, several studies reported the use of the MMPI[30] with IVF patients.[31] The MMPI-2 is the recent revision of the MMPI. It has 567 true/false items in ten clinical scales and five validity scales that are designed to detect psychopathology.[30] Scale scores of sixty-five or higher on any of the clinical scales are indicative of psychopathology and may be indicative of a psychological disorder, but there is no one-to-one correlation between MMPI-2 scores and the presence of psychiatric illness. The MMPI-2 has been translated and validated in more than twenty languages, including Chinese, Dutch, German, French, Spanish, and Hebrew. In a series of 200 IVF couples, Freeman and coworkers[8] found that 20% of men and women had at least one elevated clinical scale suggesting dysfunctional emotional distress or personality difficulties. Approximately 50% of the sample also had high levels of ego strength, indicating that they had a fair amount of emotional resilience to deal with the stress of the treatment. Alternatively, Haseltine and colleagues[28] reported no major personality disorders or psychological dysfunction on abbreviated MMPIs given to seventy-five couples in an IVF program. Keye and associates[32] found normal MMPI scores among all twenty-two women entering an IVF program, but 17% of the male IVF participants had abnormal MMPI profiles. In general, the MMPI has been used with IVF couples as a pretreatment screening tool to detect the small percentage of patients who may have preexisting psychopathology that might impact their ability to participate in treatment. As Mazure and Greenfeld[29] noted, "the single most important finding has been that, in general, IVF/ET participants score within normal limits on measurements of preexisting psychopathology. Furthermore, the data do not support the notion of an increased incidence of psychiatric diagnoses or psychosexual disorders in IVF participants." A recent large study of German couples confirms this view.[33]

Other psychologically relevant constructs have also been studied among infertility patients, with again most studies focusing on IVF participants. Using a variety of measures, studies have looked at the incidence of depression,[12,34,35] anxiety,[7,12,28,34–37] marital adjustment,[37,38] sexual functioning,[8,9,39] and ways of coping.[34,38] These studies have helped characterize the psychological state of couples undergoing IVF treatment but are limited in generalization to other infertility patients because IVF patients represent a small, self-selected group who may differ from others who decide to stop treatment to pursue adoption or remain childless, or those couples who get pregnant without assisted reproductive technologies.

The clinical recommendations regarding the use of psychological tests have been relatively sparse. The use of personality testing among infertility patients as a screening device seems to have indicated that infertility patients have no greater incidence of personality disorders than that found in the general population. Findings from other construct-specific tests, such as depression and anxiety inventories, have produced mixed results, indicating that infertility patients may be depressed or anxious at times during the treatment. Other tests have addressed coping styles, marital adjustment, and sexual functioning in relationship to infertility and, with the exception of a few studies,[12,38,40,41] have not linked pretreatment test findings to posttreatment adjustment. In addition, there have been no studies comparing the predictive utility of clinical interview data with that of testing data in predicting outcome among infertility patients. Furthermore, numerous methodological flaws, such as limited patient selection, participation rates, and attrition, make generalization from these studies difficult. Finally, the relationship between a given test result at time one and its relationship to an outcome of interest at time two has not been demonstrated. If a measure such as a pretreatment depression instrument was helpful in identifying those women who would develop a clinical depression after their third cycle of infertility treatment, then that test would have a high clinical utility. There have been few studies addressing the relationship between pretreatment psychological status and posttreatment outcomes. Those that have been done have been interesting and have indicated that there are relationships between pretreatment coping style and posttreatment adjustment[38,40] and pretreatment depression and posttreatment depression,[12] but further studies of this kind are needed to demonstrate the clinical utility of specific psychological measures.

Use of Psychological Testing

Although the research on psychological testing as a screening tool for infertility patients is emerging, it is common practice for psychological tests to be used in clinical evaluation. Psychological testing provides an additional measure to support clinical impressions and can additionally be used as a treatment intervention when the results are reviewed with the patient. If the infertility counselor is using psychometric testing, a few caveats should be kept in mind. Psychometric testing (particularly the MMPI) must be administered by a mental health professional qualified and trained to administer, score, and interpret the psychometric testing. Historically, this has been primarily psychologists, but other mental health professionals can and do pursue training qualifications in psychometric testing. Furthermore, it is the responsibility of the mental heath professional to ensure that the all appropriate testing procedures are followed (including administering the test according to testing regulations, standardized instructions, and testing in person).

Prior to testing, it is good practice to review with the patient the purpose of the testing, how the test results will be used, and how the patient will be informed of the test results. For example, in the case of screening gamete donors, the MMPI-2 is often used in conjunction with a clinical interview. The prospective donor should be informed that the test results will or will not be provided to her (depending on the practice of the clinic) and delineate whether the test results will be shared with the prospective recipient. Patients should also be told that if their test results fall outside of the bounds of normal limits, they will not be eligible to participate in the gamete donation process.

The major challenges with administering psychological tests are being prepared to: (1) use the information once it is obtained, and (2) to terminate the process if the patient's testing indicates and/or validates a problem. An invalid profile means the testing cannot be interpreted because the test-taker is being deceptive, has not completed all the questions, is being defensive, or otherwise has systematically biased the results. On the MMPI-2, a T-score is specified for each validity scale that would likely indicate an invalid profile. Additionally, the T-scores levels on the various clinical scales are often associated with clinically significant psychopathology. Unfortunately, the infertility counselor may not know why the abnormal results are found, but he or she must be prepared to terminate the process or provide psychological intervention because abnormal results are a contraindication for participation in infertility treatment. It may be difficult to terminate the patient's participation in infertility treatment based on psychological testing results but, from a risk management perspective, allowing the individual to continue despite the presence of abnormal test results puts the practitioner and the clinic in a precarious position. If there is an adverse outcome and the interview and testing results are reviewed, the mental health professional should be prepared to explain why the treatment process continued in the face of nonnormative information from the testing. If the mental health professional is not a member of the infertility treatment team, and recommends that the patient not be offered services, they should state their opinion and their rationale in writing and provide it to the treatment team. If the treatment team provides services and there is an adverse outcome, then the mental health professional has documented his or her position on the case.

FUTURE IMPLICATIONS

As the provision of assisted reproductive technologies grows, it is likely that the role of the mental health professional in providing consultation to patients will also grow, driven by the highly complex third- and fourth-party reproduction practices among nontraditional patients, (e.g., single women, gay and lesbian couples) as well as traditional couples seeking nontraditional treatment (PGD for social reasons, posthumous reproduction and embryo disposition). The complexity of these types of cases requires input from the mental health professional.

An additional possibility in the future will be psychological studies with representative samples of infertility patients to determine whether psychological tests can substantially add to the pretreatment screening information or can predict outcomes of clinical importance, such as the occurrence of depression, marital discord, length of treatment, or pregnancy. The further refinement of the integration of psychological testing with the clinical interview presents a challenge to mental health researchers. At present, the skilled clinician must determine how and when to interface psychological testing into the clinical evaluation process.

SUMMARY

▥ **Infertility treatment is psychologically stressful; therefore, many programs offer consultation with a trained mental health professional prior to treatment, 'as needed,' or in the context of specific treatments.**
▥ **The MHPG of ASRM and Psychology and Counseling Special Interest Group of ESHRE have developed guidelines for qualifications and services of mental health professionals providing infertility-related services (see Appendix 1).**
▥ **The purpose of the interview is to educate and prepare couples for the treatment and to detect the presence of any psychosocial problem that would be a contraindication for infertility treatment or impact participation in treatment.**
▥ **The Comprehensive Psychosocial History for Infertility (CPHI) is an excellent structured interview to use with infertility patients (see Appendix 3).**
▥ **Criteria for exclusion from treatment include the presence of an active, major psychiatric disorder, severe relationship discord, cognitive impairment, or inability to resolve legal and ethical issues around third-party reproduction.**

■ While numerous psychological tests have been used with infertile samples, there is not yet enough research-based evidence to support the routine use of psychological tests to predict outcomes of interest among infertility patients.

REFERENCES

1. Boivin J, Appleton TC, Baetens P, et al. Guidelines for counselling in infertility: Outline version. *Hum Reprod* 2001; 16:1301–4.

2. Speroff L, Glass RH, Kase NG. *Clinical Gynecologic Endocrinology and Infertility*, 4th ed. Baltimore: Williams & Wilkins, 1989.

3. American Society for Reproductive Medicine, *Mental Health Professional Group Bibliography*. Birmingham, AL: American Society for Reproductive Medicine, 1996.

4. Mahlstedt PP. The psychological component of infertility. *Fertil Steril* 1985; 43:335–42.

5. Klock SC, Maier D. Guidelines for the provision of psychological services at the University of Connecticut Health Center. *Fertil Steril* 1991; 56:680–5.

6. Christie GL. The psychological and social management of the infertile couple. In: RJ Pepperell , B Hudson, C Wood, eds. *The Infertile Couple*. New York: Churchill Livingstone, 1980; 229–47.

7. Mazure CM, Del'Aune W, De Cherney AH. Two methodological issues in the psychological study of in vitro fertilization/embryo transfer participants. *J Psychosom Obstet Gynaecol* 1988; 9:17–21.

8. Freeman E, Boxer As, Rickels K, et al. Psychological evaluation and support in a program of in vitro fertilization and embryo transfer. *Fertil Steril* 1985; 43:48–53.

9. Baram D, Tourelot E, Muechler E, et al. Psychosocial adjustment following unsuccessful in vitro fertilization. *J Psychosom Obstet Gynaecol* 1988; 9:181–90.

10. Micioni G, Jeker L, Zeeb M, et al. Doubtful and negative psychological indications for AID: A study of 835 couples. *J Psychosom Obstet Gynaecol* 1987; 6:89–99.

11. Downey J, Yingling S, McKinney M, et al. Mood disorders, psychiatric symptoms, and distress in women presenting for infertility evaluation. *Fertil Steril* 1989; 52:425–32.

12. Newton CR, Hearn MT, Yuzpe AA. Psychological assessment and follow-up after in vitro fertilization: Assessing the impact of failure. *Fertil Steril* 1990; 54:879–86.

13. Nachtigall RD, Becker G, Wozny M. The effect of gender-specific diagnosis on men's and women's response to infertility. *Fertil Steril* 1992; 57:113–21.

14. Klock SC. Psychological aspects of donor insemination. *Infertil Reprod Med Clin North Am* 1993; 4:455–70.

15. Dennerstein L, Morse C. A review of psychological and social aspects of in vitro fertilization. *J Psychosom Obstet Gynaecol* 1988; 9:159–70.

16. Ningel K, Strauss B. Psychological diagnosis, counseling and psychotherapy in fertility medicine – an overview. In: B. Strauss, ed. *Involuntary Childlessness: Psychological Assessment, Counseling and Psychotherapy*. Seattle: Hogrefe & Huber; 19–34.

17. Human Fertilization and Embryo Authority. Code of Practice, 6th edn. 2002 London, England, 2003. www.hfea.uk.gov.

18. American Society for Reproductive Medicine. Child-rearing ability and the provision of fertility services. *Fertil Steril* 2004; 82(Suppl 1):S208–S2111.

19. Boivin J, Scanlan LC, Walker SM. Why are infertile patients not using psychosocial counseling? *Hum Reprod* 1999; 14:1384–91.

20. Emery M, Beran MD, Darwiche J, et al. Results from a prospective, randomized, controlled study evaluating the acceptability and effects of routine pre-IVF counselling. *Hum Reprod* 2003; 18:2647–53.

21. Rein MS, Schiff I. Evaluation of the infertile couple. In: KJ Ryan, RS, Berkowitz, RL Barbieri, eds. *Kistner's Gynecology: Principles and Practice*, 6th ed. St. Louis, MO: Mosby-Yearbook, 1995; 278–304.

22. Hardy RI, Fox J. Infertility treatment. In: KJ Ryan, RS Berkowitz, RL Barbieri, eds. *Kistner's Gynecology: Principles and Practice*, 6th ed. St. Louis, MO: Mosby-Yearbook, 1995; 305–30.

23. American Psychological Association. Ethical Principles of Psychologist and Code of Conduct. American Psychological Association, Washington, D.C. 2002 www.apa.org.

24. Burns LH, Greenfeld DA, for the Mental Health Professional Group. *CPHI: Comprehensive Psychosocial History for Infertility*. Birmingham, AL: American Society for Reproductive Medicine, 1990.

25. Klock SC. Privacy and disclosure in infertility treatment. In *Session: Psychotherapy in Practice* 1996; 2:55–71.

26. Reading AE., Kerin J. Psychologic aspects of providing infertility services. *J Reprod Med* 1989; 34:861–71.

27. Mazure C. What can we learn from psychological testing? In: *Clinical Assessment and Counseling in Third-Party Reproduction*. Presented at the 26th annual meeting of the American Society for Reproductive Medicine, Montreal, Quebec, Canada, October 3, 1993.

28. Haseltine FP, Mazure CM, Del'Aune W, et al. Psychological interview in screening couples undergoing in vitro fertilization. *Ann NY Acad Sci* 1985; 442:523–32.

29. Mazure CM, Greenfeld DA. Psychological studies of in vitro fertilization/embryo transfer participants. *J In Vitro Fertil Emb Transfer* 1989; 6:242–56.

30. Graham, JR. *MMPI-2: Assessing Personality and Psychopathology*, 2nd ed. New York: Oxford University Press, 1993.

31. Garner CH, Kelly M, Arnold ES. Psychological profile of IVF patients. *Fertil Steril* 1984; 41(suppl):57S.

32. Keye WR, Bensch RL, Jones KP, et al. The psychosocial evaluation of couples undergoing in vitro fertilization. *J In Vitro Fertil Emb Transfer* 1984; 1:119–26.

33. Wischmann T, Stammer H, Scherg H, et al. Psychosocial characteristics of infertile couples: A study by the Heidelberg Fertility Consultation Service. *Hum Reprod* 2001; 16:1753–61.

34. Shatford LA, Hearn MT, Yuzpe AA, et al. Psychological correlates of differential infertility diagnosis in an in vitro fertilization program. *Am J Obstet Gynecol* 1988; 158:1099–107.

35. Hearn MT, Yuzpe AA, Brown SE, et al. Psychological characteristic of in vitro fertilization participants. *Am J Obstet Gynecol* 1987; 156:269–74.

36. Thiering P, Beaurepaire J, Jones M, et al. Mood state as a predictor of treatment outcome after in vitro

fertilization/embryo transfer technology. *J Psychosom Res* 1993; 37:481–91.

37. Shaw P, Johnston M, Shaw R. Counselling needs, emotional and relationship problems in couples awaiting IVF. *J Psychosom Obstet Gynaecol* 1988; 9:171–80.

38. Litt MD, Tennen H, Affleck G, et al. Coping and cognitive factors in adaptation to in vitro fertilization failure. *J Behav Med* 1992; 15:171–87.

39. Leiblum S, Kemmann E, Lane MK. The psychological concomitants of in vitro fertilization. *J Psychosom Obstet Gynaecol* 1987; 6:65–78.

40. Morrow KA, Toreson RW, Penney LL. Predictors of psychological distress among infertility clinic patients. *J Consult Clinic Psychol* 1995; 63:163–7.

41. Boivin J, Takefman JE. Stress level across stages of in vitro fertilization in subsequently pregnant and nonpregnant women. *Fertil Steril* 1995; 64:802–10.

6 Psychopathology and Psychopharmacology in the Infertile Patient

KATHERINE E. WILLIAMS AND LAUREL N. ZAPPERT

Fortunately psychoanalysis is not the only way to resolve inner conflicts. Life itself still remains a very effective therapist.

– Karen Horney

Psychopathology is a term that denotes behaviors and experiences that are indicative of psychological impairment, distress, or mental illness. Infertility is a condition that causes great psychological distress in patients, and the relationship between psychopathology and infertility has been long debated. Furthermore, patients bring a psychological history to their infertility, which has a profound impact on how they experience, react, and respond to this condition and which may be further complicated by medications taken to treat infertility. Psychopharmacology refers to the study of medications used to remedy psychiatric conditions, which may, in turn, interact with other medications used in infertility treatment.

This chapter

■ reviews the body of literature regarding the prevalence, clinical course, and treatment of psychiatric disorders in infertility patients;
■ discusses the known effects of typically used infertility medications on mood;
■ clarifies potential drug interactions between infertility treatment medications and psychotropic medications;
■ addresses the role of the psychiatrist on the reproductive medicine team.

HISTORICAL OVERVIEW

Prior to advances in medical evaluation techniques, many researchers believed that psychological problems in both men and women (but typically women) caused infertility through ovulatory dysfunction, recurrent miscarriage, and sexual dysfunction. In her classic and influential article, "Infertility as a Psychosomatic Defense," Benedek[1] postulated that 'underlying ambivalence' and 'rejection of motherhood' caused infertility. Infertility patients were frequently described as emotionally immature and psychologically conflicted – either about their mothers, their desire to be parents, attaining adult roles, or their sexuality. As such, researchers expected to find high rates of psychiatric morbidity in this population. However, studies have not confirmed these earlier theories, and it is now thought that in the vast majority of this population, psychopathology is usually a result of the stresses and losses associated with infertility and/or exacerbation of preexisting conditions rather than a primary cause of infertility.

By the end of the twentieth century the role of psychiatry and other mental health professionals had shifted from identifying and curing psychopathology as a means of treating infertility, to a much broader role of patient care in collaboration with the reproductive medicine team. Psychiatry, as one of the major mental health professions, has had the unique perspective and contribution to patient care (particularly in the last fifty years) with the use of psychoactive medications to restore mental health. While psychiatry emerged as a specialized field of medicine through the work Freud with his emphasis on psychoanalysis, there has been an evolutionary shift away from the purely psychological treatment of psychopathology to a greater emphasis on the combination of evidence-based psychopharmacological treatment and psychotherapy. This is particularly true in the United States where many psychiatrists are more often psychopharmacologists and, as such, less likely to treat patients with psychotherapy only or with psychotherapy and psychotropic medications. This is in contrast to other parts of the world (e.g., Germany, Austria, and Switzerland) where psychiatrists are trained in both and where obstetrician/gynecologists may obtain special training and credentialing in the treatment of mental disorders with psychotherapy and psychotropic medications.

Within the field of infertility counseling, psychiatrists and specially trained obstetrician/gynecologists have taken a leading role in helping to define the field, both in providing patient care and research.

REVIEW OF LITERATURE

There has been considerable research on psychopathology and infertile patients (most commonly women); however, most of it was based on the hypothesis that infertility was caused by psychopathology, which, if treated, would improve fertility. Most of this research involved anecdotal case studies. Ultimately, the findings or conclusions of this research were not supported by more scientifically rigorous research. Recently, research has focused on the development of psychopathology in response to infertility diagnosis and treatment and, even more recently, the impact of preexisting psychopathology and its treatment on infertility diagnosis and treatment. The review of the literature that follows addresses current research on the incidence and treatment of psychopathology in infertile patients and the impact of medications for the treatment of infertility on mood and psychological functioning.

Psychopathology in Infertility Patients

Affective Disorders

Grief reactions are common in both men and women undergoing infertility treatment because infertility represents a loss on so many levels: from the loss of a sense of self and belief in the creative powers of one's own body to the loss of the chance to have and nurture one's biological child. Several studies have shown that many women identify infertility treatment as the most distressing event in their lives – more upsetting than the loss of a loved one or divorce.[2,3] Many men, as well, report significant emotional distress associated with the diagnosis and treatment of infertility.[4,5] However, studies suggest that there are gender differences in the prevalence, intensity, and duration of grief reactions that women suffer more than men after the diagnosis of infertility except for men with male-factor diagnosis[6,7] (see Chapter 3).

It is important, then, that clinicians be able to differentially diagnose the expected grief reaction seen in most infertility patients[8] from the less common and serious complication of pathological grief. As described in Chapter 1, normal grief includes the classic symptom complex of initial shock and numbness followed by intense sadness and distress, frequent anger and hostility, guilt, and self-reproach. Grief reactions are commonly classified as adjustment disorders in the *Diagnostic and Statistical Manual of Mental Disorders*[9] (DSM-IV). It is normal for infertility patients to experience some measure of grief, and it is believed that the mourning process is important for the final resolution of the crisis of infertility.[10,11] In contrast, pathological grief is considered a psychiatric illness that requires immediate evaluation and treatment. Pathological grief is consistent with the DSM-IV definition of major depression, and it is characterized by marked vegetative symptoms such as appetite, sleep, and psychomotor disturbances; anhedonia; suicidal ideation; and memory and concentration problems. Pathologic grief may also include psychotic features, such as paranoid or somatic delusions and excessive punitive thoughts.

The prevalence of major depression in infertility patients appears to be higher than previously thought. Many earlier studies failed to define important population variables such as length of infertility treatment, diagnosis, and medication usage, all of which are now known to be important contributors to depression.[12] For instance, Hearn and colleagues[13] and Downey and colleagues[14] reported that Beck Depression Inventory (BDI) scores in female infertility patients did not differ from scores in a group of healthy female controls; however, the infertility patients were pre–in vitro fertilization (IVF) treatment, and studies have shown that there may be a honeymoon period of optimism prior to the first IVF cycle.[6] Recent studies suggest that major depression is, in fact, more common in women undergoing infertility treatment than in fertile controls. Domar and associates[15] evaluated 338 infertility patients with the BDI and the Center for Epidemiological Studies Depression Scale (CES–D), comparing them with thirty-nine healthy controls, and found that depression was twice as common in the infertility patients: 37% scored in the depressed range on the BDI compared with 18% of controls. BDI scores were correlated with length of treatment. Women with a history of infertility of two to three years had higher BDI scores than women in treatment for less than one year or greater than six years. Several other studies demonstrated increased emotional distress over time in both male and female infertility patients due to repeated treatment failures.[5,16] Domar and coworkers[17] also found that symptoms of anxiety and depression in infertile women were as prevalent as in patients with other chronic medical conditions, such as hypertension and cancer.

This finding of a high prevalence of symptoms of depression in women undergoing infertility treatment is an international finding that has been reported in diverse cultures, including Japan,[18] Taiwan,[19] Korea,[20] Kuwait,[21] and multiple countries in Europe.[22–24] It is difficult to generalize and compare the incidence of psychiatric illnesses such as major depression or anxiety disorders in infertility patients across countries because studies have used varying methodologies and measures of psychopathology.

No studies have investigated the prevalence or the emergence of bipolar disorder in infertility patients. Prevalence rates of bipolar disorder in the female general population are low (0.7–1.6%), compared with prevalence rates of major depression (10–25%).[25] However, the peak years for onset of bipolar disorder coincides with a woman's reproductive years; consequently, clinicians working with infertility patients can expect to treat women with this disorder.

Anxiety Disorders

Several studies have reported that anxiety levels are often elevated in both male and female infertility patients;[17,23] and, as expected, a high incidence of adjustment disorder with anxiety has been reported in this population.[24] Many studies have focused upon stress and not used clear diagnostic criteria for anxiety disorders, or clarified whether the anxiety symptoms began before infertility diagnosis and treatment. Chen and colleagues in Taiwan conducted clinical interview with 112 consecutive women presenting for infertility treatment and reported that 23% met criteria for generalized anxiety disorder and 17% major depressive disorder.[19] The prevalence of other anxiety disorders, such as obsessive-compulsive disorder, in infertile men and women is unknown. Anxiety disorders, especially phobias, are quite common in the general population. Six-month prevalence rates for specific phobias range from 4.5% to 11.8%.[26] Blood-injury and needle phobia can lead to significant impairment in infertility treatment. Couples in whom one or both partners suffer from these specific phobias can be expected to have significant difficulty with injections, as well as greater emotional distress associated with preparation for and recuperation from surgery and other medical procedures. During treatment planning, clinicians should inquire about both a personal and a family history of blood-injury or needle phobias because these anxiety disorders appear to have a very strong genetic link.[27]

Eating Disorders

Anorexia nervosa and bulimia are common causes of ovulatory dysfunction, yet eating disorders are frequently overlooked in women presenting for infertility evaluation. In a study of sixty-six women consec-

utively presenting to an infertility clinic, Stewart and colleagues[28] found that 7.6% met DSM-III criteria for anorexia or bulimia and 16.7% for an eating disorder, not otherwise specified, as measured by the Eating Attitudes Test and a structured clinical interview. When women with menstrual irregularities were studied separately, 58% were found to have an eating disorder. It is unclear whether this finding of a high prevalence of occult eating disorders is affected by race or culture in the United States, but recent reports suggest that this occurs in Europe as well. Resch and colleagues in their evaluation of women at an infertility clinic in Hungary found similar high numbers of previously undiagnosed eating disorders.[29] Active eating disorders are associated not only with diminished fertility but also with increased perinatal morbidity, including increased incidence of miscarriage, intrauterine growth retardation and increased congenital anomalies.[30–32] Women with menstrual irregularities should be carefully screened for the presence of an underlying eating disorder, which should be treated before proceeding with infertility treatment.[33,34]

Personality Disorders

Large population studies using standardized psychometric tests such as the Minnesota Multiphasic Personality Inventory (MMPI or MMPI-2) and the Eysenck Personality Inventory showed no increased prevalence or pattern of preexisting personality disorders in women undergoing infertility treatment.[35] Nevertheless, because of the prevalence of these disorders in the general population, clinicians can expect to be faced with personality disordered patients, who can represent major challenges to the treatment team. The borderline, narcissistic, and histrionic personality disorders are especially difficult to manage, and the treatment of these cluster B patients are discussed later in the chapter.

Infertility Medications and Mood

Many of the medications prescribed for the treatment of infertility have effects on the neurotransmitter systems involved with affective regulation. Surprisingly, very few studies have investigated the psychiatric side effects of infertility medications. A brief review of the effects of gonadal hormones on mood and a review of the reports of the effects of infertility medications on mood follow. It is important for clinicians to understand the potential effects of infertility medications on mood to help patients in their decision making

TABLE 6.1. Psychiatric effects of infertility medications

Drug	Use	Psychological effects
Bromocriptine	Hyperprolactinemia	Antidepressant effects, hypomania, psychosis
Leuprolide acetate	Hypothalamic 'downregulation'	Depression, cognitive problems, fine motor problems
Progesterone	Endometrial support	Depression, decreased libido, irritability
Estradiol	Endometrial support	Antidepressant effects, induction of rapid cycling

regarding the risks and benefits of infertility treatment (Table 6.1).

Neurotropic Effects of Gonadal Hormones

Estrogen and progesterone are steroid hormones that directly and indirectly affect central nervous system neurons involved in the regulation of mood and cognition. Animal studies have shown that these hormones can influence the production of neurotransmitters and modulate the affinity of receptors for substrates.[36] Studies suggest that estradiol affects dopamine receptors and has neuroleptic properties in both animals and humans.[37] Several authors report that psychotic disorders such as schizophrenia improve in women during pregnancy,[38,39] and it is presumed that this is due to enhanced dopamine blockade with increased estrogen level.[40]

Recent studies of estrogen use in perimenopausal women suggest that estrogen may improve mood in women whose anxiety or depression is not severe enough to meet the criteria for major depression.[41] Estrogen has been shown to increase serotonin bioavailability in several ways, including displacing its precursor tryptophan from albumin-binding sites, thereby allowing more tryptophan to be converted to serotonin,[42] and decreasing monoamine oxidase, an enzyme that degrades serotonin.[43,44] Estrogen also promotes norepinephrine release,[45] which may further improve mood; however, this enhanced noradrenergic function has also been associated with the emergence or exacerbation of anxiety disorders in some women. New-onset panic attacks have been reported in women initiating estrogen replacement therapy,[46] and some women experience increased anxiety during the second and third trimesters of pregnancy when estrogen levels are highest.[47]

In rats, progesterone treatment decreases serotonin accumulation in the brain.[48] In humans, progesterone in oral birth control pills has been shown to decrease tryptophan oxygenase, and this decreased tryptophan metabolism has been correlated with depression.[49] Progesterone metabolites act in a similar manner to barbiturates to modulate γ-aminobutyric acid (GABA) receptor complexes and have sedative effects.[50,51] Consequently, many women report improvement in anxiety disorders, such as panic disorder, during pregnancy.[52]

Clomiphene Citrate

Clomiphene citrate (Clomid, Serophene) is a synthetic estrogen used to induce ovulation in anovulatory women, improve luteal phase deficiency, and increase follicle number in women.[53] Clomiphene is usually taken on days 3 to 5 of the menstrual cycle; however, it has a metabolite that can be found in the circulation for up to thirty days after the last dose.[54] Clomiphene acts directly on the hypothalamus[55] to increase gonadotropin-releasing hormone (Gn-RH) pulse frequency and amplitude.[56] Subsequent increases in luteinizing hormone (LH) and follicle-stimulating hormone (FSH) lead to the development of multiple ovarian follicles and significant increases in midcycle estradiol in clomiphene-treated cycles, as compared with control cycles, which may persist into the luteal phase and are often accompanied by increased levels of progesterone.[57]

Clomiphene is associated with menopausal symptoms, and 10% of women taking the medication complain of hot flashes.[55] No large prospective studies using validated, standardized measurements have yet been published that evaluate the effect of clomiphene on mood. However, many women report that this medication is associated with mood changes, including irritability, emotionality, and increased symptoms of premenstrual syndrome.[58] In a small pilot study, Williams and Casper[59] reported that clomiphene is associated with decreased fatigue at midcycle, at the time when the estradiol levels are highest. They hypothesized that clomiphene may be associated with more mood changes in women with a history of affective lability at times of hormonal change, such as women with a history of premenstrual dysphoric disorder (PDD). Several studies have suggested that increased estrogen levels in the luteal phase lead to increased psychiatric symptoms in women with premenstrual dysphoric disorder.[60,61]

Women with bipolar disorder are another population who may be at risk for mood changes associated with Clomipene-related hormonal changes because this psychiatric population has been shown to be at an increased risk of mood instability at other times of hormonal change, such as the premenstruum[62] and postpartum periods.[63] To date, no studies have investigated the effect of the medication on mood in patients with bipolar disorder.

Clomiphene has been associated with psychosis in three case reports cited in English language journals. [64–66] In all the cases the psychosis began during the time that the Clomiphene was being taken (days 2–7 of stimulation), thus prior to the significant rise and fall of estrogen levels. This suggests that the mechanism of action of the psychiatric side effect had to do with the direct effect of the Clomiphene on the central nervous system rather than the indirect effect of the medication on hormone levels. In all the reported cases, the psychotic symptoms rapidly abated when clomiphene citate treatment was terminated.[67]

Human Menopausal Gonadotropins

Human menopausal gonadotropins, including menotropins (Humegon, Pergonal, and Pregova) and urofollotropin (e.g., Metrodin), are composed of purified FSH and LH in varying combinations. They act directly on the ovary to stimulate folliculogenesis; but unlike clomiphene, they have no direct hypothalamic effects. While the potential physical side effects of these medications, such as hyperstimulation syndrome, are well documented, the psychiatric side effects have been overlooked. Because these medications lead to extremely elevated estrogen levels during the follicular and midluteal phase, it can be expected that they affect mood in some women in a manner similar to clomiphene. Williams and Casper[59] are currently investigating the effects of these medications on mood and anecdotally report that many women feel a burst of energy and improved mood when their estrogen levels are rising.

Bromocriptine Mesylate

Bromocriptine mesylate (Parlodel) is an ergot alkaloid structurally related to the neurotransmitter dopamine.[68] It inhibits prolactin release from the lactotroph cells of the anterior pituitary and is used in infertility treatment to treat hyperprolactinemia (elevated levels of prolactin), which is associated with ovulatory dysfunction.[53] Because of

its effects on monoamine systems associated with affective regulation, bromocriptine has been used as an antidepressant for more than twenty years. It has been shown to be as effective as imipramine and amitriptyline in the treatment of depression in several double-blind, placebo-controlled studies.[68] Bromocriptine is also an effective adjunctive treatment, turning tricyclic antidepressant nonresponders into responders.[69]

The bromocriptine dosages used in these antidepressant studies ranged from 40 mg/day to 220 mg/day, which is considerably higher than the 1.25–5 mg/day dosing commonly used in hyperprolactinemia. Nevertheless, patients with hyperprolactinemia suffer from irritability, decreased libido, and depressive symptoms that improve with low-dose bromocriptine treatment but not with placebo.[70]

Infertility patients should be counseled about the potential psychiatric side effects of bromocriptine treatment, and women on antidepressants or with a history of bipolar disorder should be cautioned about the possible emergence of hypomania or mania, when taking this medication for fertility treatment. Other adverse psychiatric side effects include hallucinations, delusions, confusion, and behavioral changes.[71]

Gonadotropin-Releasing Hormone Agonists

Gn-RH agonists, such as Lupron and tiptorelin (Decapeptyl), are used to downregulate the pituitary to prevent premature ovulation during IVF cycles[53] or can be used for an extended period (e.g., six months) for the treatment of endometriosis. When used during an IVF treatment cycle, these medications are typically begun in the midluteal phase of the preceding cycle and continued during the stimulation phase of the treatment cycle. Gn-RH agonists lead to acute hypoestrogenism, a pharmacological menopause, and women frequently report physical symptoms, such as hot flashes, headaches, and mood changes.[72] Studies investigating the effects of these medications on mood in longer-term use for conditions such as endometriosis have reported the onset of significant depressive symptoms with use of the medication for several months.[72] Warnock and colleagues reported that sixteen of twenty patients treated with a Gn-RH agonist for twenty-four weeks developed significant depressive symptoms.[73] Further studies have shown that these depressive symptoms can, in fact, be improved with antidepressant treatment.[74]

It is difficult to extrapolate this data to the shortened period of Gn-RH exposure in IVF programs; however, two studies have evaluated the effect of Gn-RH medication on mood in IVF cycles. Toren and colleagues compared depression scores in IVF patients pretreated with the Gn-RH agonist triptorelin to depression scores in a group of women undergoing IVF without downregulation. Triptorelin caused a 40% reduction in estradiol levels during the pretreatment phase, and this hypoestrogenism was associated with significantly increased symptoms of anxiety and depression compared to controls. All the subjects entering the study were euthymic, and despite increases in mood symptoms with Gn-RH administration, no subject's symptoms were so severe as to meet the criteria for major depressive disorder.[75] Similarly, Weizman and colleagues compared Hamilton depression scores and platelet serotonin transporter in nine women undergoing IVF pretreatment with the Gn-RH agonist decapetptyl to ten women treated only with human menopausal gonadotropin (Pergonal). Ovarian suppression was associated with an elevation in depression and anxiety as well as a significant decrease in platelet imipramine binding sites.[76] Thus, it is important to recognize that women with a current history of depression who are taking antidepressants may need an adjustment in their antidepressant dosage, if they experience break-through depressive symptoms during Gn-RH treatment.

Many women taking Gn-RH agonists also complain of cognitive changes (e.g., poor memory and concentration) that may or may not be accompanied by symptoms of a mood disorder. Varney and associates[77] compared neuropsychiatric tests in women prior to pre-IVF treatment with the Gn-RH agonist leuprolide, during leuprolide treatment, and at ovulation, approximately ten days after leuprolide administration. Each woman served as her own control. A significant proportion of women demonstrated impairment in performance on one or more memory tests while taking leuprolide. Similarly, Newton and colleagues reported that 44% of women taking Gn-RH agonists reported decreases in their perceived memory functioning during treatment; although memory returned to normal once Gn-RH agonists were stopped.[78] Sherwin and Tulandi[79] demonstrated significant decreases in verbal memory scores in women on leuprolide that were reversed in a group receiving add back estrogen but not in the control group. These are important findings as IVF treatment involves complex medical protocols and relies on patient compliance, self-administration of medications, and self-assessment (e.g., hyperstimulation). Keeping this in mind, caregivers have implemented a variety of patient education and preparation strategies including pretreatment psychological consultation (e.g., infertility counseling), written materials, and group training sessions to avoid medication-induced confusion

and cognitive impairment during the IVF treatment cycle.

Progesterone
Progesterone is frequently used during infertility treatment to improve luteal phase endometrial lining in clomiphene, superovulation induction, and IVF treatment cycles.[53] Progesterone in the oral birth control pill has been associated with the onset of depression in women,[80] and there have been reports of the emergence of major depression with suicidal ideation and panic disorder in women using synthetic progesterones such as levonorgestrel subdermal implants (Norplant).[81] However, some women report improvement in anxiety symptoms while on progesterone because of the sedative properties of its metabolites.[50,51]

Oral Birth Control Pills
Oral birth control pills are frequently used in infertility patients prior to an IVF cycle to downregulate the hypothalamus. Prevalence rates of depression in women taking oral birth control pills range from 5–50%, depression being most common in progesterone-dominant pills.[82] However, because of the estrogen in oral birth control pills, there have been some case reports of the induction of rapid cycling mood in women taking these medications.[82]

THEORETICAL FRAMEWORK

The theoretical approach most applicable to psychopathology, psychopharmacology, and infertile patients is a medical model of mental illness and its medical treatment. Psychopathology is generally defined as the science dealing with diseases and abnormalities of the mind, while psychopharmacology is the treatment of psychiatric illness with psychotropic medications, which are thought to improve mental health by affecting the operation of brain cells and the levels of brain chemicals (e.g., the neurotransmitters serotonin, norepinephrine, dopamine, glutamate, and GABA). Mental health disorders are defined in the United States by the Diagnostic and Statistical Manual of Mental Disorders, Fourth Edition, published by the American Psychiatric Association[9] and globally by the World Health Organization's (WHO) International Classification of Diseases and Related Health Issues, Ninth Revision (ICD-9).[83] Although there are textual differences between DSM and ICD, treaties between the United States and the WHO ensure that the diagnostic code numbers are identical to ensure uniform reporting of national and international psychiatric statistics.

A recent study of the prevalence, severity, and treatment of DSM-IV (ICD-9) mental disorders in fourteen countries (six developing, eight developed), the WHO found that the prevalence of mental health disorders in the prior year varied widely (from 4.3% in China to 26.4% in the United States), whether severe or mild.[84] The findings were based on 60,643 face-to-face interviews with adults in 13 countries (Belgium, China, Columbia, France, Germany, Japan, Lebanon, Mexico, The Netherlands, Nigeria, Spain, Ukraine, and the United States). The prevalence and severity of disorders varied widely as did treatment access. Although researchers did not attempt to diagnose schizophrenia, they reported that anxiety disorders were found in 3.2 to 18.2% of the study participants; mood disorders in 0.9 to 9.6%; impulse control problems in 0.0 to 6.8%; substance abuse and/or dependence in 0.1 to 6.4; and any disorder in 4.3 to 26.4%. In developing countries 80% of serious cases went untreated, while in developed countries 35 to 50% went untreated. In sum, this study supported earlier findings that mental health disorders are highly prevalent worldwide; often associated with serious role and/or work impairment; more often than not, untreated.

As this research highlights, the role of the psychiatrist (and other mental health professionals) in the diagnosis and treatment of infertile patients with concomitant mental diagnoses, is integral and imperative. This chapter addresses the diagnosis and treatment of psychopathology through psychopharmacology, while other chapters address psychological treatment modalities (e.g., individual psychotherapy, sex therapy, and behavioral medicine techniques) that may or may not be used in conjunction with psychotropic medications. In the psychopharmacological approach, a distinction is made between psychological disorders with emotional etiology and psychiatric illness of primarily physical etiology, such as inherited disorders or neurological changes. As brain research has increased, it has become increasingly apparent that a significant proportion of psychiatric illnesses are probably the result of the interplay between genetic vulnerability to altered brain chemistry and environmental influences.

CLINICAL ISSUES

It is beyond the scope of this chapter to address all mental health disorders in patients undergoing treatment for infertility. It is difficult to separate clinical issues of psychiatric illness and psychopathology from therapeutic interventions. Therefore, the focus here is on psychopathology and drug interactions in which the interaction of psychotropic medications and infertility treatment medications are reviewed.

Psychopathology

Psychopathology is generally defined as the science dealing with diseases and abnormalities of the mind, while psychopharmacology is the treatment of psychiatric illness with psychotropic medications, such as antidepressants. Although the exact mechanism of treatment is not completely understood, it is thought that psychotropic medications affect levels of brain chemicals (e.g., the neurotransmitters serotonin, norepinephrine, dopamine, glutamate, and GABA) or the effective operation of brain cells.

Affective Disorders

Depressive reactions to the diagnosis or treatment of infertility are common, and treatment decisions should be based on symptom severity and past psychiatric history. Adjustment disorders not accompanied by pronounced vegetative symptoms are best treated with supportive psychotherapy. Basically, the treatment of choice for depression and anxiety in infertility patients is psychotherapy rather than pharmacotherapy because these women who are attempting to conceive and may become pregnant, and also should avoid medication interactions. When women are seen on a weekly or regular basis for individual psychotherapy, particularly during IVF treatment cycles, mood changes can be carefully monitored and managed with a variety of psychotherapeutic techniques. By the same token, with regular psychotherapy, intervention with medications can occur more efficiently as dramatic mood changes are noted and intervention facilitated expeditiously. Behaviorally oriented group psychotherapy has been found to decrease anxiety and depression in female infertility patients in several studies.[85,86]

If a patient has a history of rapid relapse depression after antidepressant discontinuation or a history of severe depression with suicidality, psychosis, or dangerous vegetative symptoms, maintenance on antidepressants may be recommended or unavoidable even during medical treatment for infertility. While some women may feel better during pregnancy, studies do not support the popular belief that pregnancy protects against depressive episodes. The prevalence of major depression during pregnancy is similar to that in nonpregnant women: 10%.[87] Furthermore, risk factors for depression (e.g., prior depressive episode, reproductive loss, and genetic predisposition) must be considered. Recent prospective research has shown that 75% of women with a history of major depressive disorder relapsed during pregnancy if they discontinued or attempted to discontinue antidepressant medication, even though they were euthymic at the onset of pregnancy.[88]

Tricyclic antidepressants have been in use for more than twenty years, and to date studies do not suggest significant increases in congenital malformations in prenatally exposed infants.[89] Most studies have been retrospective and included small numbers of patients. However, a prospective study of more than 600 patients reported that tricyclics are not associated with increased rates of major fetal malformations.[90] The long-term neurobehavioral effects of these medications on offspring have only recently been studied. The two published investigations report no differences in cognitive and behavioral measures between tricyclic-exposed infants and controls at up to three years[91] and six years[92] of age. However, these medications should be used with extreme caution, and pregnant women should always be maintained on the lowest possible dosage of medication. Even so, Wisner and colleagues[93] reported that tricyclic antidepressants required dosage increases during the second and third trimesters of pregnancy; so if a patient is nonresponsive, it is important to check tricyclic antidepressant blood levels.

Similarly, studies of most SSRIs[94–99] or Venlafaxine[100] have consistently shown that infants exposed in utero do not have higher rates of congenital major malformations than children not exposed. However, a recent unpublished retrospective study by Glaxo-SmithKline (GSK) found that infants exposed to paroxetine (Paxil) during pregnancy did have an increased risk for major congenital malformations.[101] Consequently, at this time women should be counseled to avoid the use of paroxetine during pregnancy. Recent studies suggest that children exposed to antidepressants in utero are at significantly increased risk for perinatal complications. Exposure to SSRIs during pregnancy has been associated with decreased mean gestational age[95] and increased risk for preterm birth.[103] An early report of increased incidence of poor neonatal adaptation following Fluoxetine exposure during the third trimester, including lower Apgar scores and increased rates of admission to neonatal intensive care units,[104] has now been replicated in studies of other SSRIs.[95,104,105] Casper and colleagues compared children exposed to SSRIs throughout pregnancy, to those exposed during the third trimester only, and children of depressed mothers who did not take antidepressants. When the groups were compared for time of antidepressant exposure, they found that only late exposure was associated with neonatal complications.

The third-trimester-exposed infants had significantly decreased Apgar scores at one and five minutes and increased risk of admission to neonatal care units (27% versus 8% of controls and no admissions for children exposed to SSRIs in the first trimester only).[106]

Thus, research suggests that 20–30% of third-trimester SSRI-exposed infants show symptoms of poor neonatal adaptation due to either drug withdrawal or the effect of medication itself. Symptoms vary in intensity and duration, and include respiratory distress, hypotonia, or convulsions.[103,104,107] In response to the accumulating data that exposure to antidepressants during the last trimester of pregnancy increases the risk for neonatal complications, the Pediatric Advisory Committee has recommended withdrawal of antidepressants prior to the anticipated last week of pregnancy.[108] The short-term and long-term effects of antidepressant exposure in utero on neurodevelopment remains controversial and largely unknown. Casper and colleagues compared mental and motor development of children, aged six to forty months, of depressed mothers who took SSRIs with the scores of mothers who did not take SSRIs. The pediatricians and neurologists who examined the infants were blinded to the infants' exposure history. Although Bayley scales of mental development (MDI) did not show any differences, the Psychomotor Development Index (PDI) did show that prenatal SSRI exposure was associated with increased abnormalities in fine motor development in prenatally exposed children. Behavioral Rating Scale (BRS) showed significant differences in motor quality, specifically in the areas of fine motor movement. There was also a trend for increased tremulousness.[104] Similarly, Zeskind and Stephens[109] recently compared seventeen SSRI-exposed newborns to seventeen nonexposed full-birth-weight newborns without obvious medical problems and evaluated behavioral states, startles, and tremulousness for one hour between feedings. Heart Rate Variability (HRV) was assessed as well. SSRI-exposed infants had a shorter mean gestational age, were more motorically active and tremulous, showed few rhythms in HRV, had fewer changes in behavioral states, fewer different behavioral states, and more rapid eye movement sleep. After effects of gestational age were covaried, significant differences continued to be found in tremulousness and in all measures of state and sleep organization, but effects on startles, motor activity, and rhythms in HRV were no longer significant.

To date, only two SSRI neurodevelopment follow-up studies have been completed. As previously described, Nulman and colleagues compared children fifteen to seventeen months of age who had been exposed to TCAs (n = 80) or Fluoxetine (n = 55) to a control group of unexposed children of nondepressed mothers (n = 84). They found no differences in IQ, language, behavior, or temperament.[90] These investigators recently replicated their findings with a study, which followed a cohort of children exposed to fluoxetine (n = 47) and TCAs (n = 47) for the entire pregnancy and found no neurobehavioral problems.[110] To our knowledge, no other follow-up studies have yet been completed. Animal models have shown that serotonin has important, although poorly understood, developmental effects on the brain.[111] Recently, Ansorge and colleagues have reported that inhibition of 5HTT with fluoxetine during early development led to abnormal emotional behavior in adult mice. The effect of exposure to fluoxetine in utero mimicked the behavior of mice genetically deficient in 5HTT expression; specifically, the animals demonstrated decreased exploratory behavior and impairment in shock avoidance.[112] Thus, at this time, the follow-up data of children exposed to antidepressants in utero remain sparse, and therefore it cannot be concluded that these medications may not have long-lasting neurobehavioral effects.

Women taking fluoxetine and planning to discontinue medication once they have a positive pregnancy test should be switched to another SSRI such as sertraline (Zoloft) that has a shorter half-life. Fluoxetine's active metabolite, norfluoxetine, remains in the body for nearly two weeks after the last dose, which prolongs the period of fetal exposure to the medication.[113] Women who plan to abruptly discontinue their SSRI medication should be cautioned about the possible emergence of a flu-like syndrome with antidepressant withdrawal, which does not appear to be dangerous but may exacerbate pregnancy symptoms such as nausea, malaise, and headaches.[114] Infertility patients taking antidepressant medications should also be warned about recent reports of SSRI-induced galactorrhea and hyperprolactinemia (nonpregnancy-related milk production and lactation). Several case reports have emerged in the literature, suggesting that sertraline,[115,116] paroxetine,[117] and fluoxetine,[118] may, in rare cases, be associated with increased prolactin levels. The mechanism of action is not clear, but it is postulated that SSRIs may elevate serum prolactin through serotonergic activation of prolactin-releasing factors.[119] Because prolactinemia is associated with subfertility, it is important that women on SSRIs examine themselves for the onset of breast discharge, have their prolactin levels carefully checked, and consider switching to a tricyclic antidepressant.

Men on antidepressants should also be warned about the possible connection between these medications and subfertility. Initiation of the antidepressants trimipramine, clomipramine, and nefazadone has been associated with decreased spermatogenesis and sperm motility in case reports and small studies, and no data exist regarding the SSRIs or other newer antidepressants.[120] Furthermore, antidepressants may decrease fertility in men by their adverse effects on sexual function. Rates of these side effects vary among studies, and clearly an estimate of the true incidence is obscured by issues in reporting. The SSRIs and Venlafaxine are the medications most frequently associated with decreased libido, erectile dysfunction, and anorgasmia and rates range from 30–60%.[121]

Finally, it is important that clinicians warn infertility patients considering antidepressant continuation or initiation about the ongoing controversy regarding whether these medications are associated with miscarriages. For instance, a recent meta-analysis of six cohort studies of 1,534 antidepressant exposed women and 2,033 nonexposed women found that exposure to antidepressants was associated with a significant increase in rates of spontaneous abortion (3.9%). No differences were found among classes of drug.[122] Only one study exists to date investigating whether the use of SSRIs in pregnancy is associated with differential outcomes in IVF treatment.[123] In this retrospective chart review study, IVF outcome measures were compared for women taking SSRIs and women not taking SSRIs. The groups were matched for type of infertility diagnosis and the following IVF variables were compared: peak estrogen level, number of oocytes retrieved, number of oocytes fertilized on day 1 and percentage of zygotes reaching eight-cell stage on day 3, percentage reaching blastocyst on day 5 or day 13, and day 15 hCG levels. Although no statistical differences were found between the two groups on IVF laboratory measures, 40% of women taking SSRIs had ongoing pregnancies compared with 51% of women not taking medication. It is important to note that treatment outcome of IVF in patients taking an SSRI compared with patients not taking an SSRI may have been related to the presence of depression itself, as the control group was not matched for depression scores.

Thus, another conundrum in counseling women regarding risks versus benefits of antidepressant exposure is the question of whether underlying depression is associated with an increased risk for infertility. Two studies have reported that women with infertility of unknown origin had higher lifetime prevalence of major depression and that the depression frequently predated the diagnosis of infertility.[124,125]

Recently, researchers have attempted to clarify whether the presence of current depressive symptoms affects the outcome of fertility interventions. Thiering and colleagues'[126] prospective study of IVF patients reported that women with elevated depression scores at the start of treatment had significantly lower pregnancy rates than women who were not depressed. However, interpretation of this study was limited by a lack of clarification of important IVF outcome variables in the two groups, such as number of high-quality blastocystes transferred. Demyttenaere and colleagues[127] did control for these IVF variables and reported that women with a higher Zung depression score at the beginning of the IVF cycle, and greater depressed coping score, had significantly lower pregnancy rates. In another prospective study, 291 women were evaluated for depression prior to IVF with and without ICSI. After age and number of previous pregnancies were controlled for, depression scores were significantly negatively correlated with pregnancy.[128]

As Rubinow and Roca[129] hypothesized, depression may affect behaviors associated with fertility, such as loss of libido leading to decreased sexual activity, or the underlying hypothalamic dysregulation associated with depression may compromise reproductive mechanisms and events. For instance, two recent studies have shown that women with major depression demonstrated abnormal regulation of luteinizing hormone (LH) pulses when compared with nondepressed controls.[130,131] Furthermore, the hyperactivity of the hypothalamic pituitary adrenal system (HPA) in major depression may also play a role in subfertility. Recently, Weber and colleagues[132] reported that hypercortisolemic women with severe major depression also had higher androstenedione and testosterone levels compared with age-matched controls. Thus, the neuroendocrinologic mechanisms by which major depression may affect fertility are complex and controversial, and further studies are needed to evaluate this intriguing relationship. At this time, we can only counsel patients that the long-term effects of untreated depression on fertility are not known, but clearly affect behavior and quality of life.

Women taking mood stabilizers, such as lithium for bipolar disorder, should be counseled about the high rates of relapse with abrupt medication withdrawal.[133] In addition, the abrupt changes in hormones postpartum have been shown to be associated with increased risk for bipolar relapse.[134] While no studies have yet been done evaluating the effects of infertility medications on mood in women with bipolar disorder, it may be expected that hormonal changes during IVF may increase relapse risk. Mood stabiliz-

ers, such as lithium, have been associated with an increased risk of congenital malformations, so the risks of maintaining a woman on medication should be carefully weighed against the risk of withdrawing medication. Women without a history of severe illness can be tapered off their medication, while women with a history of dangerous relapses may be maintained on the lowest possible dose of lithium. The risk of cardiac defects with lithium is less than previously thought, approximately 0.1%; however, this estimate is still ten to twenty times greater than the risk in the general population.[89]

Because valproic acid is now a first-line treatment for mania in bipolar disorder,[135] clinicians may increasingly see women on these medications presenting for infertility treatment. First-trimester exposure to valproic acid is associated with a 1–5% risk of spina bifida, while exposure to carbamazepine is associated with a 1–1.5% risk. Therefore, it may be safest to switch women taking these anticonvulsant mood stabilizers to lithium.[89]

It has been repeatedly documented that the postpartum period is associated with an increased risk of relapse in bipolar disorder patients,[136] so patients should be counseled about the benefits of resuming mood stabilizer medication immediately postpartum and relinquishing breast-feeding.[134,136,137]

While the above-mentioned medications, antidepressants, and mood stabilizers remain the primary pharmacologic agents for the treatment of affective disorders, it is important to mention the emerging body of literature on the use of omega-three fatty acids for the treatment of both unipolar and bipolar depression. Omega-three fatty acids (n3FA) are a subset of polyunsaturated fatty acids (PUFA) present in cell membranes and which have an important role in affecting cell structure and function. Omega-three fatty acids include eicosapentaenoic acid (EPA), docosahexaenoic acid (DHA), and alpha-linolenic acid (ALA). Significant decreases of plasma n3FA and/or increases in the omega 6/omega 3 plasma ratio have been implicated in the development of mood disorders because these alterations have been found in the plasma and erythrocytes of patients with major depression,[138–140] and in patients who have attempted suicide.[141]

Recently, omega-three fatty acids have been identified as having a possible role in the etiology, treatment, and prevention of antenatal and postpartum depression. A large epidemiological study reported that the point prevalence of postpartum depression was inversely related to maternal consumption of seafood rich in omega-three fatty acids and specifically to higher concentrations of DHA.[142] In two studies of women without a history that would lead to an increased risk for postpartum depression, plasma phospholipid DHA levels have been correlated with depression levels postpartum.[143,144] To date, treatment studies of n3FA in postpartum depression have achieved mixed results[145–147] and research is needed to clarify whether n3FAs are a viable treatment alternative for major depressive disorder during pregnancy and the postpartum period. These nutritional supplements are ideally suited for pregnancy because of their multiple health benefits to both fetus and mother. Specifically, preliminary reports suggest that n3FA supplementation during pregnancy may lengthen pregnancy duration,[148] improve cognitive development,[149] and reduce the risk of developing allergic disorders[150] in children exposed to supplementation in utero.

Anxiety Disorders

The effect of infertility treatment on anxiety disorders has not been studied. Because anxiety disorders, such as obsessive-compulsive disorder (OCD), typically increase during times of stress, it can be expected that patients with these disorders will experience exacerbations of their symptoms during the process of infertility diagnosis and treatment. Patients with contamination obsessions and cleaning rituals may experience increased anxiety due to the responsibility of sterile technique associated with injections. These patients may find that they experience excessive hand washing before and after injections, and they will need extra guidance and reassurance regarding sterile technique. Behavioral strategies for managing their symptoms should be implemented, such as strict time limits on hand washing prior to and after injections and thought-stopping for obsessive, intrusive thoughts.

Infertility treatment with the Gn-RH agonists requires injections; therefore, it may be an overwhelming proposition to a patient with needle phobia. Because needle phobia is the most common specific phobia in the general population,[20] clinicians should inquire about the presence of this disorder prior to assuming that a patient or her partner can assume responsibility for injections. If a patient does experience needle phobia, treatment should consist of desensitization exercises. However, some needle phobia anxiety maybe successfully addressed via the new ovulation induction medication dispenser.

The effect of anxiety disorders on pregnancy remains controversial. As previously discussed, progesterone metabolites interact with the GABA receptors in a manner similar to barbiturates,[40] so theoretically the increased progesterone in pregnancy may be associated with decreased anxiety. However, not all women report an improvement in anxiety during pregnancy, and studies have shown that panic and OCD symptoms may in fact emerge or worsen during pregnancy.[31] As with bipolar disorder, the postpartum period appears to be the time of greatest risk for relapse or escalation of symptoms in panic disorder and OCD patients.[151]

Infertility patients taking benzodiazepines for their anxiety should attempt to taper off these medications because therapeutic doses have been associated with an increased risk of cleft abnormalities.[89] Patients who are benzodiazepine dependent should be counseled that these medications should be tapered over time and not abruptly discontinued because of the risk of a unpleasant withdrawal syndrome similar in presentation to alcohol withdrawl with tachycardia, unstable blood pressure, and gastrointestinal complaints. Tricyclic antidepressants or SSRIs may be substituted for anxiolytics in women who are unable to manage without medications. Cognitive behavior therapy should always be the first-line treatment in infertility patients, pregnant women, and nursing mothers.[152]

Personality Disorders

Borderline Personality Disorder

The most common and troubling personality disorders challenging the infertility treatment team and therapist are the 'cluster B' patients; borderline, narcissistic, and histrionic personality disorders. The use of primitive defenses by individuals with borderline personality disorder can be a major obstacle to infertility treatment. Projection of poor self-esteem and fears of abandonment may disrupt patients' relationship with infertility caregivers. Patients may perceive rejection in a clinician's hurried appointment or delayed call-back, leading to intense, disruptive rage reactions and splitting. Frequently, the physician will remain the 'good object' because these patients often have intense, idealized transference reactions. Patients believe their primary caregivers have the ultimate power over their fertility and reproductive treatment plans. Clinic support staff, such as nurses, receptionists, and administrative personnel, more often bear the brunt of these patients' angry outbursts. It is extremely important that infertility treatment personnel become educated about such primitive defenses, so that they can approach patients in a dispassionate, clinical manner to minimize splitting. Clinical staff should be educated and/or reminded that these patients will not change their personalities but respond to limit setting and consistency. Angry rebuttals to such patients' rage will only fuel the projective fires and lead to canceled or disrupted cycles and staff disturbances.

Persons with borderline personality disorder have problems with boundaries and entitlement that may also pose major problems for medical staff. These patients desperately need clear, articulated, and immutable boundaries. For instance, if they keep calling after hours for questions that could be addressed earlier in the day, they need to be reminded in a calm, caring way that the on-call staff is only for emergencies, and criteria for emergencies should be reviewed. These boundaries often need restating several times.

Because borderline patients are already emotionally labile and frequently suffer comorbid depression,[153] they may be especially sensitive to the effects of infertility medications on mood. The dysphoria, increased anxiety, and irritability associated with some infertility medications may be frightening to these patients. Similarly, the 'rollercoaster' of emotions associated with infertility treatment may further destabilize this group of affectively labile women.

Finally, in borderline personality disorder, patients have a high prevalence of history of sexual abuse,[154] and the infertility evaluation and treatment process include many invasive, frequently painful procedures that may trigger increased anxiety, flashbacks, and intrusive memories. These patients should be carefully educated about all of the steps involved in treatment. If care is being provided at a teaching hospital, it is best that examinations and procedures be performed by one caregiver and his or her team, rather than by a 'revolving' door of students and residents, which may heighten anxiety and threaten the fragile sense of bodily integrity that these patients have. Some women who have been victims of sexual abuse prefer female gynecologists, and their requests should be met with understanding and accommodation, if possible.

Borderline patients may enter a mental health practice in two ways; self-referral because of emotional distress or referral by the infertility team because of disruptive behavior in the clinic. In both situations, mental health clinicians must adhere to a fundamental treatment principle with these patients: Compassionate limit-setting, because they will often attempt to engage their therapists in their battles with the clinic, furthering the splitting process. Initially, psychotherapy with borderline patients undergoing infertility treatment should be extremely supportive and educational. Once stabilized, these patients may benefit from the use of other treatment modalities, such as dialectical behavioral therapy, a form of cognitive-behavioral therapy.[155] Psychopharmacological interventions may be necessary for the management of comorbid major depression and anger.

Narcissistic Personality Disorder

Because infertility is by its nature a 'narcissistic injury,' patients with narcissistic personality disorder can be expected to be at risk for decompensation during infertility evaluation and treatment. Common reactions include narcissistic rage and devaluation of caregivers. Narcissistic patients may have trouble following directions because they are so humiliated at being in such a dependent position. For instance, they may choose their own treatment plan (e.g., taking more or less of a medication than recommended) to assert their autonomy and authority, and they may fail to ask questions when they are confused (in part due to their arrogance and grandiosity). When faced with such patients, infertility clinicians must continually remind themselves that these patients, at their core, suffer from tremendously low self-esteem.[156] Therapeutic management of a narcissistic patient includes friendly acknowledgment of their intelligence and fund of knowledge about infertility, but clear and firm recommendations regarding treatment plans. Clinicians can expect that angry confrontation or disavowal of a narcissist's ideas will lead to rage reactions and should be avoided, if possible. Psychopharmacological treatment is typically not helpful in these patients, who will not change because they see others as having problems, not themselves.

Histrionic Personality Disorder

Patients with histrionic personality disorder will challenge infertility clinicians with their somatization of affect. They are less likely than borderline or narcissistic patients to split their caregiving team into adversarial positions, but they may create chaos and confusion due to their over-the-top emotionality and, in so doing, disrupt their care. For instance, the histrionic amplification of symptoms may lead to excessive testing, unnecessary changes in medication dosage, excessive phone calls, and extra appointments. Clinicians will be called on to differentially diagnose histrionic complaints from true, potentially life-threatening, treatment-emergent side effects, such as ovarian hyperstimulation syndrome. Infertility clinicians can help these patients by redirecting their somatic preoccupations and facilitating the expression of their psychological distress through referral to a mental health professional. Therapy necessarily focuses on exploration of underlying psychodynamic and interpersonal conflicts and more effective methods of experiencing and communicating their feelings. Psychopharmacological interventions are typically not useful, although these patients prefer a medical explanation and treatment of their distress.

TABLE 6.2. Personality types and infertility[157]

Personality structure	Reaction to infertility
Obsessive: orderly, systematic, perfectionist, inflexible	Infertility is seen as punishment for letting things get out of control
Narcissistic: self-involved, angry, independent, perfectionist	Infertility is seen as an attack on autonomy and perfection of self
Borderline: demanding, impulsive, unstable	Infertility is seen as a threat of abandonment
Dependent: long-suffering, depressed, submissive	Infertility is seen as expected punishment for worthlessness
Avoidant: remote, unsociable, uninvolved	Infertility and its procedures are seen as a dangerous invasion of privacy
Paranoid: wary, suspicious, blaming, hypersensitive	Infertility is seen as annihilating assault coming from everywhere outside of self

Obsessive-Compulsive Personality Disorder

The disruptive nature of infertility treatment represents extended torture to many patients with OCD. Patients with this disorder long for a sense of control in their lives and normally rely on a devotion to work, schedules, rituals, and productivity to manage anxiety. Infertility diagnosis and treatment signify a loss of control because despite multiple attempts to control patients' chances for conception through procedures, the end result is ultimately out of the control of both patients and clinicians. Consequently, OCD patients can be expected to experience significantly increased stress and anxiety during infertility procedures and failed treatment cycles, which may lead to increased irritability, anger, and a need to control the medical team or treatment protocol and their own behaviors. Providing a predictable medical environment can alleviate some of the stress for these individuals. Clinicians working with OCD patients should attempt to provide consistent, timely information and engage them in clinical decision making, when appropriate. Psychopharmacological treatment is highly recommended in these patients, particularly SSRIs. Psychotherapeutic interventions are also helpful in symptom management and encouraging improved coping skills and stress management.

Avoidant and Dependent Personality Disorder

Patients with avoidant and dependent personality disorder can challenge the infertility medical team as well, although their interpersonal style is usually more subtle and insidious than the disorders just discussed. These patients may engender maternal and paternal feelings in their caregivers, which may lead to exceptional dependence. They may leave all medical decisions up to their clinicians, and caregivers should be careful to involve these patients in medical plans. It is important to note, however, that within certain cultures it is considered appropriate behavior to be deferential and/or dependent with medical caregivers. As such, this is appropriate behavior a culturally and not a personality disorder.

In summary, personality disorders and traits may have important effects on infertility patients' ability to cope and comply with treatment. It is extremely important for infertility clinicians to be aware of the varying personality types and their defensive behaviors as outlined in Table 6.2.

Drug Interactions

Drugs used in infertility treatment may interact with psychotropic medications, influencing their bioavailability and thus potentially affecting both infertility and psychiatric treatment. Synthetic estrogens are metabolized by the cytochrome P-450 system in the liver; consequently, they affect psychotropic drugs that are also metabolized by this system. As reviewed by Jensvold,[82] in general, oral birth control pills stimulate metabolism of drugs metabolized conjugatively and by glucuronidation, such as the benzodiazepines, lorazepam and oxazepam, which may be associated with decreased serum levels of these drugs. Oral birth control pills impair clearance of oxidatively metabolized drugs, such as the alprazolam, triazolam, and imipramine, thus potentially leading to increased serum levels.[63]

The mood stabilizer, carbamazepine induces cytochrome P-450, leading to increased oral birth control metabolism; thus, this medication combination may lead to failure of ovulation suppression.[82] Women taking carbamazepine should be counseled to inform their reproductive endocrinologists about their medication so that higher doses of an oral birth control pill may be used for pre-IVF down-regulation.

Bromocriptine is a dopamine agonist; therefore, combining it with other dopaminergic agents such as bupropion (Wellbutrin) or Venlafaxine (Effexor) may lead to symptoms of dopaminergic toxicity (e.g., hypertension, stereotypy, and confusion). Women taking bromocriptine who are started on a tricyclic antidepressant should be warned about the increased risk of orthostatic hypotension with the combination of these two medications.

THERAPEUTIC INTERVENTIONS

Increasingly, psychiatrists are working either *as* infertility counselors or *with* infertility counselors to improve the care and well-being of men and women undergoing treatment for infertility. They provide patient care, conduct research, and educate patients, professionals, and the public about the importance of mental health care during infertility medical treatment. As such, they are typically not the patient's sole caregiver and may or may not be aware that their patient is infertile and/or undergoing medical treatment for it. Additionally, some patients may be reproductive helpers (e.g., gestational carrier, oocyte donor, surrogate, or embryo donor) with a current or past mental health diagnosis that was or is affected by their reproductive experience (see Chapter 19). While clinical treatment of infertile patients with concomitant mental health disorders was addressed in earlier sections, this section addresses how the psychiatrist can facilitate therapeutic interventions that involve collaboration of patient care, specifically when it involves denial of treatment due to confounding mental health problems and/or psychopharmacological contraindications.

Collaboration with the Reproductive Medicine Team

Some infertility clinics recommend or require that the patient inform all caregivers (e.g., psychiatrist or any other medicating physician) that he or she is undergoing infertility treatment. This requirement improves patient care (e.g., reducing the potential for drug interactions) and reinforces a collaborative approach to infertility treatment. This is even more important when the patient also has complicating medical conditions for which they are being treated with medications. Frequently, infertile individuals do not tell the reproductive medicine team about their mental diagnosis or treatment for it because they are embarrassed about the diagnosis; fear that infertility treatment will be denied or postponed because of the diagnosis; or they do not

consider it relevant (i.e., they are unaware of the potential for drug interactions and consider the issues as 'two separate problems'). Patient education is highly important in the treatment of these patients – by both the MHP and the reproductive medicine team. Ideally, decisions about psychotropic medication usage and reproduction are made collaboratively with the patient (and partner) as educated participants in the decision-making process. One way of facilitating this process is an explicit treatment plan which the patient and psychiatrist have collaboratively designed and which specifically addresses psychotropic medications. A copy of this plan should be given to the patient and sent to the reproductive medicine team (with the patient's permission). The plan should address setbacks (whether mental health or medical, such as a failed treatment cycle), crisis intervention, and pregnancy. While the psychiatrist may write and share (with the patient's authorization) a complete report, it is helpful that the report includes a brief summary of the plan, usually at the end of the summary for easier reading and access. The summary may also include the psychiatrist's recommendations on psychotherapy (e.g., infertility-specific counseling, chemical dependency treatment, or support group); particular concerns or alerts (e.g., what may trigger setbacks, marital problems, or life stressors that may have an impact on the patient's coping); and/or other useful information (e.g., how often the patient is being seen and emergency contact numbers).

Very often infertility clinics and reproductive medicine facilities do not have formal protocols for handling patients with concomitant mental health problems. Situations are handled on a case-by-case basis even when the clinic has a non-psychiatrist MHP on staff. Or the clinic may leave all mental health issues to the non-psychiatrist MHP who may or may not be qualified to address them. Although some psychologists and nurses are trained and qualified to prescribe or monitor psychotropic medications, these mediations remain the expertise of psychiatrists, highlighting the importance of psychiatrists as caregivers, consultants, and/or referral sources. Psychiatrists can facilitate collaboration by providing educational presentations at reproductive medicine clinics; establishing a working relationship with clinic staff (particularly the MHP); and/or working with the infertility center to establish how to best meet patient care needs. As noted earlier, despite the preponderance of mental health disorders, the majority go untreated at great cost to individuals, their families, and the community at large. Infertile men and women are known to be psychologically and often physically vulnerable. It is imperative that the psychiatric needs of infertile patients be recognized and proactively addressed.

Denial or Deferment of Treatment

According to the American Society of Reproductive Medicine (ASRM) Ethics Committee Report on *Child-Rearing Ability and the Provision of Fertility Services*, fertility treatment providers may decline to treat a patient on well-substantiated conclusions that the potential parent will not or cannot safely care for a child.[157] The committee report recommends that infertility clinics have clear, written exclusion policies and use a team approach to decision making. This report also notes that the disabled (mentally or physically) should not be denied treatment except when they fall within the narrowly defined parameters outlined within the recommendations and should be applicable to all patients.

Psychiatrists must always consider this factor when treating infertile men and women – something neither caregiver nor patient may want to do. It is not easy to recognize that a patient's mental diagnosis and medication regime may be a contraindication for proceeding with medical treatment for infertility (and/or even parenthood). It is even more difficult when this fact may trigger increased patient mental (and social) distress and symptomatology. For this reason, it is imperative that the caregiver be cognizant of countertransference issues; consider the best interests of the patient, his or her partner, *and* any potential children; and take responsibility for appropriate patient care and education. Educating the patient and making them part of the decision-making process can facilitate these decisions while minimizing distress, particularly when the patient's partner recognizes and is supportive of the caregiver's concerns even though the patient is not.

Denial or postponements of treatment decisions are always best when the patient self-nominates: He or she acknowledges and accepts that their reproductive goals are in conflict with their mental health goals *at this time*. Most often, mental health disorders involve the deferment of treatment rather than categorical denial of treatment. Patients may be asked to postpone reproductive treatment to address ongoing and current mental health problem(s) such as changing to a reproductively safer psychotropic medication or completion of a chemical dependency or eating disorder treatment program. Denial or postponement decisions can be more complex when the patient is a reproductive tourist and/or reproductive helper (e.g., surrogate, gestational carrier, or oocyte donor) who may or may not be aware of a mental diagnosis prior to volunteering or recruitment. Although patients (or their partners) often react with distress, resistance, and even overt hostility to these recommendations, those who comply typically feel positively, even grateful, for the assistance.

Categorical denial of treatment due to a mental health disorder is more difficult – and should comply with professional guidelines that are very specifically defined. These situations usually involve intractable and chronic disorders that impair the patient's functioning, ability to provide informed consent, and/or endanger the patient, others, and/or a potential child. Unfortunately, in such cases, psychiatrists and other MHPs may easily recognize (and document) the mental disorder. Contraindications for proceeding with the reproductive plan are abundantly obvious. However, patients are often unable or unwilling to recognize or accept the diagnosis or clinical assessment. For this reason, it is very important to involve the reproductive treatment provider in the assessment and recommendations, to ensure careful decision making, and minimize patient hostility at a single caregiver and/or prevent a revolving door process of doctor shopping.

FUTURE IMPLICATIONS

Recent decades have seen a growing interest among clinicians and researchers in psychiatric disorders in women, their etiology, biology. Also of growing interest is the impact of reproductive hormones on psychological symptomology. The dramatic increase and wide variety of psychotropic medications providing more effective and efficient psychopharmacological treatment have improved the health and quality of life of individuals, allowing them (in some instances) to pursue reproductive choices they may have been denied in the past. Although worldwide, patients with psychiatric disorders are unlikely to see (or have access to) psychiatric treatment. Of increasing interest is how undiagnosed and/or untreated mental disorders impact reproductive ability; infertility treatment outcomes; and/or ability to comply (or proceed) with treatment.

SUMMARY

■ Personality disorders do not appear to be more common in infertility patients, but when they do occur, they can very disruptive to infertility treatment and cause problems for staff and caregivers. Clinicians should be educated regarding the diagnosis and management of primitive defenses, such as splitting and projection, in borderline, narcissistic, and histrionic patients.

■ Major depression is more common in infertility patients than previously recognized; it is as prevalent as in other chronic medical conditions.

■ Antidepressants should be used only when the risk of not treating with medication is greater than the risk of treating, such as suicidality, psychotic depression, and severe vegetative depressions.

■ Women taking antidepressants or considering starting these medications should be warned that antidepressant exposure during the first trimester of pregnancy may be associated with an increased incidence of spontaneous abortion. The increased risk, if it does exist, appears to be very small.

■ Infertility medications can affect the regulation of mood and cognition – particularly in women. Caregivers should be particularly attentive to this issue when the patient has a history of psychiatric diagnosis and/or displays psychiatric symptomatology whether mild or severe.

■ Psychiatrist can be/are important members of the reproductive medicine collaborative treatment as caregivers, consultants, and/or educators.

REFERENCES

1. Benedek T. Infertility as a psychosomatic defense. *Fertil Steril* 1951; 3:527–41.
2. Freeman EW, Boxer AS, Rickels K, et al. Psychological evaluation and support in a program of in vitro fertilization and embryo transfer. *Fertil Steril* 1985; 43:48–53.
3. Mahlstedt PP, Macduff S, Bernstein J. Emotional factors and the in vitro fertilization and embryo transfer process. *J In Vitro Fertil Emb Transfer* 1987; 4:232–6.
4. Newton CR, Hearn MT, Yuzpe AA. Psychological assessment and follow-up after in vitro fertilization: Assessing the impact of failure. *Fertil Steril* 1990; 54:879–86.
5. Baram D, Tourtelot E, Muechler E, et al. Psychological adjustment following unsuccessful in vitro fertilization. *J Psychosom Obstet Gynaecol* 1988; 9:181–90.
6. Leiblum SR, Kemmann E, Lane MK. The psychological concomitants of in vitro fertilization. *J Psychosom Obstet Gynaecol* 1987; 6:165–78.
7. Laffont I, Edelmann RJ. Psychological aspects of in vitro fertilization: A gender comparison. *J Psychosom Obstet Gynaecol* 1994; 15:85–92.
8. Greenfeld DA, Diamond MP, Decherney AH. Grief reactions following IVF treatment. *J Psychosom Obstet Gynaecol* 1988; 8:169–74.
9. American Psychiatric Association. *Diagnostic and Statistical Manual of Mental Disorders*, 4th ed. Washington DC: American Psychiatric Association, 1994.
10. Menning BE. The emotional needs of infertile couples. *Fertil Steril* 1980; 34:313–9.
11. Rosenfeld DL, Mitchell E. Treating the emotional aspects of infertility: Counseling services in an infertility clinic. *Am J Obstet Gynecol* 1979; 135:177–80.
12. Golombok S. Psychological functioning in infertility patients. *Hum Reprod* 1992; 7:208–12.
13. Hearn MT, Yuzpe AA, Brown SE, et al. Psychological characteristics of in vitro fertilization participants. *Am J Obstet Gynecol* 1987; 156:879–86.
14. Downey J, Yingling S, McKinney M, et al. Mood disorders, psychiatric symptoms, and distress in women presenting for infertility evaluation. *Fertil Steril* 1989; 52: 425–32.
15. Domar AD, Broome A, Zuttermeister PC, et al. The prevalence and predictability of depression in infertile women. *Fertil Steril* 1992; 58:1158–63.
16. Boivin J, Takefman J, Tulandi T, et al. Reactions to infertility based on extent of treatment failure. *Fertil Steril* 1995; 63:801–7.
17. Domar AD, Zuttermeister PC, Friedman R. The psychological impact of infertility: A comparison with patients with other medical conditions. *J Psychosom Obstet Gynaecol* 1993; 14:45–52.
18. Matsubayashi HT, Hosaka T, et al. Emotional distress of infertile women in Japan. *Human Reprod* 2001; 16: 966–9.
19. Chen T, Chang S, Tsai C, et al. Prevalence of depressive and anxiety disorders in an assisted reproductive clinic. *Human Reprod* 2004; 19:2313–8.
20. Kee BS, Lee SH. A study on psychological strain in IVF patients. *J Assist Reprod Genet* 2000; 17:445.
21. Fido A. Emotional distress in infertile women in Kuwait. *Int J Fertil Womens Med* 2004; 49:24–8.
22. Oddens BJ, den Tonkelaaer I, et al. Psychological experiences in women facing fertility problems – a comparative survey. *Human Reprod* 1999; 14:255–61.
23. Beutel M, Kupfer J, Kirchmeyer P et al. Treatment-related stresses and depression in couples undergoing assisted reproductive treatment by IVF or ICSI. *Andrologiz* 1999; 31:27–35.
24. Guerra D, Llobera A, Veiga A, et al. Psychiatric morbidity in couples attending a fertility service. *Human Reprod* 1998; 13:1733–6.
25. Robins LN, Regier DA, eds. *Psychiatric Disorders in America: The Epidemiological Catchment Area Study*. New York: The Free Press, 1991.
26. Stoudemire A, ed. *Clinical Psychiatry for Medical Students*, 2nd ed. Philadelphia: Lippincott, 1994.
27. Fyer AJ, Mannuzza S, Gallops MS, et al. Familial transmission of simple phobias and fears: A preliminary report. *Arch Gen Psychiatry* 1990; 47:252–6.
28. Stewart DE, Robinson GE, Goldbloom DS, et al. Infertility and eating disorders. *Am J Obstet Gynecol* 1990; 163:1196–9.
29. Resch M, Nagy J, Pinter J, et al. Eating disorders and depression in Hungarian women with menstrual disorders and infertility. *J Psychosom Obstet Gynecol*. 1999; 20:152–7.
30. Stewart DE. Reproductive functions in eating disorders. *Ann Med* 1992; 24:287–91.
31. Bulik CM, Sullivan PF, Fear JL, et al. Fertility and reproduction in women with anorexia nervosa: A controlled study. *J Clin Psychiatry* 1999; 60:130–5.
32. Abraham S. Sexuality and reproduction in bulimia nervosa patients over 10 years. *J Psychosom Res* 1998; 44:491–502.

33. Abraham S, Mira M, Llewellyn-Jones D. Should ovulation be induced in women recovering from an eating disorder or who are compulsive exercisers? *Fertil Steril* 1990; 53:566–8.

34. Norre J, Vandereycken W, Gordts S. The management of eating disorders in a fertility clinic: Clinical guidelines. *J Psychosom Obstet Gynaecol* 2001; 22:77–81.

35. Mazure C, Greenfeld DA. Psychological studies of in vitro fertilization/embryo transfer participants. *J In Vitro Fertil Emb Transfer* 1989; 6:242–56.

36. McEwan BS. Neural gonadal steroid actions. *Science* 1981; 211:1303–10.

37. Van Hartesveldt C, Joyce JN. Effects of estrogen on the basal ganglia. *Neurosci Biobehav Rev* 1986; 10:1–14.

38. Chang SS, Renshaw DC. Psychosis and pregnancy. *Compr Ther* 1986; 12:36–41.

39. McNeil TF, Kaij L, Malmquist-Larsson A. Women with non-organic psychosis: Pregnancy's effect on mental health during pregnancy. *Acta Psychiatr Scand* 1984; 75:140–8.

40. Seeman MV, Lang M. The role of estrogens in schizophrenia gender differences. *Hosp Community Psychiatry* 1990; 16:185–94.

41. Williams KE, Casper RC. Reproduction and psychopathology. In: RC Casper, ed. *Women's Health: Hormones, Emotions and Behavior*. Portchester, NY: Cambridge University Press, 1997; 14–35.

42. Aylward M. Plasma tryptophan levels and mental depression in postmenopausal subjects: Effects of natural piperazine oestrone sulphate. *J IRCS Med Sci* 1973; 1:30–4.

43. Luine VN, Khylchevskaya RI, McEwen BS. Effect of gonadal steroids on activities of monoamine oxidase and choline acetylase in rat brain. *Brain Res* 1975; 86:293–306.

44. Klaiber EL, Broverman DM, Vogel W, et al. Estrogen therapy for severe persistent depressions in women. *Arch Gen Psychiatry* 1979; 36:50–4.

45. Etgen A, Karkanias GB. Estrogen regulation of noradrenergic signaling in the hypothalamus. *Psychoneuroendocrinology* 1994; 19:603–10.

46. Price WA, Heil D. Estrogen induced panic attack. *Psychosomatics* 1988; 29:433–5.

47. Verburg C, Griez C, Meijer J. Increase of panic disorder during second half of pregnancy. *Eur Psychiatry* 1994; 9:260–1.

48. Krey LC, Luine VN. Effect of progesterone on monoamine turnover in the brain of the estrogen-primed rat. *Brain Res Bull* 1987; 19:195–202.

49. Shaaraway M, Fayad M, Nagui AR, et al. Serotonin metabolism and depression in oral contraceptive users. *Contraception* 1985; 26:193–204.

50. Majewski M, Harrison N, Schwartz R, et al. Steroid hormone metabolites are barbiturate-like modulators of the GABA receptor. *Science* 1986; 232:1024–7.

51. Morrow A, Suzdak P, Paul S. Steroid hormone metabolites potentiate GABA receptor mediated chloride ion flux with nanomolar potency. *Eur J Pharmacol* 1987; 142:483–5.

52. Klein DF. Pregnancy and panic disorder. *J Clin Psych* 1994; 55:293–4.

53. Speroff L, Glass RH, Kase NG. *Clinical Gynecology, Endocrinology and Infertility*, 5th ed. Baltimore: Williams & Wilkins, 1994.

54. Glasier AF. Clomiphene citrate. *Baillières Clin Obstet Gynaecol* 1990; 4:491–501.

55. Kerin JF, Liu JH, Phillipou G, Yen SSC. Evidence of a hypothalamic site of action of clomiphene citrate in women. *J Clin Endocrinol Metab* 1985; 61: 265–8.

56. Martikainen H, Ronnberg L, Ruokonen A, et al. Gonadotropin pulsatility in a stimulated cycle: Clomiphene citrate increases pulse amplitudes of both luteinizing hormone and follicle stimulating hormone. *Fertil Steril* 1991; 56:641–5.

57. Randall JM, Templeton A. The effects of clomiphene citrate upon ovulation and endocrinology when administered to patients with unexplained infertility. *Hum Reprod* 1991; 6:659–64.

58. Brenner JL. Clomiphene-induced mood swings. *J Obstet Gynecol Neonatal Nurs* 1991; 20:321–7.

59. Williams KE, Casper RC. Personal communication.

60. Hammarbachk S, Damber JF, Backstrom T. Relationship between symptom severity and hormone changes in women with premenstrual syndrome. *J Clin Endocrinol Metab* 1989; 68:125–30.

61. Dhar V, Murphy GE. Double-blind randomized crossover trial of luteal phase estrogens (Premarin) in the premenstrual syndrome (PMS). *Psychoneuroendocrinology* 1990; 15:489–93.

62. Rasgon N, Bauer M, Glenn T, et al. Menstrual cycle related mood changes in women with bipolar disorder. *Bipolar Disorder* 2003; 5:48–53.

63. Chaudron LH, Pies RW. The relationship between postpartum psychosis and bipolar disorder: a review. *J Clin Psychiatry* 2003; 64:1284–92.

64. Cashman FE. Clomiphene citrate as a possible cause of psychosis. *Can Med Assoc* 1982; 15:118.

65. Altmark D, Tomaer R, Sigal M. Psychotic episode induced by ovulation-initiating treatment. *Isr J Med Sci* 1987; 23:1156–7.

66. Siedntopf F, Horskamp B, Stief G, et al. Clomiphene citrate as a possible cause of a psychotic reaction during infertility treatment. *Human Reprod* 1997; 12: 706–7.

67. Siedntopf F, Kentenich H. Future use of clomiphene in ovarian stimulation. Psychic effects of clomiphene citrate. *Human Reprod* 1998; 11:2986–7.

68. Sitland-Marken PA, Wells BG, Froemming JH, et al. Psychiatric applications of bromocriptine therapy. *J Clin Psychiatry* 1990; 51:59–82.

69. Inoue T, Tsuchiya K, Miura J, et al. Bromocriptine treatment of tricyclic and heterocyclic antidepressant – resistant depression. *Biol Psychiatry* 1996; 40: 151–3.

70. Koppelman MCS, Parry BL, Hamilton JA, et al. Effect of bromocriptine on affect and libido in hyperprolactinemia. *Am J Psychiatry* 1987; 144:1037–41.

71. Diehl DJ, Gershon S. The role of dopamine in mood disorders. *Compr Psychiatry* 1992; 33:115–20.

72. Henzl MR. Gonadotropin-releasing hormone (GnRH) agonists in the management of endometriosis: A review. *Clin Obstet Gynecol* 1988; 31:840–56.

73. Warnock JK, Bundren JC. Anxiety and mood disorders associated with gonadotropin-releasing hormone agonist therapy. *Psychopharmacol Bull* 1997; 33: 311–6.

74. Warnock JK, Bundren JC, Morris. Sertraline in the treatment of depression associated with gonadotropin releasing hormone agonist therapy. *Biol Psychiatry* 1998; 43:464–5.

75. Toren P, Dor J, Mester R, et al. Depression in women treated with a gonadotropin-releasing hormone agonist. *Biol Psychiatry* 1996; 39:378–82.

76. Weizman ES, Toren P, Dor Y, et al. Chronic GnRH agonist administration down-regulates platelet serotonin transporter in women undergoing assisted reproductive treatment. *Psychopharm* 1996; 125:141–5.

77. Varney NR, Syrop C, Kubu CS, et al. Neuropsychologic dysfunction in women following leuprolide acetate induction of hypoestrogenism. *J Assist Reprod Genet* 1993; 10:53–7.

78. Newton C, Slota D, Yuzpe AA, et al. Memory complaints associated with the use of gonadotropin-releasing hormone agonists: A preliminary study. *Fertil Steril* 1996; 65:1253–5.

79. Sherwin BB, Tulandi T. 'Add-back' estrogen reverses cognitive deficits induced by a gonadotropin-releasing hormone agonist in women with leiomyomata uteri. *J Clin Endocrinol Metab* 1996; 81:2545–9.

80. Culberg J. Premenstrual symptom patterns and mental reactions to medication – a latent profile analysis. *Acta Psychiatr Scand Suppl* 1972; 236:9–86.

81. Wagner KD, Berenson AB. Norplant-associated major depression and panic disorder. *J Clin Psychiatry* 1994; 55:478–89.

82. Jensvold MF. Nonpregnant reproductive age women. Part II: Exogenous sex steroid hormones and psychopharmacology. In: MF Jensvold, U Halbreich, JA Hamilton, eds. *Psychopharmacology and Women: Sex, Gender and Hormones*, Washington DC: American Psychiatric Press Inc., 1996; 171–90.

83. *International Classification of Diseases and Related Problems*, 9th ed. Geneva: World Health Organization, 1992.

84. WHO World Mental Health Survey Consortium, *JAMA* 2004; 291:2581–90.

85. Domar AD, Siebel MM, Benson H. The mind/body program for infertility: A new behavioral treatment approach for women with infertility. *Fertil Steril* 1990; 53:246–9.

86. Domar AD, Zuttermeister PC, Seibel M, et al. Psychological improvement in infertile women after behavioral treatment: A replication. *Fertil Steril* 1992; 58:144–7.

87. O'Hara MS, Zekoski EM, Phillips LH, et al. Controlled prospective study of postpartum mood disorders: A comparison of childbearing and non-childbearing women. *J Abnorm Psychol* 1990; 99:3–15.

88. Cohen LS, Nonacs RM, Bailey JW, et al. Relapse of depression during pregnancy following antidepressant discontinuation: A preliminary prospective study. *Arch Women Ment Health* 2004; 7:217–21.

89. Altshuler LL, Cohen L, Szuba MP, et al. Pharmacologic management of psychiatric illness during pregnancy: Dilemmas and guidelines. *Am J Psychiatry* 1996; 153:595–606.

90. McElhatton PR, Garbis HM, Elefant E, et al. The outcome of pregnancy in 689 women exposed to therapeutic doses of antidepressants: A collaborative study of the European Network of Teratology Information Services (ENTIS). *Reprod Toxicol* 1996; 10:285–94.

91. Misri S, Sivertz K. Tricyclic drugs in pregnancy and lactation: A preliminary report. *Int J Psychiatry Med* 1991; 21:157–71.

92. Nulman I, Rovet J, Stewart DE, et al. Neurodevelopment of children exposed in utero to antidepressant drugs. *N Engl J Med* 1997; 336:258–62.

93. Wisner KL, Perel JM, Wheeler SM. Tricyclic dose requirements across pregnancy. *Am J Psychiatry* 1993; 150:1541–2.

94. Hendrick V, Smith LM, Suri R, et al. Birth outcomes after prenatal exposure to antidepressant medication. *Am J Obstet Gynecol* 2003; 188:812–5.

95. Simon GE, Cunninham ML, Davis Rl. Outcomes of prenatal antidepressant exposure. *Am J Psychiatry* 2002; 159:2055–61.

96. Ericson A, Kallen B, Wiholm BE. Delivery outcome after the use of antidepressants in early pregnancy. *Eur J Clin Pharmacol* 1999; 55:503–8.

97. Kulin N, Pastuuszak A, Sage S, et al. Pregnancy outcome following maternal use of the new selective serotonin reuptake inhibitors: A prospective controlled muticenter study. *JAMA* 1998; 279:609–10.

98. Goldstein DJ. Effects of third trimester fluoxetine exposure on the newborn. *J Clin Psychopharmacol* 1995; 15:417–20.

99. Pastuszak A, Schick-Boschetto B, Zuber C, et al. Pregnancy outcome following first-trimester exposure to fluoxetine. *JAMA* 1993; 269:2246–8.

100. Einarson A, Ratoye B, Sarkar M, et al. Pregnancy outcome following gestational exposure to venlafaxine: a multicenter prospective controlled study. *Am J Psychiatry* 2001; 158:1728–30.

101. Williams M, Wooltorton E. Paroxetine (Paxil) and congenital malformations. *CMAJ* 2005; 173:1320–1.

102. Kallen B. Neonate characteristics after maternal use of antidepressants in pregnancy. *Arch Pediatr Adolesc Med* 2004; 158:312–6.

103. Chambers CD, Johnson KA, Dick LM, et al. Birth outcomes in pregnant women taking fluoxetine. *N Engl J Med* 1996; 335:1010–15.

104. Casper RC, Fleisher BE, Lee-Ancaias JC, et al. Follow up of children of depressed mothers exposed or not exposed to antidepressant drugs during pregnancy. *J Pediatr* 2003; 142:402–8.

105. Costei AM, Kozer E, Ho T, et al. Perinatal outcome following third trimester exposure to paroxetine. *Arch Pediatr Adolesc Med* 2002; 156:1129–32.

106. Casper RC, Fleisher BE, Lee-Ancais JC, et al. Late pregnancy exposure to SSRIs is associated with neonatal adjustment problems and subtle motor changes in infancy compared to early pregnancy exposed to SSRI or no drug exposed. *Neuropharmacology Abstracts*. 2004 ACNP 43 annual meeting. Supplement 1: 102.

107. Oberlander TF, Misri S, Fitzgerald CE, et al. Pharmacologic factors associated with transient neonatal symptoms following prenatal psychotropic medications exposure. *J Clin Psychiatry* 2004; 65:230–7.

108. American Academy of Pediatrics Committee on Drugs. American Academy of Pediatrics. *Pediatrics* 2004.

109. Zeskind PS, Stephens LE. Maternal selective serotonin reuptake inhibitor use during pregnancy and newborn neurobehavior. *Pediatrics* 2004; 113:368–75.

110. Nulman I, Rovet J, Stewart DE, et al. Child development following exposure to trictyclic antidepressants or fluoxetine throughout fetal life: A prospective, controlled study. *Am J Psychiatry* 2002; 159:1189–95.

111. De Ceballos ML, Benedi A, Urdin C, et al. Prenatal exposure of rats to antidepressant drugs down-regulates beta adrenoreceptors and 5-HT receptors in cerebral cortex. Lack of correlation between 5-HT receptors and serotonin-mediated behavior. *Neuropharmacology* 1985; 24:947–52.

112. Ansorge MS, Zhou M, Lira A, et al. Early life blockade of the 5HT transporter alters emotional behavior in adult mice. *Science* 2004; 306:878–81.

113. Schatzberg AF, Cole JO. *Manual of Clinical Psychopharmacology*. Washington DC: American Psychiatric Press Inc., 1991.

114. DeBattista C. *Medical Management of Depression*. Durant, OK: Emis Inc, 1997.

115. Bronzo M, Stahl S. Galactorrhea induced by sertraline. *Am J Psychiatry* 1993; 150:1269–70.

116. Lesaca T. Sertraline and galactorrhea (letter). *J Clin Psychopharmacol* 1996; 16:333–4.

117. Amsterdam JD, Garcia-Espana F, Goodman D, et al. Breast enlargement during chronic antidepressant therapy. *J Affect Disord* 1997; 46:151–6.

118. Iancu J, Ratzoni G, Weitaman A, et al. More fluoxetine experience. *J Am Acad Child Adolesc Psych* 1992; 31:755–6.

119. Emiliano AB, Fudge JL. From galactorrhea to osteopenia: Rethinking serotonin-prolactin interactions. *Neuropsychopharm* 2004; 29:833–46.

120. Hendrick V, Gitlin M, Altshuler L, et al. Antidepressant medications, mood and male fertility. *Psychneuroendocrinology* 2000; 25:37–51.

121. Gregorian RS, Golden KA, Bahce A, et al. Antidepressant induced sexual dysfunction. *Ann Pharmacother* 2000; 36:1577–89.

122. Hemels ME, Einarson A, Koren G, et al. Antidepressant use during pregnancy and rates of spontaneous abortions: A meta-analysis. *Ann Pharmacother* 2005; 39:803–9.

123. Klock SC, Sheinin S, Kazer R, et al. A pilot study of the relationship between selective serotonin reuptake inhibitors and in vitro fertilization outcome. *Fertility and Sterility* 2004; 82:968–9.

124. Lapane KL, Zierler S, Thomas M, et al. Is a history of depressive symptoms associated with an increased risk of infertility in women? *Psychosom Med* 1995; 57:509–13.

125. Meller W, Burns LH, Crow S, et al. Major depression in unexplained infertility. *J Psychosom Obstet Gynaecol* 2002; 23:27–30.

126. Thiering P, Beaurepaire J, Jones M, et al. Mood state as a predictor of treatment outcome after in vitro fertilization/embryo transfer technology (IVF/ET). *J Psychosom Res* 1993; 37:481–91.

127. Demyttenaere K, Bonte L, Gheldof M, et al. Coping style and depression level influence outcome in in vitro fertilization. *Fertility and Sterility* 1998; 69:1026–33.

128. Smeenk JMJ, Verhaak CM, van Minnen A, et al. The effect of anxiety and depression on the outcome of in-vitro fertilization. *Human Reprod* 2001; 16:1420–3.

129. Rubinow DR, Roca CA. Editorial comment: Infertility and depression. *Psychosom Med* 1995; 57:514–6.

130. Meller WH, Zander KM, Crosby RD, et al. Luteinizing hormone pulse characteristics in depressed women. *Am J Psychiatry* 1997; 154:1454–5.

131. Meller WH, Grambsch PL, Bingham C, et al. Hypothalamic pituitary gonadal axis dysregulation in depressed women. *Psychoneuroendocrinology* 2001; 26:253–9.

132. Weber B, Lewicka S, Deuschle M, et al. Testosterone, androstenedione and dihydrotestosterone concentrations are elevated in female patients with major depression. *Psychoneuroend* 2000; 25:765–71.

133. Viguera AC, Nonacs R, Cohen LS, et al. Risk of recurrence of bipolar disorder in pregnant and nonpregnant women after discontinuation of Lithium. *Am J Psychiatry* 2000; 157:179–84.

134. Yonkers KA, Wisner KL, Stowe Z, et al. Management of bipolar disorder furing pregnancy and the postpartum period. *Am J Psychiatry* 2004; 161:608–20.

135. Keck PE, McElroy SL, Tugrul KG, et al. Valproate oral loading in the treatment of acute mania. *J Clin Psychiatry* 1993; 54:305–8.

136. Stewart DE, Klompenhauwer JL, Kendell RE, et al. Prophylactic lithium in peurperal psychosis: The experience of three centers. *Br J Psychiatry* 1991; 158: 393–7.

137. Cohen LS, Sichel DA, Robertson LH, et al. Postpartum prophylaxis for women with bipolar disorder. *J Clin Psychiatry* 1995; 55:289–92.

138. Maes M, Smith R, Christophe A, et al. Fatty acid composition in major depression: Decreased 3 fractions in cholesteryl esters and increased C20:46/C20:53 ratio in cholesteryl esters and phospholipids. *Journal of Affective Disorders* 1996; 38:1–71.

139. Adams PB, Lawson S, Sanigorski A, et al. Arachidonic acid to eicosapentaenoic acid ration in blood correlates positively with clinical symptoms of depression. *Lipids* 1996; 32:157–61.

140. Edwards M, Peet M, Shay J, et al. Omega-3 polyunsaturated fatty acid levels in the diet and in red blood cell membranes of depressed patients. *J. Affect. Disord* 1998; 48:149–55.

141. Huan M, Hamazaki K, Sun Y, et al. Suicide attempt and n-3 fatty acids levels in red blood: A case control study in China *Biol Psychiatry* 2004; 56:490–6.

142. Hibbeln J. Seafood consumption, the DHA content of mother's milk and prevalence of rates of postpartum depression: A cross-sectional, ecological analysis. *J. Affect. Disorders* 2002; 69:15–21.

143. Otto S, de Groot RH, Hornstra G. Increased risk of postpartum depressive symptoms is associated with slower normalization after pregnancy of the functional docosahexaenoic acid status. *Prostaglandins Leukot Essent Fatty Acids* 2003; 69:237–43.

144. De Vriese SR, Christophe AB, Maes M. Lowered serum n-3 polyunsaturated fatty acid (PUFA) levels predict the occurrence of postpartum depression: Further evidence lowered n-PUFAs are related to major depression *Life Sci* 2003; 73:3181–7.

145. Llorente AM, Jensen CL, Voigt RG, et al. Effect of maternal docosahexaenoic acid supplementation on postpartum depression and information processing. *Am J Obstet Gynecol* 2003; 188:1348–53.

146. Marangell L, Martinez J, Zboyan H, et al. A double-blind, placebo-controlled study of the omega-3 fatty acid

docosahexaenoic acid in the treatment of major depression. *Am J Psychiatry* 2003; 160:996–8.

147. Freeman MP, Hibbeln J, Wisner K, et al. Double blind dose finding study of omega-3 fatty acids for postpartum depression. *Neuropharmacology Abstracts* 2004 ACNP 43 annual meeting. Supplement 1: 102.

148. Olsen S, Sorensen J, Secher N, et al. Randomized controlled trial of effect of fish-oil supplementation on pregnancy duration. *Lancet* 1992; 339:1003–7.

149. Helland I, Smith L, Saarem K, et al. Maternal supplementation with very-long-chain n-3 fatty acids during pregnancy and lactation augments children's IQ at 4 years of age. *Pediatrics* 2003; 111:39–44.

150. Dunstan JA, et al. Fish oil supplementation in pregnancy modifies neonatal allergen-specific immune responses and clinical outcomes in infants at high risk of atopy: A randomized, controlled trial. *J Allergy Clin Immunol* 2003; 112:1178–84.

151. Williams KE, Koran L. Obsessive compulsive disorder in pregnancy, premenstruum and postpartum. *J Clin Psychiatry* 1997; 58:330–4.

152. Miller LJ. Psychiatric medication during pregnancy: Understanding and minimizing the risks. *Psychiatr Ann* 1994; 24:69–75.

153. Perry JC. Depression in borderline personality disorder: Lifetime prevalence at interview and longitudinal course of symptoms. *Is J Psychiatry* 1985; 142:15–21.

154. Herman JL, Perry C, van der Kolk BA. Childhood trauma in borderline personality disorder. *Am J Psychiatry* 1989; 146:490–5.

155. Linehan MM. *Cognitive-Behavioral Treatment of Borderline Personality Disorder*. New York: Guilford Press, 1993.

156. Kohut H, Wolff ES. The disorders of the self and their treatment: An outline. *Int J Psychoanal* 1978; 59:413–25.

157. Ethics Committee of the American Society of Reproductive Medicine. Child-rearing and the provision of fertility services. *Fertil Steril* 2004; 82:51.

158. Goldfarb JM, Rosenthal MB, Utian WH. Impact of psychological factors in the care of the infertile couple. *Semin Reprod Endocrinol* 1985; 3:93–9.

7 Evidenced-Based Approaches to Infertility Counseling

JACKY BOIVIN

By some small sample we judge of the whole piece.
– Cervantes

Despite some forty years of endorsement for psychosocial interventions in infertility, there is poor integration of evidence and research into professional practice. Indeed, research shows that practitioners are unlikely to engage in research at postqualification level, tend to rank research as a lower priority than clinical commitments, and tend to regard the research literature as irrelevant to their professional practice. This is a risky stance because there is increasing pressure from third-party payers, government agencies, and professional organizations on practitioners to demonstrate both the effectiveness and efficiency of their services. Infertility counselors need to find a way to integrate research and research findings into their everyday practice if they are to meet these new challenges.

This chapter presents the need for evidence-based approaches to the practice of infertility counseling and provides a framework for clinicians to meet this challenge.

This chapter

■ summarizes recent findings on effectiveness of counseling in infertility;
■ describes frameworks relevant to the integration of research and practice, and the execution of evaluation studies;
■ discusses the application of research in everyday practice;
■ examines research issues in private practice.

HISTORICAL OVERVIEW

The provision of psychosocial interventions for infertile couples has been strongly recommended since the consumer advocacy work of Barbara Eck Menning[1] directed clinical and research attention to emotional distress as a consequence of infertility rather than, as had been the emphasis until then – a cause of fertility problems. Her recommendation to provide psychosocial services to infertile couples has been reiterated by regulatory bodies in several countries, various associations involved in the care of infertile couples both at a professional and community level as well as those of numerous mental health professionals working with infertile couples. Moreover, the recommendation is consistent with the interest infertile people themselves have expressed in receiving more psychosocial help.

In response to these recommendations, numerous interventions have been developed from a range of theoretical perspectives, for example, theories of grief and loss and crisis, or cognitive-behavioral theory. The therapeutic goals in these interventions have been in accordance with the negative effects observed in clinical work and empirical studies, namely, the reduction of distress, enhanced coping skills, improvement in quality of life and interpersonal relationships, and/or increased pregnancy rates.[2] The sustained interest in psychosocial interventions is also due to compelling research demonstrating that psychological factors can have a negative impact on the course of treatment.[3–6]

Despite some forty years of endorsement for psychosocial interventions in infertility, it is surprising to find that only twenty-five to thirty independent studies have evaluated the effectiveness of psychosocial interventions. Indeed, there is a staggering disparity in the percentage of published counseling studies recommending specific interventions (i.e., 94%) and those evaluating their effectiveness (i.e., 6%).[7] However remarkable this disparity may be, it is reflective of the poor integration of evidence and research into professional practice shown in all professions concerned with mental health.[8] Indeed, research shows that practitioners are unlikely to engage in research at postqualification level, tend to rank research as a lower priority than clinical commitments, and tend to regard the

117

research literature as irrelevant to their professional practice.[9] While the inequality between investment in research and practice has, until now, been tolerated as an inevitable reflection of the priorities of the practitioner, the application of evidence-based principles to medicine and the pressures of the managed healthcare industry in the United States and other countries make this tolerant attitude increasingly risky.[10]

Managed healthcare means growing demands from third-party payers, government agencies, and professional organizations on practitioners to demonstrate both the effectiveness and efficiency of their services.[11,12] The influence of these commissioners on practice cannot be underestimated. In a 1995 report by Division 12 of the American Psychological Association (APA), eighteen psychological therapies were pronounced effective (i.e., 'empirically validated') to counter the increasing preference of insurers to fund only evidence-based biological therapies (e.g., antidepressants) for psychological disorders.[13] While this approach stopped the ebb of funding for listed therapies, it practically killed the practice of those not on the list (see Larner[10]). In the United Kingdom, the National Institute of Clinical Excellence (NICE) has similarly recommended specific 'evidence-based' treatments for psychological disorders and only those treatments are expected to receive funding from the National Health Service (NHS).[14] These examples show that current legislative emphasis has significantly influenced therapeutic decision making, from intuition and clinical judgment toward the use of research findings and empirical evaluation.[12]

It would be a mistake to think that such systematic comparisons of performance (so-called 'league tables') are far removed from the field of infertility. In its recent guidelines on evidence-based infertility treatment, NICE recently recommended against the mandatory provision of psychosocial counseling for infertility on the basis of its mixed evidence base. Thus, however politically or financially motivated one perceives these league tables to be (see, for example, Larner[10]), all practitioners in the field of infertility should consider the impact of this climate change on their practice, and, in light of these precedents, should be motivated to ensure that counseling makes it into the club of exclusive evidence-based interventions in infertility. In order to do that, there needs to be a far better integration of research and practice in this field.

Even if one wishes to ignore political issues, greater integration between research and practice is warranted because recent reviews[7,15] show that some interventions are not effective and that others vary significantly in their effectiveness, indicating a need to modify current approaches to infertility counseling. The Code of Practice for many helping professions requires that practitioners undertake ongoing efforts to develop and maintain their competence and ensure that they are up-to-date with current best practice (e.g., American Psychological Association[16]). Thus, the research-practice issue is also one concerned with the ethics of practice.

In light of these considerations, two important goals for the field in the next decade should be: (1) the generation of evaluation research on psychosocial interventions used in infertility, and (2) the integration of this and other research (empirical and clinical) in practice. Fortunately, infertility counselors can learn from decades of psychotherapy research in meeting both these goals.

REVIEW OF LITERATURE

The published work dealing with psychosocial interventions in infertility has recently been reviewed; therefore, only key findings from this review will be presented here (see Boivin[7] for a detailed analysis). In this review, a systematic literature search procedure was undertaken to identify all studies evaluating the effect of a psychosocial intervention on at least one outcome in people with fertility problems (between the years 1966 and 2001). A total of thirty-five studies were identified, and of these only twenty-five were independent evaluations. It should be noted that the studies varied dramatically in their quality and only eleven could be said to meet current criteria for evidence-based medicine, that is, studies that used a control group and that either used random assignment to groups or a pre-to-post design to account for the influence of uncontrolled factors on intervention effects. Furthermore, the patient, therapists, and settings varied significantly among studies. Most clients were patients in treatment; most interventions were delivered to couples or groups; and the average duration of interventions varied from one to thirty-two weeks (average nine weeks), with an average follow-up period of just over six months.

Despite this heterogeneity, it was possible to group the psychosocial interventions into two broad classes, counseling and educational interventions.[1] The feature that distinguished these classes was the therapeutic objective. Educational interventions were designed to

---

[1] In the original review, educational interventions were further subdivided into focused (only one skill taught) or comprehensive (more than one skill taught), but as the results did not differ according to this distinction, it is omitted here.

impart knowledge (e.g., medical, lifestyle) and provide skills training, for example, improve stress management,[17] coping skills,[18] or a combination of skills (e.g., Domar et al.[19]; Clark et al.[20]). In contrast, the main goals in counseling were emotional expression and support, and/or discussion of thoughts and feelings related to infertility (as cause or consequence). Counseling could be further classified into psychodynamic (e.g., Kemeter & Fiegl[21]), cognitive-behavioral (e.g., Liswood[22]), or infertility-focused counseling (e.g., Wischmann et al.[23]). It was acknowledged that the educational and counseling classes were not wholly independent and that information could be provided in counseling and emotional expression in educational programs. However, the interventions were sufficiently different in their emphasis to warrant separation into these respective classes.

The Boivin[7] review highlighted the kinds of therapeutic goals that could realistically be achieved with the types of psychosocial interventions used with infertile people. Reducing emotional distress (especially anxiety) and improving domains known to be negatively affected by infertility (e.g., sex during the fertile period and infertility-specific distress) were goals more likely to be achieved than making changes to traits or altering interpersonal relations (i.e., improved marital or social relationships) or pregnancy rates. These conclusions were based on the finding that about 49% of analyses on negative affect (e.g., anxiety, depression) showed positive intervention effects compared with 27% of analyses on traits and interpersonal functioning (e.g., personality features, marital functioning). Furthermore, comparisons in studies with pregnancy as an outcome were equivocal, as 62.5% of studies did not find a positive intervention effect. These findings were robust, as they were found overall and in better-quality studies. The importance of negative affect (e.g., anxiety, infertility-specific distress) as an outcome was consistent with emotional distress being a frequent presenting complaint, but with it being a reasonable outcome to target in the short duration of interventions typically offered to infertile people (e.g., six months). It should be noted that infertility-specific assessments tools were more sensitive to treatment effects than were global assessments.

The most successful interventions had a strong educational and skills training component and lasted about twelve weeks with a follow-up period of at least six months. The types of skills taught included relaxation training (e.g., Stewart et al.[24]), sex techniques,[25] or coping skills[18] whereas information mainly concerned procedural information about upcoming medical tests and treatments (e.g., Takefman et al.[26]), and

the impact of lifestyle factors (e.g., Domar et al.[19] or other health problems (e.g., obesity[20]) on fertilit In contrast, counseling interventions that focused primarily on emotional expression and support were less effective.

Several hypotheses were offered to account for the difference in effectiveness between educational programs and counseling interventions (see Boivin[7] for detailed exploration). First, most educational programs were group programs whereas counseling was almost exclusively delivered to couples. Groups may have features that are especially important to this patient group (e.g., validation and normalization) or, alternatively, aspects of counseling, for example, the male partner being reluctant to participate, may have been detrimental. It is also possible that the therapeutic goals in educational programs (e.g., increased frequency of sex during the fertile period,[25] and improved relaxation techniques[24]) can be more easily achieved or detected at assessment than the more diffuse goals of counseling (e.g., working through grief[27]). Finally, counseling may be more useful with certain types of patients, and the lack of differentiation among patient groups in the review may have obscured these results. For example, most patients were in treatment so that the strains they were facing may have lent themselves well to techniques used in educational programs (e.g., stress of waiting for test results, decision making about particular treatments) whereas other patient groups, for example, those ending treatment, may be facing other issues (e.g., "Can I have a meaningful life without children?") that lend themselves better to a [couple] psychotherapeutic counseling format.

Men and women benefited equally from interventions despite the fact that men were generally less interested or willing to participate in psychosocial counseling. However, each may have benefited for different reasons. For example, women report support groups to be useful because of the sense of belonging and validation of their reactions, whereas men report the groups to be useful because of the practical information and advice they receive.[28] Similar findings have been obtained for gender differences in the perception of telephone counseling.[29]

It should be noted that a recent meta-analytic analysis of the studies examined in the Boivin[7] review was carried out by de Liz and Strauss.[15] The conclusions from both reviews were consistent. De Liz and Strauss additionally proposed that the timing of interventions and assessments might be particularly important to their effectiveness.

Overall, the review was important in bringing together, for the first time, the outcome studies that examined the effectiveness of counseling, and in demonstrating support for the use of psychosocial interventions in this field. However, the systematic search also showed that too little attention had been devoted to the evaluation of the interventions available and, importantly, that practitioners were continuing to use interventions that were not producing concrete gains for people. These findings have implications for practitioners and researchers, as noted previously. For the practitioner, the findings point to the need to integrate research findings into everyday practice. For the researcher, the final recommendation of the review was that attention be directed toward the 'who,' 'what,' 'when' questions of counseling. That is, future evaluation studies need to yield relevant information for the practitioner about what kinds of change are produced by what kinds of interventions, for what kind of patients, by what kinds of therapists, and under what kinds of conditions.[31]

THEORETICAL FRAMEWORKS

The two theoretical frameworks applied here are the scientist-practitioner model and psychotherapeutic outcome model. The scientist-practitioner model describes a framework of principles to guide the application of research findings to practice. The psychotherapy outcome models provide approaches for the evaluation of interventions in psychotherapy.

The scientist-practitioner (S-P) or Boulder model[32] is the most common training model in clinical psychology, and since its conception in 1949, has been adopted by many more mental health professions (see, for example, in counseling[12]). Individuals trained under this framework are expected to carry out particular tasks that will ensure an evidence-based practice. Practitioners are expected to: (1) regularly read and apply research findings to their practice; (2) follow a scientific approach to clinical decision making and practicing; (3) regularly evaluate their practice; and (4) conduct clinically meaningful research, either on their own or in collaboration with researchers.[33] By clinically meaningful, it was meant that research should develop a better understanding of human beings, as well as improve the effectiveness and reliability of diagnostic procedures, interventions, and methods to promote mental health and prevent maladjustment.[32] There has been much debate about how these goals and tasks can be achieved in various contexts (a point returned to later), and whether training under this framework versus any other makes a difference to research output.[33] Despite these debates, the continued endorsement of this model in psychology and increasingly in other fields, suggests

that the principles of the S-P model target objectives that are desired by many mental health professions, that is practice should be influenced by research developments and vice versa.[11]

Models of psychotherapy outcome research have yielded two approaches to carrying out evaluation studies. The first approach, which is intervention-focused, assumes that an intervention is effective in producing a benefit (e.g., decreased fear response) because of its unique techniques (e.g., desensitization) derived from a unique theoretical perspective (i.e., self-efficacy theory). The questions addressed by this approach are whether an intervention is effective, and if so, to what extent it is compared to untreated or differently treated groups. In terms of research designs, the gold standard for this approach is the randomized controlled trial (RCT), where consecutive patients are randomly assigned to the experimental and control conditions. This type of design is the least biased form of evidence because it controls for nonspecific factors that may influence the responses of experimental and controls groups on outcome measures and, consequently, ensures that differences between groups treated and alternatively treated groups on outcome measures are due to intervention effects rather than to other factors not controlled as part of the experiment.[34]

Practitioners interested in specific interventions can evaluate entire intervention packages as they are ordinarily administered or 'dismantle' the intervention in an effort to determine which aspect of treatment is the active ingredient. For example, in early work, Domar et al.[35] found that a mind–body program was effective in reducing emotional distress and increasing pregnancy rates in people who had been infertile for about two years. This mind–body program (adapted for infertile women from a program targeting other medical conditions) combines relaxation training, peer support, and lifestyle changes to effect positive change in a range of domains. This uncontrolled research was followed-up with an RCT, which compared the mind–body program against a group that received peer support only and a group that did not receive any intervention. In this second dismantling study, it was found that while the mind–body program was superior to support or control conditions on some psychological variables (e.g., stress-management skills, state anxiety, vigor[19]), it was equivalent to the support group when it came to pregnancy rates, and both were superior to the control group.[36] Another form of outcome research examines varying the parameters of an intervention (e.g., number of sessions, number of clients in the group) to discover how to maximize the benefits of a specific intervention.[31] Many other designs can apply to this

TABLE 7.1. Factors that are common across different types of therapies that may be responsible for positive therapeutic effects[40]

Domain	Examples
Client characteristics	Positive expectations, initial client distress, help-seeking behavior
Practitioner qualities	Warmth, empathic understanding, socially sanctioned healer, expertise
Change processes	Opportunity for catharsis/ventilation, provision of a rationale or explanation for the problem, acquisition and practice of new behaviors; emotional/interpersonal learning
Treatment structure	Use of techniques/rituals, a healing setting, communication, defined roles
Therapeutic relationship	Development of an alliance, transference, engagement

approach, but the main point is to focus on evaluating individual therapies and their unique characteristics. Research emanating from this approach has probably contributed most to the league tables of empirically supported [psychological] treatments described earlier, as well as to the generation of detailed 'how to' psychotherapeutic manuals (i.e., so-called manualization) of many interventions.[37]

The second approach to evaluation studies focuses on what makes interventions similar and how that explains positive change. This approach arises from the paradoxical findings of several meta-analyses showing that despite technical and theoretical diversity, psychotherapy interventions all yield more or less the same level of benefit.[38,39] Such findings suggest that it is not the uniqueness of the intervention that is important in generating benefits, but a set of general clinical principles that must underlie all interventions aimed at helping people. The integrationist perspective[2] (or 'common-factors' approach) seeks to determine the core ingredients shared by different therapies to develop more efficacious treatments based on these commonalities. Grencavage and Norcross[40] identified five domains of commonality across therapies (see Table 7.1) and examined the extent of agreement among therapists practicing from different perspectives about the importance of these domains. They found that the common factors most therapists listed as essential for positive change were the development of a therapeutic alliance, opportunity for catharsis, acquisition and practice of new behaviors, and the

client's positive expectations. It has been argued that a significant proportion of variance in therapy outcome can be attributed to these common factors rather than to unique features of interventions.[41]

Practitioners who carry out research under this approach are more likely to use process research and qualitative methodologies than the randomized controlled trial. In process research, the researcher is interested in the phenomenology of the therapeutic relationship with a focus on examining how elements of that relationship (e.g., empathy, positive expectations, setting) contribute to the overall gains made by the patient.[31] In a review of evaluation research in counseling, it was found that 45% of studies investigated the effect of a common factor and about a third of studies used a descriptive approach or qualitative approach to explain therapeutic gains.[41]

From the types of designs used in evaluation studies in infertility, it cannot yet be determined which approach (unique or common factors) will or should dominate this field in the future. It should be noted, however, that the area appears to have spawned its own unique type of counseling, referred to as infertility counseling, and this may lend itself more to a common factors perspective. This intervention focuses directly on reactions to infertility and on discussions about the impact of infertility on various domains, for example, marital and sexual relations, or on feelings of masculinity or femininity. As practiced, it would seem to be a form of eclecticism that evolved organically from a humanist approach,[1] which has assimilated techniques relevant to coping with fertility from other perspectives (e.g., mourning from grief and loss theory, or reality testing from cognitive-behavioral approaches). Given this developmental history, it would be difficult to argue for the proposal that infertility counseling is helpful because of its unique features.

CLINICAL ISSUES

How can these theoretical frameworks and perspectives help achieve the goals of integration and generation of evaluation research? In this section, the application of the five scientist-practitioner principles to practice are discussed including methods to evaluate interventions in private practice.

---

[2] It should be noted that this perspective is not the same as technical eclecticism that recognizes virtues of different techniques and samples from them as needed to effect therapeutic change.

Practitioners Need to Regularly Read Research

To read research, practitioners must have access to it. Boivin[7] found that approximately 2,000 studies had been published on psychosocial aspects of infertility in the past thirty-five years, which would amount to reading one paper per week. This is a reasonable task, even for a busy practitioner – but only when the studies are available. The studies examined in the review had been published in about twenty psychology or medical journals, making the time and financial costs of accessing the information significantly more demanding. Fortunately, three electronic developments more or less help to overcome such difficulties. First, electronic services make access to information easier, more efficient, and, in many cases, free. Access to abstracts from many journals is easy with free electronic search engines available via the internet (e.g., PubMed). Many journals now have online alerts that send the table of contents for each issue to individual email accounts, reducing search time (and providing a helpful cue to keep on top of new research, editorials, and commentaries). Some journals devote themselves to integrating research findings by only publishing reviews or research syntheses (e.g., *In Session: Psychotherapy in Practice; Human Reproduction Updates*), and signing up to their table of contents service may be useful. Searching online bookshops using relevant key words also allows easy access to recently published books nationally and internationally. A second important electronic tool is email. Email now makes it possible to obtain published work directly from authors, quickly and with relatively little cost. Increased use of mail groups and networking among practitioners and researchers increases opportunities to receive and discuss new research. Finally, the greater precision of search engines (e.g., Google) now makes it possible to efficiently search for online help to better understand the published research being read, whether that is to find out about statistical tests, specific questionnaires, or regulations about treatment in different countries. In combination, these approaches can and should help practitioners keep on top of new work (whether clinical or research).

Practitioners Need to Follow a Scientific Approach to Clinical Decision Making and Practice

The scientist-practitioner model encourages practitioners to adopt a scientific approach to clinical decision making, although it fails to define or delineate what that really means. The impression is that decisions should be based on the application of research findings that improve best practice, but how one evaluates these find-

ings or implements 'best practice' is not addressed.[42] The principles of evidence-based medicine (EBM) were designed to meet that goal, in that they offer a framework to guide the search for and appraisal of clinically relevant information. The need for the principles espoused in EBM arose as a result of several factors in clinical medicine that, not surprisingly, extend to mental health professionals. There is a need for valid, up-to-date information about assessment and therapeutic interventions for a broad range of clients and problems, but most clinicians are unable to spend more than a short period of time per week on study and research.[43]

The process of EBM is fairly straightforward and can be practiced by mental health professionals concerned with the implementation of clinical decisions that have empirical support. There are five basic steps (see Sackett et al.[43] for detailed instructions of each step including practice exercises) that can be briefly illustrated with the following example. Suppose a forty-three-year-old Egyptian woman contacts a counselor in Western Europe because she has been experiencing acute distress since she and her husband decided to end infertility treatment and remain child-free.

First, the need for information is converted into an answerable question (e.g., "In Egyptian women facing permanent childlessness, is infertility counseling more effective in reducing acute distress than an educational group program?").

Second, the best evidence with which to answer that question is found. This would normally involve a search of relevant databases or access to valid reviews. For this example, one review found that educational programs were superior to counseling interventions in reducing acute distress.[7]

Third, the evidence is critically appraised for its validity, impact, and applicability. In the review, none of the interventions were with Egyptian women or women who had stopped treatment and only one study examined the effect of the intervention according to pretreatment distress.[7] That study showed that while infertility counseling was not effective overall, it was beneficial to *highly* distressed women.[44] This examination of research suggests that the findings of the review may not be applicable to this patient, and therefore more relevant sources of information for the case at hand need to be examined. Such findings indicate, for example, that the transition from 'not yet pregnant' to 'never going to be pregnant,'[45] is slow and acutely distressing because it involves addressing existential issues about core beliefs and values. For example, the process involves redefining the self and constructing a meaningful life.[46] It was also found that acute distress was more common at the beginning of the transition process, and when couples could not imagine a future life without children or disagreed about future parenting options.[46]

These findings were based on prospective empirical studies of people who had just ended treatment, and data were analyzed according to well-validated quantitative and qualitative methods. It was also found that in Egypt, infertility was highly stigmatizing and associated with much abuse of women, even if the woman was not the source of the fertility problem (e.g., van Rooij et al.[47]) (see Chapter 4).

Fourth, the critical appraisal is integrated with the clinician's clinical expertise and with their patients' unique psyche, values, and circumstances. The choice of an effective treatment plan is hampered by the limited evaluation of interventions on samples similar to the presenting client. Nevertheless, a counseling format was chosen, given that the client was most likely to be facing existential issues whose exploration required a less structured format than would be offered in educational programs. Research findings suggested that a couple approach would be most appropriate and this would be offered to the client, even though cultural stigma about psychological therapy made it unlikely that the husband would be willing to take up this offer.

The final step in the EBM process requires that clinicians evaluate their effectiveness and efficiency in executing the EBM process and try to find ways to improve them. For this example, the process of finding information about this case showed a gap in knowledge about this cultural group and people ending treatment.

While the EBM process was briefly reviewed here, it illustrates, basically, the expectation is that high-quality research will be used to inform all clinical decisions. It is expected that over time the clinician becomes familiar with much of the research that affects their particular area of expertise and practice so that the search for information is less onerous and more expeditious. In cases where gaps in knowledge exist, practitioners must rely on their clinical judgment and practice guidelines that also encourage collaboration with other professionals working in the field and clinical supervision. Although gaps in knowledge present a limit on the effectiveness of the EBM process, they do serve to direct future research activity.

Practitioners Need to Regularly Evaluate Their Practice

Most codes of practice urge clinicians to examine regularly and consistently whether the interventions they provide are helpful. Monitoring effectiveness in a clinical setting always provides a challenge because it typically occurs on a case-by-case basis rather than via randomized controlled trials (RCTs). However, the validity of the single-case analysis can be increased by making the process of assessment more systematic and in line with the more controlled assessment of evaluation studies or RCT.

First, response to therapy should be assessed in at least three relevant domains (e.g., behavioral, physiological, cognitive, emotional).[31] The multimode approach is important because some intervention effects may be missed because they are specific to a particular mode. For example, the positive effects of psychosocial interventions in infertility were more likely to be found in reducing acute distress than in changing how people related to their partners or social network.[7] As noted earlier, the most common goals of interventions used in infertility were for the reduction of distress, enhanced coping skills, and improvement in quality of life, interpersonal relationships, and/or increased pregnancy rates.[2] Whichever is the target of a given intervention, it is clear that the outcome measures should be consistent with the expected change, and/or assess several domains to ensure that changes are captured.

Second, outcomes need to be measured along criteria that reflect both the client perspective and the therapeutic standard. In the infertility review, all therapies were perceived by participants to be effective on 'helpfulness ratings,' but not all interventions were associated with actual changes in distress or presenting problem.[7] Although client satisfaction is an important criterion, some situations may require gains from therapy to be assessed against independent standards (e.g., clinical cut-off scores). For example, Stewart et al.[24] found that for women participating in an intervention consisting of peer support and relaxation training, mean scores on depression, as measured by two clinical inventories, decreased below clinical threshold level. However, to make such comparisons, assessment must be made on the basis of well-validated measures. As noted previously, infertility-specific instruments have been developed (see Appendix 4) but only a few provide normative data, which may or may not be relevant to a new population (e.g., see Newton et al.[48] for scores on population of Canadian people with fertility problems). Therefore, it may be necessary at this time to additionally use a global standardized instrument.

An additional set of outcome criteria that should be considered in the monitoring process is connected to efficiency, cost, and cost effectiveness (resources consumed versus outputs produced), because this type of outcome is increasingly used by those who pay for healthcare in their decision making about which interventions to fund. For example, outcome criteria may include duration of therapy, cost of administering treatment (e.g., individual versus group), and client costs (e.g., negative effects of therapy, time, costs).[31] Thus, even if an individual program in stress relaxation is effective, it may be more costly to deliver individually than the equally effective group program (e.g., Domar et al.[19,36]; Stewart et al.[24]). Other costs that need to be considered are those connected to *not* implementing interventions. For example, there is good evidence that emotional distress reduces the chances of success in treatment[3,5] or increases rates of treatment dropout.[49]

Data for monitoring can be derived from both quantitative measures (e.g., self-report questionnaires and biological assays) and qualitative measures (e.g., interviews and narratives) provided all are scored according to well-validated techniques. Taking a more systematic approach to the monitoring of individual practice not only provides the practitioner with more information about their practice but also, when accumulated over many cases, can provide important insights into what is more effective among their own patient population.

Practitioners Need to Carry Out Clinically Meaningful Research Alone or in Collaboration with Researchers

This is undoubtedly the most difficult S-P principle to implement in practice. Many research designs (e.g., surveys, RCT) can be carried out in clinical or medical settings that have a large population of patients, and these approaches can be used to address many questions of theoretical and clinical interest to the counselor. For such large-scale studies, the individual practitioner can partner with other like-minded professionals and researchers to work together collaboratively (e.g., all contributing data to expand the research base). Such collaboration is typically initiated when practitioner and researcher discover common questions or 'blind spots' and both are motivated to find answers. Such recent collaborations have led to research on: the effects of prior trauma on current infertility reactions; the effectiveness of group support for couples on IVF waiting lists, and fertility-treatment beliefs of Middle-Eastern migrants (see PsycLit database, 2005). Practitioner–researcher partnerships are important because they ensure that research is addressing clinically meaningful issues. The development of mail groups, special interest groups

in professional associations, and other forums regularly attended by practitioners and researchers are good places to start such partnerships.

Many practitioners will not have access to such large populations, and many others will not have the resources (e.g., time, money), or desire, to invest in protocols that go much beyond their own case load. This means that whatever research contribution they make needs to be based on the single-case study. The uncontrolled single-case study is often viewed as an inferior contribution to the research base because it is a methodology from which scientific inference cannot be made (i.e., due to a lack of control).[31] However, research using the single-case study *can* make an important contribution to research, provided assessment is more systematic. Whether one is interested in the unique features of an intervention or the aspects that make it similar to others, only a systematic approach can provide good evidence on effectiveness. In the previous section, discussion focused on the outcomes to be assessed, whereas this section discusses how to make the timing and replication of assessments more systematic.

First, the outcomes should be assessed repeatedly to provide a more reliable estimate of the effectiveness of whatever intervention is being administered. In the most basic single-case study, the A/B design, multiple assessments are taken before and after an intervention, and there is often a follow-up period six or eighteen months later (see Hayes[50] for other single-case designs). Second, assessments should be taken at time points that allow change to have taken place. Boivin[7] found that changes to interpersonal relationships were less likely to be reported following psychosocial interventions than changes in emotional functioning. However, this finding could have been due to the fact that many studies had very short follow-up periods (i.e., <6 months) that may not have allowed sufficient time for changes to emerge. To illustrate, suppose a couple requests help because of sexual problems that developed as a result of the investigation and diagnosis of their fertility problem, as commonly reported.[26] Assessment could take the form of specialized inventories for sexual functioning, classification according to well-established clinical criteria (e.g., DSM-IVR), or physical assessments (e.g., hormones and physiological arousal using erectile plythemosgraphy). In this case, one might assess couples prior to, and immediately after, the initiation of a cognitive-behavioral intervention (see, for example, Tuschen-Caffier et al.[25]). However, to realistically capture the effects of the intervention, further assessments would need to take place three, six and twelve months after the intervention.

Third, the accumulation of a few cases from the same practitioner, documenting similar patterns of change over time, can substantially increase the validity of case study findings. This is more so if replicated changes are large, as this will increase the likelihood that the findings can be generalized to other patient groups.[50] Replication and large effect sizes would also make it more likely that findings based on single cases would be published. Raphael-Leff[51] reported on the experiences of nineteen patients with fertility problems undergoing psychoanalytic intervention. The grouped case reports allowed the issues commonly faced by infertile people to emerge, from violation of the expectation of generativity to the heightened emotional attachment experience toward those who contributed to the individual's eventual fertility success. Although the clinical presentation was based on relatively few cases, the themes provided a starting point for the investigation of the dynamics of fertility problem stress. Furthermore, the detailed presentation of a single case, Eve, enabled the reader to better understand the clinical genesis of the contribution.

The changes suggested in this and the preceding section strengthen the validity of data from the single-case study. By adopting these changes as part of their monitoring process, practitioners can strengthen the validity of this process, and also increase the possibility that findings from their own practice can be fed back to the research community where they can influence the future direction of outcome research and RCTs. Single-case studies are published in many journals (e.g., *Professional Psychology: Research and Practice, Psychotherapy; British Journal of Clinical Psychology; Counseling Psychologist; Journal of Counseling; Human Reproduction; Fertility and Sterility*). One study found that 5% of studies evaluating particular counseling interventions were based on the single-case design, and that a further 40% of studies used data partly drawn from observations made in the single-case context.[42] Practitioners should not, therefore, be deterred from carrying out research when the only design available to them is the single-case study.

THERAPEUTIC INTERVENTION

The skills needed to integrate research into clinical practice have been discussed. These are not novel skills for the practitioner, as most practitioners will have received training in research. Moreover, this chapter has discussed methods to access, apply, and participate in research with minor deviations from usual clinical practice. Finally, whatever additional skills are required can be acquired from books, online resources, continuing

education workshops, or can be overcome by collaborating with researchers. Thus, most researchers will already have acquired the main skills needed to achieve the goals set out in this chapter.

However, other issues requiring further development and/or adopting a different perspective may need to be considered to implement some of the suggestions already provided. Many practical issues have not been addressed, for example, the lack of financial support, time constraints, or the lack of reinforcement for research activities from within clinics or organizations (Asay et al. [11]). These are barriers that even practitioners fully committed to research face and must creatively resolve. It should be noted, however, that the generation of compelling research evidence on the importance of psychosocial factors makes medical communities, government agencies, pharmaceutical companies, and other potential research sponsors want to invest in research and counseling programs. For example, the recent publication of data showing that psychosocial factors were critical in patient dropout from fertility treatment (see, for example, volume 81, issue 2, 2004 *Fertility and Sterility* for a series) prompted at least two pharmaceutical companies to fund research into the psychological aspects of decision making among infertile people. Therefore, producing research will attract funding, and *relevant* research will make clinics more willing to support the activities of their practitioners.

Some practitioners would like to contribute to research but do not feel confident that they can identify relevant gaps in knowledge. Most clinical questions arise from central issues about caring for people, and it is as a result of gaps in this knowledge that research is initiated. Therefore, any clinical situation that calls for knowledge we do not possess is an opportunity to identify relevant literature and, where lacking, initiate research. Sackett et al.[43] identified ten central issues in clinical work (see Table 7.2) that could help in the formulation of clinically relevant research questions. For example, concern about how best to gather and then interpret findings from a patient history might lead to a search for interview guides. This search would reveal the Comprehensive Psychosocial History of Infertility (CPHI) interview,[52] which was designed specifically for history-taking with infertile people. However, the search would also reveal that the CPHI has not been validated. Given the need for an interview schedule, this gap might cause one to work on validating the CPHI.

Many practitioners are not interested in participating in research because scientist-practitioner models or similar frameworks clash with their work ethos or

TABLE 7.2. Central issues in clinical work, where the clinical questions that often arise can be used to stimulate further research[43]

Domain	Type of question
Clinical findings	How to properly gather and interpret findings from the patient history and psychological examination
Etiology	How to identify the causes for the disorder (e.g., depression, sexual problem)
Clinical manifestation	Knowing the symptoms associated with various disorders or problems and how to use this information to decide on the clinical focus
Differential diagnosis	When considering the possible *causes* of our client's clinical problem, how to select those that are likely, serious, and responsive to treatment
Diagnostic tests	How to select assessment tools and interpret their findings, in order to confirm or exclude a diagnosis, based on their psychometric properties (e.g., accuracy, sensitivity, and expense)
Prognosis	How to estimate our client's likely clinical course over time and anticipate likely complications
Therapy	How to select interventions to offer our clients that do more good than harm and that are worth the efforts and costs of using them
Prevention	How to reduce the chance of disorder, distress and other complications, by identifying problems early and identifying and modifying risk factors
Experience and meaning	How to empathize with our clients' situations, appreciate the meaning they find in the experience, and understand how this meaning influences their healing
Self-improvement	How to keep up-to-date, improve clinical and other skills and run a better, more efficient clinical practice

beliefs and values about what they do, and how they do it. These different perspectives may come about through personality traits that make people choose practice over research, the philosophical underpinnings of different approaches to mental health (e.g., psychology versus counseling versus social work,[37]) learning (e.g., beliefs of supervisors and mentors[42]), or variations in individual life history.[9,53] While there is indeed great diversity in approaches to research, research itself and its application to practice are always perceived as being compatible with best practice guidelines. Nevertheless, the alienation some practitioners experience is genuine, and occurs because practitioners are not part of the research process and, therefore, do not influence the direction of research, or how meaningful and relevant the research produced is to what they do.[9] Thus, the best way to resolve these legitimate concerns is for practitioners to become involved in research.

Practitioners will also vary in their reactions to changes in their practice. Adopting a new perspective on research and its role in practice, as welcomed as it may be, means investment in new goals and relinquishing other options, and familiar ways of working. For mental health professionals, this may include adjusting to a closer working relationship with traditionally more science-oriented professionals; loss of a former sense of freedom to implement professional values in a more spontaneous or idiosyncratic way; or having to

work with a model of professional practice that seems incongruent with the value system underlying their own profession.[12] It can be expected, therefore, that the process of integrating research into practice will involve adjustment.

FUTURE IMPLICATIONS

The future of evidence-based infertility counseling relates to those connected with the integration of research into practice and those of carrying out meaningful research on the effectiveness of psychosocial interventions. How can we facilitate communication between practitioners and researchers, and facilitate the implementation of research in practice? In this field, many researchers *are* practitioners; therefore, it may be more a question of finding ways of facilitating research or facilitating collaborative research. As a result, we need information about the barriers that may be limiting the research output of professionals in the field. In other fields of mental health research, networks have been established to facilitate exchange, collaboration, and trouble-shooting among researchers (whether practitioners or not). It might be a good idea to have such a network for mental health professionals interested in the psychosocial aspects of infertility and infertility counseling.

Aside from the issues that have to do with integrating research, there are many other issues that need to be addressed in the actual evaluation studies. The field of infertility counseling is young compared to that of psychotherapy, and psychotherapy outcome research offers much insight into the sorts of questions we need to ask. So far, we know that interventions are beneficial but that some are more so than others.[7,15] However, we do not know what ingredients make useful interventions useful or what ingredients make unhelpful interventions unhelpful. We also do not know very much about who benefits from different interventions. While educational programs may be beneficial for people in treatment where distress is caused mainly by procedural events (e.g., waiting for test results, failed treatment), they may not be so useful when people are dealing with more existential issues (e.g., what they will do with the rest of their life if they end treatment and decide to remain childless). Clearly, many questions need to be addressed so that the field as a whole can produce maximally effective interventions.

SUMMARY

■ It is clear that pressure will continue to be exerted on practitioners to demonstrate the effectiveness of their practice by those who pay for psychosocial interventions (e.g., patients or clients, governments, and insurers).

■ Empirically supported interventions are increasingly the only interventions these sponsors are willing to fund. The question for counselors in this field is how best to respond to that pressure.

■ In this chapter, ways of integrating research into practice have been discussed. Research is part of the code of practice of many mental health professions. The scientist-practitioner model provides some guiding principles about how research can become an everyday part of practice.

■ Various approaches to outcome research have been also discussed. Even if practitioners cannot become involved in large surveys or randomized control trials, research based on their own caseload can contribute meaningfully to the general knowledge base.

■ Many issues will need to be addressed before such models and frameworks are adopted. These include practical (e.g., lack of time or funding) and existential (e.g., value of research to the individual) concerns.

REFERENCES

1. Menning, BE. The emotional needs of infertile couples. *Fertil Steril* 1980; 34:313–19.
2. Ningel K, Strauss B. Psychological diagnosis, counselling and psychotherapy in fertility medicine. In: B Strauss, ed. *Involuntary Childlessness: Psychological Assessment,* *Counselling and Psychotherapy*. Seattle: Hogrefe & Huber, 2002;19–34.
3. Boivin J, Schmidt L. Infertility-related stress in men and women predicts treatment outcome one year later. *Fertil Steril* 2005; 83:1745–52.
4. Klonoff-Cohen H. Female and male lifestyle habits and IVF: What is known and unknown. *Human Reprod Update* 2005; 11:180–204.
5. Lancastle DS, Boivin J. Dispositional optimism, trait anxiety and coping: Unique or shared effects on physical health? *Health Psychol* 2005; 24:171–8.
6. Smeenk JMJ, Verhaak CM, Eugster A, et al. The effect of anxiety and depression on the outcome of in vitro fertilisation. *Human Reprod* 2001; 16:1420–3.
7. Boivin J. A review of psychosocial interventions in infertility. *Soc Sci Med* 2003; 57:2325–41.
8. Cullari S. Psychotherapy practice questionnaire. *The Independent Practitioner* 1996; 16:140–2.
9. Corrie S, Callahan MM. Therapists' beliefs about research and the scientist–practitioner model in an evidence-based healthcare climate: A qualitative study. *Br J Med Psychol* 2001; 74:135–49.
10. Larner G. Family therapy and the politics of evidence. *J Fam Therapy* 2004; 26:17–39.
11. Asay TP, Lambert MJ, Gregersen AT, et al. Using patient-focused research in evaluating treatment outcome in private practice. *J Clin Psychol* 2002; 58:1213–25.
12. Corrie S, Callahan MM. A review of the scientist–practitioner model: Reflections on its potential contribution to counselling psychology within the context of current health care trends. *Br J Med Psychol* 2000; 73:413–27.
13. Sanderson WC, Woody S. Manuals for empirically validated treatments: A project of the task force on psychological interventions. Oklahoma City, OK: American Psychological Association. 1995.
14. National Institute of Clinical Excellence (NICE: Department of Health). *Treatment Choice in Psychological Therapies and Counselling: Evidence Based Clinical Practice Guidelines*. London: Department of Public Health, 2001.
15. de Liz TM, Strauss B. Differential efficacy of group and individual/couple psychotherapy with infertile patients. *Human Reprod* 2005; 20:1324–32.
16. American Psychological Association. Ethical principles of psychologists and code of conduct. *Amer Psychologist* 2002; 47:1060–73.
17. O'Moore AM, O'Moore RR, Harrison RF, Murphy G, Carruthers ME. Psychosomatic aspects in idiopathic infertility: Effects of treatment with autogenic training. *J Psychosom Res* 1983; 27:145–51.
18. McQueeney D, Stanton A, Sigmon S. Efficacy of emotion-focused and problem-focused group therapies for women with fertility problems. *J Behav Med* 1997; 20:313–31.
19. Domar AD, Clapp D, Slawsby EA, et al. Impact of group psychological interventions on pregnancy rates in infertile women. *Fertil Steril* 2000; 73:805–11.
20. Clark AM, Ledger W, Galletley C, et al. Weight loss results in significant improvement in pregnancy and ovulation rates in anovulatory obese women. *Human Reprod* 1995; 10:2705–12.
21. Kemeter P, Fiegl J. Psychosomatically oriented counselling in relation to infertility treatment – A quantification of the main topics in the interviews and therapeutic

strategies [German]. *Journal für Fertilität und Reproduktion* 1999; 9:23–31.

22. Liswood MP. *Treating the crisis of infertility: A cognitive-behavioural approach* (Doctoral dissertation, University of Toronto, 1995). *Dissertation Abstracts International Section A: Humanities and Social Sciences, 1995; 55,* (12-A), 4006.

23. Wischmann T, Stammer H, Scherg H, et al. Couple counselling and therapy for the unfulfilled desire for a child: The two-step approach of the "Heidelberg Infertility Consultation." In: B Strauss, ed. *Involuntary Childlessness: Psychological Assessment, Counselling and Psychotherapy* Seattle:Hogrefe & Huber Publishers, 2002;127–50.

24. Stewart DE, Boydell KM, McCarthy K, et al. A prospective study of the effectiveness of brief professionally-led support groups for infertility patients. *International J Psychiatry in Med* 1992; 22:173–82.

25. Tuschen-Caffier B, Florin I, Krause W, et al. Cognitive-behavioural therapy for idiopathic infertile couples. *Psychotherapy Psychosom* 1999; 68:15–21.

26. Takefman JE, Brender W, Boivin J, Tulandi T. Sexual and emotional adjustment of couples undergoing infertility investigation and the effectiveness of preparatory information. *J Psychosom Obstet Gynaecol* 1990; 11:275–90.

27. Pengelly P, Inglis M, Cudmore L. Couples' experiences and the use of counselling in treatment centres. *Psychodynamic Counselling* 1995; 1:507–24.

28. Lentner E, Glazer G. Infertile couples' perceptions of infertility support-group participation. *Health Care for Women International* 1991; 12:317–30.

29. Bartlam B, McLeod J. Infertility counselling: The ISSUE experience of setting up a telephone counselling service. *Patient Education and Counselling* 2000; 41:313–21.

30. Kazdin AE. Treatment research: The investigation and evaluation of psychotherapy. In: M Hersen, AE Kazdin, AS Bellack, eds. *The Clinical Psychology Handbook*. New York: Pergamon, 1986; 265–88.

31. Raimy, VC. *Training in Clinical Psychology*. Englewood Cliffs, NJ: Prentice Hall, 1950.

32. Baker DB, Benjamin LT. The affirmation of the scientist-practitioner: A look back at Boulder. *Amer Psychologist* 2000; 55:241–7.

33. Rodolfa ER, Kaslow NJ, Steward AE, et al. Internship training: Do models really make a difference. *Prof Psychol: Res Prac* 2005; 36:25–31.

34. Khan KS, Riet G, Popay J, et al. Study quality assessment. In Khan, Riet, Glanville, Sowden, Kleijnen, eds. *Undertaking Systematic Reviews of Research on Effectiveness: CRD's Guidance for Those Carrying Out or Commissioning Reviews. CRD Report number 4* (2nd ed.). York: NHS Centre for Reviews and Dissemination. 2001; 1–20.

35. Domar AD, Seibel M, Benson H. The mind/body program for infertility: A new behavioral treatment approach for women with infertility. *Fertil Steril* 1990; 53:246–9.

36. Domar AD, Clapp D, Slawsby E, et al. The impact of group psychological interventions on distress in infertile women. *Health Psycho* 2000; 19:568–75.

37. Sexton TL. The relevance of counselling outcome research: Current trends and practical implications. *J Counsel Develop* 1996; 74:590–600.

38. Shadish WR, Matt GE, Navarro AM, et al. The effects of psychological therapies under clinically representative conditions: A meta-analysis. *Psychol Bull* 2000; 126:512–29.

39. Wampold BE, Mondin GW, Moody M, et al. A meta-analysis of outcome studies comparing bona fide psychotherapies: Empirically, "All must have prizes." *Psychol Bull* 1997; 122:203–15.

40. Grencavage LM, Norcross JC. Where are the commonalities among the therapeutic common factors? *Prof Psychol: Res Pract* 1990; 21:372–8.

41. Sexton TL, Whiston SC. Integrating counselling research and practice. *J Counsell Develop* 1996; 74:588–9.

42. Lampropoulos GK, Goldfried MR, Castonguay LG, et al. What kind of research can we realistically expect from the practitioner. *J Clin Psychol* 2002; 58:1241–64.

43. Sackett D, Straus SE, Richardson WS, et al. *Evidence-based Medicine: How to Practice and Teach EBM* (2nd ed.). Edinburgh: Churchill Livingstone, 2000; 3–4.

44. Holzle C, Brandt U, Lutkenhaus R, et al. Solution-focused counselling for involuntarily childless couples. In: B Strauss, ed. *Involuntary Childlessness: Psychological Assessment, Counselling and Psychotherapy*. Seattle: Hogrefe & Huber Publishers, 2002; 105–26.

45. Throsby K. No-one will ever call me mummy: Making sense of the end of IVF treatment. *New Working Paper Series* 2001; 5:1–12.

46. Daniluk JC. Reconstructing their lives: A longitudinal, qualitative, analysis of the transition to biological childlessness for infertile couples. *J Counsel Devel* 2001; 79:439–49.

47. van Rooij FB, van Balen F, Hermanns JMA. A review of Islamic Middle Eastern migrants: Traditional and religious cultural beliefs about procreation in the context of infertility treatment. *J Reprod Infant Psychol* 2004; 22:321–31.

48. Newton CR, Sherrard W, Glavac I. The Fertility Problem Inventory: Measuring perceived infertility distress. *Fertil Steril* 1999; 72:54–62.

49. Smeenk JMJ, Verhaak CM, Stolwijk AM, et al. Reasons for dropout in an in vitro fertilization/intracytoplasmic sperm injection program. *Fertil Steril* 2004; 81:262–8.

50. Hayes SC. The role of the individual case in the production and consumption of clinical knowledge. In: M Hersen, AE Kazdin, AS Bellack, eds. *The Clinical Psychology Handbook*. New York: Pergamon, 1986; 181–96.

51. Raphael-Leff J. The baby makers: An in-depth single-case study of conscious and unconscious psychological reactions to infertility and 'Baby-Making' technology. *Brit J Psychother* 1992; 8:266–77.

52. Burns, LH, Greenfeld, DA (for the Mental Health Professional Group). *CPHI: Comprehensive Psychosocial History for Infertility*. Birmingham, AL: American Society for Reproductive Medicine, 1990.

53. Beutler LE, Moleiro C, Talebi H. How practitioners can systematically use empirical evidence in treatment selection. *J Clin Psychol* 2002; 58:1199–212.

8 Individual Counseling and Psychotherapy

LINDA D. APPLEGARTH

> *...counselling requires two elements to be...effective: the personal qualities of the counsellor and the acquisition of skills within a theoretical framework.*
>
> – Mack and Tucker[1]

The rapid scientific and medical advances in the assisted reproductive technologies and the growth of fertility clinics around the world have led to a greater understanding and appreciation of the psychosocial concerns and emotional needs of individuals who suffer from infertility. As the available technology has developed along with the vicissitudes of fertility treatment, patients have turned to mental health professionals for help in dealing with the many stresses inherent in diagnostic procedures and treatment, and for assistance in decision making relative to treatment protocols and alternative parenting options.

This chapter focuses on three general areas:
■ a global, historical perspective of infertility counseling and a brief consideration of some key psychological issues that are also commonly a part of the infertility struggle. The literature review is intended to provide some basic educational and theoretical constructs on which individual counseling and psychotherapy can most effectively occur;
■ several theoretical treatment approaches that may be particularly appropriate to infertile individuals. These approaches will be presented in some detail with discussion of their clinical applicability to infertility;
■ a discussion about the infertility counselor per se, with emphasis on the need for solid knowledge of medical treatments and parenting options as well as a focus on specific qualities of the therapist. In addition to one's theoretical background and treatment style, it is imperative to recognize countertransference issues that may arise for psychotherapists working with patients whose powerful and painful desire for a child can be especially palpable. These issues will be detailed along with how transference and countertransference can occur among patients and mental health professionals as well as other healthcare workers involved in the field of infertility.

HISTORICAL OVERVIEW

Infertility counseling had its beginnings with infertile couples seeking support and education from their medical and mental health professionals. More than thirty years ago, in the United States, a consumer advocacy group, Resolve the National Infertility Association, was established to provide professional and peer support to those struggling with the many emotional aspects of infertility. The writings of the founder of Resolve also led to increased attention to the important psychological issues inherent in the condition of infertility.[2,3] In recent years, other similar consumer organizations have arisen in other countries such as the United Kingdom, Australia, New Zealand, Germany, France, Spain, Italy, Mexico, and Japan. Gradually, mental health clinicians, medical professionals, and researchers around the world began to consider the psychological components of the infertility experience and to recognize patients' need for emotional support, psychoeducation, and, on occasion, psychiatric intervention. Additionally, as assisted reproductive technologies became an integral part of infertility treatment, mental health professionals from around the world began to consider the many psychosocial complexities and challenges facing the infertile population. Along with the burgeoning of more complex reproductive technologies also came ethical dilemmas, social policy issues, professional standards of care, and government oversight and/or regulations. These factors have also had an impact on the role of the mental health professional as an integral member of the team of professionals who treat infertile men and women.

In 1986, the Mental Health Professional Group (MHPG) of the American Society for Reproductive Medicine (ASRM) was formed to provide a forum for professionals working in reproductive medicine

129

to exchange theories, research findings, and clinical experience. Continuing education programs (postgraduate courses) were developed as a means of providing more formalized instruction to mental health specialists within or entering the field. Shortly after the establishment of the MHPG, the British Infertility Counselling Association (BICA – 1988) and the Australia and New Zealand Infertility Counsellors Association (ANZICA – 1989) were organized to address the psychosocial needs to infertility patients and to respond to government legislation that mandated the provision of counseling for all individuals seeking fertility treatment or third-party reproduction at licensed facilities. In 1993, the Psychology and Counselling Special Interest Group was formed as part of the European Society for Human Reproduction and Embryology (ESHRE). Recently similar professional organizations of mental health professionals working in reproductive medicine have been organized in Canada, Germany, Greece, Japan, Spain, Switzerland, and Latin America. In an effort to establish ongoing communication and coordination between these professional organizations, the International Infertility Counseling Organization (IICO) was also established in 2003. IICO's goals include (but are not limited to) the promotion of a comprehensive and ethical approach to the care of people affected by or involved with infertility as well as the establishment of global professional standards and practice guidelines for the provision of psychological care regarding reproductive issues.

Ultimately, the primary aim has been to enhance theoretical understandings, as well as to fine-tune the clinical skills of mental health practitioners as they work with this special population. In recent years, the role of the mental health professional has been clarified and expanded within the area of reproductive medicine.[4–6] The primary functions delineated include assessment, treatment, education, consultation, collaboration, and research. The field of infertility counseling presents new and continuing challenges to mental health practitioners around the world and offers limitless rewards in working with health professionals as well as with patients.

REVIEW OF LITERATURE

There are literally thousands of papers, articles, and books written about individual counseling and psychotherapy; however, infertility counseling is a new area and the data needed to guide psychological intervention and treatment recommendations are not readily available. Leiblum[7] pointed out that the role of the mental health clinician in counseling individuals and couples seeking treatment with assisted reproductive technologies is complicated. She noted that, "it often feels like negotiating rocky terrain without a map or without any certainty of arriving at a desirable destination."[7] Although the experience of infertility is not uncommon, Leon[8] suggested that there appears to be something about it that interferes with undertaking both long- and short-term psychoanalytic psychotherapy. He added that even when medical interventions have ended and emotional wounds endure, psychoanalytic psychotherapy is rarely chosen as a treatment option. Rather, it seems that most infertility patients enter counseling or psychotherapy to obtain symptom relief, to develop better coping mechanisms, to obtain assistance with decision making, or to deal with issues of loss. They may choose a more cognitive-behavioral approach or seek out grief counseling rather than ask for intensive psychotherapy aimed at personality change. Some infertile patients look to marriage and family therapy for assistance, particularly when infertility has an impact on marital functioning or relationships with extended family, or couples may seek problem specific treatment, such as sex therapy.

As recently as 1987, a body of psychiatric and gynecological literature has emerged, pointing to a dynamic psychogenic basis for infertility.[9–11] This condition was thought to be the result of intrapsychic conflicts around femininity or a conflicted or ambivalent relationship with the 'maternal object.' Sandler[12] has suggested that infertility was a sign of an intrapsychic conflict between motherhood and career for some women. Men and women were both seen as experiencing psychosexual maladjustments that resulted in the inability to conceive.[13] Recently, data have appeared that question these ideas about psychogenic causes of infertility.[14,15] Downey[16] pointed out that the significant decrease of so-called 'psychogenic infertility' from more than 50% of cases to less than 5% over the past thirty years underscores how what was originally attributed to psychological disturbances can now be explained by physical causes. The latest research, in fact, indicates that there are a number of predictable and apparently normal emotional responses to infertility and its treatment for which counseling can be especially helpful. Leiblum and Greenfeld[17] noted, in fact, that from a counseling perspective, attention has shifted recently to supporting infertile individuals and minimizing the destructive emotional components of this medical condition versus attributing psychopathology within the individual as a causal factor of his or her infertility.

Although there has been a shift away from dynamic, psychogenic bases for the failure to reproduce, many patients and health professionals have begun to question the impact of stress on fertility, particularly as the treatment failures occur and efforts to conceive are prolonged. An increasing number of researchers worldwide have suggested that decreasing psychological stress improves conception and pregnancy rates.[18,19] Several researchers have concluded that there may be an interactive effect in which it makes sense to consider psychosocial stress as a cause as well as a result of fertility disorders. As a result, a number of infertility clinics have now established stress management programs to help patients cope more effectively with the many fears and anxieties inherent in the treatment process. For example, Florin et al.[20] developed a stress reduction approach in Germany for couples with idiopathic infertility, and in the United States, Domar and colleagues[18] have developed a specific cognitive-behavioral (mind–body) intervention program for infertility patients. Some programs in Europe, North America, and Asia have introduced acupuncture, massage, nutrition, and other complementary medicine techniques as part of the IVF cycles to reduce stress with the hope of increasing pregnancy rates.

The Meaning of Reproduction

To better understand the context in which counseling or psychotherapy occurs, it is important to explore the range of psychological and emotional sequelae that individuals experience after their expectations, values, and beliefs are challenged by difficulties in achieving reproduction. It has been pointed out that, for most people, to have a child is to continue the human life cycle; it is seen as a renewal of life, as a form of immortality.[5] Mack and Tucker[1] note that there is a common desire to reproduce that has its basis in the conscious and unconscious of the individual and society. They comment that "a pregnancy belongs to everyone; it ensures the continuity of the individual's genetic heritage and secures the family and the society for the future." Because it is a source of pain for the individual and a source of concern for the wider society, the inability to bear a child precipitates a generally unanticipated life crisis for which many individuals and couples lack sufficient coping skills.

For most women and men, the ability to conceive and give birth to a child is paramount to their lifelong notions of femininity and masculinity, to gender identity, and ultimately to the meaning of life. Bearing children and parenting reflect Erickson's[21] concept of 'generativity' and are often one of the foundations around which a couple builds their relationship. Benedek[22] and Bibring[23] also described how pregnancy brings with it a new developmental phase and

that deprivation of the opportunity to parent because of infertility may lead to a break in development, resulting in stagnation. When efforts to achieve parenthood fail, life is put on hold, and many infertile people are left with deep personal feelings of guilt, self-blame, and inadequacy. There is often a fruitless but constant review of past life events that are seen as having led to the infertility. This retrospective may be coupled with private dialogues with the self that frequently commences with the phrase, "If only . . . ".

For women, Klempner[24] suggested that, in psychoanalytic thinking, maternal identification provides a background for parenting and infertility disrupts the opportunity to recapitulate or make reparation for early maternal failures. She added that when identifications with maternal objects are disrupted for women, there is an alteration of self and object representations. Notman and Lester[25] noted that a woman's knowledge that she is able to bear children is essential for the development of a notion of femininity, gender identity, and self-esteem. Conversely, Bassin[26] pointed out that although the use of reproductive technology can be a situational trauma for a woman, it need not have destructive symbolic meaning for her. The dependency or requirement of reproductive medical technology to become a mother can be a temporary insult to a woman's narcissism in that it interferes with her expectations of the natural unfolding of a life process within her body. Nonetheless, women may respond differently to the infertility experience depending on their internal psychological organization or sense of themselves as female.[26]

In addition, many women both consciously and unconsciously feel that motherhood can be reparative. Benedek[27] pointed out that parenthood allows adults to reexperience and gain mastery over early developmental states as they go through them with their children. For some women, the act of creation and the process of motherhood lead to a reidentification with positive aspects of their mothers that were denied during earlier attempts to separate from them.

Data suggest that as fertility problems arise, women worry more, are more self-blaming, and take a more active responsibility to solve their fertility problems with increasing medical treatment or other restorative attempts.[28] For example, Souter and colleagues[29] surveyed a large infertile population and found that a significant number of women in the early stages of treatment could be more at risk of developing clinically relevant mental health problems. The authors stressed that psychological aspects of infertility should be addressed as part of a more holistic approach to management of these patients. In addition, during the various phases of infertility, men and women seem to use different coping strategies.

Lee[30] stressed that men also have special psychological issues and feelings about male infertility that must be better understood and addressed. Certainly, much has been written about the female psychosocial experience of infertility[31–33] but little about the male viewpoint. Lee posited that men do not enter psychotherapy to work on crisis or bereavement issues, but rather to get help in dealing with the stresses of treatment or narcissistic injury, particularly if they have a male-factor diagnosis. It is also this author's opinion that men seek out counseling because of difficulties in understanding and effectively managing their partner's angst and emotionality about the infertility. It is therefore not the crisis of infertility itself, but the resulting crisis in the relationship that leads many men to an initiation of psychotherapy, whether individual or couples therapy.

Nonetheless, when struggling with male-factor infertility, men also may suffer from low self-esteem, loss of self-confidence, and feelings of incompetence, isolation, loneliness, guilt, fear, anger, shame, or frustration.[30,34] Not only is the diagnosis of male infertility a shock, but also male ideology is challenged. Thus, the entire idea of being a man (manhood) is challenged, and a man's belief system is threatened, placing him in a state of emotional distress or crisis.

In spite of advances in the feminist movement, there continues to be clear cultural and social factors that influence women's and men's views of themselves as parents. Regardless of other chief goals and expectations, the social message is clear: Motherhood is the primary role in a woman's life, in fact, a role every woman expects or should aspire to regardless of her other life roles and/or expectations. For men, expectations regarding fatherhood and family are more ambiguous. Newton and Houle[28] and others[35,36] have reported that men appear to be more accepting of possible childlessness and more willing than women to consider an end to treatment, even when infertility is the result of male-factor diagnosis – although this may be less generalizable across cultures than expectations about women's role as mothers. It seems that male responses to infertility approximate those of women only if infertility is attributed solely to a male factor[37] or if their culture strongly defines masculinity and virility in terms of fertility and reproduction.

Infertility: Attachment and Loss

The concepts of attachment and loss are integral to the infertility struggle.[38] The attachments can be to a fantasy child or to the gestating fetus, and are often enhanced as a person dreams about the ways that a baby will change one's lifestyle, envisions the physical characteristics that the child may have, or how the new baby will have an impact on the lives of and relationships with extended family members. These fantasies and others can occur well before a baby is conceived.[39] Women clients, for example, often describe their girlhood in terms of fantasies about future motherhood. The interruption of the emotional attachment to a dream child, either through infertility or pregnancy loss, can be devastating.

This loss of fertility or the loss of an unborn child generally goes unrecognized in society[38] as well as in most cultures and religions. Thus, infertility is a silent loss, usually lacking rituals to legitimize the grief of a couple who mourn their dream child. In addition, many find that the attachment to the unconceived or unborn child is often not shared by anyone else. Shapiro[38] suggested that as soon as there is a realization that infertility is a real problem, a process of *anticipatory* mourning begins for the offspring that may never be. Anticipatory mourning thus represents an emotional distancing from those initial attachments to the fantasy child. This type of mourning can lead to depression. Mahlstedt,[40] citing research on losses occurring in adulthood as factors causing depression, compared them to the losses of infertility. These include real or potential losses of a relationship, health, status or prestige, self-esteem, or self-confidence, as well as the loss of a fantasy, the hope of fulfilling an important fantasy, and the loss of someone or something of a great symbolic value. As such, the experience of infertility involves each of these losses illustrating how infertility involves not a single loss (the potential, dreamed-for child) but a whole host of losses, that can impact every aspect of the individual and couple's life.

It is not surprising therefore that most infertility patients become depressed and anxious to some degree. They have lost a sense of control over their lives and life plans. Infertility is a life crisis. It is frequently this crisis state (usually prolonged) that precipitates a movement into psychotherapy to obtain emotional relief and regain some sense of psychological equilibrium.

Counseling and Psychotherapy

Although some writers and mental health practitioners may differentiate the terms 'counseling' and 'psychotherapy,' they are used interchangeably in this chapter. Some may view psychotherapy as a more in-depth form of treatment aimed at significant psychiatric disorders using a broad variety of techniques. On the other hand, counseling may be considered supportive work or as a venue for providing advice or guidance to clients. No such distinction will be made here, and the reader may determine which term is preferable or most appropriate, based on his or her professional training, theoretical orientation, and treatment approach. Furthermore, while this chapter provides a review of therapeutic interventions that may be useful for working with infertile men and women, it is not intended as a substitute for the knowledge and skill that come from professional experience and training in a specific mental health field, reproductive medicine, or as a qualified infertility counselor. In addition, it should be noted that counseling and psychotherapy is influenced by the social and cultural milieu in which it occurs, and will be viewed differently within different cultures (see Chapter 4).

THEORETICAL FRAMEWORKS

Many infertile persons seek out counseling because their circumstances create feelings, thoughts, and actions that are frequently restrictive, painful, or repetitive. Primarily through talk, psychotherapy provides support, understanding, and new experiences that can result in learning and behavioral changes. There is no debate here about whether psychotherapy works; rather, it is more important for the reader to consider which psychotherapy (or combination thereof) is best for which infertile patient.

All individual counseling or psychotherapies share a general definition: a two-person interaction, primarily verbal, in which one person is designated as the help-giver and the other, the help-receiver. The goal is to elucidate the patient's characteristic problems of living, with the hope of achieving behavioral change.[41] Integral to therapeutic change is the ability of the therapist and the individual to establish a rapport (therapeutic alliance) that becomes the foundation for and fundamental to the goals of therapy and the therapeutic interventions.

Different psychotherapy orientations target different aspects of psychological functioning for change. The duration of treatments can be from hours to years, depending on the therapist's own theoretical orientation, as well as the patient's request for treatment, financial resources, description and severity of the problem(s), and mental health status.

This section summarizes a large body of information regarding a number of treatment approaches including:

- psychodynamic psychotherapy;
- cognitive-behavioral therapy;
- strategic/solution-focused brief therapy;
- crisis intervention;
- grief counseling.

Psychodynamic Psychotherapy

In psychodynamic psychotherapy, behavioral change occurs primarily through two processes of the treatment: (1) understanding the cognitive and affective patterns (defense mechanisms) derived from childhood and (2) understanding the conflicted relation(s) one had with significant childhood figures as it is reexperienced in the therapist–patient relationship (transference).[41] Of great importance to the success of psychoanalytically oriented psychotherapy is the need for patients to feel engaged in the work and to trust the relationship with the therapist.

The losses associated with the inability to conceive or give birth to a child often can reawaken unresolved issues and conflicts from the past. Patients may describe themselves as feeling underappreciated for their efforts to conceive or misunderstood with respect to their emotional pain, or they may relate to people (spouses, friends, and medical personnel) partly on the basis of expectations formed by early childhood experience. Clarifying character styles and restructuring defense mechanisms may become part of the therapist's focus in psychodynamic treatment relative to how patients react to their infertility.

Psychodynamic therapy can be brief or long-term, but much of the treatment intervention is based on psychoanalytic principles. Cooper[42] stressed, however, that the concepts of brief and long-term therapy are routinely ill-defined solely in terms of elapsed calendar time or total number of visits. He noted that "in practice, long-term treatment is often intermittent; while technically brief therapies may occur episodically over years with challenging problems such as severe abuse or trauma."[42] More specifically, brief psychodynamic psychotherapy relies more heavily than longer-term therapy on patients' ability to generalize and apply what is gained in the therapeutic work to expand the therapy's effects.

From a psychodynamic viewpoint, the importance of the therapist's role is also underscored. Psychotherapists treating infertility patients can effect healing of both the narcissistic wound and the object-relational loss, if they serve as consistently empathic figures who depend less on interpretation of unconscious conflicts than on resonating with conscious and preconscious affective states. Clearly, this is a less ambitious treatment form than psychoanalytic psychotherapy.

Interestingly, Freud's early work involved analyses that lasted three to six months. Over time, however, treatment became a much longer process. Franz Alexander was one of the first clinicians to describe brief psychodynamic psychotherapy. Recently, the works of David Malan, Peter Sifneos, James Mann, and Habib

Davanloo form the basis of this treatment theory. It has also been emphasized that long-term and brief treatments share many common processes. These include specific therapist activities such as the use of interpretation and a clear treatment focus, as well as nonspecific factors such as support and reassurance.[43] The brief psychotherapies can be especially difficult to describe and define because currently more than fifty forms exist.[42,43] Yet most brief psychotherapies share some essential characteristics and a common value system along with several common principles[44,45] which will be discussed in a later section of this chapter and elucidated in relation to infertility.

Historically and cross-culturally, the growth in the demand for counseling and psychotherapy, the community mental health movement, and the cost-consciousness of evidence-based medical practice has lead to a greatly increased demand for brief psychotherapy. As a result, "brief psychotherapy is now a necessary part of every clinician's skills."[41]

In general, long-term psychotherapy seems less applicable to the needs of patients suffering from infertility and pregnancy loss. In psychoanalytic psychotherapy, the patient's task of developing a working alliance with the therapist, learning free association, recognizing the disappointment of the opening phase of treatment, developing an understanding of transference, defenses, resistance, and learning how to work with dreams may feel overwhelming, as well as unnecessary. As Leon[8] speculated,

Ultimately, people seeking emotional help in the midst of reproductive loss are not looking – unconsciously as well as consciously – to change in fundamental ways who they are. They have endured so much recent upheaval in their self-definition and self-esteem – and essentially have changed so much in that process – that they long to regain some earlier sense of well-being and stable identity. They are less receptive to analyzing conflictual parts of themselves than seeking and needing to feel whole again...a flexible approach seems to work best with this population.

With this in mind, the short-term dynamic psychotherapies may offer infertility patients an opportunity for reflective exploration and a search for meaning in experience. Self-awareness, understanding, and personal control are promoted rather than a resolution of symptoms, although symptomatology often recedes with the resolution of internal and interpersonal conflicts and the growth of insight.[46]

Cognitive-Behavioral Therapy

In contrast to psychodynamic psychotherapy, cognitive-behavioral theories emphasize assessment and relief of current problems and use a number of empirically based techniques to achieve mutually determined goals.[47] Brief therapies, associated with Aaron Beck and Albert Ellis, primarily stress the importance of changing cognitive processes and structures to achieve a desired outcome. Cognitive-behavioral therapy strives for self-efficacy and relief of problems through challenging faulty cognitions and their behavioral correlates.[42] It can be a particularly appropriate treatment for infertility patients who present as anxious, depressed, or fearful of medical interventions. Furthermore, cognitive-behavioral therapy can often be as effective or better for the treatment of these conditions than psychopharmacological medications, especially for women who are attempting to achieve pregnancy.

Essentially, cognitive-behavioral therapy bases its theory on an interactionist perspective regarding the determinants of human behavior and psychological well-being.[48] The core belief of this perspective is that the interaction between the individual and the environment continuously determines behavior, cognitions, and affect. Private thoughts and intrapersonal factors act on the environment, just as environmental factors influence these same intrapersonal factors. Furthermore, intrapersonal factors affect an individual's perceptions of environmental forces. What emerges therefore is a three-factor model – environment/person/behavior – that in turn affects the person/situation interaction. Bandura[49] labeled this as *reciprocal determinism*. Understanding and accepting the principle of reciprocal determinism vastly increases the range of available therapeutic options and enhances the therapist's sensitivity to a wide variety of data.

Cognitive-behavioral therapy emphasizes the learning process and encourages clients to acquire new skills during the course of therapy.[50] Coping skills in particular are stressed as patient problems can often be understood as stemming from inadequate coping skills. Lehman and Salovey[48] emphasized the primary goals of this treatment approach and pointed to the importance of client–therapist collaboration to attain these goals. They include the following:

■ providing cost-effective treatment for a wide range of client problems;
■ altering clients' interpretations of themselves and their environment by changing their behavior, their environment, or their cognitions directly;
■ increasing clients' available store of coping skills; and
■ increasing the likelihood that therapeutic gain will be maintained once therapy is terminated.

Given the integrative framework of cognitive-behavioral therapy, a therapist working with infertility patients can effectively attend to thoughts, feelings, and behaviors and can intervene at any point in the person/environment/behavior triangle. Specifically, infertility therapists often incorporate stress management and relaxation response strategies, along with helping the patient minimize negative cognitions during infertility treatment that can result in increased depression, anxiety, or anger. The goal is to increase the experience of personal control and the reduction of helplessness.[20]

In sum, cognitive-behavioral therapy is widely recognized as an effective therapy for the treatment of a variety of conditions, including infertility-related distress and depression. The emphasis on cognition in a number of therapy approaches has led to a new interest in understanding and assessing the processes of change that occur throughout all forms of psychotherapy. Interestingly, there is some evidence that "a new rapprochement between behavioral and psychodynamic perspectives appears to be underway, taking its strength from the interactive approach afforded by cognitive-behavior therapy."[48]

Strategic and Solution-Focused Psychotherapy

Strategic therapy has built a great deal of its foundation on the works of Milton Erikson, Gregory Bateson, and Jay Haley, who also contributed significantly to family systems therapy. Erikson deemphasized psychopathology and used a directive (and metaphorical) style based on hypnotic paradigms. These paradigms were further elaborated in Haley's pragmatic, problem-solving approach, and in Minuchin's 'structural' approach to family treatment that emphasized resolution of specific immediate problems by "altering the transactional process that reveals and maintains" the problem.

The term *strategic* refers to the therapist's task of developing a strategy, or a plan, to interpret the client's unsuccessful attempted solution at eliminating or ameliorating his or her own distress. A primary task is to motivate clients to implement the therapist's strategic intervention/solution. The purpose of this counseling approach is to resolve the original complaint to the client's satisfaction.[51] Change is therefore effected principally through treating a presenting problem or specific symptom. The treatment is implicitly systemic and interpersonal.

Rosenbaum[52] reported that strategic therapy is not a particular orientation or therapy; rather, it can refer to any therapy in which the counselor willingly assumes responsibility for influencing people and takes an active role in planning a strategy for promoting change. He adds, however, that strategic psychotherapy does have major distinguishing characteristics that are particularly relevant. Some of these characteristics are:

■ Strategic therapists work with a systemic epistemology;
■ Strategic therapy focuses on problems and their solutions;
■ Strategic therapists tend to see client problems as maintained by their attempted solutions;
■ Strategic therapy requires only a small change;
■ Strategic therapists use whatever clients bring to help them make a satisfactory life;
■ Strategic therapy is brief therapy.

Solution-focused therapy is an important variation of strategic therapy[42] that emphasizes building on exceptions to the presenting problem and making transitions rapidly to the identification and development of solutions intrinsic to the client or problem. As opposed to considering the question "What maintains the problems?" often asked in the strategic therapy mode, the solution-focused counselor asks, "How do we construct solutions?" Walter and Peller[53] pointed out that the presuppositions within this question are that:

■ there are solutions;
■ there is more than one solution;
■ solutions are constructible;
■ 'we' (therapist and client) can do the construction;
■ we 'construct' or 'invent' solutions rather than discover them;
■ this process or these processes can be articulated and modeled.

There are essentially three steps to constructing solutions in this treatment approach:[53] (1) Define what the client wants rather than what he or she does not want; (2) Look for what is working and do more of it; and (3) If what the client is doing is not working, have him or her do something different.

Solution-focused brief therapy is seen as a total model, described specifically by such practitioners as O'Hanlon, Berg and Miller, Quick, and Walter and Peller. It is not a collection of techniques or an elaboration of a technique; rather, it reflects fundamental ideas about change, interaction, and reaching goals.[51–53]

A strategic solution-focused approach to working with infertility patients may involve the use of 'coping questions.' Quick[51] stated that coping questions ask how the client goes on in the face of a difficult, painful situation. An example of a coping question might be: "Given what this past year of failed infertility treatment has been like for you, how have you managed to get through it?" Clients may answer by describing simple behaviors or saying, "I just do it." Thus, even if the coping behavior did not seem to be the result of an active choice, the therapist may gently point out that the client *did* have a choice and that he or she chose a coping alternative.[51] Identifying coping behaviors and encouraging and amplifying healthy ones (while noting behaviors that are less useful or healthy) are important tools in solution-focused therapy. This approach is intended to help patients continue the healthy coping and increase their tolerance for distress. This treatment process can be extremely helpful to infertility patients, particularly when the therapist is also able to interrupt unsuccessful coping solutions by redirecting clients' efforts into more productive and satisfying behaviors.

In Germany, for example, Holzle et al.[54] developed a solution-focused counseling program for infertile couples with a focus on increasing the ability of clients to cope with involuntary childlessness as a transitory life crisis, with the goal of improvement of life satisfaction, independent of pregnancy. Holzle and her colleagues concluded that, based on patient reports, a significant reduction of psychological and somatic complaints could be reached within a framework of about seven sessions. They noted, however, that this treatment approach should not be used with people who demonstrate serious mental health disorders, and stressed the importance of a differential diagnosis at the time of intake.

Crisis Intervention

The term *crisis intervention* originated in relation to people with stable personalities and a history of adequate coping resources, who are facing important but transitory difficulties.[55] Although infertility patients fall into this general category, it is also common that, in most cases, the difficult infertility experience is seldom transitory. However, infertile individuals often experience 'crises within the crisis,' particularly when they are confronted by an unexpected event such as failed fertilization, premature ovarian failure, a pregnancy loss, or the sudden recommendation to end treatment.

Although the precise goals of crisis intervention depend on the specific nature of the crisis, crisis-oriented treatments do share a number of general goals.[56] These include:

- relieving the client's symptoms;
- restoring the client to his or her previous level of functioning;
- identifying the factors that precipitated the crisis;

- identifying and applying remedial measures;
- helping the client connect the current stresses with past life experiences;
- helping the client develop adaptive coping skills that can be used in future situations.

According to Rapoport,[56] the first four goals are the minimum goals of all types of crisis intervention, while the last two are considered optional or feasible only in certain situations. Understanding and developing coping behaviors appear to be a key component of crisis intervention. Lazarus and Folkman[57] suggested that coping is a process and that is situation-specific.

Infertility patients are known to use a combination of coping mechanisms, but in certain circumstances, they often fail to do so because of a number of factors: The infertility problem may seem too overwhelming or too unfamiliar; the person may use maladaptive coping methods; coping may be limited by physical or mental illness; or support from friends or family that would otherwise enable a person to cope is unavailable. All too often, infertile patients revert over time to one or two (adaptive or maladaptive) coping strategies instead of expanding their coping repertoire in response to increased stressors.

When coping fails, one may observe what Caplan[58] described as four phases of crisis:

1. Arousal and efforts at problem-solving behavior increase;
2. With increased arousal or tension, functional impairment ensues with associated disorganization and distress. Arousal reaches a point at which coping is hindered: The person is too anxious or too angry or unable to sleep properly and so on;
3. Emergency resources, both internal and external, are mobilized and novel methods of coping tried;
4. Continuing failure to resolve the problem leads to progressive deterioration, exhaustion, and decompensation.

Psychotherapeutic intervention can be made at any point during these four phases. Bancroft and Graham[55] noted that there is much scope for skill and experience in practicing crisis intervention. It requires empathy and sensitivity; therapists also often rely on the skillful use of common sense rather than highly specialized techniques. Although it has been difficult to reach a conclusion about the effectiveness of crisis intervention because of the range of approaches for which the term is applied, this should not deter the counselor from using an approach that is based on caring, common sense, and practical suggestions.[55] Infertility patients appear to respond well to crisis intervention and often benefit from having the opportunity to mobilize their coping skills and support systems.

Grief Counseling

Because bonds of attachment often develop before a child is conceived or delivered, it is important to acknowledge that the breaking of these bonds either through loss or disruption can create intense emotional pain. In the face of these reproductive losses, many infertility patients need to grieve or mourn. Here, grief and mourning are defined as the intellectual and emotional processes that gradually lessen the psychological bond to the lost loved one, enabling the bereaved to accept the loss and move forward.[59]

Grief counseling for individuals unable to conceive takes a different form from that of individuals who have experienced a pregnancy loss or perinatal death. For both groups, it is imperative that the reality of the loss be acknowledged: The loss of a child, real or fantasized, is a brutal shock and feels like an assault on self-worth and the meaning of one's life. The counselor's role is to encourage patients to accept the loss.

Second, bereaved infertility patients must also be helped to experience the pain of grief. This crucial aspect of grief consists of expressing in words the intense feelings that accompany the loss.[59] Leon[8] added that, in working with the bereaved, it is also necessary to challenge directly the therapist's own discomfort with and pathologizing of grief.

Third, the counselor can be helpful in assisting individuals who have experienced a perinatal death to commemorate the loss. Often, these people need assistance in finding an acceptable way to honor and remember the baby's death. This can be particularly important when there is a significant burden of guilt in relation to the death.[59]

Fourth, the therapist may also play an important role in helping bereaved persons let go of the loss. The bereaved ultimately must withdraw their emotional investment in the loss in order to go forward with life.

Lastly, the therapist may also be called on to assist bereaved individuals to move on. Crenshaw[59] pointed out that this can be very difficult because it involves relinquishing the hopes, dreams, plans, and aspirations that revolved around the lost dream child. At times, the resistance to moving on may result from anger that life has dealt the bereaved a cruel blow. Similarly, some grievers tend to identify themselves as tragic figures,

gaining gratification from the solicitations of family and friends. As a result of these secondary gains, they have difficulty becoming active participants in life and letting go not only of the lost loved one, but also of the role of the bereaved.

In sum, grief counseling can be a very meaningful intervention for patients who experience reproductive loss. Often, the feelings of pain can be extremely heavy to bear and must be shared, in part, by the therapist and managed supportively. In this way, the counseling intervention provides a secure base and a normalizing experience for the bereaved.

CLINICAL ISSUES

Transference and Countertransference

Although transference and countertransference are intrinsic parts of every patient–therapist relationship, it is crucial for infertility counselors to be mindful of powerful and compelling countertransference issues when working with patients experiencing infertility and pregnancy loss.

It is not uncommon, for example, for counselors working in this field to have had some form of personal experience with infertility and its associated losses. This position can have positive and negative, effects. Countertransference, broadly defined as the therapist's total response to a patient, both conscious and unconscious, can be useful in understanding the experience of the patient.[60] The infertility crisis can be laden with profound feelings for both counselors and clients about gender identity, self-image, and wishes for nurturance. The feelings that arise within therapists vary greatly depending on how they have resolved their own issues about infertility and pregnancy loss. Unless there is some form of resolution about this aspect of the therapist's life, it will be profoundly difficult to explore childbearing problems and decisions with patients while maintaining a 'neutral' stance. Subtle and not-so-subtle conflicts can therefore come into play in clinicians' relationships with clients. As a therapist personally struggles with painful, unresolved issues (e.g., feelings about becoming a parent, guilt, ambivalence, and anger) can interfere with patients' efforts at working through their conflicts and concerns about infertility and loss. In some cases, the infertile patient may not only be impacted by the psychotherapist's countertransference but also by countertransference issues that come from the medical treatment team. There is often an unconscious connection between doctors and patients, nurses and patients, as well as between administrative staff and patients.

Kentenich and colleagues[61] noted that doctors and therapists have characteristics and personality styles that may influence their reactions to patients. For physicians especially, there is a tendency to be proactive with patients on an ongoing basis so that there is no time for grief or disappointment. The "unconscious unity (between doctor and patient) defends them from emotions as, for example, they both want to quickly 'forget' failures (no pregnancy, miscarriage)." Kentenich and his colleagues, thus, argue that it is this unity that explains why psychological considerations are often not permitted in the treatment of infertility or, at minimum, avoided.[61]

Self-disclosure by psychotherapists is another important countertransference issue in infertility counseling. The question often arises regarding how much to self-disclose, if at all, and to which patients. This issue must be carefully considered because revealing personal pain can potentially be manipulative and self-indulgent rather than serving to further a patient's growth. Leibowitz[62] believed that the key to self-revelation to a patient is based on a sense of how open a therapist and patient have been with one another and how much trust and connection have been established in the therapeutic alliance. In any case, self-disclosure by therapists must be used in a thoughtful, purposeful way so as to benefit or assist a client (not the therapist) even though a therapist's personal experience with infertility may, in some cases, increase his or her ability to empathize with clients' pain and anger. Self-disclosure can also be a way to model effective behaviors and to close the perceived distance between therapist and client, thereby facilitating greater trust and openness.[63] In other cases, however, a therapist's own infertility issues may be projected onto the client's infertility experience, potentially interfering with the client's coping abilities and efforts to resolve this difficult and painful experience. From a broader perspective, Rosen and Rosen[64] discussed the effects of infertility patients' complex psychological dilemmas on the emotional lives of mental health professionals. They address, with the assistance of experienced colleagues in the field, how psychotherapists' reactions may "limit or help psychotherapy" with this unique population.

Lastly, the psychotherapist's pregnancy is a real and obvious event for both clinician and patient.[65] Although it can allow for very important therapeutic effects to occur, it unquestionably allows for critical transference and countertransference issues. A treatment crisis can ensue that can potentially lead to humiliation on the part of the infertile patient. For even the most experienced therapist, this may be an important time for her to obtain supervision.

THERAPEUTIC INTERVENTIONS

We are told that although theoretical differences in treatment approaches definitely exist, it is unclear as to the extent to which these differences are purely applied in practice. Experienced clinicians are likely to use interventions that are similar in utility and intent, if not form, but that also reflect their own unique personalities and experience, as well as situational demands.[42]

Energetic efforts to distinguish approaches from one another also risk unfairly dichotomizing and limiting them. For example, the highly interpersonal and implicit nature of strategic therapy is often ignored in favor of its technical components. Similarly, most psychodynamic approaches now consider interpersonal factors in psychotherapy to be as important as intrapsychic ones.

Because it appears that infertility patients primarily seek out short-term or brief counseling or psychotherapy, it is important to outline some essential characteristics and common principles. It is also useful to point out a common value system that most brief psychotherapies share.[42–44,66] These include:

Technical features
■ maintenance of a clear, specific treatment focus
■ conscious and conscientious use of time
■ limited goals with clearly defined outcomes
■ emphasis on intervening in the present
■ rapid assessment and integration of assessment within treatment
■ frequent review of progress and discarding of ineffective interventions
■ high level of therapist–patient activity
■ pragmatic and flexible use of techniques

Shared values
■ emphasis on pragmatism, parsimony, and least intrusive treatment versus cure
■ recognition that human change is inevitable
■ emphasis on client strengths and resources and the legitimacy of presenting complaints
■ recognition that most change occurs outside of therapy
■ commitment that a patient's outside life is more important than therapy
■ a stance that therapy is not always helpful
■ a belief that therapy is not timeless.

Leon[67] noted that of twenty cases of women presenting with emotional problems following pregnancy loss, six women left treatment during the consultation or soon after therapy began. Of the six, five were also dealing with infertility before or after their loss.

Most remarkably, however, those five who left treatment early were the only infertile women in his total sample. Other clinicians appear to have had similar experiences with infertility patients. For this reason, it would seem especially important to emphasize the significance of the first session, because it may be the *only* session.

Cooper[42] pointed out that it is helpful if the clinician considers each session as a whole in and of itself. To do this effectively, he described at least six first-session tasks that can serve multiple purposes:

1. *Form a positive working relationship. Spend a few moments constructively getting acquainted:*
   - Do some therapy education.
   - Ask how you can be helpful.
   - Use active listening, empathy, and language that demonstrates respect for each client's point of view.
   - Find a one-sentence summary to repeat to clients that reflects your understanding of their problem.
   - Find at least one thing to like or respect about each patient or his or her coping and call attention to it.
   - Create an expectation of improvement.
2. *Find a treatment focus:*
   - Ask what brought the patient to treatment now rather than earlier or later.
   - Ask what improved since the appointment was made that patients would like to continue improving.
   - Determine at the beginning what would be tangibly different for clients at the end of successful treatment.
   - Define problems in specific terms conducive to change.
   - Determine the meaning or significance of a problem to a patient.
   - If multiple problems are identified, focus first on the most important to the client.
3. *Negotiate criteria for a successful outcome:*
   - Put solutions in positive, specific, achievable terms, using client language to facilitate change.
   - Make goals/solutions achievable, and place goals within the patient's control.
4. *Distinguish clients from nonclients. Not every person who presents in therapy is a candidate for change:*
   - Clients are characterized by the acknowledgment of a problem and a willingness to work on it.
   - Nonclients may acknowledge a problem exists but do not see themselves as part of the solution.
5. *Identify patient motivational levels, and tailor interventions accordingly.*
6. *Do something that makes a difference immediately:*
   - Listen actively and empathetically.
   - Help patients understand that most of their reactions to infertility are normal and predictable.
   - Discuss the process of achieving desired solutions.
   - Conceptualize or reframe problems in ways that suggest solutions.

The focus of treatment in individual counseling with infertility patients can be collaboratively developed with them and is closely related to the ideas of assessment and diagnosis. It is therefore important to have sound diagnostic skills while working within an infertility patient's perception of the problem. A helpful diagnostic framework describing personality structures and reactions to infertility is presented in Table 8.1. Along with understanding the psychological components of infertility, it is also imperative to assess the presence of personality disorders, substance abuse or dependency, sexual abuse, domestic violence, sociopathy, and other significant mental health disorders/problems, as well as the patient's cultural experience and milieu.

It is clear that individual counseling with infertility patients requires special expertise and an understanding of and appreciation for the many psychosocial and medical components relative to this condition. A commentary by Hart[68] also supports this notion. Appendix 1 delineates qualification guidelines for mental health professionals working in reproductive medicine and stresses the need for a solid knowledge of family-building options, such as adoption, third-party reproduction, and childlessness. In addition, an understanding of the potential sociocultural, religious, and ethical implications of these choices is critical.

In sum, the treatment modalities discussed in this chapter can be extremely useful when counseling infertile patients. Most psychotherapists use a combination of interventions to meet clients' needs in the most effective and efficient way. These approaches, however, are only as effective as the therapist who makes use of them. Kottler[63] pointed out a number of common characteristics or qualities of successful psychotherapeutic outcomes, including a counselor's personality, skillful thinking processes, good communication skills, and the ability to establish an intimate and trusting relationship.

TABLE 8.1. Personality types and infertility[69]

Personality structure	Reaction to infertility
Obsessive: orderly, systematic, perfectionist, inflexible	Infertility is seen as punishment for letting things get out of control
Narcissistic: self-involved, angry, independent, perfectionist	Infertility is seen as an attack on autonomy and perfection of self
Borderline: demanding, impulsive, unstable	Infertility is seen as a threat of abandonment
Dependent: long-suffering, depressed, submissive	Infertility is seen as expected punishment for worthlessness
Avoidant: remote, unsociable, uninvolved	Infertility and its procedures are seen as a dangerous invasion of privacy
Paranoid: wary, suspicious, blaming, hypersensitive	Infertility is seen as annihilating assault coming from everywhere outside of self

FUTURE IMPLICATIONS

There is a clear future for mental health professionals treating infertile individuals. At the same time, one of the goals of this chapter has been to emphasize the importance of having a sound knowledge of the psychosocial experience of infertility and an appreciation of the numerous medical interventions available, the high financial and emotional costs involved, and the range of parenting alternatives from which patients might ultimately choose. It is only with this solid background that a psychotherapist can best apply his or her theoretical and clinical expertise to assist individuals struggling with losses and concerns associated with infertility. From a global standpoint, however, the need for a clear understanding of cultural traditions, needs, and experiences will significantly impact how the mental health professional practices his or her craft. Clinical interventions thus must be tailored not only to the psychological needs of the infertile patient but also to his or her social and cultural needs.

In light of the complexities of all forms of reproductive loss, it appears that professional training programs and postgraduate courses may, in the future, choose to incorporate or develop specific curricula that address the psychosocial components of infertility. The rapid growth of the assisted reproductive technologies and the psychological and ethical implications inherent in them require that formal clinical programs be established to provide training in this increasingly important arena. Credentialing in infertility counseling, through specific country or international professional organizations, may also help establish appropriate qualifications and expertise in the field. Subspecialties can be developed that focus on reproductive health, as well as on perinatal issues including not only pregnancy loss but also pregnancy and parenting after infertility as well as the long-term impact of assisted reproduction on children and families.

SUMMARY

■ Historically, infertility and reproductive loss were often considered by mental health professionals as having a dynamic, psychogenic basis. Recently, there has been a significant shift to supporting infertile individuals and minimizing the destructive emotional components of this medical condition. This shift has occurred among clinicians and researchers on an international level.

■ The five theoretical treatment approaches presented may be useful in working with individuals struggling with infertility. These include psychodynamic psychotherapy, cognitive-behavioral therapy, strategic and solution-focused psychotherapy, crisis intervention, and grief counseling.

• Clinical issues of countertransference and the role of the therapist who works with this special population need to be understood, especially because many therapists working in the field have had personal experience with infertility.

■ Many infertile individuals request and/or require only brief psychotherapeutic intervention.

• All infertility counselors can apply several specific tasks when meeting a new client for the first time. These tasks can serve several important purposes and include:

– forming a positive working relationship
– finding a treatment focus
– negotiating criteria for a successful outcome
– distinguishing clients from nonclients
– identifying patient motivational levels and tailoring interventions accordingly
– doing something that makes a difference immediately.

■ The treatment approach is only as effective as the therapist who employs it.

■ Individual counseling and psychotherapy with infertility patients is an area that deserves our special attention. The psychosocial needs of those who struggle to build families are compelling and require clinical expertise and a clear understanding of the underlying emotional issues involved.

REFERENCES

1. Mack S, Tucker J. *Fertility Counselling*. London: Bailliere Tindall, WB Saunders & Company, 1996; 101.

2. Menning BE. RESOLVE: A support group for infertile couples. *Am J Nurs* 1976; 76:258–9.

3. Menning BE. Counseling infertile couples. *Contemp Obstet Gynecol* 1979; 13:101–8.

4. Applegarth LD. The psychological aspects of infertility. In: WR Keye, RJ Chang, RW Rebar, MR Soules, eds. *Infertility: Evaluation and Treatment*. Philadelphia: Saunders, 1995; 25–41.

5. Applegarth LD. Emotional implications. In: EY Adashi, JA Rock, Z Rosenwaks, eds. *Reproductive Endocrinology, Surgery, and Technology*. Philadelphia: Lippincott-Raven, 1996; 2:1954–68.

6. Covington SN. The role of the mental health professional in reproductive medicine. *Fertil Steril* 1995; 64:895–7.

7. Leiblum SR, Introduction. In: SR Leiblum, ed. *Infertility: Psychological Issues and Counseling Strategies*. New York: Wiley, 1997; 3–19.

8. Leon IG. Reproductive loss: Barriers to psychoanalytic treatment. *J Am Acad Psychoanal* 1996; 24:341–52.

9. Jeker L, Micioni G, Ruspa M, et al. Wish for a child and infertility in 116 couples. 1. Interview and psycho-dynamic hypothesis. *Int J Fertil* 1987; 33:411–20.

10. Benedek T. Infertility as a psychosomatic defense. *Fertil Steril* 1952; 3:527–35.

11. Deutsch H. *The Psychology of Women*. New York: Grune & Stratton, 1944.

12. Sandler B. Infertility of emotional origin. *J Obstet Gynaecol Brit Emp* 1961; 68:809–15.

13. Seibel MM, Taymor ML. Emotional aspects of infertility. *Fertil Steril* 1982; 37:137–45.

14. Mai FM, Munday RN, Rump EE. Psychiatric interview comparisons between infertile and fertile couples. *Psychosom Med* 1972; 12:46–59.

15. Paulson JD, Haarmann BS, Salerno RL, et al. An Investigation of the relationship between emotional maladjustment and infertility. *Fertil Steril* 1988; 49:258–62.

16. Downey J. The new reproductive technologies: Psychological issues for female patients. Presented at the 35th winter meeting of the American Academy of Psychoanalysis, New York, December, 1991.

17. Leiblum SR, Greenfeld DA. The course of infertility: Immediate and long-term reactions. In: SR Leiblum, ed. *Infertility: Psychological Issues and Counseling Strategies*. New York: Wiley, 1997; 83–92.

18. Domar AD, Clapp D, Slawsby E, et al. The impact of group psychological interventions on distress in infertile women. *Health Psychol* 2000; 19:568–75.

19. Greil AL. Infertility and psychological distress: A critical review of the literature. *Soc. Sci Med* 1997; 45:1679–704.

20. Florin I, Tuschen-Caffier B, Krause W, Pook M. Psychological therapy in idiopathic infertility: A stress reduction approach. In: B Strauss, ed. *Involuntary Childlessness: Psychological Assessment, Counseling and Psychotherapy*. Seattle: Hogrete & Huber Publishers, 2002; 63–78.

21. Erickson E. *Childhood and Society*. New York: Norton, 1950.

22. Benedek T. Parenthood as a developmental phase. *J Am Psychoanal Assoc* 1959; 7:389–417.

23. Bibring G. Some consideration of the psychological processes in pregnancy. *Psychoanal Study Child* 1959; 14:113–21.

24. Klempner L. Infertility: Identification and disruptions with the maternal object. *Clin Soc Work J* 1992; 20:193–8.

25. Notman MT, Lester EP. Pregnancy: Theoretical consideration. *Psychoanal Inq* 1988; 8:139–45.

26. Bassin D. Woman's shifting sense of self – the impact of reproductive technology. In: J Offerman-Zuckerberg, ed. *Gender in Transition: A New Frontier*. New York: Plenum, 1989; 191–202.

27. Benedek T. Parenthood as a developmental phase: A contribution to libido theory. *Psychoanal Study Child* 1960; 15:60–76.

28. Newton CR, Houle M. Gender differences in psychological response to infertility treatment. *Infertil Reprod Med Clin North Am* 1993; 4:545–58.

29. Souter VL, Hopton JL, Penney GC, et al. Survey of psychological health in women with infertility. *J Psychosom Obstet Gynaecol* 2002; 23:41–9.

30. Lee S. *Counseling in Male Infertility*. London: Blackwell Science, 1996.

31. Crawshaw M. Offering woman-centered counseling in reproductive medicine. In: S Jennings, ed. *Infertility Counseling*. Oxford: Blackwell Science, 1995; 38–65.

32. Freeman EW, Rickels K, Tausig J. Emotional and psychosocial factors in follow-up of women after IVF-ET treatment. *Acta Obstet Gynecol Scand* 1987; 66:517–25.

33. Lalos A, Lalos O, Jacobson L, et al. Depression, guilt and isolation among infertile women and their partners. *J Psychosom Obstet Gynaecol* 1986; 5:197–206.

34. Mason MC. *Male Infertility – Men Talking*. London: Routledge, 1993.

35. Greil AL, Porter KL, Leitko TA. Sex and intimacy among infertile couples. *J Psychol Hum Sex* 1989; 2:117–23.

36. Ulbrich PM, Tremaglio Coyle A, Llabre MM. Involuntary childlessness and marital adjustment: His and hers. *J Sex Marital Ther* 1990; 16:147–58.

37. Nachtigall RD, Becker G, Wozny M. The effects of gender-specific diagnosis on men's and women's response to infertility. *Fertil Steril* 1992; 57:113–21.

38. Shapiro CH. *Infertility and Pregnancy Loss: A Guide for Helping Professionals*. San Francisco: Jossey-Bass, 1988.

39. Raphael B. *The Anatomy of Bereavement*. New York: Basic Books, 1983.

40. Mahlstedt PP. The psychological component of infertility. *Fertil Steril* 1985; 43:335–46.

41. Ursano RJ, Sonnenberg SM, Lazar SG. *Psychodynamic Psychotherapy*. Washington, DC: American Psychiatric Association Press, 1991.

42. Cooper JF. *A Primer of Brief Psychotherapy*. New York: Norton, 1995.

43. Koss MP, Butcher JN. Research on brief therapy. In: SL Garfield, AE Bergin, eds. *Handbook of Psychotherapy and Behavior Change*, 3rd ed. New York: Wiley, 1986; 627–70.

44. Bloom BL. *Planned Short-Term Psychotherapy: A Clinical Handbook*. Boston: Allyn & Bacon, 1992.

45. Wells RA. Clinical strategies in brief psychotherapy. In: RA Wells, VJ Gianetti, eds. *Casebook of the Brief Psychotherapies*. New York: Plenum, 1993; 3–17.

46. Hobbs M. Short-term dynamic psychotherapy. In: S Bloch, ed. *An Introduction to the Psychotherapies*, 3rd ed. New York: Oxford University Press, 1996; 52–83.

47. Peake TH, Borduin CM, Archer RP. *Brief Psychotherapies: Changing Frames of Mind*. Beverly Hills, CA: Sage, 1988.

48. Lehman AK, Salovey P. An introduction to cognitive behavior therapy In: RA Wells, VJ Gianetti, eds. *Handbook of the Brief Psychotherapies*. New York: Plenum, 1990; 239–59.

49. Bandura A. The self in reciprocal determinism. *Am Psychol* 1978; 33:344–58.

50. Mahoney MJ. Personal science: A cognitive learning theory. In: A Ellis, R Grieger, eds. *Handbook of Rational Psychotherapy*. New York: Springer, 1977; 3–33.

51. Quick EK. *Doing What Works in Brief Therapy: A Strategic Solution-Focused Approach*. San Diego, CA: Academic, 1996.

52. Rosenbaum R. Strategic psychotherapy. In: RA Wells, VJ Gianetti, eds. *Handbook of the Brief Psychotherapies*. New York: Plenum, 1990; 351–403.

53. Walter JL, Peller JE. *Becoming Solution-Focused in Brief Therapy*. New York: Brunner/Mazel, 1992.

54. Holzle C, Brandt U, Lutkenhaus R, et al. Solution-focused counseling for involuntarily childless couples. In B Strauss, ed. *Involuntary Childlessness: Psychological Assessment, Counseling and Psychotherapy*. Gottingen, Germany: Hogrete & Huber Publishers, 2002; 105–26.

55. Bancroft J, Graham C. Crisis intervention. In: S Bloch, ed. *An Introduction to the Psychotherapies*. 3rd ed. New York: Oxford University Press, 1996; 134–47.

56. Rapoport L. Crisis intervention as a mode of brief treatment. In: RW Roberts, RH Nee, eds. *Theories of Social Casework*. Chicago: University of Chicago Press, 1970; 77–98.

57. Lazarus RS, Folkman S. *Stress, Appraisal, and Coping*. New York: Springer, 1984.

58. Caplan G. *An Approach to Community Mental Health*. London: Tavistock, 1961.

59. Crenshaw DA. *Bereavement: Counseling the Grieving Throughout the Life Cycle*. New York: Continuum, 1990.

60. Tansey MJ, Burke WF. *Understanding Countertransference – From Projective Identification to Empathy*. Hillsdale, NJ: Analytic, 1989.

61. Kentenich H, Henning K, Himmel W, et al. Practical therapy in sterility – A manual for gynecologists from a psychosomatic point of view. In B Strauss, ed. *Involuntary Childlessness: Psychological Assessment, Counseling and Psychotherapy*. Seattle: Hogrete & Huber Publishers, 2002; 175–86.

62. Leibowitz L. Reflections of a childless analyst. In: B Gershon, ed. *The Therapist as a Person: Lift Crises, Life Choices, Life Experiences and Their Effects on Treatment*. Hillsdale, NJ: The Analytic Press, 1996; 71–87.

63. Kottler JA. *The Compleat Therapist*. San Francisco: Jossey-Bass, 1991.

64. Rosen A, Rosen J. Introduction. In A Rosen, J Rosen, eds. *Frozen Dreams: Psychodynamic Dimensions of Infertility and Assisted Reproduction*. Hillsdale, NJ: The Analytic Press, 2005: xvi.

65. Sayres Van Niel M. Pregnancy: The obvious and evocative real event in a therapist's life. In JH Gold, JC Nemiah, eds. *Beyond Transference: When the Therapist's Real Life Intrudes*. Washington, DC: American Psychiatric Press, Inc., 1993.

66. Pekarik G. Rationale, training, and implementation of time-sensitive treatments. Presented to the executive directors, MCC Companies, Inc., Minneapolis, MN, January, 1990.

67. Leon IG. *When a Baby Dies: Psychotherapy for Pregnancy and Newborn Loss*. New Haven: Yale University Press, 1990.

68. Hart VA. Infertility and the role of psychotherapy. *Issues Ment Health Nurs* 2002; 23:31–41.

69. Goldfarb JM, Rosenthal MB, Utian WH. Impact of psychologic factors in the care of the infertile couple. *Semin Reprod Endocrinol* 1985; 3:97.

9 Counseling the Infertile Couple

CHRISTOPHER R. NEWTON

There can be no disparity in marriage like unsuitability of mind and purpose.

– Charles Dickens

The advent of assisted reproductive techniques such as in vitro fertilization (IVF) placed much of the burden for treatment on women, and, not surprisingly, much of what has been written about treatment stress and infertility has been derived from the experience of women. In contrast, attention has only recently been directed toward the male response to infertility, yet men's reactions to infertility remain less understood. Studies assessing infertile couples have typically compared male and female levels of psychosocial distress[1] but less frequently have examined the ways in which couples' relationships are affected. Similarly, in terms of counseling, a recent review of the literature identified only thirteen published intervention studies with infertile couples.[2] By necessity, then, this chapter draws on a growing body of empirical literature about the individual effects of infertility. It also incorporates current understanding of the relationships between stress and coping on dyadic functioning. The chapter highlights some of the key clinical issues that confront infertile couples and provides an overview of different therapeutic approaches used internationally to address these problems. A pervasive theme throughout this chapter is a need for couples (and therapists) to recognize and respect gender differences. Effective couple therapy involves more than just encouraging couples to engage in emotion sharing. For example, the marital literature suggests that couples who can learn to regulate emotions under difficult circumstances are likely to be less vulnerable to relationship distress. Recent marital enrichment programs that have educated couples about both individual and dyadic strategies to manage stress have shown promise.[3] An important premise of this approach is that love and attraction alone are not enough to sustain a relationship. In the face of major obstacles in life's path, new skills may be needed. This seems particularly apropos with respect to infer-

tility. House-sized boulders seem to pepper the trail of unwary couples, who often need to learn a variety of new skills to cope with the sometimes unique demands placed on their relationship.

This chapter

- reviews current research on the impact of treatment on couples and assessment tools;
- provides a framework for assisting couples with problems created or exacerbated by infertility.

HISTORICAL OVERVIEW

Thirty-five years ago, the field of marital therapy was described as "a technique in search of a theory,"[4] where therapy with couples consisted of a hodgepodge of clinical interventions based on partial and sometimes tenuous theories.[5] Therapy with infertile couples appears to be at a similar stage; the number and range of interventions is growing but the field faces the same theoretical challenges.

Interventions with infertile couples have fallen into two broad and overlapping categories. In the first category, efforts have been made to address psychological factors that might be hindering pregnancy, particularly when infertility is unexplained. Early theories of infertility were heavily influenced by psychodynamic and psychoanalytic formulations. In this context, couples therapy consisted of attempts to uncover unconscious conflicts and work through unresolved emotional issues that might be affecting fertility. For example, Sarrel and DeCherney[6] offered couples with unexplained infertility a single psychotherapeutic interview. At follow-up, 60% of interviewed couples had achieved pregnancy in comparison to 11% of a no contact group. While the identification of previously unrecognized conflict was suggested as the mechanism of change, it was unclear to what extent other important issues concerning the marriage or the sexual relationship might also have been addressed in therapy, thereby facilitating pregnancy. Recently, interventions with infertile couples have attempted to both optimize conception rates and reduce the stress of infertility and its treatments through psychodynamic,[7] cognitive-behavioral,[8] and solution-focused approaches.[9] More comprehensive mixed interventions combining educational, behavioral, supportive, and experiential components have also been reported.[10]

In the second category, interventions have broadly targeted either treatment-related or infertility-specific stress. These have included education to reduce the stress of treatment,[11] cognitive-behavioral approaches to foster greater personal control and enhance marital and sexual satisfaction,[12] solution-focused therapy for stress relief,[13] and systemic couple therapy to facilitate communication and coping with infertility stress.[14]

While the number and range of reported interventions with couples are growing, it should be noted that actual studies vary widely in experimental quality. Many studies lack control conditions for comparison and some lack objective, standardized measures of outcome. In addition, some interventions involve the couple, but the focus is, to a considerable extent, on the individual (e.g., teaching methods of stress reduction) rather than on the dyadic interaction.

THEORETICAL FRAMEWORKS

A theoretical framework that seeks both to explain and to make testable hypotheses about the impact of infertility on couples' relationships is still lacking. Instead, theoretical descriptions of the impact of infertility on couples are often, in reality, theories of the individual, that are assumed to apply generally but often ignore gender differences and add little to our understanding of important interactional patterns.

In the past twenty-five years, concepts of grief and loss, together with stage theories, have heavily influenced thinking about the infertility experience. In fact, marriage itself has been characterized as involving sequential stages of expansion and promise, contraction and betrayal, and finally resolution. It has then been argued that infertility serves to magnify the hurt and disappointment that couples experience during the normal developmental sequence.[15] Individuals (and therefore couples) are assumed to move through certain emotional stages, for example, shock, denial, anger, guilt, grief, and resolution.[16] In conjunction

with treatment, couples have been described as moving through phases of engagement (dawning of awareness or facing a new reality), immersion (intensified treatment efforts or growing emotional distress), and disengagement (ending treatment or finding a new focus).[17]

In a similar vein, systemic couple therapy has been melded with stage theory resulting in the identification of five key phases of infertility (dawning, mobilization, immersion, resolution, and legacy). The issues facing the couple at each phase can differ and, it is assumed, require different therapeutic approaches.[14] While reports from this group are rich with clinical material and offer sophisticated dyadic techniques and strategies, the model awaits testing.

Infertility has also been characterized as involving a "transition to non-parenthood."[18] On the basis of this model, therapeutic suggestions often involve helping couples work through the grief process.[19] Unfortunately, despite its theoretical and clinical appeal, the stage theory of grief has received little empirical support. Response to loss may be more variable than has been acknowledged, and assumptions that distress is necessary and that loss must always be processed to achieve effective recovery and resolution might not be universally correct.[20] The danger therefore is that clinicians may either create or reinforce inaccurate expectations for a couple about appropriate ways to react and respond both to the stress of infertility and to each other.

At this stage, much of the published intervention literature on couples counseling has not been theory-driven, although work on control,[21] coping and appraisal,[22] and social support[23] is beginning to illustrate both the intricacy in couples' reactions and the need to recognize gender differences in planning treatment interventions. The complex interaction between stress, coping, and marital satisfaction has been highlighted in a recent review.[3] For example, when couples are faced with infertility stress, there are actually several competing agendas at play. Each partner needs to regulate his or her own emotional distress, tend to the emotional needs of the partner, be sensitive to the needs of the relationship, and consider the practical demands of the situation. At times, individuals need to engage in protective buffering through disengagement strategies of denial, distraction, and withdrawal. Where active engagement with a spouse leads to repeated negative interactions, such disengagement may also smooth over potential relationship conflicts and benefit the relationship in the short term. In fact, a failure to attend to individual emotion-focused strategies may undermine relationship functioning by creating a spillover of individual stress into a marriage. However, in the long term, persistent withdrawal might decrease marital intimacy and increase marital distress. As such, couples and therapists need to attend to both individual coping strategies and relationship interactions.

REVIEW OF LITERATURE

Effects of Infertility

There is a considerable body of evidence that men and women are affected differently by the experience of infertility. Women are more likely to worry that something is wrong even before seeking treatment, more likely to initiate discussion with their partners, and more likely to assume personal responsibility when efforts to conceive prove unsuccessful.[24] A recent review found that during infertility investigations or treatment, women reported higher levels of distress than men on measures of anxiety (seven of thirteen studies), depression (four of seven studies), self-esteem (three of four studies), and psychological adjustment (six of fourteen studies).[25] In terms of the above measures, none of the studies found infertile men to be more distressed than infertile women.

How the couple as a unit is affected remains unclear. As a group, infertile couples reported levels of marital adjustment in the normal range.[26–28] However, some couples complained of deterioration in marital functioning,[29] while others reported that the crisis of infertility improved marital communication and consequently emotional intimacy.[30] Still others suggested that sexual functioning was disturbed but that marital satisfaction remained intact.[31] One of the few studies to examine the dyadic process rather than the individuals separately highlighted the importance of what has been termed *congruence*, that is, a sense of agreement between a couple in their perception of the severity of infertility stress. Couples who experienced similar levels of social stress related to infertility were found to have higher levels of marital satisfaction compared with couples where partners experienced different levels of social stress. Similarly, when the couple expressed different views on the importance of parenthood or on the impact of infertility on their relationship, women were found to be at higher risk for depression.[32]

Impact of Medical Treatment

In the assessment of the impact of infertility on a couple's relationship, it appears that the stage of medical treatment may be a contributing factor. While the initial phase of infertility diagnosis and treatment is often characterized as an acute stress, research findings on the impact of this stage are mixed. For example, Daniluk et al.[33] presented data on couples attending an infertility clinic in which the couples reported marital and sexual functioning in the normal range and no change from the first visit to six weeks postdiagnosis. However, a similar study described a decrease in marital adjustment over the diagnostic period.[11] The results of studies examining the effects of longer infertility treatment on a couple's relationship are similarly ambiguous. In a longitudinal study, Benazon et al.[34] followed infertile couples over the course of eighteen months of treatment. Although women who failed to conceive reported increased sexual dissatisfaction over this time period, marital satisfaction remained normal and unchanged for both men and women. However, prolonged infertility treatment may well be a source of chronic relationship strain. Berg and Wilson[28] found that for couples in advanced stages of treatment (greater than three years), indices of marital and sexual satisfaction were at the lowest overall level, and marital adjustment scores were near the maladjusted range.

Rather than the length of time spent in treatment, the repeated experience of treatment failure may be more important. Women who had experienced a moderate amount of treatment failure reported greater marital distress than women who had never experienced treatment failure, and more distress than those who had experienced the most treatment failure.[35] These findings were seen as support for a stage theory, that is, the experience of infertility is a process and individual and marital distress (at least for women) is a necessary part of an evolution toward acceptance of their infertility and improved marital functioning.

Effectiveness of Couple Counseling

In a recent comprehensive review of individual, couple, and group interventions for infertility, Boivin concluded that couple counseling has been more effective in reducing individual negative affect than improving relationship functioning.[2] Studies using a variety of approaches (educational, psychodynamic/counseling, solution-focused and cognitive-behavioral interventions) have reported reductions in individual infertility distress but no measurable effect on conception rates, partner, or relationship satisfaction.[9,11,13,36] At the same time, couple therapy has resulted in a decrease in intensity of desire for a child[7,9,13] and a greater tolerance for the ambiguity created by infertility.[7] However, a single study using a measure developed to assess marital domains affected by infertility, reported a positive impact of couples counseling on relationship variables. In an eight-month sex therapy program for couples with idiopathic infertility, the authors reported that a cognitive-behavioral approach resulted in improved sperm concentration and both increased sexual satisfaction and decreased marital distress.[8]

CLINICAL ISSUES

Assessment

The assessment of the couple prior to treatment with advanced reproductive technology (ART) can serve one of three purposes. First, the clinician might wish to assess the extent to which a fertility problem is creating relationship stress in the form of marital or sexual dissatisfaction. This might serve as a springboard for individual or couples infertility or sexual counseling. Second, the clinician might wish to identify couple-specific concerns related to treatment participation. For example, is the couple in agreement about treatment participation, the extent of treatment involvement, or other options for parenthood, if necessary? Does the couple feel able to provide each other with necessary emotional and tangible support? Such information might determine whether couple counseling could be beneficial to facilitate treatment participation and/or manage the aftermath of treatment failure. Finally, and most controversially, as a gatekeeper, the assessor might be required to address the couple's suitability for treatment or for parenthood.

Particularly in the United States, there has been considerable resistance to the notion of placing limitations on who should receive treatment with ART. Concerns have been raised that restrictions impinge upon fundamental freedoms, infertile couples would be held to a higher standard than couples conceiving naturally, inconsistencies in standards between clinics might create inequalities in access, and the slippery slope argument that reasonable restrictions might ultimately lead to discriminatory or even eugenic practices.[37] Nevertheless, there are limits in place and a recent survey of American clinics indicated that 71% collect information concerning the stability of the relationship and 70% believe it is appropriate to assess parenting capacity.[37] Recently, the American Society for Reproductive Medicine Ethics Committee released a position paper proposing that the welfare of any offspring is a valid consideration that might be taken into account, but that clinics are not morally obligated to withhold services.[38] The report also suggests that the mental health counselor, as part of the treatment team, should have an active role in this decision-making process and

that the decision should not be made by a single caregiver. This stance is similar to that taken internationally. In Canada, recent government legislation enacted in 2004 states that "the health and well-being of children born through the application of assisted human reproductive technologies must be given priority...."[39] In the United Kingdom, regulatory guidelines require that treatment centers have clear criteria for assessing the welfare of any child or children and that criteria "include the importance of a stable and supportive environment...."[40] Several European countries (e.g., Austria, Norway, France, Sweden, and the Swiss cantons) restrict access to in vitro fertilization treatment to married couples or heterosexual couples in a stable relationship.[41] In continental Europe, the guidelines for counseling issued by the European Society For Human Reproduction (ESHRE) incorporate both assessment and counseling activities under the rubric of 'counseling' but acknowledge that, "In some countries assessment of suitability prior to treatment... [which] aims to ensure that the welfare of all parties involved, especially the child..." is conducted.[42] Somewhat skirting the issue, ESHRE guidelines further state that, "patients...who present with either a severely disturbed marital relationship and/or irresolvable discord..." are considered to be at risk and likely to need counseling.

In summary, international legislation, regulations and guidelines related to criteria for assessment are framed in terms of broad principles, requiring clinics to address the best interests of the potential child, but are noticeably lacking in specifics. Thus, the nature and severity of relationship problems that might preclude treatment participation remain a matter of clinical judgment for the mental health counselor and the rest of the treatment team. Furthermore, it is often difficult to assess the significance of individual issues (e.g., serious mental health problems) in isolation from the partner and the relationship. For example, when the stability of one partner is a concern, the clinician might also need to ask to what extent the healthy partner will be an active caregiver and can (and will) act as a buffer between the less healthy parent and the potential child. Relationship problems that might well lead to postponement or denial of treatment include ongoing physical or emotional abuse, a history of perpetrating abuse on others, or a documented history of inadequate parenting with other children. There is also considerable research demonstrating that conflict and hostility between parents is associated with negative consequences for the child; thus, serious ongoing marital conflict would indicate a need to at least postpone treatment until relationship problems could be addressed.

Finally, the welfare of the child is a consideration susceptible to wide interpretation and is not necessarily synonymous with the concept of the ideal family. In considering the best interests of the child, Pennings[43] has outlined the possible ethical and philosophical principles that might underlie this evaluation. For example, the 'maximum welfare principle' implies that a child should not be brought into the world under less than ideal circumstances. Unfortunately, this would likely exclude the majority of the population. The 'minimum threshold principle' implies that minimal standards exist and that certain characteristics of the potential parents (e.g., severe marital strife, history of child abuse or neglect) are unacceptable, but otherwise, adequate criteria to determine parenting capacity are lacking. Thus, clinicians can and should only prevent procreation in situations where the child's quality of life would be very low. Pennings has suggested an intermediate 'reasonable welfare' principle, whereby the standard is not a perfectly happy child. Instead, the provision of medical services is considered acceptable when the potential child could anticipate a reasonably happy life.

In assessing the effects of infertility on a relationship, clinicians need to be mindful of several factors that may influence a couple's presentation. Couples referred for medical treatment using assisted reproductive technologies such as IVF may have suffered a series of demoralizing treatment failures in the recent past, resulting in both increased emotional turmoil and relationship tension. However, referral to these new programs can produce an upsurge of optimism and a temporary sense of well-being.[44] As a result, couples may portray both the stress of infertility and its impact on the relationship as a past problem, now largely resolved. Similarly, couples may engage in positive-impression management, minimizing or denying difficulties in order not to jeopardize their acceptance into the infertility treatment program. Even when couples seek counseling, relationship problems may be relatively circumscribed, and couples may maintain a reserve of goodwill toward each other. This may lead some couples to try to protect each other by engaging in self-blame and avoiding overt criticism of the other's behavior. Finally, most couples (infertile or not) have difficulty thinking of relationship problems in systemic terms, and as a result, offer rather vague definitions or explanations – often in terms of communication difficulties when asked about the nature of relationship troubles.

Unfortunately, standardized measures that are infertility-specific and provide an objective measure of relationship problems are few. Alternatively, more general measures of marital relationship functioning often lack sensitivity to infertility concerns. However, tests with good reliability, validity, and norms for comparison can be useful both in determining the severity of relationship complaints and offering clinical leads for further inquiry. Among tests used primarily by psychologists and marriage or family therapists, the following measures can contribute to the assessment.

Locke–Wallace Marital Adjustment Scale

Locke and Wallace's[45] Marital Adjustment Scale (MAS) is a fifteen-item self-report instrument that inquires about the extent of disagreement on eight sub-areas (e.g., mutual activity and mutual decision making). The lack of a conceptual plan in selecting items raises doubts about the comprehensiveness (content validity) of the MAS. Item wording is dated, and the 'husband' and 'wife' format is not suitable for other dyads.

Dyadic Adjustment Scale

A thirty-two-item self-report scale, the Dyadic Adjustment Scale (DAS)[46] taps marital satisfaction in four areas: (1) consensus on matters important to the relationship, (2) degree of tension, (3) agreement over affection/sex, and (4) satisfaction with verbal communication and companionship activities. The DAS is probably the best brief screening device available and is a good indicator of overall relationship stress.

Marital Satisfaction Inventory

The Marital Satisfaction Inventory (MSI)[47] is a 280-item self-report inventory developed to assess global marital satisfaction and individuals' attitudes and beliefs regarding specific areas of the relationship. It is suitable for couples with or without children. The eleven scales were constructed on a rational basis and tap areas of the relationship such as: affective communication, problem-solving communication, time together, sexual dissatisfaction, and disagreement over finances. A validity scale assesses the tendency to describe the marriage in socially desirable terms. Particularly in cases where problems seem to extend beyond the bounds of infertility-related concerns, the MSI provides useful information in terms of areas of the relationship needing change. While its comprehensiveness is a strength, couples may be reluctant to complete such a lengthy instrument unless they have serious concerns about their relationship – or the therapist does.

The Fertility Problem Inventory

The Fertility Problem Inventory is a forty-six-item self-report inventory developed to measure the degree of infertility-specific stress experienced by individuals.[48] While not exclusively a measure of relationship satisfaction, two scales on the questionnaire assess perceptions of the extent to which fertility problems have strained the couple's overall relationship and specifically their sexual relationship. It provides a quick screen for relationship strain by specifically tapping infertility-related issues and offers norms based on a large sample of infertility patients active in treatment.

THERAPEUTIC INTERVENTION

Goals in Counseling the Couple

There are numerous potential goals in providing couples counseling, which can often partially overlap with the goals of individual counseling. The goals of couples counseling regarding infertility fall into three broad categories:

- Facilitating the couple's management of treatment as a team by
  - increasing awareness of treatment implications;
  - addressing decision conflict;
  - reducing stress on the relationship;[2]
  - encouraging more active participation in decision making;
  - improving or facilitating communication between the couple and medical staff.[10]
- Facilitating the management of infertility as a couple through identifying
  - differences in motivation for having children;
  - differences in reaction to infertility and in coping styles;
  - problems in constructive communication.
- Assisting in dealing with infertility strains on the relationship related to infertility or its treatment through
  - support for grief work;
  - help for the couple in identifying alternatives and new life perspectives.[7]

Particularly in the early stages of infertility and treatment, a more focused approach with couples in terms of providing information and new skills might be of more benefit than sessions with greater emphasis on emotion sharing. A recent review of interventions with couples noted that informational and skills based interventions yielded more positive changes than emotion-focused interventions. In one study, couples rated skills training more helpful than reflecting on emotional aspects of infertility.[2] However, it is quite conceivable that at later stages of infertility treatment and at treatment end, emotion-focused approaches might become more beneficial. This possibility remains to be tested.

Early Consultation

Many infertility treatment programs, particularly those offering assisted reproductive technologies such as IVF, either provide the opportunity for, or require couples to participate in, an assessment and or counseling process prior to treatment. This provides the opportunity to screen for individual problems (anxiety, depression, substance abuse) or relationship concerns that might compromise a couple's ability to cope, comply with, or agree about treatment.

At this stage, counseling often has a significant psycho-educational component in terms of ensuring that couples understand the implications of treatment and the treatment process, while concurrently helping them identify and address potential stressors associated with treatment procedures. Issues might include understanding treatment success rates, arranging time away from work, whom to tell and how much to tell about treatment, the possible impact of medications on the woman's mood and hence the relationship, dealing with treatment failure, and couple agreement on goal setting in terms of the extent of treatment participation. In fact, the very act of going to counseling together may foster a sense of teamwork and enhance intimacy,[14] which can be further enhanced if the couple is encouraged to develop a 'treatment coping plan,' whereby they identify individual and couple activities that are enjoyable and relaxing. Couples are instructed to 'coordinate' their coping strategies (e.g., her individual coping technique of distraction via shopping may not be beneficial for him). Finally, they are encouraged to incorporate their coping plan into their treatment plan.

This phase has been identified as a time where the task of clarification can be important.[7,9] This can involve helping the couple to clarify their motives for treatment and the importance of children, as a way to stabilize their commitment to treatment. It is also a phase where it is important that couples begin (if they have not already) to develop a tolerance for ambiguity,[7] in other words, an ability to actively entertain the possibility that treatment might not work and to begin to envision other options. From a solution-focused approach, this has been characterized as helping couples begin to entertain new themes or stories for the future of the relationship.[13] An inability to do so often can be seen in couples as unrelenting optimism on the part of one or both partners; a reluctance to discuss or think about program success rates; and an unwillingness to contemplate treatment cycle failures. This inability to prepare for, or even discuss, potential setbacks or failures increases the couple's vulnerability. In addition, sometimes the clinician needs to tactfully counter the couple's notion of 'the earned child' – that through conscientious planning and hard work, a pregnancy is now deserved.[13] The overarching goal in addressing these issues is to encourage the couple to take an active role in making decisions. Clarification of the different ways that infertility affects them and their different coping strategies, sets the stage for a discussion of ways to manage stress as a couple and allows identification of resources, both internal to the couple (e.g., use of humor) and external (e.g., use of key social supports).

Role of Gender Differences

While most couples may not report marital dissatisfaction or conflict at early stages of treatment, this time represents an important opportunity to prevent or minimize potential future problems. This may be particularly important if couples have markedly contrasting coping styles. In reacting to a diagnosis of infertility, women seem to be affected more personally than men. Women describe feelings of role failure[30] and diminished self-esteem[49] regardless of the locus of impairment, whereas men's reactions seem to be similar to women only when infertility is due to a male factor. Even when one partner is the sole diagnosed cause of the problem, women report a greater sense of responsibility than men.[49] As a result, when infertility treatment fails, intense feelings of guilt and self-blame can place some unique strains on a couple's relationship. Although women's tendency to accept responsibility (even when infertility is unexplained) can be problematic, in some situations it may reflect an adaptive coping response. In attributing the cause of infertility to herself, a woman may be achieving what has been described as 'interpretive control,' that is, giving a threatening, largely uncontrollable, situation meaning or purpose.[21] While some women feel 'relieved' when perceiving themselves as responsible for a fertility problem, this actually might suggest an attempt to protect a partner. It also might reflect a degree of success in reestablishing some sense of control. Thus, men and women may not need to hold identical explanations for a fertility problem, and a therapist might need to weigh the importance and benefits of trying to change such attributions (see Chapter 3).

Among infertile couples, women are more likely to reach out for social support and to use certain escape or avoidance strategies (wishing, hoping, fantasizing, and social avoidance) than men. Men, by contrast, are more likely to engage in distancing through cognitive distraction, to engage in emotional self-regulation, and to view infertility in a pragmatic, problem-solving fashion.[22] In short, men have been described as engaging in 'fight or flight' responses, whereas women engage in efforts to 'tend and befriend.'[3]

Adding to the complexity, coping styles apparently vary with socioeconomic status. When faced with stress, blue-collar couples increase the use of humor during marital interactions while the expression of humor among white-collar couples decreases. Similarly, encouraging men to express their emotions during therapy was beneficial for middle-class husbands but detrimental for lower-class husbands, who may hold different attitudes about showing emotional vulnerability.[3] Adding further to this mix, gender difference in coping styles may be more or less acceptable to the couple based upon their cultural background. Whatever the socioeconomic class or culture, it is crucial for the therapist to recognize that men and women are likely to have different vulnerabilities that may require different coping strategies. For example, couples in which one partner is experiencing problems of depression may benefit from greater emotional support, while couples who are prone to rapidly escalating negative exchanges might benefit more from learning better communication and conflict-resolution skills.[3]

Couples who fail to recognize and adjust to such differences may misinterpret each other's reactions and give negative attributions to their partner's response. For example, a husband may cope through cognitive avoidance, emotional distancing, and self-control, while his wife may cope by seeking discussion and expressing her feelings. As a result, when treatment fails, he may perceive her as overreacting and conclude that she is too preoccupied with infertility and undervalues their relationship. She, in turn, may regard him as emotionally unaffected and therefore insensitive, uncaring, or uninvolved.

Managing Conflict

Promoting Acceptance

Because women are more likely than men to use social support as a means of coping, complaints about communication difficulties are often made by female partners. As counseling implicitly assumes a relationship model, when such a complaint is made, it is tempting to immediately provide a venue for more open discussion. Although this model is likely to be attractive to many women, when a husband is clearly a reluctant participant and or uncomfortable with emotion sharing, this approach might be a strategic error. An immediate and unplanned discussion of infertility may simply serve to perpetuate cross-complaining and the negative interactional cycle already played out at home.

Instead, it may be worthwhile to adopt a wider perspective. For example, differences or incompatibilities that might have lain dormant throughout the marriage, may surface and become issues in the face of infertility. Often one partner requests and then increasingly demands change, while the other partner struggles to maintain the status quo or reciprocates with his or her own requests for change. Even when some differences are truly irreconcilable (e.g., one partner wishes to adopt and the other does not) and cannot be problem-solved or compromised away, this does not prevent couples from trying to change each other. These change efforts and resistance to change can lead to a polarization in the couple's relationship, where conflict increases rather than decreases.[50] Rather than trying to facilitate further change efforts (particularly when differences are irreconcilable), the clinician's role can be to promote acceptance of these differences. In fact, it has been suggested that a complete approach to couple therapy needs to integrate strategies for fostering both acceptance and change.[50] In this case, acceptance does not mean submitting begrudgingly to the status quo. Instead, problems or differences become a vehicle for greater intimacy rather than for eradication. Through techniques such as 'empathic joining,' couples may build a closer relationship because of problems, rather than in spite of them, and the goal is to help partners let go of the struggle to change each other. For example, couples come to recognize and understand why and how they differ in ways of dealing with infertility and to accept these differences. Empathic joining can be facilitated in a number of ways; for example, by the clinician who prompts softer disclosures of hurt, disappointment and vulnerability rather than the typical hard exposures of frustration, anger and resentment, or by the couple themselves, who might be asked to switch roles figuratively or literally during the session. Ironically, when couples stop demanding changes of each other, change often then occurs.

Facilitating Communication

I feel like I'm talking to a brick wall.

In the beginning I understood and accepted her unhappiness. But it never seemed to stop. Gradually I withdrew because I didn't know what to say and I couldn't stand to watch her crying all the time.[51]

When an infertile couple seeks counseling, one party (more typically the woman) may complain that when it comes to infertility, her partner avoids discussions, fails to listen, or fails to self-disclose. As a result, the complainant feels angry, isolated, unloved, or a burden on the relationship. This pattern, in which one spouse (the pursuer) attempts to engage in problem discussion, often resorting to pressure and demands, while the other spouse (the distancer) attempts to withdraw from the discussion, has been identified as a particularly destructive style of marital interaction.[52,53] Interestingly, the potential seriousness of this problem depends on which partner engages in withdrawal. While husbands' withdrawal has been shown to be predictive of wives' hostility, wives' withdrawal has not been found to not predict husbands' hostility.[54]

Similarly, among infertile couples, it appears that discussion needs to meet a certain threshold of frequency for women's marital satisfaction but it need not be balanced. For example, women more frequently report initiating communication about infertility with husbands than men report initiating such discussions with their wives. Women also report receiving more emotional support from husbands than husbands report receiving from them. Nevertheless, both sexes describe satisfaction with this arrangement.[55] At the same time, women's and men's perceptions of the amount of support and disregard given and received from a spouse have been found to be only moderately related, suggesting that many couples are not communicating effectively with each other.[56]

Outbursts of frustration and anger may well be interpreted by a partner as unfair blaming, if not expressed clearly. In these situations, couples may need help in identifying and conveying feelings more accurately, expressing complaints more constructively, and developing better conflict-resolution skills. Couples can learn to translate vague complaints into specific behavioral descriptions by encouraging the use of 'videotalk.'[57] In other words, complainants are taught to describe a partner's behavior minus attributed meanings or interpretations. For example, the therapist might ask, "What kinds of things would I see him doing when he is acting 'insensitive'?" In expressing complaints, couples can learn to incorporate positive statements about a partner, to avoid derogatory labels, to talk about specific behavior, to incorporate 'I' language rather than 'you' in statements of feelings, and to accept partial responsibility for problems.

Improving a couple's ability to offer each other effective support also may involve striking a balance between some women's needs for discussion and some men's needs to maintain distance and emotional control. In other words, when one partner can accept that his or her partner has legitimate and understandable reasons for coping differently, this actually may free the other partner from defensively maintaining the status quo and foster change. Empathic joining and acceptance can be facilitated in a number of ways. One option might involve teaching couples to use better active-listening skills. Basic nonverbal skills (posture, facial expressions, eye contact, and tone of voice), if neglected, leave a partner feeling unheard and often negate any other efforts made by the listener to provide support. On a cautionary note, however, there are no universal rules for good communication and, in fact, active listening while feeling angry with a partner is not typical even of happily married couples.[35] Hence, as an alternative to teaching new communication skills, the clinician can play a key role in interpreting, reformulating, and prompting softer emotional disclosures from each partner. Such soft disclosures need not lead to offers of behavioral change, but can cause each partner to experience the relationship differently.[58]

Because men are more likely to use problem-solving strategies, they often offer support in terms of suggesting solutions to the problem or ways in which women can regain emotional control. Although well intended, problem solving or attempting to cheer up a partner, are often perceived as unhelpful when emotional support is wanted or the problem is not readily amenable to change.[59] Over time, men may feel increasingly helpless to provide effective support, but subsequent avoidance of discussion then produces increasing emotional disengagement. Learning to summarize ideas heard and to reflect feelings provides couples with better listening skills and affords the opportunity to give effective support without having to generate solutions to a problem over which they have little control. At the same time that communication is encouraged, men's needs for distance and control can be incorporated by emphasizing the importance of mutual agreement on the time and place for discussion. Couples can also agree to set specific time limits on such discussions and may follow these by sharing a mutually enjoyable activity.

Once both partners feel better heard and understood, it may be easier for each to accept that the other is affected quite differently by infertility. In therapy, couples have a tendency to tell stories about each other and then to argue about their accuracy. By learning the skill of emotional validation (showing empathy for a partner's feelings without necessarily being in agreement), couples can hold quite different perceptions of the infertility experience while still be mutually supportive.

Decision Making after Treatment

The decision to end unsuccessful medical treatment for infertility can trigger a complex series of issues for a couple. One partner may be ready to end treatment before the other. Couples may be in disagree-

ment about the acceptability of alternative methods to build a family, such as adoption. Similarly, the prospect of remaining childless may be more acceptable or attractive to one partner. These are issues that might not be amenable to a problem-solving approach, nor can they necessarily be compromised away. Nevertheless, one partner might fear long-term relationship strain unless he or she acquiesces to the other partner's wishes, even though such agreements made under pressure can potentially create risk of long-term resentment. When solutions are not evident, it becomes important to focus on the process of decision making rather than the outcome. A crucial aspect at this stage is to encourage the couple to slow down the decision-making process and explore their feelings about their different options.[60] Again, techniques of empathic joining can help couples to understand, their differences, the origins of these differences, and their mutual pain. For example, a wife's fears of a future without parenthood might be juxtaposed with her husband's fears of forever losing emotional closeness to her, if he does not agree to adoption. By encouraging disclosure of emotional vulnerability, the goal is to foster mutual empathy and emotional closeness. If the couple ultimately cannot reach a mutually satisfactory solution, the hope is that they can accept and respect their differences.

Facilitating Long-Term Adjustment

When the decision is made to discontinue treatment and other options to build a family are rejected, couples confront a future without children. Stage theories characterize this phase as one of grief, as individuals acknowledge the permanence of their infertility and fully confront the loss of pregnancy, childbirth, and parenting experiences. Currently, there seems to be general agreement among clinicians that the final stages of acceptance and resolution are achieved when grief feelings are acknowledged and expressed, and that the avoidance of such feelings may prevent resolution. For example, the resolution phase has been characterized as involving three overlapping tasks: (1) ending medical treatment, (2) mourning the loss of a genetically related child, and (3) refocusing or moving past the infertility through a focus on adoption or child-free living.[14] For some couples, the end of treatment is mostly a medical decision largely beyond their control, and while an emotional blow, triggers little personal ambivalence about the decision. Other couples may disagree with each other over the decision, triggering requests for counseling. Other couples may simply drift away from medical intervention or seek out second and third opinions as a means of maintaining the status quo and avoiding grief. Whether the lack of any clear end point hinders resolution remains unclear.

Deconstruction

If stage theory is correct, helping couples deconstruct the infertility experience by encouraging them to discuss their loss and to express the full range of feelings associated with grief should facilitate the mourning process. Counseling tasks might include: helping couples understand feelings of loss and lack of control, recognizing and accepting gender differences in ways of coping, and communicating with each other effectively and constructively.[61] It has been suggested that partners might grieve separately but not necessarily as a couple, and that without shared grieving, there is a risk that grief reactions might be misunderstood and lead to growing emotional distance.[14] Similarly, from a cognitive-behavioral perspective, there is evidence that repeated exposure to a traumatic event through recall can be beneficial. Through emotionally processing (i.e., repeated access and partial re-experience of difficult emotions), certain experiences have been shown to lose their emotional impact.[62] While such interventions have proved effective in cases of morbid grief,[63] their utility in managing normal grief has not been demonstrated.

At the same time, the stages of a grief reaction have not been clearly validated, and there is some evidence that effective recovery can occur without prior apparent emotional processing.[20] In addition, the process by which couples reach a degree of closure on treatment efforts seems to be more lengthy and difficult for women than men.[64] As a result, one partner may be having greater difficulty adjusting to this new reality than the other, and the clinician must decide whether to recommend individual or conjoint counseling. To what extent the presence in therapy of the less distressed partner is facilitative is unclear, and at present there is no outcome evidence to guide this decision. However, some clinicians have advocated the importance of grieving as a couple to ensure that grief reactions are not misunderstood. Furthermore, with individual therapy, there is a risk that the therapist might come to serve as the surrogate partner and that problems between partners could persist or worsen.[14] As a compromise, the clinician might recommend individual therapy for the partner in distress, with his or her partner included for discussion of particular relationship issues. When both partners are experiencing significant emotional distress and or if problems in adjustment are creating relationship distress, couple therapy would be clearly indicated.

Reconstruction

As couples deconstruct the old reality, there is a need to construct a new reality and a new future together. The therapist must strike a balance between validating the couple's past painful experience while not ignoring the possibilities for change. Too much emphasis on acknowledging emotional pain may either encourage preoccupation with negative feelings or give a message that the situation cannot improve. At the same time, premature emphasis on making changes could give the impression that the therapist is insensitive to the couple's distress.[57] Solution-focused approaches to therapy[65,66] offer interesting, but as yet relatively untested, ways in which the therapist can validate the couple's distress, while at the same time encouraging progression. Perceptions of infertility as global and unchangeable can be challenged by highlighting and amplifying exceptions that often go unnoticed by the couple. The experience of loss (i.e., 'the problem') can be restated as specific to certain times or places rather than generally present, and questions about what makes the problem better or worse begin to restore some sense of control. In addition, a solution-focused approach can be used to help couples to reconsider and redefine life-goals. For example, parenthood may be sought with any number of goals in mind: to fulfill needs to nurture, because children might bring more spontaneity or variety into a couple's relationship, or because parenthood allows access to a child-centered social community. Holzle et al. have described a three-month intervention to facilitate coping with infertility as a transitory life-crisis.[9] Couples were encouraged to identify solutions that were positive, specific and attainable, and which offered alternative ways besides parenthood to meet their goals. Among highly distressed participants, this led to a significant reduction in the intensity of the wish for a child. However, the authors caution that this approach may not be appropriate for couples who show serious mental health disorders.

Because infertility can be such a blow to self-esteem, one or both partners may exhibit what has been termed a 'spoiled identity.'[66] Rather than having a problem, the individuals define themselves as the problem; that is, 'we are infertile.' In this situation, the clinician can assist the couple in externalizing and localizing a fertility problem that then creates possibilities for the couple to generate solutions. Using this approach in couple therapy together with other solution-focused techniques, Wischmann et al. observed a decrease in infertility distress and a reduced intensity of desire for a child.[13] The appropriate use of metaphor with the couple can also facilitate this perceptual shift; for example, infertility has been characterized as 'a hurricane' that threatens the marital home, with a consequent need to strengthen it (via communication skills) so that the home can weather the storm.[67] Alternatively, couples (women in particular) have a history of struggling long and hard to overcome infertility, and this history can be used to encourage a different 'hero' identity in which the person is valued for his or her strengths and for standing up to the fertility problem.[66]

In constructing a new reality, couples often need to reexamine the basis for their relationship. At the time of marriage, a couple may have held certain assumptions about their individual roles and the role of children in their marriage. This is a time when the infertile partner may have unexpressed fears of abandonment, or fears that feelings of blame and resentment may create a permanent distance in the relationship. The therapist can elicit these concerns and help the couple share and discuss their future priorities. Sometimes it is beneficial to have the couple step back and evaluate the personal qualities that triggered the initial mutual attraction and the actual reasons underlying their choice of a marital partner.

Ritual

Finally, to mark and facilitate a transition from infertility patient to what is sometimes termed 'child-free status,'[68] the use of a special ceremony or ritual is often advocated.[69] In the design of a ritual with the couple, 'linked objects' (symbols physically associated with infertility) can be used to generate rituals of passage[38] – medications for disposal, baby items to be given away. Alternatively, couples sometimes wish to create symbols that facilitate mourning (a letter to the unrealized child) or to memorialize their loss (making regular donations to a certain charity or planting a tree).

However, if the ritual is to accomplish a sense of ending, couples need to feel that enough discussion, emotional expression, and exploration of feelings have first taken place. As yet, the optimal timing of such rituals is not well defined. In addition, because infertile couples use diverse and, at times, contrasting coping strategies, it remains unclear which couples are likely to benefit from ritual and to what extent men and women find this process similarly helpful.

FUTURE IMPLICATIONS

A combination of research findings and clinical observations has begun to identify certain factors that can give rise to relationship distress. These include repeated treatment failure and gender differences (both in terms of lack of perceived agreement between partners on the severity of infertility stress and in the use of contrasting coping strategies). However, at this stage, a number of questions remain. First, it is unclear whether relationship distress among infertile couples differs in any important ways from more general relationship distress. Second, while we have identified external risk factors, such as treatment experience, it is still unknown whether there are critical relationship factors that reliably differentiate distressed couples from nondistressed couples. Similarly, it is unclear whether there are aspects of a relationship that serve to buffer infertile couples from marital distress and increase the likelihood of successful long-term adjustment.

Despite the stress of infertility and treatment involvement, marital satisfaction scores for infertile couples generally fall within the normal range. However, these findings are derived largely from studies of couples before and during infertility treatment, and a clear picture is still lacking of post-treatment marital adjustment and the incidence of marital breakdown. The number of intervention studies with couples is slowly increasing, and these have reported some benefit. However, post-treatment gains have occurred largely at the individual level and it has proven harder to achieve or measure positive changes in the relationship. Efforts to answer these questions would certainly be aided by the development of psychological and or relationship measures that are more sensitive to infertility issues.

Finally, while stage theories have proved extremely clinically rich in conceptualizing both infertility and the medical treatment experience, they are unable to incorporate the complexity of a couple's interactions or to account for gender differences in adjustment to infertility. At this time, there is a need to continue evaluating the potential contribution of other theoretical models for understanding and counseling infertile couples.

SUMMARY

■ Clinical understanding of an individual's adjustment to infertility has been heavily influenced by stage theories, and similar theoretical assumptions are being used in approaches to counseling infertile couples.

■ Until empirically tested theories emerge, clinicians need to be cognizant of gender differences and remain flexible in their clinical approach to counseling infertile couples.

■ Assessment tools for the study of infertile couples are currently lacking, and clinicians will need to rely on more general instruments to evaluate relationship functioning.

■ Both the frequency of experience with treatment failure and incongruity in the experience of infertility distress appear to be risk factors in predicting relationship dissatisfaction.

■ Counseling objectives can vary considerably according to culture, a couple's degree of experience with infertility, and with infertility treatment.

■ Infertile couples in conflict are often characterized by their inability to understand and accept gender differences in reaction to infertility, together with an inability to provide each other with effective social and emotional support.

■ In assisting couples to manage relationship distress, clinicians need to consider whether change or acceptance strategies are more appropriate.

■ With couples facing final treatment failure, clinicians need to strike a balance between validating feelings of loss and inviting couples to be future-oriented and to focus on solutions.

REFERENCES

1. Wright J, Allard M, Lecours A, et al. Psychosocial distress and infertility: A review of controlled research. *Int J Fertil* 1989; 34:126–42.
2. Boivin J. A review of psychosocial interventions in infertility. *Soc Sci & Med* 2003; 57:2325–41.
3. Storey LB, Bradbury TN. Understanding marriage and stress: Essential questions and challenges. *Clin Psych Rev* 2004; 23:1139–62.
4. Manus GI. Marriage counseling: A technique in search of a theory. *J Marriage Fam* 1966; 28:449–53.
5. Gurman AS, Jacobson NS. Marital therapy: From technique to theory, back again, and beyond. In: NS Jacobson, AS Gurman, eds. *Clinical Handbook of Marital Therapy*. New York: Guilford Press, 1986; 1–9.
6. Sarrel PM, DeCherney AH. Psychotherapeutic intervention for treatment of couples with secondary infertility. *Fertil Steril* 1985; 43:897–900.
7. Strauss B, Hepp U, Stading G, et al. Focal counseling for women and couples with an unfulfilled desire for a child: A three-step model. In: B Strauss, ed. *Involuntary Childlessness: Psychological assessment, counselling, and psychotherapy*. Seattle: Hogrefe & Huber, 2002; 79–103.
8. Tuschen-Caffier B, Florin I, Krause W, et al. Cognitive-behavioral therapy for idiopathic infertile couples. *Psychother Psychosom* 1999; 68:15–21.
9. Holzle C, Brandt U, Lutkenhaus R, et al. Solution-focused counseling for involuntarily childless couples. In: B Strauss, ed. *Involuntary Childlessness: Psychological assessment, counselling, and psychotherapy*. Seattle: Hogrefe & Huber, 2002; 105–26.
10. Lemmens GMD, Vervaeke M, Enzlin P, et al. Coping with infertility: A body-mind group intervention programme for infertile couples. *Hum Reprod* 2004; 19:1917–23.
11. Takefman JE, Brender W, Boivin J, et al. Sexual and emotional adjustment of couples undergoing infertility investigation and effectiveness of preparatory information. *J Psychosom Obstet Gynaecol* 1990; 11:275–90.
12. Florin I, Tuschen-Caffier B, Krause W, et al. Psychological therapy in idiopathic infertility: A stress reduction

approach. In: B Strauss, ed. *Involuntary Childlessness: Psychological assessment, counselling, and psychotherapy*. Seattle: Hogrefe & Huber, 2002; 79–103.
13. Wischmann T, Stammer H, Gerhard I, et al. Couple counselling and therapy for the unfulfilled desire for a child: The two-step approach of the Heidleberg Infertility Consultation. In: B Strauss, ed. *Involuntary Childlessness: Psychological assessment, counselling, and psychotherapy*. Seattle: Hogrefe & Huber, 2002; 79–103.
14. Diamond R, Kezur D, Meyers M, et al. *Couple Therapy for Infertility*. New York: Guilford, 1999.
15. Cooper-Hilbert B. *Infertility and Involuntary Childlessness: Helping Couples Cope*. New York: Norton, 1998.
16. Menning BE. The emotional needs of infertile couples. *Fertil Steril* 1980; 34:313–19.
17. Blenner JL. Passage through infertility: A stage theory. *Image J Nurs Sch* 1990; 22:153–5.
18. Mathews R, Mathews AM. Infertility and involuntary childlessness: The transition to non-parenthood. *J Mar Fam Ther* 1986; 48:641–9.
19. Mahlstedt PP. The psychological component of infertility. *Fertil Steril* 1985; 43:335–46.
20. Wortman CB, Silver RC. The myths of coping with loss. *J Consult Clin Psychol* 1989; 57:349–57.
21. Tennen H, Affleck G, Mandala R. Causal explanations for infertility: Their relation to control appraisals and psychological adjustment. In: AL Stanton, C Dunkel-Schetter, eds. *Infertility: Perspectives from Stress and Coping Research*. New York: Plenum, 1991; 109–31.
22. Stanton A. Cognitive appraisals, coping processes, and adjustment to infertility. In: AL Stanton, C Dunkel-Schetter, eds: *Infertility: Perspectives from Stress and Coping Research*. New York: Plenum, 1991; 87–108.
23. Abbey A, Andrews FM, Halman JL. The importance of social relationships for infertile couples' well being. In: AL Stanton, C Dunkel-Schetter, eds. *Infertility: Perspectives from Stress and Coping Research*. New York: Plenum, 1991; 61–86.
24. Newton CR, Houle M. Gender differences in psychological response to infertility treatment. *Infertil Reprod Med Clin North Am* 1993; 4:545–8.
25. Wright J, Duchesne C, Sabourin S, et al. Psychosocial distress and infertility: Men and women respond differently. *Fertil Steril* 1991; 55:100–8.
26. Freeman EW, Rickels K, Tausig J, et al. Emotional and psychosocial factors in follow-up of women after IVF-ET treatment. *Acta Obstet Gynecol Scand* 1987; 66:517–21.
27. Newton CR, Hearn MT, Yuzpe AA. Psychological assessment and follow up after in vitro fertilization assessing the impact of failure. *Fertil Steril* 1990; 54:879–86.
28. Berg BJ, Wilson JF. Psychological functioning across stages of treatment for infertility. *J Behav Med* 1991; 14:11–26.
29. Leiblum SR, Kennan E, Lane MK. The psychological concomitants of in vitro fertilization. *J Psychosom Obstet Gynaecol* 1987; 6:165–78.
30. Greil AL, Leitko TA, Porter KL. Infertility: His and hers. *Gender Soc* 1958; 2:172–99.
31. Lalos A, Lalos O, Jacobson L, Von Schoutz B. The psychosocial impact of infertility two years after completed surgical treatment. *Acta Obstet Gynecol Scand* 1985; 64:599–604.
32. Peterson B, Newton CR, Rosen K. Examining congruence between partner's perceived infertility-related stress and

its relationship to marital adjustment and depression in infertile couples. *Family Process* 2003; 42:59–70.

33. Daniluk JC, Leader A, Taylor P. Psychological and relationship changes of couples undergoing an infertility investigation: Some implications for consultants. *Br J Guid Couns* 1987; 15:29–36.

34. Benazon N, Wright J, Sabourin S. Stress, sexual satisfaction, and marital adjustment in infertile couples. *J Sex Marital Ther* 1992; 18:273–84.

35. Boivin J, Takefman J, Tulandi T. Reactions to infertility based on extent of treatment failure. *Fertil Steril* 1995; 63:801–7.

36. Connolly KJ, Edelmann RJ, Bartlett H, et al. An evaluation of counselling for couples undergoing treatment for in vitro fertilization. *Hum Reprod* 1993; 8:1332–8.

37. Gurmankin AD, Caplan AL, Braverman AM. Screening practices and beliefs of assisted reproductive technology programs. *Fertil Steril* 2005; 83:61–7.

38. Ethics Committee of the American Society for Reproductive Medicine. Child-rearing ability and the provision of fertility services. *Fertil Steril* 2004; 82S:s208–s216.

39. The Assisted Human Reproduction Act Available at http://www.hc-sc.gc.ca/English/media/releases/2002/2002_34bk4.htm. Accessed March 2005.

40. Human Fertilisation and Embryology Authority. Code of practice, 6th edition. Available at http://www.hfea.gov.uk/HFEAPublications/CodeofPractice. Accessed March 2005.

41. Mumford SE, Corrigan E, Hull MGR. Access to assisted conception: A framework of regulation. *Hum Reprod* 1998; 13:2349–55.

42. European Society of Human Reproduction and Embryology: Guidelines for Counselling in Infertility. Available at http://www.humrep.oupjournals.org/cgi/content/full/16/6/1301. Accessed March 2005.

43. Pennings G. Measuring the welfare of the child: In search of the appropriate evaluation principle. *Hum Reprod* 1999; 14:1146–50.

44. Reading AE, Kerin J. Psychologic aspects of providing infertility services. *J Reprod Med* 1989; 34:861–71.

45. Locke HJ, Wallace KM. Short marital adjustment and prediction tests: Their reliability and validity. *Marriage Fam Living* 1959; 21:251–5.

46. Spanier GB. Measuring dyadic adjustment: New scales for assessing the quality of marriage and similar dyads. *J Marriage Fam* 1976; 38:15–28.

47. Snyder DK. Multi-dimensional assessment of marital satisfaction. *J Marriage Fam* 1979; 41:812–23.

48. Newton CR, Sherrard WS, Glavac I. The Fertility Problem Inventory: Measuring perceived infertility stress. *Fertil Steril* 1999; 72:54–62.

49. Nachtigall RD, Becker G, Wozny M. The effects of gender-specific diagnosis on men's and women's response to infertility. *Fertil Steril* 1992; 57:113–21.

50. Jacobson NS, Christensen A. *Acceptance and Change In Couple Therapy*. New York: Norton, 1996.

51. Salzer LP. *Infertility: How Couples Can Cope*. Boston: GK Hall, 1986.

52. Heavy C, Layne C, Christensen A. Gender and conflict structure in marital interaction: A replication and extension. *J Consult Clin Psych* 1993; 61:16–27.

53. Notarius CI, Pellegrini DS. Differences between husbands and wives: Implications for understanding marital discord. In: K Hahlweg, MJ Goldstein, eds. *Understanding Major Mental Disorder: The Contribution of Family Interaction Research*. New York: Family Process, 1987; 231–49.

54. Gottman JM, Krokoff LJ. Marital interaction and satisfaction: A longitudinal view. *J Couns Clin Psychol* 1989; 57:47–52.

55. Berg BJ, Wilson JF, Weingartner PJ. Psychological sequelae of infertility treatment: The role of gender and sex role identification. *Soc Sci Med* 1991; 33:1071–80.

56. Abbey A, Andrews, FM, Hartman J. Provision and receipt of social support and disregard: What is their impact on the marital life quality of infertile and fertile couples? *J Pers Soc Psychol* 1995; 68:455–69.

57. O'Hanlon-Hudson P, Hudson-O'Hanlon W. *Rewriting Love Stories: Brief Marital Therapy*. New York: Norton, 1991.

58. Greenberg LS, Johnson S. *Emotionally Focused Therapy for Couples*. New York: Guilford, 1988.

59. Gottlieb BH, Wagner F. Stress and support processes in close relationships. In J Eckenrode, ed. *The Social Context of Coping*. New York: Plenum, 1991; 165–88.

60. Weinshel M. Helping couples make decisions about ART. In: *Mental Health Professional Group Newsletter*, American Society for Reproduction. Winter, 2004.

61. Myers M, Weinshel M, Scharf C, et al. An infertility primer for family therapists: II. Working with couples who struggle with infertility. *Fam Process* 1995; 34:231–40.

62. Rachman S. Emotional processing. *Behav Res Ther* 1980; 18:51–60.

63. Sireling L, Cohen D, Marks I. Guided mourning for morbid grief: A controlled replication. *Behav Ther* 1988; 19:121–32.

64. Baram D, Tourtelot Z, Eberhard M, et al. Psychosocial adjustment following unsuccessful in vitro fertilization. *J Psychosom Obstet Gynaecol* 1988; 9:181–90.

65. De Shazer S. *Keys to Solution in Brief Therapy*. New York: Norton, 1985.

66. O'Hanlon WH, Weiner-Davis M. *In Search of Solutions: A New Direction in Psychotherapy*. New York: Norton, 1988.

67. Atwood JD, Dobkin S. Storm clouds are coming: Ways to help couples reconstruct the crisis of infertility. *Contemp Fam Ther* 1992; 14:385–403.

68. Carter JW, Carter M. *Sweet Grapes: How to Stop Being Infertile and Start Living Again*. Indianapolis, IN: Perspectives Press, 1989.

69. Becker G. *Healing the Infertile Family: Strengthening Your Relationship in the Search for Parenthood*. New York: Bantam, 1990.

10 Group Approaches to Infertility Counseling

SHARON N. COVINGTON

We are held in place by the pressure of the crowd around us. We must lean upon others. Let us see that we lean gracefully and freely and acknowledge their support.

– Margaret Collier Graham

It is safe to say that groups have existed since the beginning of mankind. Throughout the centuries, people have gathered together to share their experiences and possessions to learn, support, protect, and grow. The saying 'it takes a village' implies that there is strength and wisdom in numbers, and underscores the power of groups.

Generally, group therapy is a process used to treat problems of personality, life experiences, and difficulties in daily living; it may range in duration from very brief (a session or few) to long-term (years); it can vary in focus from education to self-analysis; and can occur in a variety of settings, from hospitals, clinics, and private offices of mental health professionals to businesses and schools. It is the cohesive nature of groups which is the force that binds members together, allowing the change process to take place. In effect, the group influences the individual member's perception of self, thus facilitating change. Although a relatively recent modality of treatment (the past 100 years), it has proven effective, efficient, and beneficial in terms of behavioral change, financial cost, and time management.

Group therapy is one of the various treatment modalities traditionally and successfully used by infertility counselors. This chapter provides a framework of group counseling approaches that are relevant to reproductive medicine. It includes:

■ an historical perspective of the evolution of group counseling and its application to infertility;
■ a review of research as to the power and effectiveness of groups specifically with the infertile population;
■ a theoretical orientation to infertility group work;
■ a description of the clinical issues in providing infertility group counseling such as membership, structure, themes, and stages of group process;

■ an overview of group therapeutic interventions particularly useful in reproductive medicine from cognitive-behavioral, emotive-interactional, psycho-educational, technology-generated, and staff groups; and
■ implications for the future with infertility groups.

HISTORICAL OVERVIEW

The historical power of groups has relevance in reproduction and fertility. In recent years, popular books such as the *Red Tent*[1] describe how women gathered privately together to share, celebrate, and, at times, mourn the reproductive plight of their group. In this book, the biblical image of women gathering under a tent to share their experiences during their cycles of menses, miscarriage, birthing, and barrenness is reminiscent of the evolution of the first infertility support group when women gathered in the Boston kitchen of Barbara Eck Menning in the early 1970s and Resolve, The National Infertility Association was founded.[2] Throughout the world, other patient-centered infertility support groups started under similar circumstances – patients (usually women) gathering together to share their pain, struggle, and wisdom to minimize isolation, maximize knowledge and coping strategies, and to grow past the experience of infertility.

Interestingly, nearly seventy years earlier in Boston, the concept of group psychotherapy is believed to have begun under similar circumstances of attempting to help patients deal with medical illness. In 1905, Joseph Hersey Pratt, a Boston internist working with indigent tubercular patients, started classes to teach healthcare methods, an approach that revealed broader therapeutic value. Through weekly group meetings of approximately twenty-five patients, he taught practices to improve their disease, recorded gains made by patients on a blackboard, and used successful patients' testimonials to inspire compliance. He discovered that cohesiveness and mutual support developed within the class, which appeared helpful in combating depression and isolation common to tubercular patients.[3, p. 499]

Considered the father of contemporary group psychotherapy, Pratt realized the relationship between psychological and physical health, and began offering 'thought control classes' using behavioral techniques for other chronic diseases and, eventually, for psychosomatic problems.[4] Within a few years, psychiatrists Cody Marsh and Edward Lazell were using his methods for hospitalized psychiatric patients, including psycho-education groups for hospital personnel.

Although it is generally agreed group psychotherapy started in the United States, early developments were occurring simultaneously in Europe.[5] In 1921, Sigmund Freud, whose infamous Wednesday evening meetings in Vienna may have been a group precursor, published a single article on group psychology and, for unknown reasons, failed to delve further into the subject.[6] The same year, Alfred Adler, Freud's collaborator, began using 'collective therapy' with children and adults at his Viennese clinic. Rudolf Driekurs, his student, later brought these methods to the United States and, along with others, applied principles of 'member influence' (Driekurs, 1932), 'here and now focus' (H. C. Syz, 1928), and 'group analysis' (Trigan Burrows, 1927) to the practice of group psychotherapy.[5] These early beginnings in the use of groups were vastly accelerated during World War II, out of necessity, as there were few military psychiatrists available to treat the large numbers of psychiatric casualties. Groups provided a more economic mode of treatment, both in time and manpower, and the development of group psychotherapy practice during World War II was considered a major contribution to the psychiatric field.[4]

There was a virtual explosion of group psychotherapy during the next fifty years. Psycho-educational groups, human development groups, self-help/mutual-help groups (e.g., Twelve-Step programs, such as Alcoholics Anonymous), Encounter groups of the 1960s, Transcendental Mediation groups of the 1970s, and the more recent cognitive-behavioral groups are just a few examples. While these groups were often referred to as group therapy their approach, context, and leadership training (or lack thereof) could be vastly different. Despite these variances, a core belief was/is universal – groups can be powerful agents for change. Thus, over the years, it was through the systematic application of groups to help people improve their well-being, both physically

and psychologically, that the field of group psychotherapy became established in the twentieth century.

REVIEW OF LITERATURE

As group therapy has evolved, there has been recognition of the dual relationship between research and application to the knowledge base. With this recognition, a fundamental feature appears clear: Groups do work. Barlow and associates[5] conducted an extensive review of the empirical literature relating to the efficacy of group psychotherapy and deduced:

…the general conclusion to be drawn from approximately 730 studies that span almost three decades is that the group format consistently produced positive effects with a number of disorders using a variety of treatment models.[5, p. 122]

Despite differences in approach, setting, leadership, treatment disorders or focus, groups help people adapt, adjust, and/or modify their behavior to improve well-being. Furthermore, with the early influence of Dr. Pratt, the therapeutic value of groups for patients struggling with medical illness has been well-documented in the literature.[7] Substantial research exists on the use of group modalities to help patients dealing with a variety of medical conditions such as cancers, coronary heart disease, irritable bowel syndrome, diabetes, asthma, organ transplants, and HIV/AIDS, to name a few.

In the past thirty-five years, research has also included group interventions with infertility patients with similar positive conclusions. In 2003, Boivin conducted a systematic review of research over this time period on effect of psychological interventions, divided into counseling or educational programs, on at least one outcome of patients with fertility problems.[8] She found that the most successful intervention had a strong educational component, and almost universally approached in a group or class format. It was surmised that groups have features that are especially important to infertility patients, such as validation and normalization, and may offer structure and skill-building opportunities that are particularly suited for this population. For purposes of this literature review, the research will be viewed according to diagnostic conditions, treatment approaches, and pregnancy outcome.

Diagnostic Condition

Several studies have looked at effect of group intervention for women dealing with infertility-related medical conditions. Weijenborg and ter Kuile[9] in The Netherlands looked at seventeen women at a gynecology clinic who had Rokintansky-Kuster-Hauser (RKH) syndrome, congenital absence of the vagina, aplasia or hypoplasia of the uterus and fallopian tubes, with normal-functioning ovaries and external genitalia. These women often struggle with feelings of defectiveness, inferiority, and lack of femininity, leading to psychological distress. They attended a semistructured program of seven 2-hour group sessions and were accessed pre- and post-group for depression, anxiety, and interpersonal sensitivity. Significant improvement in these areas was noted and the program was deemed valuable in helping in ways that clinicians usually are unable to do. Of note is that one of the group leaders, a clinic social worker, also had RKH and, while helpful, the authors did not believe it is necessary in this type of group.

In a study examining the role of self-help groups in patients' perception of care, Wingfield and associates found that endometriosis patients in Australia were significantly more satisfied with care when they had contact with a counselor from the Endometriosis Association while visiting the clinic. The researchers concluded that there was a significant demand for and greater patient satisfaction with an integrated approach to the care of endometriosis, particularly one that included the provision of counseling and availability of a patient self-help group.[10]

Groups to help infertile individuals lose weight have become more popular and relevant, particularly as obesity has been identified as significantly contributing to reduced fertility and/or complicated pregnancies. Galletly and colleagues reported on a group treatment program for thirty-seven obese, infertile women over twenty-four weeks that included regular exercise and group discussion on topics such as nutrition, effects of obesity on reproductive physiology, and the psychological impact of infertility and obesity.[11] There was significant weight loss of group members and overall improvement in self-esteem, anxiety, depression, and general health. Most notable, twenty-nine women became pregnant during the program or follow-up period of three years, and only six women who wished to become pregnant did not. The researchers concluded that active measures to improve mood and self-esteem, along with better nutrition and weight reduction through diet and exercise, can produce considerable improvement in pregnancy outcome for obese, infertile women. As illustrated by this example, increasingly infertility counselors are offering groups to facilitate health behavior change for a variety of conditions including smoking cessation, prema-

ture ovarian failure (POF), medically complicating conditions, anorexia, and/or alcohol/chemical dependency to improve quality-of-life and overall health, or maximize fertility and/or treatment outcomes.

Treatment Approaches

A number of different studies have looked at group intervention for patients undergoing assisted reproductive technologies (ARTs) as well as general infertility treatments. Short-term professionally led groups were found effective in diminishing anxiety and depression,[12–16] social stigma,[17] grief,[18] and generalized stress from infertility treatment.[13,15,19–23] While many of these groups focused on women going through treatment, men who participated in groups also found them beneficial.[15,21]

Several researchers have examined the effectiveness of cognitive-behavioral group approaches, or what is more commonly referred to as mind–body groups. These groups usually are time-limited (six to twelve sessions) and have a specific format to teach cognitive-behavioral techniques (CBT) from relaxation methods with verbal and nonverbal expressive modalities. Lemmens and associates detailed a structured mind–body program for infertile couples in Belgium that was found useful in minimizing distress and improving coping.[24] In Italy, Tarabusi and colleagues developed a cognitive-behavioral group treatment program for fifty couples waiting for ART, a time period often associated with distress.[25] They found that CBT minimized the waiting stress and decreased psychological uneasiness, especially in women, as well as provided support and understanding of the waiting couples. Domar and associates developed a structured group behavioral treatment program using mind–body techniques[26] and have found that these groups decreased depression[12] and overall distress[27], as well as improved conception rates in participants.[22]

With a different approach, McQueeney and colleagues[13] tested the relative effectiveness of training infertile women in six treatment sessions to use emotion-focused versus problem-focused coping skills to manage the stress of infertility. Problem-focused training produced improvements in general distress and infertility-specific well-being at treatment termination, while emotion-focused training resulted in greater improvement one month later. Furthermore, they found that at eighteen months' follow-up, the problem-focused group members were more likely to have a child than other group participants. These findings led the researchers to promote the efficacy of both interventions in women's adjustment to infertility.

The internet is increasingly becoming an outlet for support and information for infertile people, taking on the role of a virtual support group. Epstein and colleagues looked at demographic characteristics, medical status, and psychological well-being of participants whose only outlets for talking about infertility were internet medical and support forums compared to infertile individuals who had 'additional outlets' for support.[28] Almost 600 people completed surveys at the website of an international infertility organization, including the Beck's Depression Inventory (BDI). Both groups were comparable in their medical history and education, although only outlet participants were less educated, wealthy, and more likely to be homemakers. Additionally, only outlet individuals were more depressed, received less real-world support, although they felt more supported by the internet than did study participants who had additional outlets. The researchers concluded that the internet provides group support by educating, empowering, and diminishing feelings of depression and isolation. However, they cautioned that the internet might also be used inappropriately to withdraw from real-world interactions, enhancing feelings of isolation and depression.

Pregnancy Outcome

In determining effectiveness of group intervention, several researchers have used pregnancy as an outcome measurement. Early research in the field showed promising indications that support groups could and did positively impact pregnancy rates and improve treatment outcomes. In a frequently cited study, Domar and associates[22] compared women in a ten-week cognitive-behavioral group, a traditional ten-week support group, and randomly assigned controls to determine pregnancy rates at one-year follow-up. The researchers found that viable pregnancy rates in the cognitive-behavioral and support group members were virtually the same (55%, 54%) and significantly higher than the control group (20%) for those participants who remained in the program. The researchers concluded that group psychological interventions were both efficient and cost-effective, and may positively affect pregnancy rates. A Japanese study looked at the effect of psychiatric group intervention on the emotions, natural-killer (NK) cell activity, and pregnancy rate.[29] Thirty-seven women completed a five-session intervention program and were compared with the same number of controls. Psychological discomfort and NK activity decreased significantly for the intervention group, whereas no change was noted in the control group. At one-year follow-up, the intervention group

had a significantly higher pregnancy rate than that of the controls (37.8% versus 13.5%). Other researchers have found similar results of increased pregnancy rates in women who participate in group psychological intervention.[11,13,14,16,30] However, Boivin's review found only one scientifically rigorous study (i.e., comparing controls with group participants) identified a positive pregnancy correlation with group intervention. As such, Boivin determined no conclusions could be drawn.[8]

In short, groups may be helpful for a variety of reasons such as improved social support, health behavior change, and improved stress management, all of which may have a mediating effect on health and fertility. However, based on current data it is too early to conclude that groups in general or infertility-specific group therapy can and/or will improve fertility, pregnancy rates, or treatment outcomes.

THEORETICAL FRAMEWORK

Theoretical models that apply to groups can encompass a multitude of psychological theory from earlier works such as the Freudian psychodynamic model to a more modern approach of Ellis' group rational-emotive and cognitive-behavioral theory.[4] However, the approach of Irving Yalom, author of long-held standard text in the field for over three decades and four editions, focuses on correcting 'here-and-now' interpersonal relationships that are particularly relevant to infertility group counseling. Whatever the therapeutic approach of a group (e.g., cognitive-behavioral or traditional emotive support), the basis for all groups is Yalom's theory of 'curative factors' in group therapy.[3] The ten 'curative factors' are interdependent, neither occur nor function separately, and are not necessarily universally applicable to all groups, although they are based on the premise that the group process promotes improved well-being.[3, p. 100] The factors forming the foundation of Yalom's group theoretical approach and its application to infertility group work include:

1. ***Instillation of hope*** – hope combined with a conviction and confidence in treatment modality, brings people into therapy and keeps them there, enabling the therapeutic process to occur. Hope is the elixir of infertility treatment. Like many self-help groups, infertility groups use personal testimonials that can offer inspiration for successfully managing the stresses and strains of infertility and treatment. Hope is offered by the infertility counselor's conviction in the efficacy of group treatment, as well as group members'

experiences as both providers and recipients of hope and encouragement in the achievement of their goals (i.e., improved quality of life, coping skills, diminished anxiety and depression).

2. *Universality* – individuals usually enter group therapy with the belief that their painful struggles with infertility are unique and their self-perception damaged by feelings of stigma and isolation. Interactions with group members facilitate universality through the realization that others have similar feelings and experiences – often a member's first experience of feeling truly understood and accepted. Group therapy provides universality through normalizing the feelings of infertility, providing an arena for catharsis, and acceptance by others grappling with infertility, the demands of treatment, and decisions about family-building.

3. *Imparting information* – another curative factor of groups is the sharing of information through exchange of information among group members, didactic instruction, and/or educational process regarding medical and/or psychological issues relevant to infertility. Typically, infertility-specific groups impart information about the medical and emotional aspects of impaired fertility that is integral to the therapeutic process. The psycho-educational component may involve learning new skills (e.g., cognitive-behavioral techniques), highlighting the power of knowledge, and helping infertile individuals gain a greater sense of control.

4. *Altruism* – in therapy groups, individuals receive through giving, not only by participating in the group process but also via the intrinsic act of giving. Group members offer support, sharing, reassurances, suggestions, insight, and other gentle acts of kindness and generosity of spirit that facilitate the healing of others as well as their own healing, boosting self-esteem, and confidence. All too often, the wisdom and the experiences of the infertility group members are more beneficial and therapeutic than that of the infertility counselor.

5. *The corrective recapitulation of the primary family group* – frequently individuals entering an infertility group have family-of-origin issues that can significantly impact behavior, reactions, and roles in the group, as the group can resemble or be experienced as the family-of-origin. Because infertility is a multigenerational family system crisis, family issues often emerge particularly around issues of grief, emotional support,

envy, and jealousy of family pregnancies. However, family-of-origin issues in infertility-specific groups may be less relevant because group members are more invested in future relationships (e.g., 'wished-for' child) than reworking past family relationships. Nonetheless, groups often provide the warm, supportive, and understanding 'chosen family' that their family-of-origin cannot.

6. *Development of socializing techniques* – learning skills that help one interact appropriately with others (i.e., social skills) is another curative factor of groups. Infertility groups frequently help members learn how to deal with issues that come up with family, friends, work, clinic staff, and other relationships over the course of treatment. Members often help each other by providing suggestions, feedback, or role-playing opportunities (e.g., practice) to help manage difficult interpersonal situations and/or conflicts with the fertile world or treatment team.

7. *Imitative behavior* – sometimes referred to as 'spectator therapy,' groups provide social learning opportunities by allowing group members to observe and imitate the healthy behaviors of the therapist and other group members. The group allows members to 'try on' new behaviors in a safe environment and in a manner not usually available in other therapies. Members often talk about using some of the behaviors they have seen or heard other group members use when dealing with difficult situations or relationships.

8. *Interpersonal learning* – group is a social microcosm in which members obtain insight into themselves, their relationship with others, and how they interact with others. As such, it is a corrective emotional experience offered in a psychosocially safe relationship. Infertility-specific groups can be particularly helpful arenas for interpersonal learning opportunities and healing because infertility is socially isolating and stigmatizing.

9. *Group cohesiveness* – is a complex process of solidarity, fundamental to group therapy, in which individual members become attached to the group and develop a sense of 'we-ness' or 'group-ness.' Infertility-specific groups typically vary in their degree of cohesiveness for a variety of reasons including group structure, type, and frequency of group meetings. However, the universal experience of involuntary childlessness typically contributes to strong feelings of cohesion.

10. *Catharsis* – is the process of expression of strong emotion or affect and, while a curative factor, is

not a primary therapeutic goal of group therapy. Nevertheless, infertility-specific groups usually provide a strong cathartic experience for most members, which is both healing and hopeful. The facilitation of catharsis by the infertility counselor may be through deliberate techniques (e.g., guided imagery) or group members may relate a particularly painful experience within the group that facilitates catharsis, exorcizing the pain of infertility or the infertility experience.

Group work with infertile people promotes change through a combination of mastery of skills and the operation of Yalom's curative factors. This theoretical approach for group practice provides a framework in understanding the clinical issues and therapeutic interventions for a variety of infertility groups.

CLINICAL ISSUES

While the term group is used throughout this discussion to identify treatment process, it is important to examine the differences between what is meant by therapy groups and support groups, the model most often used with infertility patients. According to Lederberg, support groups and therapy groups have marked differences in technical method.[31] In support groups, anxiety is defused, regression headed-off, confrontation between members carefully modulated, and transference reactions to the leader recognized but not interpreted, while in a therapy groups these issues are encouraged and processed. Outside-of-group contact between members is usually strongly discouraged in therapy groups, while outside contact between group members is usually allowed and often encouraged in support groups. Leaders of support groups tend to be more active, more directive, and provide more structure to relieve anxiety and channel group affect. In addition, support group leaders may be more self-disclosing and ready to use themselves as models to minimize fantasy or as a mechanism of hope (i.e., when the leader has experienced similar pathos such as infertility, pregnancy loss, or genetic condition). Nevertheless, both therapy and support groups have the capacity to help people change behavior and facilitate coping. It should be noted that, at times, support group leaders may not be mental health professionals and, as such, their sole qualification may be shared experience of infertility (or some other experience). However, group leaders in therapy groups are mental health professionals typically with special training in group therapy. While infertility patients may be involved in either therapy groups or support groups, this chapter focuses on the support and therapy groups led by mental health professionals.

Infertility groups use a variety of modalities to promote change. Some groups may be symptom-focused (i.e., reduce anxiety, stress, and relaxation) and apply cognitive-behavioral techniques in a psycho-educational format to teach skills. Other groups encourage the expression and exploration of affect to promote a sense of commonality, hope, and catharsis. Many use a combination of both emotive-interactional and cognitive-behavioral to address feelings, beliefs, and behaviors that have disrupted the patient's life in the pursuit of parenthood. Despite differences in therapeutic approach, there are a number of clinical issues that are common in an infertility group.

Group Structure

A primary consideration at the outset for the group leader is the group's structure and membership. The ideal size for most groups is between five and ten members. With three or four members, the group tends to operate less as a group and more as individual therapy. More than twelve members affect group dynamics and the leader must be more active to ensure that all members have an opportunity to talk and no single member dominates the group process or session. Another consideration for the group leader is whether the group will be 'open-ended' (i.e., members may join and leave the group throughout the life of the group) or 'closed' (i.e., members commit to participate in the group for the duration of the group and new members are not allowed to join). For example, informal, drop-in groups (i.e., monthly support) are usually open-ended, while time-limited groups (i.e., a specific number of sessions) are usually closed. The length of time for the group session will need to be identified and is usually most productive between one and a half and two hours. Additionally, the issue of outside group contact between group members is typically addressed during the initial session. Some leaders allow, even encourage outside of session contact, particularly with infertility-specific groups.

Another consideration will be if there is a financial charge for the group. In some clinics, periodic groups are offered as a service to patients for no fee. Time-limited, focused groups, such as cognitive-behavioral instruction, usually are fee-for-service. There is a therapeutic value to fee groups, even a very minimal amount, as members make a commitment to participating for the duration of the group by paying for it. As has been found in other therapeutic relationships, patients see more value in a service they have to pay for rather than one that is free.

Membership

Another clinical issue concerns membership and the heterogeneity or homogeneity desired in the group. Will the group be open to all infertility patients or to a specific treatment group (i.e., IVF, donor recipients, miscarriage, endometriosis, or secondary infertility patients)? Will it be directed to couples or gender-specific? Will length of time in treatment be a consideration, such as members who are new to treatment versus those who have been in treatment for years? While patients often express an interest in being a group with others just like themselves (i.e., a homogeneous group), it is often therapeutic to have a more heterogeneous membership to add greater depth to the wisdom and experience of the group.

Screening of group members through a clinical interview is not always possible with infertility support groups, especially drop-in type groups. It is ideal for the group leader to have some contact and information about participants before the group begins – general social and treatment history, presenting concerns, and what they hope to gain from attending the group. Formal collaboration with a present or current mental health professional can be helpful, particularly if the potential member has a mental health diagnosis and/or is taking psychotropic medications. Group members should have the capacity to emphasize, be open to self-disclosure, and have sufficient ego strength to take-in group process without decompensating or exacerbating preexisting mental health diagnosis. If a group member exhibits significant psychopathology which cannot be addressed or contained in the group, such as serious depression or borderline personality disorder, it is best for the leader to counsel the member out of group and into individual therapy where their issues are better served. If one member's issues dominate the group process, the leader takes the risk of losing other members who may drop out due to frustration or fear. It is the responsibility of the group leader to preserve the integrity and safety of the group and all its members.

Confidentiality

Confidentiality is essential in any therapeutic relationship, be it medical or psychological, and a key component of the group process. Patients must feel safe and secure that any information and affect shared in the context of therapy will be protected. Some infertility groups may be offered within the structure of a repro-

ductive medical practice where the patient is receiving treatment. Patients may be struggling with difficulties with their physician, nurse, or other staff and need the assistance of the group to find solutions to these interpersonal relationships that impact their treatment experience. Consequently, it is important for the therapist to reassure group members that information they share will *not* be communicated to clinic staff. However, it is also important that the therapist control discontent so that the focus of the group does not become a gripe session and subvert group process. If concerns are raised that the therapist feels may be important for staff to know (either specific or generalized issues), patients need to be informed that their expressed permission will be obtained prior to any communication. If the therapist will be communicating a general summary of group content with staff, such as when a time-limited support group ends, patients need to be informed that this information will be nonidentifying and for the primary purpose of promoting better understanding of infertile patients' needs. Specific information regarding a patient may be done through a formal letter, with the patient's authorization for release of information attached, and a copy of which may or may not be sent to the patient.

Confidentiality also applies to group members. They need to understand the importance of holding information they learn about other members private and discuss only their own personal information with others outside of group. It may be helpful to point out that whether in a large urban community or rural area, there is a small town mentality that needs to be in everyone's consciousness. Sharing even nonidentifying information about other group members, even in the most innocent of situations, may have detrimental consequences.

Group Development

All groups, whether a single session or years long, have a beginning, middle, and end stage. It is the leader's responsibility to recognize, acknowledge, and facilitate this process. Ulman describes the therapist's role as shaping the process of group development "...by promoting creation of group norms of support, validation, respect, and curiosity, and by encouraging quiet members to speak."[32, p. 356] In the beginning phase, members get to know each other, develop a sense of commonality, and shared purpose. After a level of cohesion has been established, during the middle phase the work of the group takes place. Members identify goals or issues with which they need assistance and look to the support of others to achieve a higher level of mastery and understanding. In the final phase, time is spent saying goodbye, acknowledging skills gained, and recognizing new connections that have been made. The leader helps the group know how to hold on to what they have learned, what others have offered, and what they have provided each other. Again, these phases – formation, work, and termination – need to occur in all groups.

In single session groups, such as an open-ended, monthly emotion-focused support group, the three-phase processes takes place rapidly and are facilitated by the group leader, with formation and work phases usually occurring simultaneously. In time-limited, or short-term groups (typically between six and twelve weeks), the beginning formation phase is approximately one-quarter of the sessions, the middle work phase is approximately one-half of the meetings, and the termination phase the last quarter of the sessions. Time-limited structure works particularly well with infertility groups. The role of the infertility counselor/group leader is to clarify boundaries, expectations, maintain focus, forestall a member's premature termination, and reinforce the timeframe by keeping the group phases in the consciousness of the group and as an integral part of the group functioning process.[33]

Group Themes

There are a number of themes that tend to emerge in most infertility groups. This list is not meant to be inclusive of all issues that may occur in infertility-specific groups but rather an overview of common themes of groups addressing reproductive issues.

Grief

Grief is a normal response to infertility. Feelings of shock, sadness, anger, guilt, blame, shame, depression, and hopelessness are common emotional responses and take a great deal of energy to manage. Anger is an affect that may permeate these groups and may be expressed at family members or friends, other pregnant women, the medical staff, God, work, spouses, other group members and/or the leader. It is also an emotion that may be expressed as a defense against feelings of profound sadness and loss. For many members, especially women, anger is an emotion with which they are very uncomfortable and unable to manage. Furthermore, when anger is projected inward toward the self, it becomes depression. Members need to learn how to manage and express these strong feelings in helpful ways. While the expression of feelings of grief is necessary and often cathartic, the impact of strong affect on group process can be potentially deleterious. Bonanno and Kaltman point out that the continuous expression of negative affect tends to irritate, frustrate, and alienate other group members, while the expression of positive affect tends to increase contact and support from group members.[34]

The implication for leaders facilitating infertility groups is important. McCallum and associates investigated the variables of early group process as predictors of patient dropout rates in short-term therapy groups for complicated grief.[35] They found that the first session was crucial in determining follow-through in the group and in setting the tone for future sessions. They point out that for patients to benefit from the experience, they need to feel positively toward it. More often than not, however, mental health professionals tend to focus on negative feelings when assessing the value of a therapy session, emphasizing negative affect and the pain of grief and loss. As a result of their research, McCallum and associates concluded that "when working with loss patients, perhaps the therapist should be as attentive to encouraging positive affect as/she is to negative affect, group cohesion, group climate, and positive therapeutic alliance."[35, p. 252] It is suggested that group members may be invited to identify positive experiences that occurred during the week before leaving a group session, a form of cognitive restructuring, reframing, and encouraging transcendence/transformation of the infertility experience.

Loss of Control

One of the most common feelings infertility patients express is a sense of loss of control that permeates a variety of areas of their lives – loss of control over their hopes, dreams, bodies, life goals, sex, relationships, finances, and so forth. The feeling of being out of control heightens a sense of anxiety, worry, and fears. Often group members need these feelings acknowledged while being able to identify things in their lives that, in reality, they *do* have control over (i.e., job choices or where they live) and what they *do not* (when they will have a baby or treatment outcome).

Gender Differences

Another common area of discussion, whether in couples groups or gender-specific groups, is the differences between the ways men and women feel and deal with infertility. Men and women experience infertility differently, a fact that has been covered in other chapters of this book. However, 'different' is not a judgment or indication of a behavior being 'better' or 'worse,' only 'not the same.' In couples groups, it is normalizing experience for women to hear men other than their husbands, express similar feelings or describe behaviors they have heard from their spouse, and vice versa. Furthermore, it is an excellent opportunity for infertility counselors to educate group members about gender differences and infertility.

Interpersonal Relationships

Group members frequently need assistance with issues that arise in interpersonal relationships regarding their infertility. Difficulties with family members or friends, problems at work with colleagues, or upsetting interactions with acquaintances or even strangers may precipitate painful feelings. Group members usually have a wealth of experience to draw upon, often with more credibility than what the leader may offer.

Dealing with Treatment Team

A frequent topic in infertility support groups concerns ways to deal effectively and collaboratively with the physician, nurse, and other clinic staff. Patients may need help in communicating with their doctor or nurse; stating their needs; asking for realistic support; realizing the limits of their doctor or nurse's ability; and planing and strategizing for making these relationships work. At times, other group members may be able to help by sharing what they have found effective in dealing with similar issues. Although it is ideal for the group to assist a member to find a solution to any communication problems or difficulties, the group leader may also act as an advocate if the patient requests. Helping the group come up with tips on working with the medical team is a useful and therapeutic task.[36]

Stress and Coping

Finding ways to deal with the distress of infertility is a common reason people join these groups. Cognitive-behavioral techniques are often an educational component providing skills to diminish stress and increase coping. Learning and practicing such skills as breathing techniques, cognitive restructuring, and meditation give patients tools to use during treatment. Humor is, also an effective coping mechanism and one that works well in groups. Being able to laugh about oneself with others, as well as the struggles of infertility, is a cathartic and cohesive experience. Group members often appreciate the levity humor brings and express how it lightens the load of infertility.

Decision Making

Patients join groups at various stages of medical treatment, thereby making decisions along the way. Some members may be facing decisions about treatment options, such as moving from IUI to IVF, while others may be at a point of ending treatment and moving toward alternative family building, such as donor gametes, donor embryos, or adoption. Others may seek support in coming to terms with childlessness as a permanent state. Group therapy offers the opportunity to explore treatment options in a supportive, nonjudgmental setting with people who understand the seductive nature of the evolving technology. With more options come more choices that often makes it confusing to change treatment, or difficult to leave it entirely. Group offers a safe place to explore decision-making options and make peace with one's decisions.

Pregnant Members

It is possible, and often likely, that a member or members may become pregnant during the group sessions. While this is the goal of all infertility group members, it nonetheless brings up feelings within the group when someone is no longer 'one of us' but has, instead, become 'one of them'. Furthermore, this transition from 'us' to 'them' can be difficult, as the pregnant, formerly infertile woman feels more isolated: disconnected from both infertility support systems and pregnancy-specific support systems. The group leader should address the issue of a group member becoming pregnant early in the formation of group and help the group decide how they want to handle it. Group members need to understand that a positive pregnancy test does not necessarily mean a successful and safe pregnancy and delivery of a healthy baby and, as such, does not eliminate all worries and fears about having a baby. As such, the member may still need the group. On the other hand, a pregnant group member may feel guilty to have succeeded when others are still struggling with the pain of infertility and may want to drop out. Or some members may feel too uncomfortable with a pregnant member continuing in group. While there is no right answer, discussing this issue is often a very therapeutic process because dealing with pregnant women is an experience group members face on a daily basis. Furthermore, the group may be an opportunity to try on new behaviors that assist with systematic desensitization regarding pregnant women.

THERAPEUTIC INTERVENTION

There are several modalities of infertility groups, which provide a framework for therapeutic intervention. These include: cognitive-behavioral, emotive-interactional, psycho-educational, technology-mediated, and staff groups.

Cognitive-Behavioral Groups

The inherent nature of stress during infertility has given rise to an explosion of interest in helping patients find ways to manage these feelings. As indicated throughout the literature, cognitive-behavioral techniques have been both popular and proven effective with this population, and are now commonly referred to as mind–body groups. Benson, in the early 1970s, wrote about stress and its impact on health.[37] Noting that stress induces the fight-or-flight response, physiologically connected to prehistoric times when cavemen had to fight or run from danger, Benson studied behaviors that directly counteracted this reaction. He noted that these techniques, when practiced on a regular basis, produced a profound and automatic antidote to stress, called the 'relaxation response' (RR). In the early 1990s, Domar, Benson and associates wrote about the application of these techniques and their effectiveness in a formalized group program for infertility patients.[26]

The structure and format of these groups have been documented in a number of articles and books.[24,32,37,38] Generally, the time-limited model involves teaching patients about relaxation response and the various ways to illicit it, including: diaphragmatic breathing; associated breathing exercises; cognitive restructuring; journaling; meditation; mindfulness; spirituality; yoga; massage; and lifestyle choices (nutrition, exercise, and nonsmoking). Art and music therapy techniques may also be a component. While cognitive-behavioral training is a major focus of the group, and often the reason members join, a portion of the session is emotive-interactional, operating as a traditional support group. Building connectedness, cohesion, and relatedness to other infertile people is fundamental to the healing process. Frequently, when members end group, they report that the skills learned continue to help them cope with other life challenges, yet the relationships made are the greatest gift (and sometimes biggest surprise), often lasting a lifetime.

Emotive-Interactional Groups

Although all infertility groups involve the sharing of feelings and experiences to some degree, the traditional support group's focus and foundation is an emotive-interactional model. These groups may be facilitated by either a mental health or healthcare professional (i.e., a clinic nurse) or, at times, by other infertile people on a formal or informal, peer-led basis. When facilitators have no professional mental health training, they need to be cognizant of their abilities and limitations. Patient support organizations that offer peer-led groups usually have instructions on the facilitator's role and responsibilities.

Professionally led support groups may be time-limited, regularly scheduled (i.e., monthly or weekly), or episodic on an 'as needed,' or 'as requested' basis. The role and responsibility of the leader have been outlined previously, and involve helping the group form cohesion, sharing their feelings in a safe environment, and problem-solving in a positive manner. Brief, professionally led support groups for infertility patients have been found to be a highly acceptable and effective intervention in alleviating psychological distress.[39]

Psycho-Educational Groups

Many infertility groups are specifically psycho-educational groups or have psycho-educational components as part of other forms of groups. For example, clinics may offer classes that are either treatment-oriented and/or wellness-oriented that provide specific information to patients (e.g., injection training, weight loss, and smoking cessation). Patients who are about to undergo IVF or donor gametes/embryos may attend pretreatment classes that give an overview of the medical process, what to expect along the way, and how to work with treatment team members. An overview of the emotional experience, including counseling and support services available to patients, also help to educate patients that infertility is as much a psychological as it is a physiological experience. Wellness-oriented programs promote healthy lifestyle practices such as yoga, exercise, and nutrition. In a different venue, these classes may be open to patients and staff members, both dealing with the consequences of infertility-related stress, and promote a positive, collaborative experience. Clinics that have offered these psycho-educational classes have had very positive feedback from patients, who find the groups instructive and supportive.

Another approach to psycho-educational groups is Thorn and Daniels' seminar model for donor insemination (DI) recipients.[40] The group setting provides comprehensive information on medical, legal, and psychosocial aspects of DI presented by experts in the field. Additionally, a family built by DI discusses their experience, providing a role model for group participants. Attendees also have an opportunity to talk about their ideas, attitudes, and concerns with others going through the process. Thorn and Daniels found that all three aspects (information, sharing with others, and exposure to a role model) helped to reduce feelings of stigmatization and marginalization, and better prepared DI recipients for the future. This model may be adapted for other groups of patients who are considering alternative family-building.

Technology-Mediated Groups

Communication technology has had a profound effect on modern life, including the potential for groups of people to interact without ever seeing each other. Without the limits of time and/or territory, the telephone and, more recently, computers linked together (the internet) offer infertile people, as well as their caregivers, the opportunity to send and receive support and information. It is a virtual space with no boundaries, creating both potential and challenge for those who use technology-mediated groups. A feature of most infertility-focused websites is a discussion list, which is a 'virtual group' of people who electronically discuss issues of common interest and concern.

The internet is considered one of the major communication developments in decades, yet the understanding of group phenomena on the internet and the implications for group work is limited. A discussion list, or listserve, behaves as a small group, with similar dynamics, where members try to understand their responsibility in a faceless, anonymous situation. Weinberg outlines discussion group dynamics regarding contract (usually vague), boundaries (often blurry and meaningless in cyberspace), extra-list communication (common), group norms (varies from list to list), members joining and leaving the group without notice, and whether the list focuses on content versus process.[41] The challenges in managing the dynamics for the discussion group leader are evident, and yet these virtual groups have been shown to be helpful in diminishing the sense of isolation infertility patients feel, while empowering them with knowledge and normalization. These same issues exist for infertility counselors and listserves, such as the Mental Health Professional Group of American Society of Reproductive Medicine with over 300 members. Nonetheless, they provide an important forum for group communication among infertility counselors.

Staff Groups

As mentioned earlier, staff support groups have a long history of assisting medical staff with the stresses and pressure of dealing with patients struggling with medical conditions. Reproductive medicine is considered a high-stress occupation, dealing with patients who may be highly anxious, demanding, controlling, and investing a great deal to be cured. In addition, medical staff members are adapting and adjusting to rapidly changing science that requires new, highly technical knowledge and techniques. Burnout in reproductive medicine is a continuing problem, for clinical to administrative staff. The stress level often trickles down from physi-

cians, nurses, and laboratory staff to front-line support personnel who handle scheduling, front desk operations and phones. Staff members who handle finances, billing, and insurance often get the brunt of patients' anger and frustration, and are least prepared to deal with it. The 'trickle down effect' is reflective of the 'pecking order' or hierarchy in the clinic imagined by patients (and often reality-based), and those staff members who are perceived to be least threatening to their care often get the force of patients' negative transference with the treatment process.

Staff groups offer an opportunity for infertility counselors to use their skills to support, educate, problem solve, and teach coping strategies for dealing with the stress to the caregivers. Many of the same cognitive-behavioral techniques that are used with and taught to infertility patients are just as helpful for staff. Groups can meet on a regular basis (i.e., weekly or monthly), time-limited (eight to twelve weeks), or as needed. Some issues of importance in dealing with patients include dealing with the 'difficult' patient (demanding, highly anxious, angry, or noncompliant); delivering bad news (whether medical, administrative, or financial); managing large caseloads; and resolving personal and ethical dilemmas related to treatments and technology. Other issues that may come up relate to interpersonal difficulties and demands between colleagues, supervisors, and other staff members. While the focus of a staff group pertains to work matters, some staff members may be dealing with family struggles and/or personal psychological problems (i.e., depression and anxiety) that may affect group dynamics and need to be addressed by the leader outside the group sessions.

The goal of these groups is to improve staff well-being. As in other groups, the limits and boundaries of the staff group need to be clarified and maintained. The leader also needs to be aware of, and assist the group in understanding, what can be changed and what cannot so that the group does not become a gripe session. The challenge for the group facilitator is to be compassionately engaged, without succumbing to the unhappiness and helplessness that burned-out staff members may generate. For further reference, Lederberg[31] presents a useful model for the leader's role and structure of staff support groups for high-stress medical environments.

FUTURE IMPLICATONS

Groups for infertility patients have proven effective and efficient, in both time and cost. With the continuing shift in financial coverage for healthcare, insurance-managed, or state-run socialized medicine, the need for psychological services that can be offerd to the greatest number of people, for the least cost, will grow. Not all infertility counselors are comfortable or feel trained to lead groups, and the necessity for skilled group clinicians will require training programs that serve this need.

As the world has become smaller and patients are traveling long distances, sometimes across continents for treatment, the use of computer-mediated groups will likely increase. More research needs to be conducted on the implication of the internet, discussion groups, and listserves on group dynamics, function, and effectiveness. While the internet is currently a faceless community, in the future video technology will allow members to participate in a manner similar to other groups. In the future, computer translation technology will likely offer the opportunity for people who speak different languages to communicate and participate in internet infertility groups, where previously, language served as a barrier.

SUMMARY

■ Group counseling began a century ago, founded on principles of assisting patients improve health and well-being, when struggling with serious medical conditions, and has come full circle to assisting infertility patients.

■ Research has shown infertility group treatment to be both effective and cost-efficient.

■ Despite differences in approach, setting, leadership, treatment disorders or focus, group counseling helps people adapt, adjust, and/or modify their behavior to improve well-being.

■ The theoretical framework of Yalom's curative factors[3] applies to a variety of infertility counseling groups, especially instillation of hope, universality, cohesion, information sharing, and catharsis.

■ There is a difference between support groups and therapy groups, which patient and leader need to understand. Although psychological issues of infertility and the psychological history a patient brings into it may be treated in a psychotherapy group, most groups associated with a medical treatment program are support groups.

■ Mental health professionals running infertility counseling groups need to be aware of clinical issues including group structure, development, membership, confidentiality, and common themes.

■ Therapeutic interventions in infertility group counseling include cognitive-behavioral, emotive-interactional, psycho-educational, technology-mediated, and staff groups.

■ There will continue to be a growing need for skilled infertility group counselors and group services for patients.

REFERENCES

1. Diamant A. *The Red Tent*. St. Martin's Press, 1997.
2. Menning BE. RESOLVE: A support group for infertile couples. *Am J Nurs* 1976; 76:258–9.
3. Yalom ID. *The Theory and Practice of Group Psychotherapy*. 4th ed. New York: Basic Books, 1995.
4. Scheidlinger S. The group psychotherapy movement at the millennium: Some historical perspectives. *Int J Group Psychother* 2000; 50:315–39.
5. Barlow SH, Burlingame GM, Fuhriman A. Therapeutic application of groups: From Pratt's "thought control classes" to modern group psychotherapy. *Group Dyn* 2000; 4:115–34.
6. Freud S. Group psychology and the analysis of the ego. In: J Strachey, ed. and trans. *The Standard Edition of the Complete Psychological Works of Sigmund Freud*. London: Hogarth Press, 1921; 18:67–145.
7. Stern MJ. Group therapy with medically-ill patients. In: A Alonso, H Swiller, eds. *Group Therapy in Clinical Practice*. Washington, DC: American Psychiatric Press, 1993;185–99.
8. Boivin, J. A review of psychosocial interventions in infertility. *Soc Sci Med* 2003; 57:2325–41.
9. Weijenborg P, ter Kuile MM. The effect of a group programme on women with the Mayer-Rokintansky-Kuster-Huster Syndrome. *Br J Obstet Gynecol* 2000; 107:365–8.
10. Wingfield MB, Wood C, Henderson LS, et al. Treatment of endometriosis involving a self-help group positively affects patients' perception of care. *J Psychosom Obstet Gynaecol* 1997; 18:255–8.
11. Galletly C, Clark A, Tomlinson L, et al. Improved pregnancy rates for obese, infertility women following a group treatment program. An open pilot study. *Gen Hosp Psychiatry* 1996;18:192–5.
12. Domar AD, Zuttermeister PC, Seibel MM, et al. Psychological improvement in infertile women after behavioral treatment: A replication. *Fertil Stertil* 1992; 58:144–7.
13. McQueeney DA, Stanton AL, Sigmon S. Efficacy of emotion-focused and problem-focused group therapies for women with fertility problems. *J Behav Med* 1997; 20:313–31.
14. Domar AD, Zuttermeister PC, Friedman R. Distress and conception in infertile women: A complementary approach. *J Am Med Womens Assoc* 1999; 54:196–8.
15. McNaughton-Cassill ME, Bostwick JM, Arthur NJ, et al. Efficacy of brief couples support groups developed to manage the stress of in vitro fertilization treatment. *Mayo Clin Proc* 2002; 77:1060–6.
16. de Liz TM, Strauss B. Differential efficacy of group and individual/couple psychotherapy with infertile patients. *Hum Reprod* 2005; 20:1324–32.
17. Bergart A. Group work as an antidote to isolation of bearing an invisible stigma. *Soc Work Groups* 2003; 26:33–43.
18. Lukse MP. The effect of group counseling on the frequency of grief reported by infertile couples. *J Obstet Gynecol Neonatal Nurs* 1985; 14:67s–70s.

19. Goodman K, Rothman B. Group work with infertility treatment. *Soc Work Groups* 1984; 7:79–97.

20. Christianson C. Support groups for infertile patients. *J Obstet Gynecol Neonatal Nurs* 1986;15:293–6.

21. Lenter E, Glazer G. Infertile couples' perceptions of infertility support group participation. *Health Care Women Int* 1991;12:317–30.

22. Domar AD, Clapp D, Slawsby E, et al. The impact of group psychological interventions on pregnancy rates in infertile women. *Fertil Stertil* 2000; 73:805–11.

23. McNaughton-Cassill ME, Bostwick JM, Vanscoy SE, et al. Development of brief stress management support goups for couples undergoing in vitro fertilization treatment. *Fertil Stertil* 2000;74:87–93.

24. Lemmens GM, Vervacke M, Enzlin P, et al. Coping with infertility: A body–mind group intervention programme for infertile couples. *Hum Reprod* 2004;19:1917–23.

25. Tarabusi M, Volpe A, Facchinetti F. Psychological group support attenuates distress of waiting in couples scheduled for assisted reproduction. *J Psychosom Obstet Gynaecol* 2004; 25:273–9.

26. Domar AD, Seibel MM, Benson H. The mind–body program for infertility: A new behavioral treatment approach for women with infertility. *Fertil Stertil* 1990; 53:246–9.

27. Domar AD, Clapp D, Slawsby E, et al. The impact of group psychological interventions on distress in infertile women. *Health Psychol* 2000; 19:568–75.

28. Epstein YM, Rosenberg HS, Grant TV, et al. Use of the internet as the only outlet for talking about infertility. *Fertil Stertil* 2002;78:507–14.

29. Hosaka T, Matsubayashi H, Sugiyama Y, et al. Effect of psychiatric group intervention on natural-killer cell activity and pregnancy rate. *Gen Hosp Psychiatry* 2002; 24:353–6.

30. Christie G, Morgan A. Individual and group psychotherapy for infertile couples. *Int J Group Psychother* 2000; 50:237–50.

31. Lederberg MS. Staff support groups for high-stress medical environments. *Int J Group Psychother* 1998; 48:275–304.

32. Ulman KH. An integrative model of stress management groups for women. *Int J Group Psychother* 2000; 50:341–62.

33. Mackenzie KR. Time-limited group psychotherapy. *Int J Group Psychother* 1996; 46:41–60.

34. Bonanno GA, Kaltman S. Toward an integrative perspective on bereavement. *Psychol Bulletin* 1999; 125:760–6.

35. McCallum M, Piper WE, Ogrodniczuk JS, et al. Early process and dropping out from short-term group therapy for complicated grief. *Group Dyn* 2002;6:243–54.

36. Covington SN, Burns LH. *Working with your medical team: Tips on changing from the difficult patient to the perfect patient.* Resolve Family Building Magazine; Spring 2002.

37. Benson H. *The Relaxation Response.* New York: Morrow, 1975.

38. Domar AD, Kelly AL. *Conquering Infertility: Dr. Alice Domar's Mind/Body Guide to Enhancing Fertility and Coping with Infertility.* New York: Penguin Books, 2004.

39. Steward DE, Boydell KM, McCarthy K, et al. A prospective study of the effectiveness of brief professionally-led support groups for infertility patients. *Int J Psychiatry Med* 1992; 22:173–82.

40. Thorn P, Daniels K. A group–work approach in family building by donor insemination: Empowering the marginalized. *Hum Fertil*, 2003; 6:46–50.

41. Weinberg H. Group process and group phenomena on the internet. *Int J Group Psychother* 2001; 51:361–78.

11 Behavioral Medicine Approaches to Infertility Counseling

CHRISTIANNE VERHAAK AND LINDA HAMMER BURNS

The reason why a sound body becomes ill, or an ailing body recovers, very often lies in the mind.

– Gaub, 1747

During the late twentieth century, behavioral medicine emerged as an interdisciplinary field concerned with the development and integration of behavioral and biomedical science, knowledge, and techniques relevant to health and illness, and the application of this knowledge to prevention, diagnosis, treatment, and rehabilitation. Behavioral medicine has been integral in improving disease prevention, diagnosis, treatment, and rehabilitation.[1] At the same time, medical and health psychology emerged as a specialty within the field of psychology devoted to the promotion and maintenance of health; the prevention and treatment of illness; the identification of etiologic and diagnostic correlates of health, illness, and related dysfunction; and the improvement of healthcare systems. An important contribution of medical psychology was patient education and support as well as improving patient compliance and the identification of psychosocial issues that may impact patient well-being, the disease or treatment process, or treatment outcome.[2] Behavioral health and health psychology as well as medical psychology, clinical health psychology, psychosomatic medicine, healthcare psychology, and collaborative healthcare all are based on the concept of a mind–body connection and, as such, all diseases and conditions (whether of the mind or the physical body) must be treated as if they have both been affected.

Behavioral medicine and health psychology have three areas of focus: (1) the prevention of future health problems, (2) change behaviors that contribute to current or future health problems, and (3) the improvement of quality-of-life. Behavioral medicine mental health professionals, health psychologists, and, as such, infertility counselors use a variety of techniques to implement these goals, many of which are addressed in other chapters. As such, the focus of this chapter is on stress and coping techniques found to be effective in the care and treatment of infertile men and women as well as the various roles and treatment interventions available to the infertility counselor.

In recent decades, behavioral medicine and health psychology have rapidly expanded, in part due to burgeoning scientific evidence linking psychosocial factors with important aspects of health and illness, as well as empirically demonstrated success of psychosocial interventions applied to disease treatment and promotion for a variety of illness and health behaviors. This has been the case in reproductive medicine as evidenced by the once emergent and now widely recognized and respected field of infertility counseling, also known as reproductive health psychology, reproductive behavioral medicine, or psychosomatic obstetric and gynecology. Although these fields may have distinct or specific applications, all use various principles and practices developed by or adapted from behavioral medicine.

The application of behavioral medicine to infertility has involved a variety of applications focusing on the relationship between psychological, social, and biological factors to protect or maximize current fertility; use stress and coping techniques for the management of infertility and/or treatment-related distress; and/or improve the outcome of specific fertility treatments. Within this context improving outcomes is not restricted to biological parameters (e.g., pregnancy and live births) but involves improved psychosocial outcomes (e.g., emotional adjustment to the experience of infertility, reduced stress, diminished depression and anxiety, etc.). As such, the behavioral medicine approach recognize the importance of a multidimensional approach to infertility that considers biological, psychological, and social (environmental) factors that have an impact on the infertile individual and/or couple's experience of and adjustment to infertility and treatment for it. Behavioral medicine and health psychology have been useful in exploring the mind and body connection in infertility, facilitating the understanding of the emotional consequences of infertility and development of coping and stress management interventions, while providing a foundation for research theory and design.

This chapter

■ provides a brief historical overview of the psychosomatic approaches to the psychology of infertility and the biopsychosocial model of infertility;
■ examines research regarding stress and coping during infertility;
■ outlines illustrative theoretical frameworks of behavioral medicine and health psychology, as they apply to the psychology of infertility;
■ describes stress management and coping interventions;
■ discusses clinical applications of stress and coping theory for aiding couples as they confront the psychosocial demands of infertility.

HISTORICAL OVERVIEW

Throughout history and across cultures, caregivers have recognized the interconnectedness of the human mind and body, although this has been more prominent in some cultures (e.g., Chinese) than in others. Hippocrates, considered the founder of Western medicine, acknowledged with other Greeks of the time (e.g., Socrates) the importance of including the human spirit in conjunction with physical illness. However, during the early seventeenth century, French philosopher Rene Descartes contended that the human mind and body were separate entities requiring separate and distinct treatments. The 'Cartesian dualistic approach' referred to two forms of dualism: mind–body separation and the dualism of patient–caregiver roles. Accordingly, physicians took paternalistic responsibility for the diagnosis and development of a treatment regime while the patient role was one of deference and obedient compliance. Cartesian dualism influenced Western medicine until the middle of the twentieth century during which mind–body processes moved from the province of philosophy and religion to the domain of respectable scientific inquiry. During this time, *psychosomatic medicine* emerged as a formalized field based on a combination of psychodynamics and psychophysiologic theories. The psychodynamic approach was based on psychoanalytic

theory and Franz Alexander's *nuclear conflict theory* that contended unresolved unconscious conflicts produced specific somatic disorders. The psychophysiologic approach of the psychosomatic medicine was based on Harold G. Wolfe's research on the effects of psychological stimuli on physiological processes. *Psychosomatic medicine* was originally intended to acknowledge and recognize the unity of mind–body relationships but came to convey psychological causation of physiological disorders.[3]

The diagnosis of *psychogenic infertility* was based on psychosomatic medicine principles and referred to intrapsychic conflicts (typically within women) that caused or contributed to involuntary childlessness and sterility. Accordingly, a woman's deep-seated neurotic anxiety; conflicted feelings about parenthood, sexuality, and/or adult roles; fears of childbirth; and/or intrapsychic conflicts regarding her own mother were considered feasible explanations for infertility.[4] *Psychogenic infertility* was a popular diagnosis at a time when 'unexplained' infertility was more prevalent and widespread. However, the attribution of idiopathic infertility to psychological factors became less appropriate as advances in reproductive medicine increased diagnostic accuracy. Furthermore, research failed to substantiate theories of specific personality characteristics in infertile patients or a higher incidence of psychopathology in infertile individuals compared with that of the general population or individuals with other medical conditions.[5–7] While the psychosomatic approach recognized mind–body connectedness and the relevance of psychosocial factors in disease development, experience, and treatment, by the 1970s, the concept of *psychogenic infertility* had fallen into disfavor. Psychological distress was no longer thought to be the *cause* of infertility, but rather the *result* of the stress of infertility and the treatments for it.

The significance of stress as a mediating factor in health emerged with the original work in 1936 of Canadian endocrinologist Hans Selye, who identified the body's reactions to real or perceived threats (stressors) with a variety of physiological responses including increased metabolism, heart rate, blood pressure, rate of breathing, and blood flow to the muscles as well as the release of catecholamines (i.e., adrenalin and noradrenalin).[8] Selye described stress as a nonspecific response by the body to a demand in which distress (negative stress) triggered the *general adaptation syndrome* (also known as the *stress syndrome*). Accordingly, the body responds to stress in a predictable pattern in three stages: (1) *alarm reaction*, in which the body responds to the external distress with initial short-term stage of alarm; (2) *adaptation*, in which the body engages defensive countermeasures against the stressor involving a longer period of resistance; and (3) *exhaustion*, in which the body begins to run out of physiological defenses for managing the stressor. In 1941, American neurologist Walter Cannon described this cascade of physiological responses to stress as the 'fight or flight' response which prepared the individual to either confront (fight), the perceived or actual threat, or to flee it.[9] This became the basis for investigations into the impact of stress on fertility, in that emotional stress, either directly or by releasing adrenaline, was thought to centrally inhibit or prevent the secretion of oxytocin or counteract its action.[10] Personality factors and a recurring pattern of 'situation-stress-symptom' were also considered causes of infertility.[11] Recently researchers have investigated mechanisms by which stress may impair fertility by impacting functioning of the hypothalamic-pituitary-adrenal axis thereby deregulating the reproductive process in both women and men.[12,13] Despite growing evidence for relationships between stress, endocrine and immunological factors and infertility, there is still little insight into the mechanism of this process and/or how it exactly operates.

Subsequently, American physician Herbert Benson developed the 'relaxation response' based on transcendental mediation and his research that found meditation (even sitting quietly in a room and/or restructuring an individual's thoughts) produced significant physiological changes.[14] The 'relaxation response' became a counter mechanism to the 'fight or flight' physiological stress response and was applied to a variety of medical conditions including infertility. Stress management, coping techniques, and relaxation-based interventions significantly contributed to the understanding of the psychosocial dynamics of infertility and, as such, were a basis for the emerging field of infertility counseling. Even though these important applications significantly contribute to improved patient quality-of-life, no randomized controlled trials have examined the efficacy of any of these techniques with infertile patients specifically, although there have been some efforts along these lines recently. Research on stress, coping, and patient responses (positive and negative) to infertility became instrumental in the emergence of patient care models (e.g., the biopsychosocial, health psychology, and collaborative medicine models), all of which eliminated mind–body dualism and physician–patient dualism and encouraged caregiver–patient collaboration in improving treatment outcomes and improving patient satisfaction and quality-of-life.

During the late twentieth century, increased patient awareness, participation in health maintenance, and a self-help consumer movement also marked the move away from dualistic physician–patient roles. At the same time, an awareness of the bidirectional nature of stress and infertility supported a more collaborative approach to patient care that emphasized the role of infertility counselors and patient participation in treatment, including active involvement in maximizing health and well-being.

REVIEW OF LITERATURE

As noted, the initial focus of research on stress and infertility was based on the *psychogenic hypothesis* (i.e., infertility caused by psychological factors) and then on the *psychological consequences hypothesis* (i.e., the psychological consequences of infertility). Recently, research has focused on a related hypothesis, which contends that stress may be a causal factor in infertility, particularly in terms of the impact of stress on treatment outcomes.[7] This may be referred to as the *psychological outcome hypothesis*. Research regarding infertility and behavioral medicine will be reviewed by examining the ways stress and coping affect: psychological reactions to infertility, gender differences, responses to assisted reproductive technologies, and treatment outcomes.

Psychological Reactions to Infertility

In a comprehensive review of available research on psychological reactions to infertility, Dunkel-Schetter and Lobel investigated both descriptive and empirical research.[15] Their conclusion on descriptive reports was that a greater focus was placed on the emotional effects of infertility than on loss of control, changes in identity or esteem, or social effects. In terms of the empirical research, they concluded that the evidence *did not* clearly indicate that negative effects accompany infertility, although there is some evidence of adverse effects in a few studies. Furthermore, Dunkel-Schetter and Lobel concluded "that the average infertile individual does not experience severe or clinically significant distress, marital problems, sexual problems, or other psychological difficulties, or is there evidence for a set sequence of emotional reactions." In a more recent review of the literature, Greil's findings were similar to the earlier literature review by Dunkel-Schetter and Lobel in that descriptive literature on the psychological consequences of infertility often presented infertility as a psychologically devastating experience for individuals, although empirically sound research found no significant differences between infertile individuals and others in terms of psychopathology or self-esteem. Greil's research did find that there was some evidence that infertility was a stressful experience, typically more so for women than men.[7] In a similar review of research on stress and infertility, no solid evidence was found that infertility patients demonstrate more psychopathology than controls, although modest evidence was found of an association between distress during treatment and the outcome of the treatment itself.[16] More positive adjustment to infertility seems to be related to better self-esteem, internal (versus external) locus of control, higher socioeconomic status, and moderate age, while higher levels of anxiety and distress are associated with low self-esteem, undifferentiated sex role identity, and advanced age. Actual and perceived duration of infertility have also been found to relate to psychological reactions to infertility.[17]

Psychological Responses in Men versus Women

In a review of empirical research on gender differences, Wright and colleagues as well as other researchers concluded that women tended to be more distressed by the infertility experience and its medical treatment than men, even when the infertility diagnosis was not attributable to her or when the diagnosis was ambiguous.[7,18–20] Women appear to experience greater levels of distress, depression, anxiety, and poor self-esteem.[5,21,22] Although women appear to experience more infertility-specific distress than men, men experience greater psychological distress when the cause of infertility is male-factor. Men with male-factor infertility experience more negative emotions including more feelings of stigma, anxiety, loss, and poor self-esteem.[19,23] Men with male-factor infertility tend to make more self-denigrating remarks. In addition, although some research indicates that men are less affected than women by the process of infertility evaluation and over the course of treatment, other research found that men experienced more infertility-specific distress over the course of treatment, specifically when treatment was more than seventeen months and was related to specific treatment (e.g., testicular biopsy).[23,24] Finally, predictors of distress in infertile men were: an anxious disposition; a general tendency to appraise situations as stressful; an avoidant coping style; and failure to seek social support.[25]

Gender differences have also been found in that different aspects of infertility are stressful to men versus women, and men and women use different coping techniques. Women are more likely to use a wider array of coping strategies (e.g., information seeking), and women may be better able to identify and access other areas of potential social support outside of their marriages.[26,27] Women tend to use more coping behaviors (e.g., self-controlling, seeking social support, and escape-avoidance) to deal with infertility and treatment than did their husbands, who were more likely to use confronting the problem, accepting responsibility, and escape-avoidance as coping strategies.[20] Davis and Dearman identified six coping strategies commonly used by women to cope with infertility: (1) increasing the space or distancing oneself from reminders of infertility; (2) instituting measures for regaining control; (3) acting to increase self-esteem by being the best (e.g., control weight or appearance); (4) looking for meaning in infertility; (5) giving in to feelings (expressing emotions); and (6) sharing the burden with others.[28].

In contrast, men are more likely to use coping strategies that involve denial, distancing, avoidance, and withdrawal and are less likely to seek social support, counseling, or discussions with caregivers.[18,27] One longitudinal study of infertile men found that a man's coping strategy with earlier phases of infertility impacted his long-term adjustment to it: Men who substituted an object (e.g., house, pet, or garden) or a child (e.g., leading a church youth group) to nurture during unfertility treatment were more likely to achieve generativity and parenthood, while those who used self-centered substitutes (e.g., body building) failed to achieve either generativity or fatherhood by midlife.[29] While men and women may experience different aspects of infertility as stressful, another factor in the emotional impact of infertility-related stress on couples may be the congruence (e.g., agreement) between partners regarding the experience of infertility. To infertile couples in whom there was high congruence in their perception of infertility-specific stress, higher levels of marital adjustment were found.[30]

Finally, infertility-specific distress may be influenced by cultural factors. In a review of qualitative studies from African countries, infertility was found to be an overwhelmingly negative and distressing experience associated with high levels of psychological distress in women. For women in cultures in which male-factor infertility diagnosis is socioculturally unacceptable, the burden of infertility may have more than psychological consequences in that women may be at increased risk of abuse, abandonment, divorce, or social stigma.[31] In addition, lack of a husband's support has been found to increase anxiety and depression in women, adding to feelings of infertility-specific distress.[32]

Psychological Responses to Assisted Reproductive Technologies

Considerable research has addressed stress related to assisted reproductive technologies and patients' perception of ART treatment as stressful. Early research found that patients undergoing ARTs (e.g., IVF) were at no greater risk for psychological disturbances, although there was some evidence of greater anxiety, distress, and grief if the procedure was unsuccessful. Nevertheless, ARTs patients scored within normal limits on measurements of preexisting psychopathology.[33] Factors contributing to grief reaction following unsuccessful ARTs included a belief that the treatment was the couple's last chance at having a biological child, preexisting psychological illness, and overestimation of success rates.[34,35] Recent research has shown that mood (anxiety, depression, or distress) probably fluctuates in both men and women over the course of ARTs cycles: anxiety and depression increasing on oocyte-retrieval day, decreasing on embryo-transfer day, and rising again on pregnancy-testing day. However, severity of response appears to diminish with repeated cycles.[34,36,37] In general, oocyte retrieval and pregnancy test(s) seem to be the most stressful aspects of the IVF treatment cycle.[38,39] In accessing perceived infertility-specific stress at twelve months and twenty-four months posttreatment, self-esteem was the only factor associated with increased stress over the course of treatment regardless of treatment method and number of treatment cycles.[22]

Other research has shown, however, that even though most women appear to adjust well to unsuccessful treatment, a considerable proportion continue to experience substantial distress over time when ARTs is unsuccessful.[40] Not surprisingly, anxiety and depression have been found to be significantly higher in women who experienced failed IVF cycles and in initial stages of treatment (<3 years).[41] In fact, women who experienced infertility of medium to long duration were found to have significantly lower state anxiety but higher state anxiety following failed treatment cycles.[42] Perceived helplessness and marital dissatisfaction were found to be risk factors, while acceptance and perceived social support were found to be protective factors, in the development of anxiety and depression after a failed fertility treatment[43]. In a study comparing psychological adjustment of patients pursuing parenthood via (1) ARTs; (2) surrogacy; and (3) adoption, women seeking ART were younger (thirty-three years old) than women pursuing surrogacy (thirty-seven years old) and adoption (thirty-seven years old). Women pursuing ART and/or who remained childless were more likely to use distancing and denial coping strategies.[44] By contrast, patient optimism prior to an ART treatment cycle was found to be predictive of less distress following a failed first treatment cycle (specifically IVF and ICSI).[40]

In contrast, men appear to experience no change in infertility-specific distress (e.g., anxiety and depression) whether or not ARTs treatment is successful or unsuccessful.[40] However, long waits before beginning assisted reproduction increased anxiety levels, particularly for male partners.[45] Prior to treatment, women were found to be more anxious than their partners and were less positive than men about their marital and sexual relationships, although these feelings diminished or reversed when the treatment cycle was successful. During the IVF, women experienced highest levels of distress after embryo transfer and negative pregnancy testing. First and last treatment cycles were associated with greatest levels of anxiety and distress. [46–49]

In short, individuals undergoing assisted reproduction appear to be at no greater risk for psychological disturbances, although there may be a greater risk of anxiety, distress, and grief, especially if the procedure is unsuccessful.[34]

Impact of Psychosocial Interventions on Treatment Outcome

The impact of psychological interventions, particularly stress reduction and relaxation techniques, has become an increasing focus of research in behavioral medicine as researchers and clinicians strive to determine whether psychosocial interventions positively affect endocrine and immune function – and ultimately positively impact treatment outcomes. In a review of research on stress and infertility, no solid evidence was found that infertility patients demonstrated more psychopathology than controls, although modest evidence was found of an association between distress during treatment and the outcome of the treatment itself.[16] In a more comprehensive review of research on the effectiveness of interventions to improve psychosocial well-being and pregnancy rates, Boivin found that psychosocial interventions were more effective in reducing negative affect than in changing interpersonal functioning (e.g., marital and social functioning), although pregnancy rates were unlikely to be affected by psychosocial interventions. Group interventions that emphasized education and skills training (e.g., relaxation training) were significantly more effective in producing positive change across a range of outcomes than counseling interventions that emphasized emotional expression and support and/or discussion about thoughts and feelings related to infertility. In addition, men and women were found to benefit equally from psychosocial interventions, although again these changes did not seem to impact treatment outcomes.[50]

In a Danish study that examined separate and joint effects of male and female infertility-specific stress and the source of stress (e.g., personal, social, or marital) on treatment outcome, researchers found that infertility-specific stress *was* associated with poorer treatment outcomes in women (i.e., lower pregnancy rates). Women who reported *more* infertility-specific stress related to personal and marital issues (versus social problems) were more likely to have lower treatment outcomes. In short, women reported more marital distress and took more treatment cycles to conceive (median 3) than women reporting less marital distress (median 2). The findings provide evidence that infertility-related stress has direct and indirect effects on treatment outcome.[51] Higher levels of anxiety or depression were associated with lower pregnancy rates.[52] Infertile women were found to have elevated levels of cortisol compared with fertile controls, while lower levels of adrenaline at oocyte retrieval and embryo transfer were found to be associated with higher pregnancy rates.[13,53] In addition, differences in immune factors were found between women who achieved pregnancy following IVF treatment and women who did not.[12] In a study evaluating treatment outcomes comparing ARTs procedural-specific stress versus infertility-specific stress, higher expectations of pregnancy (optimism) were found to be associated with greater numbers of oocytes fertilized and embryos transferred. Baseline (acute and chronic) stress affected biologic end points (i.e., number of oocytes retrieved and fertilized) as well as pregnancy (e.g., live birth delivery, birth weight, and multiple gestations), whereas procedural-specific stress only influenced biologic end points.[38]

Increasingly, research has focused on the assessment of the physiological stress response on fertility, treatment outcomes, and specific interventions to reverse infertility-specific stress to improve fertility and/or treatment outcomes. One study investigated the association between stress hormones (i.e., adrenaline, noradrenaline, and cortisol), mood, and IVF/ICSI treatment outcome using urine samples to assess stress hormones and questionnaires to measure anxiety and depression. In women with successful treatment, lower concentrations of adrenaline at oocyte retrieval and lower concentrations of adrenaline and noradrenaline at embryo transfer were found, leading the researchers to conclude that adrenal hormones could be a factor in the complex relationship between psychosocial stress and treatment outcome.[13] Stress levels of women undergoing IVF and a control group of fertile women were assessed using blood tests to measure circulating prolactin and cortisol levels and questionnaires to measure mood and personality traits. Infertile women were found to have more suspicion, guilt, and hostility compared with fertile women, which the researchers speculated was in response to their infertility. The researchers concluded that the infertile women's psychological stress negatively affected the IVF treatment outcome in that their state-anxiety levels were higher than women who had become pregnant following IVF.[48] In an investigation of a possible correlation between immunological changes and implantation rates in patients undergoing IVF, questionnaires were used to assess mood and blood samples to measure circulating T-helper and T-suppressor lymphocytes. Prolonged stress was found to decrease adaptability and cause transitory anxiety that was found to be associated with higher levels of activated T-cells in peripheral blood. These researchers found reduced implantation rates in women undergoing IVF who had elevated T-cells.[12] In short, there is evidence that infertility-specific stress physiologically impacts fertility and treatments outcomes negatively, perhaps through deregulation of the endocrine and/or immune response or through a complex interplay of factors, and that specific interventions may help to improve treatment outcome.

THEORETICAL FRAMEWORK

The *biopsychosocial model* and s*tress and coping theory* are two theoretical frameworks that are particularly relevant to a behavioral medicine/health psychology approach to infertility counseling. Both perspectives build on the developments in medicine and infertility during the twentieth century offering theoretical perspective as well as the identification of clinical issues and therapeutic interventions contributing to improved patient care and patient satisfaction by addressing the physical and psychosocial needs of the patient(s). A new and developing theoretical framework is the *biopsychosocial model of infertility*, which incorporates principles from both the biopsychosocial model and stress and coping theory. These theories provide different perspectives for understanding the multifaceted and complex experience of infertility; the unique stressors of the experience of infertility and treatment for it; and the expanding role of infertility counselors in identifying clinical issues, developing effective therapeutic interventions, and conducting research to improve patient well-being, treatment outcomes, and effective psychotherapeutic interventions. The application of the biopsychosocial model, stress and coping theories, and the biopsychosocial models of infertility have provided greater understanding of the determinants of distress experienced by infertile men and women, as well as suggesting research directions and clinical applications for therapeutic interventions to mitigate distress and improve treatment outcomes. As such, these theories guide professional practice by helping to target specific coping strategies for therapeutic intervention, tailoring them to specific patient needs, contexts, and resources.

Biopsychosocial Model

The *biopsychosocial model* of health and illness represents an alternative to the conventional Western biomedical model in that it recognizes and incorporates biological, psychological, and social influences on the onset, course, and treatment of disease and medical conditions.[1] The biopsychosocial model was developed by Engel in the 1970s based on general systems theory.[54] It takes into consideration the wide array of issues impacting an individual's experience of health and illness as well as cultural, familial, and other interpersonal factors in the complex and reciprocal interplay among body, mind, and environment. The biopsychosocial model emphasizes the importance of the physician and patient as collaborators in the diagnosis, treatment, and health maintenance by encouraging caregivers and patients to see themselves as equal partners. Aims of this approach are to bolster patients' sense of control and self-efficacy; promote health-enhancing behaviors; and work collaboratively with cultural and religious factors and other contextual factors influencing the patients' experience of illness and orientation toward treatment. As such, this model emphasizes the importance of the patient–physician relationship in achieving optimum medical treatment and health.

The biopsychosocial model recognizes the potential impact of stress and coping as well as other psychosocial factors as potentially significant factors in the experience of infertility and in treatment outcomes. Relevant constructs of this approach include illness behavior, acute versus chronic illness; adaptation and maladaptation to illness; and the importance of individual cognition, self-awareness, self-efficacy, and self-control. Illness behavior or what is expected or appropriate response to a health condition is mediated by a number of factors including the medical condition itself, individual personality characteristics, and cultural beliefs about health and/or illness. Interestingly, the most important determinants of assuming the status of being ill seem to be sociological and cognitive.[55] Both acute and chronic disorders symptoms may be modified by emotions and beliefs. For some infertile men and women, infertility is an acute diagnosis, although for the majority of infertile individuals, infertility represents a chronic condition, which may or may not have a specific, identifiable diagnosis despite ongoing, long-term treatment. However, any chronic illness requires reorganization and adaptation on a variety of levels (e.g., physical, psychological, and social).

Taymor and Bresnick were the first to refer to infertility as a *biopsychosocial crisis* because it involves interaction among physical conditions predisposing to infertility; medical interventions addressing infertility; reactions of others; and individual psychological characteristics.[56] All too often, infertile individuals (more commonly women) attempt to adjust to infertility by *not* adjusting – attempting to function socially or occupationally at preinfertility levels – a near impossible feat. One reason for this may be beliefs about illness behavior, but another may be that without a specific diagnosis many infertile individuals do not perceive themselves (nor do others perceive them) as being ill or being a patient despite the extensive medical treatment they are undergoing. Impaired fertility may not be viewed as life-threatening or dangerous, thereby not requiring support or adaptation. Cognition is an important mediator in the experience of illness in that how individuals think about and interpret their condition has an impact on their illness behavior and adjustment. Typically, addressing cognitions includes identifying underlying assumptions or attributions that cause distress; restructuring negative thought patterns; and/or providing evidence or an environment for reinterpretation (cognitive reframing). Fundamental to the biopsychosocial model is the patient's participation in treatment, which is thought to improve the patient's feelings of control; facilitates participation in decision making; and improves treatment compliance through self-care. Self-efficacy behavior enhances individual health behavior changes, improving health and facilitating adaptation and coping.

Stress and Coping Theory

Fundamental to stress and coping theory is the individual's perception of the stressor, other stressful life events, coping skills, resilience, and social support.

Variables in the response to stress include personality, cognition, social environment, gender, and culture. *Stress* refers to events in which demands of the internal or external environment challenge or exceed an individual's adaptive resources.[55] Stress has also been conceptualized as a stimulus, with stressors from major life events (e.g., illness, divorce) or daily hassles. In short, although stress is a universal life experience, it may be positive or negative in that each individual perceives and experiences an event (even the same event) differently. What is threatening and stressful to one person may not be stressful to another individual and, in fact, may even be experienced as enjoyable (e.g., sky diving). As such, stress (whether a positive or negative experience) challenges an individual's resources and requires adaptation. These physiological changes enable an individual to respond to threat(s), whether the threat is a perceived or actual danger. Negative stress is typically referred to as *distress*. Additionally, stress may be acute or chronic. An *acute stressor* typically is sudden or abrupt, requiring immediate adaptation with an expectation of short-term adjustment and a rapid return to previous functioning. By contrast, a *chronic stressor* may occur abruptly or over time but requires long-term, persistent adjustment and adaptation that may or may not involve a return to prior level of functioning. *Coping* refers to the process by which a person takes some action to manage external or internal demands that cause stress and tax the individual's inner resources. It involves the individual's deliberate efforts or techniques to effectively respond to threats or challenges or, specifically, an individual's adaptability when confronted with difficult circumstances. Coping may be *adaptive* or *maladaptive* (i.e., effective or ineffective), and although coping responses are neither uniformly adaptive nor maladaptive, some coping strategies (e.g., denial and disengagement) are associated with maladjustment because they can cause or increase distress – typically in another arena in the individual's life.

In the 1980s, Lazarus and Folkman proposed a *cognitive-phenomenological theory of stress* that addressed the interactive effect of stress and coping. Their definition of stress involved "a relationship between the person and the environment that is appraised by the person as taxing or exceeding his or her resources and endangering his or her well-being."[57] According to *cognitive-phenomenological theory*, an individual's appraisal of an experience is integral in the experience of stress and to the individual's ability to manage or cope with the stressor.[57] This relational perspective emphasized the importance of an individual's perception, life experiences, personality, and the context in which the negative stressor is experienced. In short, an individual's adaptability and adjustment to stress can be predicted by his or her cognitive appraisal and coping strategies. The negative consequences of stressful encounters are assessed in terms of morale; social or interpersonal functioning; physical health; and individual perception or interpretation of the stressful event. Cognitive appraisal and coping processes are central to *cognitive-phenomenological theory of stress*, as individuals assess the potentially harmful and beneficial aspects of a stressful experience (i.e., primary appraisal) as well as their ability to influence its outcome (i.e., secondary appraisal). According to this theory, three primary coping strategies were identified: appraisal-focused coping, problem-focused coping, and emotion-focused coping.

Appraisal-focused coping (also referred to as meaning-based coping) involves attempts by the individual to define or redefine the meaning of the stressful situation and includes logical analysis; cognitive redefinition (i.e., active meaning-based coping); and cognitive avoidance (i.e., passive meaning-based coping). *Problem-focused* coping is the modification or elimination of the source of stress and seeking information or advice, taking problem-solving action, and developing alternative rewards. *Emotion-focused* coping involves managing the emotions aroused by stress or stressors, enabling the individual to maintain affective equilibrium. Emotion-focused strategies include affective regulation, resignation, acceptance, and emotional discharge.[58]

Stanton and Dunkel-Schetter applied stress and coping theory to infertility, suggesting that infertility is characterized by the very dimensions that individuals find most stressful: unpredictability, negativity, uncontrollability, and ambiguity.[59] As such, infertility is a stressor that takes place over an extended period of time; is beyond the control of the individuals involved; and entails negative consequences, responses, and outcomes that are unknown and unpredictable. Coping techniques for managing the crisis involve not only assessment of the individual's and couple's resources, personality, perceptions of the stressor, and response to the stress but also how these are applied to the stressor (infertility) to achieve adaptive adjustment.

Infertility can be conceptualized as a stressful experience, in that the individual's appraisal of an experience is integral: If parenthood is not an important goal, then infertility carries fewer negative consequences and thus is not perceived as particularly stressful. Whereas if an individual (or couple) feels that major life goals and roles are thwarted by involuntary childlessness, then

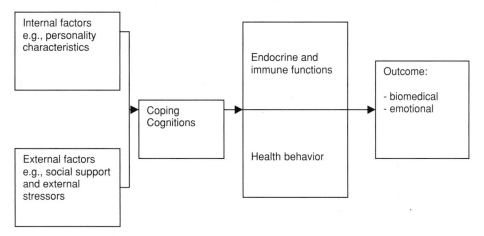

Figure 11.1. Biopsychosocial model of infertility

infertility may be experienced as extraordinarily stressful. It is the latter individuals who are at particular risk for negative emotional outcomes. As such, stress and coping theory provides a basis for defining the circumstances under which infertility is perceived or experienced as stressful; the factors that facilitate or impede adjustment for infertile couples; and what constitutes successful psychological adjustment to infertility.

Using stress and coping theories as a foundation, Stanton and Dunkel-Schettter noted that infertile couples typically perceive infertility as carrying the potential for both harm (e.g., loss of a central role) and benefit (e.g., strengthening of the marital relationship).[59] Infertile couples typically perceive some aspects of infertility as relatively uncontrollable (e.g., attaining conception) and others as more controllable (e.g., deciding for or against engaging in diagnostic tests and treatment).[60] Additionally, stress and coping theories suggest that the effectiveness of coping partly depends on the timeframe and the controllability of the stressor. Additionally, personal and situational attributions regarding infertility as well as the appraisal process can be instrumental in the initiation as well as the effectiveness of specific coping strategies. As a result of their research, Stanton and Dunkel-Schetter recommended that professionals working with infertile couples should enhance perceptions of control; discourage avoidance; and promote positive reappraisal of infertility. Furthermore, patients should be encouraged to improve their overall quality-of-life through maintaining individual health and well-being (e.g., exercise and abstinence from tobacco and alcohol) and nurturing their couple relationship (e.g., communication, intimacy, and humor).[61]

The stress and coping approach has become instrumental in attempts to determine which behavioral techniques (e.g., relaxation and expression of emotion) may facilitate conception and parenthood, in what some have considered a recycling of the psychogenic infertility model. While cognitive-behavior theory provides conceptualization and therapeutic direction for individuals experiencing infertility, Stanton and Dunkel-Schetter[21] suggest that it provides little direction for furthering our knowledge of systematic variability in adjustment. However, they also suggest that the application of stress and coping theory to infertility provides a greater understanding of: (1) the conditions under which infertility is likely to be perceived as stressful; (2) factors most likely to facilitate or impede adjustment in infertile couples or individuals; and (3) guidance in defining what constitutes successful psychological adjustment to infertility.

Biopsychosocial Model of Infertility

The *biopsychosocial model of infertility* (Figure 11.1) developed by Verhaak is based on a combination of the biopsychosocial model and principles from stress and coping theories. It identifies the reciprocal nature of the array of factors that can and do impact emotional responses to infertility and biomedical outcomes of infertility treatment. The biopsychosocial model of infertility makes a distinction between internal, stable, dispositional factors (e.g., personality characteristics) and external factors (e.g., life events, social support, and illness-related stressors) that can impact the outcome of infertility and psychosocial adjustment to the experience of infertility. The relationship between the internal and external factors and health outcome is mediated by appraisals or cognitions and coping. Lack of social support and marital discord are risk factors for maladjustment to severe stressors, next to the existence of one or more severe external stressors. Appraisals or cognitions refer to the way individuals perceive and evaluate the stressful infertility-related situation. This model emphasizes coping strategies that are problem-focused and emotion-focused. Both appraisals and other coping strategies are assumed to impact infertility treatment outcome via two different pathways: (1) endocrine and immune responses, and (2) the infertile patient's own health behavior.

Later research acknowledged more differentiations in coping dimensions involving cognitive attempts to change the meaning of the stressor: Trying to change the meaning of a problem can make it less harmful.[57,62] The effectiveness of coping depends partly on the characteristics (controllability) and the time-frame of the stressor (short-term versus long-term). To fully understand the emotional impact of infertility and how to cope with it, the entire process – from diagnosis of infertility to either positive treatment or termination of treatment – helps to explain how infertility is (or becomes) a *chronic stressor*. Infertility as a chronic stressor consists of different aspects: the invasive treatment including physical and emotional strenuous aspects; the uncertainty about the treatment outcome; the uncontrollability of fertility problems; and the loss of hope for a pregnancy when infertility is definitive.[15,63] Coping with infertility as a chronic stressor requires the completion of major adaptive tasks for men, women, and couples that includes maintaining: (1) emotional equilibrium; (2) a positive sense of self from sense of self as infertile; and (3) good relationships with family and friends as well as (4) preparing for the future such as defining new life goals and a marital relationship without children.[58] These tasks must be accomplished while dealing with the physiological consequences of fertility treatment, treatment schedules, the clinic environment, and an array of healthcare workers.

CLINICAL ISSUES

Infertility counselors work to improve quality-of-life and change behaviors that may contribute to improved treatment outcomes. As such, several clinical issues regarding a behavioral medicine approach to infertility counseling are of significance, and include: (1) identifying and assessing typical psychological responses to infertility and medical treatment; (2) understanding the complex role of stress and coping in the experience of infertility; and (3) engaging the highly distressed but resistant infertility patient in the psychosocial treatment process.

Identifying Infertility-Specific Stress

The goals of assessment in infertility counseling are gaining an understanding of the individual's physical and social environment; relevant strengths and weaknesses; evidence for psychopathology; the infertility diagnosis and treatment; and coping skills being used individually and by the couple.[3] The best and most universally used assessment technique is the clinical interview. An example of an infertility-specific clinical interview is the Comprehensive Psychosocial History of Infertility (CPHI, see Appendix 3). Using either a standard clinical interview or the CPHI, professionals gain additional information on stress and coping through infertility-specific questions such as, "What is the most stressful part of infertility for you?"; "How would you rate your level stress at this time?"; "What do you find helpful for coping with infertility?"; "Is there any coping technique that your partner uses that you find stressful?" The genogram is another means of augmenting the clinical interview in that it provides a structure for gathering information about the individual's family system, social support, and religious and cultural backgrounds as well as identifying factors that may intensify or mediate the stresses of infertility (see Chapter 4).

Often infertility counselors supplement the clinical interview with objective data gained from standardized psychometric measures, questionnaires, and/or daily diaries that may or may not be infertility-specific. Objective measures provide a means of quickly assessing a patient's current state; confirming information from the clinical interview; and providing a basis in therapy for psycho-education, intervention, and treatment. Typically, measures of stress and coping have been based on self-report taking one of the following perspectives: stimulus-oriented, response-oriented, or interactional viewpoint. From the *stimulus-oriented view* of stress, assessment involves those aspects of the environment that are demanding or disorganizing for the individual, stress him or her. The *response-oriented* perspective, based on Selye's work, assesses the individual's response to stressful events in the environment. From the *interactional* perspective, characteristics in the individual and the environment as well as the individual's response to the environmental stressors are assessed. Examples of inventories that measure multiple psychological symptoms include the Minnesota Multiphasic Personality Disorder-2 (MMPI-2) and Symptom Checklist-90 (SCL-90), while examples of measures that assess a single psychological symptom include the Beck Depression Inventory (BDI) and State-Trait Anxiety Inventory (STAI). An example of a measure that assesses coping methods is the Ways of Coping Checklist (WCC), while an example of a coping measure that assesses task-oriented coping, emotion-focused coping, and avoidance-oriented coping is the Coping Inventory for Stressful Situations (CISS). The administration of some standardized psychometric tests (e.g., MMPI-2) is restricted in use to trained mental health professionals (typically psychologists), while other measures (e.g., BDI) are available for use by any mental health or medical caregiver.

Over the years, there has been an increase in the development and use of infertility-specific measures including standardized psychometric measures, questionnaires for research or clinical use, and daily/weekly rating scales. (see Appendix 4) Objective measures are often used in research but can be clinically useful in identifying those individuals and/or couples at risk of emotional maladjustment to the infertility experience and/or treatment, allowing early identification and psychotherapeutic intervention. Newton and colleagues developed a standardized objective measure that addresses infertility-specific stress (Fertility Problem Inventory), which assesses social, sexual, and relationship concerns as well as rejection of child-free lifestyle, the need for parenthood, and global stress. It is a forty-six-item measure using a Likert scale that includes questions on stressful aspects of infertility and has a global measure of stress.[64] Boivin and Takefman investigated psychosocial responses to infertility using an infertility-specific Daily Record Keeping Sheet in which patients rated their emotions and reactions each day of a treatment cycle (starting at day 1 and ending the day of report of the pregnancy test results).[65] They found that distress levels remained the same during the first half of the treatment cycle, during which ovulation induction and ovum retrieval occurred. However, significant increase in distress was noted at the end of the treatment cycle, just prior to the pregnancy test. In a study investigating infertility-specific psychological strain in couples in which weekly diary ratings were used, there was a general lack of distress or strain, even in response to medical investigations and diagnosis, except in individuals with preexisting psychopathology (e.g., depression or anxiety) as assessed by pretreatment standard psychometric measures. For these individuals, diary ratings did reflect elevated levels of distress over the course of diagnosis and treatment.[66] The use of daily rating scales has been applied to a variety of conditions in behavioral medicine but may have more research than clinical applications in that patient compliance has been found to be problematic. Recently, Schmidt and colleagues developed an infertility-specific coping inventory, based on the same Ways of Coping Questionnaire of Lazarus and Folkman and on qualitative interviews with infertile couples about infertility-specific distress and coping. The nineteen-item coping inventory is part of the Copenhagen Multicentre Psychosocial Infertility (COMPI) research program questionnaire administered to 2,250 women and men.[57,67] The inventory consists of four scales: active avoidant coping (e.g., avoid being with pregnant women or children), active confronting coping (e.g., ask other childless people for advice), passive avoidant coping (e.g., hope a miracle will happen), and meaning-based coping (e.g., find other life goals or gain meaning of pain and suffering of infertility).

Infertility-Specific Stress and Coping

Infertility often begins as an acute crisis, which individuals expect to be a time-limited stressor yet usually evolves into a chronic stressor experienced over an extended period of time. For the majority, infertility is not a discrete event but an evolving process initially involving a potential threat or loss that expands over time from a potential threat to a real threat (e.g., a future of childlessness, chronic illness, repeated medical treatments).[15] This evolutionary process typically involves an accumulation of losses both minor (e.g., uncomfortable medical diagnostic procedure) and major (e.g., miscarriage or diagnosis of a life-threatening genetic disorder). Infertility is stressful in that it is an unpredictable experience, which is negative, uncontrollable, and ambiguous. As such, the psychosocial strain of infertility involves an acute stressor during initial diagnosis and treatment that becomes a chronic strain over time and extended medical treatment trials. However, when levels of distress approach clinical significance or persist over an extended period of time, individuals typically experience psychological impairment of role functioning, mood, and self-esteem or diminished or impaired couple functioning.[15] In fact, infertile couples experience moderately elevated emotional strain during the initial stages of infertility diagnosis and treatment, which often returns to near normal levels in the second year of treatment. However, emotional well-being and relationship stability typically deteriorate significantly after the third year of treatment.[68] It is also important to note infertility is not experienced in a vacuum and that individuals and couples have other stresses occurring in their life besides infertility. Job pressures, family problems (e.g., illness and/or death of family members or friends), and national or international events (e.g., terrorism, hurricanes) are but a few life events that may impact the perception of stress and distress during infertility.

Neither patients nor caregivers can know or predict with accuracy individual or couple psychosocial responses to an infertility diagnosis; individual or couple resilience or ability to manage the stresses of infertility or treatment; and/or the outcome of treatment. Furthermore, the personal meaning of infertility is unique and idiosyncratic as are the thoughts (cognitions) individuals have about the experience. The meaning (attributions) and cognitions individuals have about infertility may, in and of themselves, be a source of stress. For some individuals, the experience of infertility violates deeply held beliefs about the world and their place in it. Infertility can (and does) challenge assumptions about a stable and predictable world and their beliefs in a benevolent and just world. Some may come to believe that life without children is meaningless and/or they are unworthy, if they are infertile or childless. Because infertility involves potential or actual loss of control over an important life goal and one's future, individual appraisals of the experience and their personal control within the context of infertility are significant to their experience of infertility and their adaptation to it.[60]

The Distressed but Resistant Infertile Patient

Most often reluctant and/or hostile patients present because the counseling session is required pretreatment preparation and educational counseling, or as a result of a referral by a medical caregiver of patients who have been identified as distressed, ill-prepared, or for some other reason. The reasons for the patient's hostility and resistance may vary, and Belar and Deardorff have described some common causes: (1) the patient was not told the reason for the referral or that it was to a mental health professional; (2) the patient has negative perceptions about psychological interventions, preferring to have infertility strictly defined in medical terms; (3) the patient is being asked to shift to a biopsychosocial model of infertility and treatment requiring more patient–caregiver collaboration and cooperation; (4) the patient is resistant or openly opposed to the behavioral changes recommended by the medical treatment team (e.g., weight loss, smoking, alcohol, and/or chemical cessation); and (5) patients rarely self-refer to a infertility counselor, thus tending to be more skeptical about the initial session than those individuals who have self-initiated contact with a mental health professional.[3]

Of these, the most typical source of reluctance is the individual focused on the medical aspects of infertility and treatment, and angry about what they perceive as the physician's implication that the problem is 'all in your head' or that the patient has to 'jump through hoops' with a mental health professional who they view as unqualified and irrelevant to their goal: pregnancy. Some indications of patient reluctance or hostility include: (1) refusal to schedule an appointment or to return for subsequent appointments; (2) anger and bewilderment during the initial session about the reason for the referral or refusing to discuss the problem; (3) polite cooperation during the initial session but then refusing to collaboratively address the issues and/or taking personal exception to what has been discussed; and/or (4) clear expression of their belief that pursuing medical treatments is a priority and counseling is not, even if/when it is required, recommended, or strongly encouraged by the treatment team.

Adapted from Belar and Deardorff, the following suggestions are recommendations and ideas for the infertility counselors to facilitate reduction of patient reluctance, hostility, and resistance in infertile patients referred to a mental health professional:[3]

Establish rapport. The infertility counselor should begin with a self-introduction that clearly states their name and position. Establish good eye contact with the patient(s), when possible, sit down while talking, and ask the patient to explain his or her understanding of the referral. Use this opportunity to clarify the purpose of the interview and dispel any misconceptions.

Ask open-ended questions. Yes–no questions are usually not questions but statements in disguise. The reluctant patient quickly assumes that the mental health professional has already determined a diagnosis or position, making the patient's input irrelevant and unnecessary.

Define the organic verus functional myth. As this is addressed in other chapters, it is probably most useful to begin with a discussion of the patient's feelings and thoughts about seeing a mental health professional about a medical issue and to discuss the infertility counselor's relationship with the medical treatment team. It is crucial to allow the patient to acknowledge the real aspects of the medical condition to reduce the patient's anxiety. Yet this discussion should be as abbreviated as possible to focus on more useful short-term goals that support adaptive behaviors and improve coping and stress management.[55]

Avoid 'psychologizing' the patient's symptoms. Many patients are not psychologically minded or insightful, or even interested in viewing things differently. As such, it is important to give the patient something concrete during the first interview such as some explanation of biopsychosocial aspects of infertility, a rationale for infertility counseling, or a plan for cognitive restructuring or implementing stress reduction strategies.

Shape adequate beliefs rather than challenge misconceptions. While the initial interview should focus primarily on listening and encouragement, acknowledging but not overtly challenging the patient's reluctance to participate can facilitate the patient's willingness to return, if warranted.

Present the treatment strategy in a positive, collaboratively developed plan, rather than as a last resort. Very often patients (or even caregivers) perceive a referral to the infertility counselor as a 'last resort' when no other medical treatment options are readily available. Patients may feel they have 'failed' or that the medical system has 'failed' or 'rejected' them. The infertility counselor may be helpful in facilitating caregiver communication as well as helping patients define (or redefine) their goals regarding treatment or other family-building alternatives.

Foster realistic expectations about treatment. Many infertile patients are ill-prepared for the time commitment of infertility and even less prepared for the time commitment of psychotherapeutic interventions. Providing a clear rationale and treatment plan can help patients remain hopeful and realistic while providing emotional support and encouraging healthy coping strategies. It is also helpful during this session to address any expectations of an 'instant' or 'sudden' cure (e.g., "I wouldn't be stressed if I were just pregnant"); that the patient's role is more active and participatory; and that there will be 'ups and downs' in infertility counseling just as there are in infertility treatment.

Clarify other treatment roles. The infertility counselor should be prepared to educate the patient about how psychological treatment will interface with ongoing infertility treatment. Part of the infertility counselor's role may be provision of patient education as well as stress management, support, and facilitation of communication between patients and caregivers. While the patient should expect confidentiality, within behavioral medicine practice the separation of roles and responsibilities may be redefined. One of the dilemmas of infertility counseling is the distressed patient who lacks insight into how their distress is impacting them; their social relationships; their treatment; and/or their interactions with members of the treatment team. All too often these patients (and their caregivers) are so

intensely focused on their reproductive goals and medical treatment that the very real and obvious distress is minimized and ignored, despite clear warning signs in the patient and by caregivers. Referrals for assistance to an infertility counselor at this point often become more crisis intervention and are all the more challenging as the expectation from the patient and medical team is an 'instant cure' despite the patient's hostility, resistance, and reluctance to address the circumstances that brought them to this crisis state of distress.

THERAPEUTIC INTERVENTIONS

Infertility counselors use a wide array of therapeutic techniques and interventions. Whatever the therapeutic intervention used, the goal is to improve patient emotional health and well-being; promote healthy coping strategies; provide a supportive environment for the expression of feelings; support the acquisition of healthy emotional skills and/or behavioral changes; improve stress management; and, ultimately, to possibly improve fertility treatment outcome. Although the infertility counselor may use any or all of these strategies in one form or another, it must be noted that some of these interventions require specialized training and/or certification or licensure (e.g., hypnosis and biofeedback). The focus of this section is on psychoeducational counseling, psychotherapeutic interventions, and health behavior change interventions that improve coping strategies and facilitate stress reduction.

Psychoeducation

The primary aim of psychoeducation is enhancing patient education, preparation, and knowledge of their medical diagnosis, treatment, and any concomitant or relevant psychosocial implications, thereby enhancing patient control and diminishing feelings of helplessness. Patient information is an integral part of infertility counseling that enhances patient understanding and improves psychosocial and physical well-being. Infertility counselors provide information about health behavior; diagnosis and treatment protocols of procedures; typical emotional and marital responses to infertility and/or treatment for it; effective coping strategies; relaxation techniques; and how to access appropriate medical or psychological care. Infertility counselors also educate patients about health behaviors that can improve their general health as well as preserve and/or enhance their fertility or treatment outcomes (e.g., obesity, smoking, and alcohol use). Psychoeducational information may be provided through a variety of mediums including patient education handouts and booklets. In addition to these traditional forms of patient education, videos, computer-facilitated learning, and the internet can all play an important role in providing patient education, particularly if and when patients are directed to appropriate internet sites.

An assumption of patient education approaches is that if healthcare professionals can assist individuals in knowing what to expect regarding diagnostic or treatment procedures, patients will benefit as a result of an enhanced sense of control and more informed decision making. Certainly, some infertile individuals are active information seekers; however, information alone often is insufficient for decreasing stress.[69] Its effects may vary substantially as a function of characteristics of the information offered (e.g., information regarding the medial procedure itself, potential psychological response, or recommended coping strategies); the nature of the stressor (e.g., its controllability); and patient characteristics (e.g., preference for information). This seems to be particularly important in that patients using assisted reproductive technologies have been consistently found to *overestimate* personal likelihood of success, despite patient education about treatment success rates.

There is significant evidence that preparatory (pre-treatment) information can be beneficial to infertility patients both during and after treatment, although it is important to differentiate between the different kinds of information provided and patient preferences regarding education and information. Takefman and colleagues randomly assigned couples beginning medical investigation of infertility to one of three interventions: (1) information videotape regarding procedural aspects of diagnostic tests only; (2) videotape on diagnostic procedures as well as the emotional aspects of the medical procedure; and (3) videotape on diagnostic procedures and emotional strains as well as an information pamphlet on relationships issues.[70] Decreased infertility-specific negative feelings and increased infertility knowledge were found to be most significant in the group receiving the procedural information only. Furthermore, groups that received the enhanced information did not demonstrate significant benefit across the course of the medical investigation. Although a no-treatment control group was not included, suggestive evidence that information provision is useful comes from Connolly and colleagues.[71] Couples undergoing a first IVF attempt were assigned randomly to a single session of oral and written information provision regarding IVF treatment procedures or to an information session plus three sessions of nondirective counseling across a treatment cycle. State anxiety dropped significantly over the course of treatment; however, counsel-

ing did not enhance anxiety reduction over information provision alone.

Further evidence of positive effects of patient education, at least when combined with other interventions, was provided by Newton and associates.[49] Highly anxious women preparing for oocyte retrieval were assigned randomly to relaxation training alone or to relaxation training plus education (a booklet) regarding the retrieval procedure, the accompanying sensory experience, and coping mechanisms. Those who received relaxation training along with information reported less anxiety and pain surrounding the retrieval procedure than did women who received relaxation training alone. It is difficult to determine what specific aspect of the information provision was beneficial and whether the benefit was attributable to enhanced professional attention provided to those in the more comprehensive intervention or the specific relaxation or coping strategies themselves. However, these results suggest that information to enhance infertile patients' understanding of particular medical procedures, offered within the context of training in techniques to cope with the procedure, may be beneficial. Although men are generally less likely to access patient educational materials, one study found that for men undergoing infertility treatment, educational materials may be beneficial, at least in a subgroup of men, in facilitating treatment compliance and reducing treatment-specific distress.[72]

In recent years there has been an impressive and growing array of patient education resources for infertile patients, influenced in part by consumer demand but also by increased access to multimedia means of information dissemination. Patient education materials have become a small industry including videotapes, audiotapes, internet websites and self-help books addressing both the medical and psychological aspects of infertility, pamphlets from pharmaceutical companies, multilingual materials from local and international support organizations, and professional organizations providing patient education. Patients are also educating themselves through radio, television, telephone and internet help-lines, and the internet. Additionally, the development of multimedia approaches (e.g., videos, CDs) has been found to be useful in offering a broad range of information on infertility diagnosis, treatment, emotional response, and coping strategies as well as easily accessible educational and support opportunities.[73]

Individuals and couples using assisted reproduction have been found to be more likely to use the internet as a source of information about infertility than couples involved in other forms of fertility treatment.[74,75]

Additionally, women seem to be more active internet users in both seeking fertility-related information and emotional support. Furthermore, the internet can be a potential source of patient education materials for infertility counselors as it allows the infertility counselor to tailor the information to a specific patient's needs as well as educate patients about how to use the internet as a resource and which sites are more appropriate for their needs than others. Nevertheless, some information obtained through these patient education sources (e.g., the internet and organizations or companies with a specific 'agenda') may provide inaccurate or misleading information or may be misunderstood by patients. As such, the infertility counselor can be helpful in guiding patients toward appropriate websites and educating them on how to carefully evaluate and assess information sources. A belief that more information is better is naïve, as some patients actually do worse with more information. Thus, the clinician must have a strong understanding of the literature he or she is recommending to practice effectively.[3]

In short, patient preparation for infertility treatment should contain, at minimum, information on the treatment procedure. Additionally, educational and/or supportive information should be tailored to the needs of the specific patient. This is particularly relevant as individual personality and coping styles can and do impact information processing. Individual coping styles vary in that not all patients are active information seekers, and forcing information on patients who prefer a more avoidant coping approach is not appropriate nor clinically helpful. In contrast, patient self-efficacy can be supported by facilitating and guiding information seeking through educational materials or pretreatment information packets that include information on treatment procedures, psychological factors, and additional resources that patients can use selectively in concurrence with their coping style.

Psychotherapeutic Interventions

The benefits of infertility-specific psychotherapeutic interventions including individual, marital, sex, and group therapies are addressed in other chapters. However, there is increasing evidence of the usefulness of psychotherapy for stress reduction with infertile individuals. Even though psychological counseling can improve quality-of-life, any suggestion that it can or will confer biological advantage (i.e., increase treatment success or improve pregnancy rates) must be interpreted cautiously. Typically, infertility-specific psychotherapy rarely involves a single therapeutic approach but, rather, an eclectic use of a variety of treatment modalities in which a variety of interventions are

TABLE 11.1. Adaptive tasks for managing crisis and stress of infertility[76]
Establish meaning and personal significance of infertility for each partner and for the couple
Confront reality of infertility and respond to the requirements of medical treatment and psychosocial distress
Sustain personal relationships with family members, friends, and others who may be helpful
Maintain reasonable emotional balance (i.e., morale)
Preserve a satisfactory self-image and sense of competence

engaged to facilitate the therapeutic process. Whatever the form of psychotherapeutic intervention or treatment modality, the goals of the intervention should be healthy adaptation to infertility. Defining and addressing systematically the central adaptive tasks for managing the stresses of infertility enhances a sense of control and mastery over the infertility experiences for both individuals and couples[76] (see Table 11.1).

Relaxation Techniques

There are a wide variety of relaxation techniques that have been useful in inducing the relaxation response which interrupts the cascade of negative physiological responses to stress (e.g., increased heart rate, blood pressure, respiratory rate, and muscle tension). Relaxation techniques include diaphragmatic breathing; progressive muscle relaxation (PMR); autogenic relaxation training; imagery (e.g., guided imagery and covert sensitization); hypnosis; biofeedback; systematic desensitization; modeling skills training; behavioral rehearsal; and exercise. One study found that group interventions that emphasized education and skills training (e.g., relaxation training) were significantly more effective in producing positive change than counseling interventions that emphasized emotional expression and support and/or discussion about thoughts and feelings related to infertility. Men and women were found to benefit equally from psychosocial interventions.[50] Furthermore, there is some evidence that interventions based on the principles of the relaxation response and mind–body programs specifically adapted for infertile women are beneficial in improving quality-of-life and may be helpful in improving fertility rates and/or treatment outcomes.[77]

Whether relaxation training is a specific goal of psychotherapy or a patient 'homework' assignment, patient preparation regarding the importance of relaxation training in infertility treatment is important. Relaxation is thought to positively affect the endocrine and immune systems, which could explain a possible positive relation to fertility and some evidence that relaxation may modify immune responses under hypnosis, by expression of emotion or by relaxation training.[78] Hypnosis based on imagery and a relaxation strategy may be beneficial in modifying attitude, increasing optimism, and facilitating mind–body interaction as well as possibly improving treatment outcomes.[79,80] Some infertility counselors are properly trained and/or certified to include hypnosis, biofeedback, massage therapy, or yoga in their treatment interventions while others refer patients who would benefit from these treatments to qualified professionals (preferably with some expertise in reproductive medicine). Another example of a relaxation technique that is easily introduced and potentially beneficial is meditation, which has been found to have many healing and relaxing effects on the body. Meditation is a private activity that is about disciplining the mind to focus or concentrate on peace and tranquility. Infertility counselors can introduce the basics of medication including its purpose (e.g., relief from chaotic, stressful thoughts and feelings) and principles (e.g., focus on calm breathing, a sound, or a simple, peaceful thought). Some patients prefer to term this form of relaxation as 'purposeful meditation' while others find spirituality or prayer more applicable to them.

Cognitive Restructuring

Cognitive restructuring is a construct or therapeutic intervention based on cognitive-behavioral theory, which is a unique combination of behaviorism and cognitive psychology: Behaviorism focuses on changing overt behaviors rather than on understanding subjective feelings, unconscious processes, or motivations, while cognitive psychology involves changing thought processes. Cognitive psychology applies social learning principles based on three basic propositions: (1) cognitive activity affects behavior, (2) behavior can be monitored, and (3) behavioral changes can be effected through cognitive changes. Cognitive-behavioral application to infertility emphasizes current behavior, thoughts, and feelings about the medical situation rather than long-term, in-depth discussions of early childhood experiences; unconscious motivations; or inner psychic conflicts as causal factors of infertility

Cognitive therapy encourages patients to see that their stress does not always come from an outside event or situation (e.g., infertility treatment) – it may have much more to do with how they perceive their situation (e.g., thoughts that they will remain childless forever). Accordingly, stress is the perception of a threat to an individual's physical or psychological well-being

and the perception that one is unable to cope with that threat.[81] While individuals may be unable to alter the stressful situation, they can change their perception of that stress and their thoughts about it. The basic principles of cognitive therapy are: (1) an individual's thoughts and cognitions create most of his or her moods and emotions; (2) when people are depressed or anxious, their thoughts are primarily negative; and (3) negative thoughts almost always contain distortions and exaggerations and are, as such, irrational. Cognitive restructuring, a technique of cognitive therapy, helps individuals change the *way* they think and *what* they think. It provides a means of recognizing that stress is often caused by negative thoughts and that these thoughts create moods or emotions which, in turn, can affect physical symptoms and behaviors.[82] The goals of cognitive restructuring are to train patients to: (1) identify negative automatic thoughts; (2) recognize the connection between their thoughts and their feelings; (3) identify the thoughts and attitudes that are distorted, exaggerated, or illogical; (4) challenge these automatic thoughts; (5) substitute more realistic and positive thoughts and beliefs, which will reduce painful feelings (narrative repair); (6) practice *in vivo*; and (7) prepare for relapse.

Cognitive appraisal of the infertility experience is central to psychosocial interventions and applications of stress and coping theories with infertile couples. In short, the personal meaning(s) of infertility for each individual and couple defines the experience (e.g., what is specifically stressful about infertility for them) and, ultimately, determines adaptation and adjustment (e.g., effectiveness of their coping strategies) over the long term. Extensive research has found that patients experience considerable emotional distress when fertility treatment is unsuccessful, which may be related to thoughts and expectations that define the experience and, perhaps, the outcome. In fact, research has indicated significantly increased levels of depression, anxiety, and distress after only *one* unsuccessful treatment cycle.[37,47] While cognitions of helplessness have been related to unsuccessful treatment outcomes, more positive thoughts about one's ability to manage the demands of infertility and treatment (e.g., emotional equanimity) have been found to be related to more positive adjustment and better treatment outcomes.[18,40,83–87]

Increasingly, research in infertility has focused on identifying relationships between physiological factors and psychosocial interventions. Of particular interest has been the identification of the role of 'stress hormones' such as cortisol levels in reproduction, particularly in women. Berga and associates found that

---

TABLE 11.2. Cognitions regarding infertility (adapted from Evers)[129]

To what extent do you agree with the following items (1 = strongly disagree to 5 = strongly agree)? Scores of helplessness and acceptance are obtained by sum of scores on the six items of both scales. Higher scores mean more helplessness and more acceptance. Mean scores on helplessness in Dutch population: 11.5 (SD = 5.3) and acceptance: 13.6 (SD = 4.9) (N = 386)

Helplessness:

   My infertility frequently makes me feel helpless

   My infertility limits me in everything that is important to me

   My infertility controls my life

   Because of my infertility, I miss the things I like to do most

   My infertility prevents me from doing what I would really like to do

   My infertility makes me feel useless at times

Acceptance:

   I have learned to accept my infertility

   I have learned to live with my infertility

   I can accept my infertility well

   I can cope effectively with my infertility

   I think I can handle the problems related to my infertility even if they will not be solved

   I can handle the problems related to my infertility

---

cortisol secretion was higher in women with functional hypothalamic amenorrhea than in women with other causes of anovulation or eumenorrheic women.[88, 89] An association between increased hypothalamic-pituitary-adrenal activity and reduced Gn-RH drive supports the concept that functional hypothalamic amenorrhea develops in response to stress-induced alterations in central neural function that modify hypothalamic function. The researchers used cognitive-behavior interventions (specifically cognitive restructuring) to minimize problematic attitudes linked to hypothalamic allostasis; mediate stress; and reduce cortisol levels. Within twenty weeks of beginning cognitive-behavioral therapy, 87% of the women had regained ovulation compared to 25% of the control group women. These researchers concluded that prompt ovarian response to cognitive-behavioral therapy as a behavioral intervention may provide an efficacious treatment option for some women, particularly those for whom pharmacological modalities may be inapplicable or unacceptable.[88,89]

Based on a similar approach, cognitions with respect to infertility have been shown to be predictive of short-term as well as long-term emotional adjustment to unsuccessful fertility treatment.[90] Cognitions of helplessness seem to be related to worse posttreatment adjustment, while cognitions of acceptance seem to be related to better adjustment to unsuccessful IVF (see Table 11.2). Addressing helplessness and acceptance during treatment provides opportunities for restructuring of cognitions that are maladaptive (i.e., helplessness) into adaptive cognitions (i.e., acceptance in terms of feeling able to successfully manage the stresses of infertility). An example of the application of cognitive-behavioral therapy in the field of infertility is a ten-week group program for women that includes relaxation, stress management, cognitive restructuring, nutritional education, and body work. Outside of the group, participants perform relaxation exercises daily. This structured patient education, relaxation, and psychotherapeutic program (e.g., cognitive-behavioral therapy) improved stress management skills and positive mood compared with a counseling support and a control group.[91] In another study involving couples undergoing six months of cognitive-behavioral therapy, researchers reported decreased thoughts of helplessness; decreased marital distress; and improved sexual satisfaction.[92] The program was designed to alleviate infertility-specific anxiety; to dispel maladaptive cognitions; and to encourage behavior likely to improve chances of conception. The study reported higher conception rates and less distress in the treatment group, but the lack of a control group does not permit firm conclusions.

Coping Strategies

When confronting infertility as a stressful situation, individuals use two component cognitive appraisal processes enabling them to assess the situation and their ability to manage it and maintain well-being.[61] *Primary appraisal* addresses the question: 'What is at stake in this encounter?' and, as such, the infertile individual evaluates the nature and magnitude of infertility-specific threats and challenges as well as any other life stressors. In *secondary appraisal* the question is 'What, if anything, can I do about it?,' which involves the initiation of the infertile individual's coping strategies. Coping is active, multidimensional, and, for the most part, situation-specific.[57] As such, coping represents an individual's constantly changing and evolving cognitive and behavioral efforts to manage the external and/or internal demands of a specific stressor.[57] However, avoidance and self-blame coping techniques have been found to contribute to greater infertility-specific distress, while garnering emotional support has been found to be associated with more positive adjustment.[61]

Coping strategies were identified earlier as: (1) *emotion-focused*, (2) *problem-focused*, and (3) *appraisal or meaning-focused*. *Emotion-focused* coping such as venting distressing feelings, seeking social support, or managing feelings through self-control can be calming, comforting, and a means of gaining control of overwhelming emotions. By contrast, *problem-focused* coping strategies such as conscious problem-solving, information gathering, and contingency planning can mediate the painful experiences of infertility by taking action. Infertility counselors can facilitate *appraisal-focused* coping through gentle questions that encourage reappraisal while acknowledging the painful distress of infertility (e.g., 'Has anything positive come out of this experience for you?'; 'Has going through this experience together strengthened your relationship in any way?'; 'Has anything happened during this very stressful time that made you feel more positive about yourself or your relationship?').[76]

Encouraging and bolstering adaptive coping skills is an important therapeutic goal even though no coping strategy is inherently and universally adaptive or maladaptive. Table 11.3 identifies coping strategies suggested by clinical or empirical literature. Coping is most effective when the strategy is responsive to contextual demands and congruent with an individual's personality, culture, and personal values. Studies on the effectiveness of coping with infertility-specific stress have revealed equivocal results with some studies, indicating problem-focused coping as helpful.[87,93] Others have found no specific coping strategy more beneficial than another. Differences in results may be the result of the earlier stated principles of stress and coping in that what is stressful is idiosyncratic and no coping strategy is universally effective or applicable across all stressful situations.[43,94] As such, acknowledging and addressing individual differences may be the most effective therapeutic intervention available. Simply asking each partner to articulate the top three most stressful things about infertility for you at this time can be helpful in setting the foundation for the next coping stage: what to do.

Avoidance and self-blame coping techniques have been found to contribute to greater infertility-specific distress, while garnering emotional support has been found to be associated with more positive adjustment.[61] Problem-solving strategies seem to be more effective for specific situations and/or alterable aspects of infertility (e.g., whether to pursue a specific treatment or form of family-building) while emotion-focused coping strategies seem to be more useful for uncontrollable aspects of infertility (e.g., grief following treatment failure). Consistently, meaning or appraisal-focused coping strategies have been found to be useful as both short-term and long-term coping strategies. Appraisal-focused coping is a form of cognitive restructuring, reappraisal, and giving meaning to a situation that is unpredictable, uncontrollable, and existentially challenging. As such, it can be palliative over the short and long term.[67,93]

A study by Schmidt and colleagues found that difficulties in partner communication significantly predicted high infertility-specific stress for both men and women. Active-avoidant coping (e.g., avoiding being with pregnant women or children; using alcohol, drugs, or gambling as self-distraction/reward) was also found to be a significant predictor of high infertility-specific stress. Among men, high use of active-confrontive coping (e.g., gathering information about treatment alternatives, exercise, or sports) predicted low infertility-specific stress, while for women, medium or high use of meaning-based (garnering social suport and emotional venting) coping significantly predicted low infertility-specific stress.[95] Women undergoing ART were more likely to use distancing and denial as coping strategies than women pursuing motherhood through adoption or surrogacy. General physical and psychosocial well-being and negative coping strategies seemed to be predictive of long-term well-being as well as treatment outcome. Women who remained childless were more likely to use distancing and denial coping strategies than women pursuing adoption or ARTs. Younger women used different coping strategies than older women to process and overcome infertility-specific distress.[96] Among both men and women, difficulties in partner communication predicted high infertility-specific stress. These findings provide some guidance on what coping strategies are most helpful for men and women, particularly after medical treatment has been unsuccessful over time.[95]

TABLE 11.3. Sample patient coping strategies suggested by clinical or empirical literature[76]

Use relaxation audiotapes, videotapes, compact discs

Improve decision-making and problem-solving skills

Take treatment holidays

Learn and use self-hypnosis or guided imagery

Learn the benefits of physical well-being (e.g., exercise and massage)

Pay attention to nutrition and eating a balanced diet (reduce or gain weight if necessary)

Eliminate recreational drugs, alcohol, tobacco; eliminate or cut down on caffeine

Get plenty of sleep

Learn and practice positive reappraisal

Use relaxing music during specific medical procedures

Reduce daily hassles and minor stressors (e.g., improve time management)

Get assertiveness training if needed

Increase pleasurable activities

Seek information on infertility and/or coping through books, videos, organizations, or the internet that are accurate respected

Enhance spirituality (e.g., prayer, meditation, religious services, rituals, or pastoral counseling)

Learn to manage hostility and anger

Expand support system by confiding in a trusted friend or joining a support group

Find enjoyment in the company of loved ones and friendships

Learn to decrease worry and anxiety through relaxation, meditation, or progressive relaxation

Laugh more and look for humor

Try to maintain a realistic yet positive and hopeful attitude

Get a pet or spend time with animals

Refute irrational ideas

Learn thought-stopping and how to refute illogical fears

Turn to nature for comfort (e.g., plant a garden, visit parks)

Volunteer and find time for kindness to others

Structure infertility treatment as much as possible (i.e., manage what you can)

Find ways to soothe yourself daily

Take frequent brief weekends to relax and enjoy life and your partner

Establish realistic goals and expectations of treatments or success rates

Improve management of financial matters

Identify stress responses and successful coping techniques

Improve communication skills

In short, maladaptive coping strategies (e.g., distancing and denial) may be less useful and couples should be encouraged to consider strategies that encourage dealing with the psychological distress (e.g., problem-solving), which may not only facilitate goal attainment (i.e., parenthood), but also increase self-efficacy and self-esteem. Individuals and couples should be encouraged to expand upon their coping strategies, using a variety that include acknowledgment and expression of emotion; active, problem-solving coping; stress management; self-control; emotional expression; relaxation techniques; and cognitive restructuring that involves reappraisal, meaning, and acceptance. Finally, the infertile individual and couple may have to be in a constant process of rearranging, recycling, and reevaluating their coping strategies over the course of their infertility experience and treatment. Different coping strategies for coping with infertility are presented in Table 11.4.

Health Behavior Change Interventions

Health behavior interventions and health efficacy behaviors are relevant in infertility, particularly in

TABLE 11.4. Strategies for coping with infertility[130]

Meaning-based or appraisal-focused coping
　Be mentally prepared
　Accept and redefine
　Keep busy, avoid, and deny

Problem-focused coping
　Seek information and support
　Take action to be a problem solver
　Look to alternative rewards

Emotion-focused coping
　Calm acceptance of emotions
　Emotional discharge
　Resigned acceptance

regard to health behavior changes that may impact fertility by improving overall health and/or treatment outcomes (e.g., patients with weight, smoking, alcohol, or other lifestyle problems). Self-efficacy beliefs are based on the premise that an individual is capable of accomplishing a particular behavior, task, or goal including a particular behavior change regarding health. Self-efficacy beliefs help determine how much *effort* people are willing to expend on an activity, how long they will *persevere* when confronting obstacles, and how *resilient* they will be in the face of adverse situations. The higher the sense of self-efficacy, the greater the effort, persistence, and resilience.

Regarding patients with fertility problems, addressing weight, smoking, and alcohol/drug use is important because these issues have been shown to have a significant impact overall health as well as fertility. Tech-

niques to support patients in changing health behavior are motivational interviewing or patient-centered approaches to the consultation. Patients who judge the behavior change as important, and have confidence to achieve them will be more ready to change their behavior and are more likely to succeed.[97] Healthcare providers have to pay attention to these three aspects in the consultation. Both motivational interviewing and patient-centered techniques rely heavily on the communication techniques of the healthcare provider. In general, clinicians have to recognize the patient's phase in the process to change health behavior and adjust interventions accordingly. There are four phases:

(1) precontemplation: not seriously considering behavior change;
(2) contemplation: having some thoughts about changing;
(3) action: initial behavioral change;
(4) maintenance: maintaining behavior change.[98]

For some patients, supportive initiatives by their healthcare providers are enough for them to adopt more healthy behaviors, while others need more substantial support encouragement. Behavioral medicine approaches to change health behaviors have shown to be effective in smoking cessation and weight loss in general populations. Cognitive-behavioral therapy interventions generally consist of comparable elements that are presented in Table 11.5.

The American Public Health Service suggested five A's as a golden standard for smoking cessation treatment that can also be adapted to other health behavior: (1) ask about smoking (or weight problem) at every opportunity; (2) advise all smokers to stop or all obese patients to lose weight; (3) assess willingness to stop

TABLE 11.5. Cognitive-behavioral therapy strategies for changing health behavior such as weight loss and smoking cessation[101,111]

Daily self-monitoring with respect to problem behavior and exercise patterns	Recording amounts and types of food eaten and frequency, intensity, and type of physical activity; recording smoking frequency, time, and circumstances
Stimulus control	Keeping high-calorie foods out of the house; limit times and places of eating; removing ashtrays, removing cigarettes in the house, avoiding places that provoke smoking
Stress management	Eating or smoking may alleviate stress in short term; change coping style by training in other coping strategies: meditation and relaxation
Contingency management	Reward self for actions that support the change in eating or smoking behavior
Cognitive restructuring	Changing unrealistic goals and irrational cognitions with respect to weight loss and body image: > I had that snack, but I can still follow my diet the rest of the day.
Developing social support	Family, friends, and colleagues can assist a patient in maintaining motivation and providing positive reinforcement; some patients may benefit from support groups.

TABLE 11.6. BMI normal/Obesity cutoffs

18.5–24.9 = normal weight

25–29.9 = pre-obese

30+ = obesity

Obesity class I = 30–34.9

Obesity class II = 35–39.9

Obesity class III (extreme obesity) = 40+

or to change behavior; (4) assist patients in stopping or changing health behavior (including use of pharmacotherapy); and (5) arrange follow-up visits.

Obesity and Malnutrition

BMI is a measurement of obesity developed during the 1980s and adopted by the World Health Organization (WHO) as an inexact measurement enabling comparison and assessment of obesity globally. The body mass index (BMI), based on height and weight, is calculated using a formula in which weight is divided by the square of the height:

$$\mathrm{BMI} = \frac{weight}{height^2}$$

The BMI is a calculation of normal/obesity cutoffs calculated using kilograms and meters (http://nhlbisupport.com/bmi/bmi-m.htm) or pounds and inches (http://nhlbisupport.com/bmi/bmicalc.htm). WHO guidelines for normal (ideal) weight is BMI = 18.5 to 24.9. A body mass index (BMI) of 25 to 29.9 is considered overweight, and obesity is defined as a BMI of 30 or above. Additionally, WHO guidelines make distinctions based on body type, for example, WHO normal/overweight threshold for Asians is BMI = 23. As noted in Table 11.6, obesity is categorized in terms of normal weight and obesity cutoffs.

Obesity, as both a health concern and a reproductive risk factor, has gained increasing attention worldwide. Obesity, being underweight, poor nutritional habits, and disordered eating have been shown to negatively impact overall health, fertility, and the outcome of fertility treatment, particularly in women.[99–101] In the United States one-quarter of all women of childbearing age are obese (BMI > 30).[101] In Europe, the prevalence of obesity among women varies from less than 10% in France, Italy, and The Netherlands to about 20% in Germany, United Kingdom, and Finland.[102] Fertility issues in women who are overweight or obese include increased incidence of infertility; irregular or infrequent menstrual cycles; miscarriage; and decreased success with fertility treatments. Poten-

tial pregnancy complications due to obesity include increased risk of high blood pressure; diabetes; birth defects; high birth-weight babies; and Cesarean section. Weight loss of 5–10% can dramatically improve ovulation and pregnancy rates; improve health including reducing the risk of diabetes, high blood pressure, and heart disease; and improve overall quality-of-life.[103] In short, obesity defined as a BMI > 25 is a risk factor that has an impact on fertility and the outcome of treatment in both men and women, but particularly for women during infertility treatment and pregnancy.

An example of the interrelationship between obesity and fertility problems in women is Polycystic Ovarian Syndrome (PCOS), which causes increased androgen and hyperinsulinemia, contributing to weight gain and obesity. For PCOS women, losing weight (maintaining a BMI between 20 and 30) decreases androgen and increases ovulation.[104,105] Little attention has been given to the impact of weight and nutritional factors on male fertility although there is some evidence that nutritional deficiencies may cause impaired male reproduction, although the mechanisms for this are not clearly understood.[106]

Underweight is defined as a BMI lower than 19. Underweight women (BMI < 20) have been found to have higher incidence of amenorrhea and/or annovulation and reduced IVF success rates. Additionally, less than ideal weight not only impairs fertility, but it is also a risk factor for pregnancy complications.[100] Malnutrition in both men and women is a treatable and preventable condition that can and does impact reproduction in men and women.[107] Whether underweight due to acute malnutrition (e.g., famine) or self-imposed weight loss (e.g., anorexia nervosa), low BMI is associated with a dramatic decrease in fertility. In developing countries, weight-related amenorrhea and delayed menarche are largely the result of nutritional deprivation from borderline body weight in women. However, reduced weight in Western countries is more often the result of disordered eating (e.g., bulimia and anorexia nervosa). In fact, self-imposed weight loss is the most common single cause of secondary amenorrhea in the developed world. Simple weight loss of more than 30% of body fat can cause impaired fertility. Although there is currently no clearly defined threshold between impaired fertility and normal reproduction in men and women, there is now significant evidence that optimal weight levels can and do impact fertility and the success of treatment outcomes.

The reality is that the majority of obese infertile patients visiting healthcare professionals are not counseled or educated about the importance of weight loss and the impact of weight (under or over) on fertility and fertility treatment outcome.[108,109] Clinicians tend to avoid addressing the issue of health behavior change regarding weight with patients for a variety of reasons including: time constraints; perceived lack of professional expertise; respect for the patient's privacy; avoidance of patient distress or conflict with the patient; and pessimism about the effectiveness of interventions.[110] Generally, the best treatment approach for weight issues (under or over) is to *not* avoid the issue and to address weight in the same calm, nonjudgmental, clinical manner used to address other health concerns. The clinician should allow sufficient time to address this issue with the patient and be prepared for resistance, emotional distress, and even psychopathology (e.g., disordered eating). If there are clinical parameters or protocols regarding weight and infertility treatment, these should be addressed as well. Patient education materials should be made available as well as referrals and/or resources to address the weight issue (e.g., weight loss program and psychological care for disordered eating). The patient should be reassured that the caregiver's focus and goals are the same as the patient's: protecting the patient's health and well-being; maximizing their fertility; and facilitating a healthy pregnancy for the mother and the birth of a healthy baby. The optimum treatments for obesity are behavioral therapy programs that include reduced caloric intake; increased physical activity; and educational and behavioral support services.[111] The behavioral therapy approach has been shown to be more effective in long-term weight reduction than pharmacological treatments, bariatric surgery, or 'fad diets.' Few studies have evaluated the effect of psychosocial interventions for pretreatment weight reduction to enhance fertility. However, one study showed positive effects of a weight reduction program on factors related to reproductive outcome such as blood glucose, insulin, androstenedione, dihydrotestosterone, and estradiol concentrations in women with fertility problems[104]. Clark and colleagues found direct positive effects of weight loss programs on reproductive outcome.[105,112] They reported increased ovulation and pregnancy rates in women who had completed a weight loss program to maximize fertility compared to women who had dropped out of the weight loss program.

Smoking and Tobacco Use

As with weight, there has been a growing awareness of the negative impact of smoking and tobacco usage on reproduction in both men and women. Currently, one in three adults, or 1.2 billion people, use tobacco worldwide.[113] In the United States, 30% of women of reproductive age smoke compared to 35% of men. The available biologic, experimental, and epidemiological data indicate that up to 13% of infertility may be attributable to cigarette smoking.[114] Smoking in women appears to accelerate the loss of reproductive function and may advance the time of menopause by one to four years. It is also associated with increased risk of miscarriage and ectopic pregnancy. Furthermore, smoking impairs fertility by reducing the number and quality of oocytes as well as ovarian stimulation, fertilization, implantation, and pregnancy. Apart from pregnancy complications due to smoking, fetuses born to smoking mothers are at risk for low birth weight and other complicating conditions.[115–118] In men, smoking impairs sperm quality and IVF treatment outcomes.[119,120] Semen parameters and results of sperm function tests have been found to be generally poorer in smokers than nonsmokers. However, results of a meta-analysis examining the outcome of ART cycles indicated that smokers required nearly twice the number of IVF attempts to conceive as nonsmokers.[114,121] Although smoking has been found to have an impact on male fertility, the use of tobacco can also cause male-factor infertility. In a study that examined the use of chewing tobacco by men undergoing infertility evaluation, researchers found decreased sperm quality and, to a lesser extent, oligospermia and/or azoospermia.[122]

While there is a greater understanding of the detrimental effects of smoking on reproduction, the majority of infertile patients are not advised by their healthcare providers to stop smoking, even though clinicians can facilitate smoking cessation by providing education, monitoring, and consistent individualized support.[110] There are a variety of smoking cessation approaches including nicotine replacement, behavioral therapy, hypnotherapy, and antidepressants, all of which have been shown to be effective. A drawback of nicotine replacement is that it remains a nicotine delivery system and, as such, is less than optimum for infertile patients pursuing conception, particularly via ART. Hence, antidepressants and behavioral therapy that focuses on health behavior change and includes a variety of techniques such as hypnosis, patient education, caregiver/self-monitoring, and support programs may be more optimal smoking cessation approaches for infertile men and women.[114]

Alcohol and Drug Usage

It is estimated that 70 million people in the world have alcohol use disorders, including harmful use and dependence – 78% of whom remain untreated. The rate of alcohol use disorder for men is 2.8% and for women 0.5%. An estimated 5 million people worldwide use illicit drugs.[113] However, there is now evidence of a relationship between excessive use of alcohol (>2 units daily) and reduced fertility in both women and men, although the exact causal mechanisms have yet to be clarified.[99,123]

Heavy alcohol consumption in men has been found to cause impotence, infertility, reduced testosterone, and impaired sperm maturation[124]. Chronic alcohol consumption has a detrimental effect on male reproductive hormones and on all parameters of semen quality.[125] High alcohol consumption has been found to be equally detrimental to fertility in women by impairing hormonal functioning and lowering rates of first and second pregnancies.[123] This is in addition to the negative impact of alcohol use during pregnancy on fetal development.

Recreational drug (e.g., cannabis, lysergic acid diethylamide or LSD, amphetamines, cocaine) exposure in women has been found to contribute to primary infertility. Women who reported smoking marijuana had a slightly elevated risk for infertility due to an ovulatory abnormality. The risk was greatest among women who had used marijuana within one year of trying to become pregnant. The risk of infertility due to tubal abnormality was found to be greatly increased by cocaine use in women.[126] Similarly, drug use among men, particularly the use of cocaine, was found to contribute to male-factor infertility. Men who had used cocaine within two years of their first semen analysis were found to be twice as likely to have lower sperm counts. Furthermore, the duration of cocaine use for five or more years was found to lower sperm motility and poor sperm morphology.[127] Further, marijuana has been consistently found to reduce sperm counts and impair sperm quality.[128]

While drug and alcohol abuse is prevalent, many infertile men and women are unaware of how their patterns of usage may be negatively affecting their fertility. Whether drug and alcohol abuse represents a lifestyle choice, coping mechanism, or genetic predisposition to addiction, it can trigger other health and relationship problems. However, as with obesity and smoking, healthcare providers typically fail to address the issue of chemical abuse or addiction despite the availability of effective treatment measures and the obvious negative impact on fertility and overall health. Although traditional medicine can offer supportive medical care, detoxification, treatment of concurrent problems, and medications (e.g., Antabuse), the most successful long-term treatments involve inpatient or outpatient rehabilitation often based on the Twelve-Step Program of Alcoholics Anonymous.

FUTURE IMPLICATIONS

Behavioral medicine and stress and coping theory have become the foundation for much of the clinical issues and therapeutic interventions of infertility counseling. They have been the basis for research for decades, although the focus of that research has shifted away from psychogenic factors toward practical applications of stress and coping that improve patient health and well-being. The focus of research now includes an emphasis on quality-of-life, patient education, and behaviors and/or interventions that improve fertility and/or treatment outcome. Still, the exact mechanism or interrelationship between psychological and biomedical factors; between distress and maximizing fertility and medical treatment outcomes; and/or the influence of endocrine and immune factors remains unclear.

The biopsychosocial model of infertility emphasizes the importance of health behavior in psychological factors and biomedical outcome as evidenced by health efficacy behavior as an important contributor to the reproductive process as well as the efficacy of cognitive-behavioral interventions and health behavior change.

Behavioral medicine has become the bulwark of infertility counseling practice whether it involves stress management, patient education, skills training, or health behavior change. As such, infertility counselors are using an ever-increasing array of therapeutic interventions to meet the needs of patients and infertility clinics to maximize patient care, satisfaction, and the success of treatment outcomes.

SUMMARY

■ Psychosocial and biomedical factors both contribute to the emotional response to infertility and physiological responses to stress that negatively affect fertility and infertility treatment outcome. Coping and cognitions, endocrine and immune factors, as well as health behavior change all contribute to mediating this process by improving fertility, coping, and treatment outcomes.

■ The actual physiological mechanisms of the endocrine and immune systems that impact fertility and treatment outcome have not been identified although there appears to be significant evidence of the complex interplay of these factors.

■ While the stresses of infertility have been more clearly identified for both men and women, coping approaches and strategies that are most effective may differ.

■ Helplessness with respect to fertility problems and a lack of social support are important risk factors for problematic adjustment to unsuccessful fertility treatment.

■ Patients should be encouraged to consider and use a wide array of coping strategies that are adaptable to their particular situation and stage of infertility and infertility treatment.

■ To date, cognitive-behavioral therapy (particularly cognitive restructuring) seems to be the most effective intervention that can be generalized and applied across infertility diagnosis and treatment to couples and individuals.

■ Smoking, alcohol consumption, drug abuse, obesity, and malnutrition have all been identified as important in contributing to infertility and impacting treatment outcome. As such, the infertility counselor working within a framework of behavioral medicine can provide patient education, support, and therapeutic interventions to positively affect health behavior.

REFERENCES

1. Schwartz GE, Weiss SM. Behavioral medicine revisited: An amended definition. *J Behav Med* 1978; 1:249–51.
2. Matarazzo JC. Behavioral health's challenge to academic, scientific, and professional psychology. *Am Psychol* 1982; 37:1–14.
3. Belar CD, Deardorff WW. *Clinical Health Psychology in Medical Settings: A Practitioner's Guide*. Washington, DC: American Psychological Association Press, 1999.
4. Kroger WS, Freed SC. Psychosomatic aspects of sterility. *Am J Obstet Gynecol* 1950; 59:867–74.
5. Wisschman TH. Psychogenic infertility. *J Ass Reprod Genet* 2003; 20:485–94.
6. Batstra L, van de Wiel HBM, Schuiling GA. Opinions about 'unexplained subfertility.' *J Psychosom Obs Gyn* 2002; 23:211–14.
7. Greil AL. Infertility and psychological distress: A critical review of the literature. *Soc Sci Med* 1997; 45:1679–704.
8. Selye H. *The Stress of Life*. New York: McGraw-Hill, 1978.
9. Cannon WB. The emergency function of the adrenal medulla in pain and the major emotions. *Am J Physiology* 1941; 33:356.
10. Karahasanoglu A, Barglow P, Growe G. Psychological aspects of infertility. *J Reprod Med* 1972; 9:241–7.
11. Sandler B. Emotional stress and infertility. *J Psychosom Res* 1968; 12:51–9.
12. Gallinelli A, Roncaglia R, Matteo ML, et al. Immunological changes and stress are associated with different implantation rates in patients undergoing in vitro fertilization-embryo transfer. *Fertil Steril* 2001; 76:85–91.

13. Smeenk JMJ, Verhaak CM, Vingerhoets AJJM, et al. Stress and outcome success in IVF: The role of self-reports and endocrine variables. *Hum Reprod* 2005; 20:991–6.
14. Benson H, Beary JF, Carol MP. The relaxation response. *Psychiatry* 1974; 37–45.
15. Dunkel-Schetter C, Lobel M. Psychological reactions to infertility. In: AL Stanton, C Dunkel-Schetter, eds. *Infertility: Perspectives from Stress and Coping Research*. New York: Plenum Press, 1991; 29–57.
16. Wilson JF, Kopitzke EJ. Stress and infertility. *Curr Womens Health Rep* 2002; 2:194–9.
17. Koropatnick S, Daniluk J, Pattinson HA. Infertility: A non-event transition. *Fertil Steril* 1993; 59:163–71.
18. Wright J, Duchesne C, Sabourin S, et al. Psychosocial distress and infertility: Men and women respond differently. *Fertil Steril* 1991; 55:100–8.
19. Nachtigall RD, Quiroga SS, Tschann JM, et. al. Stigma, disclosure, and family functioning among parents with children conceived through donor insemination *Fertil Steril* 1997; 68:1–7.
20. Hsu YL, Kuo BJ. Evaluations of emotional reactions and coping behaviors as well as correlated factors for infertile couples receiving assisted reproductive technologies. *J Nurs Res* 2002; 10:291–302.
21. Benyamini Y, Gozlan M, Kokia E. Variability in the difficulties experienced by women undergoing infertility treatments. *Fertil Steril* 2005; 83:275–83.
22. Schneider MG, Forthofer MS. Associations of psychosocial factors with the stress of infertility treatment. *Health Soc Work* 2005; 30:183–91.
23. Dhaliwal LK, Gupta KR, Gopalan S, et al. Psychological aspects of infertility due to various causes – prospective study. *Int J Fertil Womens Med* 2004; 49:44–8.
24. Pook M, Krause W. The impact of treatment experiences on the course of infertility distress in male patients. *Hum Reprod* 2005; 20:825–8.
25. Walker I, Broderick P. Correlates of psychological distress in relation to male infertility. *Australian Psychologist* 1999; 34:38–44.
26. Edelmann RJ, Connolly KJ. Stress and infertility in women. *J Comm Applied Soc Psychology* 1998; 8:303–11.
27. Abbey A, Andrews FM, Halman LJ. Gender's role in responses to infertility. *Psychol Women Q* 1991; 15:295–316.
28. Davis DC, Dearman CN. Coping strategies of infertile women. *J Obstet Gynecol Neonatal Nurs* 1991; 20:221–8.
29. Snarey J, Son L, Kuihne, et al. The role of parenting in men's psychosocial development: A longitudinal study of early adulthood infertility and midlife generativity. *Dev Psychol* 1987; 23:593–603.
30. Peterson BD, Newton CR, Rosen KH. Examining congruence between partners' perceived infertility-related stress and its relationship to marital adjustment and depression in infertile couples. *Fam Process* 2003; 42:59–70.
31. Dyer SJ, Abrahams N, Mokoena NE, Lombard CJ, van der Spuy ZM. Psychological distress among women suffering from couple infertility in South Africa: A quantitative assessment. *Hum Reprod* 2005; 20:1938–43.
32. Matsubayashi H, Hosaka T, Izumi S, et al. Increased depression and anxiety in infertile Japanese women resulting from lack of husband's support and feelings of stress. *Gen Hosp Psychiatry* 2004; 26:398–404.

33. Mazure CM, Greenfeld DA. Psychological studies of in vitro fertilization/embryo transfer participants. *J In Vitro Fertil Emb Transfer* 1989; 6:242–56.

34. Boivin J, Takefman JE, Tulandi T, et al. Reactions to infertility based on extent of treatment failure. *Fertil Steril* 1995; 63:801–7.

35. Greenfeld D, Haseltine F. Stress in females as compared with males entering in vitro fertilization treatment. *Fertil Steril* l992; 57:350–6.

36. Merari D, Feldberg D, Elizur A, et al. Psychological and hormonal changes in the course of in vitro fertilization. *J Assist Reprod Technol Genet* 1992; 9:161–9.

37. Beaurepaire J, Jones M, Theiring P, et al. Psychosocial adjustment in infertility and its treatment: Male and female responses at different stages of IVF/ET treatment. *J Psychosom Res* 1994; 38:229–40.

38. Kolonoff-Cohen H, Chu E, Natarajan L, et al. A prospective study of stress among women undergoing in vitro fertilization or gamate intrafallopian transfer. *Fertil Steril* 2001; 76:675–87.

39. Yong PC, Martin C, Thong J. A comparison of psychological functioning in women at different stages of in vitro fertilization treatment using the mean affect adjective check list. *J Assist. Reprod Gen* 2000; 17:553–6.

40. Verhaak CM, Smeenk JM, van Minnen A, et al. A longitudinal, prospective study on emotional adjustment before, during and after consecutive fertility treatment cycles. *Hum Reprod* 2005; 20: 2253–60.

41. Kee BS, Jung BJ, Lee SH. A study on psychological strain in IVF patients. *J Ass Rep Gen* 2000; 17:445–8.

42. Ardenti R, Campari C, Agazzi L, et al. Anxiety and perceptive functioning of infertile women during in-vitro fertilization: Exploratory survey of an Italian sample. *Hum Reprod* 1999; 14:3126–32.

43. Verhaak CM, Smeenk JM, Evers AW, et al. Predicting emotional response to unsuccessful fertility treatment: A prospective study. *J Behav Med* 2005; 28:181–90.

44. van den Akker OBA. Younger women may have more difficulty coping with infertility than older women. *Patient Education Counseling* 2005; 57:183–9.

45. Tarabusi M, Volpe A, Facchinetti F. Psychological group support attenuates distress of waiting in couples scheduled for assisted reproduction. *J Psychosom Obstet Gynaecol* 2004; 25:273–9.

46. Slade P, Emery J, Lieberman BA. A prospective, longitudinal study of emotions and relationships in in-vitro fertilization treatment. *Hum Reprod* 1997; 12:183–90.

47. Newton CR, Heaern MT, Yuzpe AA. Psychological assessment and follow-up after in vitro fertilization: Assessing the impact of failure. *Fertil Steril* 1990; 54:879–86.

48. Csemiczky G, Landgren BM, Collins A. The influence of stress and state anxiety on the outcome of IVF-treatment: Psychological and endocrinological assessment of Swedish women entering IVF-treatment. *Acta Obstet Gynecol Scand* 2000; 79:113–8.

49. Newton CR, Sherrad W, Houle M. Preparing women for oocyte retrieval (OR): A comparison of psychological interventions. *Fertil Steril* 1994:S27.

50. Boivin J. A review of psychosocial interventions in infertility. *Soc Sci Med* 2003; 57:2325–41.

51. Boivin J, Schmidt L. Infertility-related stress in men and women predicts treatment outcome 1 year later. *Fertil Steril*. 2005; 83:1745–52.

52. Demyttenaere K, Bonte L, Gheldof M, et al. Coping style and depression level influence outcome in in vitro fertilization. *Fertil Steril* 1998; 69:1026–33.

53. Sanders K, Bruce NW. Psychosocial stress and treatment outcome following assisted reproductive technology. *Hum Reprod* 1999; 14:1656–62.

54. Engel GL. The need for a new medical model. *Science* 1977; 196:129–36.

55. Tunks E, Bellissimo A. *Behavioral Medicine: Concepts and Procedures*. New York: Pergamon Press, 1991.

56. Taymor ML, Bresnick E. Emotional stress and infertility *Infertility* 1979; 2:39–47.

57. Lazarus RS, Folkman S. *Stress, Appraisal, and Coping.* New York: Springer, 1984.

58. Moos RH, Schaefer JA. Coping resources and processes: Current concepts and measures. In: L Goldberger, S Breznitz, eds. *Handbook of Stress: Theoretical and Clinical Aspects*. New York: Free Press, 1994; 234–57.

59. Stanton AL, Dunkel-Schetter C. Psychological adjustment to infertility: An overview of conceptual approaches. In: AL Stanton, C. Dunkel-Schetter, eds. *Infertility: Perspectives from Stress and Coping Research*. New York: Plenum Press, 1991; 3–16.

60. Campbell SM, Dunkel-Schetter C., Peplau LA. Perceived control and adjustment to infertility among women undergoing in vitro fertilizations. In: AL Stanton, C. Dunkel-Schetter, eds. *Infertility: Perspectives from Stress and Coping Research*. New York: Plenum Press, 1991; 133–56.

61. Stanton AL. Cognitive appraisals, coping processes, and adjustment to infertility. In. AL Stanton, C. Dunkel-Schetter, eds. *Infertility: Perspectives from Stress and Coping Research*. New York: Plenum Press, 1991; 87–108.

62. Holahan CJ, Moos RM. Risk, resistance, and psychological distress: A longitudinal analysis with adult and children. *Abn Psycholol* 1987; 96:3–13.

63. Domar AD, Zuttermeister PC, Friedman R. The psychological impact of infertility, a comparison with patients with other medical conditions. *J Psychosom Obstet Gyn* 1993; 14:45–52.

64. Newton CR, Sherrard W, Glavac I. The Fertility Problem Inventory: Measuring perceived infertility-related stress. *Fertil Steril* 1999; 72:54–62.

65. Boivin J, Takefman JE. Stress levels across stages of in vitro fertilization in subsequently pregnant and non-pregnant women. *Fertil Steril* 1995; 64:802–10.

66. Hansell PL, Thorn BE, Prentice-Dunn S, et al. Psychological state and psychological strain in relation to infertility. *J Clin Psychology Med Settings* 1998; 5:133–45.

67. Schmidt L, Christensen U, Holstein BE. The social epidemiology of coping with infertility. *Hum Reprod* 2005; 20:1044–52.

68. Berg BJ, Wilson JF. Psychological functioning across stages of treatment for infertility. *J Behav Med* 1991; 14:11–26.

69. Parker JC. Stress management. In: PM Nicassio, TW Smith, eds. *Managing Chronic Illness: A Biopsychosocial Perspective*. Washington, DC: American Psychological Association, 1995; 285–312.

70. Takefman JE, Brender W, Boivin J, et al. Sexual and emotional adjustment of couples undergoing infertility investigation and the effectiveness of preparatory information. *J Psychosom Obstet Gynaecol* 1990; 11:275–90.

71. Connolly KJ, Edelmann RJ, Barlett H, et al. An evaluation of counseling for couples undergoing treatment for in-vitro fertilization. *Hum Reprod* 1993; 8:1332–8.

72. Pook M, Krause W. Stress reduction in male infertility patients: A randomized, controlled trial. *Fertil Steril* 2005; 83:68–73.

73. Cousineau TM, Lord SE, Seibring AR, et al. A multimedia psychosocial support program for couples receiving infertility treatment: a feasibility study. *Fertil Steril* 2004; 81:532–8.

74. Haagen EC, Tuil W, Hendriks J, et al. Current internet use and preferences of IVF and ICSI patients. *Hum Reprod* 2003; 18:2073–8.

75. Weissman A, Gotlieb L, Ward S, et al. Use of the internet by infertile couples. *Fertil Steril* 2000; 73:1179–82.

76. Stanton AL, Burns LH. Behavioral medicine approaches to infertility counseling. In LH Burns, SN Covington, eds. *Infertility Counseling: A Comprehensive Handbook for Clinicians*. New York: Parthenon, 1999; 129–47.

77. Domar AD, Zuttermeister PC, Friedman R. The relationship between distress and conception in infertile women. *J Am Med Womens Assoc* 1999; 54:196–8.

78. Tschuggel W, Berga SL. Treatment of functional hypothalamic amenorrhea with hypnotherapy. *Fertil Steril* 2003; 80:982–5.

79. Gravitz MA. Hypnosis in the treatment of functional infertility. *Am J Clin Hypn* 1995; 38:22–6.

80. Mikesell SG. Infertility and pregnancy loss: Hypnotic interventions for reproductive challenges. In: LM Hornyak, JP Green, eds. *Healing from Within: The Use of Hypnosis in Women's Health Care*. Washington, DC: American Psychological Association Press, 2000; 191–212.

81. Webster A. *Cognitive Therapy and Emotions. Skills Training for Mind/body Change*. Mind/Body Institute Harvard Medical School. Boston, MA. 2001.

82. Benson HR, Stuart EM. *The Wellness Book: A Comprehensive Guide to Maintaining Health and Treating Stress Related Illness*. New York: Fireside, 1993.

83. Eugster A, Vingerhoets AJJM. Psychological aspects of in vitro fertilisation. *Soc Sc Med* 1999; 48:575–89.

84. Edelmann RJ. Emotional aspects of in vitro fertilization procedures: Review. *J Reprod Inf Psychol* 1990; 8:161–73.

85. Visser AP, Haan G, Zalmstra H, et al. Psychological aspects of in vitro fertilization. *J Psychosom Obstet Gyn* 1994; 15:35–43.

86. Connolly KJ, Edelmann RJ, Cooke ID, et al. The impact of infertility on psychological functioning. *J Psychosom Res* 1992; 36:459–68.

87. Hynes GJ, Callan VJ, Terry DJ, et al. The psychological well-being of infertile women after an unsuccessful IVF attempt: The effects of coping. *Br J Med Psychol* 1992; 65:269–78.

88. Berga SL, Marcus MD, Loucks TL, et al. Recovery of ovarian activity in women with functional hypothalamic amenorrhea who were treated with cognitive behavior therapy. *Fertil Steril* 2003; 80:976–81.

89. Berga SL, Daniels TL, Giles DE. Women with functional hypothalamic amenorrhea but not other forms of anovulation display amplified cortisol concentrations. *Fertil Steril* 1997; 67:1024–30.

90. Facchinetti F, Tarabusi M, Volpe A. Cognitive behavioral treatment decreases cardiovascular and neuroendocrine reaction to stress in women waiting for assisted reproduction. *Psychoendocrinology* 2004; 29:162–73.

91. Domar AD, Clapp D, Slawsby EA, et al. Impact of group psychological interventions on pregnancy rates in infertile women. *Fertil Steril* 2000; 73:805–11.

92. Tuschen-Caffier B, Florin I, Krause W, Pook M. Cognitive-behavioral therapy for idiopathic infertile couples *Psychother Psychosom* 1999; 68:15–21.

93. Terry DJ, Hynes, GJ. Adjustment to a low-control situation: Reexamining the role of coping responses. *J Pers. Soc Psychol* 1998; 74:1078–92.

94. Lukse MP, Vacc NA. Grief depression, and coping in women undergoing infertility treatment. *Obstet Gyn* 1999; 93:245–51.

95. Schmidt L, Holstein BE, Christensen U, et al. Communication and coping as predictors of fertility problem stress: cohort study of 816 participants who did not achieve a delivery after 12 months of fertility treatment. *Hum Reprod* 2005; 20:3248–56.

96. van den Akker OB. Coping, quality of life and psychological symptoms in three groups of sub-fertile women. *Patient Educ Couns* 2005; 57:183–9.

97. Miller WR, Rollnick S. *Motivational Interviewing: Preparing People for Change*. New York: Guilford Press; 1991.

98. Sarafino EP. *Health Psychology, Biopsychosocial Interventions*. New York: Wiley, 1998.

99. Hassan MAM, Killick SR. Negative lifestyle is associated with a significant reduction in fecundity. *Fertil Steril* 2004; 81:384–92.

100. Nichols JE, Crane MM, Higdon HL, et al. Extremes of body mass index reduce in vitro fertilization pregnancy rates. *Fertil Steril* 2003; 79:645–7.

101. Cogswell ME, Perry GS, Schieve LA, Dietz WH. Obesity in women of childbearing age: Risks, prevention, and treatment. *Prim Care Update Ob/Gyn* 2001; 8:89–105.

102. Obesity: Prevention and managing the global epidemic. WHO: 2000. www.heartstats.org.

103. ASRM Patient's Fact Sheet: Weight and fertility. www.asrm.org.

104. Hollmann M, Runnebaum B, Gerhard I. Effects of weight loss on the hormonal profile in obese infertile women. *Hum Reprod* 1996; 11:1884–91.

105. Clark AM, Ledger W, Galletly C, et al. Weight loss results in significant improvement in pregnancy and ovulation rates in anovulatory obese women. *Hum Reprod* 1995; 10:2705–12.

106. Wong WY, Thomas CMG, Merkus JMWM, et al. Male factor subfertility: Possible causes and the impact of nutritional factors. *Fertil Steril* 2000; 73:435–42.

107. Van Der Spuy ZM, Jacobs HS. Weight reduction, fertility and contraception. *IPPF Med Bull* 1983; 17:2–4.

108. Nawaz H, Adams ML, Katz DL. Weight loss counseling by health care providers. *Am J Public Health* 1999; 89:764–7.

109. Galusk DA, Will JC, Serdula MK. Are health care professionals advising obese patients to lose weight? *JAMA* 1999; 282:1576–8.

110. Schroeder SA. What to do with a patient who smokes? *JAMA* 2005; 294:482–7.

111. Wadden TA, Foster GD, Letizia KA. One year behavioral treatment of obesity: Comparison of moderate and severe caloric restriction and the effects of weight maintenance therapy. *J Cons Clin Psychol* 1994; 62:165–71.

112. Clark AM, Thornley B, Tomlinson L, et al. Weight loss in obese infertile women results in improvement in reproductive outcome for all forms of fertility treatment. *Hum Reprod* 1998; 13:1502–5.

113. World Health Organization. Mental and neurological disorders. Fact Sheet No. 265, 2001. http://www.who.int/mediacentre/factsheets/fs265/en/.

114. The Practice Committee of the American Society for Reproductive Medicine. Smoking and infertility. *Fertil Steril* 2004; 81:1181–6.

115. Chia I, Hruba D, Fiala J, et al. The outcome of infertility treatment by in-vitro fertilization in smoking and non-smoking women. *Cent Eur J Publ H* 2001; 9:64–8.

116. El-Nemr A, Shawaf T, Sabatini L, et al. Effect of smoking on ovarian reserve and ovarian stimulation in in-vitro fertilization and embryo transfer. *Hum Reprod* 1998; 13:2192–8.

117. Klonoff-Cohen H, Natarjan L, Marrs R, Yee B. Effects of female and male smoking on success rates of IVF and gamete intra-fallopian transfer. *Hum Reprod* 2001b; 16:1382–90.

118. Paszkowski T, Clarke RN, Hornstein MD. Smoking induces oxidative stress inside the Graafian follicle. *Hum Reprod* 2002; 17:921–5.

119. Vine MF, Tse CK, Hu P, Truong KY. Cigarette smoking and semen quality. *Fertil Steril* 1996; 65:835–42.

120. Zitzmann M, Rolf C, Nordoff V, et al. Male smokers have a decreased success rate for in vitro fertilization and intracytoplamic sperm injection. *Fertil Steril* 2003; 79:1550–4.

121. Lintsen AM, Pasker de Jong PC, de Boer EJ, et al. Effects of subfertility cause, smoking and body weight on the success rate of IVF. *Hum Reprod* 2005; 20:1867–75.

122. Said TM, Ranga G, A. Relationship between semen quality and tobacco chewing in men undergoing infertility evaluation. *Fertil Steril* 2005; 84:649–53.

123. Eggert J, Theobald H, Engfeldt P. Effects of alcohol consumption on female fertility during an 18-year period. *Fertil Steril* 2004; 81:379–3.

124. Emanuele MA, Emanuele NV. Alcohol's effects on male reproduction. *Alcohol Health Res World* 1998; 22:195–201.

125. Muthusami KR, Chinnaswamy P. Effect of chronic alcoholism on male fertility hormones and semen quality. *Fertil Steril* 2005; 84:919–24.

126. Mueller BA, Daling JR, Weiss NS, et al. Recreational drug use and the risk of primary infertility. *Epidemiology* 1990; 1:189–92.

127. Bracken MB, Eskenazi B, Sachse K, et al. Association of cocaine use with sperm concentration, motility, and morphology. *Fertil Steril* 1990; 53:315–22.

128. Whan LB, West MC, McClure N, et al. Effects of delta-9-tetrahydrocannabinol, the primary psychoactive cannabinoid in marijuana, on human sperm function in vitro. *Fertil Steril* 2006; 85:653–60.

129. Evers AWM, Kraaimaat FW, Lankveld W van, et al. Beyond unfavorable thinking: The illness cognition questionnaire for chronic diseases. *J Consult Clinl Psychol* 2001; 69:1026–36.

130. Callan VJ, Hennessey JF. Emotional aspects and support in in vitro fertilization and embryo transfer programs. *J In Vitro Fert Embryo Transf* 1988; 5:290–5.

12 Complementary and Alternative Medicine in Infertility Counseling

JACQUELINE N. GUTMANN AND SHARON N. COVINGTON

This is one of those cases where the imagination is baffled by the facts.

– Winston Churchill

A number of terms have been applied to describe complementary and/or alternative treatments that fall outside the range of conventional medicine. Terms for these adjunctive treatments include nontraditional, unconventional, holistic, natural, unorthodox, unproven, and new age. The use of these treatments to heal a variety of conditions and maladies has received wide attention worldwide, as evidenced by the increasing array of national and international organizations considering the use (and abuse) of adjunctive therapies and remedies.

Definitions for complementary and alternative medicine (CAM) vary from clinics to countries to cultures, causing confusion as to what patients and practitioners are referring to when discussing treatments beyond 'traditional' methods. For example, according to the World Health Organization (WHO), 'traditional medicine' refers to "health practices, approaches, knowledge and beliefs incorporating plant, animal- and mineral-based medicines, spiritual therapies, manual techniques and exercises, applied singularly or in combination to treat, diagnose, and prevent illnesses or maintain well-being."[1] In the United Kingdom, the Cochrane Collaboration's definition of CAM is "a broad domain of healing resources that encompasses all healthy systems, modalities, and practices and their accompanying theories and beliefs other than those intrinsic to the politically dominant health systems of a particular society or culture in a given historical period."[2] The definition of CAM in the United States by the National Center for Complementary and Alternative Medicine (NCCAM), a component of the National Institutes of Health, is similar to that of the United Kingdom in that CAM is defined as "a group of diverse medical and health care systems, practices and products that are not presently considered part of conventional medicine and are used together with or as

an alternative to conventional medicinal treatment."[3] While using different terms, the WHO and NCCAM consider 'integrated medicine' an approach that combines mainstream treatment with CAM therapies for which there is some high-quality scientific evidence of safety and effectiveness.

Integral to the care of infertile men and women is the importance of optimum care, patient safety, and quality assurance (efficacy) issues. It is, therefore, paramount that the infertility counselor be well aware of not only a patient's use (and/or abuse) of CAM procedures but also of the potential benefits and limitations of these treatments. According to the WHO, unregulated or inappropriate use of CAM treatments and practices can have negative or dangerous effects. A complete and comprehensive discussion of CAM that includes an overview of current practice, research, and applications of CAM in reproductive medicine worldwide is beyond the scope of this chapter. As such, this chapter focuses on those modalities most commonly used by patients and practitioners involved in the treatment of infertility. Mind–body interventions and issues of culture and spirituality are addressed in separate chapters. For the purposes of this chapter, all nontraditional, unconventional, holistic, natural, adjunctive, complementary, and/or alternative remedies or treatments will be referred to as CAM.

This chapter

■ Briefly reviews the history of CAM and its resurgence in recent years;
■ Examines current research on CAM treatments used by infertility patients;
■ Identifies a theoretical framework to understand CAM in the context of infertility treatment;
■ Describes CAM therapies and their efficacy in reproductive medicine; and

■ Suggests therapeutic interventions for infertility counselors and their patients considering or using CAM methods.

HISTORICAL OVERVIEW

From prehistoric times and for centuries, humans have used a wide array of remedies for treating ailments, many of them based on cultural beliefs about health and illness, available herbs, plants and potions, traditional healers, and/or traditional belief systems. The advent of modern medicine has brought scientific investigation, advanced medical technologies, and evidence-based approaches that have evolved modern medicine from an art to a science. Nevertheless, many cultures continue to rely on various forms of traditional remedies and culturally specific solutions to cure health problems – remedies or cures that may or may not be backed by any scientific support.

While traditional medicine remains a popular and familiar (comfortable) approach to the treatment of medical ailments, including infertility, the reality is over one-third of the population in developing countries lack access to essential medicines and/or medical caregivers. The provision of safe and effective CAM therapies could become a critical tool to increase access to healthcare as well as an effective adjunctive and/or palliative care approach in collaboration with modern medicine. In fact, 25% of modern medicines are made from plants first used traditionally. Acupuncture has been proven effective in relieving postoperative pain, nausea during pregnancy, nausea and vomiting resulting from chemotherapy, and dental pain with extremely low side effects. It can also alleviate anxiety, panic disorders, and insomnia.

Although CAM methods have been around since the beginning of mankind, there has been a dramatic change in attitude, interest, and use in Western cultures in the last fifteen years. According to the WHO, while CAM has maintained its popularity in all regions of the developing world, there is rapid and increasing use within industrialized countries. In Europe, North America, and other industrialized regions, more than 50% of the population has used complementary or alternative medicine at least once and there is some evidence that the number of visits to alternative care providers exceeds the number of visits to physicians. In Canada, 70% of the population has used complementary medicine at least once, while in Germany, 90% of the population has used a natural remedy at some point in their life. Consequently, more doctors undertaking special training in CAM (10,800 between 1995 and 2000) and people are spending more money on CAM ($17 bil-

lion in the United States and $230 million in the United Kingdom in 2000). In addition, the global market for herbal medicines currently stands at more than $60 billion annually and is growing steadily.[1]

In a 2002 survey in the United States, through the Center for Disease Control and Prevention's (CDC) National Center for Health Statistics (NCHS), more than 31,000 adults were interviewed. Researchers found that more than 62% of individuals over the age of eighteen had used some form of CAM therapy during the past twelve months, when the definition of CAM therapy included prayer specifically for health reasons.[4] When prayer was excluded, the number decreased to 36%, which represented 72 million U.S. adults.[5] National survey data do not support the view that the use of CAM therapy in the United States primarily reflects dissatisfaction with conventional care. In fact, almost 80% of those surveyed perceived that the combination of CAM and conventional therapy is superior to one or the other alone.[6] Survey data suggest that among American women, CAM users tend to be older, Caucasian, have more education, and are of a higher socioeconomic status. They are also more likely to be of poorer health.[7]

In the United Kingdom, a BBC telephone poll of 1,204 randomly selected members of the general population, in 2000, found that 20% reported using CAM during the proceeding year. The most commonly used CAM was herbalism (34%); aromatherapy (21%); homeopathy (17%); acupuncture (14%); reflexology (6%); and massage (6%).[8] A postal survey the following year of randomly selected men and women found that 13.6% had visited a CAM therapist in the preceding twelve months and 28.3% had bought an over-the-counter CAM remedy and/or seen a CAM therapist.[9]

In an Australian study that compared the characteristics of CAM users and nonusers among women, a postal questionnaire was mailed to 41,817 women, aged eighteen to seventy-five, who were selected randomly from a health insurance database. Women in middle age [45–50] were most likely (28%) to have used CAM therapies during the previous year, while younger women aged eighteen to twenty-two (19%) and older women aged seventy to seventy-five (15%) were less likely to have used CAM. Furthermore, women in nonurban Australia were more likely to use CAM, although in conjunction with conventional health services.[10]

In Japan, in a nationwide, random-sampled, and population-weighted telephone survey, 1,000 individuals were questioned on their use of CAM during the previous twelve months, out-of-pocket expenditures for CAM therapies, and the use of conventional medicine. Although more respondents had used CAM therapies

(76%) than conventional medicine (65.5%), this was not a dramatic difference, particularly considering cultural factors. The most common CAM therapies were nutritional supplements (43%); dietary supplements (43%); health-related appliances (21%); herbs (17%); massage or acupressure (15%); chiropractic or osteopathy (7%); acupuncture (7%); and homeopathy (3%). The majority of the respondents (60%) stated that their reason for using CAM was that their condition was not serious enough to warrant the use of conventional medicine, while 49% used CAM therapies to promote health and prevent disease. Interestingly, out-of-pocket expenses for CAM therapies were half as much as the cost of conventional medicine.[11]

In summary, CAM is increasingly being used by patients throughout the world as an adjunct to traditional treatment rather than conventional approaches. As modern technology has influenced the course and direction of medicine, what has been thought of as unorthodox or even primitive with these methods, is now considered by many to be conventional. Despite this growth and interest, there must be high-quality scientific evidence as to the efficacy and safety of these therapies for CAM to be integrated into standard medical care.

LITERATURE REVIEW

While there is growing research on the use of CAM for various medical conditions and procedures, studies reviewing its use by infertile people are limited. In the United Kingdom, a questionnaire was used to assess CAM employed by infertile men and women presenting for treatment at two facilities: a private practice clinic and a National Health Service (NHS) facility. Respondents included 157 patients (120 women, 37 men) from the private clinic and 181 (124 women, 57 men) from the NHS clinic. In general, women (63%) were more likely than men (25%) to use CAM, regardless of the treatment facility. Women at the private clinic (40%) had the highest users of CAM, while the usage rate for men at both facilities was comparable. Of the respondents who had used CAM, 10% thought it had been helpful for infertility, 13% felt it had helped them psychologically and that they had done everything possible, and 22% felt it had helped them relax. This study found that the most commonly used CAM remedies were: nutritional advice; reflexology; acupuncture; traditional Chinese medicine; herbalism; hypnosis; and spiritual healing. An interesting finding of this study was that under additional comments, several respondents indicated that they would have liked advice from their doctor specifically about CAM and infertility. Addi-

tionally, respondents described their encounters with a CAM provider in terms of someone who was "really interested"; "listened really carefully to what I was saying"; and "seemed to understand how I feel."[12]

In a study of the use of CAM in Pakistan, researchers noted that 70% of the developing world's population continues to depend on complementary and alternative medical systems for a variety of reasons including cultural beliefs and practices; proximity; availability of traditional (faith) healers and/or unavailability of modern medical caregivers; affordable fees; and family and community pressure. Interestingly, the researchers noted that CAM therapies (including spiritual healers, clergy, hakeems, homeopaths, and quacks) were the *first choice* for infertility and other ailments (e.g., epilepsy and depression). These researchers concluded that given the health-seeking behavior and cultural traditions, particularly in developing countries, modern medicine has a responsibility to be available for back-up referral to ensure that all CAM healers are properly trained and their facilities properly maintained. This approach will ensure a positive interaction between the two systems, working toward the common goal of improving health for all people.[13]

In Iceland, CAM therapists and allopathic caregivers were found to provide a holistic approach to infertility treatment that patients preferred. CAM treatments for infertility were used to address stress; hormonal imbalances in both men and women; amenorrhea; and/or other menstrual irregularities. The most common CAM remedies were nutritional advice; traditional Chinese medicine; herbalism; aromatherapy, homeopathy, and Ayrvedic treatments.[14]

In a U.S. survey of sixty-six women and six men who were members of an infertility patient support organization, 86% of respondents used a combination of conventional and CAM treatments. Only 1% used neither, 4% used only CAM treatments; and 8% used conventional medical treatments only. While 32% reported that conventional medical treatment had been helpful, 43% reported that CAM therapies had been helpful. The most frequently used CAM therapies were vitamins (71%); mind–body techniques (49%); and herbs (49%). Other CAM therapies included acupuncture, prayer, massage, yoga, chiropractic, nutrition, ayurveda, reflexology, aromatherapy, and homeopathy. Reasons for using CAM therapies included dissatisfaction with conventional medical treatment; assistance with getting pregnant; a means of regaining control; means of feeling healthier; and a personal belief in the efficacy of the approach. Additionally, respondents felt that CAM was a means of feeling that they had tried everything. The researcher concluded that there is a greater need to evaluate and integrate CAM therapies into conventional fertility therapy.[15]

In an Australian study that examined how women with endometriosis coped with the disease and infertility, sixty-one women attended focus groups during which they described the experience of endometriosis as a chronic illness with multiple losses. All but one of the women in this study found complementary therapies vital, with some of the women replacing traditional medical care with CAM therapies. The women felt that the use of CAM therapies was a mechanism for regaining control of their lives, the disease, and even fertility. These women also complained that the worst part of the experience was encounters with health professionals who trivialized and dismissed their symptoms.[16,17]

Although research on how infertility patients perceive and use CAM is sparse, several themes can be interpreted from these studies. Patients want more information and assistance from their medical providers on complementary therapies, and need to feel their caregiver is open and knowledgeable to discuss it. In addition, using CAM therapies may help infertility patients regain some sense of control that is lost in conventional medical treatment and provide benefits that help to alleviate the associated stress. It is clear, however, that more research is needed on how infertility patients perceive and use CAM therapies, as well as how their physicians understand and address these approaches as a part of their treatment protocols for infertility.

THEORETICAL FRAMEWORK

Several theoretical frameworks are applicable to the use of complementary medicine in reproductive medicine including biopsychosocial theory, collaborative medicine approach, and cultural traditions. All of these theories are covered in greater depth in other chapters. However, the theoretical approach of social cognition theory with an emphasis on self-efficacy behaviors provides a different perspective. It helps explain patient beliefs, roles, and effectiveness in managing the crisis of infertility; implementing health behaviors that maximize fertility and treatment success; as well as how CAM therapies may be used as an effective coping mechanism that enhances feelings of control, self-efficacy, and self-esteem. In addition, another approach that may be applicable when considering CAM therapies is expectancy theory and the placebo effect. In this sense, there is power in patients' beliefs and expectations that certain therapies will help them feel better, or perhaps cure their infertility. Both theories offer a different perspective on the growing interest and use of CAM with infertility patients.

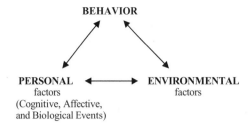

Figure 12.1. Bandura's social cognition theory[19]

Social Cognition Theory and Self-Efficacy Behaviors

Social cognition theory was first presented by Canadian psychologist Bandura in 1977.[18] It is based on a view of human functioning that views people proactively rather than reactively, using self-organization, self-reflection, and self-regulation rather than being driven by unconscious inner impulses or shaped by environmental forces. From this theoretical perspective, human functioning is viewed as the product of a dynamic interplay of personal, behavioral, and environmental influences. The foundation of Bandura's concept of *reciprocal determinism* is how people interpret the results of their own behavior informs and alters their environments and behavior.[19] In sum, (a) personal factors in the form of cognition, affect, and biological events; (b) behavior; and (c) environmental influences create interactions that result in a *triadic reciprocality* (see Figure 12.1). Bandura altered the label of his theory from social learning to social cognition both to distance it from prevalent social learning theories of the day and to emphasize that cognition plays a critical role in people's capacity to construct reality, self-regulate, encode information, and perform behaviors.

The reciprocal nature of the determinants of human functioning in social cognitive theory makes it possible for therapeutic and counseling efforts to be directed at personal, environmental, or behavioral factors. Strategies for increasing well-being can be aimed at improving emotional, cognitive, or motivational processes, increasing behavioral competencies, or altering the social conditions under which people live and work.[20]

Self-Efficacy Beliefs and Behaviors

At the foundation of social cognitive theory are *self-efficacy* beliefs or "people's judgments of their capabilities to organize and execute courses of action required to attain designated types of performances."[21] Briefly, if people believe that their actions can produce their desired outcomes, individuals are more motivated to act or persevere in the face of difficulties. This is particularly true for infertile individuals for whom the challenges are significant but the desired outcome (parenthood) is a significant motivator. There is significant evidence that self-efficacy beliefs impact virtually every aspect of people's lives – whether they think productively, self-debilitatingly, pessimistically, or optimistically; how well they motivate themselves and persevere in the face of adversities; their vulnerability to stress and depression; and the life choices they make. This being the case, its application to the experience of infertility and involuntary childlessness seems even more appropriate. Self-efficacy is also a critical determinant of self-regulation. Self-efficacy perceptions help determine what individuals do with the knowledge and skills they have – as well as why people's behaviors are sometimes incongruent with their actual capabilities, and/or their behaviors differ despite having knowledge and skills. More often, self-efficacy beliefs help determine the outcomes one might expect. Confident individuals anticipate successful outcomes.

Self-efficacy beliefs are based on the core belief that one has the capability to accomplish a particular behavior, task, or goal. Self-efficacy beliefs also help determine how much *effort* people are willing to expend on an activity, how long they will *persevere* when confronting obstacles, and how *resilient* they will be in the face of adverse situations. People with a strong sense of personal competence approach difficult tasks as challenges to be mastered rather than as threats to be avoided. All too often infertile individuals may be very motivated about pursuing infertility treatment but are unaware of what they can and should do in terms of their own behaviors to reach their goals or maximize their efforts. Self-efficacy can be an integral concept for infertile men and women, particularly those who turn to CAM therapies as a means of implementing self-efficacy behaviors. Self-efficacy beliefs also influence an individual's *thought patterns and emotional reactions*, and many CAM therapies target this – a means of reducing emotional distress and reactivity while maximizing emotional regulation and relaxation.

According to social cognition theory, obscure aims and ambiguous goals make it difficult to predict the impact of self-efficacy in predicting behavioral outcomes. Basically, ambiguous goals and situations make it difficult for individuals to have a clear idea of how much effort to expend, how long to sustain it, and how to correct missteps and misjudgments. This is particularly evident in infertility when the goal is often not specifically defined (e.g., mastery of injection training) but more vaguely defined as getting pregnant. Typically, infertile couples do not even define their goal as becoming parents until after a significantly negative diagnosis or repeated treatment failures. As such, CAM remedies may be specific and clearly defined behaviors and goals (e.g., yoga to improve relaxation) and thereby, more readily achievable than getting pregnant. In general, researchers have established that self-efficacy beliefs and behavior changes and outcomes are highly correlated. Self-efficacy has proven to be a more consistent predictor of behavioral outcomes than have any other motivational constructs. Clearly, it is not simply a matter of how capable one is, but of how capable one believes oneself to be.

Placebo Effect and Expectancy Theory

In examining the benefits of CAM therapies, one possibility to be considered is the placebo effect. Placebo effects have traditionally been attributed to the recipient's belief in the efficacy of a substance or procedure – and CAM therapies are often viewed by patients as self-efficacy efforts. The archetypal placebo event occurs in a medical setting: A physician gives a patient a treatment (i.e., a sugar pill) that is a placebo. Presently, the patient's health improves, apparently because the patient believes that the pill (placebo) was a pharmacological agent, effective for the treatment of his or her condition. This is the placebo effect. Placebo effects are effects that, though attributable to the administration of a substance or procedures, are not due to the inherent powers of the substance or procedure.[22]

Although the placebo effect is typically viewed with derision and/or discounted as a myth, in actuality it is a very real, very impressive phenomenon that has existed for centuries. Throughout history, placebos have been used to treat thousands of ailments and been tested in more clinical trials than any other treatment. Placebos are the standard against which all other medications are compared, yet are safe enough to be administered to infants, the elderly, and even pregnant women. Nevertheless, the placebo effect has been often relegated to the role of a control procedure and characterized as a treatment that is ineffective.[22] Overall, the evidence favors the view that the placebo effect is a genuine phenomenon and not merely a product of misattribution or misperception.[23]

The main theories of the placebo effect are expectancy theory and classical conditioning (see Figure 12.2). Although these approaches are sometimes thought to be competing models, in actuality they provide different perspectives and, as such, greater understanding of the placebo effect. Most placebo effects are linked to expectancies, and classical

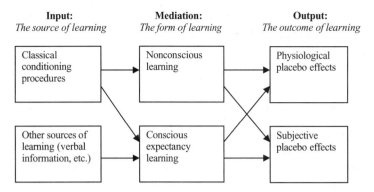

Figure 12.2. The roles of classical conditioning procedures and expectancy in the production of placebo effects[22]

conditioning is one factor (but not the only factor) by which these expectancies can be produced and altered. According to classical conditioning theory, placebo effects are conditioned responses. Conditioned placebo effects without expectancies exist but are relatively rare in humans. The adaptive advantage of cognition is increased response flexibility. For it to convey that benefit, however, it must be capable of overriding the influence of simpler automatic processes.[22]

According to expectancy theory, placebo effects are mediated by explicit (consciously accessible) expectancies. A placebo produces an effect because the recipient expects it to: The placebo elicits an expectation for a particular effect, and the expectation produces that effect. Expectancies are at the core of most placebo effects in human beings. Infertility patients seek CAM treatments because they believe they will help them and their expectation of receiving some benefit, be it reduced anxiety or getting pregnant, may be an important influence on outcome. According to expectancy theory, placebo effects are a subcategory of expectancy effects, and placebos, an expectancy manipulation. Despite expectancy accounting for some measure of placebo effects, there remains the possibility that the therapeutic relationship, the provider's expectations, or sociocultural factors may also account for the placebo effect.[24] In short, the relationship between the patient and the practitioner, in which the practitioner is supportive and positive, may provide more benefit to the patient given a placebo – or standard treatment – than a practitioner who fails to establish a positive therapeutic relationship with the patient.[25] This issue is relevant as infertility patients may perceive their CAM providers as more emotionally in tune or sympathetic to their needs than their physicians, and be a factor in benefits they receive from CAM treatment.

Both social cognition theory and expectancy theory provide a framework for the enormous role cognitions and expectations play in behavior and outcome, particularly in how they may apply to infertility patients using CAM therapies. Most infertility patients are driven to do whatever they can to achieve their wished-for child, and CAM offers other options and opportunities to reach this goal.

CLINICAL ISSUES

Patients and practitioners considering CAM therapies may be overwhelmed by the many different options being used and offered that are specifically directed at infertility and reproductive health problems. Determining the efficacy of these treatments is an even more daunting task. Although there is not complete consensus on classification systems for CAM, the NCCAM classifies CAM therapies into five categories:[1]

(1) *Alternative Medical Systems*, as exemplified by homeopathic and naturopathic medicine, are based on complete systems of theory and practice. Homeopathic and naturopathic medicines are examples of alternative medical systems that have developed in Western cultures. Traditional Chinese medicine is an example from a non-Western culture.

(2) *Mind–Body Interventions* use a variety of techniques designed to enhance the mind's capacity to affect bodily function and symptoms including support groups, cognitive-behavioral therapy, meditation, prayer, and hypnosis.

(3) *Biologically Based Therapies* are based on the use of substances (typically ingested or injected) that are found in nature such as herbs, foods, and vitamins.

(4) *Manipulative and Body-Based Methods* are based on manipulation and/or movement of one or more parts of the body exemplified by chiropractic manipulation and massage.

(5) *Energy Therapies and Biofield Therapies* are intended to affect energy fields that purportedly surround and penetrate the human body by

applying pressure and/or manipulating the body as exemplified by gigong, reiki, and therapeutic touch, or the more unconventional use of electromagnetic fields.

Alternative Medical Systems

Traditional Chinese Medicine

One of the most commonly used alternative medical systems has been traditional Chinese medicine (TCM). It is based on the belief that health is the result of a delicate balance between the ying and the yang. When balance exists, the life force (qi) is able to flow smoothly through the body along invisible channels called meridians. In the absence of balance, qi can be disturbed and disease may set in. To restore balance, herbal preparations are administered and acupuncture, in which specifically designed needles are inserted at points along meridians, is used. Stimulation with the acupuncture needles can be achieved manually or with electrical current (electroacupuncture).[3] TCM has been applied to the treatment of male and female infertility for thousands of years.

There are thousands of herbal substances used in TCM, usually prescribed in combinations of eight to twenty different herbs. It is common for formulations to vary from patient to patient, making the evaluation of the efficacy of these treatments in well-controlled trials almost impossible. A few uncontrolled studies have demonstrated improvement in menstrual function and correction of luteal phase defects.[26–29] Commonly used preparations for the treatment of menstrual irregularity include Hachimijiogan and Guyin decoction. TCM practitioners also use iontophoresis, a method of transdermal drug delivery using electrical current, to administer herbal preparations. A small uncontrolled trial demonstrated an improvement in fertility using iontophoresis of peach kernel mixture.[30] Moxibustion, a procedure in which small quantities of herbal mixtures are burned over the body, has been used to increase circulation in the pelvis and promote healing and follicular development. There are no data to support this practice.

Herbal mixtures have also been used to treat male infertility. Results from uncontrolled studies claimed that use of Guizhi-Fuling-Wan, Ju Jing powder, and Hoccheukkito resulted in improvement in seminal parameters.[31,32] A double-blind, placebo-controlled, randomized trial evaluated the effects of Y virilin in forty patients with oligospermia. A significant improvement in sperm count was found two to three months after initiation of therapy. No change in motility was seen.[33]

Acupuncture

According to Chinese medicine, the etiology of gynecologic dysfunction is kidney deficiency, liver-chi stagnation, and liver-blood deficiency.[34] Acupoints are then chosen to treat these conditions. Acupuncture has been demonstrated to impact the central nervous system, the hypothalamic-pituitary-ovarian axis, and the pelvic organs. Acupuncture increases β endorphin levels.[35] This may explain the decrease in stress and anxiety that has been reported with acupuncture treatment.[36] The alteration in β endorphins impacts gonadotropin-releasing hormone (Gn-RH) secretion and the menstrual cycle. Treatment with acupuncture has been shown to normalize Gn-RH secretion and gonadotropin levels.[37] Acupuncture has also been demonstrated to induce changes in gonadotropin levels and ovarian steroid concentrations in both ovulatory and anovulatory women.[38,39] Acupuncture has been used to trigger ovulation during ovulation induction.[40] A series of studies evaluating the efficacy of auricular acupuncture in the treatment of ovulatory dysfunction demonstrated adequate ovulation, as defined by a temperature increase in basal body temperature of at least eleven days, in 75% of treated women. Fifty percent of these women conceived during the acupuncture treatment.[41] In another study, electroacupuncture improved ovulatory function in 30% of women with polycystic ovarian disease. Patients who responded had lower body mass index (BMI), waist-to-hip circumference ratio, androgen levels, and basal insulin levels.[42]

In addition to the central modulation of the hypothalamic-pituitary-ovarian axis, acupuncture appears to have peripheral effects. Electroacupuncture has been shown to increase blood flow through the uterine arteries in women,[43] although it does not appear to reduce endometrial motility.[44] In an animal model, blood flow to the ovaries was also increased after electroacupuncture.[45]

A number of studies have evaluated the role of acupuncture in in vitro fertilization (IVF). A few retrospective studies have demonstrated improved outcome with IVF in patients receiving acupuncture. [46–48] A single, small matched-control study did not find an increase in pregnancy rate when patients who received acupuncture were compared with those who did not.[49] There was a large randomized controlled trial evaluating the use of acupuncture in patients undergoing IVF.[50] In the treatment group, acupuncture was performed in eighty patients twenty-five minutes before and after embryo transfer. The clinical pregnancy rate was 42.5% in the treatment group and 26.3% in the control group. The authors concluded that acupuncture seemed to be a useful tool for improving pregnancy rate after IVF. The lack of a placebo/control group certainly weakens this conclusion, although the underlying physiologic changes produced from acupuncture treatment do support a possible role for acupuncture in the treatment of female infertility. Other smaller prospective trials have confirmed this finding.[51,52]

Acupuncture has also been applied to the treatment of male-factor infertility. The mechanism of action is likely secondary to both central and peripheral effects as seen in women. A number of uncontrolled trials have shown an improvement in sperm count, motility, and fertilization rate in IVF.[53,54] A small controlled trial demonstrated an improvement in the ultrastructural integrity of sperm with acupuncture treatment.[55] Two randomized controlled trials also demonstrated a positive effect on seminal parameters with acupuncture treatment.[56,57] In a randomized placebo-controlled blinded study evaluating acupuncture and moxa treatment in nineteen patients with oligoasthenospermia, sperm morphology was significantly improved in those men receiving treatment.[58] Clearly, more data are required to assess the role of acupuncture in male infertility.

The risk of serious events occurring in association with acupuncture is quite low, and indeed below that of many common medical treatments. Evidence from twelve prospective studies, which surveyed more than a million treatments, found the risk of a serious adverse event with acupuncture to be 0.05 per 10,000 treatments and 0.55 per 10,000 patients.[59] The most common complications include hepatitis, pneumothorax, infection to the outer ear, and drowsiness. As such, acupuncture should only be performed by properly trained, licensed, or certified professionals.

Homeopathy

Homeopathy is an alternative medical system pioneered by Samuel Hahnemann, a physician who, beginning with an article published in a German medical journal in 1796, founded homoeopathic medicine. The premise behind homeopathy is the law of similars or 'like heals like.' Hence, a substance that produces a certain symptom in a healthy person can cure a sick person with the same symptoms. Administration of the treatment is believed to stimulate the body's own healing functions to reorganizing it into a state of balance. Homeopathy uses only minute doses of substances such as arsenic, venom, and dandelion. In fact, it is believed that the more dilute the substance, the greater the potency. There are more than 200 homeopathic remedies proposed for the treatment of infertility and 170

for the treatment of miscarriage. An uncontrolled clinical trial reported that individual homeopathic therapy improved sperm count.[60] Although probably safe because of the extremely dilute nature of the administered substance, there is the potential for interaction with other medications, for example, ovulation induction medications. In addition, there exists a risk of adverse outcome as a result of delaying allopathic treatment.

Mind–Body Interventions

Mind–body medicine uses a variety of approaches to enhance the capacity of one's mind to positively affect bodily functions. This, in part, is based on the belief that psychological symptoms including depression and anxiety may interfere with conception. These techniques may include cognitive-behavioral therapy, meditation, hypnosis, prayer, and guided imagery.

There are little data evaluating the role of hypnosis in reproductive medicine. In one study, a single session of hypnosis was administered to patients with hypothalamic amenorrhea. Seventy-five percent of women experienced a menses within twelve weeks.[61] There is a report of two pregnancies occurring after hypnosis.[62] The authors postulated that pregnancy might have resulted from a reduction in muscular tension in the fallopian tube allowing for passage of the oocyte. They also felt that hypnosis helped modify the patient's expressed attitude, self-confidence, and sense of optimism, impacting somatic function. Clearly, more data are required.

Transcendental meditation has been shown to reduce blood pressure and cortisol production.[63] There is a single case report of pregnancy occurring with the use of transcendental meditation.[64] Autogenic therapy, which is a series of simple mental exercises designed to diminish the stress response and enhance the relaxation response, was evaluated in patients with unexplained infertility.[65] A small uncontrolled trial demonstrated a reduction in mean anxiety score and three patients achieved pregnancy.

Biologically Based Therapies

These treatments are based on the use of substances found in nature such as herbs, vitamins, and foods. Herbal therapies, as used in traditional Chinese medicine, have indirect evidence of safety and efficacy. However, the traditional application of herbal therapy differs from the way it is used in Western cultures. For example, in traditional use, ephedra is used safely in low doses, combined with other herbs, in the treatment of asthma and other respiratory diseases. In nontraditional use, ephedra was used for weight loss, body building, and recreational purposes in very high doses leading to complications and even death. Given that the use of these approaches differs so greatly, they are considered separately in this chapter.

Female infertility

A number of herbs have been recommended to treat female infertility. Vitex, or chastetree berry, has been used to treat ovulatory dysfunction. In an uncontrolled study of its effects on the gonadotropin-releasing hormone and thyrotropin-releasing tests, prolactin and ovarian hormones, only early follicular phase estradiol and prolactin concentrations were increased.[66] A case report suggested that a disturbed ovulatory response to gonadotropins may have been the result of concurrent Vitex consumption.[67] Recently, a small double-blind placebo-controlled study evaluated the use of a nutritional supplement containing Vitex and green tea extracts as well as L-arginine, vitamins, and minerals. After three months, those in the treatment group had higher luteal progesterone and a longer luteal phase. After five months, five of fifteen treated women conceived as opposed to none in the placebo group.[68] The impact of each agent in the fertility blend cannot be assessed. There are claims that other herbal preparations, including black cohash, dong quai, false unicorn root, nettle leaves, evening primrose oil, red raspberry leaves, crampbark, blue cohash, wheatgrass and bromelain, increased female fertility. It has been suggested that topical application of St. John's Wort over the abdomen will reduce adhesions. There are no data to support any of these claims. In fact, black cohash, dong quai, false unicorn root, and nettle leaves may cause uterine contractions. Blue cohash has been associated with a risk of fetal anomalies.

Because phytoestrogens act on the estrogen receptor, there is concern that excessive phytoestrogen consumption, for example, soy, may impede conception. In cows, data suggest that a diet high in red clover improves fertility[69] but another report states that fertility is decreased with such a diet.[70] The role of phytoestrogens supplementation in maximizing conception in women is unclear. A randomized trial found that supplementation with high-dose phytoestrogens increased endometrial thickness in women treated with clomiphene citrate.[71] Another randomized trial found that luteal phase supplementation with high-dose phytoestrogens in women undergoing IVF was associated with a higher pregnancy rate.[72] These studies would appear to contradict those who recommend restricting soy intake to maximize fertility. Clearly, more research is required.

Other nutritional supplements have been evaluated regarding their role in female reproductive function and fertility. Nitric oxide has vasodilatory properties, which are believed to enhance folliculogenesis. It was postulated that supplementation with L-arginine, which is converted to nitric oxide, would improve fertility. L-arginine supplementation has shown to improve outcome in a randomized trial of poor responders undergoing IVF.[73] Another randomized trial performed by the same authors evaluating normal responders found that women treated with L-arginine had poorer quality embryos and a lower pregnancy rate.[74] The dose of L-arginine administered was the same.

Vitamin C supplementation was shown to enhance the ovulation-inducing effects of clomiphene citrate in an uncontrolled trial.[75] A recent randomized trial of patients with luteal phase defect found that supplementation with vitamin C significantly increased progesterone levels and pregnancy rate.[76] However, another randomized placebo-controlled study evaluating luteal supplementation with vitamin C, even at very high doses, failed to find an impact.[77] Use of vitamin C supplementation in the follicular phase has also been evaluated in patients undergoing IVF. This study found higher levels of ascorbic acid in the follicular fluid and an increase in the pregnancy rate in those patients who received vitamin C supplementation.[78] In the absence of a true deficiency, supplementation with other vitamins or minerals does not appear to increase final fertility. In addition, excessive vitamin A increases the risk of fetal congenital abnormalities and high doses of vitamin B6 are associated with peripheral neuropathy.

It has also been postulated that dietary modification in the absence of supplements may improve fertility. In her book, *The Infertility Diet: Get Pregnant and Prevent Miscarriage*, Reiss makes several recommendations including avoidance of white flour, processed sugar, red meat, and dairy; increased usage of foods high in essential fatty acids and kelp; and the use, if possible, of organically grown food.[79] Although there are no data to support that adoption of this diet will improve reproductive outcome, there is considerable evidence that a diet that is nutritionally sound and well-balanced maximizes general health and well-being, while dieting itself or a diet that is nutritionally unbalanced can have a negative impact on reproductive health, particularly in women. Furthermore, although others have advocated minifast purification and cleansing regimens, there are no data to support such practices, which may be unsafe. Finally, the issue of dieting and slimming regimens must be carefully assessed and evaluated in terms of their potential for triggering disordered eating, impairing the effectiveness of fertility treatments, and/or triggering stress and anxiety by overattending to food versus healthy nutrition.

Male Infertility

Herbal preparations have also been used to treat male infertility. In an uncontrolled study, Pychnogenol (French maritime tree bark extract) improved sperm morphology and mannose receptor binding.[80] In another uncontrolled trial, ginseng administration enhanced sperm number and motility as well as increased testosterone and gonadotropin levels.[81] Although there are no data available, there are claims that saw palmetto and gingko strengthen the male reproductive system. Interestingly, sperm, when exposed to saw palmetto or gingko in vitro, have demonstrated a reduction in motility.[82] Exposure to gingko, as well as the commonly used St. John's wort and echinacea, resulted in decreased oocyte penetration in the zona free hamster test.[83] Sperm, when exposed to St. John's wort or echinacea, also experienced DNA denaturation.

Isoflavones may also impact male infertility. In one study, genestein induced hydrogen peroxide-induced DNA damage in sperm.[84] In another study, in vitro exposure of sperm to low-dose genestein induced capacitation and the acrosome reaction. Higher doses, however, impaired sperm function.[85] This suggests that isoflavones may be beneficial in facilitating male fertility, but there is much to learn before advocating its use.

There are a number of nutrients that appear to improve seminal parameters. L-carnitine is essential for transport of fatty acids into the mitochondria. Administration of L-carnitine has been demonstrated to improve sperm count, motility, and morphology in double-blind placebo-controlled trials.[86,87] Uncontrolled trials have found that arginine, which is a precursor to compounds essential in sperm motility, increases sperm count and motility.[88,89] Glutathione, a small protein molecule, is an integral part of the mid-piece of the sperm. Glutathione therapy was used in a randomized double-blind placebo-controlled trial to improve sperm motility in patients with abnormal semen analysis.[90]

Certain minerals have also been shown to be beneficial in improving semen parameters. Zinc is essential to spermatogenesis. Zinc supplementation was shown to improve semen parameters in uncontrolled studies.[91,92] A recent randomized blind trial found that zinc and folic acid supplementation resulted in an increase in sperm numbers when administered together.[93] Neither substance was effective when given alone. Selenium, like glutathione, is present in the mitochondrial capsule of the mid-piece of the sperm. The data regarding selenium are quite mixed. A ran-

domized controlled study evaluating the impact of dietary selenium on semen analysis demonstrated no effect.[94] Another randomized double-blind controlled trial found a significant increase in sperm motility with selenium supplementation.[95]

Vitamin supplementation has also been evaluated in the treatment of male infertility. A placebo-controlled randomized trial found that high-dose supplementation with vitamin B12 resulted in a significant increase in sperm count.[96] As high concentrations of free radicals are detrimental to sperm cells, antioxidants could have a role in improving sperm function. A randomized placebo-controlled trial of vitamin C supplementation demonstrated a significant improvement in sperm quality.[97]. Another randomized trial demonstrated a 140% increase in sperm count after one week of supplementation.[98] However, given that sperm turnover is much longer than one week, the results of this study must be called into question. Vitamin E, another antioxidant, has been shown to improve sperm motility in an uncontrolled trial.[99] A randomized crossover trial demonstrated that supplementation with vitamin E enhanced the sperm function in the zona binding assay.[100] On the other hand, a randomized placebo-controlled trial failed to demonstrate any effect after eight weeks of vitamin C and E supplementation.[101] Another antioxidant, coenzyme Q10, was shown in an uncontrolled study to improve fertilization rate with intracytoplasmic sperm injection (ICSI).[102] Another series found that sperm motility was improved with coenzyme Q10 treatment.[103]

There are several controlled studies that have found an improvement in seminal parameters with the use of some herbal, nutritional, and dietary supplements. Unfortunately, pregnancy was not typically evaluated as an end point. As improvement in sperm count and motility do not always correlate with an increase in pregnancy rate and/or live birth, the need for controlled studies that evaluate pregnancy rates and/or live births cannot be overstated.

Manipulative and Body-Based Methods

Yoga is a classical Indian practice that is built on the foundation of ethics (yama) and personal discipline (niyama). It has been suggested that in addition to providing exercise and flexibility, yoga can alter brain and body chemistry.[104] Although there are clear benefits to yoga, there are no data supporting claims that it enhances fertility or conception.

Others have suggested that various types of massage improve female fertility. There are claims that femoral massage and hip rotation increase pelvic blood flow. Others have proposed rolfing, or intense manual massage, as a treatment for infertility. Deep tissue work in the pelvic area is reported to increase blood flow and neuronal response. Clinics performing this technique have claimed a 75% success rate in treating infertility. There are no data to support these claims.

'Clear Passage Therapies' is a program that uses soft tissue physical and massage therapy to decrease adhesions and increase the function of the fallopian tubes. The owners of the patent for this report a pregnancy rate of greater than 60% as a result of their therapy. They have published a case series of selected individual testimonies attributing conception to this therapy.[105] Unfortunately, the research has several epidemiologic and statistical flaws in addition to flawed research design. Correction of vertical alignment and subluxation is also claimed by some practitioners of these approaches to treat infertility, although there are no data to support these claims.

Energy Therapies

According to reflexology, the feet are the maps to the body's organs. By applying pressure to certain parts of the feet, reflexologists can reroute the body's life force. Reflexologists recommend rubbing tender spots on either side of the ankles in different directions to induce menses. At present, there are no scientific data to support the use of energy therapies in the treatment of infertility. In the only study published evaluating energy healers, it was found that the healer was unable to distinguish the presence or absence of infertility in the study subjects.[106] At present, energy therapies are only occasionally used to treat infertility.

THERAPEUTIC INTERVENTIONS

Infertility counselors, like all members of the infertility treatment team, are likely to encounter an increasing number of patients using CAM therapies either in conjunction with conventional reproductive technologies as a primary treatment for infertility, or to facilitate conception. As in any situation, patient motivations and psychosocial circumstances should be considered. A further consideration is patient expectations regarding CAM therapies – particularly their health beliefs, self-efficacy health behaviors, and cultural circumstances. Additionally, if patients are using CAM in conjunction with conventional reproductive medicine, the infertility counselor may be in a unique position to facilitate communication and collaboration between the patient and physician regarding the use of CAM. Finally, the infertility counselor may be professionally trained as a practitioner of one or more CAM therapies and, as such, may be able to offer adjunctive care via CAM therapies

in collaboration with the reproductive medicine treatment team.

Helping Patients Explore Motivations for Using CAM

As documented earlier, the number of patient visits to CAM providers exceeds the number of visits to primary care providers, highlighting the increasing popularity and importance of CAM therapies. Infertile patients represent a unique patient population in that many do not perceive themselves as sick and may not have an actual medical diagnosis. Motivations for pursuing CAM therapies are varied. Many infertile men and women perceive the use of some CAM therapies (e.g., vitamins, yoga, spirituality) as a means of maximizing their general health and well-being. Others may actively pursue exacting CAM treatment regimes (e.g., specific herbal remedies and/or manipulative methods) in dogged pursuit of conception, while others consider CAM therapies a means of enhancing or improving treatment outcomes in assisted reproductive technologies (ARTs). Cultural mores or traditions (including pressure from family and friends) may be a reason for pursing CAM therapies for some couples – a motivation that may or may *not* be acceptable to one or both partners. Some infertile couples feel they must pursue every avenue in their quest of conception and pregnancy and, as such, are motivated to use CAM therapies to minimize future regret. Finally, an increasing number of infertile individuals are pursuing CAM therapies to improve emotional well-being and quality-of-life as evidenced by mind–body groups.

Careful exploration of motivations for pursuing CAM treatments can be useful (even necessary) to ensure that the individual's (and couple's) motivations and expectations are realistic, accurate, and congruent. Some of these therapies are costly and can put further strains on an already financially strapped couple, who may have invested a great deal of money on conventional infertility treatment. Partner disagreement about the importance and value of CAM therapies has the potential for creating undue stress due to couple conflict. Cultural issues may also warrant special attention, again to avoid coercion or social pressure to pursue CAM therapies or cognitive dissonance when CAM therapies are rejected. Patients should be encouraged to optimize self-care and self-efficacy, while avoiding unrealistic expectations or hopes. A primary goal for the infertility counselor is helping patients approach CAM therapies as a means of improving quality-of-life and enhancing self-efficacy (e.g., taking control) rather than engaging in a wide array of CAM therapies *solely* to ensure conception and pregnancy.

Assistance in Decision Making and Assessment of Treatment Efficacy

As the availability of CAM therapies and the increasing promotion of CAM therapies as remedies or cures for infertility make their way into the public arena, infertile patients are faced with the dilemma of what are legitimate practices and what are frauds, shams, quacks, or charlatans. Infertility patients, as a consumer group, are potentially vulnerable to exploitation in their quest for a baby. As such, infertility counselors may be called upon to provide patient education albeit consumer protection by helping patients find qualified, competent practitioners who are properly credentialed and licensed. Infertility counselors (as all professionals) must be careful not to advocate the use of untested and/or ineffective therapies, particularly to vulnerable individuals who will try everything to achieve a pregnancy.[15]

Toward that end, in 2002 the WHO launched its first ever, comprehensive traditional medicine strategy designed to assist countries to:[1]

■ develop national policies on the evaluation and regulation of CAM practices;
■ create a stronger evidence base on the safety, efficacy, and quality of the CAM products and practices;
■ ensure availability and affordability of CAM including essential herbal medicines;
■ promote therapeutically sound use of CAM by providers and consumers;
■ document traditional medicines and remedies.

Because scientific evidence from randomized clinical trials is only strong for acupuncture, some herbal medicines, and some manual therapies, the WHO recommends further research to ascertain the efficacy and safety of other forms of CAM therapies. Because of the limited scientific evidence about CAM's safety and efficacy, the WHO has recommended that governments worldwide:

■ formulate national policy and regulations for the proper use of CAM and its integration into national healthcare systems in line with the provisions of the WHO guidelines;
■ establish regulatory mechanisms to control the safety and quality of products and of CAM practice;
■ create awareness about safe and effective CAM therapies among the public and consumers.

Keeping these recommendations in mind, it is a responsibility of infertility counselors as well as all medical caregivers to help infertile men and women accurately assess claims of success, efficacy, cost-effectiveness, and benefits of all CAM therapies. This is particularly important for patients using CAM therapies as an adjunct to assisted reproduction. Furthermore, many patients feel it is the responsibility of conventional medicine caregivers to ensure that CAM providers they refer to are properly trained. An ideal approach for patients is one that ensures a positive interaction (integration) between conventional medicine and CAM therapies, working together to improve the health and well-being of infertile patients and maximizing the goal of conception and pregnancy.[13]

As the field of reproductive medicine and CAM therapies grows, anxious vulnerable infertile patients may look to their physicians and reproductive health providers to provide referrals to competent and qualified CAM providers. As such, infertility counselors along with all members of the reproductive medicine team must be aware of CAM therapies, evidence-based research on their efficacy, application, and reliability. Furthermore, reproductive treatment teams should be aware of the qualifications and credentialing of various CAM providers as well as a system for vetting the qualifications, training, and credentialing of CAM providers so as to best protect consumers and maintain quality assurance of patient care.

Facilitating Communication with Caregivers

A dilemma for many CAM therapy users is whether or not to tell their physicians about the CAM therapies they are using and, if so, how. As reported earlier, infertile patients reported that they would have liked advice from their physician about CAM therapies.[12] However, many infertile patients are reluctant to discuss the use of CAM therapies because of cultural differences or because they fear (or accurately assess) that their conventional medical caregiver will not discuss the use of CAM therapies in a respectful and open manner. Interestingly, many infertile patients perceived the CAM provider as more interested, understanding and attentive, so it may be these qualities that the infertile patient is not receiving from the conventional caregiver that they seek in a CAM provider.[12]

As a member of the collaborative treatment team, the infertility counselor may have the opportunity to facilitate communication among the caregivers and with the patient, particularly regarding CAM therapies. Because some of these therapies may impact or interact with conventional medication or treatments, it is crucially important that infertility counselors encourage patients to be honest and forthright with their physician about the use of CAM. Infertility counselors may also be in a position to provide the treatment team with appropriate CAM practitioners within the community, who are suitably trained and licensed (if required).

Infertility Counselor as CAM Provider

Some CAM therapies are particularly well-suited for the mental health profession. Thus, infertility counselors may also be a CAM provider. There are a number of CAM therapies that infertility counselors may have integrated into their practice. For example, hypnotherapy may be used as a part of psychotherapy or as an adjunct to behavioral treatment, such as with smoking cessation. In addition, many infertility counselors use mind–body treatments, such as relaxation and breathing exercises, guided imagery and visualization, as part of therapy or a structured mind–body group program. Some counselors may be trained in yoga, healing touch, or massage therapy and use these techniques with their patients. The important consideration for infertility counselors providing CAM services is that they be well-trained and certified in the treatments they are promoting and providing. Many of these areas require extensive training programs with many hours of practice to be eligible for certification. As advocates for consumer protection, infertility counselors must be held to the same standard of care and competency as others practicing in the field.

FUTURE IMPLICATIONS

While CAM modalities have been around since the beginning of mankind, only recently has it come into popularity as part of conventional infertility treatment. The use of CAM therapies will continue to grow as infertility patients seek supportive and alternative means to help maximize fertility and ensure pregnancy. Individuals experiencing infertility use a variety of CAM therapies. At present, there are some data to support the use of acupuncture and nutritional supplementation containing Vitex and green tree extract, in increasing female fertility. Acupuncture, antioxidants, mineral supplements, and L-carnitine appear to be of greatest benefit in improving seminal parameters. Clearly, the greatest need in the future is for much more high-quality research to evaluate the efficacy of these therapies. In addition, the medical community has a responsibility to see that unproven methods and untrained practitioners are not allowed or encouraged to prey upon an emotionally vulnerable group, infertility patients. Sound, evidence-based medical practice requires scientifically rigorous research that meets consistent standards, and CAM must be evaluated under the same conditions. This is the challenge of the future.

SUMMARY

■ CAM is defined as a group of diverse medical and healthcare systems, practices and products that are not presently considered part of conventional medicine and are used together with or as an alternative to conventional medicinal treatment.

■ While many CAM therapies have been used for centuries, controlled studies evaluating their efficacy in infertility treatment are limited.

■ The use of CAM by infertility patients is increasing and patients must be encouraged to communicate with their physicians regarding their use of CAM therapies, especially regarding herbal preparations that may interact with other medications or be contraindicated in pregnancy.

■ Patients need to be cautioned when choosing CAM practitioners as an entire industry has developed targeting the infertile populations, often at great cost, by soliciting patients with unsubstantiated claims of success.

REFERENCES

1. World Health Organization Fact Sheet 134, 2003. www.who.int/mediacentre/factsheets/fs134/en.
2. *House of Lords*, House of Lords Science and Technology Sixth Report, 2000.
3. Get the Facts. What is complementary and alternative medicine (CAM)? Available at: http://nccam.nih.gov/health/whatiscam/.
4. Barnes PM, Powell-Griner E, McFann K, et al. Complementary and alternative medicine among adults: United States, 2002. *Adv Data* 2004; 343:1–19.
5. Tindle HA, Davis RB, Phillips RS, et al. Trends in use of complementary and alternative medicine by US adults: 1997–2002. *Altern Ther Health Med* 2005; 11: 42–9.
6. Eisenberg DM, Kessler RC, Van Rompay MI, et al. Perceptions about complementary therapies relative to conventional therapies among adults who use both: Results from a national survey. *Ann Intern Med* 2001; 135:344–51.
7. Upchurch DM, Chyu L. Use of complementary and alternative medicine among women. *Women's Health Issues* 2005; 15:5–13.
8. Ernest E, White A. The BBC survey of complementary medicine use in the UK. *Complemt Ther Med* 2000; 8:32–6.
9. Thomas KJ, Nicholl JP, Coleman P. Use and expenditure on complementary medicine in England: A population-based survey. *Complemt Ther Med* 2001; 9:2–11.

10. Adams J, Sibbritt DW, Easthope G, et al. The profile of women who consult alternative health practitioners in Australia. *Med J Aust* 2003; 15:297–300.

11. Yamashita H, Tsukayama H, Sugishita C. Popularity of complementary and alternative medicine in Japan: A telephone survey. *Complement Ther Med* 2002; 10:84–93.

12. Coulson C, Jenkins J. Complementary and alternative medicine utilization in NHS and private clinic settings: A United Kingdom survey of 400 infertility patients. *J Exp Clin Assist Reprod* 2005; 2:5.

13. Shaikh BT, Hatcher J. Complementary and alternative medicine in Pakistan: Prospects and limitations. *Evid Based Complement Alternat Med* 2005; 129–42.

14. Veal L. Complementary therapy and infertility: An Icelandic perspective. *Complement Ther Nurs Midwifery* 1998; 4:3–6.

15. Galst JP. Alternative medicine and infertility: What infertility patients are using and why. *Fertil Steril* 1999; 72:S130.

16. Cox H, Henderson L, Wood R, et al. Learning to take charge: Women's experiences of living with endometriosis. *Complement Ther Nurs Midwifery* 2003; 9:62–8.

17. Cox H, Henderson L, Anderson N, et al. Focus group study of endometriosis: Struggle, loss, and the medical merry-go-round. *Int J Nurs Pract* 2003; 9:2–9.

18. Bandura A. Self-efficacy: Toward a unifying theory of behavioral change. *Psychological Rev* 1977; 84: 191–215.

19. Bandura A.*Social Foundations of Thought and Action: A Social Cognitive Theory*. Englewood Cliffs, NJ: Prentice Hall, 1986.

20. Pajares Overview of social cognitive theory and of self-efficacy. 2002. Retrieved: 9/25/2005 from http://www.emory.edu/EDUCATION/mfp/eff.html.

21. Bandura A, ed. *Self-Efficacy in Changing Societies*. New York: Cambridge University Press, 1995.

22. Kirsch I. Conditioning, expectancy, and the placebo effect: Comment on Stewart-Williams and Podd. *Psychological Bulletins* 2004; 130:341–3.

23. Stewart-Williams S. The placebo puzzle: Putting together the pieces. *Health Psychology* 2004; 23:198–206.

24. Stewart-Williams S, Podd J. The placebo effect: Dissolving the expectancy versus conditioning debate. *Psychological Bulletin* 2004; 130:324–40.

25. Mayo Clinic College of Medicine. A center for patient oriented research publication. *Patient Oriented Research* 2005; 3:1–15.

26. Fang L. TCM treatment of luteal phase defect. An analysis of 60 cases. *J Tradit Chin Med* 1991; 11:115–20.

27. Chen X, Chen D, Dong G. Guyin decoction in the treatment of immuno-sterility and its effect on humoral immunity. *J Tradit Chin Med* 1995; 15:259–61.

28. Luolon Z. Observation on the result of treatment of female infertility in 343 cases. *J Tradit Chin Med* 1986; 6:175–7.

29. Usuki S, Kubota S, Usuki Y. Treatment with hachimijiogan, a non-ergot Chinese herbal medicine, in two hyperprolactinemia infertile women. *Acta Obstet Gynecol Scand* 1989; 68:475–8.

30. Banchi P, Wenqian Y, Zhoujun S. Observation of effect of iotophoresis of traditional Chinese drug in female infertility. *J Tradit Chin Med* 1984; 4:259–60.

31. Ishikawa H, Ohashi M, Hayakawa K, et al. Effects of Guizhi-Fuling-Wan on male infertility with varicocele. *Am J Chin Med* 1996; 24:327–31.

32. Zhai Y, et al. TCM treatment of male infertility due to seminal abnormality – a clinical observation of 82 cases. *J Tradit Chin Med* 1990; 10:26–9.

33. Rege NN, Date J, Kulkarni V, et al. Effect of Y virilin on male infertility. *J Postgrad Med* 1997; 43:64–7.

34. Maciocia G. *Obstetrics and Gynecology in Chinese Medicine*. New York: Churchill Livingstone, 1998.

35. Petti F, Bangrazi A, Liguori A, Reale G, et al. Effects of acupuncture on immune response related to opioid-like peptides. *J Tradit Chin Med* 1998; 18:55–63.

36. Chen A. An introduction to sequential electric acupuncture (SEA) in the treatment of stress related physical and mental disorders. *Acupunct Electrother Res* 1992; 17:273–83.

37. Lin JH, Liu SH, Chan WW, et al. Effects of electroacupuncture and gonadotropin-releasing hormone treatments on hormone changes in anoestrous sows. *Am J Chin Med* 1988; 16:117–26.

38. Aso T, Motohashi T, Murata M, et al. The influence of acupuncture stimulation on plasma levels of LH, FSH, progesterone and estradiol in normally ovulating women. *Am J Chin Med* 1976; 4:391–401.

39. Mo X, Li D, Pu Y, et al. Clinical studies on the mechanism of acupuncture stimulation of ovulation. *J Trad Chin Med* 1993; 13:115–9.

40. Cai X. Substitution of acupuncture for human chorionic gonadotropin in ovulation induction. *J Tradit Chin Med* 1997; 17:119–21.

41. Gerhard I, Postneek F. Auricular acupuncture in the treatment of female infertility. *Gynecol Endocrinol* 1992; 6:171–81.

42. Stener-Victorin E, Waldenstrom U, et al. Effects of electro-acupuncture on anovulation in women with polycystic ovary syndrome. *Acta Obstet Gynecol Scand* 2000; 79:180–8.

43. Stener-Victorin E, Waldenstrom U, Andersson SA, et al. Reduction of blood flow impedance in the uterine arteries of infertile women with electro-acupuncture. *Hum Reprod* 1996; 11:1314–7.

44. Paulus WE, Zhang M, Strehler E, et al. Motility of the endometrium after acupuncture treatment. *Fertil Steril* 2003; 80:131.

45. Stener-Victorin E, Kobayashi R, Watanabe O, et al. Effects of electroacupuncture stimulation of different frequencies and intensities on ovarian blood flow in anesthetized rats with steroid induced polycystic ovaries. *Reprod Biol Endocrinol* 2004; 2:16–24.

46. Magarelli PC, Cridennda DK, Cohen M. Acupuncture and good prognosis IVF patients: Synergy. *Fertil Steril* 2004; 82:S80–S81.

47. Magarelli PC, Cridennda DK. Acupuncture and IVF poor responders: A cure? *Fertil Steril* 2004; 81:20.

48. Khorram NM, Horton S, Sahakian V. The effect of acupuncture on outcome of in vitro fertilization. *Fertil Steril* 2005; 84:S364.

49. Wang W, Check JH, Liss J, et al. A matched controlled study to evaluate the efficacy of acupuncture for improving pregnancy rates following in vitro fertilization-embryo transfer. *Fertil Steril* 2005; 83:S24.

50. Paulus EW, Zhang M, Strehler E, et al. Influence of acupuncture on the pregnancy rate in patients who undergo assisted reproduction therapy. *Fertil Steril* 2002; 77:721–4.

51. Zhang M, Paulus WE, Strehler E, et al. Increase of pregnancy rate in assisted reproduction therapy by acupuncture. *Fertil Steril* 2001; 76:S75.

52. Quintero R. A randomized, controlled, double-blind, cross-over study evaluating acupuncture as an adjunct to IVF. *Fertil Steril* 2004; 81:11–12.

53. Zheng Z. Analysis on the therapeutic effect of combined use of acupuncture and medication in 297 cases of male sterility. *J Tradit Chin Med* 1997; 17:190–3.

54. Zhang M, Huang G, Lu F, et al. Influence of acupuncture on idiopathic male infertility in assisted reproductive technology. *J Huazhong Univ Sci Technolog Med Sci* 2002; 22:228–30.

55. Pei J, Strehler E, Noss U, et al. Quantitative evaluation of spermatozoa ultrastructure after acupuncture treatment for idiopathic male infertility. *Fertil Steril* 2005; 84:141–7.

56. Siterman S, Eltes F, Wolfson V, et al. Effect of acupuncture on sperm parameters of males suffering from subfertility related to low sperm quality. *Arch Androl* 1997; 39:155–61.

57. Siterman S, Eltes F, Wolfson V, et al. Does acupuncture treatment affect sperm density in males with very low sperm count? A pilot study. *Androl* 2000; 32:31–9.

58. Garfinkel E, Cedenho AP, Yamaura Y, et al. Effects of acupuncture and moxa treatment in patients with semen abnormalities. *Asian J Androl* 2003; 5:345–8.

59. White A. A cumulative review of the range and incidence of significant adverse events associated with acupuncture. *Acupunct Med* 2004; 22:122–33.

60. Gerhar I, Wallis E. Individualized homeopathic therapy for male infertility. *Homeopathy* 2002; 91:133–44.

61. Tschugguel W, Berga JL. Treatment of functional hypothalamic amenorrhea with hypnotherapy. *Fertil Steril* 2003; 80:983–5.

62. Gravitz MA. Hypnosis in the treatment of functional infertility. *Amer J Clin Hypn* 1995; 38:22–6.

63. Jevning R, Wilson AF, Davidson MK. Adrenocortical activity during meditation. *Hormones Behav* 1978; 10:54–60.

64. Lovell-Smith HD. Transcendental meditation and infertility. *New Zealand Med J* 1985; 98:922.

65. Harrison RF, O'Moore RR, O'Moore AM. Stress and fertility: Some modalities of investigation and treatment in couples with unexplained infertility in Dublin. *Int J Fertil* 1986; 31:153–9.

66. Neumann-Kunhelt B, Steif G, Schmiady H, et al. Investigations of possible effects of the phytotherapeutic agent Agnus castus on the follicular and corpus luteum phases. *Hum Reprod* 1993; 8:110.

67. Cahill DJ, Fox R, Wardle PG, et al. Multiple follicular development associated with herbal medicine. *Hum Reprod* 1994; 9:1469–70.

68. Westphal LM, Polan ML, Trant AS, et al. A nutritional supplement for improving fertility in women: A pilot study. *J Reprod Med* 2004; 49:289–93.

69. Morley FH, Axelsen A, Bennett D. Recovery of normal fertility after grazing on oestrogenic red clover. *Aust Vet J* 1966; 42:204–6.

70. Kallela K. Heinonen K, Saloniemi H. Plant oestrogens: The cause of decreased fertility in cows. A case report. *Nord Vet Med* 1984; 36:124–9.

71. Unfer V, Casini ML, Costabile L, et al. High dose of phytoestrogens can reverse the antiestrogenic effects of clomiphene citrate on the endometrium in patients undergoing intrauterine insemination: A randomized trial. *Fertil Steril* 2004; 27:1509–13.

72. Unfer V, Casini ML, Gerli S, et al. Phytoestrogens may improve the pregnancy rate in in vitro fertilization-embryo transfer cycles: A prospective, controlled randomized trial. *Fertil Steril* 2004; 6:1509–13.

73. Battaglia C, Salvatori M, Maxia N, et al. Adjuvant L-arginine treatment for in vitro fertilization in poor responder patients. *Hum Reprod* 1999; 14:1690–7.

74. Battaglia C, Regnani G, Marsella T, et al. Adjuvant L-arginine treatment in controlled ovarian hyperstimulation: A double-blind, randomized study. *Hum Reprod* 2002; 17:659–65.

75. Igarashi M. Augmentative effect of ascorbic acid upon induction of human ovulation in clomiphene-ineffective anovulatory women. *Int J Fertil* 1977; 22:168–73.

76. Henmi H, Endo T, Kitajima Y, et al. Effects of ascorbic acid supplementation on serum progesterone levels in patients with a luteal phase defect. *Fertil Steril* 2003; 80:459–61.

77. Griesinger G, Franke K, Kinast C, et al. Ascorbic acid supplement during luteal phase in IVF. *J Assist Reprod Genet* 2002; 19:164–8.

78. Crha I, Hruba D, Ventruba P, et al. Ascorbic acid and infertility treatment. *Cent Eur J Public Health* 2003; 11:63–7.

79. Reis F. *The Infertility Diet: Get Pregnant and Prevent Miscarriage*. Boston, MA: Peanut Butter and Jelly Press 2004.

80. Roseff SJ. Improvement in sperm quality and function with French maritime pine tree bark extract. *J Reprod Med* 2002; 47:821–4.

81. Salvati G, Genovesi G, Marcellini L, et al. Effects of Panax Ginseng C. A. Meyer Saponis on male fertility. *Pan Minerva Med* 1996; 38:249–54.

82. Ondrizek RR, Chan PJ, Patton NC, et al. Inhibition of human sperm motility by specific herbs used in alternative medicine. *J Assist Reprod Genet* 1999; 16:87–91.

83. Ondrizek RR, Chan PJ, Patton WC, et al. An alternative medicine study of herbal effects in the penetration of zona free hamster oocytes and the integrity of sperm deoxyribonucleic acid. *Fertil Steril* 1999; 71:517–22.

84. Sierens J, Hartley JA, Campbell MJ, et al. In vitro isoflavone supplementation reduces hydrogen peroxide-induced DNA damage in sperm. *Teratog Carcinog Mutagen* 2002; 22:227–34.

85. Kumi-Diaka J, Townsend J. Toxic potential of dietary genistein isoflavone and beta-lapachone on capacitation and acrosome reaction of epididymal spermatozoa. *J Med Food* 2003; 6:201–8.

86. Lenzi A, Sjro P, Salacone P, et al. A placebo controlled blind randomized trial of the use of combined L-carnitine and La-cetyl carnitine treatment in men with asthenospermia. *Fertil Steril* 2004; 81:1578–84.

87. Cavillini G, Curavett AP, Giamorol L, et al. Cinnoxicam and L carnitine/acetyl carnitine treatment for idiopathic

and varicocele associated oligoasthenospermia. *J Androl* 2004; 5:761–70.

88. Schachter A, Goldman JA, Zukerman Z. Treatment of oligospermia with the amino acid arginine. *J Urol* 1973; 110:311–13.

89. Scibona M, Meschini P, Capparelli S, et al. L-arginine and male infertility. *Minerva Urol Nefrol* 1994; 46:251–53.

90. Lenzi A, Culasso F, Gandini L, et al. Placebo controlled, double blind, cross-over trial of glutathione therapy in male infertility. *Hum Reprod* 1993; 8:1657–62.

91. Netter A, Hartoma R, Nahoul K. Effect of zinc administration on plasma testosterone, dihydrotestosterone, and sperm count. *Arch Androl* 1981; 17:69–73.

92. Tikkiwal M, Ajmera RL, Mathur NK. Effect of zinc administration on seminal zinc and fertility of oligospermic males. *Indian J Physiol Pharmacol* 1987; 31:30–4.

93. Wong WY, Merkus HMWM, Thomas CMG, et al. Effects of folic acid and zinc sulfate on male factor subfertility: A double-blind, randomized, placebo-controlled trial. *Fertil Steril* 2002; 77:491–8.

94. Hawkes WC, Turek PJ. Effects of dietary selenium on sperm motility in healthy men. *J Androl* 2001; 22:764–72.

95. Scott R, MacPherson A, Yates RW, et al. The effect of oral selenium supplementation on human sperm motility. *Br J Urol* 1998; 82:76–80.

96. Kumamoto Y, Maruta H, Ishigami J, et al. Clinical efficacy of mecobalamin in the treatment of oligospermia-results of double-blind comparative clinical study. *Hinyokika Kiyo* 1988; 34:1109–32.

97. Dawson EB, Harris WA, Rankin WE, et al. Effect of ascorbic acid supplementation on the sperm quality of smokers. *Fertil Steril* 1992; 58:1034–9.

98. Dawson EB, Harris WA, Rankin WE, et al. Effect of ascorbic acid on male fertility. *Ann NY Acca Su* 1987; 498:312–23.

99. Suleiman SA, Ali ME, Zaki ZM, et al. Lipid peroxidation and human sperm motility: Protective role of vitamin E. *J Androl* 1996; 17:530–7.

100. Kessopoulou E, Powes HJ, Sharma KK, et al. A double-blind randomized placebo cross-over controlled trial using the antioxidant vitamin E to treat reactive oxygen species associated with male infertility. *Fertil Steril* 1995; 64:825–31.

101. Rolf C, Cooper TG, Yeung CH, et al. Antioxident treatment of patients with asthenospermia or moderate oligoasthenospermia with high dose vitamin C and vitamin E: A randomized, placebo controlled double blind study. *Hum Reprod* 1999; 14:1028–33.

102. Lewin A, Lavon H. The effect of coenzyme Q-10 on sperm motility and function. *Mol Aspects Med* 1997; 18:S213–S19.

103. Balercia G, Mosca F, Mantero F, et al. Coenzyme Q(10) supplementation in infertile men with idiopathic asthenospermia: An open, uncontrolled pilot study. *Fertil Steril* 2004; 81:93–8.

104. Khalsa HK. Yoga, an adjunct to infertility treatment. *Fertil Steril* 2003; 80:546–81.

105. Wurn BF, Wurn LJ, King CR, et al. Treating female infertility and improving IVF pregnancy rates with a manual physical therapy technique. *Med Gen Med* 2004; 6:51.

106. Eisenberg DM, Davis RB, Waletzky J, et al. Inability of an "energy transfer diagnostician" to distinguish between fertile and infertile women. *Med Gen Med* 2001; 22:E4.

13 Sexual Counseling and Infertility

LINDA HAMMER BURNS

The child will never lie in me, and you will never be its father. Mirrors must replace the real image, make it true so that the gentle lovemaking we do has powerful passions and a parent's trust.

– Elizabeth Jennings

Sex is an important means of expressing feelings of sharing and commitment, as well as strengthening the bonds between a man and a woman. Sexuality and sexual activity represent a unique combination of physical, emotional, and social expression bringing individuals together to be close, procreate, and play, as well as to express lust, desire, and need. Sexuality is influenced by social mores, religious beliefs, laws, emotions, relationships, and a myriad of physical factors, not the least of which is the brain. In addition, sexual activity is influenced by health and well-being, availability of a partner, self-concept, sexual stimuli, social setting, and prior sexual experiences. Sexuality also represents one of the most unique, intimate, and rewarding of human experiences.

However, for many infertile couples, the pleasurable experience of sexual intimacy is altered, so that sex becomes methodical, predictable, and unexciting. No longer a way of communicating intimacy and sharing, the meaning of sex focuses on procreation only. Frequently, self-perceptions are impacted: Research indicates that men may feel less virile and women less feminine or incomplete when they are infertile.[1] Common feelings of infertility, such as loss, anger, guilt, despair, depression, shame, and anxiety, often overshadow the usual feelings of warmth, affection, and emotional connection that are the natural prerequisites of enjoyable sexual encounters. Furthermore, infertility can be a melancholy reminder of the child that should be, past procreative failures, and the myriad of 'insults' imposed by medical treatment. Gone is lovemaking that is primarily spontaneous, adventuresome, tender, and thrilling.

Sexual health is a multidimensional phenomenon that generally encompasses three essential elements: (1) capacity to enjoy and control sexual and reproductive behavior in accordance with social and personal values; (2) freedom from fear, shame, guilt, myths, and other psychological factors that inhibit sexual response and impair sexual relationships; and (3) freedom from organic disorders, diseases, and deficiencies that interfere with sexual and reproductive functions.[2] In short, sexual health is considered the physical and emotional state of well-being that enables sexual enjoyment and acting on sexual feelings.

By contrast, sexual dysfunction involves an interruption in an individual's or couple's enjoyment or performance of sexual activity. Sexual dysfunction is defined as any impairment or disturbance in one or more of the phases of the sexual response cycle: desire, arousal, orgasm, and satisfaction. A *primary* (lifelong) dysfunction has always been present, while a *secondary* (acquired) dysfunction is one that occurs after a period of normal, healthy sexual functioning. Dysfunctions are further specified as *generalized* when they occur in all situations and with all partners or *situational* when the sexual problem is limited to certain situations or partners. The three categories of sexual dysfunctions are: disorders of sexual desire, disorders of arousal, and disorders of orgasm. In the 1970s, Walker[3] was one of the first to suggest that "sexual functioning is subject to disruption from physical, cultural, and psychological forces . . . and as well as *causing* infertility, sexual dysfunction may *result* from the work-up and treatment procedures such as 'sex-on-demand.'" Riddick[4] expanded on this premise, suggesting that sexual impairment in infertile couples was due to planned sex, extensive and painful tests, intense feelings of anxiety, and the highly personal matter of sexuality being turned over to the external control of a physician. The interactive effect of infertility treatment and sexual functioning appears to provide the best understanding of the complexities of infertility: Severe sexual dysfunction can cause infertility; just as psychological

TABLE 13.1. Impact of infertility on sexual practices and function[37]

Effect on sexual practices

Increased frequency at midcycle

Decreased frequency in luteal phase

Decreased variety of sexual expression

Change in who initiates sex

Effect on sexual function

Occasional periovulatory impotence or retarded ejaculation

Occasional periovulatory orgasmic dysfunction due to 'spectatoring'

disturbance often impairs sexual functioning, as well as responses to infertility treatment (Table 13.1).

At times, infertility highlights long-standing sexual or relationship problems which existed before infertility. In some instances, sexual difficulties may be the *cause* of the inability to conceive by either preventing or interrupting coitus, preventing conception. However, most often, sexual difficulties for infertile individuals are the result of scheduled sex, the pressure to perform on demand, the psychological presence of the medical team in the bedroom, and/or the couple's own internal pressure to conceive.

This chapter

■ provides an outline of sexual dysfunctions within the context of infertility;
■ identifies etiology and treatment for men and women.

It does not include issues related marital problems, which are addressed in other chapters.

HISTORICAL OVERVIEW

Early primitive humans did not understand the correlation between sex and reproduction (or the role of the male in procreation), probably due to the time delay between sexual intercourse, obvious pregnancy signs, and birth. During the prehistoric era from 25,000–3,000 BCE in which humans were primarily hunter-gatherers, matrilineality was the norm, gods were feminine, and children 'belonged' to the mother's kinship group. Women, as a result of their procreative ability, were thought to have magical powers and reproduction was often attributed to spirits or mystical powers.[5] An example of these myths that still have an impact on the lives of modern men and women are the Pilaga peoples of Argentina, who continue to have a more mythic notion of reproduction in which the

womb is thought to be a bag in which the embryo develops. Conception and pregnancy are believed to result from intervention of spirits called *payak* acting in concert with human actions (sometimes sexual intercourse but not always). The souls of children to be born are sent to the mother's body and the *payak* provide men with supplemental strength during coitus. Sterility is always attributed to the female and may be due to bad intentions of a *payak*, which comes in the form of a small insect that ties off her womb so that the embryo cannot receive the deposits of semen which contribute to the embryo's development and growth. Sterility can sometimes be cured by interventions of a shaman who attempts to persuade the *payak* to leave the woman alone. If unsuccessful, her continued sterility will end her marriage.[6]

Over time, humans gradually made the connection between sexual activity and males' contribution to procreation, probably through animal husbandry and the development of agrarian lifestyles. As a result, not only was the man's reproductive role recognized, but it also became revered as exemplified by the early Egyptian ankh (a cross and oval thought to represent the phallus and testes). Although women clearly had a role in reproduction (pregnancy and birth), in ancient Greece it was the male's contribution that was considered more valuable. According to Aristotle (384–322 BCE), reproduction was the result of man contributing his 'seed,' producing an embryo which was nourished in the 'soil' of menstrual blood.[5] Women (and children) were the property of men and Greek wives competed sexually for their husband's attention with prostitutes and male slaves. Homosexuality (particularly older men with young boys) was widely practiced as evidenced in Greek art and the ancient saying, women are for business, boys are for pleasure. These behaviors were based on a belief that semen was a source of knowledge and, as such, sexual relations, a means of passing on wisdom. In ancient Roman civilization, Roman emperor Augustus (27 BCE–14 CE) decreed that men between the ages of twenty-five and fifty must marry and were given rewards if they created the 'ideal family': three children.[7]

Judaism emerged before the ancient Egyptian, Greek, or Roman Empires, 2,000 years before the birth of Jesus in a region now known as the Middle East. It is based on the religious text, the Torah (also referred to as the Old Testament), and principles that promote study and knowledge as a pathway to correct behavior and closeness to God, a single deity. According to Jewish tradition, asceticism for its own sake is ingratitude to God and sexuality, as such, is a gift from God. According to Jewish tradition, a man is expected to bring pleasure to his wife, and is doubly blessed to do so on the Sabbath. Examples of other traditions that impact sexuality or behavior are *bris* (i.e., religious ceremony and celebration in which male newborns are circumcised); *mikva* (i.e., an Orthodox Jewish custom prohibiting sexual intercourse when the wife is 'unclean,' a period of time that includes menses and seven days after the last sign of vaginal bleeding); and *onanism* (i.e., ejaculation outside the vagina), which is forbidden because it allows the spilling of seed and prevents conception.[8] According to Jewish tradition, marriage is a sacred contract and, as noted earlier, sexual pleasure for both partners is a shared expectation.

Islam, which emerged during the seventh century also in the Middle East, is based on the prophet Muhammad and the religious text, the Koran (Qur'an). It is a monotheistic religion that promotes self-control, devotion to family, diligence to work, charitable giving, and modest dress for both men and women. Homosexuality is forbidden.[9] Female virginity is highly valued and *zina* (female sexual activity outside of marriage including unmarried sexual liaisons, adultery, and rape) is reason for public physical punishment (e.g., stoning to death).[10] Marriages are often arranged and are not a sacrosanct commitment for the husband, who can leave the marriage at will, either by abandoning or divorcing his current wife or by taking additional wives about whom his current wife may or may not be aware. In traditional Islamic marriages, it is expected that the bride will become pregnant within the first year, providing her husband with progeny that will ensure his well-being in this life and the next.[10] Although the Koran teaches that a husband should give his wife the right of sexual pleasure, in fact, sexual dysfunction in women is common because brides are almost universally virgins and piously uneducated about sex.[9] There are reports that 60% of Islamic women do not have sexual intercourse on their wedding night out of fear.[10] Men value a woman for her sexual purity, ability to meet her husband's sexual needs, and her reproductive capacities. Like many patrilineal, masculine-centric cultures, male-factor infertility is a difficult if not unacceptable diagnosis and, as such, polygamy affords a man psychosocial protection against the stigma of childlessness while the wife is subject to social stigma, abandonment, and/or physical maltreatment.

In medieval Europe, it was believed that the womb could move up and down within the body and that the consequences of this motion were of great medical significance, a belief dating from Hippocrates's description of uterine movements (probably what is known today as prolapsed uterus). In sexual relations, women were thought to enjoy two kinds of sexual pleasure: that of receiving the male seed, drawn by the 'attractive virtue' of the vulva, and that of ejaculating her own female seed. Womanhood involved 'excess humidity' enabling a woman to indulge in unlimited sex and, as a result, it was thought women were impossible to sexually satisfy.[11] With the advent of Christianity in medieval Europe, marriage was considered a religious 'sacrament' with the purpose of sanctioning sexual intercourse and the production of children who were (with wives) the chattel property of men. Restricting sexual behavior to the confines of the marriage bed was important not only morally but also to ensure the 'legitimacy' of a man's heirs – a principle that continues to remain relevant in many parts of the world today. St. Augustine (345–450 AD) was one of the more influential Christian moralists of his time contending that sex had no pleasurable purpose and abstinence from sex was the ultimate good a man could achieve. Sex was justified for the purpose of procreation because God had declared 'be fruitful and multiply.'[12] The missionary position was the only acceptable position, masturbation was prohibited, and sexual desire qualified as the same level of sin as actual sinful sex acts. Birth control or sexual intercourse for pleasure (or avoidance of procreation) was (and remains) unacceptable according to Roman Catholic tradition, as is homosexuality.

In contrast to medieval Christian Europe, Asia took a much more open and straightforward approach to sexuality and sexual relations. Asian literature and art openly and vividly described explicit heterosexual and homosexual relations; romantic interludes; 'sex toys'; and graphic erotica. In short, sexual pleasure was considered integral to the human experience; openly acknowledged by society; and pursued by both men and women despite patriarchy and sexism that valued women more as sex objects than for their reproductive abilities. A glaring example is the centuries-long custom of foot-binding in China that began with an emperor who had a foot fetish and sexual predilection for tiny feet in his women. As a result, women did what they have done across time and all cultures; they altered their bodies to meet the cultural standard of 'sexy.'

A comparable custom exists in a large portion of Africa today: female circumcision (also referred to as infabulation), which is a social (not religious) custom based on a belief that infabulation eliminates or controls female sexual desires and/or behaviors and is more hygienic. It is also has a long history as an initiation rite based on cultural beliefs that all newborns have elements of both sexes: the foreskin of the penis is the female element, while the clitoris, the male element. When an adolescent reaches puberty, these elements must be removed to clarify the individual's gender and/or sexual identity. According to this custom, infabulation is performed on girls between the ages of twelve and fourteen; however, it also is customarily done to girls aged four to eight. Typically, female elders perform the procedure (from mild 'trimming' of the labia to the removal of the clitoris and labia and/or closing the vagina with stitches) without anesthetic using rudimentary instruments (e.g., shards of glass). As a result, girls are at risk for urinary and reproductive tract infections; scarring; infertility; and birth complications.[13] Female circumcision is closely associated with a young woman's marital potential, in that if only one or a few families in a community 'deprive' their daughters of the procedure, her chances of finding a husband are significantly reduced – as was the case with foot-binding in China.

During the Renaissance in Europe, the concept of marriage changed from one of religious duty or social necessity to 'companionate marriage' based on conjugal compatibility, affection, and mutual sexual attraction (versus arranged marriages). Ideal wifely behavior included the provision of emotional warmth as well as sexual satisfaction (excitement) which had previously been provided by mistresses and/or prostitutes. This change became the foundation for the concept of marriage as it is known/practiced in much of the world today.[14] Arranged marriages continue in many societies (e.g., India).

Despite the advent of the 'companionate marriage' based on love and sexual attraction, during the eighteenth and nineteenth centuries, the 'ideal wife' was defined as a pious and virtuous symbol of hearth and home. According to distinguished English physician William Acton, a woman "seldom desire[s] any sexual gratification for herself. She submits to her husband's embraces, but principally to gratify him."[7] French doctor Auguste Debay, who published the first popular marriage manual, advised, "O wives! Follow this advice. Submit to your husband's needs ... force yourself to satisfy him, put on an act and simulate the spasm of pleasure; this innocent deception is permitted when it is a question of keeping a husband."[7] American physician William A. Alcott recommended that married couples have sex no more than once a month as any greater frequency was "prostitution of the matrimonial life." In short, women raised during the Victorian era believed that sex was beastly, all women hated it, and all men's brutal lusts were the chief obstacle to marital happiness.[15]

Early in the twentieth century, women particularly in the developed world, sought greater freedom (politically, educationally, and socially) and had different expectations of the 'companionate marriage': emotional and sexual intimacy, conjugal unity as well as a recognition of each partner's individuality. Marriage advice following World War I made sex the centerpiece of marriage and the sexual adjustment of both partners, the principal measures of marital harmony.[16] By the middle of the twentieth century, women (and their partners) had more control of their reproductive lives via reliable birth control (i.e., birth control pills and legalized abortion in some countries), enabling both partners to enjoy sex without the fear or reality of pregnancy. This set the stage for a fundamental and irrevocable shift: the separation of sexuality, sexual intercourse, and procreation.[17] While these advancements had worldwide impact, their implementation was culturally adapted. For instance, the long history of patriarchy and ancestor worship, common in many Asian cultures, continued the preference of male offspring over female children. China used modern birth control measures to implement a 'one child per couple' policy to stem population growth during the middle of the twentieth century. Still, the preference for male offspring perpetuated a long-standing practice of infanticide and/or abandonment of female children (e.g., India and China) that has been facilitated by modern medicine and/or international adoption. In the Islamic world, modern medicine has facilitated patriarchal parenthood and pronatalist agendas, while in the developing world the challenges of treatment for unwanted pregnancies (e.g., reliable birth control and abortion) compete with treatment for wanted pregnancies (i.e., infertility) for limited resources and accessible treatment facilities. Still, in the early twenty-first century, elective reproduction and companionate marriage remain the ideal, although not universal, despite soaring divorce rates; postponed (elderly) reproduction; 'repeat' parenthood (children after remarriage); complex reproductive technologies; reproductive tourism; and stratification of reproductive services. Sexual mores, as always, fluctuate and evolve so that now homosexuality, illegal in many parts of the world even in the recent past, is now not only accepted, but also condoned by marriage laws and facilitated parenthood, albeit controversial globally and religiously.

REVIEW OF LITERATURE

Sexual functioning and infertility have not, until recently, been the subject of scientific study. Early analyses of sexual functioning and infertility were most often based on unique clinical cases and/or theoretical speculations that focused on emotional barriers (especially in women) as an explanation for impaired fertility. At a time when 50% of infertility could not be explained by a medical diagnosis, it was the contention of early psychoanalytic theories that infertility was caused by psychological or emotional disturbances. Termed *psychogenic infertility*, it was thought to be caused by a woman's unconscious fear of pregnancy; history of frigidity, childhood timidity, or unsocial behavior; poor psychosexual development; rejection by or hatred of her mother; and fear that the infertile woman would kill her child if she had one.[18–22] In a man, psychogenic infertility was thought to be due to a controlling, unaffectionate, rigid, and moralistic mother; ambivalence about parenthood; insecure masculinity; and anger toward his spouse.[3,23–25] These theories contended that a man or woman's psychological problems either directly caused infertility or interrupted sexual activity sufficiently to impair reproduction. In fact, one early researcher[4] concluded that tubal spasming in tense and nervous women (a 'relatively permanent' condition) resulted in sexual dysfunction and infertility because infertile women were extremely preoccupied "with female sex organs in a disturbed way." Although these theories have fallen into disfavor over the past thirty years, different versions continue to resurface in various forms, influencing theory, practice, and research.

Early research on sexual functioning in infertile couples focused on evidence of neurotic conflicts or personality traits that prevented normal sexual functioning. Recently, research has focused on the incidence and type of sexual dysfunctions in infertile couples; the impact of infertility on sexual functioning in women or in comparison to men; and the impact of specific infertility diagnosis or treatments (most often assisted reproductive technologies) on sexual functioning. Eisner[26] described the causes of sexual dysfunction in infertile couples as: (1) psychosexual problems masquerading as cases of infertility; (2) incidental findings of psychosexual disturbances in cases of infertility; and (3) infertility causing psychosexual problems. Common sexual dysfunctions in women resulting from the stresses of medical treatments (most often directed at women regardless of the etiology of the infertility) include problems with loss of libido, anorgasmia, and disturbance of sexual identity. Several researchers have found that infertility treatment contributed to feelings of loss of control, intimacy, privacy, and esteem and decreased sexual desire, response, and activity in women.

Sexually Transmitted Infections as a Cause of Infertility

Although often overlooked, the most common preventable cause of infertility for both men and women is infection due to sexually transmitted infections (STIs). In some parts of the world, infection-related infertil-

ity is so widespread that it constitutes not only a personal health problem but a public health crisis.[27–30] Although research has progressed on the prevention and treatment of STIs, patient barriers still include misconceptions about the impact of STIs on fertility; silent (asymptomatic) infections; shame and embarrassment; reluctance to seek medical care and support; fear of the impact on partner(s); and lack of ready access to medical care.[27,28] Infertility due to STIs has not only significant reproductive health consequences but also significant psychosocial ramifications, often highlighting an individual's lifestyle, personal history, and/or cultural factors.

The most common STIs resulting in infertility are syphilis, gonorrhea, chlamydiosis, human papilloma virus (HPV), mycoplasmosis, genital herpes, trichomoniasis, and human immunodeficiency virus (HIV).[31,32] STIs adversely affect fertility through several mechanisms: (1) pregnancy loss; (2) neonatal deaths; (3) obstruction of either male or female reproductive ducts; (4) impaired semen parameters; and (5) the risk of transmission of HIV to a partner and/or offspring.[27,28,33,34] STIs cause infertility by infecting the genital tract of men and women, although this is a less frequent mechanism of infertility in men. Portals of entry for STIs include genitalia, urinary tract, mouth, rectum, and skin.[31]

STIs resulting in infertility require examination of personal decisions, especially those regarding sexual behavior; partner choice; cultural circumstances; domestic environment; drug and alcohol use/abuse; social life; and availability/usage of quality medical care.[31,35,36] It is widely recognized that the distress of infertility results in feelings of anger, depression, isolation, guilt, self-reproach, and diminished self-esteem. These feelings can be significantly intensified when infertility is caused by one's own sexual behavior or that of one's partner, and therefore potentially are preventable. Not only is the individual vulnerable to significant feelings of loss, guilt, and self-reproach, but the marital relationship may also be disturbed or threatened by the diagnosis, especially if it intimates extramarital sexual contacts.

Sexual Dysfunction in Infertile Couples

In an early study of couples, Keye[37] determined that sexual problems in conjunction with infertility arose for the following reasons: dyspareunia; progesterone-inhibited sexual desire; 'sex-on-demand'; unrealistic sexual demands; rigid or routinized approach to sex; poor body image; depression; guilt; and ambivalence. The three areas of sexual difficulty were (1) the actual physical condition causing infertility or resulting from treatment; (2) sexual intercourse becoming only a means of reproduction rather than intimacy or pleasure; and (3) the global psychological impact of the infertility experience. However, in a review of literature on the psychosocial impact of infertility and ART treatment on marital sexuality, Coeffin-Driol and Gianmi[38] noted that the literature on infertile couple's sexual satisfaction was mostly descriptive and presented infertility as a deleterious experience for both men and women regardless of gender-specific diagnosis or couple functioning. Furthermore, many of the studies were qualitative and culturally specific (i.e., Anglo-Saxon). The studies showed equivocal or contradictory results from which no conclusions could be made.

In a study of infertile women, Boivin and colleagues[39] found that one-third experienced feelings of discomfort and nervousness during postcoital testing and 20% with normal sexual functioning reported an unfavorable sexual response to sexual intercourse prior to postcoital testing. Furthermore, the majority of the women reported lower levels of postcoital sexual satisfaction as compared to sexual relations at other times. The authors concluded that the inherent pressure of the postcoital situation may be stressful for women, contributing to decreased sexual enjoyment and poor sexual response, resulting in poorer physiological results, although they found no significant relation between erectile difficulties and female sexual satisfaction, arousal, and orgasm. Women reported severe marital strain, as well as sexual inhibitions, anorgasmia, and reduced interest in sex. Andrews and associates[40] found that infertility-specific stress had a stronger negative impact on women's sense of sexual identity and self-efficacy than it did on men.

A few studies have investigated the impact of a specific infertility diagnosis or a treatment protocol on male sexual functioning. In a study assessing stigma in infertile couples with male-factor infertility,[41] Nachtigall and colleagues reported that men with male-factor infertility experienced greater stigma than men who did not have it. Berg and Wilson[42] evaluated couples across different stages of the infertility investigation (years 1, 2, and 3) and found that over time infertile couples experienced increased marital and sexual problems, with men reporting less ability to control ejaculation and less satisfaction with their sexual performance in general. In a study comparing infertile men and a control group, Kemer and colleagues[43] found that infertile men reported lower self-esteem; higher anxiety; more somatic symptoms; and greater sexual inadequacy, as well as more depression, which, in turn, had a impact on negative erectile functioning. In a

study[44] of infertile men in Germany, age of partners; attitudes toward sexuality; treatment duration; duration of the partnership; the duration of the desire for a child; and gender-specific diagnosis were found to have no impact on sexual satisfaction. The researchers found that treatment duration and duration of the desire for a child may not necessarily be connected to lowered sexual satisfaction in infertile males, and that coitus frequency did not impact sexual satisfaction. However, this is in contrast to a similar study by the same researchers which found that a short-lasting partnership and high sexual dissatisfaction prior to the diagnosis of infertility caused more distress in infertile men whereas being in a longer-lasting and sexually satisfying partnership seemed to have a buffering effect with regard to sexual distress and infertility.[45]

Sexual Dysfunction and ARTs

A few researchers have evaluated sexual dysfunction in couples requesting or completing IVF, an interesting approach because the success or failure of the IVF protocol is not contingent on sexual intercourse, eliminating the pressure and marital strain that many infertile couples experience as a result of other infertility treatments. In a study[46] comparing perceptions of men and women following IVF, researchers found fewer gender differences regarding couples' sexual relationship and both men and women felt that IVF decreased the female partner's sexual desire. In short, the high-technology treatment of IVF does not appear to dramatically affect sexual functioning in couples as a whole or in men in particular, but women (who receive the greatest portion of treatment during IVF) may experience a slightly increased risk of diminished sexual satisfaction or desire. In a study involving women undergoing IVF and sexual functioning, researchers[47] examined the impact of coping strategies. They found that positive reinterpretation and active coping strategies had a positive impact on sexual functioning while planning and self-restraint coping had an adverse effect on sexual functioning. Interestingly, being sexually active and adaptive coping strategies during the IVF treatment cycle were found to be positively associated with a positive outcome (i.e., successful pregnancy). Research[48] to assess overall marital and sexual adjustment after the completion of infertility treatment involved three groups of women: (1) post-IVF women with children; (2) unsuccessful IVF women who adopted; and (3) unsuccessful IVF women who remained childless. There were no significant differences between the three groups on the standardized measures of marital and sexual satisfaction.

Several studies have addressed the impact of stress on semen quality. Hammond and colleagues[49] investigated men undergoing IVF and AIH to assess semen quality in infertility treatments associated with heightened performance anxiety. The researchers found no significant differences in either group of men. In fact, some of the men who had begun health-seeking behaviors (e.g., reduced hot baths and reduced use of alcohol and tobacco) had improved semen quality, leading the researchers to conclude that performance anxiety does not appear to be detrimental to semen quality. Saleh and colleagues found that among men undergoing infertility evaluation, 11% failed to collect semen by masturbation for a second semen analysis after repeated (two to four) attempts; 20% were able to collect semen using vibratory stimulation; and 31% experienced problems with erection or orgasm in addition to severe anxiety during attempts to masturbate and during sexual contact with their partners.[50]

THEORETICAL FRAMEWORK

The Human Sexual Response

Sexuality is a term used to refer to a person's gender identity, feelings, sexual orientation, and attitudes, and is distinct from sexual behavior. It encompasses the most intimate feelings of individuality; the need for emotional closeness to another human being; and a fundamental aspect of one's humanity. Sexual health includes a knowledge of sexual functioning; a positive body image; self-awareness about attitudes regarding sex: understanding the appreciation of one's sexual feelings; a well-developed and usable value system; the ability to create effective and rewarding relationships; and emotional comfort, interdependence, and stability within sexual encounters. It is these qualities of personal awareness, values, and relationships that contribute as much to sexual health and well-being as hormones, genitalia, and brain centers.

The human sexual response is not much different from other human interactions: It follows a pattern of response involving biological responses to psychological and sensory input. It represents the interplay of physiological, psychological, and social influences that determine behavior. Masters and Johnson,[51] with their landmark work that scientifically documented the human physiological sexual response, identified four phases of human sexual response: excitement, plateau, orgasm, and resolution. Masters and Johnson's work marked the emergence of the modern era of sex therapy, offering specific treatment protocols and identifying the role of anxiety, specifically 'spectatoring' and

performance anxiety. However, they did not address the problematic issue of sexual desire. Kaplan[52] built on the work of Masters and Johnson, noting that the excitement phases consist of sexual arousal and last until orgasm begins. Accordingly, Kaplan[52] offered three phases of human sexual response cycle, *desire, excitement (arousal)*, and *orgasm*. The *desire phase* is influenced by a wide variety of environmental stimuli, including psychosocial and cultural factors and physiology, allowing initiation or receptivity to sexual activity. During the *excitement (arousal) phase* of sexual response, various factors come together, allowing one to either initiate or respond to sexual activity. Vaginal lubrication in women and penile erection in men are the most noticeable signs of increased excitement during the arousal phase. In women, this phase also involves internal vaginal expansion (ballooning) and erection of the nipples and clitoris. Vasocongestion results, in women, in swelling of the outer portion of the vagina and the labia and, in men, an increase in scrotal size, with the scrotum pulling up against the body. *Orgasm* in both men and women involves a series of muscular contractions that diminish in intensity and rapidity. In women, these contractions involve the vagina, uterus, and anal sphincter, while in men orgasm involves the prostate and seminal vesicles and the contractions are followed by ejaculation. Following orgasm, the body returns to its resting or preexcitement state as vasocongestion is relieved. In men, this is marked by loss of erection, while in women it involves decrease in clitoral size and diminished vaginal width and length. In summary, *desire* is mediated by the brain, *excitement (arousal)* involves physiological vasodilation, and *orgasm* is essentially a muscular reflex contraction.

Basson[53] further expanded on these theories with a theoretical perspective that addresses desire and arousal in women. According to this theoretical approach, women seek sexual experiences for intimacy as well as sexual gratification and may be receptive to or seek out sexual stimuli to eventually enhance intimacy. Biological and psychological factors can contribute to the processing of these stimuli, enhancing arousal and desire simultaneously. It is a multifactorial approach to human sexual response that has been adapted to infertility.

While men have a refractory period after orgasm during which ejaculation and orgasm cannot occur, this is not the case for women. Failure to experience orgasm in both men and women can result in pelvic and genital discomfort when vasocongestion is not relieved. Contrary to popular belief, orgasmic response in women is the same whether it is the result of clitoral or vaginal stimulation.

TABLE 13.2. Taking a sexual history[52]

Chief complaint

Sexual status examination

Assessment of medical status

Assessment of psychiatric status

Family and psychosexual history

Evaluation of the relationship

Assessment of Sexual Dysfunction

The most common and useful assessment tool is the sexual history interview developed by Masters and Johnson.[51] It is a semistructured, extended face-to-face interview, often lasting several hours. Masters and Johnson's approach focuses on exploration of the current sexual problem with attention to environmental influences on sexual functioning. Kaplan's[52] adaptation of this method provides a means of evaluation and consideration of sexual dysfunctions that uses a 'conflict-oriented' approach for investigating psychodynamic phenomena (Table 13.2). Kaplan's model was the basis for the Comprehensive Psychosocial History for Infertility by Burns[54] and Greenfeld (see Appendix 3), a semistructured interview tool that includes sections on sexual dysfunction and marital adjustment. Most researchers and clinicians using assessment measures of sexual adjustment rely on available standardized measures, even though none to date has been adapted to the infertility population (see Chapters 7 and 9).

CLINICAL ISSUES

Impact of Culture and Religion on Sexuality and Infertility

Culture and religion, as noted earlier, have and continue to impact the sexual behavior of individuals and couples. Infertility may be a global problem, but the etiology of infertility is demographically different globally.[55] For instance, in many developed countries a significant causal factor for female-factor infertility is advanced maternal age, while in the developing world (particularly sub-Saharan Africa) the primary cause of infertility is sexually transmitted infections, particularly HIV.[56–58] Furthermore, while the desire for a child is a universal human experience, available treatments to remedy the condition are not universally available.[59] Compounding these issues for infertile men and women is that infertility is a narcissistic injury in which the individual and couple experiences bereave-

ment for an ambiguous loss; social stigma and isolation; and marital distress – all within the context of their culture and often with an overlay of religious or spiritual beliefs that may ameliorate or exacerbate their distress. In short, infertility is a private trauma – and so are sexual problems. For the majority of people, more so in some cultures than others, talking about the private intimacies of their lives while undergoing invasive treatments of their private parts compounds an already gaping wound. An additional confounding variable is the infertile couple who travels across borders (reproductive tourists) to obtain reproductive assistance away from home. Within this 'culture shock' the couple may find discussing their private sexual problems extremely helpful because there is a buffer of quasi-anonymity being away from home, or they find such discussions inappropriate, shocking, and uncomfortable. Against this backdrop, the challenge for the infertility counselor is to provide culturally-sensitive counseling that understands and respects their unique cultural and/or religious circumstances (see Chapter 4).

Sexual Dysfunction Causing Infertility

For a small percentage of infertile couples, sexual problems in one or both partners will be the primary cause of infertility. Sexual difficulties are the cause of infertility when sexual dysfunction prevents or interrupts coitus, preventing conception. The exact number of men and women affected by this type of infertility is not known, primarily because these patients may not seek infertility treatment or disclose the problem to caregivers, or because caregivers fail to investigate it and little research has been devoted to it. Sexual dysfunctions in men contributing to infertility are: impotency (both general and organic); too frequent sexual activity (resulting in reduced sperm count); or too infrequent sexual activity (no ejaculation, premature ejaculation, and failure of intromission). One study that examined the prevalence of erectile dysfunction in infertile men found that androgen deficiency (congruent with andropause) and erectile dysfunction were significantly higher than in the general population.[60] Additional reported causes of infertility due to sexual dysfunction include unconsummated marriage (failure to ever have sexual intercourse); vaginismus (vaginal muscle spasms that prevent penile penetration); infrequent sexual intercourse; mid-cyle male impotency; inability to achieve coitus for postcoital examination; or refusal (inability) to submit a semen sample. In addition, some sexual practices related to a sexual dysfunction may cause infertility, such as use of vaginal lubricants that are spermicidal.

Psychological problems or psychiatric disorders as an antecedent or contributing factor to sexual dysfunctions causing infertility may also be a consideration. Although rare, deviant sexual activities may cause infertility; these include exclusively oral and/or anal sex, bondage, cross-dressing, fetishism, sadomasochism, or partner swapping. Conflicted gender identity, homosexuality, and bisexuality are other potential causes of infertility, especially if a partner is unaware or unwilling to acknowledge his or her sexual orientation and sexual identity or is being intentionally deceptive. However these issues arise, they usually precipitate a personal crisis, serious marital disruption, and interference with infertility treatment.

Sexual Dysfunctions in Both Men and Women

Loss of sexual desire or libido, also referred to as *hypoactive sexual desire disorder*, is shared by both men and women, representing dysfunction in the first phase of the sexual response (desire, arousal, and orgasm).[61] Low libido may be an isolated sexual problem that is episodic or situational; a long-standing malady; or a symptom of a problem that is not primarily sexual in nature, such as depression, physical illness (e.g., heart disease or hypertension), or social problems (e.g., job stress or social isolation). Additionally, an increasing number of men and women presenting for infertility treatment are older and, as such, are more likely to have age-related sexual dysfunction issues such as low sexual desire; vaginal dryness; erectile dysfunction: and/or sexual problems attributable to an underlying illness, condition, or treatment (e.g., diabetes and obesity). The proportion of sexual desire disorders has risen steadily and dramatically in recent decades and now accounts for the largest group of complaints voiced by patients seeking sex therapy.[61,62] Traditionally, loss of sexual desire was more common in women, but today, low libido is more prevalent in men.

The desire phase of sexual functioning represents interest in sexual contact and the need for sexual intimacy in both men and women. Diagnostic criteria of disordered sexual desire include presence or absence of sexual fantasies; masturbation; noncoital sexual activity; coitus with a partner; any non-partner-related sexual activity; and initiation of sexual activity versus partner receptivity.[61,63] Sexual desire disorders rarely occur in isolation; the context and mediating factors include age; number of years married; socioeconomic status; religiosity; marital happiness; physical well-being; previous sexual appetite; and current social stressors.

Hypoactive sexual desire disorder is low libido; loss of sexual interest or mood; and diminished desire or sexual appetite, which may be *generalized* to all real or potential sexual partners or specific to one's current partner, usually indicating relationship problems or dissatisfaction with this partner. *Primary* hypoactive sexual desire disorder is the total absence of sexual desire, feelings, thoughts, fantasies, or interest, and typically becomes apparent in adolescence or early adulthood. It is generally a lifelong problem that is very difficult to treat, as its etiology is usually a combination of physical and psychological factors. *Secondary* hypoactive sexual desire disorder, occurring after a period of normal sexual desire, is marked by absence of sexual desire, feelings, thoughts, fantasies, or interest.

Low libido or diminished sexual desire may be the result of relationship problems; alcohol or other drugs; illness; sexual boredom; inadequate sexual information; restrictive upbringing; or body-image problems. Sometimes loss of sexual interest is due to psychological problems such as depression, stress, history of traumatic sexual experiences, or insecurity about one's psychosexual role – all influencing sexual responsiveness and enjoyment. For infertile men and women, disorders of sexual desire are usually episodic or situational responses to the emotional distress or physical strains of infertility or a specific medical treatment. As the focus of sexual activity continues to emphasize procreation, infertile men and women may feel depressed, lose interest in 'sex-on-demand,' or find it difficult to feel sexual when they feel chronically frustrated and unhappy due to childlessness. Chronic health problems or the invasiveness of medical treatment for infertility often dampen erotic thoughts and feelings, resulting in sexual intercourse becoming a less appealing source of affection and more a necessary reproductive chore. Finally, another common culprit in loss of sexual interest in men and women is medications such as oral contraceptives, medroxy-progesterone contraceptive injection (Depo-Provera), gonadotropin-releasing hormone agonists, ovulation-induction medications, antihypertensives, and antidepressants that interfere with sexual response and/or interest by changing hormone levels; affecting sexual appetite or arousal; or altering the experience of orgasm.

Relationship problems such as poor communication, anger, rejection, avoidance of commitment, and confused priorities often masquerade (or at least present) as sexual complaints regardless of the presence or absence of infertility. Intrapsychic issues such as concealed homosexuality; participation in extramarital sex; excessive masturbation; or compulsive sexual activity (e.g., excessive internet sex activity and/or pornography) are

TABLE 13.3. Sexual problem diagnostic grid[64]

Influencing factors	Focus of problem		
	Orgasm	Arousal	Desire
Contextual	1	1	1,2
Relational I (simple conflict communication)	1,2	2	2,3
Relational II (underlying structural ssues)	2,3	3	3,4
Relational III (commitment)	3	3,4	4
Intrapsychic	3,4	4	4

Key: **1**, low severity: educational/behavioral treatment, including self-help methods; **2**, moderate severity: behavioral treatment with additional counseling likely; **3**, high severity: behavioral treatment by a sex therapist in conjunction with personal or relational counseling; **4**, extreme severity: behavioral treatment only an adjunct to intensive personal and/or relational psychotherapy.

not problems of sexual desire as they are presented, but actually represent problems within the individual or the relationship. Persistent marital difficulties in infertile couples may be indicative of earlier conflicts either within the marriage or within the individuals. In some couples, partners blame themselves or each other for infertility (irrespective of actual etiology) or medical diagnosis, resulting in anger that interferes with sexual desire and functioning. Lack of emotional closeness may masquerade as sexual problems when the actual problem is inappropriate or destructive behaviors such as violence, abuse, or boundary violations. In such cases, treatment for sexual dysfunction is less important than resolution of more significant marital issues (see Chapter 9).

One approach for determining whether a presenting sexual complaint is primarily sexual or relationship-related was designed by Sanderson and Maddock[64] and includes a diagnostic and treatment planning guide, as well as a helpful taxonomy of relationship difficulties (Table 13.3). The sexual complaint is assessed in terms of the phase of sexual functioning (desire, arousal, and orgasm) and three 'influencing variables': *context* (immediate context of the erotic contact); *relationship* (general interaction of the partners); and *intrapsychic* (psychological makeup of the individual). As a general rule, the longer the duration of sexual complaints, the more resistant they are to treatment. Relationship difficulties are defined in terms of three subgroups: (1) problems involving minor difficulties that may affect sexual interaction but do not threaten the overall structure of the

relationship (e.g., simple conflicts or stylistic communication differences); (2) more severe conflicts impacting every aspect of the overall relationship, as well as relationship dynamics (e.g., inability to trust each other, power struggles, or differing levels of need for intimacy); and (3) problems involving partner commitment and psychological presence in the relationship affecting the fundamental stability of the relationship (e.g., extramarital affairs, homosexuality, and sexual addictions).

Even couples who never encounter major or disrupting sexual problems often experience periodic diminished sexual desire and satisfaction at some point during medical treatment for infertility. Episodic loss of libido in one or both partners is not particularly disruptive and can usually be addressed with minimal education and reassurance. However, consistent and extensive diminished sexual desire in infertile men and women is more problematic and usually multifactorial: a common side effect of feelings of sexual unattractiveness or defectiveness, guilt or shame, depression or anger. Loss of libido may be the result of the conditions contributing to infertility or the result of a specific medical treatment for infertility. Or it may be due to the stresses and demands that infertility places on the marriage, social relationships, work life, or financial resources. All these factors contribute to loss of sexual desire or interest in infertile men and women, resulting in diminished sexual functioning. Individuals may respond with silent resignation; anger or blame directed at self, spouse, infertility or medical caregivers; help-seeking; or self-treatment. Silent resignation is the abandonment of sexual satisfaction or desire by one or both partners, who learn *not* to expect physical or emotional rewards from their lovemaking and consider sexual intercourse a reproductive duty to be endured. This is often more common and easier to disguise in women. Self-treatment includes not only a variety of over-the-counter medical remedies or gadgets but also various self-defeating sexual behaviors such as excessive masturbation; additional intimate relationships (i.e., extramarital affairs); obsessive search for sexual thrills; sexual release without emotional entanglement; sexual addiction behaviors; pornography with or without excessive internet sex; or parenthood without one's infertility partner. Rarely do infertile men or women actually seek help for sexual problems, unless the difficulty is clearly interfering with their reproductive agenda or medical treatment plan. This lack of help-seeking behavior may represent a desire to avoid further boundary violations (maintaining as much of the privacy around their intimate relationship as possible), or a belief that sexual problems are unimportant to their caregivers or that their caregivers cannot/are unable to provide assistance.

Response to treatment of a sexual desire disorder is contingent on its etiology, whether it is generalized or situational, and how long the desire disorder has continued without treatment. Disorders of sexual desire have traditionally been notoriously difficult to treat, primarily because men and women have learned to involuntarily and automatically focus on negative or distracting thoughts that suppress sexual feelings while simultaneously not responding to sexual stimuli. Research on the treatment of sexual desire disorders has shown that standard sex therapy usually fails to raise sexual desire.[65] However, treatments that focus specifically on low sexual desire have been found to be more effective, especially those using a combination of cognitive-behavioral treatment programs involving the following principles: (1) *affectional awareness* in which patients become aware of negative attitudes, beliefs, and cognitions regarding sex; (2) *insight-oriented* therapy in which patients gain understanding of their negative thoughts or feelings; (3) *cognitive therapy* which assists alteration of irrational thoughts that inhibit sexual desire; and (4) *behavioral interventions* that focus on behavioral assignments which evoke positive sexual feelings during experiential/sensory awareness and change nonsexual behaviors that may be maintaining the sexual difficulty.[63] Successful treatment involving behavioral tasks and a nondemanding, reassuring environment removes common obstacles to sexual pleasure such as poor communication, anxiety, unrealistic expectations, or mechanical sex. Other treatment suggestions include hormonal therapy (testosterone) for men and women or medications (e.g., sildenafil) for men; anxiety reduction; increasing sensory awareness; enhancing positive sexual/sensual experiences; modifying the inhibition of erotic impulses; and facilitation of erotic responses.

Sexual Dysfunction in Women

Regardless of the cause of infertility, research has consistently shown that in response to infertility, women experience greater emotional distress than men and often assume more personal responsibility, while enduring a disproportionate share of medical treatment (see Chapter 3). More often women initiate medical treatment for infertility; are more invested in having a child; more aware of the limits of their reproductive life; and more willing to consider extreme or alternative measures to achieve parenthood. For women, reproduction and sexuality may be more intrinsically intertwined

than they are for men, so that disturbances in one area necessarily reverberate into other areas. In short, infertility clearly impacts the sexual functioning and sexual health of women in myriad ways.

Current research indicates that the most common female sexual dysfunction is arousal phase disorders, followed by orgasm phase disorders of vaginismus and dyspareunia.[52,66] However, there has been a recent effort to expand the classifications of female sexual dysfunction to include psychogenic and organic causes of desire, arousal, orgasm, and sexual pain disorders to include a 'personal distress' criterion and a new category of noncoital sexual pain disorder.[67] As such, infertility clearly qualifies as 'personal distress' having an impact on sexual functioning. Sexual dysfunction in women may be due to hormonal changes, anatomical or physical factors (e.g., endometriosis, ovarian cysts, or uterine fibroids), or organic conditions (e.g., illness and diseases affecting general well-being and sexual health). Medications, disease, or physical problems can, and often do, affect sexual pleasure and sexual functioning. *Hormonal changes*, including loss of hormones with menopause, premature ovarian failure, or surgical removal of the ovaries, may lead to diminished sexual appetite; loss of vaginal lubrication; painful intercourse; decreased sexual sensation and arousal; and less intense orgasms. *Anatomical* reasons for sexual dysfunction include surgical outcomes and congenital malformations of the reproductive tract, such as congenital absence of the vagina or biforate uterus. *Organic conditions* include endometriosis, ovarian cysts, pelvic disorders, STIs (e.g., herpes or HPV infection), obesity, myomas, diabetes, alcoholism, neurological conditions, or other illnesses that can cause painful intercourse and sexual dysfunction.

Arousal Phase Disorders

The arousal phase of sexual excitement occurs in response to sexual stimuli and results in vaginal lubrication and expansion. Arousal disorders are defined as impaired female excitement or the persistent and recurrent lack of response to sexual stimuli and activity, resulting in lack of vaginal lubrication and engorgement. Estimates of the prevalence of arousal disorders in the general population vary between 11% and 48%.[65] Causes of arousal problems include pelvic vascular disease; neurological conditions; hormonal changes; and psychosocial factors, such as stress, prior history of sexual trauma, painful intercourse, or relationship problems.

Arousal disorders in women are often difficult to treat. Cognitive restructuring can be helpful in changing involuntary, automatic negative thoughts that suppress sexual feelings.[52,67] Other treatment suggestions include sensate-focus exercises (see Table 13.6); anxiety reduction; education about normal physiological sexual responses; increased sensory awareness; enhancing sexual/sensual experiences; facilitation of erotic responses; increased use of fantasy and/or erotica; and masturbation.[68,69] Female sexual arousal disorders constitute a varied spectrum of difficulties, ranging from the total absence of any physical arousal or emotional pleasure to physiological arousal without emotional feelings of sexual desire, pleasure, and/or orgasm. 'Spectatoring' is a common phenomenon in which the individual is physically engaged but emotionally detached – watching themselves during sexual encounters. The most common complaint is the absence of subjective sexual excitement or pleasure despite adequate physical arousal (e.g., lubrication). Pharmacological and physical treatments include the use of hormones (i.e., estrogen, testosterone, oxytocin, progesterone, and vasodilators), lubricants, vibrators, antidepressants, and various herbal remedies.[70] Psychological therapy addresses inhibitions as well as interpersonal and motivational factors. Hypnosis and relaxation techniques have also been suggested as measures that reduce anxiety and cognitive restructuring as a technique to eliminate 'spectatoring' and negative thought process, typically related to past sexual trauma.[71]

Orgasm Phase Disorders

Impaired or inhibited orgasm, or anorgasmia, is the total absence of orgasm or the persistent, recurrent delay of orgasm following normal and sufficient arousal. Historically referred to as frigidity, disorders of orgasm were once considered the most common sexual problem in women. Today about one-third of young women experience orgasm phase disorder. *Primary* anorgasmia is never having experienced orgasm either alone or with a partner following any kind of stimulation. *Secondary* anorgasmia is the absence or delay of orgasm after previously having been orgasmic. Most often, a woman can achieve orgasm with masturbation, manual stimulation, or cunnilingus but is unable to do so with intercourse. In the past, there was some controversy about whether failure to orgasm with intercourse alone was actually a 'dysfunction' in women; however, this issue is not a concern today.

Orgasmic dysfunction in infertile women is common, at least episodically, and is attributable to several factors including medical conditions (e.g., diabetes, estrogen deficiency, anatomical problems, and gynecological conditions); medications (including psychotropic drugs, alcohol, 'recreational' drugs, and certain pain medications); and psychosocial factors (e.g., depression or relationship conflict). Although anorgasmia is frequently attributed to psychological disturbances, there are few psychological factors that consistently relate to the inability to achieve orgasm. Because orgasm is not necessary for natural procreation in women, preoccupation with pregnancy and a willingness to relinquish orgasm often have an impact on sexual responsiveness during infertility. This is more likely to become a marital problem than a psychosexual problem. Women may surrender orgasm as penance for past sexual misdeeds; in trade for the 'baby at any price'; or for the sake of minimizing the impact of infertility on their own or their partner's life. Sometimes women and their partners, in an attempt to proceed with intercourse and circumvent natural sexual response, use various commercial lubricants (most of which are spermicidal) to facilitate intercourse. However, they are usually unaware that this is a counterproductive self-help solution.

Treatment techniques for anorgasmia in women focus on increasing sexual response by providing increasing awareness of arousing environmental cues and her body's responses to sensation, often with the assistance of masturbation. Treatment must necessarily address the issue of 'relinquishing orgasm' for procreative purposes, and the woman's willingness to recognize and alter this practice. Treatment that focuses on satisfying her male partner is usually not successful, although attention to relationship and interaction issues and her partner's sexual response and sensitivity to her are usually beneficial. Additional treatment interventions include relaxation training; cognitive restructuring; pelvic exercises; relaxation and biofeedback; and increased tolerance for normal feelings of arousal and excitement. Treatment of female orgasm disorders has been quite successful, although the definition of success has often been an issue: If orgasm with their partner is the criterion, the success rate is 85–95%, but only 30–50% if orgasm during intercourse is the criterion.

Vaginismus

Vaginismus is defined as recurrent and persistent involuntary vaginal spasms or muscle contractions that make entry into the vagina impossible or painful. Although the woman is sexually aroused and capable of experiencing an orgasm, the vaginal muscles close tightly, preventing penile or digital entry into the vagina. Vaginismus may be localized to sexual intercourse or may be generalized to include any attempt to enter the vagina, including digital foreplay; cunnilingus; self-examination with fingers; tampon insertion; or pelvic examinations by a physician. Vaginismus may be *primary* (inability to tolerate penetration and present in all encounters) or *secondary* (occurring in specific relationships or situations). Women with vaginismus typically experience sexual arousal and sexual pleasure in response to foreplay and are often able to have pleasurable and plentiful sexual activity, even though they are unable to have sexual intercourse. However, it should be noted that while sex therapists and the ICD/DSM-IV distinguish between vaginismus and sexual pain disorder, there are no published diagnostic studies that have demonstrated that a gynecologist or mental health professional can reliably diagnose vaginismus or distinguish it from dyspareunia. Research reviews have led to the conclusion that this diagnosis is questionable due to the high rate of comorbitity for dysparenia and vaginismus.[72,73]

Vaginismus may be caused by physical problems, emotional trauma, or psychosocial stressors but is less likely to be due to physical etiology. Typically, women present requesting and/or expecting treatment for a physical condition and are resistant or openly reject the suggestion of a psychological intervention. However, while this condition generally is thought to be psychological in nature, physical factors cannot be ruled out. Possible physiological causal factors include congenital deformity of the vagina; infections; hormonal abnormalities; sexual trauma; insufficient lubrication as a result of inadequate foreplay or poor sexual technique; allergic reactions; or other physical etiology.[74] Understandably, vaginismus often causes significant relationship problems, sometimes triggering erectile dysfunction in partners, particularly if the man becomes impatient, angry, or guilty, or feels responsible for his partner's problem.

Treatment of vaginismus usually involves a comprehensive program of physical evaluation, psychotherapy, and behavioral interventions aimed at modifying or altering the immediate cause of the conditioned response (tightening of the vaginal muscles).[75] Treatment often includes pelvic exercises, dilators, biofeedback, psychotherapeutic interventions, or physical therapy. Finally, treatment for vaginismus can take a fair bit of time, requiring the woman's commitment and compliance, as well as the patient cooperation of her partner. The time demand can be an additional stressor for infertile couples who often do not want to delay their pursuit of pregnancy to address a sexual problem they have learned to live with or accommodate. However, vaginismus has the highest rates of treatment success (Table 13.6).

Dyspareunia

Painful intercourse, or dyspareunia, may be the result of lack of arousal but is most often due to physical factors such as pelvic infection; anatomical conditions; congenital deformities; or vaginal atrophy due to inadequate estrogen exposure. Female sexual pain disorder can or may become the *cause* of infertility, if not the result, when pain is so intense as to limit or halt sexual intercourse. [72,74,76]. Other factors causing painful intercourse include side effects of medications; insufficient hormones; scarring from pelvic infections or surgeries; myomas; cancer; and STIs such as HPV infection and genital herpes. In infertile women, dyspareunia may be the result of ovarian cysts; side effects of ovulation-induction medications; ovarian hyperstimulation; infection; surgical adhesions; and endometriosis. Lubrication problems, or failure of the vaginal walls to provide adequate secretion to moisten the vagina and facilitate penile penetration, can be another common cause of painful intercourse and may be due to inadequate hormone levels; injury to the vaginal walls; lack of adequate sexual arousal; or poor sexual technique. Inadequate lubrication may also be due to attempts to proceed with sexual intercourse when a woman is not sufficiently aroused, an all too common occurrence in infertile couples who wish to get the reproductive chore over.

The optimum treatment for dyspareunia is contingent on etiology and involves a multimodal assessment and treatment protocol that addresses the following: behavior, affect, sensation, imagery, cognition, interpersonal relations, and medications.[72] Pain during intercourse can be treated medically (e.g., pain medications, leuprolide for endometriosis, or hormone-replacement therapy) or surgically (e.g., removal of pelvic adhesions or myomas). Psychotherapy involves relaxation techniques; desensitization; pain management; biofeedback; specialized physical therapy; and reeducation focusing on recognition of pelvic, genital, and muscular sensations. Alteration or adaptation of sexual positions, with the woman taking more control of the sexual encounter to avoid painful sites or positions, has also been found helpful, especially for women with endometriosis or other pelvic conditions. Physical therapy involving site-specific, manual soft-tissue therapy has also been found to be effective for reducing dyspareunia and increasing orgasm, particularly in women with a history of abdominal adhesions.[76]

Sexual Dysfunction in Men

Myths about male sexual functioning – such as men are ready, willing, and able to engage in sexual activity at any time or any place – have contributed to cavalier and unrealistic expectations regarding sexual functioning in men, and infertile men in particular. Such assumptions and perfunctory attitudes toward male sexuality are often the biggest impediment in the identification and treatment of sexual dysfunction in infertile men. Traditionally, sexual functioning in infertile men has focused on sexual disorders preventing impregnation or impacting infertility treatment plans, and less on sexual satisfaction or men's feelings about sexual performance or reproductive ability. However, infertility (especially male-factor infertility) frequently triggers feelings of failure; sexual inadequacy; diminished masculinity; loss of potency or power; and altered sense of self – all contributory factors in male sexual dysfunction.[41] During infertility, sexual intercourse for many men becomes obligatory, repetitive, and routine, providing few emotional rewards and little excitement. Many men develop performance anxiety, sexual avoidance, or even aversion to sex, especially if sex is for 'procreation purposes only' and their partner is sexually unresponsive or impassive. Frequently, infertile men complain of feeling like 'stud service' (that all his partner wants from him is his sperm) or of the 'queen bee syndrome' (his sole importance is to fertilize his partner).[77] Such feelings can be further intensified if the man equates sperm production with ejaculation, even though the two are distinct physiological functions.

The most common sexual dysfunctions in men are erectile dysfunction, traditionally referred to as impotence (inability to achieve or maintain an erection adequate for sexual intercourse); premature ejaculation (inability to exert voluntary control of ejaculatory reflex); and retarded or inhibited ejaculation (inhibition, delay, or absence of ejaculation). For men, erectile disorder is the most common presenting problem in sex therapy clinics, whereas premature ejaculation is more widespread in the community. Inhibited male orgasm is less common both in community and clinical settings. Causes of sexual dysfunction in men include hormonal changes (e.g., diminished testosterone with age); physical factors (e.g., injury or congenital anomaly); or organic conditions (e.g., illness and diseases such as diabetes or hypertension).

Erectile Dysfunction

Primary erectile dysfunction is never having had the ability to achieve and/or maintain an erection sufficient for vaginal penetration or successful coitus. This is a very rare condition most often due to physical or organic factors but, in rare situations, to psychological factors as well. Although rare, when it does occur, primary erectile dysfunction whether due to psychologi-

cal or physiological factors is a direct cause of infertility. Treatment success rates for primary erectile dysfunction are the lowest among all sexual disorders in men and women. *Secondary* or *acquired* erectile dysfunction is partial or weak erections; total absence of an erection; or the inability to sustain an erection long enough for vaginal penetration and/or intravaginal ejaculation. Most men experience some form of episodic, transient erectile dysfunction at some point in their lifetime. A significant number of men suffer from chronic erectile dysfunction especially as they age, although it affects men of all ages. In the past, it was believed that 90% of erectile dysfunction disorders were due to psychological factors, but it is now believed that this is an overestimate and that 50% of erectile dysfunction problems have a physical (or organic) etiology.[78,79] Causes of impotence include organic factors (e.g., endocrine or neurological problems; medications, alcohol, tobacco, and recreational drugs); hormonal changes (e.g., hormonal therapy including medications used to treat infertility); physical factors (e.g., injury, cancer, urological, or vascular problems); and psychological or relationship difficulties.

Erectile dysfunction is the most important cause of male-factor infertility due to sexual dysfunction, although men (and/or their partners) rarely disclose this problem to caregivers.[80] This may be because many men generally have difficulty discussing their sexual problems or because it is difficult to discuss these problems with infertility physicians (who are typically gynecologists). Erectile dysfunction due to psychological factors is generally believed to be the result of the man's blocking sexual arousal and focusing instead on nonsexual or antisexual cues.[78] A variety of psychosexual issues may account for erection problems in men, involving not only his feelings about himself but also his feelings about his health (e.g., semen analysis), relationships, sexuality, and life situation. Relationship issues, especially those involving conflict and anger, have been found to be a major factor in erectile dysfunction.[79] Intrapersonal dynamics, such as ambivalence about parenthood; threatened masculinity or self-esteem; or fear of intimacy or commitment, can surface during the crisis of infertility and become influential issues in a man's sexual functioning.

Erectile dysfunction, like vaginismus in women, often contributes to considerable marital tension, especially in terms of infertility, in which the husband's healthy sexual functioning is a prerequisite to procreation as well as many infertility treatment protocols. Inability to perform sexually (intercourse or produce a sperm specimen) may not be simply embarrassing but financially expensive; culturally reprehensible; religiously unacceptable; emotionally distressing; and relationship-damaging. Conflicts or disagreements about medical treatments; family-building options; personal agendas; or relationship dynamics can, and often do, contribute to erectile dysfunction problems in infertile couples.

Treatments for secondary erectile dysfunction have had mixed success rates, although medications (e.g., sildenafil citrate) have been found to be very effective. Furthermore, in addition to reversing anxiety and stress-induced transitory impotence, sildenafil improved seminal parameters (e.g., sperm motility).[81] Furthermore, sildenafil was found to be helpful in increasing compliance in men using procreation to conceive or pursuing infertility treatments that required semen collection.[82] Treatment usually begins with a physical examination that evaluates hormone levels, nerves, and blood vessels and assesses nocturnal tumescence (rigidity of the penis during sleep). There are two general types of nocturnal tumescence devices: the snap gauge cuff and the nocturnal penile tumescence monitor.[83] When erectile dysfunction is determined to be organic and not reversible (e.g., in the case of injury or disease), treatment usually involves medical (oral or injectable medications) or surgical interventions such as penile injections, penile prostheses, and/or penile implants. Medications, penile injections, penile prostheses, and penile implants all facilitate erections and sexual intercourse, thereby improving quality-of-life. However, these treatments usually do not and cannot improve or restore fertility.

Psychological treatments for erectile dysfunction include decreasing performance anxiety; eliminating 'spectatoring'; increasing awareness of erotic sensations; and disputing irrational beliefs and myths. Psychodynamic-depth approaches that do not include behavioral or cognitive interventions have been found to be ineffective in the treatment of erectile dysfunction,[78] while guided imagery and sensate-focus exercises (see Table 13.6) have been found to be helpful in deemphasizing sexual performance and refocusing on sensation and pleasure. Cognitive restructuring, sexual education, and relaxation techniques are successful for redirecting negative and automatic thoughts while increasing comfort with feelings of sexual arousal. For infertile couples, marital counseling addressing relationship issues, husband's sexuality, and couple sexual functioning can be beneficial.[79] Whether erectile dysfunction is due to physical or emotional factors, counseling can help the man and his partner maintain realistic expectations about treatment outcomes and provides a supportive environment for discussing the problem.

Premature Ejaculation

Premature ejaculation, or inadequate ejaculatory control, is the inability to exert voluntary control over the ejaculatory reflex, so that once a man reaches a certain level of sexual arousal or excitement, he ejaculates reflexively and rapidly soon after or even before vaginal penetration. It should be noted that in some cultures this is *not* considered a sexual problem because the woman's involvement and/or response during sexual intercourse is irrelevant and unimportant. Nevertheless, premature ejaculation is defined as a problem when the man is unable to delay ejaculatory reflex for sufficient time during intercourse to satisfy a responsive partner during 50% of their coital experiences.[84,85] Premature ejaculation is problematic for infertile couples, particularly when they pursue intercourse with insufficient lubrication causing significant pain for the woman. Premature ejaculation is usually not situational; it typically occurs with *all* partners because the man has not learned to voluntarily control his ejaculatory reflexes. Diagnostic criteria for premature ejaculation are contingent on the length of coitus; sexual attitudes of both partners; and sexual expectations often defined by sociocultural issues. Although rare, there can be physical causes for premature ejaculation, especially when loss of control is not associated with significant stress or a change in the man's sexual relationship.[52] Organic causes of premature ejaculation involve congenital conditions; neurological problems; side effects of medications; and other health problems, including hormonal changes (especially hormone medications used for infertility treatment). Psychological factors (apart from learned response) may be related to infertility with its emphasis on sex for procreation; the man's (or couple's) attempts to make the sexual encounter as brief as possible; or habituated rapid ejaculation to provide specimens for infertility treatment.

Premature ejaculation has the highest rates of treatment success (see Table 13.4). Psychological interventions in which couples are taught either the stop-start or squeeze technique have had fairly high success rates, although they are less successful when both partners are overconcerned with reproduction and underconcerned with sexual pleasuring or lovemaking. Medical treatment of ejaculatory problems is often difficult, although there are numerous medications that can help delay ejaculation. The most effective psychosexual treatment for premature ejaculation combines multiple strategies such as physiological relaxation; muscle training; cognitive and behavioral pacing strategies; and the involvement of the partner in the therapy.[86] Other treatment interventions include promoting couple communication and couple

TABLE 13.4. Success rates for treatment of sexual dysfunction[68]

Premature ejaculation and vaginismus	90–95%
Absolute female orgasmic dysfunction (no orgasm ever)	85–95% if orgasm with partner is criterion, but only 30–50% if orgasm during intercourse is criterion
Partial female orgasmic dysfunction (patient seldom orgasmic or orgasmic only with solo masturbation)	70–80%, but only 30–50% if criterion is during intercourse
Secondary erectile dysfunction (patient has had erections in past)	60–80%
Primary erectile dysfunction (no erections ever in sexual situations)	40–60%
Retarded or blocked ejaculations	50–82%
Low or inhibited sexual desire	no reliable outcome studies of sex therapy; sporadic success at best after much longer therapies

cooperation; teaching the man to concentrate on his genital sensations; and facilitating his mastery of a series of tasks that progressively provide more intense genital stimulation while he learns to control his ejaculatory response.

Inhibited or Delayed Ejaculation

Inhibited or delayed ejaculation or orgasm (sometimes referred to as retarded ejaculation) is the persistent and recurrent inhibition of orgasm, manifested by delay or absence of ejaculation following adequate sexual excitement. It is commonly defined as difficulty or inability to ejaculate during sexual intercourse or masturbation. Although failure to orgasm is fairly common in women, delayed or absence of orgasm in men is fairly rare. Inhibited male orgasm or delayed ejaculation ranges from mild situational delays in ejaculation to excessively long periods of intravaginal thrusting without orgasm. Historically, physical causes have been rare, although delayed ejaculation may be symptomatic of underlying medical conditions or due to physical conditions such as spinal cord injury. Recently, delayed ejaculation has been identified as a common side effect of some antidepressant medications, particularly SSRIs. Psychological etiology may be due to performance anxiety; depression; anger; guilt regarding sex in general or with certain partners; relationship problems; traumatic sexual history; religious orthodoxy; prolonged fear of pregnancy leading to conditioned response; history of withdrawal method of birth control; gender identity issues; cultural factors; and/or partner unresponsiveness. Recently it has been suggested that delayed or retarded ejaculation is due to a combination of insufficient arousal to reach orgasm in intercourse and reflex inhibition.[87]

Treatment of inhibited male orgasm or delayed ejaculation has been notoriously difficult and time-consuming, with success often followed by relapse.[87] Medical treatment for delayed ejaculation usually entails addressing underlying medical conditions, the removal of medications and/or alcohol, tobacco, and recreational drugs. Psychological treatment of delayed ejaculation using sensate-focus techniques has been successful by increasing the man's awareness of his sexual sensations and arousal responses. Psychological interventions aim at overcoming ejaculatory inhibitions; reducing fear and anxiety; improving couple interactions; and resolving underlying psychological conflicts, aggression, and problems. In fact, it has been suggested that treatment be redefined from introvaginal orgasm to something less – avoiding a rigorous treatment regime and thereby avoiding or enhancing ever-present performance anxiety.[87] When delayed ejaculation affects fertility, electroejaculation or testicular biopsy can be used to obtain sperm for insemination of the female partner or use in IVF. However, this solution is only recommended when psychosocial causes have been ruled out or successfully treated, although most infertile couples resist psychosocial treatments in their relentless pursuit of pregnancy and their aversion to 'wasting time' in that pursuit. Furthermore, given the possible etiology of 'learned response' and the rather dismal treatment success rates, it may be unrealistic to defer infertility treatment to address adequately this sexual dysfunction. At best, the goal for the infertility counselor may be effectively and confidently ruling out dissatisfaction and/or loss of desire for the partner and/or partnership before proceeding with family-building medical treatments with this partner.

Sexual Pain Disorders in Men

Disorders in men involving any form of pain during sexual activity (also termed male dyspareunia) are usually categorized on the basis of the point in the sexual act during which pain occurs: pain with erection; pain on intromission; or pain accompanying ejaculation. Sexual pain disorders in men are typically uncommon and are usually due to physical factors such as infection, tight foreskin, or spasm of the perineal muscles.[79,88] When no physical etiology can be identified, treatment usually consists of empirical medical remedies; reassurance of anatomical normalcy; and investigation of psychological factors.[79] Psychological interventions focus on adaptation to physical factors in pain disorder; the secondary gains of pain; illness behaviors; relaxation and behavioral-cognitive interventions; and relationship issues.

THERAPEUTIC INTERVENTIONS

Treatment of Sexual Dysfunction

Most couples are reluctant to discuss the private sexual aspects of their relationship, but even more so when sexual functioning may be problematic and/or involve behavior that is embarrassing or atypical for either one or both partners.[89] Infertile couples appear to be even more reluctant to discuss sexual dysfunction if they fear that it will interrupt medical treatment. Even so, no clinician working with infertile couples should *assume* that a couple is having regular sexual intercourse sufficient for reproduction or ignore the possibility of unusual sexual practices that interfere with conception and/or medical treatment plans. The first issue in any medical and/or sexual history, especially regarding infertility, must address whether or not the couple is having sexual intercourse that involves penile ejaculation into the vagina on a regular basis (i.e., at least twice a month).

Treatment success rates vary according to the specific sexual dysfunction: Premature ejaculation and vaginismus have the highest rates of treatment success, while primary erectile dysfunction has the lowest treatment success rate (see Table 13.4). Female orgasm disorders can be treated with considerable success, depending upon the definition of success: 85–95% success rate if orgasm with partner is the criterion but 30–50% success rate if orgasm during intercourse is the criterion. Erectile dysfunctions have mixed success rates, with secondary erectile dysfunctions having higher rates of success than primary erectile dysfunction. Mixed success is also the case for delayed ejaculations. In general, the most difficult sexual dysfunction to treat is diminished sexual desire.[75] Finally, successful outcomes in sex therapy have been found to be influenced by the diagnosis of sexual dysfunction; the pretreatment quality of a couple's general relationship; the quality of their pretreatment sexual relationship; their motivation for

TABLE 13.5. P-LI-SS-IT model[90]	
P	Permission to talk about sexual issues, reassurance and empathy, and the acknowledgment that we are sexual beings
LI	Limited information, including sex education; clarification of sexual myths and stereotypes; and bibliography with suggested related books
SS	Specific suggestions, such as Kegel exercises, squeeze technique, or sensate focus
IT	Intensive therapy, individual or conjoint, including focus on relationship dynamics and psychological concerns and other complex issues

treatment and/or unproved sexual functioning; medical diagnosis of infertility; type of sex therapy; and extent of progress made by the third treatment session.[52]

Clinicians treating sexual problems can intervene on several different therapeutic levels. Annon and Robinson's[90] P-LI-SS-IT model of sexual counseling identifies four levels of intervention: (1) permission; (2) limited information, (3) specific suggestions, and (4) intensive therapy (Table 13.5). This behavioral therapy model is based on a continuum of less intense to increasingly intensive interventions. Initial interventions involve encouraging discussions of the sexual problem; the provision of basic information about sexual functioning; definition and explanation of the specific sexual problem; and education about how infertility impacts sexual functioning. More intense therapeutic interventions and formal treatment may involve referral to a trained sex therapist or collaborative work between an infertility counselor and sex therapist.

Almost all approaches for the treatment of sexual dysfunction incorporate strategies of sexual reeducation designed to eliminate sexual myth and misinformation; attitude-changing techniques; marital and communication enhancement methods; and specific prescriptions for behavior change.[91] The basic behavioral techniques include:

■ *anxiety-reduction techniques*: progressive relaxation; systematic desensitization; methohexital sodium (Brevital, a fast-acting muscle relaxant); and assertiveness training procedures

■ *directed masturbation*: treatment for both anorgasmia in men and women

■ *orgasmic reconditioning*: directed fantasy in conjunction with masturbation to modify the kinds of sexual stimuli associated with arousal

■ *imagery techniques*: assessment and rehearsal of desired sexual responses

TABLE 13.6. Sensate-focus exercises

Pleasuring without direct attempts to produce arousal/erection

Penile erection/arousal through genital pleasuring

Extravaginal orgasm

Penetration without orgasm

Full coitus with orgasm

■ *explicit homework assignments*: massage, self-stimulation, or couple communication exercises
■ *sensate-focus technique*: exercises designed to help couples enrich their ways of touching each other initially and increasing their awareness of pleasurable feelings. Touch is initially nongenital, eventually leading to genital touching (Table 13.6).

At times, sex therapy includes the use of various devices, such as the vacuum constriction device and penile prosthesis, antidepressants for male anorgasmia, and vibrators for female anorgasmia or vaginismus. Medications (e.g., sildenafil or antidepressants) may be used for erectile dysfunction or sexual desire disorders. Devices and medications may be used alone or in combination with medical or surgical therapies, couples counseling, physical therapy, hypnosis, or interpersonal therapy.[70,71,76] In all treatment of sexual dysfunction, cultural and/or religious restrictions, foreplay, and timing of sexual intercourse should be considered, as well as persistent marital difficulties, including preexisting marital disturbance, unrealistic sexual expectations, prior sexual trauma or victimization, and performance pressures. In truth, individuals often find the suggestions of homework, reading, medications, or devices alarming or offensive. Finally, the success of treatment is contingent on diagnosis; motivation of the patient and his or her partner; the type of therapy; and the qualifications of the therapist, as well as the fundamentals of sexual intimacy – equality, mutuality, and reciprocity.

Prevention of Sexual Dysfunction in Infertile Couples

One of the goals of infertility counseling is the prevention of disturbance whenever possible, a goal that is particularly important to an infertile couple's sexual relationship (see Table 13.7). Prevention of sexual dysfunction may involve targeting either issues related to the medical treatment or the couple's relationship. Demands of medical treatment that strain sexual functioning include producing a sperm specimen for medical treatments; the requirement of mid-cycle sexual intercourse; and sexual intercourse followed by postcoital testing. It is important to carefully assess with a couple (and medical caregivers) the pros and cons of a treatment procedure in terms of its potential for contributing to or exacerbating sexual difficulties. For example, if a couple already has problems with sexual intercourse, the medical information provided by postcoital testing may be minimal, compared to the deleterious effect on the couple's sexual relationship. By the same token, every effort should be made to accommodate medical treatment plans to a couple's sexual problems and religious or cultural proscriptions. For men with problems producing a sperm sample, assistance may involve allowing his wife to participate; providing special semen collection condoms to be used during intercourse; or making environmental accommodations (e.g., providing erotica, sound machines, earphones, and a more secluded 'collection' room). If the clinic cannot make logistical accommodations, it may be useful for these men to bring a tape player with ear plugs to block out clinic sounds. For couples with female sexual pain problems (perhaps related to endometriosis or ovulation induction), changing sexual positions; the use of over-the-counter pain medication *before* sexual intercourse; or preintercourse relaxation exercises, massage, and hot baths may be beneficial.

Sometimes, the most effective means of preventing sexual dysfunction is simply addressing with the couple the importance of their sexual relationship and specifically asking each partner about common sexual problems, such as painful intercourse, 'sex-on-demand,' and problems with specimen collection. Couples usually respond with relief at being given permission to discuss these problems, especially men who are often too embarrassed to admit problems such as shyness about specimen production; mid-cycle sexual problems; or sex causing or increasing pain in their partners. For these couples, preventing problems may involve basic education; offering helpful tips; or encouraging them to discuss the problems with their physician, infertility counselor, and/or a sex therapist. This can also normalize sexual problems for the infertile couple, minimizing guilt and stigma, while helping them understand the nature of common sexual problems in infertility. In this manner, the importance of their sexual relationship is validated, and they are encouraged not to 'sacrifice' sexual rewards for the sake of a pregnancy, parenthood, or infertility treatment.

Prevention of sexual problems also involves addressing relationship issues and giving couples education and support regarding sexual matters. If the

---

TABLE 13.7. Tips for infertile couples on keeping sex enjoyable

For female sexual disorders: change sexual positions (woman on top or side by side); use over-the-counter pain medication before sexual intercourse; try preintercourse relaxation exercises, and/or hot baths

For problems with sperm collection: bring an audiotape player with ear plugs or ask to use the clinic video machine and bring own videotape with ear phones

Discuss sexual problems with physician or other caregivers

Educate oneself about normal sexual functioning and typical sexual problems of infertility

Don't 'sacrifice' rewarding sexual encounters or intimacy for infertility treatment

For marital problems (in addition to sexual difficulties): seek help from qualified infertility counselor

Take turns planning special sex 'dates' at nonfertile times

Practice 'nonintercourse' sexual pleasuring

Plan treatment 'holidays' with focus on renewing physical intimacy and warmth

Plan a hotel date or special time away from home for 'distraction-free' sex

Renew commitment to each other

Devote time to activities and interests you as a couple really enjoy

Try sexual 'play,' as you did early in your relationship

Be creative and inventive

Take your time

When interest wanes, try erotic books, board games, or videotapes

---

sexual problems reflect more fundamental relationship problems, it may be that marital issues must take precedence over further infertility treatment. This is especially important if there is evidence of an extramarital affair or sexual behavior that is likely to precipitate a marital crisis, such as homosexuality; illegal sexual behavior (e.g., victimization or use of prostitutes); sexually addictive behaviors (e.g., excessive masturbation, pornography with or without internet sexual activity); or deviant sexual behaviors (e.g., partner swapping). These problems may be a serious mental health problem involving at risk behaviors either causing infertility; destabilizing the relationship; or potentially exposing the child to a harmful environment.

For less serious problems, prevention may simply involve encouraging couples to keep their sexual relationship rewarding, interesting, and enlivened (see Table 13.8). For couples complaining of lost spontaneity, the benefits of planned, special sex dates at nonfertile times may be explored, or they may be given homework in which each partner takes responsibility for planning a sexual surprise. Couples may wish to explore nonintercourse sexual expression, such as massage or sensate-focus exercises (see Table 13.6) that emphasize physical closeness and nongenital pleasuring. Taking treatment holidays is always helpful, encouraging the couple to use the holiday to renew

physical intimacy and warmth by spending an evening at a hotel or away from home; renewing their commitment to each other; devoting time to activities that they as a couple find particularly enjoyable; and learning to 'play' with each other again as they did early in their relationship together. For couples who have a difficult time being creative, using books, videotapes, or educational materials may be beneficial, especially those that give ideas on how to be intimate and close. These can, but need not be, actual erotica. For couples complaining of loss of interest or desire (and there is no evidence of depression or other psychological or physical factors), discussions may focus on increasing awareness of sexual cues and what the couple finds erotic or arousing. Homework may involve erotic reading materials, board games, or videotapes that increase the individual's or couple's awareness of what they find exciting and arousing.

Although prevention of sexual distress should be a primary goal for all infertility caregivers, it often is not. And worse, it may not be a priority for the infertile couple who is singularly focused on having a baby, after which they believe all their problems will be solved and their sexual relationship will return to its 'preinfertility' level of satisfaction. Of course, this is one of the myths that the infertility counselor must address, helping couples understand that postinfertility

---

TABLE 13.8. Therapeutic recommendations

Ask about sexual functioning and satisfaction; then ask again later

Look for evidence or indications of sexual problems

Watch for signs in spouse or marriage of excessive difficulties coping

Watch for signs of marital conflict and disturbance

Encourage discussion and improved communication between partners about sexual issues

Encourage couple to become educated about normal sexual functioning and sexual activity

Recommend against ritualized, mechanistic, procreation approaches to sex

Suggest planning sexual activities that are not for procreation only

Encourage sexual activities that are playful, enjoyable, or interesting, especially during nontreatment times

Provide educational materials about sexual functioning

Inquire about how stressful patient perceives medical treatments

Be aware of mood disorders that may affect sexual functioning

Make referrals to appropriate sex therapy professional

Encourage patient or couple to discuss the sexual problem with infertility caregiver

---

(especially when they are parents) will have its own challenges and prevention at this time is worth a pound of cure later on.[92]

Ethical Dilemmas

One of the ethical dilemmas of sexual dysfunction in couples undergoing medical treatment for infertility is the patient or couple who requests medical interventions to avoid sexual intercourse or treatment of a sexual dysfunction. This may include the patient with primary sexual dysfunction who wishes to have a family or the couple who develops sexual problems secondary to infertility treatment. A couple with an unconsummated marriage, sexual aversion, primary impotence, or vaginismus, while acknowledging the dysfunction and refusing appropriate treatment, may present desiring inseminations, IVF, or third-party reproduction to become pregnant. Some couples will develop mid-cycle impotence or vaginismus, sexual avoidance, inability to produce sperm specimen for IVF or inseminations, or other sexual problems over the course of treatment and request treatments, such as husband insemination, that will accommodate their sexual difficulties. The ethical dilemma is that the sexual problem may mask more severe psychological or marital problems, while at the same time additional medical treatment may further strain individual or couple functioning which may be further exacerbated by pregnancy and parenthood. Will assisting these couples in achieving pregnancy further impair individual, couple, or family functioning? Should couples be assisted in achieving pregnancy when there is evidence of a disturbance that may impact or impair family or parental adjustment, such as in cases of disturbed gender identity or latent homosexuality? Should medical treatment for infertility proceed unchecked even when patients refuse psychological or sexual treatment, although they have acknowledged the existence of significant problems? What about the well-being of the 'whole' patient or couple and comprehensive care? These questions often pose very real dilemmas for medical caregivers and for infertile couples, especially if their avoidant coping style and/or fixation on parenthood clouds their judgment about the health and well-being of their marriage, family, their potential children, and themselves.[93]

It seems advisable that, in accordance with the ethical principle of 'to do no harm,' patients with acknowledged primary sexual dysfunction causing infertility should not proceed with medical treatment for infertility, especially as a means of avoiding more appropriate treatment. In addition, although some patients may proceed with infertility treatment in the presence of some sexual dysfunctions, medical treatment should be in conjunction with psychotherapy and/or sex therapy, emphasizing the importance of sexual health and well-being in infertile couples.

Role of the Infertility Counselor

Whether sexual dysfunction is a preexisting condition or an unwelcome side effect of infertility treatment, it can be a devastating and discouraging blow, compounding the disappointment of childlessness and the distress of medical treatment. Although at some point in infertility treatment sex may become regulatory, obligatory, and uninspired, not all infertile couples experience sexual difficulties. Nevertheless, changes in sexual practices or behavior may often occur, such as the initiator of sexual encounters; preferred sexual positions; reduced sexual activity during the luteal phase; or increased mid-cycle frequency. Adaptation to these changes not only contributes to a couple's self-confidence in managing the crisis and stresses of infertility but can also improve communication and marital satisfaction. When infertility results in relationship disturbance or sexual problems, the support and intervention of caregivers are paramount. All too often, the sexual problems of infertile couples are ignored or minimized in a belief that they will dissipate on their own or will have few long-term consequences. Unfortunately, these beliefs are myths. Although some sexual problems may disappear when the pressures of infertility treatment end, sexual difficulties typically linger or become more problematic after treatment ends or parenthood is achieved.[94,95]

Most infertility counselors are not certified sex therapists and are therefore not qualified to provide sex therapy as such. However, sexual problems can be integrated into psychotherapy by providing sexual education specific to infertility, brief interventions, and marital counseling (see Table 13.7). The infertility counselor should, at a minimum, become familiar with the sexual problems relevant to infertility, treatment methods, success rates, and typical as well as atypical psychosexual responses to infertility treatment.[92,94] Also important is an awareness of available resources, organizations, and sex therapists in the area with expertise or special interest in treating infertile couples or willingness to collaborate with the infertility counselor in the treatment of the infertile couple or individual with sexual problems.

FUTURE IMPLICATIONS

As our understanding of sexual functioning has increased dramatically even in the past decade, so too has our understanding of the interface of sexual functioning and infertility. Once thought to be fairly straightforward, with the advent of assisted reproductive technologies and the plethora of new medications and treatments for sexual dysfunction, there are now new ways to overcome sexual problems as well as new ways of creating or contributing to them. Leiblum and Rosen identified major trends in the practice of sex therapy in 1989 that seem all the more relevant today, particularly when applied to the treatment of infertility: (1) a trend toward greater 'medicalization'; (2) increasing emphasis on pharmacological interventions; and (3) greater attention to desire disorders.[96]

Despite considerable research dispelling longstanding myths and inaccuracies about infertility and sexual functioning (e.g., that failure to orgasm in women or tubal spasms cause infertility or that sperm quality or production is not affected by environmental or ingested chemicals), culture and ignorance remain problematic – particularly in the developing world. Furthermore, there remains a need for well-designed research in the area of sexual functioning and infertility: What is the actual incidence of sexual dysfunction among infertile men and women as compared with the general population? What is the incidence of sexual dysfunction causing infertility? What is the incidence of specific sexual dysfunctions within the context of infertility and which are more common? Is the incidence of diagnosable sexual dysfunction more common in infertile women or men? Are there specific infertility diagnoses or treatments that are more detrimental to sexual functioning in infertile couples? What are the circumstances that make it easier for patients to bring up sexual problems with their caregivers?

As treatment of infertility involves higher rates of technology use, as such making sexual intercourse less relevant for procreative purposes, sexual dysfunctions secondary to infertility may become less problematic. However, they also may mask sexual disorders allowing couples to 'bypass' their sexual problem and go directly to parenthood without having to have sex or address the sexual dysfunction. Furthermore, increased reliance on assisted reproductive technologies may represent the technologizing of our society and interpersonal relationships, allowing more distance, mechanization, and reserve, impeding intimacy, warmth, and connections. By the same token, the use of ART without sexual intercourse for procreation lessens 'performance anxiety' and distress, allowing sexual intercourse to be valued for the intimacy and relationship rewards that it has always provided.

SUMMARY

■ The ability to reproduce is intimately tied to sexuality, self-image, and self-esteem. The extent to which this is important varies with cultural expectations, religious beliefs, individuals, and the impact of medical conditions and treatment.

■ Although sexual problems can occur during infertility, sometimes even causing infertility, sexual difficulties are not universally experienced by infertile couples. The majority of infertile couples do not develop diagnosable sexual problems requiring intensive treatment, although they may experience episodic, transient problems, warranting education and support.

■ The medical assessment and treatment for infertility may interfere with the infertile couple's sexual pleasure due to performance demands, treatment requirements, or emotional response to treatment or infertility diagnosis.

■ A large percentage of sexual problems may be addressed by the infertility counselor educated about the impact of infertility on sexual functioning. Professional attention and education regarding sexual difficulties during infertility can minimize the impact and even prevent sexual difficulties.

■ Because most couples do not volunteer sexual problems, caregivers must specifically ask questions about sexual behavior as part of a comprehensive medical and social history, particularly whether the couple is actually having sexual intercourse on a regular basis.

■ When sexual dysfunction is the presenting cause of infertility, assessment and therapy for the individual or couple is necessary and should preclude medical treatment for infertility.

REFERENCES

1. Edelmann RJ, Humphrey M, Owens DJ. The meaning of parenthood and couples reactions to male infertility. *Br J Med Psychol* 1994; 67:291–9.
2. Fogel CI, Lauver D. *Sexual Health Promotion*. Philadelphia: Saunders, 1990.
3. Walker HE. Psychiatric aspects of infertility. *Urol Clin North Am* 1978; 5:481–8.
4. Riddick DH. Sexual dysfunction: Cause and result of infertility. *Fem Patient* 1982; 7:45–8.
5. Potts M, Short R. *Ever since Adam and Eve: The Evolution of Human Sexuality*. New York: Cambridge University Press, 1999.
6. Idoyaga Molina A. Hermeneutic approach to ideas about conception, pregnancy and birth among the Pilago of the Central Chaco. *Scr Ethnol* 1977; 4:78–98.
7. Yalom M. *A History of the Wife*. New York: Harper Collins, 2001.
8. Petok WD. *A Brief History of Sex and Sex Therapy: Evolution and Revolutions*. ASRM Postgraduate Course #4: Male and female sexual dysfunction: Contemporary thought and interventions. October 16–17, 2004, Philadelphia, PA.
9. Hendrickx K, Lodewijckx E, Van Royen P, et al. Sexual behavior of second generation Moroccan immigrants balancing between traditional attitudes and safe sex. *Patient Educ Couns*. 2002; 4:89–94.
10. Goodwin J. *The Price of Honor: Muslim Women Lift the Veil of Silence on the Islamic World*. Boston: Little, Brown & Co, 1993.
11. Thomasset C. The nature of women. In: C Klapish-Zuber, ed. *A History of Women in the West: II: Silences of the Middle Ages*. Cambridge, MA: Harvard University Press, 1992; 41–69.
12. *The New English Bible*. Cambridge, UK: Cambridge University, 1970. Genesis 1:22.
13. Obermeyer, Carla Makhlouf. The health consequences of female circumcision: Science, advocacy, and standards of evidence. *Medical Anthropology Quarterly* 2003; 17:394–412.
14. Grieco SFM. The body, appearance, and sexuality. In: NZ Davis, A Farge, eds. *A History of Women in the West: III: Renaissance and Englightment Paradoxes*. Cambridge, MA: Harvard University Press, 1993; 46–85.
15. Walker BG. *The Woman's Encyclopedia of Myths and Secrets*. New York: HarperCollins, 1983.
16. Cott NF. The modern woman of the 1920s American style. In. F Thebaud, ed. *A History of Women in the West:V: Toward a Cultural Identity in the Twentieth Century*. Cambridge, MA: Harvard University Press 1994; 76–91.
17. Thebaud F, ed. *A History of Women in the West: V: Toward a Cultural Identity in the Twentieth Century*. Cambridge, MA: Harvard University Press 1994; 494.
18. Benedek T. Infertility as a psychosomatic defense. *Fertil Steril* 1952; 3:527–41.
19. Benedek T, Ham GC, Robbins FP, et al. Some emotional factors in infertility. *Psychosom Med* 1953; 15:485–98.
20. Fischer IC. Psychogenic aspects of sterility. *Fertil Steril* 1953; 4:466–71.
21. Rubenstein BB. An emotional factor in infertility: A psychosomatic approach. *Fertil Steril* 1951; 2:80–6.
22. Belonoschkin B. Psychosomatic factors and matrimonial infertility. *Int J Fertil* 1962; 7:29–36.
23. de Watteville H. Psychologic factors in the treatment of sterility. *Fertil Steril* 1957; 8:12–24.
24. Rutherford RN. Emotional aspects of infertility. *Clin Obstet Gynecol* 1965; 8:100–14.
25. Cohen HR. The psychosomatic factor in infertility. *Int J Fertil* 1961; 6:369–73.
26. Eisner BB. Some psychological differences between fertile and infertile women. *J Clin Psychiatry* 1963; 19:391–5.
27. World Health Organization: From bench to bedside: Setting a path for translation of improved sexually transmitted infection, diagnostics into health care delivery in the developing world. WHO/TDR/Wellcome Trust. Geneva:29–30 January, 2001.
28. Aral SO. Sexually transmitted diseases: Magnitude, determinants and consequences. *Int J STD AIDS* 2001; 12:211–5.
29. Fugate KA, McCluskey MM. The impact of sexually transmitted diseases on fertility: A review of literature and nursing opportunities. *Infertil Reprod Med Clin North Am* 1996; 7:521–34.
30. Lande R. Sexual and reproductive health: What are the possibilities? *Plan Parent Chall*. 1993; 2:19–21.
31. Cates W Jr, Rolfs RT Jr, Aral SO. Sexually transmitted diseases, pelvic inflammatory disease, and infertility: An epidemiologic update. *Epidemiol Rev* 1990; 12:199–220.
32. Sexually transmitted diseases and reproductive health. *Prog Hum Reprod Res* 1992; 21:6–7.
33. van Leeuwen E, van Weert JM, van der Veen F, et al. The effects of the human immunodeficiency virus on semen parameters and intrauterine insemination outcome. *Hum Reprod* 2005; 20:2033–4.
34. Umapathy E. STD/HIV association: Effects on semen characteristics. *Arch Androl* 2005; 51:361–5.
35. Arya R, Mannion PT, Woodcock K, et al. Incidence of genital Chlamydia trachomatis infection in the male partners attending an infertility clinic. *J Obstet Gynecol* 2005; 25:364–7.
36. Pitts M, Shields P Access to infertility investigations and treatment for HIV+ people: A survey of Australian infertility clinics. *Aust N Z J Public Health* 2004; 28:360–2.
37. Keye WR. The impact of infertility on psychosexual function. *Fertil Steril* 1980; 34:308–9.
38. Coeffin-Driol C, Gianmi A. The impact of infertility and its treatment on the sexual life and marital relationships: Review of the literatue. *Gynecol Obstet Fertil* 2004; 32:624–37.

39. Boivin J, Takefman JE, Brender W, et al. The effects of female sexual response in coitus on early reproductive process. *J Behav Med* 1992; 15:509–18.

40. Andrews FM, Abbey A, Halman J. Stress from infertility, marriage factors, and subjective well-being of wives and husbands. *J Health Soc Behav* 1991; 32:238–53.

41. Nachtigall RD, Becker G, Wozny M. The effects of gender-specific diagnosis on men's and women's response to infertility. *Fertil Steril* 1992; 57:113–21.

42. Berg BJ, Wilson JF. Psychological functioning across stages of treatment in infertility. *J Behav Med* 1991; 14:11–26.

43. Kemer P, Mikulincer M, Nathanson YE, et al. Psychological aspects of male infertility. *Br J Med Psychol* 1990; 63:73–80.

44. Muller MJ, Schilling G, Haidl G. Sexual satisfaction in male infertility. *Arch Androl* 1999; 42:137–43.

45. Schilling G, Muller MJ, Haidl G. Sexual dissatisfaction and somatic complaints in male infertility. *Psychother Psychosom Med Psychol* 1999; 49:256–63.

46. Laffont I, Edelmann RJ. Psychological aspects of in vitro fertilization: A gender comparison. *J Psychosom Obstet Gynecol* 1994; 15:85–92.

47. Bar-Hava M, Azam F, Yovel I, et al. The interrelationship between coping strategies and sexual functioning in in vitro fertilization patients. *J Sex Marital Ther* 2001; 27:389–94.

48. Leiblum SR, Aviv A, Hamer R. Life after infertility treatment: A long-term investigation of marital and sexual function. *Hum Reprod* 1998; 13:3569–74.

49. Hammond KR, Kretzer PA, Blackwell RE, et al. Performance anxiety during infertility treatment: Effect of semen quality. *Fertil Steril* 1990; 53:337–40.

50. Saleh RA, Ranga GM, Raina R, et al. Sexual dysfunction in men undergoing infertility evaluation: A cohort observational study. *Fertil Steril* 2003; 79:909–12.

51. Masters WH, Johnson VE. *Human Sexual Response* Boston: Little, Brown, 1966.

52. Kaplan HS. *Evaluation of Sexual Disorders: Psychological and Medical Aspects*. New York: Brunner/Mazel, 1983.

53. Basson F. Human sex-response cycles. *J Sex Marital Ther* 2001; 27:33–43.

54. Burns LH. An overview of the psychology of infertility: Comprehensive psychosocial history of infertility. *Infertil Reprod Med Clin North Am* 1993; 4:433–54.

55. Inhorn MC, van Balen F, eds. *Infertility Around the Globe: New Thinking on Childlessness, Gender, and Reproductive Technologies*. Los Angeles, CA: University of California Press, 2002.

56. Folkvord S, Odegaard OA, Sundby J. Male infertility in Zimbabwe. *Patient Educ Couns* 2005; 59:239–43.

57. Araoye MO. Epidemiology of infertility: Social problems of the infertile couples. *West Afr J Med* 2003; 22:190–6.

58. Chikovore J, Mbizvo MT. Beliefs about sexual relationships and behavior among commercial farm residents in Zimbabwe. *Cent Afr J Med* 1999; 45:178–82.

59. Dyer SJ, Abraham N, Hoffman, van der Spuy ZM. 'Men leave me as I cannot have children': Women's experiences with involuntary childlessness. *Hum Reprod* 2002; 17:1663–8.

60. O'Brien JH, Lazarou S, Deane L, et al. Erectile dysfunction and andropause symptoms in infertile. *J Urol* 2005; 174:1932–4.

61. LoPiccolo L. Low sexual desire. In: SR Leiblum, LA Pervin, eds. *Principles and Practice of Sex Therapy*. New York: Guilford Press, 1980; 27–64.

62. Spector IP, Carey MP. Incidence and prevalence of the sexual dysfunctions: A critical review of the empirical literature. *Arch Sex Beh* 1990; 19:389–408.

63. Schover LR, LoPiccolo J. Treatment effectiveness for dysfunctions of sexual desire. *J Sex Marital Ther* 1982; 8:179–97.

64. Sanderson MO, Maddock JW. Guidelines for assessment and treatment of sexual dysfunction. *Obstet Gynecol* 1989; 73:130–5.

65. Reading AE. Sexual aspects of infertility and its treatment. *Infertil Reprod Med Clin North Am* 1993; 4:559–67.

66. Meana M, Binik YM, Khalife S, et al. Dyspareunia: More than bad sex. *Pain* 1997; 71:211–2.

67. Basson R, Berman J, Burnett A, et al. Report of the international consensus development conference on female sexual dysfunction: Definitions and classifications. *J Urol* 2000; 163:888–93.

68. LoPiccolo L. Sexual dysfunction. In: LW Craighead, WE Craighead, AE Kazdin, et al., eds. *Cognitive and Behavioral Interventions: An Empirical Approach to Mental Health Problems*. Boston: Allyn & Bacon, 1994; 183–96.

69. Leiblum SR. Arousal disorders in women: Complaints and complexities. *MJA* 2003; 178:638–40.

70. Bartlik B, Goldberg J. Female sexual arousal disorder. In: SR Leiblum, RC Rosen, eds. *Principles and Practice of Sex Therapy*, 3rd ed. New York: Guilford Press, 2000; 85–117.

71. Araoz D. Hypnosis in human sexuality problems. *Am J Clin Hypn* 2005; 47:229–42.

72. Binik YM, Bergeeron S, Khalife S. Dyspareunia. In: SR Leiblum, RC Rosen, eds. *Principles and Practice of Sex Therapy*, 3rd ed. New York: Guilford Press, 2000; 154–80.

73. Leiblum SR. Vaginismus: A most perplexing problem. In: SR Leiblum, RC Rosen, eds. *Principles and Practice of Sex Therapy*, 3rd ed. New York: Guilford Press, 2000; 181–202.

74. Bachman GA. Dyspareunia and vaginismus. In: Sexual Dysfunction: Patient Concerns and Practical Strategies, 24th annual postgraduate course of the American Fertility Society, 1991.

75. Heiman JR, LoPiccolo L, LoPiccolo J. The treatment of sexual dysfunction. In: AL Gurman, D Kniskern, eds. *Handbook of Family Therapy*. New York: Brunner/Mazel, 1981; 592–630.

76. Wurn LJ, Wurn BF, King CR, et al. Increasing orgasm and decreasing dyspareunia by a manual physical therapy technique. *MedGenMed* 2004; 14:47.

77. Mazor M. Emotional reactions to infertility. In: MD Mazor, HF Simon, eds, *Infertility: Medical, Emotional, and Social Considerations*. New York: Human Sciences Press, 1984; 23–35.

78. Althof SE. Erectile dysfunction: Psychotherapy with men and couples. In: SR Leiblum, RC Rosen, eds. *Principles and Practice of Sex Therapy*, 3rd ed. New York: Guilford Press, 2000; 242–75.

79. Weeks GR, Gambescia N. *Erectile Dysfunction: Integrating Couple Therapy, Sex Therapy and Medical Treatment*. New York: Norton, 2000.

80. Andrews FM, Abbey A, Halman J. Stress from infertility, marriage factors, and subjective well-being of wives and husbands. *J Health Soc Behav* 1991; 32:238–53.

81. Jannini EA, Lobardo F, Salacone P, et al. Treatment of sexual dysfunctions secondary to male infertility with sildenafil citrate. *Fertil Steril* 2004; 81:705–7.

82. Lenzi A, Lombardo F, Salacone P, et al. Stress, sexual dysfunction, and male infertility. *J Endocrinol Invest* 2003; 25:72–6.

83. Metz ME, McCarthy BW. *Coping with Erectile Dysfunction*. Oakland, CA: New Harbinger Press, 2004.

84. Polonsky D. Premature ejaculation. In: SR Leiblum, RC Rosen, eds. *Principles and Practice of Sex Therapy*, 3rd ed. New York: Guilford Press, 2000; 305–32.

85. Zilbergeld B. *The New Male Sexuality*. New York: Bantam Books, 1999.

86. Metz ME, Pryor JL. Premature ejaculation: A psychophysiological approach for assessment and management. *J Sex Marital Ther* 2000; 26:293–320.

87. Apfelbaum B. Retarded ejaculation: A much misunderstood syndrome. In: SR Leiblum, RC Rosen, eds. *Principles and Practice of Sex Therapy*, 3rd ed. New York: Guilford Press, 2000; 205–41.

88. Bain J. Sexuality and infertility in the male. *Can J Hum Sex* 1993; 2:157–60.

89. Bachmann GA, Leiblum SR, Grill J. Brief sexual inquiry in gynecologic practice. *Obstet Gynecol* 1989; 73: 425–7.

90. Annon J, Robinson C. Behavioral treatment of sexual dysfunctions. In: A Sha'Ked, ed. *Human Sexuality and Rehabilitation Medicine: Sexual Functioning Following Spinal Cord Injury*. Baltimore: Williams & Wilkins, 1981; 104–18.

91. Leiblum SR, Previn LA. The development of sex therapy from a sociocultural perspective. In: ST Leiblum, LA Previn, eds. *Principles and Practice of Sex Therapy*. New York: Guilford Press, 1980; 1–26.

92. Burns LH. Infertility and the sexual health of the family. *J Sex Educ Ther* 1987; 14:30–4.

93. Anderson, KM, Sharpe M, Rattray A, Irvine DS. Sexual problems associated with infertility, pregnancy, and ageing. *J Psychosomatic Res* 2004; 54:353–5.

94. Burns LH. An overview of sexual dysfunction in the infertile couple. *J Fam Psychother* 1995; 6:25–46, 74.

95. Boxer AS. Infertility and sexual dysfunction. *Infertil Reprod Med Clin North Am* 1996; 7:565–75.

96. Leiblum SR, Rosen R. Introduction: Sex therapy in the age of AIDs. In: S Leiblum, R Rosen, eds. *Principles and Practice of Sex Therapy*. New York: Guilford Press, 1989; 1–16.

14 Patients with Medically Complicating Conditions

DONALD B. MAIER, SHARON N. COVINGTON, AND LOUISE U. MAIER

> *Perfect health, like perfect beauty, is a rare thing: And so it seems, is perfect disease.*
>
> – Peter Mere Latham

Infertility patients with medically complicating conditions often confront complex psychological issues. Medical conditions such as diabetes, hypertension, obesity, and endometriosis have always affected some patients seeking infertility services. While patients with these and other medical problems have been a relatively small percentage of the infertile population in the past, their numbers are increasing. There are several reasons for this trend. First, due to better medical treatment, there are now more people living with chronic diseases such as human immunodeficiency virus (HIV) and cancer in remission. Second, the trend toward delaying pregnancy has resulted in older infertility patients, and people are more likely to develop medical problems as they age. Third, new reproductive treatment options, such as oocyte donation, intracytoplasmic sperm injection (ICSI), and gestational carrier, make pregnancy and biological parenthood possible for many patients whose medically complicating condition had prevented traditional reproduction. This chapter

■ describes the medical conditions that cause infertility or impact infertility treatment; and
■ discusses the psychological and counseling issues that arise for infertility patients with chronic medical conditions.

HISTORICAL OVERVIEW

A variety of medical conditions have historically had an impact on fertility and the ability to procreate. The first section of this chapter reviews these medical conditions. The impact of such conditions can be direct, where the medical condition causes infertility, or indirect. In the latter category (indirect) are diseases in which treatment for the medical condition impairs fertility, the desire for fertility alters treatment of the medical condition, genetic traits or the disease itself may be passed to the offspring, or pregnancy outcome is altered by the disease (Table 14.1). It is important to consider the impact of medical conditions on both the couple's fertility and their subsequent pregnancy.

It is possible to group the interactions between medical conditions and fertility into five categories (see Table 14.1). The first category includes diseases or syndromes that cause infertility, and the second involves diseases whose treatment causes infertility. The third category includes diseases that have several possible treatments, the choice of which may be influenced by a patient's desire for fertility and/or reproduction. The fourth group, one of increasing importance, includes diseases in which genetic traits or the disease itself may be transmitted along to the offspring. Finally, there are diseases in which the main impact is not on conception but on the resultant pregnancy; either the disease or its treatment may be affected by a pregnancy or the pregnancy may be adversely affected by the medical condition. Some medical conditions will interact with fertility in many ways, and these groupings may be helpful to therapists in categorizing the difficulties faced by some infertile individuals.

Genetic and Congenital Causes of Infertility

Klinefelter's syndrome is a chromosomal disorder affecting males born with a karoytype of 47, XXY (or an extra X chromosome) resulting in such symptoms as small testes, absence of sperm, enlarged breasts, high levels of FSH (follicle-stimulating hormone), mental retardation, and/or behavioral problems. Klinefelter's syndrome is the most common chromosomal disorder in men with primary testicular failure and small testes typically causing infertility due to azoospermia. Reproductive technologies such as ICSI may help these men

TABLE 14.1. Categories of relationships between medical conditions and infertility

1. **Medical conditions that may cause infertility**
   Endometriosis
   Premature ovarian failure
   Cancers – testicular, ovarian, Hodgkin's disease
   Klinefelter's syndrome
   Turner's syndrome
   Rokitansky-Küster-Hauser syndrome
   Weight extremes – obesity and underweight

2. **Medical conditions whose treatment may cause infertility**
   Male hypertension
   Cancers – testicular, uterine, ovarian, cervical, breast, Hodgkin's disease
   Endometriosis, inflammatory bowel diseases

3. **Medical conditions in which the patient's choice of treatment may be influenced by his or her desire for fertility**
   Endometriosis
   Hodgkin's disease
   Breast cancer
   Borderline ovarian cancers

4. **Medical conditions in which genetic traits or the disease itself may be passed along to offspring**
   Cystic fibrosis
   Severe male infertility
   Breast cancer
   HIV/AIDS

5. **Medical conditions in which the primary impact is on the pregnancy**
   Diabetes
   Asthma
   Lupus
   Heart disease

reproduce although there is some evidence that they may transmit the disorder to their offspring.

Recent advances in the use of ICSI for severely oligospermic males (men with very low sperm counts) have raised a new concern. Approximately 13% of these cases appear to be caused by a genetic factor, specifically a deletion in a gene on the Y chromosome called azoospermia factor gene.[1] While these men may now be able to produce children, their sons may be at a high risk for themselves having infertility because they will inherit this abnormal gene. Preimplantation genetic diagnosis (PGD) may be used to select female embryos for transfer. Mak and Jarvi[2] reviewed this rapidly evolving area (see Chapter 15).

Turner's syndrome is a chromosomal disorder in women marked by the absence of all or part of one of the two X chromosomes. The effects of this condition include absence of menstrual onset, webbing of the neck, short stature, and/or aortic coarctation. In most but not all cases, women with this condition have very early loss of all oocytes, so that at birth the residual ovarian tissue is small (streak ovaries) and nonfunctional. Because the fallopian tubes, uterus, cervix, and vagina are formed independently from the ovaries, pregnancy is a viable option for women with this condition as long as donor oocytes are used. However, women with Turner's syndrome may be at increased risk for some potentially fatal cardiovascular complications of pregnancy, so a thorough medical evaluation should be conducted before proceeding with assisted reproduction.[3]

Rokitansky-Küster-Hauser syndrome is a congenital defect of the female reproductive tract in which the ovaries are normal but the uterus, cervix, and most of the vagina are abnormal or absent. Women with this disorder have all of the secondary external characteristics of womanhood including breasts, clitoris, and vulva. Typically, a young woman is not diagnosed with this disorder until adolescence when she fails to menstruate or encounters acute pain during a pelvic exam or sexual activity. Treatments are available to enlarge the vaginal pouch either through the use of dilators or surgery allowing her to have a normal sexual life. Because she has normally functioning ovaries, these women can have a child through assisted reproductive technologies (ARTs) and a gestational carrier who carries a pregnancy for her.

Medical Conditions Affecting Males

Male infertility is infrequently caused by medical conditions. Overall, approximately 1% of men referred for urological evaluation because of a low sperm count are found to have a serious medical condition.[4] Diseases impacting male fertility include hypertension (high blood pressure), diabetes, cystic fibrosis, Hodgkin's lymphoma, and testicular cancer. With other medical problems such as HIV/AIDS and genetic causes of infertility, transmission of the disease to others is the primary concern.

Hypertension

Hypertension does not cause infertility, but its treatment may. Erectile dysfunction is a side effect of some antihypertensive medications. Understandably, such difficulties may cause infertility by preventing sexual intercourse. In addition, medications can interfere with a man's ability to ejaculate at specific or stressful times, such as at ovulation or when a semen specimen is required. In the latter situation, sperm cryopreservation may be helpful in allowing a man to produce a semen sample under less stressful conditions, with the sample being used later, if or when needed. Alternatively, a change in medications may be necessary if medications are available to control the man's blood pressure without these or other negative side effects.

One group of antihypertensive medications, calcium channel blockers, can interfere with male fertility more subtly. These medications interfere with the acrosome reaction, a process by which sperm acquire the capacity to fertilize oocytes.[5] When men taking these medications are treated with a different medication, their sperm undergo the acrosome reaction at a normal rate. Because this fertilization problem cannot be detected through a routine semen analysis, it is unclear how many men on calcium channel blockers have impaired fertility. Until there is an adequate test for fertilization, it is prudent to have infertile men use another medication. This side effect of these calcium channel blockers is not commonly known, and a counselor may be the first healthcare professional to bring this connection to a patient's attention. In addition, these medications are also used for prevention of migraine headaches.

Cancer

Cancer or its treatment may cause male infertility. Testicular cancer and Hodgkin's lymphoma are two of the more common cancers in young men.

Testicular cancer is a serious cause of male infertility, and many men have been found to have low sperm counts even prior to diagnosis, perhaps due to an autoimmune process.[6] This process is probably confined to a few months prior to diagnosis although, unfortunately, it can limit the usefulness of sperm banking at the time of diagnosis for some men.[7] While the cure rate is high with removal of the affected testicle, fertility may be impaired by subsequent chemotherapy.[8] With surgical removal of the affected testicle, azoospermia or severe oligospermic is found in 30% of survivors. Those with metastatic disease cured by multidrug chemotherapy are also at risk for diminished reproductive capacity, although, as with Hodgkin's disease survivors, a proportion (approximately 10–15%) are rendered permanently infertile by the effects of the disease itself, prior to any chemotherapy.[9]

Sperm cryopreservation should be discussed with all men diagnosed with testicular cancer, even if they are adolescents and/or have no immediate plans for reproduction. With the advent of ICSI, even a few barely motile sperm may be sufficient to establish a pregnancy. Unfortunately, this option is not always presented to men with testicular cancer prior to chemotherapy.[10]

Whether or not sperm retrieval directly from the testicles would isolate sperm from men with no sperm in their ejaculate after chemotherapy is not presently known. Even if this were possible, it is an invasive procedure that would result in the use of sperm exposed to mutagenic drugs; therefore, cryopreservation of sperm prior to chemotherapy is clearly preferable. Nevertheless, if sperm was not preserved prior to treatment, the outcomes of ICSI treatment using sperm after chemotherapy is encouraging.[10]

Hodgkin's lymphoma is another cancer that commonly occurs in young individuals. As with testicular cancer, sperm quality may be abnormal at the time the disease is diagnosed and may be decreased by chemotherapy, especially mechlorethamine, vincristine [Oncovin], procarbazine, and prednisone (MOPP). However, treatment with doxorubicin [Adriamycin], bleomycin, vinblastine, and dacarbazine (ABVD) has much less of an impact on future fertility and has as good a cure rate.[11] Regardless of the type of therapy that is planned, pretreatment sperm cryopreservation should be discussed with these men.

Cystic Fibrosis

Males with cystic fibrosis (CF) are generally infertile as a result of aberrant development of Wolffian duct derivitives, more commonly known as full or partial absence of the vas deferens.[12] This condition is referred to as congenital bilateral absence of the vas deferens (CBAVD) and is sometimes referred to as genital cystic fibrosis as reproductive problems may be the only symptom or indication of the disease. Approximately 50% of apparently healthy men with an absent vas deferens have mutations in the cystic fibrosis gene.[13] With recent advances in microsurgical epididymal sperm aspiration (MESA), sperm can now be retrieved from the epididymis and used in IVF. However, there are two important counseling considerations: counseling regarding the dual diagnosis of a chronic medical condition (CF) and infertility, and the need for genetic testing and counseling regarding CF transmission risk. Some men with cystic fibrosis may be asymptomatic, and, as such, unaware of having cystic fibrosis until they are evaluated and determined to be azoospermic. In this situation, the patient is confronted with the simultaneous diagnosis of two unsuspected conditions. Other men with CBAVD are carriers of cystic fibrosis. If their female partners are also carriers, they have a 25% chance of having a child with this typically very serious disease and a 50% chance of having a child who is also a carrier. These couples warrant genetic testing and counseling, they need to be aware of the risk of genetic transmission of the disease. With this information they are better able to make an informed decision about their reproductive alternatives: donor insemination, ICSI, or PGD (see Chapter 15).

HIV

Today, more than 30 million people worldwide are infected with HIV and most are heterosexual adults of reproductive age.[14] HIV does not impair male fertility until the more advanced stages of AIDS, and its effects may be lessened with antiviral therapy.[15] The primary concern is disease transmission to the partner or child. If the couple has not been practicing safe sex, attempts to conceive will put the woman at risk. It is unclear to what extent this risk can be reduced by sperm preparation that may remove the human immunodeficiency virus (HIV). Semprini and colleagues[16] were the first to report a series of twenty-nine HIV-positive men whose sperm was used for intrauterine insemination after having been prepared to eliminate viral contamination. Seventeen pregnancies occurred in fifteen women, and none of the women inseminated became HIV-positive. The same author has recently summarized the present status of all types of assisted reproductive technologies in the treatment of couples where the male is HIV-positive.[17]

Increasingly, HIV-positive couples (typically an HIV-positive husband with an HIV-negative wife) want to have biological children and seek the assistance of ART programs not only to conceive but also to reduce the risk of HIV transmission to the noninfected partner. This can be accomplished through intrauterine insemination or IVF. Studies have found no transmission of the disease in HIV-infected couples treated at ART programs,[16,18] while couples who practiced repeated unprotected intercourse for the purpose of conceiving were reported to transmit the disease in 5% of the cases.[19] Current research has led to a different perspective on the treatment of HIV-positive couples and pointed toward the need for developing strict protocols, informed consent, and counseling of HIV-infected couples.[20]

Diabetes

Diabetes can affect male fertility in two ways. Neurological damage may cause difficulties with erection or ejaculation. Retrograde ejaculation occurs when there is interruption of normal muscle function and the semen is directed back into the bladder. This situation can sometimes be corrected medically. Alternatively, sperm can be collected from the urine, processed, and used for insemination. In addition, sperm counts may be decreased in men with diabetes. This may result from occlusions in small blood vessels that decrease blood flow to the testicles. Treatment options

would be the same as for any man with a reduced count.

Medications

In addition to the antihypertensive medications mentioned above, other medications can affect male fertility, a side effect frequently not recognized as a problem by prescribing physicians. Medications that can reduce sperm counts or motility include sulfasalazine (Azulfidine), used to treat inflammatory bowel disease; cimetidine (Tagamet), an antiulcer medication; nitrofurantoin (Furadantin, Macrobid, and Macrodantin, etc.), an antibiotic that is toxic only at high doses; and spironolactone (Aldactone), a diuretic.

Medical Conditions Affecting Females

Medical conditions are more likely to impact female than male fertility and fertility treatment. Some of the diseases that are described next are more common in women than in men, affect female but not male fertility, or have effects on the potential pregnancy. These conditions can affect the reproductive system directly, their treatment can damage the ovaries, or they may primarily complicate pregnancies that may already be at high risk because of infertility treatments.

Premature Ovarian Failure

Premature ovarian failure (POF) was at one time referred to as premature menopause because it was thought to represent the development of irreversible ovarian failure and, as such, the end of a woman's ability to reproduce. However, the condition is not always irreversible, and is more accurately referred to as hypergonadotropic hypogonadism. In this condition, the ovaries fail to respond normally to stimulation leading to low or absent ovarian hormones and ovulatory failure or irregularity. Some clinicians prefer the term ovarian insufficiency to describe this condition because about 5–10% of women with POF conceive without treatment, sometimes many years after the diagnosis. Ovarian failure is considered premature when it occurs before age forty.

Ovarian failure may either be primary (the woman has never menstruated) or secondary (ovarian function stops after some menstruation has occurred). Women may have nonfunctioning or absent ovaries for multiple reasons. Turner's syndrome is a common cause of absent ovarian function from birth. Secondary POF may occur from surgery, radiation, chromosomal abnormalities, or autoimmune diseases. In most cases, however, the cause is unknown. Some women may either be born with fewer oocytes than usual or there may be an accelerated loss of oocytes over time for unknown reasons.

It is important to realize that premature ovarian failure (POF) is more than infertility. The condition induces an estrogen-deficient state that may be associated with 'hot flashes,' night sweats, sleep disturbance, and vaginal dryness. Also, women with this condition are at increased risk for developing deficiencies of thyroid hormone (hypothyroidism) and adrenal hormone (adrenal insufficiency). Furthermore, most women find the diagnosis emotionally traumatic, and it has been suggested that psychological care should be provided as part of the management of POF. While women whose ovaries stop functioning at any time can use donor oocytes to conceive and carry a pregnancy, it is recommended that women address the physical and emotional aspects of their health before making decisions about family building.[21]

Hodgkin's Disease

As with men, treating women who have Hodgkin's disease with ABVD is much less likely to cause gonadal failure than treating them with MOPP.[22] Typically, a woman cannot have oocytes cryopreserved prior to chemotherapy, whereas a man can have his sperm frozen. Unfortunately, oocyte freezing is currently not a well-accepted or very successful technique nor is cryopreservation of ovaries or ovarian tissue, and/or ovarian transplant. Van der Elst has summarized the progress and pitfalls of this technique.[23] Therefore, the main hope for maintaining fertility for women with cancer rests in the development of less toxic chemotherapy regimens. Rarely, it may be possible to perform IVF prior to the initiation of chemotherapy and cryopreserve the resultant embryos for implantation after chemotherapy is completed.

Breast Cancer

Breast cancer victims often present with fertility concerns, because 10–20% of breast cancers occur in reproductive-age women.[24] While in most cases, breast cancer does not require removal of any reproductive organs, it can profoundly affect fertility. Chemotherapy is commonly used and can result in temporary cessation of menses or permanent ovarian failure. The class of drugs that is most effective against breast cancer, the alkylating agents, are unfortunately especially toxic to the ovaries. Toxicity and ovarian failure are worse and may be permanent if the dosages are high, the treatment is prolonged, or the woman is older. Even with younger women, rates of ovarian failure are high: It is estimated that 50% of women younger than thirty-five will experience ovarian failure or cessation of menses after chemotherapy for breast cancer.[25] At present, there are no good alternatives for a woman facing chemotherapy who would like to increase her chances for subsequent fertility. Unlike the situation with Hodgkin's disease, there are no alternative chemotherapy treatment regimens that have a lesser impact on ovarian function.

It is important to distinguish between women who have already been treated for breast cancer and those who have been recently diagnosed and not yet treated. The options for preserving fertility in a woman about to undergo a potentially fertility-compromising treatment remain limited. In theory, there might be several possibilities. One possibility is the removal of part or all of an ovary for cryopreservation. The ovary or ovarian tissue could later be thawed and transplanted into the woman's body, where it could resume oocyte production. While this treatment option has been attempted in a few cases, there are, to date, no undisputed successes. The limiting factor at present is the technology of freezing ovarian tissue. Similarly, freezing of oocytes is still primarily experimental. This is especially true of immature oocytes. At present, to obtain oocytes that have the potential for being successfully frozen and thawed, the oocytes must be stimulated to develop to maturation. While the one oocyte that a woman normally produces each month could be collected and frozen, the very low success rate with this procedure mandates that many oocytes be collected. This requires the woman undergo IVF, with the resultant high hormone levels and time delay. If she does not have a partner to provide sperm for fertilizing the oocytes and creating embryos, she is in a situation where the chance for successfully freezing ovarian tissue or oocytes is small. For a woman newly diagnosed with breast cancer, there is the option of performing IVF prior to chemotherapy to retrieve oocytes, which can then be fertilized. The resultant embryos are then frozen for potential transfer after successful therapy. The whole topic of preserving fertility for women with cancer has recently been well reviewed by Sonmezer and Oktay.[26]

If a breast cancer survivor wants to conceive, it is important for her to consider the possibility that she might have a recurrence of her disease during pregnancy or postpartum. Breast cancer is more difficult to diagnose and treat in pregnancy. Because most cases of aggressive disease will recur within two years of diagnosis, the current recommendation is that women with breast cancer wait at least two years before attempting to conceive. It is important to note that there are no reports of any increase in either miscarriages or birth defects in pregnancies conceived by women previously treated with any form of chemotherapy.

Several other issues need to be considered. Besides the initial problem of the effect of disease treatment on fertility, there is also the question of possible effects of fertility treatments or pregnancy on disease recurrence. Many breast cancers are estrogen-sensitive, and it is known that removal of the ovaries or treatment with antiestrogens such as tamoxifen citrate (Novaldex) or aromatase inhibitors such as letrozole (Femara) will decrease the recurrence risk in these women. Hormonal therapies that enhance conception (superovulation, IVF) and pregnancy itself results in high estrogen levels. Whether these increased hormone levels would increase the chance for a cancer recurrence is an important question. There are no data that specifically address the issue of fertility treatments and breast cancer recurrence, although there has been considerable research on the whether there is an increased risk of first-time breast cancer from use of clomiphene citrate[27](Clomid or Serophene) and following IVF.[28] Rossing and associates[27] found no increased risk of breast cancer in women who had taken clomiphene, compared to the rate in the general population. Similarly, Venn and coworkers[28] found no increase in the incidence of breast cancer in 5,564 women who had IVF, compared with 4,794 infertile controls who had not. Despite the large number of subjects, this study had a relatively short follow-up period and did not address the question of the recurrence-risk faced by a woman with a history of breast cancer.

More reassuring are the data concerning the risk of later recurrence in women who have a spontaneous pregnancy following breast cancer treatment. A recent review of the literature found no differences in survival rates in breast cancer survivors who conceived compared with similar women who did not.[22] However, the studies were small and not well-designed. Ideally, women whose cancers are estrogen-receptor positive would need to be studied to have accurate information for counseling women with a history of infertility regarding her reproductive future and choices.

Another medical consideration for breast cancer survivors who still have ovarian function is the increased risk that their daughters will contract breast cancer. It is apparent that counseling this group of women is a complex task. In the absence of any large, long-term studies, patients, physicians, infertility counselors, and genetic counselors are left without data that can help in answering many of their important questions.

Cancer of the Reproductive System

Cervical cancer is the second most common cancer worldwide among women although the mortality from cervical cancer has dramatically declined, a trend attributable to the advent of cervical cytology screening using the Papanicolaou (Pap) test.[29] Cervical cancer occurs most commonly in reproductive-age women, and its treatment can be altered if the woman desires fertility. Human papillomavirus (HPV) is a major cofactor in the development of cervical cancer. HPV is a sexually transmitted disease in which the infected individuals are frequently asymptomatic and therefore unaware they are infected. While patient screening is important in the diagnosis and treatment of cervical cancers, patient education regarding prevention of HPV and its status as a sexually transmitted disease are important.

For early-stage cervical cancer, surgery has replaced ovary-damaging radiation therapy. This treatment may involve removal of all or part of the cervix leaving the uterus intact allowing future pregnancies – although pregnancy complications still may be a risk. Initial results of this new procedure have been quite promising.[30] Alternatively, treatment may involve a hysterectomy in which the cervix and uterus are removed but the ovaries remain intact. Women who have had a hysterectomy can become mothers by having embryos created from their oocytes implanted into a gestational carrier.

Ovarian cancer most commonly occurs in women beyond the reproductive years and is therefore an infrequent cause of infertility. When it does occur in younger women, removal of both ovaries is often necessary, as the disease usually is not diagnosable in early stages and therefore has typically spread. There are some types of borderline tumors of lower malignant potential where removal of one ovary may be curative. Because ovarian cancer like some breast cancers may be a genetic disorder, it is suggested that these women have genetic counseling and that the other ovary be removed when they are finished with childbearing. Fernandez and Frydman[31] described two women with ovarian cancer who, at the time of oophorectomy, had oocytes retrieved for IVF that were fertilized and cryopreserved as embryos; however, no similar cases have been reported. If ovarian tissue cryopreservation becomes a reality, treatment options for women with cervical or ovarian cancer facing immediate loss of ovarian function may be dramatically increased.

Endometrial cancer (cancer of the uterine lining) is very uncommon in reproductive-age women. Precancerous lesions can usually be treated medically and subsequent reproduction is not impaired. However, because these women are at risk for recurrence, they may be advised to complete their families early and then have a hysterectomy to ensure their long-term health.

Endometriosis

Endometriosis is a common cause of infertility and may create difficult decisions for the woman, her physician, and her counselor. Endometriosis causes both infertility and pain, and the methods to treat one of these symptoms can worsen the other. Except for pain medications, all medical therapies for pain from endometriosis interrupt ovulation, preventing conception. Definitive surgical therapy for pain involves removal of the ovaries and/or other reproductive organs affected by the disease. Alternatively, most treatments to enhance fertility in women with endometriosis involve administration of ovulation-induction medications such as clomiphene or human menopausal gonadotropins. These medications stimulate the ovaries but also increase estrogen levels. It has not been established whether these treatments accelerate the growth of endometriosis, but they may increase pain levels during the cycles in which they are taken. Therefore, a woman may have to choose between treatment for pain and treatment for infertility. One exception is conservative surgical treatment, commonly using laparoscopic therapy. This can relieve pain, while either improving fertility or at least not worsening it.

Many questions still remain about the effects of endometriosis therapy. These questions include whether surgical treatment of minimal endometriosis improves fertility; whether use of medical suppression either pre- or post-operatively improves surgical outcome; and whether suppressive medical therapy or removal of endometriosis from the ovaries improves IVF success rates. For the woman trying to conceive, the lack of definitive information on these subjects can be very frustrating, as she must decide between taking medication and delaying pregnancy for three to six months, or attempting pregnancy knowing that her long-term outcome may be worsened. The counselor should be aware that endometriosis is a chronic disease as well as a chronic pain condition of unknown etiology, with no absolute cure. All available treatments merely suppress or remove existing endometriosis without preventing its recurrence. Patients often undergo multiple surgical and medical therapies in the course of their disease and may eventually undergo removal of the ovaries and hysterectomy.

HIV

Infertile HIV-positive women present an especially difficult challenge for clinicians and counselors. Perhaps the most difficult issue is the possibility of disease transmission to the offspring. In one study, the rate of transmission from untreated mothers was 25%. This rate dropped to 8% in women treated with antiviral therapy during their pregnancy.[32] However, even this rate may be considered unacceptably high, and long-term follow-up on these children is not yet available. Other important issues to consider are the potential effects of

pregnancy on the woman's chance for long-term survival, the issue of the amount of parenting that will be available to the child because of the woman's potentially shortened life expectancy (with the same issue applying to the child's father if he is HIV-positive), and the reluctance of some healthcare providers to treat these patients if they present with infertility (see Olaitan and colleagues[33] for a discussion). However, in the United States, HIV-positive persons are protected by the American with Disabilities Act and are entitled to medical services unless it can be demonstrated that there is significant risk of infection transmission.[34]

Diabetes

Prior to the discovery of insulin, it was very uncommon for diabetic women to conceive; uncontrolled diabetic women usually are anovulatory. With modern diabetic management, these women have a much better chance for conception and normal pregnancy. Diabetes should therefore not be a common cause of infertility in women whose disease is well-controlled.[35] Nonetheless, there are several aspects of pregnancy in diabetic women that can affect treatment of infertile women regardless of the cause of infertility. Women with elevated blood sugars who conceive have a higher chance of having a miscarriage or a baby with birth defects. They are also at risk for worsening of diabetic complications (eye or kidney damage, for example) or difficult delivery of large infants. Adequate blood sugar control before conception typically reduces these risks. Although infertility therapy per se will not alter blood sugar levels or insulin requirements, the additional stress from involved therapies such as IVF may distract the diabetic from closely monitoring herself. Diabetes can also decrease the blood flow to the placenta, potentially resulting in intrauterine growth retardation, premature delivery, and long-term neurological defects in the baby. Such problems are important for the infertile diabetic woman to consider, especially treatments such as IVF that increase the risk of multiple gestations in which the adverse effects of impaired blood flow are even more harmful. In addition as obesity is a growing health risk in younger women worldwide and is a causal factor for diabetes and PCOS, it can be anticipated that there will be an increase in the number of diabetic women undergoing infertility treatment.

Weight

A woman's weight may be important in three ways. Women with significantly low or high weight may have hormonal imbalances or ovulatory dysfunction. Even if they are ovulatory, these women may have a worse response to infertility therapies. Finally, pregnancy may be complicated by extremes of body weight.

While most obese women will ovulate normally, there may an increased rate of ovulatory abnormalities such as polycystic ovarian syndrome in obese women. Obesity contributes to the insulin insensitivity that is one of the causes of this disease. In women with minimal body fat, ovulation may be suppressed through changes in the central nervous system that results in a woman not having any periods (hypothalamic amenorrhea). This may be seen with overt psychological diagnoses such as anorexia and bulimia, or may be seen in women without any apparent psychological problems. In women with eating disorders, treatment of those problems should precede infertility therapy, as correction of low body weight may restore normal ovarian function.

When over or underweight women undergo infertility therapy, the results may be worse than what is seen in women with normal weight. One retrospective study found a significant reduction in pregnancy rates in women undergoing IVF who were underweight or obese, despite being younger than the normal weight group.[36] Obese women also usually require higher doses of ovulation-induction medications. Finally, many pregnancy complications are increased in obese women, such as high blood pressure, gestational diabetes, preterm delivery, and difficult deliveries due to larger babies.

Women at either body weight extreme need to be counseled medically and psychologically regarding the impact of their weight not only on successful treatment outcome but also during pregnancy as well. As such, they need to be encouraged to normalize their weight before infertility treatment in general, as well as before IVF. Even in women with normal weight and without overt eating disorders, counseling may be beneficial in treating subclinical conditions. Berga et al.[37] used a combination of cognitive-behavior therapy and dietary counseling to treat eight women with hypothalamic amenorrhea. Six of these women had partial or total resumption of ovulatory function, compared with two in a control group. Women with abnormal weight will benefit from a combined medical and psychological approach to enhance their fertility and their response to treatment (see Chapter 11).

Other Conditions

Many other medical conditions may coexist with infertility. These conditions may have little impact on fertility or on infertility therapy but can impact the success of pregnancy. These diseases include systemic lupus erythematosus, multiple sclerosis, asthma, and heart or kidney disease. These diseases may increase the chance for miscarriage or may worsen during pregnancy as the increased metabolic demands of pregnancy stress already compromised organs. The more advanced reproductive technologies, such as IVF, result in an increased rate of multiple births and place the woman at additional risk. In women whose bodies would have difficulty in handling the increased demands from a single pregnancy, even twins may create a risk of serious medical complications that may endanger the mother's life. These factors must be kept in mind as a patient decides what treatments to pursue. A couple should be encouraged to talk with their infertility specialist or an expert in high-risk pregnancies (perinatologist) and other specialists to make sure that there will be no interaction between a medical condition and either the conception or the completion of a planned pregnancy.

Women with inflammatory bowel diseases (e.g., ulcerative colitis or Crohn's disease) frequently require removal of the colon or other major abdominal surgeries to treat these conditions. These surgeries could result in significant pelvic adhesions and resultant infertility. These consequences might not have been discussed with the patients at the time of their surgery, and these women understandably may be depressed to learn that a disease they had thought was treated now has unwanted sequellae of infertility and chronic pain.

REVIEW OF LITERATURE

The literature on infertility and medically complicating conditions has become an increasing focus of research for a variety of reasons. Recently, there has been a move toward a more collaborative approach to patient care and a greater recognition of the physiological as well as psychosocial interactive effect of reproduction on chronic health conditions. Furthermore, an awareness of the psychosocial issues relevant to infertility and chronic illness has increased investigation into the impact of patients' experiences of chronic medical conditions and/or infertility as well as health efficacy behaviors, treatment compliance, coping strategies, and the reaction to chronic illness and/or infertility of partners and families. An early study that compared psychological distress of women with infertility to other medical conditions involved 149 patients with infertility, 136 with chronic pain, 22 undergoing cardiac rehabilitation, 93 with cancer, 77 with hypertension, and 11 with HIV-positive status. The researchers found that infertile women had global symptom scores equivalent to the cancer, cardiac rehabilitation, and hypertension patients, but lower scores than the chronic pain and HIV-positive patients. The anxiety and depression scores of the infertile women were significantly lower than those of chronic pain patients but not statistically different from the other groups.[38] These researchers suggest that standard psychosocial interventions for serious medical illness should also be applied to infertility treatment. However, this study also highlights, perhaps inadvertently, the complex and challenging issues facing patients with both conditions as well as their caregivers in addressing the unique physical and psychosocial needs of these patients and their partners.

Cancer

As an increasing number of men and women are surviving cancer, postcancer life goals change from survival to quality-of-life and family building. Two studies have investigated the motivation for parenthood in young men and women cancer survivors. Schover[39] found that the majority felt that cancer had increased the value of family ties and the importance of having children. However, 17% of women had unrealistically high anxiety about pregnancy causing cancer recurrence and even greater percentages of survivors fear that their children would be at high risk for birth defects or cancer. Teeter and associates[40] did a large-sample retrospective survey study of decisions about marriage and family among survivors of childhood cancer and compared cancer survivors to a control group of siblings without cancer. Although the cancer survivors were no more likely than the controls to have documented fertility problems or offspring with birth defects, they were more likely to have been told by physicians not to attempt to have children. This result suggests that childhood cancer survivors may not be acting on complete or currently accurate information in making childbearing decisions. As such, caregivers must be cognizant of providing appropriate and accurate postcancer education particularly regarding reproductive goals.

The predominant theme in the literature on male cancer patients and infertility has been the importance of sperm banking prior to treatment for testicular cancer or Hodgkin's disease.[41–47] Cella and Najavits[48] found that denial of infertility – that is, unrealistic optimism about being spared treatment-induced infertility – resulted in decisions not to cryobank sperm. Thus, addressing denial may be important in helping men make fully informed decisions and prevent future regret. Several authors[45,46] noted the sensitive issue of discussing sperm banking with adolescent males. Counseling issues include the need for professional discussion of the issues, the provision of accurate information about the differences between infertility and impotence, and the usefulness of having

the counselor meet with adolescents alone rather than with their parents present.

Urological cancer survivors reported significant distress and anxiety about infertility and sexual performance.[42–44] Several authors have emphasized the ethical and psychosocial importance of discussing treatment alternatives that have a lesser impact on future fertility, and noted that oncologists have become increasingly aware of infertility concerns.[42–45,49] Due to the extremely high cure rates for these early-onset male cancers, quality-of-life (including future fertility) has become a focus of concern in counseling and treatment. While distress about infertility was reported by a significant number of testicular cancer survivors, its impact did not necessarily extend into survivors' psychological well-being, with no significant correlations found between fertility distress and measures of psychological well-being.[50] There is some evidence that cancer survivors feared that their infertility would create marital problems, although survivors of testicular cancer appeared best able to compartmentalize their feelings about infertility as a means of protecting their overall emotional state, particularly if they had banked sperm or if adoption was a viable option, descreasing the medical and psychological impact of infertility.[51]

Literature on female cancer patients and infertility also emphasizes quality-of-life issues.[49,52,53] Several authors urged discussion regarding the variable impact of different treatment options on ovarian suppression and future fertility, as well as the importance of acknowledging and discussing potential loss of fertility at the time of cancer diagnosis and treatment.[46,47,49,53] Lamb[53] noted that fear of infertility is a common psychological effect of cancer treatment. Lamb,[53] Dow and colleagues,[52] and Hubner and Glazer[47] discussed the importance of a thorough and responsible case-by-case discussion of options and risks. Dow and associates[52] found that women who had children after breast cancer treatment reported that family issues were an important contributor to postcancer quality-of-life and that having children contributed to a feeling of being cured and to a sense of reconnection with peers and family. Hubner[49] underscored the importance of the dual "longing for life" one's own and that of future children – expressed by female cancer patients. She recommended the identification and subsequent referral for psychosocial assessment of cancer patients at risk for infertility concerns – those with a history of miscarriage, stillbirth, or abortion, and all premenopausal women without children.

In their excellent review article, Hubner and Glazer[47] raised five important points for oncology caregivers regarding infertility: (1) issues of fertility become overshadowed in the face of crisis; (2) significance of fertility must be acknowledged; (3) patients may later experience an 'intolerance of regret'; (4) fertility must be addressed with all patients of reproductive age; and (5) discussion of fertility signifies a belief in the patient's future.

In a study comparing the psychosocial and sexual adjustment of Hodgkin's disease and acute leukemia survivors (even when other medical and sociodemographic factors were controlled), Hodgkin's disease survivors reported significantly worse sexual functioning, as well as greater psychological distress than leukemia survivors.[54] Furthermore, as infertility in Hodgkin's disease survivors increased (based on test results of perceived infertility), overall psychosocial adjustment worsened significantly. The researchers suggested that long-term problems in sexual functioning due to infertility may possibly have been mitigated by survivors who already had children at the time of diagnosis, and partial resolution of problems in psychosexual adjustment by one year after treatment completion, the minimum time for entry into this study.

Obesity

In an Australian study that addressed obesity in infertile women, the researchers designed a group treatment program for obese infertile women.[55] The twenty-four-week program included regular exercise and group discussion of topics such as coping with the psychological impact of infertility; developing health eating patterns; and the effects of obesity on reproductive physiology. There was a significant weight loss (mean weight loss 6.2+/−4.5 kg, $p < .001$) and improvement on measures of self-esteem, anxiety, depression, and general health. Twenty-nine of the thirty-seven women in the group became pregnant during the follow-up period (twenty-one to thirty-six months). Two women were avoiding pregnancy, and only six of the women who had completed the group program had not conceived by the end of the follow-up period. A further five women did not complete the program as they became pregnant while attending the group.

Cystic Fibrosis

Several studies have investigated the psychosocial issues involved in the diagnosis of cystic fibrosis (CF). In an interesting study of CF patients aware of their diagnosis from childhood, researchers in Scotland sent questionnaires investigating patient attitudes about fertility and the information healthcare professional gave

them about future fertility.[56] All but two men (eighty-two men; fifty-four women) knew they were likely to be infertile; fourteen women and five men had children. Interestingly, 85% of men and 72% of women stated that having children was important or would be in the next ten years; however, 43% of men and 26% of women had never had any discussion of fertility issues with healthcare professionals. The researchers noted that men, in particular, were reluctant to introduce the topic of reproduction even though it was very important to them, leading the researchers to conclude that caregivers should initiate fertility discussions with CF patients in early adulthood. Similar findings were reported in an Australian study of men with CF.[57] Researchers found that the majority of the men with CF (94%) were aware the CF reduced fertility but the men reported first hearing about infertility later than they desired and only 53% heard from their preferred source. Interestingly, 53% of the men in the study had undergone semen analysis and 68% of men who had not been tested wanted semen analysis. Furthermore, 73% believed semen analysis should occur before the age of eighteen, but youngest testing in this group was twenty-four years. Some of the men in this study had become parents by natural conception ($n = 1$), micro-epididymal sperm aspiration (MESA) ($n = 6$), donor sperm ($n = 9$), and through stepchildren ($n = 1$). However, 66% of the men wanted more information on reproductive options and 84% wanted children. These studies reveal the significance of reproductive ability and concomitant infertility in patients with CF.

Endometriosis

A study that examined the clinical characteristics of women attending a clinic specializing in endometriosis in Australia was used to determine patient satisfaction with clinic services.[58] Patient histories and a postal questionnaire were used to assess women who had attended the clinic during a one-year period. For 70% of the women, the diagnosis of endometriosis had been made elsewhere while the remainder of the women attended the clinic for a second opinion or information. The majority of the women (86%) presented for issues related to symptoms of endometriosis, 6% for issues of endometriosis symptomatology and infertility, while 8% presented primarily for issues related to infertility. Interestingly, 97% of the women felt that consultation with a counselor who had specific knowledge of the physical and psychosocial consequences of the disease was a major source of satisfaction. The researchers concluded that there was a significant demand for and greater patient satisfaction with an integrated approach to the care for endometriosis, particularly one that included the provision of counseling and availability of a patient self-help group. In a study in the United Kingdom that addressed quality-of-life issues in women with endometriosis, the women rated infertility, pain, physical functioning, social functioning, emotional well-being, and sexual intercourse among their concerns.[59] These researchers noted that the impact of endometriosis was multidimensional and complex impacting the women's life on a variety of levels.

THEORETICAL FRAMEWORK

The theoretical framework used in approaching infertility patients with medically complicating conditions can be viewed from a biopsychosocial model of chronic illness, which promotes collaborative healthcare. In addition, stigma theory provides a perspective of the psychological consequence for patients with a dual diagnosis of impaired fertility and impaired health.

Biopsychosocial/Chronic Illness Theory

Each illness has its unique psychosocial issues and challenges, whether episodic or chronic, progressive or life-threatening. Regardless of the unique characteristics of any given illness, a biopsychosocial approach to diagnosis and treatment provides a basis for understanding the illness and the patient's experience of it. It also provides an integrated approach to treatment by taking into consideration the psychological, social, and biological factors that impact the illness as well as the patient's adjustment, individually and socially. Individual well-being depends on a dynamic balance among these three levels of functioning: individual physical functioning, individual psychological functioning, and family/social/marital functioning. Examples of imbalance in patients with chronic illness and infertility issues include a spouse focusing on reproductive issues while discounting or ignoring the impact of a chronic illness on reproductive ability or, in contrast, the partner with the illness focusing on health rehabilitation or maintenance without regard to current or future reproductive goals. The ability of an individual or couple to maintain a healthy balance is influenced by a number of factors. These factors include healthy coping strategies (e.g., good communication, healthy efficacy behaviors, and social support); the ability of the individual and/or marriage to adapt and accommodate the demands of the chronic illness and treatment; individual and/or marital functioning prior to the diagnosis of the illness; other stressors (e.g., economic, cultural, religious, and legal); and the tendency

for maladaptive individual and/or marital patterns to interfere with disease management (e.g., impeding compliance).

Chronic illness is differentiated from acute illness in that it involves progressive deterioration with increasing symptoms, functional impairment, and disability over an extended period of time. It is long-term, progressive, and requires ongoing care. The onset of chronic illnesses may be gradual, involving a long latency period during which the disease process has begun, but the individual is asymptomatic. Alternatively, diagnosis of the disease may be acute, involving a medical crisis in which the individual's health or life is jeopardized. Each chronic illness has specific, known pathological manifestations. Typically, chronic illness profoundly influences an individual as well as his or her partner, family, and social network, including friends and workplace colleagues. The trajectory of chronic illness illustrates not only the physiological changes but also the psychosocial, self-identity alternations, life consequences, and efforts to manage the disease. Although each chronic illness has a unique trajectory or course, in general, individuals with chronic illness experience an onset or crisis phase (depending on the circumstances of diagnosis), a chronic phase (that may involve relapses or reoccurrence), and a terminal phase that may be delayed by decades after initial diagnosis, and may be not be the primary cause of death but a contributing factor in undermining the individual's health over the lifetime. The specific illness, understandably, impacts how the individual experiences the chronic illness. Other factors having an impact on the individual's experience and functioning include the individual's coping strategies, age, gender, overall psychosocial adjustment prior to diagnosis, family support, and social factors.

In short, the heterogenous nature of any chronic illness must be considered within the family and social context in which the individual experiences it. Disease-related factors, individual characteristics, and the family and social environment all impact how the illness trajectory unfolds. As such, all caregivers (physicians, nurses, and mental health professionals) must take into consideration the complex nature of the chronic illness experience in helping individuals and their families cope. It is imperative to give the chronically ill individual, and his or her family, choices, support, and autonomy in managing the various challenges of his or her chronic illness.[60,61]

Infertile patients with medically complicating conditions are, in effect, dealing with two chronic illnesses that entwine with each other – the medical condition and impaired fertility. Both are concerned with loss, be it health and all that is associated with it, and fertility with all the hopes and dreams of a child. With most chronic illness, the focus for patients is on adaptation as opposed to recovery or cure. Patients experience a recurring cycle of shock, suffering, and then adaptation as they deal with issues related to their health condition and/or infertility. With each cycle, feelings of grief and loss may be rekindled, creating a 'chronic sorrow' in which the pain is periodically remembered and mourned.[62]

Stigma Theory

Stigma theory is the experience of the individual in regard to any personal trait that clearly distinguishes the individual from others and which constitutes or is assumed to constitute a physical, psychological, or social disadvantage, for example, chronic illness and/or infertility. According to stigma theory, failure to comply with individual developmental tasks or with societal expectations typically causes feelings of embarrassment, social disapproval, abnormality, shame, and isolation. As Goffman explained, "Given that the stigmatized individual in our society acquires identity standards which he applies to himself in spite of failing to conform to them, it is inevitable that he will feel more ambivalence about his own self."[63, p. 106] Individuals with a medical condition (particularly chronic medical conditions) and infertility feel they have a personal defect or are damaged. They are often concerned about how they are perceived by others, particularly their spouse who may be impacted by their medical condition. Feelings of guilt and shame are particularly burdensome if the medical condition is the result of the individual's own behavior (e.g., sexually transmitted disease, obesity). Because both medically complicating conditions and involuntary childlessness are experienced within a social context (marriage, family, and community), individuals face a number of challenges including coping with feelings of shame and embarrassment. They adapt social relationships to accommodate to the diagnoses – all while managing the illness, its treatment, and treatment for infertility.

CLINICAL ISSUES

The medical information and psychological literature reviewed in the following section point to several counseling needs and emotional concerns of infertility patients with medical conditions. This section begins with a consideration of the types of decisions faced by patients and the role of mental health professionals in assisting with such decisions. This is followed by a

discussion of two types of psychological issues of particular significance to these patients: (1) mortality and loss, and (2) defectiveness and abnormality, as well as how to provide assistance. A further clinical issue concerns the feelings that occur within the mental health professional, that is, 'countertransference,' while working with patients with medically complicating conditions.

Decision Making

Like other infertility patients, individuals or couples with medically complicating conditions may consult with mental health professionals for assistance with decisions about treatment options. Looked at separately, the decision-making process for either infertility or other medical conditions involves considering treatment options and balancing the potential chances for and benefits of a successful treatment outcome with the risks (physical, emotional, and financial) of the procedures. For these patients, the preferred choice for treating one condition may be detrimental to the other condition, creating a more complex decision process.

Decisions Regarding Treatment of Newly Diagnosed Cancers

A mental health professional may be consulted at the time of cancer diagnosis. If a patient is of childbearing age or an adolescent whose future fertility may be affected by cancer treatment, the oncologist may present treatment options that will differentially affect future fertility. For males with Hodgkin's disease or testicular cancer, the oncologist may recommend cryopreservation of sperm before surgery, chemotherapy, or radiation treatment. In these cases, the mode of psychological treatment is crisis-intervention counseling, in which frightened and highly stressed patients are required to make important life-impacting decisions rapidly, usually within a few days. The patient and the oncology team will want to treat the cancer rapidly and maximize disease control and life expectancy. At the same time, potentially impaired fertility as a result of cancer treatment is an important counseling consideration, and surveys of cancer patients reveal a strong desire to be informed of fertility preservation and future reproductive options.[64] Cancer patients have important needs regarding future fertility and preservation options, and the mental health professional may be called upon to counsel for both the cause and consequence of treatment.[65]

A mental health professional can assist the patient in expressing fears and feelings of loss and in clarifying the meaning and importance of parenthood in his or her life. The latter task will vary widely, depending on age, marital status, and current parenthood status of the patient. For young single patients, particularly adolescent males, parenthood may have been no more than a remote possibility before the cancer diagnosis, whereas older married patients may have definite family-building plans. The mental health professional should consult with the oncologist to obtain information on treatment choices and their impact on future fertility and cancer control. Such consultation enables the counselor to assist a distraught patient (whose capacity for memory and concentration is likely to be diminished) with the task of accurately understanding complex information. To avoid confusion, it is also important for the mental health professional to know what the oncologist's views are regarding preferred cancer treatments and what the oncologist has said to the patient in presenting options. With such information, the counselor can optimally assist the patient in a decision-making process that includes accurate risk–benefit factors.

When a diagnosis of testicular cancer is made, it is hoped that the urologist will suggest sperm cryopreservation for future inseminations. In such cases, the patient, or patient and his wife, may be referred for discussion of this option. The counselor should ensure that the patient is making an autonomous decision and giving fully informed consent to this choice, especially if it appears that his partner or parents are pressuring him. It is also important to clarify that cryopreservation is a current decision that makes possible but does not guarantee future childbearing, which will be followed by a separate future decision about whether to use that option. This may simplify the complex decision-making process by separating out and postponing the major life decision of whether to become a biological parent. It may also prevent future conflict arising from lack of clarity about the meaning of cryopreservation, in which one member of the couple or family assumes that it means a definite decision has been made to have children, while the other member does not share that assumption. The signed consent forms required by sperm cryobanking centers can promote this process of clarification and support the patient's autonomy if the man alone (and not his partner) signs the forms indicating how long his sperm will remain in storage and what the disposition of the sperm will be if he dies. In the case of a patient who has a partner, the counselor should encourage careful discussion of the issues involved in 'willing' the sperm to the man's surviving partner and the possible use of the sperm after the patient's death. These include the child's welfare, each partner's feelings, and attitudes of other family members. The com-

plex ethical and legal issues involved in posthumous reproduction have been discussed elsewhere[66,67] and are beyond the scope of this discussion (see Chapter 30).

Decision making regarding disease process control and fertility preservation is extremely complex in the case of breast cancer. The most aggressive treatment includes chemotherapy that results in ovarian suppression. However, many women with a strong desire to maintain reproductive capacity will want to choose surgical and radiation treatment without subsequent chemotherapy. The counselor, working in consultation with the oncologist, can help the patient conduct a risk–benefit analysis, address potential denial about cancer or infertility risk, obtain information about pregnancy after breast cancer, and express fears and grief.

The patient with uterine or cervical cancer may be given the options of hysterectomy with or without oophorectomy. Her decision may involve weighing potentially greater cancer prevention through ovary removal against the partial fertility-sparing option of leaving her ovaries intact to use a gestational carrier in the future. Likewise, the patient with early-stage ovarian cancer may be given the option of oophorectomy with or without hysterectomy. Her decision may involve weighing potentially greater cancer prevention against the partial fertility-sparing option of leaving her uterus intact and using donor oocytes in the future. She also may be experiencing pressure from family members to choose one of the options. Here again, the counselor's role includes advocating for an autonomous informed decision. In cases in which the oncologist recommends hysterectomy without oophorectomy, many women currently undergoing cancer treatment will be unaware of the gestational carrier option and will unnecessarily assume that they are losing any chance for future biological parenting. The mental health professional can help patients by educating oncologists about the important psychological consolation such knowledge can provide.

Cryopreservation of ovarian tissue for potential future childbearing is not currently an approved clinical treatment. Clinicians should be aware of the 2004 American Society for Reproductive Medicine (ASRM) statement on cryopreservation of ovarian tissue, which states that this technique should be used for experimental research purposes only.[68] Cancer patients faced with loss of fertility through surgery, radiation, or chemotherapy could potentially be drawn to ovarian cryopreservation if it is presented as a viable option. The clinician can help such patients by providing accurate information and by helping them accept and grieve the loss of fertility if no fertility-preserving cancer treatment options are available.

Because Hodgkin's disease usually strikes men and women in their twenties or early thirties, most of these patients will be of childbearing age. Ideally, the oncology treatment team will discuss the issue of infertility and offer patients the ABVD treatment regimen, which offers a high rate of cure combined with a high rate of future fertility. For men with Hodgkin's disease, the oncologist and mental health professional should be aware that denial of fertility impact may interfere with use of sperm cryobanking procedures.[48] A team approach can help address this denial, so that patients can optimally preserve future fertility and prevent future regret. Patient should be directed to support organizations that offer information on preserving fertility options (see Resource listing).

Decisions Regarding Treatment of Newly Diagnosed Endometriosis

Use of a common treatment for endometriosis, gonadotropin-releasing hormone agonists (leuprolide acetate [Lupron], nafarelin acetate [Synarel], and goserelin acetate [Zoladex]), results in temporary cessation of menstruation for three to six months. Many patients are unconflicted about using this treatment to relieve pain associated with endometriosis. However, other patients with feelings of feeling an urgency to conceive due to advanced maternal age or other personal factors may find it difficult to choose a treatment that precludes pregnancy for months. Decision making in this area is complicated by the fact that there is not always a clear-cut link between endometriosis and infertility; many women with endometriosis become pregnant without medical intervention. In cases of endometriosis with severe pain not relieved by medication or surgery, oophorectomy may be recommended to reduce the estrogen levels associated with ovarian function. Women may thus need to decide between preserving their fertility and relieving severe pain. Historically, a hysterectomy was often performed along with oophorectomy, in part because it was thought that this would further reduce pain and in part because fertility was already sacrificed by ovarian removal. However, with the option of donor egg or oocyte cryopreservation, oophorectomy alone allows the possibility of future pregnancy, although not genetic continuity, for the woman while potentially relieving much of the pain of endometriosis.

Decisions Regarding Treatment of Newly Diagnosed Premature Ovarian Failure

Women who are newly diagnosed with spontaneous premature ovarian failure (POF) experience a host of emotions in learning a condition that is life altering yet not life threatening. Hearing the news of the diagnosis is often described as emotionally traumatic for women, who may feel unprepared and unsupported by their physician.[69] The incongruity of diagnosis is especially disconcerting – although young, they are experiencing symptoms similar to women their mothers' age who are going through menopause, while facing the prospect of never having a biological child. The diagnosis negatively affects body image, with women feeling "old, unfeminine, less healthy, empty and worthless."[69] The term 'failure' seems to reinforce this sense of defectiveness and narcissistic injury.

Attending to the psychological needs of these patients is an important part of medical treatment. Patients first need information and resources to understand the multifaceted nature of this condition (see Resource listing). Support groups and networks offered by International Premature Ovarian Failure Association (IPOFA) provide a healing place where women find others struggling with similar feelings and experiences, as well as a wealth of information. For many women, the most distressing part of the diagnosis is infertility. Often, they need to pursue infertility treatment, often unproven, in the process of coming to terms with the diagnosis. As with other aspects of infertility, these women and their partners need the opportunity to grieve before making treatment decisions regarding alternative family building. The mental health professional can play an important role in assisting these patients by encouraging advocacy with their clinicians, providing information, directing them to support resources, and grief counseling.

Another consequence of POF is altered sexual functioning with women experiencing decreased libido, vaginal dryness, and other conditions associated with estrogen deficiency. Patients may need help in finding techniques and resources that help in achieving sexual satisfaction (see Resource listing).

Decisions Regarding Infertility Treatment When the Medical Condition Has Been Previously Diagnosed and Treated

The discussion above has focused on decision making at the initial time of disease diagnosis. A second major time of decision making occurs when the patient with a medical condition that has been diagnosed and treated in the past is currently dealing with infertility. If the infertility treatment or pregnancy will potentially make the medical condition worse or create a high-risk pregnancy, the patient and her or his caregiver face complex decisions. Once again, the role of the mental health professional is to assist patients in making decisions based on a thorough consideration of the risks and benefits of various choices. The patient may be feeling a sense of urgency about pursuing infertility treatment as soon as possible, or her or his partner may disagree about priorities, with one focused on treating infertility and the other focused on preventing disease recurrence or exacerbation. The therapist's first task may be to help the patient or couple slow down and take time for a carefully considered decision. This does not need to be quick, crisis-intervention counseling.

Male hypertension. In cases in which medications for treatment of hypertension result in impotence or reduced fertility, the patient can nearly always be switched to an alternate medication that effectively treats the hypertension without impairing infertility or they may consider a diet and exercise regime to manage this disease. Informational counseling regarding these options thus precludes the need for more complex decision making.

Diabetes and lupus. Interestingly, the desire to reproduce may become a motivator for a woman who has been lax about treating her diabetes to become more vigilant about her care. On the other hand, pregnancy for a diabetic carries the risk of shortened life, kidney damage, and loss of vision. For women with lupus or other autoimmune disorders, pregnancy can shorten life span or have other deleterious effects. The patient may thus need to make decisions that weigh the desire for reproduction against a shorter or less healthy life. In some cases, desire for a child may lead to denial or minimization of the very real health risks for the patient; such denial should be addressed in counseling.

Breast cancer. The decision to pursue pregnancy and infertility treatment after breast cancer treatment, while life-affirming, is complex. Some patients find it difficult to tolerate the recommended two-year waiting period before attempting pregnancy. Many patients are concerned that pregnancy and use of hormonal therapies will increase their chances for disease recurrence, and they must make their decision in the absence of definitive large-sample longitudinal research studies about these factors. Other patients will be willing to assume the risks associated with pregnancy and use of infertility drugs.[26] Patients with complete ovarian suppression whose only options are costly oocyte donation/IVF or surrogacy may be financially unable to use these treatments, exacerbating feelings of anger and frustration about the unfairness of cancer. Some patients who want infertility treatment encounter opposition from significant others or physicians concerned with pregnancy-caused disease recurrence or maternal death before children reach adulthood. A patient's right to autonomous decision making and her quality-of-life concerns are important factors to consider as mental health professionals help infertile breast cancer survivors explore these issues.

Decisions Regarding Infertility Treatment When a Genetic or Medical Condition May Be Transmitted to Offspring

Patients with cystic fibrosis, severe male-factor problems that are genetically caused, and breast or ovarian cancer may all be concerned with the genetic risks of passing on such conditions to their offspring. Many of these patients will meet with genetic counselors, but at times a mental health professional will be consulted about decision making. Risk factors, alternative treatments such as donor insemination and oocyte donation, and ethical issues should be included in the discussion.

Most couples are ill-prepared for a genetic diagnosis as the cause of their infertility and often emotionally bewildered and overwhelmed with the news. All too frequently, genetically-based infertility involves more than a fertility diagnosis; it can include the diagnosis of a genetic disorder with potentially life-threatening medical complications, the possibility of transmission of that genetic disorder to offspring, and the identification of a genetic disorder in other family members. Understandably, this ripple effect of consequences can have significant psychological, social, and medical consequences for individuals and couples affecting the infertile couple's quality-of-life, family-building alternatives, and healthcare.

HIV patients present with concerns about infecting offspring, as well as infecting the female partner in cases where the male partner is seropositive. Infertility doctors are increasingly seeing patients who are HIV-positive due to the increased prevalence of HIV infection in women and longer life expectancy from newly developed anti-HIV drugs. With longer survival, HIV-infected patients have broadened the focus from disease management to consideration of quality-of-life issues, including parenthood. Rojansky and Schenker[70] suggest that HIV-positive patients should be counseled regarding five issues: (1) risks of perinatal transmission, (2) possible effects of pregnancy on the maternal condition, (3) available therapy for mother and offspring, (4) preventive measures and safe-sex practices, and (5) issues related to infancy and childhood, including orphaned or infected children. Mental health professionals should clarify their own position regarding infertility treatment for HIV-positive patients before counseling such patients, and can advocate for patients by encouraging physicians to develop clear and ethical treatment policies.

Decisions Regarding Infertility Treatment in the Face of Limited Life Expectancy

With diseases such as HIV, severe early-childhood-onset diabetes, and cancers with low survival rates, patients are faced with the decision of whether to treat infertility and conceive in the face of limited life expectancy. The patient, couple, or infertility doctor may struggle with ethical dilemmas and emotional issues of creating a child whose parent is unlikely to live or to be healthy enough to care for the child until the child has reached adulthood. In this way, some of the counseling issues are identical to those presented by couples where one or both are over the age of fifty. The therapist's role may be to assist the patient or couple in facing the realities of limited life expectancy and in making provisions for the care of the child if a parent dies. This process will often include assessment of the supportive role of other family members and friends and evaluation of the family's resources. It is important to recognize and validate the strong "longing for life"[53] that exists for many patients with life-threatening illnesses, and the ways in which biological parenting may satisfy this longing.

Mortality and Loss Issues

The decision about whether to become pregnant (or to adopt a child) when one's own life expectancy is limited is only one facet of the general psychological issue of loss and mortality faced by infertility patients with a medically complicating condition. Infertility in itself involves multiple potential losses.[71] These include loss of control over reproduction, a healthy sexual sense of self, marital or sexual satisfaction, control over life planning, and an ideal family. The other medical condition can also involve multiple losses. These range from the potential loss of life (from cancer, AIDS, or lupus) to the loss of freedom to live an unrestricted life due to daily medical regimens (e.g., diabetes and hypertension) or pain (e.g., endometriosis).

When patients are facing the dual losses inherent in infertility and their other medical condition, they may respond with depression or anger at the unfairness of life. They may also experience an especially powerful longing for life fueled by the simultaneous threat of loss of life and loss of the ability to create a new life. Overcoming infertility and giving birth are seen as a powerful affirmation of patients' survival of the disease process. If patients are ultimately unable to find a cure for infertility, the grief work involved in the loss of the wished-for child may be compounded with renewed grief for the loss of a full, healthy life.

Some patients, faced with these dual losses, may become clinically depressed. The therapist may need to help a patient address previously unresolved grief regarding the medical condition. In some cases, a patient will have grieved at the time of the medical diagnosis, but a diagnosis of infertility will reopen the grieving process by adding another dimension to the meaning of the illness. In cases in which the depression requires a psychotropic medication that is contraindicated during pregnancy, a patient may need to defer infertility treatment until the depression is alleviated. This postponement, difficult for infertility patients in general, may be particularly difficult for patients with a sense of urgency to reproduce and parent within a potentially shortened life span.

Glazer and Hubner[72] noted that infertility patients with cancer often report feeling a sense of exclusion from the infertile community. They feel that others going through infertility cannot possibly appreciate what it means to face cancer as well, with its additional emotional struggles and losses. Patients may also feel a sense of disconnection from others with their medical condition who are not undergoing infertility treatment. In particular, others may criticize them for choosing to have children when the disease itself is life-threatening. Such criticism can increase these patients' sense of isolation.

Defectiveness and Abnormality Issues

Feelings of defectiveness and abnormality are common in infertility patients, as well as those with other medical conditions. A diagnosis of infertility and the process of infertility treatment can compound feelings of defectiveness associated with the other medical condition, causing loss of self-esteem and exacerbating a sense of difference from the normal world. Many of these medical conditions involve problems with sexual functioning, which influence a person's sexual relationships and sexual self-esteem prior to infertility treatment. For instance, males with diabetes or hypertension often have difficulty maintaining erections or having orgasms. Women with endometriosis may have pain with intercourse. In these patients, the infertility problem can represent an additional experience of feeling sexually abnormal or deficient. Counseling may be needed to assist in expressing such feelings, to address sexual dysfunction problems that interfere with timed intercourse or the production of semen samples, and to explore general feelings regarding femininity or masculinity. In some cases, the shame associated with feeling sexually abnormal or defective may inhibit one member of the couple from participating actively in the infertility treatment.

More generally, medical diseases can bring up thoughts and feelings of "my body is defective" and "I am abnormal," which are exacerbated by infertility. The dual narcissistic injury of infertility and other illness can lead to feelings of being betrayed by one's body. Clinicians should be particularly sensitive to issues of defectiveness in patients whose other medical condition (e.g., testicular cancer, endometriosis, diabetes, Rokitansky-Küster-Hauser syndrome) was first diagnosed in adolescence, a developmental period when difference from peers is particularly challenging to the creation and maintenance of a healthy ego. For such patients, infertility treatment can be threatening to their basic sense of self. The infertility physician can help by being sensitive to these issues and by referring patients or couples for supportive counseling.

Patients with genetic, chromosomal, or congenital conditions involving sexual abnormalities and concomitant infertility are particularly vulnerable to feelings of stigma, defectiveness, grief, and loss in addition to all of the issues involved in having a chronic medical condition. Individuals originally diagnosed in infancy or childhood (e.g., Turner's syndrome and cystic fibrosis) typically have faced psychosocial stigma and chronic illness issues throughout their lives and have, to a large extent, integrated the reality of this into their sense of self. A large portion of them may have considered reproductive issues, although research shows that many feel reproduction and sexuality issues may not have been addressed by caregivers as early as most patients would have liked. Individuals diagnosed with a congenital or chromosomal disorder in adolescence or young adulthood (e.g., Rokitansky-Küster-Hauser syndrome or Klinefelter's syndrome) face similar issues. However, an additional challenge for these individuals is the integration of the diagnosis into individual sense of self as a man or woman occurs at an age when individual identity may still be in flux. While assisted reproduction may provide parenting options, using such treatments can trigger reemergence of stigma and bereavement issues. Furthermore, while patients with these conditions may have become psychosocially accustomed to their medical condition, their spouses and/or in-laws may not, triggering a variety of emotional issues for the patient (e.g., guilt) or the couple (e.g., conflict or feelings of inequity). Like men with CBAVD, men with Klinefelter's syndrome are often unaware their fertility is impaired and only discover it in the process of trying to have a family. While dealing with feelings of infertility, men with these disorders often grapple with the feeling of not being a complete man due to the genetic/sexual abnormality. Men and women with these unique disorders often face a double threat to maintaining a healthy sexual ego while addressing feelings about their reproductive abilities. Infertility physicians and counselors should be sensitive to these issues by helping the patient and their partner explore feelings regarding sexuality, masculinity/femininity, reproduction, and family-building.

Countertransference

Throughout this discussion, reference has been made that the physician and counselor need to be aware of their personal feelings in regard to treating infertility patients with medically complicating conditions. Countertransference concerns both the unconscious and conscious awareness of thoughts, feelings, and reactions that a therapist (or other healthcare provider) experiences in the context of relationship with the patient. Goodheart and Lansing describe it as "an aid to understanding the patient's experience through the therapist's own personality filter."[73, p. 90] They identify two classes of induced countertransference responses that are of relevance to working with chronically ill patients: (1) responses to the disease impact and its usual course, and (2) responses to the individual patient's characterological reactions to the disease. Responses to the disease impact may include anxiety, fear, and discomfort around the course of disease and/or treatment primarily due to long-term health issues (i.e., death and disability), vulnerability, loss, helplessness, and failure (i.e., infertility treatment). Responses to the patient's reactions to their illness relate to therapists' feelings of liking the good patient (those that have qualities one admires such as spunk, pleasantness, trying hard, and resourcefulness) and disliking or wanting to get away from the bad patient (angry, demanding, resentful, or manipulative, etc.).

What is apparent is that healthcare professionals need to be aware of their feelings, defenses, anxieties, and other reactions to these patients to provide the best care. Helplessness, often an underlying reaction, is a difficult feeling for those in the helping professions. These feelings are, at times, reflections of the patient's own sense of helplessness in facing two chronic conditions – infertility and their medical condition. Goodheart and Lansing point to several examples of signs that countertransference issues are prominent and should be addressed.[73] They include an awareness that the therapy is not going well; being preoccupied with the patient out of the session; intense feelings persisting with the therapist; and possible feedback from other colleagues or friends regarding the therapist's preoccupation or intense feelings.[73, p. 101] Having the opportunity to understand and analyze these responses, with peers or self, will assist the therapist in helping these challenging patients.

THERAPEUTIC INTERVENTIONS

In addition to strategies discussed with clinical issues, there are several approaches that may be used in developing therapeutic interventions when working with infertility patients with medically complicating conditions. These include patient education, psychosocial support, and stress management.

Patient Education

A fundamental aspect of assisting patients involves helping them obtain sufficient medical information about their condition as well as infertility treatment options. It is the responsibility of the infertility counselor to be educated and informed about the condition so that the patient is not in the position of having to educate the counselor. With this background, the counselor will be able to provide information about what to expect with the infertility evaluation/treatment process, how to work with the treatment team, and the normal emotional responses to infertility within the context of the medical condition. Patients do best when they are well-educated, know what to expect, and are provided with sufficient information to help in decision making. This may involve assisting patients with genetic conditions to get genetic counseling to better understand their condition and its impact on reproduction.

Patient education may also include helping the medical team to understand the emotional needs of patients with medically complicating conditions. While the team may have firm knowledge on the medical needs of these patients, often they feel ill-equipped to deal with their complex emotional needs and demands. Helping the team understand the issues as well as their own countertransference to the patient will facilitate team members' sense of effectiveness.

Psychosocial Support

There are a number of ways the infertility counselor can help to provide psychosocial support. First, the patient may need assistance in addressing the psychosocial issues of the chronic illness. This may mean information on disease management and facilitating contact with support groups such as for cancer survivors, POF, PCOS, endometriosis, or genetic conditions. It may also mean helping to address feelings of stigma associated not only with the disease but also with the desire for family despite the risks, especially true with HIV patients.

Individual, couple, or group counseling are appropriate modalities for addressing the complex needs and issues of these patients. Individual counseling may be useful in managing depression and anxiety, a common consequence of chronic illness as well as infertility, and psychopharmacological assessment may be needed. It may also provide a framework for facilitating bereavement, relating to the loss issues associated with both conditions. Couple counseling is useful to address the impact of these conditions on the marital relationship while pursuing infertility treatment. It is also an opportunity to provide support to the partner, who may feel somewhat ignored as the focus is usually on the identified patient, that is, the patient with the chronic illness, as opposed to the couple. Finally, group counseling provides a safe setting to explore the issues of infertility, without the focus being on chronic illness, often a relief to these patients. Groups are a normalizing experience and usually diminish feelings of isolation, shame, stigma, and defectiveness that patients may face outside the clinic.

Stress Management

An important component in dealing with either chronic illness or infertility, both inherently stressful conditions, is stress management. While specific aspects of stress management and relaxation techniques are covered in depth in other chapters (see Chapter 11), it needs to be underscored how useful these interventions are in helping patients cope with their disease and treatment. These may include: helping patients learning how to breathe diaphragmatically to elicit the relaxation response; practicing age-old techniques of meditation and mindfulness; cognitive restructuring; learning visualization and guided imagery; journaling; making healthy lifestyle choices such as exercise and nutrition; and joining a yoga class. There is growing evidence that practicing these skills not only helps in quality-of-life issues but also may assist in remitting or healing chronic conditions, including infertility.

Another aspect of stress management concerns an oft-neglected factor in healthcare, spirituality. There is substantial amount of research on the relationship between religion, spirituality, and mental health, especially in patients with health problems.[74] This research provides evidence that spirituality and religiosity enhance positive emotions such as well-being, hope, and sense of purpose as well as diminish depression and anxiety symptomatology. It is also associated with better health habits, stronger immune function, better cardiovascular status, and longer survival. Nonetheless, it is an area that many MHPs are uncomfortable pursuing with patients. Exploring and addressing the role of religion and spirituality in a patient's life is part of his or her history, and opens the opportunity to support these beliefs and practices that are commonly used in coping as well as medical decision making.

FUTURE IMPLICATIONS

The best interests of infertility patients with medically complicating conditions will be served when there is good communication and a teamwork approach among the infertility physician, the mental health professional, oncologists, and/or other physicians treating the medical condition. By sharing information about the impact on fertility of the disease and its treatment, the impact of fertility on the disease process, and the psychological issues involved, healthcare providers can assist patients in making decisions that maximize informed consent and peace of mind and minimize the possibility of future regret and distress.

Mental health professionals working in the area of infertility can act as advocates for their patients by educating oncology treatment teams about the options of oocyte donation for patients who have lost ovarian function and gestational carrier for patients who have had hysterectomies but retain ovarian function. Knowledge of these ways to partially preserve fertility can be extremely comforting to some newly diagnosed cancer patients who otherwise might assume that their cancer means a complete loss of reproductive capacity. Likewise, mental health professionals can act as advocates by encouraging oncologists who treat males with Hodgkin's disease and oncologists/urologists who treat testicular cancer to discuss pretreatment sperm cryobanking with all patients, regardless of age or marital status.

Mental health professionals will increasingly see infertility patients with medically complicating conditions, due to increased survival of patients with cancer and other illnesses combined with improved and expanded infertility treatment techniques such as IVF, ICSI, oocyte donation, oocyte cryopreservation, and gestational carrier. All of these advanced infertility treatments are very costly, and not all patients will have the financial means to use them or access to treatment clinics. Also, none of these treatments is guaranteed to treat the infertility problems. In addition, many of these treatment options carry a risk of multifetal pregnancy, which entails higher costs and greater risks than single-ton pregnancies. Thus, healthcare providers should be thoughtful and realistic in discussing these options to avoid offering false hopes of a simple solution to infertility problems or of a solution that might be financially out of reach.

Issues that need to be clarified in the future include ovarian and oocyte cryopreservation, treatment of patients with HIV, and the passing on of genetic problems to children. While ovarian cryopreservation is currently in the early stages of development, it may become more available in the future. Furthermore, as techniques such as ICSI permit reproduction in men who previously were infertile due to genetic problems, some of these genetic problems will be passed on to the children created through infertility treatment.

SUMMARY

■ **Infertility counselors can better serve clients by obtaining general medical knowledge about medical conditions affecting infertility.**

■ **Patients experiencing infertility and a medically complicating condition are often dealing with multiple layers of chronic illness, grief, and social stigma.**

■ **Interdisciplinary teamwork among infertility specialists, mental health professionals, oncologists, and other physicians will serve the best interests of dually diagnosed infertility patients with other medical conditions. Counselors can often serve as advocates for patients.**

■ **Mental health professionals can play a vital role in assisting patients with complex decision making regarding treatment, in which risks and benefits for both disease control and fertility preservation must be considered.**

■ **Cancer treatment decision making requires rapid crisis intervention counseling. While addressing primary feelings of fear and grief regarding cancer diagnosis and potential loss of life, counselors must also bring the topic of future fertility into the discussion. Doing so conveys a sense of hopefulness about the future and helps patients avoid future regret.**

■ **The losses faced by infertility patients in general are compounded for patients with other medical conditions. These patients may experience disconnection from the general infertile population who have not confronted personal mortality issues.**

■ **The abnormality and defectiveness issues faced by infertility patients in general are intensified for patients with other medical conditions. Patients whose other medical condition was first diagnosed in adolescence are particularly vulnerable to such feelings.**

■ **Helping professionals need to be aware of their countertransference feelings and find ways to use the information to better serve these challenging patients.**

■ Therapeutic intervention strategies include patient education, psychosocial support services, and stress management.

REFERENCES

1. Reijo R, Alagappan RK, Patrizio P. Severe oligozoospermia resulting from deletions of azoospermia factor gene on Y chromosome. *Lancet* 1996; 347:1290–3.
2. Mak V, Jarvi K. The genetics of male infertility. *J Urol* 1996; 156:1245–57.
3. American Society of Reproductive Medicine. Increased maternal cardiovascular mortality associated with pregnancy in women with Turner's syndrome. *Fertil Steril* 2005; 83:1074–5.
4. Honig S, Lipshultz L, Jarow J. Significant medical pathology uncovered by a comprehensive male infertility evaluation. *Fertil Steril* 1994; 62:1028–34.
5. Benoff S, Cooper G, Hurley I, et al. The effect of calcium ion channel blockers on sperm fertilizing potential. *Fertil Steril* 1994; 62:606–17.
6. Costabile R. The effects of cancer and cancer therapy on male reproductive function. *J Urol* 1993; 149:1327–30.
7. Roth AJ, Scher HI. Genitourinary malignancies. In: JC Holland, ed. *Psycho-oncology*. New York: Oxford University Press, 1998.
8. Aass N, Fossa SC, Raghavan D, Vogelzang NJ. Late toxicity after chemotherapy of testis cancer. In: NJ Vogelzang PT, Scardino, WU Shipley, DS Cofey, eds. *Comprehensive Textbook of Genitourinary Oncology*. Baltimore, MD: Williams & Wilkins, 1996; p. 1090–6.
9. Einhorn LH, Richie JP, Shipley WU. Cancer of the testis. In: VT DeVita Jr, S Hellman, SA Rosenberg, eds. *Cancer: Principles and Practice of Oncology*. 4th ed. Philadelphia, PA: JP Lippincott; 1993; p. 1126–51.
10. Tournaye H, Goossens E, Verheyen G, Frederpckx V, DeBlock G, Devroey P, Van Steirteghem. Preserving the reproductive potential of men and boys with cancer: Current concepts and future prospects. *Hum Reprod Update* 2004; 10:525–32.
11. Ragni G, Perotti L, Viviani S, Santori A, Devizzi L, Della Serra A. Fertility outcome in men with Hodgkin's disease after four different combination chemotherapy regimens. Presented at the 52nd annual meeting of the American Society for Reproductive Medicine, Boston, MA, November 2–6, 1996.
12. Mickle J, Milunsky A, Amos J, Oates RD. Congenital unilateral absence of the vas deferens: A heterogeneous disorder with two distinct subpopulations based upon aetiology and mutational status of the cystic fibrosis gene. *Hum Reprod* 1995; 10:1728–35.
13. van der Ven K, Messer L, van der Ven H, Jeyendran RS, Ober C. Cystic fibrosis mutation screening in healthy men with reduced sperm quality. *Hum Reprod* 1996; 11:513–17.
14. Anderson DJ. Assisted reproduction for couples infected with the human immunodeficiency virus type 1. *Fert Stert* 1999;72: 592–4.
15. Politch JA, Abbott AF, Mayer KH, Anderson DJ. The effects of disease progression and zidovudine therapy on semen quality in human immunodeficiency virus type 1 seropositive men. *Fertil Steril* 1994; 61:922–8.
16. Semprini AE, Levi-Setti P, Bozzo M, et al. Insemination of HIV-negative women with processed semen of HIV-positive men. *Lancet* 1992; 340:1317–9.
17. Semprini A E, Fiore S. HIV and reproduction. *Current Opinion in Obstetrics & Gynecology* 2004; 16:257–62.
18. Marina S, Marina F, Alcolea R, et al. Human immunodeficiency virus type 1-serodiscordant couples can bear healthy children after undergoing intrauterine insemination. *Fertil Steril* 1998; 70:35–9.
19. Mandelbrot L, Heard I, Henrion-Geant E., et al. Natural conception in HIV-negative women with HIV-infected partners. *Lancet* 1997; 349:850–1.
20. Ethics Committee of the American Society for Reproductive Medicine. Human immunodeficiency virus and infertility treatment. *Fertil Steril* 2002; 77:218–22.
21. Nelson LM, Covington SN, Rebar RW. An update: Spontaneous premature ovarian failure is not early menopause. *Fertil Steril* 2005; 83:1327–32.
22. Santoro A, Bonadonna G, Valabussa P, Zucali R, Viviani S, Villani F. Long-term results of combined chemotherapy-radio-therapy approach in Hodgkin's disease: Superiority of ABVD plus radiotherapy versus MOPP plus radiotherapy. *J Clin Oncol* 1987; 5:27–37.
23. Van der Elst J. Oocyte freezing: Here to stay? *Hum Reprod Update* 2003; 9:463–70.
24. Friedlander M, Thewes B. Counting the costs of treatment: the reproductive and gynaecological consequences of adjuvant therapy in young women with breast cancer. *Intern Med J* 2003; 33:372–9.
25. Reichman B, Green K. Breast cancer in young women: Effect of chemotherapy on ovarian function, fertility, and birth defects. *J Natl Cancer Inst Monogr* 1994; 16:125–9.
26. Sonmezer M, Oktay K. Fertility preservation in female patients. *Hum Reprod Update* 2004; 10:251–66.
27. Rossing MA, Daling JR, Weiss NS, Moore DE, Self SG. Risk of breast cancer in a cohort of infertile women. *Gynecol Oncol* 1996; 60:3–7.
28. Venn A, Watson L, Lumley J, Giles G, King C, Healy D. Breast and ovarian cancer incidence after infertility and in vitro fertilization. *Lancet* 1995; 346:995–1000.
29. Bryant, LT, Lee CW, Willouby DF, Hearn HB. Human papillomavirus and cervical cancer. *Women's Health Prim Care* 2005; 8:230–41.
30. Bernardini M, Barrett J, Seaward G, Covens A. Pregnancy outcomes in patients after radical trachelectomy. *Am J Obstet Gynecol* 2003; 189:1378–82.
31. Fernandez H, Frydman R. Cancer and in vitro fertilization. *J In Vitro Fertil Embryo Transf* 1987; 4:241–2.
32. Connor E, Sperling R, Gelber R, et al. Reduction of maternal-infant transmission of human immunodeficiency virus type 1 with zidovudine treatment. *N Engl J Med* 1994; 331:1173–80.
33. Olaitan A, Reid W, Mocroft A, McCarthy K, Madge S, Johnson M. Infertility among human immunodeficiency virus-positive women: Incidence and treatment dilemmas. *Hum Reprod* 1996; 11:2793–6.
34. Annas G. Protecting patients from discrimination – The Americans with Disabilities Act and HIV infection. *N Engl J Med* 1998; 339:1255–9.
35. Selby PI, Oakley CE. Women's problems with diabetes. *Diabet Med* 1992; 9:290–2.

36. Nichols JE, Crane MM, Higdon HL, et al. Extremes of body mass index reduce in vitro fertilization pregnancy rates. *Fertil Stertil* 2003; 79:645–7.

37. Berga S, Marcus M, Loucks T, et al. Recovery of ovarian activity in women with functional hypothalamic amenorrhea (FHA) treated with cognitive behavior therapy (CBT). *Fertil Steril* 2003; 80:976–81.

38. Domar AD, Zutermeister, PC, Freidman R. The psychological impact of infertility: A comparison with patients with other medical conditions. *J Psychosom Obstet gynaecol* 1993; 14:Suppl 45–52.

39. Schover LR Motivation for parenthood after cancer: A review. *J Natl Cancer Inst Monogr* 2005; 4:2–5.

40. Teeter MA, Holmes GE, Holmes FF, Baker AB. Decisions about marriage and family among survivors of childhood cancer. *J Psychosoc Oncol* 1987; 5:59–68.

41. Sanger WG, Olson JH, Sherman JK. Semen cryobanking for men with cancer – criteria change. *Fertil Steril* 1992; 58:1024–7.

42. Schover LR. Sexuality and fertility in urologic cancer patients. *Cancer* 1987; 60:553–8.

43. Rieker PP, Fitzgerald EM, Kalish LA. Adaptive behavioral responses to potential infertility among survivors of testis cancer. *J Clin Oncol* 1990; 8:347–55.

44. Rieker PP, Fitzgerald EM, Kalish LA, et al. Psychosocial factors, curative therapies, and behavioral outcomes: A comparison of testis cancer survivors and a control group of healthy men. *Cancer* 1989; 64:2399– 407.

45. Sweet V, Servy EJ, Karow AM. Reproductive issues for men with cancer: Technology and nursing management. *Oncol Nurs Forum* 1996; 23:51–8.

46. Kaempfer SH, Wiley FM, Hoffman DJ, Rhodes EA. Fertility considerations and procreative alternatives in cancer care. *Semin Oncol Nurs* 1985; 1:25–34.

47. Hubner MK, Glazer ES. Now on common ground: Cancer and infertility in the 1990s. *Infertil Reprod Med Clin North Am* 1993; 4:581–96.

48. Cella DF, Najavits L. Denial of infertility in patients with Hodgkin's disease. *Psychosomatics* 1986; 27:71.

49. Hubner MK. Cancer and infertility: Longing for life. *J Psychosoc Oncol* 1989; 7:1–19.

50. Rieker, PP, Fitzgerald, EM, Kalish, LA. Adaptive behavioral responses to potential infertility among survivors of testis cancer. *J Clin Oncol* 1990:347–55.

51. Gritz, ER, Wellisch, DK, Wang HJ, et al. Long-term effects of testicular cancer on sexual functioning in married couples. *Cancer* 1989; 64:1560–7.

52. Dow KH, Harris JR, Roy C. Pregnancy after breast-conserving surgery and radiation therapy for breast cancer. *J Natl Cancer Inst Monogr* 1994; 16:131–7.

53. Lamb MA. Effects of cancer on the sexuality and fertility of women. *Semin Oncol Nurs* 1995; 11:120–7.

54. Kornblith AB, Anderson J, Cella DF, et al. Comparison of psychosocial adaptation and sexual function of survivors of advanced Hodgkin's disease treated by MOPP, ABVD, or MOPP alternating with ABVD. *Cancer* 1992; 70:2508–16.

55. Galletly, C, Clark A., Tomlinson L, Blaney F. Improved pregnancy rates for obese, infertile women following a group treatment program: An open pilot study. *Gen Hosp Psychiatry* 1996; 3:192–5.

56. Fair A, Griffiths K, Osman LM. Atttitudes to fertility issues among adults with cystic fibrosis in Scotland. The Collaborative Group of Scottish Adult CF Centres. *Thorax* 2000; 8:672–7.

57. Sawyer SM, Farrant B, Cerritelli B, Wilson J. A survey of sexual and reproductive health in men with cystic fibrosis: New challenges for adolescent and adult services. *Thorax* 2005; 4:326–30.

58. Wingfield MB, Wood C, Henderson, LS, Wood RM. Treatment of endometriosis involving a self-help group positively affects patients' perception of care. *J Psychsom Obstet Gynaeol* 1997; 18:255–8.

59. Jones G, Jenkinson, C, Kennedy S. The impact of endometriosis upon quality of life: A qualitative analysis. *J Psychom Obstet Gynaecol* 2004; 2:123–33.

60. Rolland, JS. Toward a psychosocial typology of chronic and life threatening illness. *Family Systems Medicine* 1984; 2:245–62.

61. Primomo, J. Chronic illnesses and women. In: CI Fogel, NF Woods, eds. *Women's Health Care: A Comprehensive Handbook*. Thousands Oak, CA: Sage Publications. 1995; 651–71.

62. Unruh AM, McGrath PJ. The psychology of female infertility: Toward a new perspective. *Health Care Women Int* 1985; 6:369–81.

63. Goffman E. *Stigma: Notes on the Management of Spoiled Identity*. Englewood Cliffs, NJ: Prentice Hall, 1963.

64. Schrover LR, Brey K, Lechtin A, et al. Knowledge and experience regarding cancer, infertility and sperm banking in younger male survivors. *J Clin Oncol* 2002; 20:1880–9.

65. The Ethics Committee of the American Society for Reproductive Medicine. Fertility preservation and reproduction in cancer patients. *Fertil Stertil* 2005; 83:1622–8.

66. Robertson JA. Posthumous reproduction. *Indiana Law J* 1994; 69:1027.

67. Ohl DA, Park J, Cohen C, Goodman K, Menge AC. Procreation after death or mental incompetence: Medical advance or technology gone awry? *Fertil Steril* 1996; 66:889–95.

68. Practice Committee of the American Society for Reproductive Medicine. Ovarian tissue and oocyte cryopreservation. *Fertil Steril* 2004; 82:993–8.

69. Groff AA, Covington SN, Halverson LR, et al. Assessing the emotional needs of women with spontaneous premature ovarian failure. *Fertil Stertil* 2005; 83:1734–41.

70. Rojansky N, Schenker JG. Ethical aspects of assisted reproduction in AIDS patients. *Assist Reprod Genet* 1995; 12:537–42.

71. Manning BE. The emotional aspects of infertility. *Fertil Steril* 1980; 34:313–9.

72. Glazer ES, Hubner MK. Coping with the double blow: Facing cancer and infertility. Resolve Fact Sheet. Boston, MA: Resolve Inc, 1992.

73. Goodheart CD and Lansing MH. *Treating People with Chronic Disease: A Psychological Guide*. Washington, DC: American Psychological Association; 1996.

74. Koenig HG. Spirituality, wellness, and quality of life. *Sexuality, Reproduction, & Menopause*. 2004; 2:76–82.

15 Genetic Counseling and the Infertile Patient

LINDA HAMMER BURNS, KRISTA REDLINGER-GROSSE, AND CHERI SCHOONVELD

We are a spectacular, splendid manifestation of life. We have language.... We have affection. We have genes for usefulness, and usefulness is about as close to a 'common goal' of nature as I can guess at.

– Lewis Thomas

During the last half of the twentieth century, there were a series of stunning advancements in reproductive medicine and genetics that, ultimately, led to the two fields of medicine becoming inextricably intertwined. Some of these medical milestones include the discovery of DNA in 1953 by Watson and Crick in Great Britain, the birth of the first baby conceived via in vitro fertilization (IVF) in 1978 in Great Britain, the birth of the first baby following preimplantation genetic diagnosis (PGD) in 1989 in Great Britain, and the completion of the mapping of the full human genome sequence in 2003 in the United States. These achievements have enabled both reproductive and genetic medicine to improve patient health and well-being while facilitating reproduction for individuals or couples previously incapable of having a genetically-shared and/or healthy, unaffected offspring. In short, the range of applications of genetics in infertility is extensive, varied, and consistently expanding contributing to the emergence of a new medical specialty: reproductive genetic medicine. While this new field increasingly enables would-be parents to have the hoped for 'perfect' baby – a baby with maximum health and minimum defects – the would-be parents all too often have unrealistic or misguided expectations of feasibility, success, and applicability of any given technology or potential treatment. Furthermore, not unexpectedly, the ability of reproductive medicine and medical genetics to facilitate the conception and/or birth of a healthy baby can be fraught with moral dilemmas and technological bewilderments for individuals as well as the family, community, and society in which they live not to mention offspring conceived or born as a result of these technological advancements.

Genetic counselors and infertility counselors as mental health professionals working in reproductive medicine deal with basic issues of reproductive health and normality/abnormality.[1,2] Increasingly, genetic and infertility counselors, as members of the reproductive medicine team, provide informational and supportive care to individuals and couples undergoing treatment for infertility and/or related genetic conditions. In reproductive medicine, genetic counselors provide educational information about genetic conditions that can, and do, impact the individual's or couple's reproductive future including known or unknown genetic disorders and the risk of transmission of genetic disorders to offspring. By contrast, infertility counselors must be cognizant of the impact of genetic diseases and disorders on reproduction and the psychosocial impact of these diagnoses on reproductive decision making and emotional and marital well-being. Both infertility and genetic counselors provide reproductive education, preparation, comfort, and support as well as address individual and couple response to genetic diagnosis; the impact of extended and/or repeated reproductive losses; impaired information processing; explore family-building alternatives (e.g., adoption and assisted reproduction); marital conflict, and individual distress while providing the opportunity to discuss feelings about genetic risk factors or transmission patterns.[2] Infertility counselors and genetic counselors provide services that dovetail; they work together as integral members of the reproductive medicine team providing comprehensive patient care to infertile couples.

This chapter

■ addresses the concepts involved in the applications of reproductive genetic counseling to infertility and infertility counseling;

■ provides an overview of the applications of genetic medicine to infertility;

■ outlines the basis for testing for the diagnosis of genetic infertility, prenatal genetic testing with applications to infertility, PGD (genetic testing done during IVF and before embryo transfer), and the genetic screening and counseling of gamete and embryo donors;

- ■ illustrates how the genetic and infertility counselors work together in meeting the complex needs of the infertile patient.

HISTORICAL OVERVIEW

The Discovery of the Concept of Heredity and Beyond

Historically, birth defects and intrafamilial disorders were (and sometimes still are) attributed to external factors such as punishment or favor by a deity; misdeed or misadventure by the parent (typically the mother); a curse; or phenomena of nature (e.g., eclipse).[3] Such beliefs remain prominent in some cultures and may be held and acted upon simultaneously with modern, scientific medical practices. Even though until recently there has been little scientific information, throughout history there are various accounts of apparently familial disorder or birth defect occurring (or recurring) in offspring. Examples include the understanding of hemophilia evidenced by Talmudic proscription against circumcising brothers of 'bleeders'; French physician Paul Pierre Broca's 1866 report of a seemingly dominant breast cancer predisposition in five generations of his wife's family; and the societal taboos against marriages between close relatives in various cultures.[3] An interesting historical example is the genetic disorder of hemophilia suffered by the only son of Czar Nicholas I and Czarina Alexandra – a condition that some have contended influenced the course of history.

Modern genetics had its beginnings in the abbey garden of Gregor Mendel, an Austrian monk, who was the first to identify 'units' (now known as genes). In addition, he developed a theory of inheritances based on a series of experiments on pea plants. Originally published in 1865, Mendel's laws became the foundation of modern genetics, beginning with the principle that inherited characteristics are controlled by genes that occur in pairs. Additional Mendelian principles include the Law of Dominance (one dominant gene in a pair masks the recessive gene, thereby preventing it from showing its effect); the Law of Segregation (each offspring receives only one factor, gene, from each parent); and the Law of Independent Assortment (different factors, genes, are inherited separately and randomly).[4]

In 1902, American biologist Walter S. Sutton and German cell biologist Theodor Boveri, and others, separately noted the parallels between Mendel's factors (genes) and chromosomes, which led to the chromosomal theory of inheritance. According to this theory, Mendelian genes have specific loci on chromosomes and it is the chromosomes that undergo segregation and independent assortment. American embryologist, Thomas H. Morgan was the first to associate a specific gene with a specific chromosome through his experimental work with fruit flies early in the twentieth century.[4] The term *genetics* (meaning the biological study of heredity) was coined in 1905 by British biologist William Bateson, and the terms *gene* and *genotype* (meaning genetic makeup) were contributed in 1909 by German scientist Wilhelm Johannsen.[3]

As the field of genetics emerged, both the scientific and general public became interested in how hereditary factors might contribute to medical conditions (e.g., mental retardation and birth defects) as well as social and behavioral conditions (e.g., poverty, crime, and mental illness). Francis Galton, an English scientist, coined the term 'eugenics' in 1883 and founded the Eugenics Society of Great Britain in 1908, which was based on a belief that humanity could be improved by encouraging the ablest and healthiest people to have more children (typically referred to as *positive eugenics*).[5] Eugenics became a popular movement early in the twentieth century. Its aim was achieving social and biological evolution through selective human breeding by encouraging or permitting reproduction of only those individuals with genetic characteristics judged desirable. The eugenics movements in the United States, Germany, Australia, and Scandinavia favored negative eugenics, which advocated preventing the least able from reproducing. In the United States, laws were passed instituting quotas limiting immigration of inferior ethnic groups as well as laws promoting sterilization and/or denying immigration or marriage of degenerates based on race, mental or physical illness or incapacity, or criminal behavior. By 1926, twenty-three of the then forty-eight United States had laws mandating sterilization of the mentally defective and more than 6,000 people had been involuntarily sterilized.[5] In some Scandinavian countries this practice persisted into the 1960s and 1970s.[6] In Australia, eugenics principles became part of a public health movement to eliminate sexually transmitted diseases and regulate indigenous peoples. Negative eugenics reached its pinnacle with the Holocaust of World War II in Germany during which millions of Jews, Gypsies, minorities, the disabled, criminals, and others were murdered en masse. In 1939, Germany legalized euthanasia for the genetically-defective resulting in the deaths of more than 70,000 people with hereditary disorders.[7] Although negative eugenics fell into disfavor after the Holocaust, various forms continue to reemerge throughout the world as exemplified by the ethnic cleansing movements in Kosovo and Central Africa; religious and/or racial pronatalism with political agendas (e.g., fundamentalist religious movements); and reproductive social reformation movements (e.g., China's 'single child' policy or high rates of female infanticide worldwide).

Although these policies may seem to be passé, they are increasingly relevant as reproductive medicine, genetics, and medical technologies have become a popular method of implementing these agendas. Historically, the eugenics movement most certainly had a negative end. The use of the eugenics movement as a theoretical basis for the implementation of public policies that resulted in widespread discrimination and genocide led to a movement away from negative genetics and toward positive genetics with its emphasis on the identification of hereditary components of health issues to improve health and the human condition.

After World War II, research focused on investigation of genes, their structure, and the genetic information stored in genes. In 1953, molecular biologists Crick and Watson announced they had discovered the structure of deoxyribonucleic acid, DNA.[8] Known as the 'double helix,' the researchers confirmed that DNA carries life's hereditary information. This discovery, coupled with the advent of sophisticated molecular genetic technologies, allowed researchers to unravel the genetic code present in all humans.

In 2003, the International Human Genome Project (HGP) (officially inaugurated in 1990) completed the mapping of the human genome: the sequencing of the entire DNA code found in human cells, or the entire complement of human hereditary material. It is this DNA code that orchestrates the functioning and development of the human body. The major rationale of the HGP was acquiring fundamental information concerning a basic understanding of human genetics and the role of genes in health and disease. The outcomes of this project led to: The development of methods for locating specific genes responsible for determining specific human traits; causing certain diseases; and or contributing to human development and behavior. Today, genetic testing can be useful for diagnostic purposes; for the assessment of genetic risk; identification of carrier status (individuals who are unaffected but carrying genes capable of causing a genetic disease or disorder in their offspring); predicting an individual's risk of adult-onset disorders; and determining genetic causes of infertility.[9] Information gained from the HGP has provided increasingly sophisticated molecular technologies, determined the genetic basis or genetic

involvement in diseases or disorders, and aided in the discovery of new opportunities for the care, treatment, and even cure of some genetic-based diseases or disorders, including those related to infertility.

A Genetics Primer

Today, approximately 3–5% of all live births worldwide will have a birth defect, chromosomal anomaly, or genetic disease. To date, more than 8,000 diseases are documented as having a genetic basis in McKusick's catalog, a reference text on single gene disorders that is updated regularly.[10] Moreover, all diseases are suspected of having some genetic involvement, including the susceptibility to infections and common conditions with adult onset such as cancer, heart disease, chemical addiction, and mental illnesses. At some level, all humans are at risk for being affected by a condition that has a genetic basis.

The basic units of inheritance are the *genes*, which are the biochemical blueprints from which cells 'read' the instructions needed for normal growth, development, and function. Scientists estimate that there are about 30,000 genes in every cell of the human body, carried in duplicate on the twenty-three pairs of chromosomes found within the cells of the body. *Chromosomes* are therefore 'packaging units' for the genes. One chromosome from each of the pairs is inherited from the mother through her egg cell (oocyte or ovum), and the other of the pair is inherited from the father through the sperm cell, for a total of forty-six chromosomes. Each of the chromosomes carries hundreds to thousands of genes, and, like the chromosomes, 50% of genes are inherited from the mother and 50% from the father. The first twenty-two pairs of chromosomes carry genes that every human has in common and that are the same in males and females. The twenty-third pair carries the genes that determine the gender of the developing fetus, as well as other information. Females normally have two chromosomes identified as X chromosomes, and males normally have one X chromosome and one Y chromosome. The typical female chromosome designation (karyotype) is 46, XX and the typical male karyotype is 46, XY. The presence of a Y chromosome with normally functioning genetic material directs the fetus to develop into a male. The absence of a Y chromosome with functioning genetic material, along with the presence of two X chromosomes with normally functioning genetic material, directs the fetus to develop into a female. Changes in the number or the structure of one or more chromosome(s) or changes in the structure and functioning of one or more gene(s) can result in infertility problems and/or the development of a child with a birth defect and/or genetic disease. These changes are the basis of testing that can help diagnose a genetic cause of infertility.

An Overview of the Field of Genetic Counseling

Genetic counseling is defined as a communication process meant to help an individual or family: (1) comprehend the medical facts, including diagnosis, probable cause, and available management of a disorder; (2) understand how heredity contributes to the disorder and risk of transmission to offspring; (3) facilitate evaluation of risks and decision making regarding treatment; and (4) assist in the adjustment to a disorder in the individual or in an affected family member.[2] Sheldon C. Reed, American Genetist Director of the Dight Institute of Human Genetics at the University of Minnesota, coined the term genetic counseling in 1947. He defined the three requirements of genetic counseling as: (1) knowledge of human genetics; (2) respect for sensitivities, attitudes, and reactions of clients; and (3) teaching and providing genetic information to the full extent known.[11] Genetic counseling was originally done by university-based research geneticists involved in research programs. As such, the emphasis was on the provision of genetic information and knowledge-based advice rather than on counseling. With the advent of genetic testing in the early 1970s, genetic counseling moved toward a more medical model of patient care, in which genetic counselors saw their responsibilities as not only providing genetic information, but also as providing supportive counseling and clinical services to patients seeking assistance in reproductive and medical care decisions, and to enable patient decision making consistent with the patient's own needs and values.[12]

As such, genetic counseling, as a fully recognized health profession, is a relatively new and still evolving profession. There are international variations in qualifications, roles, and expectations but, in general, genetic counselors are healthcare professionals with a master's level graduate degree. Although a small number of nurses have been certified by the International Society of Nurses in Genetics, the majority of genetic counselors in the United States and Canada complete formalized training through programs accredited by the American Board of Genetic Counseling. The first formal graduate program for educating genetic counselors was established in the United States in 1969 at Sarah Lawrence College in New York.[13] Graduate training and coursework in genetic counseling includes studies in human and molecular genetics, related biological sci-

ences, and psychosocial counseling with clinical application. Graduates must demonstrate clinical skills in a variety of settings with diverse patient populations to be eligible to apply for board certification, and to be certified, an applicant must pass both general and subspecialty exams.[14] Increasingly, genetic counselors are specializing in a specific field of genetic counseling such as reproductive genetic counseling, as evidenced by the addition of the Genetic Counseling Special Interest Groups to both the American Society of Reproductive Medicine (ASRM) and the European Society of Human Reproduction and Embryology (ESHRE).

In the past, nurses working with physicians and/or medical geneticists had traditionally provided genetic counseling in Australia and the United Kingdom. Recently, with the advent of master's level genetic training courses, a distinct genetic counseling profession has begun to develop in these and other countries. In Australia, accreditation is provided through the Human Genetics Society of Australia and genetic counseling training courses have expanded to training professionals in southeast Asia (e.g., New Zealand, India, and Vietnam).[15] Master's level training is also available in Mexico where genetic counselors are certified by the National Board of Medical Genetics and in Israel where master's level graduate training and clinical experience qualifies the genetic counselor for licensing by the Ministry of Health. In other parts of Europe, social workers or geneticists often provide counseling.[16] In other countries including Japan, Argentina, Chile, Italy, and China, physicians who may or may not have additional training in genetics and/or reproductive genetics have been the ones to provide genetic counseling services.[17] Prenatal or reproductive genetic counseling is often provided by obstetricians (e.g., Germany) or by midwives, with medical geneticists only involved in the diagnosis of rare disorders.[18] Likewise, in Brazil the need for genetic counseling services has been recognized, but may be provided by: genetic counselors, physicians, medical geneticists, psychologists, or social workers – all of whom may or may not have had formal training in medical genetics.[19,20] As genetic counseling has become a distinct health profession, specific organizations related to genetic counseling have been established in many countries.

Genetic counseling typically involves interactive discussions of the medical aspects of a disease or presenting problem; clarification of the genetic basis for the identified disease or disorder; assessment of genetic transmission risk; and explanation of relevant medical management and available testing options. Genetic counselors facilitate decision making regarding diagnosis, testing, or management; provide support and educational resources; and facilitate the exploration of complicated feelings and the integration of complex information all within the context of the patient's needs and values. Like the clinical interview in counseling, a fundamental tool used by genetic counselors to gather information regarding family history is the *pedigree* (see Figure 15.1) using standardized nomenclature. Information obtained from the pedigree helps the genetic counselor determine whether further testing such as chromosome analysis (karyotyping) is appropriate and, if so, he or she makes arrangements for obtaining samples for karyotyping and/or other genetic testing. Figure 15.1 is an example of a pedigree depicting a couple who is childless due to a history of multiple miscarriages. Furthermore, the pedigree provides an organizational method for collecting and organizing information; assessing familial patterns of disease and/or behaviors; and developing hypotheses about how family dynamics affect genetic diagnosis, counseling, and even decision making.[12] The use of the pedigree has been adapted by mental health professionals (including infertility counselors) to further assess family systems over a several generations. Expanding on the *pedigree/genogram*, Kenen and Peters[21] developed the Colored Ecologicaland Genetic Relational Map (CEGRM) as a conceptual approach and tool for presenting information about family relationships and stories about inherited diseases in a simple, understandable form (see Figure 15.1). It is particularly useful for genetic and infertility counselors in that patient decision making regarding reproductive plans, therapeutic intervention, lifestyle behavior, and sharing or withholding of genetic information frequently becomes enmeshed with preexisting psychosocial relationships whether biological kin, in-laws, and/or fictive kin (friends who act as family). As such, the CEGRM as a form of the pedigree/genogram makes it easier to compare different types of social interactions and the impact of the diagnosis on the individual or couple's family and social network.

REVIEW OF LITERATURE

The field of reproductive genetics is a new and evolving field and, as a result, research initially was sparse and marked by case reports of specific genetic diseases or disorders that featured infertility. Initially there was limited investigation into patient emotional response or psychological adjustment following reproductive genetic testing or diagnosis and a significant focus on specific genetic developments in reproductive medicine.

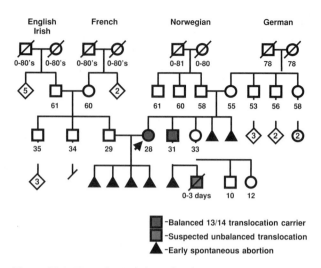

Figure 15.1. Hypothetical clinical pedigree representing infertility using recommended nomenclature. (Adapted from ref. 140, with permission)

International Perspectives on Reproductive Genetic Testing and Counseling

Over the last two decades, four models of policy development have been adopted in relation to human reproductive technologies and genetics: the market model; the human rights approach; self-regulatory mechanisms; and legislation. In a review of regulatory approaches in reproductive medicine, the human rights approach was found to be less favored due to its dependence on legal interpretation of basic rights, making it expensive, time-consuming, and cumbersome. Knoppers and Isasi[22] investigated regulatory approaches to the provision of reproductive genetic testing in eleven countries (Australia, Austria, Canada, France, Germany, India, Israel, Japan, The Netherlands, Switzerland, and the United Kingdom). Although no country had adopted a market or laissez-faire approach, the authors cited Italy as an example of a country with a long history of a permissive, laissez-faire approach in which overly restrictive legislation was recently implemented – with significant negative consequences. Despite the difficulty of making generalizations due to different regulatory systems adopted in each country, reflecting legal traditions, cultural, and socioreligious beliefs influencing public policy in each country, two different approaches were identified: *public order* (legislative, top-down approach) and *private ordering* (nonlegislative, bottom-up) approach. Limiting their analysis to countries that ranged from restrictive to pragmatic approaches, the researchers found a remarkable symmetry in both the (1) substantive requirements (i.e., gravity and health indications generally) and (2) procedural safeguards (i.e., informed consent, counseling, confidentiality, civil status, oversight, and accreditation) surrounding reproductive genetic testing. All countries in this study had a mix of the self-regulatory and legislative-specific approaches. Unitary countries, such as Austria, France, The Netherlands, and Israel, rely heavily on legislation as opposed to federal countries (e.g., Switzerland and Australia). Interestingly, countries that had adopted prohibitive legislative approaches in the 1990s (e.g., Austria and Germany) were required to develop new/adapted legal statues to accommodate new technologies. Furthermore, although professional guidelines were found to allow flexibility, the absence of efficient accreditation mechanisms and oversight bodies was found to lead to arbitrary and inconsistent interpretations and applications contributing to social inequities.

In a preliminary survey of 2,901 genetic professionals in thirty-six nations, researchers reported that the nondirective counseling approach was prominent in English-speaking countries, an aberration from the rest of the world in which a more eugenic approach to genetic counseling was prevalent. Furthermore, respect for patient autonomy was found to be greatest in the United States and least evident in China and India.[23] Most providers of genetic counseling, with the exception of China, rejected government involvement in pre-marital testing or sterilization, despite holding personal negative biases against persons with genetic disabilities. The negatively biased views led to an approach to genetic counseling based on pessimistically biased information, especially in developing nations in Asia and Eastern Europe.[24] This survey study was expanded to included 4,629 medical and nonmedical genetic counselors in thirty-six countries. Based on this larger sample, Wertz reported similar findings in that a pessimistic and prevalent view of genetic disorders influenced counseling direction and outcomes. Most providers of genetic counseling regarded educational success of a session as more important than empathy or support. Additionally, many thought their goal was to prevent the birth of children with genetic conditions, by prenatal diagnosis and elective abortion if necessary. Wertz found that except in North America, the United Kingdom, and Australia, many providers of genetic counseling reported that they would be both directive and pessimistic about a wide array of genetic disorders and diseases, especially in Eastern Europe and Asia. In the United Kingdom, 10% would counsel in favor of abortion for Trisomy 21; in Northern Europe, 34%; in Southern Europe, 47%; and in Eastern Europe, 63%. For cystic fibrosis, percentages favoring abortion were: 10% in the United Kingdom; 21% in Northern Europe; 34% in Southern Europe; and 48% in Eastern Europe.[25]

THEORETICAL FRAMEWORK

Genetic counseling uses many of the same principles and theoretical frameworks of psychology, but genetic counseling is *not* psychotherapy. Genetic counseling is based on a definition of counseling as giving advice, expert opinion, or instruction in directing the judgment or conduct of an individual, couple, or family to make autonomous decisions within the context of the medical model of patient care. As such, genetic counseling is not simply the provision of information but the empowering of patients through education, emotional support and the facilitation of information processing and decision making. Alternatively, infertility counselors (as licensed mental health professionals) are educated and trained to provide psychotherapy: the treatment of personality maladjustment or mental illness by psychological and/or psychopharmacological means as part of therapeutic relationship. While both genetic counselors and infertility counselors provide expert advice and support, only infertility counseling provides *psychological treatment* of patients. Historically, genetic counseling was based on the adaptation or application of the principles of various psychological theories including client-centered counseling, communication theories, biopsychosocial medicine approach, family systems theory, and stress theory. Only recently has there been a move to develop specific genetic counseling theoretical frameworks.

One theoretical framework fundamental to genetic counseling is *client-centered counseling* based on humanistic psychology and the work of American psychologist Carl Rogers. Accordingly, client-centered counseling emphasizes a nondirective, empathic approach in which the counselor provides a warm, accepting environment that respects the patient's perspective and provides unconditional positive regard. These principles are thought to facilitate the exploration of feelings, issues, and decision making, and, as such, provides a basis for genetic counseling that is nondirective and respects patient autonomy.[26] The basis for this approach emphasizes the "respect for client's beliefs, background and culture, and the counselor's duty to enable clients to make autonomous decisions by providing all necessary information."[26] According to the *communication approach* to genetic counseling, the genetic counselor uses the principles of communication and decision making theories that address communication processes and behaviors; information processing; and decision making as a cognitive process affected by the information provided, the method of communicating the information, and the context in which the decision is being made. Within the context of a medical model of diagnosis and treatment, caregivers and patients make collaborative decisions with the aim of minimizing risks and maximizing benefits (e.g., health and well-being) while considering all treatment possibilities (including doing nothing).[27] As such, genetic counselors provide unbiased information; assist exploration of personal views and values regarding medical treatments and available options; and facilitate individual and/or family decision making. Genetic counseling is not simply the provision of facts, but the processing and integration of information enabling an individual's autonomous decision making and assimilation of complex scientific information.[26]

The application of *family systems theory* to genetic counseling has been suggested because family systems theory deemphasizes individual psychological problems while addressing the family's strengths (e.g., resiliency) and weaknesses (e.g., chaotic functioning). Based on general systems theory, family systems theory addresses the family as a unit with predictable patterns of interactions, behaviors, and communications that impact the individual family members as well as the system as a whole. Accordingly, genetic counselors use family systems theory to address individual, intrafamilial, and intergenerational issues associated with inherited and genetic disorders.[12] Kessler[28] characterized the change in emphasis in genetic counseling as a 'paradigm shift,' describing the shift in emphasis in genetic counseling from a communication-of-information model of counseling to a preventive medicine model and, finally, the biopsychosocial medicine approach currently favored.[26]

The *biopsychosocial medicine approach* (introduced by Engel) is a patient-center approach to medical care based on general systems theory in which diagnosis and treatment of medical conditions consider a wide array of aspects (e.g., physiological, psychosocial, experiential, interpersonal, familial, and societal influences) that may potentially impact an individual's (family's) experience of the illness and treatment. Caregivers and patient are collaborators in diagnosis, treatment, and health maintenance. The biopsychosocial medicine approach emphasizes patient self-determination and the genetic and infertility counselor's role as a patient advocate, researcher, and healthcare professional providing supportive care, education, resources, and referrals.

The biopsychosocial medicine approach is the basis for a *multidisciplinary collaborative treatment approach*

that acknowledges the importance of a wide variety of medical professionals with specific expertise in providing optimum patient care. This approach minimizes rigid distinctions between fields (but not expertise), allowing genetic counselors to provide more psychological support or counseling; mental health professionals to provide more genetic education and assessment; and physicians the opportunity to address both medical genetics and emotional issues within the context of comprehensive patient care. A collaborative multidisciplinary team approach in reproductive medicine seems particularly applicable given the wide array of medical professionals: reproductive endocrinologists, urologists, perinatologists, nurses, andrologists, embryologists, laboratory technicians, mental health professionals, genetic counselors, and various support personnel (e.g., treatment coordinators).[29–31] Furthermore, a multidisciplinary collaborative approach provides a methodology for improving patient care through evidence-based medical care; the integration of research into clinical practice; and the development of system-based curriculum for training a variety of medical professionals.[32] This team approach to the care of infertile couples has gained increasing acceptance with a growing number of reproductive medicine practices using genetic counselors either as staff or consultants in North America, Europe, and Australia.

Recently there has been an effort to develop a specific *genetic counseling theoretical approach*. Using a grounded theory study approach, researchers[33] found that while the need for certainty was the most powerful factor motivating individuals to pursue genetic counseling, additional factors were the individual's lay knowledge of the condition and the ability of genetic counseling to satisfy the need for certainty. Also important was the formation of a personalized relationship between the client and the genetic counselor, which was found to significantly influence the central outcome, identified as a change in the client's psychological adaptation to the genetic condition in the family. Further formalizing the profession of genetic counseling has been the encouragement of cultural competency. To that end, genetic counselors are encouraged to (1) become aware of their personal cultural heritage and beliefs, particularly how these may impact their values and assumptions about human behavior and beliefs; (2) actively pursue training and education in multiculturalism; and (3) develop appropriate interventions skills for working with patients who are culturally differently.[34] It should be noted that although the principles of autonomy and patient-centered genetic counseling are highly valued in the North America, this is not a globally universal approach, a consideration that is important in terms of providing culturally sensitive genetic counseling (see Chapter 4).

CLINICAL ISSUES

Psychological Tasks of Reproductive Genetic Counseling

Genetic counselors use nondirective counseling to provide accurate information and identify all available options to facilitate informed decisions for individuals and/or couples.[35] Family factors (both good and bad) are often influential in the psychosocial adjustment of the infertile couple and are especially relevant if the genetic diagnosis affects the health or reproductive future of other family members. Hence, a myriad of family problems can be expected such as family secrets; dysfunctional communication patterns; inappropriate family reactions to stress and loss; boundary violations; divided family loyalties; and patterns of enmeshment and diffusions. Negative or inaccurate perceptions, religious values, or cultural beliefs about heredity, disability, and medical technologies can limit a couple's options and increase their emotional distress. Alternatively, a healthy family system; individual emotional well-being; and stable marital functioning can facilitate adjustment by reinforcing effective coping skills and encouraging adaptability and emotional warmth.[12]

The role of genetic testing, diagnosis, and treatment in reproductive medicine represents another area about which infertility counselors must be prepared to address complex biopsychosocial issues of childbearing and family-building. The couple presenting for infertility services may not know that they have a genetic disorder causing their infertility and may be predictably distressed when confronted with an unexpected *dual* diagnosis: infertility and a genetic disease. This can be even more distressing when the genetic diagnosis has health or reproductive consequences for other family members. Additionally, an increasing number of men and women seeking reproductive medicine treatments and/or infertility counseling may technically *not* be infertile and have other reasons for using assisted reproduction (e.g., during a previous marriage a partner had children and voluntary surgical sterilization). Thus, the psychosocial issues and needs of these individuals are different from the typical infertile patient. The couple with a genetic problem presenting for infertility counseling is more apt to focus on maximizing their opportunities of having a healthy, unaffected infant; exploring their feelings about raising a child affected with a genetic disease or disorder; and addressing their feel-

ings of guilt or anger at transmitting a genetic problem to their offspring. Marital or family-of-origin issues are more likely to focus expectations of 'normalcy' and 'acceptability' in babies or the impact of the diagnosis on other family members. In addition, a couple may have to consider the implications of the genetic disorder on the affected partner's health and longevity, as well as how the disorder may impact childbearing and childrearing decisions. The diagnosis of a genetic disorder that may impact the reproductive ability of other family members may make a couple's private trauma a public family drama, potentially destabilizing the family system and impairing the family's ability to support the couple and/or appropriately integrate the diagnosis into the family's identity. Finally, a healthy and enthusiastic altruistic gamete donor is, understandably, ill-prepared for the diagnosis of a problem – let alone a genetic disorder that may have major implications for his or her health, reproductive life, marital relationship, extended family, and psychosocial well-being. Understandably, these factors can and do trigger an array of psychological responses to genetic diagnosis including feelings of loss, grief, defectiveness, and or altered sense of self similar to those experienced by infertile individuals.

Deciding for or against Reproductive Genetic Counseling and Testing

There are an increasing number of reasons for reproductive genetic testing to be suggested or recommended within the context of reproductive medicine and, understandably, various reasons why individuals or couples may embrace, reject, or feel ambivalent about it. Genetic testing or counseling may be a diagnostic measure to determine or confirm the etiology of the infertility; an individual or couple may have a known family history of a genetic disorder that could be a causal factor in their infertility; or their medical history (e.g., azoospermia and repeated miscarriage) may warrant genetic testing. For many couples investigating a genetic component in the diagnosis of infertility may be viewed as just another medical test that may provide a diagnosis, and therefore, a treatment. Traumatized and stymied by the unknowns of their infertility, these couples typically look to modern medicine and technology as a source of comfort and hope. If technology can provide answers, they willingly pursue genetic testing and counseling in anticipation of gaining knowledge and control of an overwhelmingly ambiguous situation. Their approach may be that even if the information is negative, the information obtained may open other avenues of treatment and/or family building. This approach, which may be more common in the developed or Western cultures, is one in which reproductive and genetic technologies are viewed as providing hope and promise. As a result, there is the possibility of regret or social criticism if they *refuse* to use the technology.[36]

For other couples, the suggestion of genetic testing or counseling as part of the infertility diagnostic process may come as an unforeseen shock, triggering feelings of disbelief or even denial due to the implication of a deformity. These couples may be less comfortable with reproductive or genetic technologies and interpret the possibility of a genetic disorder as stigmatizing, shameful, or unlaterally unacceptable. They may prefer the 'unknown' to the 'known' for a variety of reasons including individual coping, family beliefs, religious or cultural traditions, or the social stigma of a genetic diagnosis or disorder. For these couples, information gained from genetic testing or counseling may be too costly, on too many levels and, as such, is not an option with which they can live or even realistically consider. For them, the threat of additional emotional trauma compounding those already experienced by infertility may be too overwhelming and threatening – either to the individual, their spouse, or even their marriage. Still others, ignorant of genetic counseling or testing, often find the prospect frightening and daunting and are suspicious or wary of the information gained from it. For example, couples from developing countries, traditional cultures, or with strong fundamentalist religious beliefs may be more skeptical of technology; the information it can provide; or the options available if the diagnosis is positive for a genetic disorder. They may have difficulty recognizing any personal or societal benefit in its use or may even suffer social sanctions for considering and/or using it. For these couples, the consideration or use of technological procedures may be more stressful and frightening experiences further complicated by language barriers, economic barriers, and/or lack of access to genetic counseling or testing.

Regardless of an infertile couple's approach to genetic testing, decision making about genetic counseling and testing typically triggers profound feelings of ambivalence. Fundamentally, infertility and genetic diagnoses imply flaw and/or failure, often precipitating feelings of shame, guilt, and abnormality. Inherent in genetic testing is the possibility and potential for narcissistic injury, loss of health, or negative social consequences (e.g., marriage or family) if a genetic disorder, disease, or anomaly is detected either in the individual, the couple, a pregnancy, or potential offspring. Ambivalence usually represents simultaneous feelings of security and self-protection in 'not knowing' and feelings of hope and relief in 'knowing' – having a definitive diagnosis.

Additionally, whether a couple decides for or against genetic testing or counseling, feelings of ambivalence may never completely dissipate. Ambivalence or even regret may remain after refusing testing or may remain after testing – particularly if the diagnosis is positive and has significant impact on the couple's family-building plans or a partner's health.

There is some evidence that men and women may view decisions about whether or not to pursue prenatal genetic counseling differently. One study[37] found that male partners tended to view the decision to prenatal testing as either an (1) information decision or (2) action decision. Men appeared to take a more active role in decision making when both partners viewed the decision as an action decision. For women, worry was the most important variable influencing decision making about prenatal testing. Women were also found to use more denial-using mechanisms, reporting that there could not possibly be anything wrong – even when there was evidence to the contrary.

Altered sense of self, stigma, and narcissistic injury as factors influencing decision making are apparent in a number of aspects of infertility but may be best demonstrated in male-factor infertility for two reasons: (1) there is growing evidence of genetic factors as a significant causal factor in male infertility and (2) there is considerable evidence that male-factor infertility is universally more stigmatizing to both men and women than female-factor infertility.[38] Frequently, wives may collude with their husbands to deny or minimize the male-factor infertility diagnosis or to identify a minor female-factor as the cause of the couple's childlessness. This 'protective dance' that couples do around male-factor infertility can have a significant impact on their reproductive decisions and their decision making process. Furthermore, this protective dance is often influenced by religious or cultural beliefs or traditions and has been shown to be more evident in male-dominated, traditional cultures (see Chapters 3 and 4). For example, it is common for wives to proceed with reproductive treatments with which they are uncomfortable to protect the relationship and/or the husband's sense of self or his standing in their community or family. By the same token, husbands often refuse to consider reproductive technologies that involve the relinquishment of a genetically-related offspring or refuse to acknowledge the ramifications of the male-factor infertility diagnosis, often using reassurances such as 'it only takes one sperm.' These issues become even more relevant if responses to genetic diagnosis trigger strong feelings of responsibility, guilt, and defectiveness in the identified patient, and blame, shame, and resentment in their spouse, or they are bound by cultural or religious traditions that disallow assisted reproduction remedies.

There is considerable evidence that infertile couples' reproductive decisions are less likely to be influenced by statistical probability of genetic abnormality and more likely to be influenced by qualitative factors such as a couple's or individual's interpretation or perception of risks;[39–41] desire to have a child;[39] the perceived consequences of having a disabled child, with its impact on marital, family, and the child's quality of life;[42] and the perceived burden of the genetic condition.[41] For many infertile couples, deciding to proceed with genetic testing or counseling is an excruciating decision, usually influenced by past infertility experiences; phase of mourning the losses of infertility; personal identity issues; medical recommendations or indications; and willingness of partners to acknowledge and accept a genetic component to their infertility.[1] The challenges and pressures of infertility may leave couples ill-equipped to cope with the potential losses inherent in genetic screening or testing. Already overwhelmed by grief or emotional distress, couples may engage in avoidance or have profound ambivalence reflecting their inability to assimilate or process the implications or ramifications of genetic screening or diagnosis. Acknowledging the need for self-protective measures and the normalcy of ambivalence may reduce anxiety and distress or help individuals identify and grapple with these feelings. Alternatively, profound ambivalence, avoidance, and self-protection may also reflect more deep-seated emotional or marital problems warranting psychotherapeutic intervention.

Emotional Response to Diagnosis of Genetic Disorder

Although it has been known for some time that genetic disorders and diseases can cause or impair reproduction, recent advances in genetics (e.g., mapping of the human genome) have led to the identification of an increasing number of genetic causes or factors contributing to impaired fertility in men and women. However, when genetic factors are determined to be the etiology of failed or impaired reproduction, significant emotional consequences are common. Although a genetic diagnosis may confirm an individual's infertility or sterility, providing definition to an ambiguous and distressing situation, it is typically an unexpected diagnosis having an impact on not only the infertile man or woman's health but also the health of future pregnancies and children and/or other family members.

A diagnosis of a genetic disorder or disease in an individual, partner, or potential offspring can precipitate a personal crisis and endanger the stability of a marriage and even extended family relationships. As such, assistance and interventions should be directed at help-

ing the couple cope with their acute distress, anxiety, and uncertainty as they struggle with making decisions and deal with the aftermath of the diagnosis.[43] The scarcity of support and understanding for this unique crisis and vulnerability to feelings of stigma, shame, and secrecy highlight the importance of a referral to an appropriate mental health professional (i.e., infertility counselor) and/or support group, the use of patient education materials, and collaboration or other caregivers and support networks.[43]

Family factors are often influential in the psychosocial adjustment of infertile couples and are especially relevant if the genetic diagnosis affects other family members or precipitates a family crisis. As such, the emergence of myriad family problems can be expected, such as disclosure of family secrets; dysfunctional communication patterns; inappropriate family reactions to stress and loss (particularly infertility and/or pregnancy loss); boundary violations; divided family loyalties; parental guilt for causing the genetic disorder; and patterns of enmeshment and diffusion. Negative or inaccurate family beliefs regarding heredity, illness, and disability, childbearing expectations, kinship ties, and medical technologies (e.g., genetic testing and/or diagnosis and assisted reproduction) may impair a couple's adjustment by limiting their options and increasing their distress. Alternatively, family values, expectations, and resources may facilitate a couple's adjustment by reinforcing effective coping skills; encouraging adaptability to change; providing emotional warmth and support; and modeling positive mental health habits.

Learning that one has a genetic disorder or is a carrier of one, has the potential for profoundly altering one's sense of self, altering the individual's perception of his or her genetic identity as well as social identity, health, and well-being. Ultimately, the diagnosis of a genetic disorder or carrier status can and does threaten reproductive ability and choices, impacting not only the individual's reproductive future but also relationships with his or her spouse and partners and extended family members.[44] As such, the diagnosis of a genetic disorder or disease can precipitate a crisis potentially endangering the stability of the individual, marriage, or family system. Assistance and interventions should be directed at helping the individuals and/or couple cope and manage their acute distress, anxiety, and uncertainty as they struggle with making decisions and dealing with the aftermath of the diagnosis as well as any chronic distress stemming from their decisions.[43] A scarcity of support or understanding about this unique crisis (e.g., diagnosis of a fetal abnormality or genetic cause of infertility) and vulnerability to feelings of stigma, shame, and secrecy, highlight the importance of identifying 'at-risk' individuals and a collaborative approach to patient care.

Genetic assisted reproductive technologies can be fraught with potential abuses, conflicts, discriminations, and misuses and involve legal and moral dilemmas. The majority of infertility treatment is still geared toward the woman; available to individuals with financial resources or geographic access to treatment facilities; unevenly available to minority populations; and remains personally, socially, and culturally humiliating. An increasing number of participants are using the internet to make reproductive arrangements contributing to reproductive tourism: couples and individuals crossing geographic boundaries to pursue reproductive agendas that are illegal, unacceptable, or unavailable in their homeland. However, this may lead to misuses of the technology through the devaluation and stigmatization of people with genetic disorders; the assumption that a genetic condition can and should be avoided such as cultural preference for a specific gender; and/or the use of reproductive or prenatal technologies to foster a social environment that is intolerant of disabled individuals.

The primary goals of reproductive genetic counseling are ensuring that patients considering any procedure (e.g., genetic testing, PGD, prenatal testing, assisted reproductive) understand the scope and ramifications of the testing and that they have realistic expectations of success rates, financial cost, and the timeframe of treatment. Whatever reproductive procedures the patients are pursuing, they should be informed about other reproductive and family-building alternatives. Additionally, because many patients with genetic disorders are unfamiliar with assisted reproduction and the treatment process, counseling should review all applicable forms of assisted and third-party reproduction (e.g., IVF, IVF/ICSI, PGD). The psychosocial aspects of treatment should also be reviewed including what may be stressful about treatment, and coping strategies should be introduced or reviewed. Finally, the possibility of treatment failure should be addressed and appropriate supportive and therapeutic counseling offered. This includes the offer of ongoing supportive or therapeutic counseling with an infertility counselor during treatment or as a resource in the event treatment is unsuccessful. Furthermore, patients should be provided appropriate bereavement and crisis intervention counseling, when appropriate.

THERAPEUTIC INTERVENTIONS

To aid in patient care and highlight the overlapping roles of genetic and infertility counselors, Shapiro and Djurdjinovic[1] outlined the psychosocial issues of genetic counseling for infertile couples. They pointed out how the emotional vulnerability and reproductive history of infertile couples alters their perspective on genetic and reproductive medicine, often resulting in unrealistic expectations and decisions based on hope versus reality. In fact, research has shown that infertile couples consistently *overestimate* the success rates of reproductive technologies while *underestimating* the risks of transmission or impact of genetic diagnosis. In addition, they make decisions influenced more by the perceived burden of a condition than by the actual numerical risk.[45] It is against this backdrop of high expectations, prior narcissistic wounds, lengthy history of medical treatment, and impaired information processing that genetic and infertility counselors provide assistance to individuals seeking reproductive services whether or not they have an infertility diagnosis.

Genetic counseling provides a unique structured setting for the provision of education and assessment of the risks of and/or diagnosis of genetic disorders. If a genetic disorder is suspected or has been identified, risks for recurrence or transmission and education regarding the diagnosed disorder are addressed. Options regarding prenatal screening, testing, and possible diagnosis are also typically explored. In addition, reproductive options are reviewed with the couple, including ARTs, third-party reproduction, and adoption all as viable family-building alternatives. Within this context, it is ethically and clinically responsible to facilitate exploration of religious or personal ethics, internal context reproductive goals, feasible medical treatments, availability of family support, acceptability of prenatal genetic testing, and possible test results (with perceived emotional response of the patient/family). Finally, the genetic counselor assesses the emotional response, reactivity, and receptivity of the individuals; their response as a couple and to each other; and their preparedness for pregnancy or ARTs. Working within the collaborative reproductive team, an individual or couple with a reproductive genetic issue may be referred to an infertility counselor, appropriate support organization, or other members of the reproductive treatment team (e.g., perinataologist) for additional assessment or assistance.

All too frequently, the identification of an actual or potential genetic issue as part of their reproductive treatment plan is something very few involuntarily childless couples anticipate. Typically, they are ill-prepared for a potential genetic problem let alone the diagnosis of a genetic cause of their infertility; the possibility of a health problem in addition to a genetic disorder; and/or the issue of their potential offspring having a genetic disorder. As such, referral for genetic counseling can be met with an array of emotional responses including psychological resistance, refusal, anger, denial, confusion, and alarm. Not surprisingly, spouses often react differently, further complicating the process and making information gathering, assessment, and provision of diagnostic information more challenging. Within this context, issues of recall and comprehension of information conveyed in genetic counseling; decision making processes; coping with threatening events; family dynamics; and risk perception can further complicate the experience. Psychological aspects of genetic counseling include the meaning of the genetic information and of illness/disability; patient and families' adaptation to stressful events and illness/imperfection; and reactions to uncertainty. Infertility counselors provide support and collaborate with genetic counselors in addition to providing an array of psychotherapeutic interventions.

In the past, men and women with a chromosomal problem, genetically-transmittable heritable disorder, or genetic causes of infertility had few family-building alternatives: childlessness, adoption, donated gametes, or repeated 'trial' pregnancies involving prenatal testing and termination of affected pregnancies. Today, with the availability of a wide array of ARTs including IVF, ICSI, PGD and prenatal tests, couples previously unable to reproduce or have a healthy child, have new avenues and opportunities for achieving parenthood and having healthy offspring. However, while ARTs can facilitate parenthood for a variety of conditions (both genetic and nongenetic), there is some concern that ARTs, in and of themselves, may actually cause congenital malformations. There is some evidence of genetic and congenital anomalies after IVF and/or ICSI due to identified genetic disorders *or* as a result of the procedure itself (e.g., imprinting defects). Although inconclusive, some studies have indicated that children conceived via IVF and/or ICSI may be at increased risk of major and/or rare birth defects (e.g., Angelman syndrome and Beckwith Wiedemann syndrome).[46–49] Furthermore, ARTs treatments can be expensive; not easily or universally accessible; inapplicable to a couple's unique circumstance (e.g., legally restricted or regulated); or simply unacceptable, impossible, or objectionable for a variety of reasons (e.g., culture and religion).[50] As such, the provision of genetic counseling about ARTs must include the psychosocial impact of the diagnosis as well as available assisted reproduction remedies, enabling couples to make a decision that is comfortable and appropriate for them.

In summary, although the use of ARTs for couples faced with a genetic cause of infertility is feasible, it is a complicated process and thus, genetic in addition to infertility counseling, are warranted. It is interesting to note that despite education on the genetic

risks, even in the face of possible abnormalities associated with a known genetic disorder, 71% of couples expressed *no* interest in formal genetic counseling or psychological support counseling.[51] The majority of couples were found to almost universally prefer to have a genetically-shared child, even if it involved transmitting an unknown genetic disorder, and only willing to consider the use of donated gametes for financial, cultural, or religious reasons.[51,52] This may reflect high levels of denial and defensiveness commonly seen in infertile couples and/or individuals with genetic diagnoses. However, it may also indicate that despite clinical and professional recommendations about the importance of genetic and infertility counseling in reproductive medicine, caregivers' efforts to ensure patients take part in genetic and/or infertility counseling have been inadequate or ineffective.[53,54]

Clinical applications of genetic counseling in reproductive medicine run the gamut of services with genetic counselors and infertility counselors providing a wide variety of patient care in a wide array of circumstances. Areas in which genetic and infertility counseling intertwine include:

- preconception genetic counseling;
- reproductive genetic counseling, specifically involving genetic causes of male and female infertility requiring the use of ARTs and third-party reproduction;
- prenatal genetic counseling and testing including continuing or terminating an affected pregnancy and loss of an affected pregnancy;
- gamete and embryo donor genetic screening.

Preconception Genetic Counseling

Preconception genetic counseling refers to the preparation and education about any definable increased risk for a fetal genetic disorder that may be diagnosed by one or more methods for men and women who are considering pregnancy.[55] Although some couples may or may not be aware of their fertility status before seeking genetic counseling, most often, preconception genetic counseling is sought by couples who are aware they have a genetic condition or disease or are carriers of one. As such, they want to be informed about the impact of their condition or carrier status on their reproductive ability or, most commonly, the risk of transmission of the disorder to their offspring. Additionally, there is a growing trend among older first-time parents to obtain preconception genetic counseling so as to be best informed about having the healthiest baby and/or pregnancy possible.

Some couples purposefully pursue preconception counseling because they are aware of a genetic disorder in themselves or family and, as a result, find the information obtained through the process sobering but unsurprising. Some of these couples are reassured by the information that the risk of recurrence is lower than they expected, while others interpret the same information as a significant (and alarming) risk. Other couples, particularly those with a perfunctory approach to preconception counseling, may be surprised and distressed when a significant problem is identified about which they were unaware and for which they are unprepared. Couples with no identifiable risk factors may interpret the preconception counseling as a reassuring start for their planned pregnancy, although they may also interpret this information as a guarantee of a healthy baby without any reproductive misadventures.

Performing preconception genetic counseling prior to pregnancy helps reduce the risk of having an affected child for couples who have a genetic disorder, or who are known carriers of a gene that could be transmitted to offspring. Preconception genetic counseling allows couples to consider their alternatives including remaining childless or using other family-building alternatives such as third-party reproduction, adoption, or ARTs (e.g., PGD). For other couples, preconception counseling allows them to make an informed decision to pursue a pregnancy with a 75% chance (in the case of autosomal recessive conditions) of having an unaffected child. Some of these couples may elect prenatal screening to allow preparation for having a child with a genetic condition or the termination of the affected pregnancy. These complex scenarios highlight the need for patient care that is collaborative involving infertility and genetic counselors, members of the reproductive and/or maternal/fetal medicine team, as well as medical caregivers for a specific genetic disorder.

Preconception is also the optimal time to review the importance of rubella immunity (to reduce the risk of congenital anomalies associated with exposure) and folic acid supplementation (0.4 mg/day to reduce the risk of neural tube defects; 4 mg/day if there is a history of a previously affected child). It also provides the opportunity to address the risks associated with tobacco, alcohol, recreational drug usage (e.g., cannabis), and medications (e.g., antidepressants), and to point out that all pregnancies carry a 3–5% risk of congenital anomaly. Additional risks that should be addressed include the increasing risk of fetal trisomy; miscarriage due to advancing maternal age; and the greater occurrence of certain genetic disorders within specific ethnic backgrounds (many of these disorders also have preconception screening options). Preconception counseling involves a thorough history, including the medical, social, and reproductive histories of both partners.

Family History

A family medical history is an essential part of a preconception visit. Information on birth defects, mental retardation, genetic disease, reproductive history, general health, and causes of death should be ascertained for three generations. The careful analysis of a family history allows for discussion of risk for recurrence and available genetic testing options. Regardless of the reason for preconception genetic counseling, performing this analysis prior to conception allows for discussion of all pertinent issues in the absence of the stress and time constraints of a pregnancy or in the midst of infertility treatments. When a condition is identified in the family for which testing is available, the testing process is often complex, time-consuming, and can involve multiple family members. If initiated prior to pregnancy, all reproductive options are available to the couple. If concerns are identified while assessing the family history, a referral to a genetic specialist is a consideration. Additionally, if unknown fertility concerns are discovered, the genetic counselor may work in coloboration with the infertility counselor and other members of the reproductive team to assure that appropriate referrals are made and treatments pursued. Similarly, if the pedigree analysis indicates significant risk factors, the genetic counselor may work with the reproductive treatment team to address other family-building alternatives for the couple such as third-party reproduction (e.g., donor gametes or gestational carrier), ARTs (e.g., IVF or IVF/PGD), adoption, and/or childlessness.

Age

Patient age is important, particularly the age of the female member of the couple seeking preconception counseling. As all women get older, the chance of having a child born with a chromosomal trisomy increases (see Tables 15.1 and 15.2), with trisomy 21

TABLE 15.1. Risk of having a live baby with any chromosomal problem[56]	
Age	Births per 1000
20	1.9
25	2.1
30	2.6
35	5.2
40	15.2
45	47.6

TABLE 15.2. Risk of Down syndrome live birth[56]	
Age	Risk
20	1/1923
30	1/885
35	1/365
40	1/109
45	1/32
49	1/12

(Down syndrome), trisomy 18 (Edward's syndrome), trisomy 13 (Pateau syndrome), 47, XXY (Klinefelter syndrome), and 47, XXX being the most common.[56] It is also notable that miscarriage rates also increase with maternal age, from about 15% for women under thirty to about 30–40% for women aged forty.[57] This is a factor that comes into consideration as the genetic and fertility counselors work together to offer reproductive modalities that are most appropriate for the couple. Advanced paternal age does not appear to carry the same increased risk of trisomy as advanced maternal age, although there is evidence of increased risk for autosomal dominant diseases (e.g., Marfan syndrome, neurofibromatosis, achondroplasia, and Apert syndrome). However, routine screening for these disorders is generally not recommended as practical because the risk is small in the absence of a family history.[58,59]

Most women are increasingly aware of the designator 'advanced maternal age,' usually defined as thirty-five years or older at the time of delivery, but many couples do not fully comprehend the implications of age for themselves and/or their pregnancies. There are many misperceptions, both positive and negative, about advancing maternal age. Having a clear understanding of the involved risk may actually relieve anxiety for some couples. Preconception counseling can help couples better understand the array of prenatal screening and testing options available for pregnancies in women of advanced maternal age. While some tests are performed early in a pregnancy, tests performed later in pregnancy are so distressing that discussion of testing options and timing prior to pregnancy can help couples sufficiently contemplate and consider which approach best suit their needs and values.

Ethnic Background

Individuals and/or couples from specific ethnic groups are at greater risk for genetic conditions and, as such, should be educated about and offered preconception screening. Genetic disorders common to certain ethnic backgrounds for which screening should be offered include:[55,60]

- *African ancestry* – Sickle cell anemia, beta thalassemia, Hemoglobin C trait, alpha thalassemia
- *East Asian and Southeast Asian ancestry* – beta thalassemia, Hemoglobin E, alpha thalassemia, Hemoglobin H disease
- *French Canadian and Cajun ancestry* – Tay Sachs disease, cystic fibrosis
- *Hispanic ancestry* – Sickle cell anemia, Hemoglobin C, and beta thalassemia
- *Ashkenazi Jewish ancestry* – Tay Sachs disease, Canavan disease, cystic fibrosis, familial dysautonomia
- *Mediterranean ancestry* – beta thalassemia, alpha thalassemia, sickle cell disease, structural hemoglobin variants (Hemoglobins S, D, G and Lepore)
- *Middle Eastern and South Central Asian ancestry* – beta thalassemia, alpha thalassemia, sickle cell anemia
- *European ancestry* – Cystic fibrosis, individuals with ancestors from Southern Europe may also be at increased risk for several hemoglobinopathies associated with Mediterranean ancestry

Additionally, in 2001, the American College of Medical Genetics (ACMG), along with American College of Obstetricians and Gynecologists (ACOG), recommended that carrier testing for cystic fibrosis be offered to non-Jewish Caucasians and Ashkenazi Jews, and be made available to other ethnic and racial groups.[61] Screening is complicated by the fact that the detection rate for cystic fibrosis carriers varies among individuals of differing ethnicities[62] and, therefore, a thoughtful discussion with a genetic counselor is of great necessity.

All of the above-listed conditions demonstrate autosomal recessive inheritance, meaning both members of a couple must be carriers of a specific gene in order to have a child affected with the condition although there is usually not anyone in the family history reported to be affected with the condition. Some couples may wish to pursue genetic testing to determine their carrier status. If both prospective parents are carriers for the same autosomal recessive condition, they have a 25% risk with each pregnancy of having a child affected with that condition.

In summary, preconception genetic counseling helps couples:

- comprehend the medical facts, including any genetic diagnosis, probable cause of the disorder, and available management;
- identify potential pregnancy risks;

■ appreciate the way in which heredity contributes to the disorder and the risk of occurrence or recurrence in specific relatives;

■ develop a plan of care regarding the pregnancy risks identified;

■ understand the options for dealing with the risk of recurrence including prenatal genetic diagnosis;

■ make decisions regarding risk assessment and options available;

■ make the best possible adjustment to the disorder in an affected family member and the risk of recurrence in another family member.

Preconception genetic counseling and testing has become an increasingly common part of the infertility diagnosis work-up and, as such, is potentially beneficial as both a diagnostic tool and a patient education measure.

Reproductive Genetic Counseling

Genetic Causes of Male-Factor Infertility and ARTs

The genetics of male-factor infertility can be divided into four main categories: (1) chromosome abnormalities (e.g., Klinefelter syndrome); (2) microdeletions in the Y chromosomes; (3) congenital bilateral absence of vas deferens (CBAVD)/cystic fibrosis; and (4) rare genetic syndromes. The reproductive impairment for men with genetic causes of infertility typically involves the failure to produce sperm; the failure of sperm-transport (obstruction in the male reproductive tract (vas deferens); and/or the risk of transmission of a genetic disorder to offspring. Donor sperm has a long history as an expeditious and inexpensive method of family-building that prevents the transmission of the husband's genetic disorder and allows couples to share the pregnancy experience (see Chapter 17). However, it means that the husband must to relinquish having a child to whom he is genetically-linked and who is genetically-shared with his spouse.

Today, ARTs can facilitate biological parenthood for infertile men by enabling them to have a genetically-related child; overcoming sperm penetration, count, and mobility problems; and reducing or eliminating the risk of transmitting their genetic disorder to any offspring. For men with azoospermia (no sperm) or low sperm counts (oligospermia), sperm can be retrieved through aspiration using microsurgical epididymal sperm aspiration (MESA) or testicular sperm extraction (TESE). Fertilization can be achieved through the use of sperm injection into the oocyte using intracytoplasmic sperm injection (ICSI) during IVF (i.e., IVF/ICSI). Despite these advances, assisted reproduction does not overcome the genetic disorder causing infertility: Affected men still have a chromosomal abnormality (and concomitant health problems), and, consequently, their offspring may be at risk of the disorder as well.

Genetic counseling for male-factor infertility not only involves the implications of the diagnosis but also implications for the future: pregnancies, reproduction, health, and other family members. Furthermore, although IVF/ICSI may facilitate reproduction for men with low sperm counts, there is evidence of significantly higher incidence of de-novo chromosomal abnormalities in ICSI offspring, including a higher number of sex chromosome abnormalities, structural chromosome abnormalities, and observed inherited anomalies related to a higher rate of constitutional chromosomal abnormalities in the fathers. As such, it would appear that couples considering IVF/ICSI should be informed of the risks of an abnormal chromosome and encouraged to consider genetic testing as well as prenatal testing, if conception occurs as a result of ARTs treatment.[63]

Chromosome abnormalities. Klinefelter syndrome (also known as hypogonadism) is a chromosomal disorder affecting males born with a karyotype of 47, XXY (or an extra X chromosome) resulting in a range of symptoms including small testes, absence of sperm, enlarged breasts, high levels of FSH (follicle-stimulating hormone), learning disabilities, and behavioral problems. Because of other health issues, Klinefelter syndrome is typically, but not always, a condition diagnosed before the man seeks infertility treatment. Klinefelter syndrome is the most common chromosomal disorder impacting reproduction in men, affecting 1 in 1,000, causing impaired spermatogenesis, infertility, and azoospermia due to the extra X chromosome and abnormal testicular development.

For males with chromosome abnormalities due to chromosome translocations, future pregnancies are at risk for miscarriage or congenital abnormalities should a fetus inherit an unbalanced form of the translocation. Although assisted reproduction using sperm aspiration may facilitate pregnancy, it may also facilitate the transmission of a genetic disorder that was previously undetected and/or untransmittable. Assisted reproduction does not overcome the genetic disorder causing infertility: Affected men still have a chromosomal abnormality (and concomitant health problems), and, consequently, their offspring remain at risk of inheriting the disorder or developing an unknown variation of it. They also are in need and must be made aware of ongoing medical care for their own health even after parenthood has been achieved. For men who are aware of their diagnosis and wish to use their own sperm, IVF/PGD allows them to have a genetically-linked child through technology that identifies and uses only unaffected embryos.[64]

Y-microdeletions. Another genetic cause of male-factor infertility are malformations on the Y chromosome, where several genes have been identified as playing an important role in spermatogenesis. Specifically, microdeletions of the Y chromosome, in the region of Y chromosome called AZFa, AZFb and AZFc, cause azoospermia or severe oligospermia[65] in 9–18%.[66,67] Interestingly, apart from the failed spermatogenesis or severe oligospermia, men with microdeletions of the Y chromosome have not been identified as having any other health or genetic problems. Sperm donation is one means of family-building for this condition, or couples may choose to use IVF/ICSI following sperm retrieval using MESA or TESE. However, sons conceived via this method may be at high risk of inheriting their father's same Y chromosome microdeletion. As such, it is recommended that couples considering this treatment be counseled about the possibility of transmission of the same defect to their sons and how this may impact their son's potential fertility.[50,68] Alternatively, IVF/PGD may be a treatment option for men with Y microdeletions to reduce the risk of transmission of the disorder, typically by selecting only female embryos for transfer.

Congenital bilateral absence of the vas deferens (CBAVD). CBAVD is the most common form of obstructive azoospermia, occurring in about 1–2% of all infertile men. Men with CBAVD have one or more mutations in the CFTR (cystic fibrosis transmembrane conductance regulator) gene with approximately 60–70% of men with CBAVD carrying at least one mutation of the cystic fibrosis gene and 10–20% carrying two mutations. CBAVD is sometimes referred to as 'genital cystic fibrosis' because men with the disorder are often asymptomatic of cystic fibrosis apart from azoospermia.[69] Approximately 50% of apparently healthy men with an absent vas deferens have mutations in the cystic fibrosis gene, albeit not a classical presentation of CF.[70,71] As such, these men face not only the diagnosis of cystic fibrosis but also the potential risk of transmitting cystic fibrosis (or CF gene mutation) to their offspring. Cystic fibrosis is inherited in an autosomal recessive pattern, and thus CF carrier testing should be offered to the female partner to assess the couple's risk of having a child with either classical or nonclassical cystic fibrosis. If female partners are also carriers,

couples have a 25% chance of having a child with this genetic disorder, which is typically a very serious disease, and a 50% chance of having a child who is also a carrier.

Sperm donation is one family-building alternative for men with CBAVD as is IVF/ICSI following sperm retrieval using MESA or TESE, particularly if the wife is not a CF carrier. IVF/PGD is also a viable option for couples with CBAVD as a cause of their infertility. Genetic counseling for these couples involves addressing a number of issues including: (1) the dual diagnosis of a chronic medical condition (CF) and sterility; (2) the risk that other family members may also be at risk for undiagnosed CF; and (3) the risk of transmitting CF to offspring if the couple or man decides to use his own sperm. These couples warrant genetic testing and counseling, as these individuals (and their partners) need to be aware of the risk of genetic transmission of the disease as well as potentially serious health issues.

Genetic syndromes. There are numerous other rare conditions that are associated with male infertility. These include, but are not limited to: Kartagener syndrome, myotonic dystrophy, adrenomyeloneropathy, and androgen receptor mutations seen in spinal and bulbar muscular atrophy. Typically, these conditions are diagnosed in childhood (before men reach childbearing age) as the conditions involve a variety of health concerns and treatments. As such, infertility is a secondary diagnosis and a consequence of the genetic syndrome. For example, individuals with Kartagener syndrome (a condition characterized by abnormal cilia) become symptomatic during childhood with chronic ear infections, rhinitism, and sinusitis. Thus, men are typically aware of the genetic diagnosis prior to their presentation at the infertility clinic, although they (and/or their partners) may or may not be aware of how their genetic condition can or does impact their reproductive ability. The inheritance pattern of any given genetic syndrome varies, and genetic counseling to review and/or clarify risks to future offspring is recommended. Reproductive options for these men include donor sperm, MESA/TESE for sperm retrieval, and IVF/ICSI to facilitate fertilization. Additionally, IVF/PGD may be a viable option for men with genetic syndromes in which there is an identified genetic disorder.

Genetic Causes of Female-Factor Infertility and ARTs
The genetic causes of female-factor infertility include: (1) chromosome abnormalities (e.g., Turner syndrome); (2) genetic syndromes (e.g., Rokitansky-Küster-Hauser syndrome, Fragile X); and (3) congenital adrenal hyperplasia (CAH) (e.g., polycystic ovary syndrome (PCOS).

Reproductive impairment for women with genetic causes of infertility typically involve disorders that impair the development and functioning of female organs (e.g., mullerian anomalies, feminization and ambiguous genitalia) resulting in absence of or defective reproductive organs; hormone regulation that impairs reproduction (e.g., advanced maternal age or premature ovarian failure); or genetic disorders in which pregnancy would impair the woman's health and/or the health of the pregnancy or infant due to the transmission of the genetic disorder to offspring. In the past, women with genetic conditions and/or causes for infertility had few family-building options apart from adoption. Recently, ARTs and third-party reproduction can facilitate biological parenthood for infertile women by enabling them to have a genetically-related child; and helping them overcome hormone production problems and even absent or defective reproductive organs; as well as reducing or eliminating the risk of transmitting their genetic disorder or a chromosomal anomaly due to advanced maternal age to their offspring. For women with impaired ovulatory function, medications with or without IVF can facilitate reproduction, or if the woman is unable to produce healthy oocytes due to absent or underfunctioning ovaries, donated oocytes is a family-building alternative. Although oocyte donation allows women to reproduce by experiencing pregnancy, it also means the relinquishment of a child to whom she is genetically-linked or one that is genetically-shared with her spouse (see Chapter 18). For women without a uterus or unable to carry a pregnancy, gestational carrier or surrogacy are family-building options albeit options in which she must relinquish the pregnancy experience. Using a gestational carrier, a woman is able to have a genetically-shared pregnancy with her spouse, while surrogacy allows the couple to have a child that is genetically-linked to her husband but not her (see Chapter 21). Finally, although these forms of third-party reproduction enable a woman to build a family, they do not eliminate her genetic disorder or age-related reproduction issues. As such, IVF/PGD can be helpful for identifying genetically-affected embryos and selecting unaffected embryos for transfer to the genetic mother or a gestational carrier.

While complex reproductive technologies and third-party reproduction can, and do, facilitate family-building, the fact remains that they do not alter the underlying genetic disorder or condition causing infertility and/or the risk of transmission of the disorder to offspring, if women use their own oocytes. Furthermore, none of the technologies are foolproof or fail-safe and, as such, even with these treatments, conception and/or pregnancy may not occur and the birth of a healthy child cannot be assumed. Therefore, genetic counseling and additional prenatal testing after pregnancy are warranted – although typically not considered by the majority of infertile couples who have gone to great lengths to have a child using ARTs and often feel that pregnancy, not the birth of a healthy baby, is the goal. Thus, genetic counseling for female-factor infertility (as for male-factor) involves not only the implications of the diagnosis, but also implications for the future: pregnancies, reproduction, health, and other family members.

Chromosome abnormalities. Similar to male-factor infertility, women with chromosomal abnormalities, which result in infertility, can be due to either structural rearrangements (i.e., translocations) or chromosome aneuploidy. Women who carry balanced chromosome translocations are predisposed to extremely early miscarriages, often before they are even aware of the pregnancy. Again, the diagnosis of a chromosome translocation also carries risks for first-trimester miscarriages and/or a pregnancy with multiple congenital anomalies. With these disorders, psychological issues typically involve personal identity, reproductive choices, and sexual functioning, as well as medical or surgical treatment. And while assisted reproduction may help many women with genetic disorders become biological mothers, the risk of transmission of the disorder to offspring remains an important consideration for them and their partners, especially if the women plan to use their own oocytes. If women decide to use donated oocytes, it involves not only complex medical treatments but also the relinquishment of a genetically-linked child. Additionally, many of these conditions involve other health considerations.

Turner syndrome (45, X) is a the most common genetic cause of reproductive failure in women and is associated with heart and kidney abnormalities, webbing of the neck, small stature, and primary amenorrhea. It is a chromosomal disorder marked by the absence of all or part of one of the two X chromosomes. In most but not all cases, women with this condition have very early loss of all oocytes, so that at birth the residual ovarian tissue is small (streak ovaries) and nonfunctional. Because the fallopian tubes, uterus, cervix, and vagina are formed independently from the ovaries, pregnancy is a viable option for women with this condition as long as donor oocytes are used. Women with variations (mosaic) Turner syndrome (45, X/46, XX) are often asymptomatic and normal-appearing and, as such, may present to an infertility clinic seeking services, unaware they have a genetic disorder. Women with Turner syndrome may occasionally conceive, although there is a risk of transmitting the disorder or chromosomal disorder to their offspring. For most with Turner syndrome, however, motherhood is best achieved through IVF using donated oocytes as it prevents the transmission of the genetic disorder to any offspring, yet enables family-building via pregnancy. However, pregnancy in women with Turner syndrome has been reported to increase the risk of death due to aortic rupture or dissection during pregnancy – an underlying condition that may be overlooked prior to pursuing assisted reproduction or pregnancy.[72]

With these genetic disorders, psychological issues typically involve personal identity, reproductive choices, and sexual functioning, as well as medical or surgical treatment. And while assisted reproduction may help many women with these genetic disorders become biological mothers, the risk of transmission of the disorder to offspring remains an important consideration, especially if the plan is to use the woman's own oocytes. If the woman decides to use donated oocytes, it involves not only complex medical treatments (oocyte retrieval for the donor, medical treatment for the woman, and coordination of their reproductive cycles) but also the relinquishment of a genetically-linked child. Furthermore, many of these conditions involve ongoing health concerns and treatments for the woman.

Genetic syndromes. There are numerous genetic syndromes that can result in female infertility. One example is Rokitansky-Küster-Hauser syndrome. This syndrome is a congenital defect of the female reproductive tract in which the ovaries are normal but the uterus, cervix, and most of the vagina are abnormal or absent. Women with this disorder have all of the secondary external characteristics of womanhood including breasts, clitoris, and vulva. Typically, a young woman is not diagnosed with this disorder until adolescence, when she fails to menstruate or encounters acute pain during a pelvic exam or sexual activity. Because they have normally functioning ovaries, women with Rokitansky-Küster-Hauser syndrome may achieve parenthood through the fertilization of their own oocytes via IVF and the assistance of a gestational carrier who bears the pregnancy. Although gestational carriers can provide a biological child, this method of third-party reproduction means the relinquishment of the pregnancy experience. Genetic counseling should address the risk of transmission to any offspring. Additionally, these women also have ongoing health concerns and issues apart from their reproductive goals.

Another example of female infertility due to a genetic cordation is Fragile X syndrome. Interestingly, premature ovarian failure (POF) has been associated with an increased incidence of female carriers for Fragile X syndrome.[73] Thus, women who are found to be carriers for Fragile X syndrome, often as the result of a family history of Fragile X syndrome and/or mental retardation in males, should be counseled accordingly about their risk for premature ovarian failure, as well as the risks of future sons having Fragile X syndrome. Reproductive choices for these women may be donated oocytes that would not only facilitate parenthood but also eliminate the risk of transmission of the genetic disorder to offspring. Other couples may choose to use IVF/PGD to select only female embryos for transfer to avoid the transmission of Fragile X syndrome.

Congenital adrenal hyperplasia (CAH). Congenital adrenal hyperplasia, or CAH, is an autosomal recessive genetic disorder that causes defects in the enzymes of the adrenal cortex required for cortisol production. Polycystic ovary syndrome (PCOS) a common cause of female infertility, is also associated with a nonclassical form of CAH. The clinical severity of CAH has a large range, and typically women with the nonclassical form of CAH and polycystic ovaries present with premature puberty, hirsutism, and severe cystic acne. However, women with nonclassical CAH can be at risk of having a child with a more severe form of CAH involving the inability to metabolize salt and ambiguous genitalia. Carrier screening for the woman's partner should be made available to assess recurrence risk implications. Genetic counseling regarding the diagnosis of CAH in conjunction with infertility treatment and, perhaps, the diagnosis of PCOS should address both the woman's feelings about her health concerns and reproductive options. Typically women with PCOS are treated with ovulation-stimulating hormones that may or may not involve IVF. Depending on a woman's risk factors, IVF/PGD may be the most appropriate treatment. For some women, the best treatment is the use of donated oocytes facilitating motherhood, yet eliminating the risk of transmitting a genetic disorder. However, as with many genetic disorders, health issues and ongoing medical care may be necessary even after reproductive goals have been achieved.

Preimplantation Genetic Diagnosis and Screening
Preimplantation genetic diagnosis (PGD) was developed in 1989 by British physician Alan Handyside to screen for a specific genetic disorder (i.e., Tay Sachs).[74]

PGD involves the integration of three specific medical technologies: IVF, embryo biopsy, and molecular genetic testing requiring the expertise of professionals in assisted reproductive technology, genetic and infertility counseling, embryology, and molecular genetics.[75,76] In most cases, PGD involves the analysis of one or two biopsied cells of a three-day-old embryo in an effort to avoid the transfer of IVF-created embryos with documented genetic abnormalities from couples who are carriers of a genetic disorder. Two basic techniques are used to analyze an embryo's genetic status through PGD: polymerase chain reaction (PCR) and fluorescent in situ hybridization (FISH).[76] Initially PGD was developed for the evaluation of a specific disorder, but over time its application has dramatically expanded to evaluate a wide array of genetic disorders including monogenic conditions, aneuploidy screening, and structural chromosomal aberrations.[77] Currently, PGD is recommended for monogenic disorders and chromosomal rearrangements including: autosomal recessive disorders (e.g., beta thalassemia, spinal muscular atrophy, Tay Sachs, and cystic fibrosis); X-linked recessive (e.g., fragile X, Duchenne muscular dystrophy, and hemophilia); autosomal dominant disorders (e.g., myotonic dystrophy and Huntington's disease); chromosomal rearrangements (e.g., Robertsonian translocations); and mitochondrial disorders. It is estimated that more than 6,000 clinical cycles of PGD have been performed worldwide and that approximately 1,000 cycles are completely annually.[78]

Preimplantation genetic screening (PGS) for aneuploidy is a method used to identify the most chromosomally normal embryo for transfer in an IVF/ICSI cycle. Usually five to nine pairs of chromosomes are examined. PGS has increased dramatically for use in conjunction with IVF, in which no previous familial risk of an affected offspring exists. Its aim is to improve IVF results in women: (1) of advanced maternal age; and/or (2) who have recurrent miscarriages not attributable to constitutional chromosomal aberrations or other factors.[79] Aneuploidy from nondisjunction increases with maternal age, whereas polyploidy and mosaicism appear irrespective of maternal age, and are associated with poor embryo morphology.[80,81] PGS can be enhanced by new technologies (e.g., comparative genomic hybridization) to enable full karyotyping of single cells.[82] However, PGS may lead to confusion between embryo viability screening and screening for chromosomal disorders during pregnancy. Although experience with the efficacy, reliability, and safety of PGS is increasing, it remains limited and therefore is still considered experimental. Further-

more, there is no universal agreement about the indications for PGS and the legal status of the method varies internationally.[79]

IVF/PGD was designed for the infertile couple with a high genetic risk of having an affected child, whereas IVF/PGS was developed to detect certain anomalies of the embryo which might prevent a successful pregnancy. As such, indications and applications are totally different. In PGD, the genetic defect is known and established in the parent(s) who carries the defect, whereas PGS is used to screen for aneuploidies when there is a possibility of an increased but unspecified risk.[79]

Patient attitudes. While the aim of IVF was helping infertile couples have a child, the aim of PGD is helping individuals and/or couples with genetic disorders have a healthy child. By transferring only unaffected embryos, PGD enables couples to deliver genetically-shared children, who are free of genetic disorders, helping couples avoid the rigors of 'trial pregnancies'; extensive prenatal genetic testing; and/or pregnancy termination of an affected pregnancy. By selecting embryos before they are transferred to the uterus, couples are better able to avoid moral dilemmas (e.g., abortion to avoid transmission of genetic disease) and emotional distress (e.g., repeated miscarriage of genetically-affected pregnancies).[76,79]

Research on couples considering PGD found that the majority of women considered PGD either the same or better than conventional prenatal diagnosis, particularly because it helped avoid termination of an affected pregnancy.[83] However, women were also found to underestimate the burden of PGD treatment beforehand despite a strong desire to avoid recurrent miscarriages and/or abortions. Women who had done PGD reported that the PGD cycle was extremely stressful and a major disadvantage was the low success rates, although the majority would consider doing PGD again in a subsequent pregnancy attempt.[84] The majority of couples found PGD to be a highly acceptable treatment that was morally less problematic than abortion, although the recommendation of 'back-up' prenatal testing after pregnancy was achieved was a concern for half the patients in an Australian study.[85] While the majority of women considered the practical difficulties of PGD (including IVF) a disadvantage and were more concerned than men about the possibility of damage to the embryo as a result of the procedure, they still considered it a more positive alternative than termination of an affected pregnancy.[83,86] Finally, factors predicting couples' decision to pursue parenthood via IVF/PGD were previous miscarriages and/or abortions of an affected pregnancy; absence of acceptable alternatives; and openness about the treatment.

Limitations. Although IVF/PGD is a complex, expensive, and time-consuming procedure, success rates are slightly lower (20–25%) or comparable to IVF and/or IVF/ICSI.[87] Pregnancy rates, birth abnormalities, and obstetrical outcomes are also comparable to IVF and/or IVF/ICSI, [88] with the additional concern that the biopsy process itself may have long-term impact on the embryos.[79] However, no treatment is perfect and the misdiagnosis rate with PGD is 2.2% globally, leading to the recommendation worldwide of prenatal testing (CVS or amniocentesis) as a safeguard against diagnostic error or a serious unscreened-fetal abnormality.[79] Further prenatal genetic testing for other genetic disorders may be necessary and may potentially precipitate the discovery of a different genetic or chromosomal disorder warranting pregnancy termination due to fetal anomaly.[89] Moral and religious objections to IVF/PGD are based on the fundamental nature of the procedure (destruction of affected embryos) as well as religious proscriptions against all forms of 'noncoital' reproduction.

In summary, criticisms of IVF/PGD are its limited accuracy (in comparison with other forms of prenatal genetic testing); its current ability to detect limited number of genetic disorders; its invasiveness (e.g., IVF); financial cost; limited accessibility (i.e., few treatment centers worldwide); moral, religious, cultural, or legal prohibitions; and the financial expense. However, positive indications for IVF/PGD are patient satisfaction; minimization of psychosocial trauma by limiting reproductive losses; ability to not transmit a known genetic disorder; and religious or cultural beliefs in favor of genetically-shared offspring; and improved quality-of-life by fulfilling the desire for a child.

International perspective. International use of IVF/PGD varies widely from explicit legalization (e.g., Australia, Canada, and United Kingdom) with or without a governmental regulatory agency (e.g., Norway) and with or without restriction (e.g., Denmark, Finland, France, Spain, Sweden, and The Netherlands) to a 'professional guideline' approach (e.g., Austria, Belgium, Japan, Portugal, and the United States) to legal prohibition through restrictive laws (e.g., Germany, Italy, and Switzerland).[90–92] Although some countries regulate the practice of all assisted reproduction through laws, government regulations, or licensing organizations (e.g., United Kingdom and Canada), others involve recommendations and guidelines established by pro-

fessional organizations (e.g., ESHRE Task Force on PGD). While PGD is totally banned in some countries, most countries limit the indications for PGD to serious disorders or conditions (typically the detection of the sex of the embryo to avoid serious hereditary X-linked disease).[79] Guidelines and recommendations of the ASRM, ESHRE, HGC, HFEA, PGDIS, UNESCO/IBC, and WHO are now amending the lack of generally accepted rules concerning PGD, while the European Commission, European Society of Human Genetics, and European Society of Human Reproduction and Embryology (ESHRE) recently issued a draft report on the interface between ARTs and genetics that included an overview and practice guidelines. Based on the findings of ESHRE/PGD Task Force, twenty-nine countries worldwide reported offering PGD at ninety-six medical centers ranging from the highest (19) in the United States to only one per country in Argentina, Chile, China, Columbia, Cyprus, Czech Republic, Iran, Korea, Portugal, Saudi Arabia, Slovakia, and Thailand.[79]

Counseling issues. The ESHRE Consortium of 2005 issued practice guidelines on PGD that warrant both genetic and infertility counseling to address the complexity of medical treatment and genetic information required for patient consent. Ample reproductive counseling should be available (required) for all couples considering treatment with qualified infertility and reproductive genetic counselors able to address the complicated components of PGD including the IVF treatment cycle; embryo biopsy procedure; an overview of genetic testing and risk assessment; the patient's particular genetic diagnosis warranting the use of PGD; the benefits and limitations of PGD; the reliability of PGD diagnosis; the odds of misdiagnosis and adverse outcome; and the need for prenatal testing after pregnancy has been achieved. Counseling should also address moral, ethical, cultural, religious, and legal factors influencing the couple's use of PGD as well as the individual and couple's psychosocial response and adjustment to undertaking this treatment.[76,79]

Prenatal Genetic Testing and Counseling

The experience of prenatal genetic testing has the potential for altering the experience of pregnancy for previously infertile women, their partners, and even their extended family. Whatever its form, prenatal genetic testing can both validate the existence of a baby (e.g., ultrasound, photos, and confirmation of sex) and potentially invalidate the basis for its continued existence (e.g., detection of fetal anomaly, absence of fetal

TABLE 15.3. Indications for genetic counseling and possible prenatal testing[141]

Mother over 35 years of age at expected date of confinement

High or low maternal serum AFP screen

Family history of X-linked disorder in male related to mother through female family member

Member of ethnic group in which carrier screening for common disorder is available

Maternal illness

Exposure to medications or substance use

Two or more first-trimester miscarriages

Abnormal finding on ultrasound

Parental anxiety (primarily for reassurance)

heartbeat).[93] The postinfertility pregnancy is a highly valued, purposeful pregnancy achieved after considerable investment of time, money, effort, and emotion. Prenatal testing makes 'tentative pregnancies,' in which attachment to the pregnancy and fetus is often delayed; the experience of pregnancy is altered; and expectations of parenthood are influenced.[94] It is understandable that previously infertile couples often prefer to avoid the whole arena of prenatal testing in an effort to protect against the myriad possible threats, both physical and psychological (see Table 25.1).

Prenatal genetic screening and/or testing for the purpose of detecting chromosomal abnormalities, single gene disorders, and/or structural fetal anomalies can be offered as early as ten weeks' gestation. Recommendations for prenatal genetic testing and/or screening are usually based on: (1) advanced maternal age; (2) family history of a genetic disease or previous child/pregnancy with an anomaly; (3) exposure to potentially harmful substances; and (4) abnormal ultrasound or maternal serum screen. Unfortunately, prenatal screening and testing often are not single events, but rather a process of a variety of procedures administered throughout the pregnancy. In addition, no single test is able to test for all of the causes of mental retardation, birth defects, or other abnormalities in a pregnancy. In other words, no procedure can guarantee a perfect baby. 'False positives' and ambiguous results can wreak emotional havoc, plunging expectant parents into emotional highs and lows. This may tax the couple's emotional well-being, coping abilities, and relationship stability. Additionally, invasive testing offered in pregnancy always has a risk of miscarriage and the burden of guilt felt by the infertile couple who chooses to have testing that does actually cause the pregnancy to miscarry may be hard to recover from. These risks and downsides of prenatal testing may explain why many finally pregnant infertility patients refuse prenatal testing and/or counseling. (see Table 15.3)

The most common disorders for which couples seek prenatal genetic screening and testing are the fetal chromosomal trisomies that increase with a woman's age and neural tube defects (such as spina bifida or anencephaly). As noted earlier, the chance of having a child with Down syndrome, as well as other abnormalities caused by the presence of an extra chromosome, increases with advancing maternal age (Tables 15.3 and 15.4). However, it should be noted that what is medically defined as advanced maternal age (older than thirty-five years at delivery) may not be understood by infertile couples, who are typically even older.

Neural tube defects are malformations of the central nervous system with both a genetic and an environmental component. The incidence of neural tube defects is highest in Northern Ireland, with the lowest incidence in Japan.[95] The incidence of neural tube defects is not related to the age of the mother, although if a couple has had a previous child with a neural tube defect, the risk of recurrence in each subsequent pregnancy is increased to about one in thirty.[95]

Current prenatal screening and testing options that address the above-mentioned concerns include both noninvasive screening measures, such as maternal blood screens or ultrasound, and invasive diagnostic testing (e.g., amniocentesis and CVS) that incur a risk of pregnancy loss. Prenatal screens may help assess a risk but are not diagnostic: While diagnostic testing is more definitive, it still may be inaccurate due to other contributing factors (for example, having a child born with mental retardation that is not caused by a numerical or structural chromosome abnormality and therefore not routinely detected by amniocentesis or CVS). Prenatal screening currently available includes: (1) the first-trimester biochemical and nuchal translucency screen (also known as the first-trimester screen); (2) the second-trimester maternal serum screen (also known as the 'quad' screen or multiple-marker screen); and (3) ultrasound. Diagnostic testing includes: (1) CVS (chorionic villi sampling); (2) amniocentesis; and (3) fetal blood sampling (cordocentesis).

Both the first-trimester screen and the second-trimester serum screen are noninvasive methods that allow couples to obtain more information about the risks of Down syndrome and trisomy 18 during a pregnancy. The second-trimester quad screen was developed in the 1990s and gives a couple a risk estimate for the chances of Down syndrome, trisomy 18, and open neural tube defects during a pregnancy. The risk numbers are generated through a calculation that incorporates the concentrations of four chemicals within the maternal bloodstream, the gestational age of the pregnancy, and the prior age-related risk of the mother. The four chemicals measured include: a protein produced in fetal level call alpha-fetoprotein (AFP) and three hormones produced in the placenta called human chorionic gonadotropin (hCG), unconjugated estriol (uE3), and diameric inhibin-A (DIA). This approach yields a 67–76% detection rate for fetal Down syndrome with a 5% false positive rate.[96] Second trimester screening does not give a risk assessment for the other trisomies that increase with a woman's age. Until recently, second-trimester maternal serum screening was considered the standard of care for pregnancy in North America and Europe.[97,98]

Recently, great interest has been directed toward first-trimester screening with the use of new ultrasonography (also known as sonogram and ultrasound) and serum screening markers. The first-trimester screen gives couples a risk estimate for the chances of Down syndrome and trisomy 18 within the first trimester of pregnancy. In first-trimester screening, the risk estimates are based on an ultrasound measurement of the amount of fluid at the back of the fetal neck (the nuchal translucency); the concentrations of two chemicals within the maternal bloodstream (pregnancy-associated plasma protein A and hCG); the gestational age of the pregnancy; and the prior age-related risk of the mother. First-trimester screening measures have comparable detection rates and false positive rates for Down syndrome as second-trimester maternal serum screening and may be offered as an earlier alternative to second-trimester screening, as long as strict clinical criteria are met.[97,99,100]

While both the first-trimester and second-trimester screens have the benefit of providing more information in a pregnancy without a risk of miscarriage, there are limitations to the accuracy and amount of information provided. Results may be influenced by a number of factors including maternal age, weight, diabetes, race, and current medications as well as unique properties of this pregnancy (e.g., bleeding and multiples).[101] Additionally, an abnormal screening result does not definitively determine the presence of a chromosome abnormality or open neural tube defect in a pregnancy. In fact, the only certain means of accurately determining the presence or absence of a fetal chromosome abnormality is through invasive testing, which always poses a risk of miscarriage (however minimal). When screening results indicate an abnormality, couples face an array of difficult options and decisions: having a child with a disorder; termination of an affected pregnancy; and/or additional procedures. Understandably, this inalterably changes the pregnancy experience; producing feelings of anxiety, anger, and fear; and often triggering a crisis of values and faith. For infertile couples, decision making about how to proceed with a much-wanted, potentially affected pregnancy is particularly challenging. Feelings of uncertainty, distress, confusion, and hopelessness are common. With so much at stake and both partners experiencing an array of feelings, communication, information processing, and decision making can be impaired or, at least, less than optimal.

Ultrasound (also referred to as sonography) is a diagnostic tool that detects structural birth defects and rare genetic disorders. When a family history is positive for a genetic condition that only affects males, it is helpful to identify fetal gender via ultrasound prior to invasive testing. Ultrasound is also used to evaluate fetal growth, well-being, and variations in amniotic fluid that can provide information about potential fetal anomalies. Abnormalities commonly identified on ultrasound include misshapen (club) feet; mild hydronephrosis (fluid on the kidneys); neural tube defects such as anencephaly (absence of skull and brain); hydrocephaly (increased cerebrospinal fluid in the brain); choroid plexus cysts (small pockets of fluid trapped in brain blood cells); facial clefts (e.g., cleft palate); cystic hygromas (cystic swelling in the neck); abnormalities in the heart; diaphragmatic hernia (contents of abdomen outside the chest); limb problems (e.g., dwarfism); and others.[102] Ultrasound is also used as a screening tool for subtle variations that may indicate potential problems such as fetal thigh bone measurements more than one week behind other fetal measurements indicating increased risk for Down syndrome.[103]

Chorionic villi sampling (CVS) (occasionally called placental biopsy or placentocentesis) was introduced in the mid-1980s primarily to evaluate fetal chromosomes and/or test for single gene disorders. CVS is usually done between ten and twelve weeks of pregnancy and involves the passage of a needle into the placenta to withdraw tissue (cells) into a syringe for testing. CVS may be transvaginal or transabdominal, with both methods guided by ultrasound. The risk of miscarriage following CVS is generally about 1%, and it usually takes about ten days to obtain the test results of the chromosome analysis. The use and acceptance of CVS is based almost entirely on the fact that it can be done much earlier in the pregnancy than amniocentesis and test results are more quickly available. Earlier test results facilitate earlier pregnancy termination if the fetus is determined to have any anomalies. However, there are significant drawbacks with CVS: (1) while most diseases detectable by amniocentesis can also be detected by CVS, neural tube defects cannot; (2) ambiguous test results occur in 1 of every 100 tests; and (3) limb damage to the developing fetus has been reported to occur in 1 of every 1,000 tests.[104]

Amniocentesis, introduced in the 1930s, initially involved injecting dye into the uterus to outline the fetus on x-ray examination.[95] In the 1950s, it was used to test for Rh factor or fetal blood type when the baby's blood group was incompatible with the mother's. Amniocentesis was first introduced for testing fetuses with suspected genetic diseases in 1967 and today remains the most common and reliable method used for prenatal testing. Amniocentesis was introduced before ultrasound was widely used, but with the benefit of ultrasound, the risk of miscarriage following amniocentesis is currently reported to be 0.6 in 100 pregnancies.[95] Amniocentesis involves the use of ultrasound to guide a needle into the amniotic fluid surrounding the fetus and the withdrawal of fluid containing fetal cells used for genetic testing. The most common reasons for undertaking amniocentesis are to evaluate fetal chromosomes and to detect neural tube defects. Amniocentesis is usually performed between fifteen and seventeen weeks of pregnancy, with chromosome test results available in about ten days (testing for other disorders often takes longer), allowing termination of an affected pregnancy before twenty-one-weeks gestation. However, many women and their partners find the termination of an affected fetus so late in pregnancy a significant drawback of this procedure. Even when the pregnancy is found to be normal, delayed attachment often affects a couple's enjoyment of, and attachment to, the pregnancy. For infertile couples, advanced maternal age may be the most important determining factor in their decision to proceed with amniocentesis.[105]

Infertile couples may be more likely to decline prenatal testing because they are more acutely aware of how theirs is a 'premium pregnancy' and, as such, difficult to put at risk (however small) for the potential information obtainable. Furthermore, the screening process (e.g., ultrasound) may trigger unpleasant memories of infertility treatments, further disrupting the pregnancy experience. In contrast, infertile couples who have con-

comitant genetic issues may approach genetic testing differently: as a necessary evil in their journey toward parenthood and a healthy baby. Although the experience of infertility may make them more keenly aware of how prenatal testing can both enhance and depreciate the pregnancy experience, they may also be more aware of how it can provide them with much needed information whether positive or negative.

Continuing or Terminating a Genetically Affected Pregnancy

Frequently, couples confuse the decision to pursue prenatal testing as an automatic endorsement of pregnancy termination if a genetic disorder is detected. Although elective termination of an affected pregnancy is a viable alternative, it is not a universal choice. A certain portion of couples chose prenatal testing to prepare for the care of a handicapped child. As such, prenatal testing and diagnosis can help couples emotionally prepare for a negative outcome and different parenting challenges, but it also can become a prolonged period of emotional upset and anxious waiting.[106] Accordingly, considerations of prenatal testing as preparation for the care of a handicapped child must involve explorations of the expectant parents' personal perspective. Most parents experience a mourning process following prenatal diagnosis or birth of a handicapped child, in which they grieve the loss of the expected healthy child.[107] Advanced knowledge of the problem can allow some measure of control over the events surrounding the birth of a handicapped or affected baby, benefiting long-term coping and family adjustment.[108] For couples with a history of infertility, considerations typically include issues of parental age, expectations of parenthood, perceived burden versus actual resources, and prior commitments or responsibilities, such as children from previous marriages or elderly parents.

A number of factors have been found to impact decisions about whether or not to terminate an affected pregnancy including the severity of the fetal abnormality, religiosity, maternal or parental age, other children in the family, education, and socioeconomic status. Often this is a decision couples have made or at least seriously consider before undertaking prenatal testing.[109] In a recent study in the United States that evaluated 53,000 pregnancies at a university hospital between 1984 and 1997 to assess the degree to which prenatal knowledge of fetal anomalies and sociodemographic characteristics impacted decision making about outcome,[110] researchers found that the severity of anomalies directly correlated with termination rates and that severity of central nervous system anomalies were more likely to lead to pregnancy termination.

Older and more educated mothers were more likely to terminate the pregnancy than younger, less educated mothers. In a Swiss study of parental decisions following the prenatal diagnosis of sex chromosome abnormalities, 72% decided to terminate the pregnancy. Termination rates were 100% for Turner syndrome; 73.9% for Klinefelter syndrome; 70% for 47, XYY males; and 42.9% for mosaic cases.[111] Couples undergoing IVF were significantly more likely to opt for prenatal testing if terminating a pregnancy for a severe genetic abnormality was an option for them. However, Roman Catholic couples tended to have more conservative attitudes about pregnancy termination.[112] Among Israeli Muslims predictors of pregnancy termination for a known disorder (cystic fibrosis) were: religiosity, familiarity with an affected child, and benefits of the test.[113] In short, although pregnancy termination for a genetic anomaly is common, some couples choose to continue their pregnancy after receiving a 'less than normal' diagnosis. It appears that a perspective in which termination of affected pregnancy is an acceptable option and consideration of alternatives prior to prenatal testing are helpful predictors of a couple's decision making. As such, both genetic and infertility counselors cannot facilitate these decisions by considering the couple's religiosity; prior infertility experience; cultural and family context; and their familiarity and comfort with having a child with a genetic condition.

Psychological reactions following the termination of a pregnancy due to fetal anomaly appear to be more similar to psychological responses following spontaneous miscarriage than reactions to elective termination (abortion).[43] Grief loss, sadness, depression, and psychological distress are typical responses to miscarriage, while relief is the most common response to elective abortion. Depression following termination of a pregnancy for genetic reasons can be a significant risk for both women and men even though terminating an affected pregnancy was felt to be preferable to giving birth to an affected child.[114] Nevertheless, risk factors for psychological distress following the loss of a wanted pregnancy include prior history of depression, poor social support, ambivalence or coercion about the termination, and disturbed marital relationship.[43,115] Infertility counselors should help grieving parents distinguish between the healthy child that they had anticipated and the unhealthy child actually lost.[116] Sharing the loss with a few close, nonjudgmental confidants often promotes recovery and reduces shame, as does networking with appropriate support groups. Increasingly, men and women are finding the anonymous support offered by internet resources help-

ful. Like other perinatal losses, this loss often reawakens past unresolved losses, disappointments, and/or deprivations, especially those involving elective termination of unwanted pregnancy (see Chapter 16).

Decisions regarding pregnancy termination are always challenging but are even more so when the 'elective' termination involves a wanted pregnancy following discovery of a genetic disorder or defect. Even when a couple is certain and confident that termination is the right decision for them, ending a wanted pregnancy is onerous even if it is a viable medical option for them. Adding another dimension to the loss is the variety of decisions that the couple must consider, such as termination techniques, termination facility and/or caregivers, autopsy, genetic testing of fetal tissue, and disposal of fetal remains. Some women prefer procedures that minimize the pregnancy experience and/or physical trauma, while others prefer to experience labor and delivery, recreating as much as possible a 'normal' delivery surrounded by familiar medical caregivers. Furthermore, some couples (and their families) prefer to mark the event with religious ceremonies or other memorial rituals, while others do not.

By contrast, the counseling tasks and the psychological impact of continuing a pregnancy after an abnormal prenatal diagnosis differ greatly from those associated with termination. For couples who have experienced infertility, the high emotional investment and fear (or actuality) that a future pregnancy may not be possible may strengthen their desire to continue, even after abnormal test results are obtained and in the face of a determination of 'imminent fetal demise.' However, when prenatal test results indicate a less severe prognosis or only a probability for poor outcome, the option of termination may not even be considered. Furthermore, as medical technology advances, physicians are increasingly able to treat babies, prenatally and/or postnatally, for complications of genetic disorders and birth defects. Psychological tasks for these couples often involve attachment to a fetus that is different from what they had anticipated and emotional preparation for parenting an affected (even disabled) child. Or it may be anticipatory grief and mourning a fetus that probably will die in utero or shortly after birth. In such cases, it is important to provide appropriate support and facilitate grieving while always keeping the patient firmly in the reality of the situation, not indulging in fantasies that the baby actually will be all right by some miracle.

Lamentably, prenatal testing procedures have the potential (although minimal) of precipitating a pregnancy loss. This 'preventable' pregnancy loss can be a bitter finale for infertile couples after such extensive and extraordinary efforts to achieve parenthood. These

---

TABLE 15.4. Questions for screening for genetic risk[141]

Have you or other close relatives had one or more stillbirths or early infant losses?

Did any of your close relatives die at an early age (under the age of 50), and if so, do you know why?

Did you or anyone in your family have more than two miscarriages?

Are you and your spouse related to each other in any way?

Are you and your spouse cousins or do you have relatives with the same last name?

Does anyone in your family have learning problems, or is anyone mentally retarded?

Does anyone in your family have hearing loss, vision loss, or any birth defect?

Does anyone in your family look very different from others in the family (e.g., very tall or very short)?

What country(ies) did your family originally come from?

---

couples may feel angry, guilty, and betrayed by the medical science on which they relied for help, often while personally denying the medical risks of the procedures. However, it is important to note that some of these losses may have been 'natural' miscarriages, perhaps related to the genetic disorder or factors associated with the infertility diagnosis.

Genetically-Affected Pregnancy Losses

Multiple or repeated pregnancy loss is a common reason for referral for genetic counseling. At least 10–15% of recognized pregnancies end in miscarriage, with the majority of losses occurring in the first trimester.[117,118] Additionally, many infertile couples are more closely monitoring themselves for pregnancy or as part of infertility treatment, resulting in the detection and documentation of early miscarriages. Infertile couples may be self-referred or referred by their physician as part of the infertility evaluations for recurrent pregnancy loss. In approximately 50–70% of spontaneous miscarriages, a chromosome abnormality is identified.[60,119] Chromosomal problems causing fetal losses may be present in one or both parents (thereby increasing the risk of a subsequent pregnancy loss) or may be due to an error in fertilization or in cell division during oocyte or sperm cell production ('packaging error'), known as nondisjunction. Genetic causes of miscarriage may be sporadic, chromosomally abnormal, or recurrent due to heritable chromosomal abnormalities. In fact, in approximately 4% of couples with a history of recurrent pregnancy loss, one partner has a balanced chromosomal translocation[120] that predisposes the couple not only to miscarriage, but also to an increased chance of having a live-born child with multiple congenital anomalies. Other contributing causes to recurrent miscarriage are: endocrine abnormalities; blood disorders; environmental agents; immunologic reactions; and maternal

factors (e.g., uterine anatomic malformations, myomas, cervical abnormalities, and chromosomal and single gene disorders).[121] As result, couples experiencing two or more miscarriages, a miscarriage plus a stillbirth, a malformed fetus, or live-born baby with anomalies should receive a formal genetic evaluation for recurrent pregnancy loss. Genetic evaluation usually involves chromosome studies (karyotyping) of both parents and fetal tissue, detailed family history (see Table 15.4), and when available, photographs of the fetus, radiographic studies, autopsy, laboratory testing, placenta and cord assessment, and a recommendation of additional testing.[121]

While there is increasing public awareness (in part due to public education campaigns) of advanced maternal age as a risk factor in miscarriage and repeated miscarriages, this issue can trigger a cascade of emotional responses in partners regarding further medical evaluations and family-building considerations. Very often women who have experienced an age-related miscarriage not only experience common feelings of grief and guilt, but also a complex array of feelings about aging and their own age in particular. In many parts of the world, aging in women is a cultural advantage increasing social status, wisdom, and authority. However, this is not a universal experience for women and may not apply to her reproductive ability. In many developed countries women are empowered by youth, beauty, and reproductive ability, so that a pregnancy loss due to advanced maternal age is a significant psychological and social blow. Furthermore, the loss may force a woman to come to terms with the realities of her reproductive capability, forcing her to consider other family-building alternatives (e.g., donor oocytes; see Chapters 4 and 18).

Typically, there are both practical and psychological benefits for infertile couples to pursue genetic counseling following a fetal loss, even though information may be provisional or difficult to accept or provide less than 100% accuracy.[116] Often, infertile couples feel that a pregnancy loss is a mixed blessing: The good news is they have achieved a pregnancy; the bad news is the pregnancy was lost. They (and possibly their caregivers) may have difficulty in seeing a pattern in the losses and the couple may respond with alarm when a referral for genetic evaluation is suggested. Alternatively, infertile couples may perceive genetic testing and counseling as an opportunity to reduce ambiguity and gain an explanation or greater understanding of their infertility, even though it carries with it the possibility of a genetic diagnosis. However, the results of genetic testing and even the process of genetic counseling may exacerbate a couple's grieving; reopen wounds; precipitate feelings of defectiveness; touch off a crisis with other family members; and influence future reproductive decisions.

Genetic Screening of Potential Gamete and Embryo Donors

Today, reproduction medicine, with the help of genetics, provides opportunities for family-building using donated gametes, embryos, and/or gestational carriers/surrogates. These third-party reproduction arrangements have been referred to as 'complex' reproduction, reflecting the complex medical technologies and psychosocial issues involved in bringing these families into fruition. As third-party reproduction has become an increasingly medically appropriate treatment while gaining greater social acceptance, the importance of genetic screening of donors has become more relevant and important. As such, infertile individuals, as consumers, justifiably expect gamete donors and traditional surrogates to have been 'vetted' as healthy and disease-free through a complete medical, psychological, and genetic evaluation.[122] In fact, genetic assessment of potential gamete and embryo donors as well as surrogates has become the standard of care if not the legal requirement worldwide[79,122–127] (see Chapters 19 and 21).

Genetic assessment of potential sperm or oocyte donors typically involves obtaining a family and medical history through a standard questionnaire, as well as psychological assessment, preparation, and education. At this time, worldwide most sperm banks and oocyte donation programs do not engage the services of genetic counselors or involve comprehensive genetic counseling or screening services. Although it has been recommended that genetic testing (karyotyping) be done on all potential gamete donors,[128] historically very few sperm banks offer these services, and it has not typi-

cally been included in assessments of oocyte or embryo donors or surrogates. However, more recently karyotyping of oocyte donors has been recommended in addition to genetic assessment. This is due in part to evidence that a number of women with normal physical examinations and personal and family histories tested positive for major genetic abnormalities[129] and high rates of abnormalities were found in donated oocytes.[80] Similar findings have been reported among sperm donors. Research on the quality of sperm donated to commercial sperm banks was found to have differed significantly in semen parameters in terms of the percentage of motile and progressively motile sperm.[130] These concerns have led to recommendations that all donor programs use thorough screening protocols to minimize transmission of genetic abnormalities or carrier status. It has also been recommended that donation programs and medical centers consult with a genetic specialist when establishing donor screening protocols.[129,131] Whether or not the gametes have been genetically-tested, it is now recognized that recipient couples should be assessed for potential genetic risk due to family medical and pregnancy history, particularly if the recipient and donor have similar ethnic or racial backgrounds, thereby increasing the risk of certain genetic disorders or diseases; or if the recipient couple wishes to screen for a specific genetic disorder (e.g., cystic fibrosis or Tay-Sachs disease).[132] Finally, when considering the genetic issues of donated gametes, recipients should be fully informed about: (1) the genetic screening protocols used by the gamete donation facility; (2) the *impossibility* of detecting 100% of carrier or genetic disorders; and (3) the possibility of *de novo* genetic disorders.[122,132] Based on this information (and the recipient's particular situation), prenatal genetic testing during pregnancy may be appropriate and another consideration for the recipients prior to treatment (see Chapter 19).

Toward that end, there has been increasing attention and interest in the provision of appropriate genetic assessment of donors and the gametes they provide. Currently, there is no universal code of practice globally, with international use of donor gametes and embryo varying from explicit legalization with government regulation (e.g., Australia, Canada, and United Kingdom) to the more common 'professional guideline' approach (e.g., United States and Belgium) to legal prohibition through restrictive laws (e.g., Germany, Italy, and Switzerland).[91,133,134] Other world agencies expressing interest or participating in the development of a global policy include the Human Genetics Commission (www.hgc.gov.uk), the World Health Organization (www.who.int), and the United Nation's

Educational, Scientific, and Cultural Organisation (www.portal.unesco.org).[79] Whether by government legislation or professional practice guidelines, genetic counseling along with some form of genetic screening is universally recommended for all gamete and/or embryo donors as well as surrogates. However, the specific criteria and/or recommendations of genetic counseling remain fluid and ever-evolving, an issue about which the genetic and infertility counselor should be ever cognizant. This is particularly the case when gametes or embryos are being shipped across borders for donation and/or the treatment of reproductive tourists who have different agendas and expectations, either as a donor or recipient.

Although a rare occurrence, occasionally gamete donors are diagnosed with a genetic disorder during the donation screening process. Understandably, this can be a disquieting experience and one that involves the genetic counselor's best counseling skills including delivering bad news, crisis intervention, education, empathy, and referral to appropriate support organizations, medical caregivers, and/or a mental health professional. Additionally, the genetic counselor assesses the individual's ability to cope and manage this crisis and the impact of the diagnosis on the individual's identity, marital and family relationships, health, and personal reproductive goals. This is a unique situation that truly demands a multidisciplinary team approach for the provision of optimum patient care.

Donation of embryos usually arises from the cryopreservation of 'extra' embryos from an IVF treatment cycle which the treated couple does not wish to use themselves. As with gamete donation, legal, cultural, and religious factors very much influence the feasibility of this practice. Again, there is no universal practice, with approaches varying from explicit legalization with government regulation to a professional guideline approach to legal prohibition through restrictive laws – the most common approach regarding this reproductive option. Sometimes these donation agreements are privately arranged without the input of professionals, while in other countries (most commonly the United States) embryo donation agencies facilitate these third-party assisted reproduction arrangements – again with or without professional guidance. Because IVF patients have altruistically donated the majority of these embryos, the embryos typically have not been genetically-screened, nor have the donating patients been genetically-screened or had genetic counseling. Given that the donating couple used IVF and therefore must have had some sort of fertility issue, it is highly plausible, even likely that without genetic screening, donated embryos (and the children born as a result of

them) are at risk for a genetic disorder. Additionally, it is important to note that morally, the screening of embryos differs from the screening of gametes. Some may argue against screening of an embryo postconception because it represents the screening of a human life that could/should not be endangered or destroyed if an anomaly is detected. Furthermore, congenital disability is not uniformly considered to be harmful and screening decisions may be considered by the public to have eugenic overtones[135] reflecting the vast ethical and moral dilemmas regarding the screening of embryos.

Adding to the conundrum is the perspective of the donor versus the recipient. While the embryo donors may feel genetic screening is unnecessary (and even insulting), recipients may feel it a perfectly appropriate means of assuring them of the most viable and healthiest embryos for reproduction: to assure they have the healthiest child possible. However, routine genetic screening of all IVF patients based on potential donation of unused embryos is unrealistic, impractical, and logistically impossible – at least at this point. Nevertheless, these concerns have led to recommendations that all embryo donor programs use thorough screening protocols to minimize transmission of genetic abnormalities or carrier status. It has also been recommended that embryo donation agencies and medical centers use the services of a genetic counselor when establishing donor screening protocols.[129,131] Finally, when considering the genetic issues of donated embryos, recipient couples should be made aware: (1) of the genetic screening protocols used by the embryo donation agency and/or medical facility; (2) the *impossibility* of detecting 100% of carrier or genetic disorders; and (3) the possibility of *de novo* genetic disorders.[122,132] As such, recipient couples may wish to consider the use of IVF/PGD or IVF/PGS on donated embryos or, at minimum, consider prenatal testing after pregnancy has been achieved. In short, despite the best efforts of their caregivers and their own best efforts, there is no guarantee that couples will have the 'perfect baby' they expect and deserve. Supporting unfounded expectations can lead to unnecessary psychological distress (see Chapter 20).

FUTURE IMPLICATIONS

The burgeoning technologies in reproductive medicine and genetics will no doubt continue to make available an increasingly complex array of reproductive alternatives and treatments. As a result, the decision making process, information processing, and psychosocial ramifications of these complicated reproductive alternatives will no doubt become more difficult rather than less. In future, the complexity of reproductive alternatives will no doubt contribute to more confounding ethical, cultural, and religious dilemmas impacting individuals, families, and society, particularly in terms of reproductive genetics, reproductive tourism, and the stratification of access to reproductive and genetic services. Rapidly developing technological choices (e.g., cloning, and gene therapy) highlight the conundrums faced by families considering them: whether what can be done should be done, at what cost, and for whose benefit. Finally, availability of medical technologies does not guarantee that any particular technology is feasible or accessible for the vast majority of individuals (or even one couple) or that the outcome of assisted reproduction will be the desired outcome for everyone.[136–139] Given these circumstances, both genetic counselors and infertility counselors will continue to play an increasingly important and integral role as members of the collaborative practice of reproductive and genetic medicine.

SUMMARY

■ Both infertility and genetic counselors, as well as other medical professionals, 'counsel' by advising, supporting, and instructing patients dealing with reproductive health problems. While genetic counselors are trained to provide information and support on genetic issues, infertility counselors are trained mental health professionals who provide psychological treatment with the knowledge of infertility issues. Genetic and infertility counselors work together as part of the collaborative reproductive medicine team counseling couples about their reproductive health problems and family-building alternatives.

■ Contrary to patient expectations, genetic medicine cannot detect and prevent *all* birth defects, and reproductive medicine cannot provide everyone with the flawless baby he or she wants.

■ Infertile couples (accustomed to failed effort and loss) are more likely to highly value their pregnancy and baby and, as a result, are more keenly aware of how prenatal genetic testing can both enhance and depreciate the pregnancy experience.

■ Emotional reactions to pregnancy termination of a genetically-affected fetus appear to be much more similar to reactions following spontaneous miscarriage than to elective abortion and are seldom protracted or disturbed.

■ Prenatal diagnosis of a fetal anomaly may help emotional preparation or prolong the period of emotional upset.

■ Couples who have had two or more miscarriages; a miscarriage plus a stillbirth; the birth of a malformed fetus; live-born baby with genetic anomalies; or have a family history of a genetic disorder should receive formal genetic evaluation and counseling.

■ Decisions to proceed with prenatal genetic testing are usually based on: (1) advanced maternal age; (2) family history of a genetic disease; (3) two or more unexplained miscarriages or prior pregnancies/children with birth defects; and (4) exposure to potentially harmful substances. The major prenatal testing procedures are: blood screening, ultrasound, CVS, and amniocentesis.

■ PGD allows individuals with a history of a genetic condition to screen for a genetic disorder *before* pregnancy, eliminating or at least decreasing the need for prenatal genetic testing and pregnancy termination.

■ Assisted reproduction should not be initiated in men and women with a possible or known genetic cause of infertility without prior genetic counseling and risk assessment.

■ Genetics is an extremely complicated field that is advancing at the same rapid pace as reproductive medicine. Understanding the new advances and interpreting new testing methods in genetics is fundamental to the competency and provision of competent care for infertility counselors. By the same token, an understanding of advances in reproductive medicine is increasingly important for the professional competency qualifications for genetics counselors working in reproductive genetics.

ACKNOWLEDGMENT

The authors would like to gratefully acknowledge the contribution of Mary Ahrens, MS and Bonnie LeRoy, MS in the preparation of this chapter.

REFERENCES

1. Shapiro CH, Djurdjinovic L. Understanding our infertile genetic counseling patients. In: BA Fine, EL Getting, K Greendale, et al., eds. *Strategies in Genetic Counseling: Reproductive Genetics and New Technologies*. White Plains, NY: March of Dimes Defects Foundation, 1990.

2. Shiloh S. Genetic counseling: A developing area of interest for psychologists. *Professional Psychology: Research and Practice* 1996; 27:475–86.

3. Walker AP. The practice of genetic counseling. In: DL Baker, JL Schuette, WR Uhlmann, eds. *A Guide to Genetic Counseling* 1998; 1–20.

4. Campbell NA, Reece JB. The chromosomal basis of inheritance. In: E Ang, HJ Arnott, AR Blaustein, et al., eds. *Biology*. 6th ed. San Francisco: Pearson 2002; 269–72.

5. Carr-Saunders AM. Eugenics. In: *The Encyclopedia Britannica*, 14th ed. London: Encyclopedia Britannica Company, 1929; 806.

6. Wooldridge A. Eugenics: The secret lurking in many nations' past. *Los Angeles Times*, Sept. 7, 1997.

7. Neel JV. *Physician to the Gene Poll: Genetic Lessons and Other Stories*. New York: Wiley, 1994.

8. Campbell NA, Reece JB. The molecular basis of inheritance. In: E Ang, HJ Arnott, AR Blaustein, et al., eds. *Biology*. 6th ed. San Francisco: Pearson, 2002.

9. Bartels DM, LeRoy BS, Caplan A, eds. *Prescribing Our Future: Ethical Challenges in Genetic Counseling*. New York: Aldine de Gruyter, 1993.

10. McKusick BA. *Mendelian Inheritance in Man: Catalogues of Human Genes and Genetic Disorders*, 11th ed. Baltimore: Johns Hopkins University Press, 1994.

11. Reed SC. *Counseling in Medical Genetics*. Philadelphia: Saunders, 1955.

12. Eunpu DL. Systemically-based psychotherapeutic techniques in genetic counseling. *J Genet Couns* 1997; 6:1–20.

13. Marks JH, Richter ML. The genetics associate: A new health professional. *Am J Public Health* 1976; 66:388–90.

14. American Board of Genetic Counseling. *Requirements for Graduate Programs in Genetic Counseling Seeking Accreditation by the American Board of Genetic Counseling*. Bethesda, MD: American Board of Genetic Counseling, Aug. 2003.

15. Sahbar MA, Young MA, Sheffield LJ, Aitkin M. Educating genetic counselors in Australia: Developing an international perspective. *J Genet Couns* 2005; 14:283–94.

16. Harris R. Genetic counseling and testing in Europe. *J R Coll Physicians Lond* 1998; 32:335–8.

17. Revel M. *Genetic Counseling*: United Nations Educational, Scientific, and Cultural Organization, Paris, 15 December 1995.

18. Biesecker BB, Marteau TM. The future of genetic counseling: An international perspective. *Nature Genetics* 1999; 22:133–7.

19. Ramalho AS, de Paiva e Silva RB. Community genetics: A new discipline and its application in Brazil. *Cad Salude Publica* 2000; 16:261–3.

20. Kofman-Alfaro S, Penchaszadeh VB. Community genetic services in Latin America and regional network of medical genetics. Recommendations of a World Health Organization consultation. *Comm Genet* 2004; 7:157–9.

21. Kenen R, Peters J. The colored, eco-genetic, relationship map (CEGRM): A conceptual approach and tool for genetic counseling research. *J Genet Coun* 2001; 10:289–309.

22. Knoppers BM, Isasi RM. Regulatory approaches to reproductive genetic testing. *Human Reprod* 2004; 19:2695–701.

23. Wertz DC, Fletcher JC, Nippert I, et al. In focus: Has patient autonomy gone too far? Geneticists' views in 36 nations. *Am J Bioeth* 2002; 2:W21.

24. Wertz D. Eugenics is alive and well: A survey of genetic professionals around the world. *Sci Context* 1998; 11:493–510.

25. Wertz DC. Is genetic counseling unbiased? A 36-nation survey. Abstract # 35860 130th Annual Meeting of APHA.

26. Fine BA. The evolution of nondirectiveness in genetic counseling and implications of the Human Genome Project. In: DM Bartels, BS LeRoy, A Caplan, eds. *Prescribing Our Future: Ethical Challenges in Genetic Counseling*. New York: Aldine de Gruyter, 1993; 101–18.

27. McNutt RA. Shared medical decision making: Problems, process, progress. *JAMA* 2004; 292:2516–18.

28. Kessler S. The psychological paradigm shift in genetic counseling. *Soc Biol* 1980; 27:167–85.

29. *The Genetic Self: The Impact of the Human Genome Project on You and Your Practice*. National Institutes of Health & National Human Genome Research Institute. Airlie House, Airlie, VA, June 27–29, 1997.

30. Strong C. Models for a psychosocial team approach to genetic counseling. In Course IX: The New Genetics and Reproductive Decisions: Psychosocial and Ethical Issues. *American Society for Reproductive Medicine*. Cincinnati, OH: October 18–19, 1997; 133–4.

31. Macek M, Vilimova S, Potuznikova P, et al. Medical genetics in reproductive medicine. *Cas Lek Cesk* 2002; 141:28–34.

32. Bitzer J. Quality assessment and quality in psychosomatic obstetrics and gynecology: Old wine in new bottles? *J Psychosom Ob Gyn* 2001; 22:67–8.

33. Skirton H. The client's perspective of genetic counseling – a grounded theory study. *J Genet Counsel* 2001; 10:311–39.

34. Greb A. Multiculturalism and the practice of genetic counseling. In: DL Baker, JL Schuette, WR Uhlmann, eds. *A Guide to Genetic Counseling*. 1998; 171–98.

35. Harper PS. *Practical Genetic Counselling*, 4th ed. Oxford: Butterworth-Heinemanns, 1993.

36. Sandelowski M, Harris BG, Holitch-Davis D. Mazing: Infertile couples and the quest for a child. *Image J Nurs Sch* 1989; 21:220–6.

37. Kenen R, Smith ACM, Watkins C, et al. To use or not use: The prenatal genetic technology/worry conundrum. *J Gen Counsel* 2000b; 9:203–17.

38. Nachtigall RD, Quiroga SS, Tschann JM. Stigma, disclosure, and family functioning among parents of children conceived through donor insemination. *Fertil Steril* 1997; 68:1–7.

39. Frets P, Neirmeiher M. Reproductive planning after genetic counseling: A perspective from the last decade. *Clin Genet* 1990; 38:295–306.

40. Lippman-Hand A, Fraser CF. Genetic counseling – the post-counseling period: 1. Parents' perception of uncertainty. *Am J Med Genet* 1979; 4:51–71.

41. Leonard CO, Chase GA, Childs B. Genetic counseling: A consumer's view. *N Engl J Med* 1972; 287:433–9.

42. Beeson D, Goldbus M. Decision making: Whether or not to have prenatal diagnosis and abortion after detection of fetal abnormality. *Am J Genet* 1984; 36(suppl):122s.

43. Leon IG. Pregnancy termination due to fetal anomaly: Clinical considerations. *J Infant Ment Health* 1995; 16:112–26.

44. McConkle-Rosell A, Devellis BM. Threat to parental role: A possible mechanism of altered self-concept related to carrier knowledge. *J Gen Coun* 2000; 9:285–302.

45. Plunkett KS, Simpson JL. A general approach to genetic counseling. *Obstet Gynecol Clin N Am* 2002; 29:265–76.

46. Olson CK, Keppler-Noreuil KM, Romitti PA, et al. In vitro fertilization is associated with an increase in major birth defects. *Fertil Steril* 2005; 84:1308–15.

47. Hansen M, Kurinczuk J, Bower C, Webb S. The risk of major birth defects after intracytoplasmic sperm

injection and in vitro fertilization. *N Engl J Med* 2002; 346:725–30.

48. Lie RT, Lyngstadaas A, Orstavid KH, Bakketeig LS, Jacobsen G, Tanbo T. Birth defects in children conceived by ICSI compared with children conceived by other IVF-methods; A meta analysis. *Int J Epidemiol* 2005; 34:696–701.

49. Allen C, Reardon W. Assisted reproduction technology and defects of genomic imprinting. *BJOG* 2005; 112:1589–94.

50. Stouffs K, Lissens W, Tournaye H, et al. The choice and outcome of the fertility treatment of 38 couples in whom the male partner has an Yq microdeletion. *Hum Reprod* 2005; 20:1887–96.

51. Schover LR, Thomas AJ, Falcone T, et al. Attitudes about genetic risk of couples undergoing in-vitro fertilization. *Hum Reprod* 1998; 13:862–6.

52. Levron J, Aviram-Goldring AL, Madgar I, et al. Sperm chromosome abnormalities in men with severe male factor infertility who are undergoing in vitro fertilization with intracytoplasmic sperm injection. *Fertil Steril* 2001; 76:479–84.

53. Rives N, Mousset-Simeon N, Sibert L, et al. Chromosome abnormalities of spermatozoa. *Gynecol Obstet Fertil* 2004; 32:771–8.

54. May-Panloup P, Malinge MC, Larget-Piet L, Chretien MF. Genetic male infertility and medically assisted reproduction. *Gynecol Obstet Fertil* 2001; 29:583–93.

55. Wille MC, Weitz B, Kerper P, Frazier S. Advances in preconception genetic counseling. *J Perinat Neonatal Nurs* 2004; 18:28–40.

56. Hook EB. Rates of chromosome abnormalities at different maternal ages. *Obstet Gynecol* 1981; 58:282.

57. Simpson JL, Bombard A, Bennet MJ, Edmonds DK. Chromosomal abnormalities in spontaneous abortion: Frequency, pathology and genetic counseling. In: MJ Bennett, DK Edmonds, eds. *Spontaneous and Recurrent Abortion*. Oxford: Blackwell Scientific 1987; 51–76.

58. ACOG Committee Opinion. Advanced paternal age: Risks to the fetus. Number 189, October 1997. Committee on Genetics. American College of Obstetricians and Gynecologists. *Int J Gynaecol Obstet* 1997; 59:271–2.

59. Zhu JL, Madsen KM, Vestergaard M, et al. Paternal age and congenital malformations. *Hum Reprod* 2005; 28:3173–7.

60. American Society for Reproductive Medicine. Information on commonly asked questions about genetic evaluation and counseling for infertile couples. *Fertil Steril* 2004; 82:S97–S101.

61. American College of Obstetricians and Gynecologists, American College of Medical Genetics. *Preconception and Prenatal Carrier Screening for Cystic Fibrosis: Clinical and Laboratory guidelines*. 2001; Washington, DC: American College of Obstetricians and Gynecologists.

62. Palomaki GE, FitzSimmons SC, Haddow JE. Clinical sensitivity of prenatal screening for cystic fibrosis via CFTR carrier testing in a United States panethnic population. *Genet Med* 2004; 6:405–14.

63. Bonduelle M, Van Assche E, Joris H, et al. Prenatal testing in ICSI pregnancies: Incidence of chromosomal anomalies in 1586 karyotypes and relation to sperm parameters. *Hum Reprod* 2002; 17:2600–14.

64. Sele B, Cozze J, Chevret E, et al. ICSI et syndrome de Klinefelter. *Contracept Fertil Sex* 1996; 24:581–4.

65. Chandley AC, Cooke HG. Human male fertility – y-linked genes and spermatogenesis. *Hum Molec Genet* 1994; 3:1449–52.

66. Kent-First MG, et al. The incidence and possible relevance of Y-linked microdeletions in babies born after intracytoplasmic sperm injection and their infertile fathers. *Mol Hum Reprod* 1996; 12:943–50.

67. Reijo R. Diverse spermatogenic defects in humans caused by Y chromosome deletions encompassing a novel RNA-binding protein gene. *Nat Genet* 1995; 10:383.

68. Cram DS, Ma K, Bhasin S, et al. Y chromosome analysis of infertile men and their sons conceived though intracytoplasmic sperm injection: Vertical transmission of deletions and rarity of de novo deletions. *Fertil Steril* 2000; 74:909–15.

69. Olaitan A, Reid W, Mocroft A, McCarthy K, Madge S, Johnson M. Infertility among human immunodeficiency virus-positive women: Incidence and treatment dilemmas. *Hum Reprod* 1996; 11:2793–6.

70. Roth AJ, Scher HI. Genitourinary malignancies. In: JC Holland, ed. *Psycho-oncology*. New York: Oxford University Press, 1998.

71. Aass N, Fossa SC, Raghavan D, et al. Late toxicity after chemotherapy of testis cancer. In: NJ Vogelzang, PT Scardino, WU Shipley, DS Cofey, eds. *Comprehensive Textbook of Genitourinary Oncology*. Baltimore, MD: Williams & Wilkins, 1996; 1090–6.

72. Karnis MF, Simon AE, Lalwani SI, et al. Risk of death in pregnancy achieved through oocyte donation in patients with Turner syndrome: A national survey. *Fertil Steril* 2003; 80:498–501.

73. Bretherick KL, Fluker, MR, Robinson WP. FMR1 repeat sizes in the gray zone and high end of the normal range are associated with premature ovarian failure. *Hum Genet* 2005; 117:376–82.

74. Handyside AH, Kontogianni EH, Hardy K, et al. Pregnancies from biopsied human preimplantation embryos sexed by Y-specific DNA amplification. *Nature* 1990; 344:768–70.

75. Thornbill AR, deDie-Smulders CE, Geraedts JP, et al. ESHRE PGD Consortium: Best practice guidelines for clinical preimplantation genetic diagnosis (PGD) and preimplantation genetic screening (PGS). *Hum Reprod* 2005; 20:35–48.

76. ASRM Practice Committee. Preimplantation genetic diagnosis. *Fertil Steril* 2004; 82:S1.

77. ESHRE Task Force. Best Practice Guidelines for PGD. *Human Reprod* 2005; 20:231–8.

78. Verlinsky Y, Cohen J, Munne S, et al. Reproductive genetics institute over a decade of experience with preimplantation genetic diagnosis: A multicenter report. *Fertil Steril* 2004; 82:292–4.

79. European Commission, European Society of Human Genetics, & ESHRE. The interface between medically assisted reproduction and genetics: Technical, social, ethical, and legal issues. 3 June 2005, draft. www.eshre.com.

80. Ziebe S, Lundin K, Loft A, et al. CEMAS II and Study Group. FISH analysis for chromosomes 13, 16, 18, 21, 22, X and Y in all blastomeres of IVF pre-embryos from 144 randomly selected donated human oocytes and impact

on pre-embryo morphology. *Hum Reprod* 2003; 18:2575–81.

81. Sermon K, Van Steirteghem A, Liebaers I. Preimplantation genetic diagnosis. *Lancet* 2004; 363:1633–41.

82. Wilton L. Preimplantation genetic diagnosis and chromosome analysis of blastomeres using comparative genome hybridization. *Hum Reprod Update* 2005; 11:33–41.

83. Hui PW, lam YH, Chen M, et al. Attitude of at-risk subjects towards preimplantation genetic diagnosis of alpha- and beta-thalassaemias in Hong Kong. *Prenat Diagn* 2002; 22:508–11.

84. Lavery SA, Aurrell R, Turner C, et al. Preimplantation genetic diagnosis: Patients' experiences and attitudes. *Hum Reprod* 2002; 17:2464–7.

85. Katz MG, Fitzgerald L, Bankier A, et al. Issues and concerns of couples presenting for preimplantation genetic diagnosis (PGD). *Prenatal Diagn* 2002; 22: 1117–22.

86. Snowdon C, Green JM. Preimplantation diagnosis and other reproductive options: Attitudes of male and female carriers of recessive disorders. *Hum Reprod* 1997; 12:341–50.

87. Lashwood A. Preimplantation genetic diagnosis to prevent disorders in children. *Br J Nurs* 2005; 9:64–70.

88. Soussis I, Harper JC, Kontogianni E, et al. Pregnancies resulting from embryos biopsied for preimplantation diagnosis of genetic disease: Biochemical and ultrasonic studies in the first trimester of pregnancy. *J Assist Reprod Genet* 1996; 13:254–65.

89. Verlinksy Y. Preimplantation genetic diagnosis. *J Assist Reprod Genet* 1996; 13:87–9.

90. Feichtinger W. preimplantation diagnosis (PGD) – a European clinician's point of view. *J Assist Reprod Gen* 2004; 21:15–17.

91. Takeshita N, Kubo H. Regulating preimplantation genetic diagnosis – how to control PGD. *J Assist Reprod Gen* 2004; 21:19–25.

92. Menezo, YJR, Frydman R, Frydman N. Preimplantation genetic diagnosis (PGD) in France. *Assist Reprod Gen* 2004; 21:7–9.

93. Sandelowski M. A case of conflicting paradigms: Nursing and reproductive technology. *Adv Nurs Sci* 1988; 10:35–45.

94. Rothman BK. The tentative pregnancy: Then and now. In: KH Rothenberg, EJ Thomson, eds. *Women and Prenatal Testing: Facing the Challenges of Genetic Technology*. Columbus, OH: Ohio State University Press, 1994; 260–70.

95. deCrespigny L, Dredge R. *Which Tests for My Unborn Baby?* New York: Oxford University Press, 1996.

96. Wald NJ, Kennard A, Hackshaw A, McGuire A. Antenatal screening for Down's syndrome. *J Med Screen* 1997; 4:181–246.

97. American College of Obstetricians and Gynecologists (ACOG). First-trimester screening for fetal anomalies and nuchal translucency. *ACOG Committee Opinion* No. 223. Washington, DC: ACOG; Oct 1999.

98. Driscoll DA. Second trimester maternal serum screening for fetal open neural tube defects and aneuploidy. *ACMG Policy Statement* 2004.

99. Wald NJ, Rodeck C, Hackshaw AK, et al. First and second trimester antenatal screening for Down's syndrome: The results of the serum, urine, and ultrasound screening study (SURUSS). *Health Technol Assess* 2003; 7:1–77.

100. Joint HGSA/RANZCOG. Best practice guidelines on antenatal screening for Down syndrome and other fetal aneuploidy. No. C-Obs 4 Mar 2004.

101. Ormond KE. Update and review: Maternal serum screening. *J Genetic Counsel* 1997; 6:395–417.

102. Romero R, Pilu P, Jeanty A, et al. *Prenatal Diagnosis of Congenital Abnormalities*. Norwalk, CT: Appleton & Lange, 1988.

103. Daniel A, Athayde N, Ogle R, George AM, et al. Prospective ranking of the sonographic markers for aneuploidy: Data of 2143 prenatal cytogenetic diagnoses referred for abnormalities on ultrasound. *Austral New Zealand J Obstet Gynaecol* 2003; 43:16–26.

104. Olney RS, Moore CA, Khoury MJ, et al. Chorionic villus sampling and amniocentesis: Recommendations for prenatal counseling. *CDC* 1995; MMWR 44(RR-1); 1–12.

105. Sandelowski M, Harris BG, Holditch-Davis D. Amniocentesis in the context of infertility. *Health Care Women Int* 1991; 12:167–78.

106. Zuzkar D. The psychological impact of prenatal diagnosis of fetal abnormality: Strategies for investigation and intervention. *Women's Health Rev* 1987; 12:91–103.

107. Solnit JA, Stark MH. Mourning and the birth of a defective child. *Psychoanal Study Child* 1961; 16:523–7.

108. Allen JSF, Mulhauser LC. Genetic counseling after abnormal prenatal diagnosis: Facilitating coping in families who continue their pregnancies. *J Genet Couns* 1995; 4:251–65.

109. Wertz D. How parents of affected children view selective abortion. In: H Holmes, ed. *Issues in Reproductive Technology*. New York: Garland, 1992; 161–89.

110. Schechtman KB, Gray DL, Bary JD, et al. Decision making for termination of pregnancies with fetal anomalies: Analysis of 53,000 pregnancies. *Obstet Gyn* 2002; 99:216–22.

111. Hamamy HA, Dahoun S. Parental decisions following the prenatal diagnosis of sex chromosome abnormalities. *Eur J Obstet Gynecol Reprod Biol* 2004; 10:58–62.

112. Schover LR, Thomas AJ, Falcone T, et al. Attitudes about genetic risk of couples undergoing in-vitro fertilization. *Hum Reprod.* 1998; 13:862–6.

113. Neter F, Wlowlsky Y, Borochowitz ZU. Attitudes of Israeli Muslims at risk of genetic disorders towards pregnancy termination. *Community Genet* 2005; 8:88–93.

114. Blumberg B, Golbus M, Hanson K. Prenatal diagnosis: The experience of families who have children. *Am J Med Genet* 1975; 19:729–39.

115. Zeanah C, Dailey J, Rosenblatt M, et al. Do women grieve after terminating pregnancies because of fetal anomalies? A controlled investigation. *Obstet Gynecol* 1993; 82:270–5.

116. Curry CJR. Pregnancy loss, stillbirth, and neonatal death: A guide for the pediatrician. *Pediatr Clin North Am* 1992; 39:157–92.

117. ACOG. ACOG practice bulletin. Management of recurrent pregnancy loss. Number 24, February 2001. *J Gynaecol Obstet* 2001; 78:179–90.

118. Gardner R, Sutherland G. *Chromosome Abnormalities and Genetic Counseling*, 3rd ed. New York: Oxford University Press Inc., 2004.

119. Hogge WA, Byrnes AL, Lanasa MC, et al. The clinical use of karyotyping spontaneous abortions. *Am J Obstet Gynecol* 2003; 189:397–400.

120. Warburton D, Strobino B. Recurrent spontaneous abortions. In: MJ Bennett, DK Edmonds, eds. *Spontaneous and Recurrent Abortion*. Oxford: Blackwell Scientific, 1987; 193–213.

121. Laurino MY, Bennett RL, Saraiy KS, Baumeister L, et al. Genetic evaluation and counseling of couples with recurrent miscarriage: Recommendations of the national society of genetic counselors. *J Genet Counsel* 2005; 14:165–81.

122. Jones SL. Advances in human genetics: Implications for infertility nursing practice. *Infertil Reprod Med Clin North Am* 1996; 7:577–85.

123. American Society for Reproductive Medicine. Guidelines for gamete and embryo donation: A practice committee report. Guidelines and minimum standards. *Fertil Steril* 2002; 77:Suppl 5.

124. American Society for Reproductive Medicine. Guidelines for sperm donation. *Fertil Steril* 2002; 77:Suppl 5.

125. American Society for Reproductive Medicine. Guidelines for oocyte donation. *Fertil Steril* 2002; 77:Suppl 5.

126. American Society of Reproductive Medicine. Revised minimum standards offering assisted reproductive technology. *Fertil Steril* 2003; 80:1556–9.

127. EHSRE Task Force on Ethics and Law. Gamete and embryo donation. *Hum Reprod* 2002; 17:1407–8.

128. ACOG. Committee Opinion. Genetic screening of gamete donors. 1997; Number 192.

129. Licciardi F, Jansen V, Fantini D, et al. Strict genetic screening is necessary for oocyte donors. *J Assist Reprod Genet* 1997; 14(Suppl):49s.

130. Carrell DT, Cartmill D, Jones KP, et al. Prospective, randomized, blinded evaluation of donor sperm quality provided by seven commercial sperm banks. *Fertil Steril* 2002; 78:16–21.

131. Lewis V, Saller DN, Kouides RW, Garza J. Survey of genetic screening for oocyte donors. *Fertil Steril* 1999; 71:278–81.

132. Zilberstein M, Verp MS. Genetic issues in gamete donation. In: MM Seibel, SL Crockin. *Family Building Through Egg and Sperm Donation*. Boston, MA: Jones and Bartlett, 1996; 94–109.

133. Feichtinger W. Preimplantation diagnosis (PGD) – a European clinician's point of view. *J Assist Reprod Gen* 2004; 21:15–17.

134. Menezo, YJR, Frydman R, Frydman N. Preimplantation genetic diagnosis (PGD) in France. *Assist Reprod Gen* 2004; 21:7–9.

135. Bateman S. When reproductive freedom encounters medical responsibility: Changing conceptions of reproductive choice. In E Vayena, P Rowe, eds. *Medical, Ethical and Social Aspects of Assisted Reproduction*. Geneva, Switzerland, World Health Organization, 2001; 320–32.

136. Soules MR. Human reproduction cloning: Not ready for prime time. *Fertil Steril* 2001; 76:232–4.

137. Reame N. Making babies in the 21st century: New strategies, old dilemmas. *Women's Health* 2000; 10:152–9.

138. Bonnickson A. Commentary: Unnatural deeds to breed unnatural troubles. *Fertil Steril* 2001; 76:1084–5.

139. Massey JB, Slayden S, Shapiro DM, et al. Unnatural deeds do breed unnatural troubles. *Fertil Steril* 2001; 76:1083–4.

140. Bennett RL, Steinhaus KA, Ubrich SB, et al. Recommendations for standardized human pedigree nomenclature. *J Genet Couns* 1995; 4:267–79.

141. Allen JF. A guide to genetic counseling. *J Am Acad Phys Assist* 1991; 4:131–41.

16 Pregnancy Loss

SHARON N. COVINGTON

To contain the whole of death so gently even before life has begun, and not be angry – this is beyond description.
— Rainer Maria Rilke

Infertility has been defined as the inability to conceive or carry a pregnancy to a live birth. This broad definition implies that infertility encompasses both the inability to conceive a pregnancy and the loss of a pregnancy during the perinatal period, that is, before birth. Pregnancy or perinatal loss is a catch-all phrase for the death of a conceptus, fetus, or neonate during the continuum of conception, pregnancy, and birth.

A *miscarriage*, or spontaneous abortion, occurs in the first twenty weeks of pregnancy and is the most common pregnancy loss, estimated to occur in 20–50% of all conceptions. An *ectopic pregnancy* occurs in 2–3% of pregnancies when the embryo implants and grows in the fallopian tube or anywhere outside the uterus. More rarely, *trophoblastic disease*, or molar pregnancy, happens in 1 out of 2,000 pregnancies when the fetus dies but the placenta and/or chorionic villi continue to grow rapidly in a cancer-like way. Both ectopic and molar pregnancies are medical emergencies that may affect future fertility. *Stillbirth* involves the death of a fetus in utero after twenty weeks' gestation and before birth, and occurs in approximately 1–2 of every 100 births in industrialized countries. The death of a newborn infant before twenty-eight days of life is termed *neonatal death*, occurring in about 1 out of 100 births in industrialized countries, and may involve prematurity, birth defects, or sudden infant death syndrome (SIDS). Finally, the term *elective abortion* applies to the voluntary termination of a pregnancy, whether or not the fetus is viable. Statistics of both perinatal and neonatal (as well as maternal) deaths are dramatically higher in developing countries, remain high in developed countries, and as such, a critical concern of the World Health Organization.

Assisted reproductive technologies have further broadened the definition of pregnancy loss. During in vitro fertilization (IVF), conception takes place in the laboratory, and if implantation does not result after transfer of the embryo, it may be called a *preimplantation miscarriage*. Patients may also experience symptoms of pregnancy (i.e., sore breasts, weight gain, and delayed period) due to ovulation-inducing medications, commonly known as a *chemical pregnancy*, and feel fooled into thinking they are pregnant when they are not. Furthermore, the development of genetic testing of fertilized eggs during IVF has resulted in *preimplantation termination* of genetically defective embryos before transfer. Finally, as a consequence of multiple gestation following IVF, *multifetal pregnancy reduction* (MPR), or selective reduction, was developed to terminate a preselected number of fetuses in a multiple pregnancy, to maximize the viability of the remaining fetuses and/or protect the health of the mother (Figure 16.1).

In the last twenty-five years, there has been growth in the knowledge and understanding of the psychological ramifications of pregnancy loss, which is frequently a traumatic event in family life. This chapter

- reviews research in the area;
- provides theoretical frameworks that underpin a plan for clinical intervention; and
- describes psychotherapeutic strategies and interventions for counseling couples after a pregnancy loss.

HISTORICAL OVERVIEW

Pregnancy loss is a broad term used to describe the death of a fetus or baby after conception, during pregnancy, or shortly after birth. Although pregnancy losses have existed since the beginning of mankind, the context has changed dramatically with the advent of reproductive medical technology. For centuries, the death of a baby in pregnancy or shortly after birth was a fact of life – maternal and infant mortality were high and

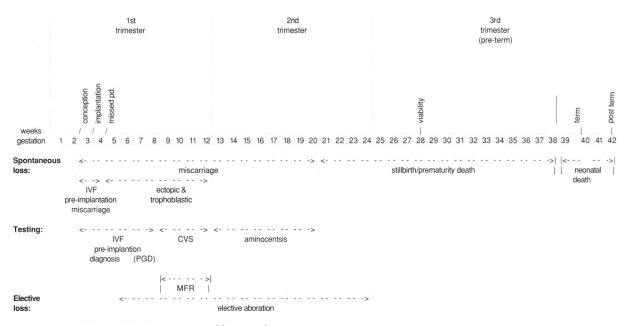

Figure 16.1. Pregnancy and loss timeline.

medical intervention almost nonexistent. Some societies and religions protected against this by bestowing 'personhood' only on infants that survived a certain period of time. For example, in China, a child is not recognized as a person until three months of age, and in traditional Judaism, religious funeral and mourning rituals are not performed before thirty days of life.

However, rapid technological growth in reproductive medicine in the past fifty years has created a picture of medicine-as-god, with the ability to create and continue life. Today, women have more control over their reproductive lives, using a variety of contraceptive devices to avoid pregnancy, advanced reproductive technologies to produce a pregnancy, therapeutic options to terminate or reduce undesired pregnancies, and extensive medical treatment to manage complicated or threatened pregnancies. However, the consequence has often been an unrealistic expectation that medical intervention can, in fact, prevent or stop losses in pregnancy.

Just as medical technology has changed, so too has the psychological approach to pregnancy loss. Prior to this century, pregnancy and infant losses were a common event and a fact of life in the community, acknowledged, grieved, and mourned in the same manner as other deaths. However, when the treatment of illness, including childbirth, moved from home to hospital, the manner in which death was dealt with changed. Death and dying became sanitized and sterilized. When a baby died, it was handled like a shameful secret, almost as if modern medicine was not suppose to let this happen. The deceased baby was often quietly disposed of with-

out being seen by parents, who were not encouraged to mourn the loss, as it was believed that the whole experience would be too upsetting for them and was better forgotten. 'Out of sight, out of mind' was the emotional approach to a pregnancy loss, and psychological support was minimal. This approach remains the same in many cultures today.

REVIEW OF LITERATURE

Early research in the area of pregnancy loss tended to be retrospective, poorly designed, and anecdotal.[1–3] However, it facilitated a growing knowledge-base that pregnancy loss is a significant psychological trauma for parents. A review of the literature covers five areas centering around grief: mourning, gestation, gender, predictors, and interventions.

Grief and Mourning

The first published study on perinatal loss appeared in 1970 when Kennell and colleagues[4] reported on their interviews with families who had experienced a stillbirth. Subsequent research supports the finding that pregnancy loss involves considerable pain and suffering for parents, with such typical symptoms as sadness, loss of appetite, sleep difficulties, irritability, preoccupation with thoughts of the baby, guilt, shame, and anger.[5–9] Grief is typically intense and begins to decline after the first year of bereavement.[10,11] In addition, there is considerable risk of disordered or pathological grief following a pregnancy loss.[11–13] *Pathological grief* is usually described in terms of psychiatric symptomatology, intense grieving extending beyond the first year, or the absence of grief. Results from these investigations suggests that a substantial number of women, possibly 20–30%, experience significant psychiatric morbidity following a perinatal loss.[2]

Grief and Gestation

A common area of interest is the relationship between grief reactions and gestation. There is substantial evidence that the intensity and the duration of grief correspond to the length of gestation.[9,14–16] However, other researchers have found no quantitative difference in the grief reactions of mothers who had miscarriages, stillbirths, or neonatal deaths.[17] A more predictive factor in the intensity of grief relates to the sense of psychological attachment to the developing fetus rather than gestational age.[9,14] For example, it has been demonstrated that grief may occur after an unsuccessful IVF cycle, when conception took place in the laboratory but did not result in pregnancy (preimplantation miscarriage).[18]

The kind of loss does not appear to be a determinant in grief and mourning. Grief occurs after ectopic and molar pregnancies, significantly impacting on self- and body-image due to the medically intrusive nature of the loss.[19,20] Planned terminations of pregnancies may be distressing and grieved, although not universally and often with no long-term psychological consequences.[21,22] Mothers of a twin who has died experience grief that is quantitatively indistinguishable from mothers who lose a singleton baby.[23] It is also evident that women who terminate a pregnancy because of fetal anomalies experience grief as intense as those who experience spontaneous pregnancy loss and may require similar clinical management.[24]

Grief and Gender

Mothers and fathers both mourn pregnancy loss but often experience grief in different ways.[23,25] Mothers tend to experience more intense grief, perhaps due to greater prenatal and postnatal attachment.[9,14] However, one study[25] found that 22% of fathers had significantly higher grief scores than mothers. Another study[26] compared grief symptomatology between men and women, with mothers experiencing more emotional and somatic distress, while fathers describing difficulty working, increasing use of alcohol, and social withdrawal. More research on the differing

patterns of mourning between mothers and fathers is needed.

Predictors of Complicated Grief

Complicated, disordered, or pathological grief concerns serious psychiatric symptomatology, the absence of grief, or intense grieving beyond the first year that affects the long-term psychological functioning of the individual. The greatest predictor of a pathological grief reaction is a history of poor psychological functioning prior to the loss.[14,27] One study[28] found that women were at five times greater risk of developing depression after a miscarriage than women in the general population. Childless women were also found to be at greater risk of developing a major depression after a perinatal loss.[27] Other risk factors identified in the literature include problematic or lack of social supports, significant life stressors during pregnancy, difficult marital relationship, and poor physical health.[10,11,14] A history of pregnancy or other reproductive loss may also affect the process of grief.[16]

Intervention and Grief

Intervention following a pregnancy loss has an impact on grief. There is substantial evidence that family involvement with the deceased baby helps facilitate the grief process.[4,11,25] Supportive, reality-enforcing interventions by caregivers to parents, such as seeing, touching, and spending time with the baby, acknowledge the loss and encouraging healthy mourning by making it real and tangible. However, one controversial study[29] questions the practices of having contact with the deceased baby suggesting higher rates of maternal depression[30], post-traumatic stress disorder[31,32] and disorganized attachment with the next-born infant.[33] Patient organizations have taken issue with this study, fearing a return to earlier times when contact with the deceased baby was denied. Nonetheless, this study may highlight the importance of patient choice and tailoring interventions versus a single approach applied to all patients.

Patients are responsive to open, compassionate, sensitive communication with caregivers and are in need of follow-up care and information, which to facilitate grieving.[34] As important, supportive counseling has been found to significantly shorten bereavement following a perinatal loss.[10,35] Even a single, follow-up phone call to parents within a few weeks of the loss, in which the grieving process is reviewed and parental concerns are addressed, has been found to significantly reduce guilt and depression several months later.[36]

THEORETICAL FRAMEWORK

Pregnancy and Pregnancy Loss Theory

The psychological impact of pregnancy loss is best understood in the context within which it occurs, that is, pregnancy. Pregnancy begins psychologically long before it occurs physically. From the time girls are little, most play with baby dolls and dream of having children and being mothers. Boys also try on the role of fatherhood in their play. Young couples often carefully plan how their family will grow and talk about their wishes for their children long before they are ready to attempt pregnancy. Thus, men and women lay the psychological and emotional groundwork for adaptation to parenthood and attachment to their child years before the actual event takes place.

Pregnancy is a crisis time when significant changes occur in a short period, and is as much a psychological experience as it is a physical condition. Women experience profound changes in body, sense of self, and in relationship with others. It is a time when psychological defenses are loosened, and unconscious material is apt to emerge. From a psychoanalytic perspective, pregnancy is a regressed state in which early conflicts are revived and repeated.[37] A pregnant woman's identification with her own mother, called maternal identification, is a crucial influence in the psychological course and outcome of pregnancy. Pregnancy is also an intensely narcissistic condition, whereby a man and a woman are recreating themselves. The developing relationship with the baby is based on fantasies, dreams, and images that are reflective of their own psychological issues. There is intense narcissistic involvement, and the pregnancy becomes a source of narcissistic pride or, if problems occur, narcissistic injury. For parents, the psychological challenge in pregnancy is to incorporate and attach to the developing baby, while differentiating the child from one's self.[38]

Bonding and attachment, which previously was believed to begin at the time of quickening, have been influenced by the use of new medical technologies.[18,22,39] Women currently have much more control over their reproductive capabilities than ever before, through birth control choices, medical treatments, and pregnancy termination. Today, blood tests can confirm a pregnancy before a menstrual period is missed. Sonography or ultrasound, much like a window into the uterus, provides an early visual image of the developing baby. Real-time moving pictures of the baby – arms, legs, face, and heartbeat – can be seen before any physical changes have occurred to make others aware of the pregnancy. Genetic testing can be done early in the laboratory on the embryo during IVF before implantation has occurred, or later with chorionic villus sampling (CVS) and amniocentesis when the genetic makeup and sex of the baby can be learned before a woman is even wearing maternity clothes. Consequently, the information learned from this technology facilitates a very early, intensified psychological involvement with both the pregnancy and the baby, which is seen as a person, not a fetus. A pregnancy loss is experienced as an assault on one's psychological foundation. It comes at a time of extreme psychological vulnerability and is, in effect, a crisis (the loss) within a crisis (the pregnancy). Leon[3] integrated the psychology of pregnancy and pregnancy loss into four areas: a new developmental stage, an instinctual process, object-seeking, and self-enhancement. Pregnancy is a *new phase in life* in which a woman renegotiates the developmental issues of separateness, autonomy, and independence from her mother. If loss occurs, it becomes an obstacle to entering the stage and can result in arrested development and psychological stagnation. Pregnancy is also an *instinctual process*, whereby strong psychological and biological drives come together. A perinatal loss creates an instinctual frustration both by depriving one of the satisfaction of powerful oral drives and by reviving earlier internalized conflicts. For example, mothers often describe a literal 'baby hunger,' a profound deprivation of the need to hold, feed, and nurture their baby. Pregnancy is also *object-seeking*, whereby the process of making a person involves internalized interactions that represent both self and others. In addition, pregnancy may be viewed as the pinnacle of both selflessness and self-involvement, a fulfillment of one's most grandiose narcissistic wishes. When a pregnancy loss occurs, there is narcissistic and object loss – the *real* loss of the baby becomes a narcissistic injury and, therefore, a *symbolic* loss of self. The loss must be understood in terms of the intrapsychic meanings of and the interpersonal responses to perinatal loss.

Bereavement Theory

A significant amount of research has focused on perinatal grief, much of which was based on the early bereavement works of Freud,[40] Lindemann,[41] Parkes,[42] and Bowlby.[43] The grief experience is a universal and predictable process, whereby an individual acknowledges the loss and gradually lets go of the psychological ties to the loved one. Although often used interchangeably, the terms *grief*, *mourning*, and *bereavement* are distinctly different. Grief is the emotional response to a loss, manifested by a host of feelings such as shock, numbness, anger, guilt, sadness, and anxiety. Mourning is the process, often culturally defined, that one goes through to deal with these emotions. Bereavement refers to the time period during which grief is being resolved. Although the mourning process occurs on a continuum of shock, emotional disorganization, and eventual reorganization, the grief experience is like a roller-coaster, where emotional reactions are unpredictable and repetitive. Hence, mourning is a complex process mediated by a wide variety of variables including previous loss, previous childbirth experiences, length of gestation, quality of marital relationship, maternal age, mental health, fertility history, religiosity, physical health, and the likelihood of a subsequent successful pregnancy.[14] The mourning process, while universal in nature, occurs within a cultural context that may forbid talking about the loss, participating in loss-related events, and/or expressing grief in public or close private circles, thus affecting grief and adaptation.[44,45]

CLINICAL ISSUES

Losing a baby in pregnancy or after birth is a unique psychological experience. Grief, mourning, and bereavement have distinctive aspects, which differ from other losses, and the grief pattern may be somewhat unpredictable. The following section describes clinical issues involved in perinatal grief counseling.

Unique Aspects of Perinatal Grief

A pregnancy loss occurs at a time of profound developmental change for a couple and may be their first experience with death. However, this death is different from that of a parent, friend, spouse, or even an older child, in which grief is *retrospective* and real memories and experiences are mourned and shared by others. With a perinatal loss, grief is *prospective*: Mourning occurs around the hopes, wishes, and fantasies of the future for a baby known only to the parents and possibly other immediate family. The loss is also *multidimensional* and reflects an individual's unique experiences. For example, it may reflect a loss of a pregnancy, baby, future relationships, innocence, health, control, reproductive capacity, hopes and dreams, and so on. Furthermore, the narcissistic nature of the loss is different and affects feelings of grief, with mothers often experiencing intense guilt, shame, envy, rage, and self-blame, which are not usually experienced with other losses.

Because the loss is different from other losses and comes at a time of extreme psychological vulnerability, several aspects make grieving particularly difficult.[14,37,39] First, there is little opportunity for antic-ipatory grieving, as the loss often occurs suddenly and without warning. Second, there is frequently an absence of any visible and publicly acknowledged object to mourn, especially in earlier losses where others may not have even been aware of the pregnancy. Furthermore, there are often few socially acceptable avenues for mourning – no funerals, rituals, or cultural traditions that help to acknowledge loss and facilitate grieving. Fourth, there is a remarkable lack of social support, and the loss is experienced as socially unspeakable, often being glossed over or minimized by others in many cultures. When the loss is not acknowledged or discussed, a deep sense of shame and personal failure is intensified, especially for mothers. Last, and probably most difficult, is the prospective nature of grieving in which fantasies of future interactions must be mourned. When memories of a life are primarily dreams, the grief takes on a new dimension – the pain of not ever knowing. The ability to resolve grief following a perinatal loss often depends on a couple's ability to find avenues to acknowledge the loss and express their emotions.

Although perinatal grief reflects the characteristics of grief identified by a number of authors, mourning is a uniquely personal experience. Each person deals with the feelings in his or her own unique way, based on personality, culture, and life experiences. Thus, husbands and wives feel and deal differently with the loss; just as they have bonded differently with the child, they grieve differently. Couples need to be aware that no two people, as close as they may be, experience the loss and deal with the feelings in exactly the same way. They also need to know that different does not mean better or worse; it only means not the same. Furthermore, gender differences in mourning are culturally defined, influencing the meaning of the experience and the process of grief.[44,46,47]

Unpredictable Pattern of Perinatal Grief

Feelings of grief are like a tidal wave that sweeps over one, growing and cresting with time. Intense feelings of shock, disbelief, anger, self-blame, rage, guilt, anxiety, and depression occur unpredictably and repetitively. In the author's clinical experience, the feelings seem to peak somewhere between three to nine months following the loss. This is problematic for parents, as it occurs at a time when social supports, if there were any, may have disappeared. It also may occur within the context of a subsequent pregnancy or other reproductive events, such as infertility. Grieving a perinatal loss takes far longer than most people anticipate, anywhere from a few months to several years.

TABLE 16.1. Risk factors for complicated grief

History of poor psychological functioning

History of reproductive loss

Medical history associated with the loss

Medical interventions to achieve or maintain pregnancy

Age

Marital instability

Social isolation

Recent crises or losses

There are also physical manifestations of grief. Symptoms may include aching breasts and arms, difficulty sleeping, nightmares, lack of appetite, heart palpitations, shortness of breath, difficulty concentrating, forgetfulness, or tiredness. Mothers also may experience their milk coming in and other physical discomforts following delivery, which may enhance the reality of there being no baby. The stress from the loss sometimes brings out physical problems such as headaches, muscle spasms, or a susceptibility to infections, colds, and other viruses. Often, grieving mothers feel as if their bodies have failed them, furthering narcissistic injury. The feeling of physical defectiveness is particularly compounded when there are difficulties or complications with physical healing, especially following an ectopic or molar pregnancy. It is also important to recognize that after giving birth, a woman may experience profound hormonal changes that may affect mood and emotions.

As the tidal wave of grief passes, swells of grief remain that are triggers and remind the parents of their loss and rekindle feelings. Peppers and Knapp[48] use the term *shadow grief* to describe this occurrence. It relates to a parent's desire never to forget the baby and also to the general inability to express the feelings to others. Like a shadow, it is always there yet requires no coping mechanisms. Feelings of sadness are often triggered around significant days and events, such as the due date, date of conception, birth date, and anniversary of the baby's death. Holidays such as Mother's Day, Father's Day, Children's Day in Japan or child-centered religious ceremonies can also be painful. Changes in the season or special places may rekindle memories. However, with time, this sadness becomes a dull ache and not the all-encompassing pain of before.

There are several factors that may adversely affect the grief response – undercurrents of grief that may impact the size and duration of the tidal wave. These are circumstances that may complicate the already dif-

ficult task of mourning (Table 16.1). As identified in the research and in this author's clinical experience, the more intense the psychological attachment to the baby, the more significant will be the loss experienced by the parents. Clinicians need to consider the following factors in assessing the risk for complicated bereavement: a history of *poor psychological functioning*, including depression, other psychiatric symptomatology, and personality disorders; a history of *reproductive loss*, including infertility, prior pregnancy losses, or elective abortions; *medical history*, including risk factors associated with the loss, such as lupus, hypertension, cervical cancer, gestational diabetes, blood-related disorders such as thrombophilia, Group B Streptococcus, or overall physical health problems; *medical interventions*, including the use of high-tech infertility treatment to achieve pregnancy, high-risk pregnancy, extended bed rest, and selective reduction or amniocentesis prior to the loss; *age*, including older women facing their reproductive biological clock and very young women lacking social support and resources to deal with the loss; *marital instability*, including absence of other children; *social isolation* including culturally defined practices of social withdrawal or stigma, and *other recent crisis or losses*, such as another death in the family, a move, or job problems. Any of these factors may influence the psychological attachment to the developing baby and intensify the grief reaction, as well as being concurrent risk factors of postpartum depression. It is important to note, however, that with recurrent pregnancy loss, not every loss will be experienced in the same way or have the same meaning. For example, an early pregnancy loss of an unplanned, unwanted pregnancy may have small emotional significance, while a loss a few years later of a planned, much desired pregnancy may be much more psychologically difficult.

Acceptance or resolution occurs when the loss has been integrated into the person's life and no longer consumes all energy. This point may coincide with a subsequent successful birth, which appears to be an important contribution to resolution of a perinatal loss for some women.[49] For many women, another pregnancy is an opportunity to redo a failed experience and, as such, regain feelings of competency and accomplishment with a successful birth. Although women often experience a profound hole in their lives following a perinatal loss, some imagine that the way to feel better is to get pregnant quickly, thereby replacing the dead baby. The pregnancy then serves as a means of avoiding grief and may affect the relationship with the subsequent child.[2] Thus, women need encouragement to allow sufficient time to heal physically and emotionally before attempting another pregnancy,

---

TABLE 16.2. Interventions after perinatal loss that may facilitate grieving

Medical

Choice of induction/delivery plan

Seeing, touching, spending time with the baby, or viewing products of conception

Naming the baby

Taking pictures (if declined by parents, stored in record for later availability)

Providing mementos (e.g., lock of hair, wrist band, foot/hand prints, length/weight certificate, symbolic representations, sonograms)

Planning for disposition of body/tissue

Funeral or memorial service

Choosing room assignment off obstetrics floor or discharge planning

Providing written materials on perinatal grief and support resources

Interim phone call from staff before follow-up office visit

Psychological

Creating a memory box or album (e.g., photographs, sonogram pictures, laboratory reports, IVF petri dish, cards, toy or item of clothing)

Memorial activities (e.g., planting a tree, selecting a garden statue, donation to special charity, books for support groups, items for neonatal intensive care unit or high-risk unit)

Self-care activities (e.g., regular exercise, proper diet, avoidance of alcohol/drugs, following a schedule/routine)

Keeping a journal, diary, or audiotape describing the loss and grief

Writing a letter or poem of goodbye to baby

Planning a memorial service, private or with others

Reaching out to a support group or family/friends

---

understanding that physical healing often occurs long before emotional healing.

THERAPEUTIC INTERVENTIONS

The goal of all interventions – whether medical or psychological – following a pregnancy loss is to facilitate positive grieving. In addition, it is to restore the patient's narcissistic equilibrium and self-esteem. Because parents mourn regardless of the kind of loss, no distinction will be made in this section between interventions for early versus later gestational losses. However, attention will be given to special situations of loss, including recurrent pregnancy loss, loss of a multiple in pregnancy, and selected cases of multifetal reduction and pregnancy termination due to a genetic defect.

Medical Approaches

Intervention at the time of loss, that is, in the hospital and with medical caregivers, can have a great effect on the course of mourning. Couples often say that the best medicine or the only medicine that helped following the loss was the compassionate, sensitive care of the medical staff. Conversely, patients' greatest complaints about

their medical care often concern feeling traumatized by the lack of sensitivity, responsiveness, communication, and concern by their medical caregivers.[34] This accelerates further narcissistic injury and the projection of rage and blame onto caregivers. It is this author's belief that most medical malpractice following a perinatal loss is *not* due primarily to medical negligence or incompetence but more often to poor and insensitive communication with the grieving couple by the physician and/or medical staff.

Patients need to be presented with reality-enforcing options and allowed to make choices that are right for them (Table 16.2), and within their cultural context. These options may include the following: choices about induction, delivery, or dilation and curettage (D &C) plan, and whether to wait for the loss to occur naturally or proceed with immediate medical intervention; being able to see, touch, and spend time with the baby or view the products of conception, with careful preparation as to what they will see; having a support person immediately available; taking pictures of the fetus/baby; being provided with mementos such as a lock of hair, wrist band, certificate with length and weight, foot and hand prints, symbolic representation of the fetus/ products of conception; naming the baby; having a religious/cultural ceremony (e.g., baptism); having a copy of an autopsy or pathology report; burial, cremation, or other form of disposition of the fetus/tissue; funeral or memorial services; and choice of hospital room assignment or discharge planning. Patients need to be carefully guided as to what to anticipate and expect in considering these options, and need to be given the opportunity to consider and later reconsider if they initially refuse a choice.[50] For example, patients often have fears associated with seeing their dead baby or fetus, yet are embarrassed to express these concerns. However, they need to understand that this will be their only opportunity to see the baby, need to be told what to expect, and advised that while some parents have found this useful in making the loss a reality others have not. If they still choose not to see the baby, pictures can be taken and placed in the chart, and the parents informed of access to the pictures later on if they change their mind. Lastly, aftercare needs to be planned, with written materials given at discharge, information provided on support groups and counseling resources, an interim phone call to offer support and understanding, and a scheduled follow-up office visit.

Psychotherapeutic Approaches

A psychodynamic and cognitive-behavioral approach is applicable to perinatal loss therapy. Leon[3] presented a psychodynamic framework in which the intrapsychic meaning of the perinatal death is considered within the context of revived conflicts and identifications occurring in pregnancy. This form of expressive psychotherapy can be used in a short-term or long-term model. Shapiro[51] described a cognitive-behavioral model in which concrete direction and advice are provided by the therapist as a means of improving coping and communication skills to manage the loss. This is a more active counseling approach to therapy that is usually short-term and focused. Both models provide useful tools for psychotherapeutic intervention. This author uses a combination of the two models, based on careful psychological assessment of the patient.

Assessment

Patients presenting for therapy following a perinatal loss are usually in tremendous emotional pain. Leon[3] pointed to the importance of being able to recognize the difference between behavior and affects that, in another context, would be viewed as pathological. For example, transient hallucinatory descriptions of hearing the baby cry are common. Nonetheless, an awareness of the danger of a pathological outcome is important, which is a matter of degree, affecting the long-range functioning of the individual and his or her relationship with others. History taking must include questions covering the areas mentioned previously regarding the risk factors for complicated bereavement and/or postpartum depression (see Table 16.1). The assessment phase usually takes from two to four sessions, at the end of which a treatment plan is discussed.

A differential diagnosis needs to be determined between primary perinatal grief and perinatal grief that is secondary to a prior depressive constellation or other mental health diagnosis. When there is evidence of pre-existing depression, it may be the tip of the iceberg to complicating borderline and narcissistic personality disorders, which cannot be treated in a short-term therapy approach. (However, specific goals that facilitate grief may still be attained.) A complete history of psychological functioning prior to the loss will also assist the therapist in determining clinical depression and true suicidality. Patients often express a wish to be with their dead baby. However, suicidal danger can be ascertained "by the usual criteria of conscious intent to harm or kill oneself, history of suicidal behavior, reality-testing, impulsivity, and existence of an actual plan."[3]

A number of studies have indicated the traumatic nature of perinatal loss and the increased risk of developing post-traumatic stress disorder (PTSD) with depression.[31,52,53] It is useful to consider how the DSM-IV diagnostic description of PTSD (#309.81) applies to perinatal loss:[54]

A person has been exposed to a traumatic event in which...[he/she] experienced a death...or a threat to the physical integrity of self...and [the] response involved intense fear, helplessness, or horror. The traumatic event is then persistently re-experienced [with]...recurrent and intrusive distressing recollections of the event, including images, thoughts, or perceptions;...recurrent and distressing dreams of the event; [and/or]...a sense of reliving the experience.

This definition accurately describes symptomatology patients often experience following a pregnancy loss: flashbacks or, what this author calls, replaying a 'psychological videotape' of the experience; intrusive and distressing thoughts of the event; nightmares; and avoidance of situations (e.g., seeing babies) that trigger feelings. In recalling the circumstances of learning and experiencing a perinatal loss, patients can often describe in vivid detail what occurred. Women who thirty or forty years earlier experienced a pregnancy loss can often give vivid descriptions of surroundings (who was there and what was said), almost as if it occurred that very morning.[55] There is often an uncontrollable need and desire to replay the psychological videotape as a means of reliving and working through the traumatic experience. In fact, as with other types of PTSD, it is necessary to be able to repeatedly remember and discuss the experience to obtain distance from it.

The use of psychotropic medication may need to be considered as an adjunct to perinatal loss therapy. Patients frequently have difficulty sleeping immediately after the loss, and their obstetrician may prescribe sleeping pills or tranquilizers to help patients relax and/or cope. However, these are short-term solutions to grief symptomatology and need to be carefully monitored so as not to circumvent mourning or precipitate other problems (e.g., history of chemical dependency or abuse). Patients having difficulty with eating, sleeping, anxiety, or depression may be helped with increasing the frequency of therapy (e.g., from weekly to twice a week), to provide more opportunity to work through feelings. They may also be helped with behavioral techniques, such as regular exercise, deep relaxation, and meditation. If, however, symptomatology does not improve and is adversely affecting daily functioning, a medication referral is warranted. This is particularly important if perinatal grief is secondary to a prior or preexisting depressive constellation or other mental health diagnosis. An experienced psychiatrist or psychopharmacologist is the ideal knowledge source for the rapidly expanding options in psychotropic medications (see Chapter 6). Patients may need assistance in understanding that medication is not a happy pill, which in effect denies and avoids their grief. Instead, it is a useful tool in alleviating depressive symptomatology, thus giving the patient more energy and cognitive clarity to deal effectively with the problems at hand and facilitate grieving.

A determination will need to be made about whether the focus of treatment will be individual, couple, or a combination. Sometimes, the decision is made when only one person presents for therapy. However, in the course of obtaining an individual and marital history, it may become apparent that marital instability was a preexisting condition that will need to be addressed. In some relationships, one person will take on the task of grieving for the two, frequently the wife for the husband, in which case both partners may need to be encouraged to participate in the therapy to restore equilibrium and avoid divisiveness. A perinatal loss has the potential of making a good marriage stronger and of destroying a problem marriage. Attention also needs to be given to additional stressors in a couple's life: other children at home; financial problems; job pressures; extended family strains, such as siblings having babies or parents who are ill; health issues, such as continued infertility treatment or the diagnosis of cancer during the pregnancy; sexual dysfunction; or the pregnancy loss representing the end of childbearing and the approach of menopause.

Setting the Stage

Important as it is in treatment to obtain a complete individual and marital history, it cannot take place before the therapist has heard the patient's story of the pregnancy loss. The first session is very important in setting the tone for therapy, and the therapist may want to schedule an extended session (one-and-a-half to two regular therapy hours) for the initial appointment. The couple needs the opportunity to describe in detail the psychological videotape of the loss – what the circumstances surrounding the pregnancy were; how they learned there was a problem; what happened at the hospital/time of loss; what reality-supporting interventions occurred; what were the availability and reactions of medical caregivers, family, and friends at the time of loss and later; what were the woman's and/or man's emotional reaction at the time and since; and what actions they have taken in response to the loss. If the couple has pictures and/or other mementos of their baby, it is very helpful for them to bring these to a session to share with the therapist. The therapist needs to give sufficient time to go over each item, have the couple talk about what each piece means to them, and offer positive feedback about the specialness of this child. This action communicates the therapist's willingness to emotionally engage in the system and validates the fetus/baby's existence as real and worthy of mourning. At the same time, it may provide the therapist with insight into the patient's emerging mental health problems when the response seems out of the norm (e.g., having a large photo of the dead fetus displayed over the living room fireplace). It also allows the therapist to gain understanding of cultural norms influencing a couple's grieving.

There are two situations in which patients may feel either bolstered or betrayed by medical technology. Infertility patients who lose a pregnancy may feel both success and failure – similar to theatrical masks with one side smiling and the other frowning. These patients often feel bolstered that they have achieved a pregnancy, while experiencing a tremendous sense of loss for the wished-for child in whom they have considerable emotional, physical, and financial investment. With repeated pregnancy loss, there is a recurring cycle of hope and despair that makes it exceedingly more difficult to grieve. On the other hand, patients who have had CVS or amniocentesis genetic testing and shortly thereafter lost a healthy pregnancy often feel betrayed by the medical technology that they thought or were told would be helpful. Understandably, feelings of anger, guilt, and blame may be accentuated and need to be worked through to avoid pathological grief and/or lingering bitterness. While feelings of anger, guilt, self-blame, and blame of caregivers are common, patients may need to be encouraged to dispel hindsight and recognize that they made the best decision at the time with the best of intentions. Often, these patients express complete naiveté about the risks associated with prenatal genetic testing, discounting information that may have been explained to them prior to the procedure. Even patients who understand the risks often cannot believe it happened to them. Consequently, patients need to be prepared for the potential for loss. They will need to recognize that if they would not terminate a problem pregnancy, then the information obtained from the procedure may not be worth the risk.

Patients often present in an emotionally vulnerable and somewhat defenseless manner. Initially, the therapist may need to help them integrate some defenses to deal with the overwhelming feelings. However, if they present in a highly defensive manner, the therapist needs to be very careful about removing any of these defenses until their meaning and purpose for patients are clear. Patients who are defensive believe that there is something that they need to defend against, possibly exposure of major mental health problems. Furthermore, following a perinatal loss, patients are highly sensitive to perceived criticism and judgment, especially if they think that the pregnancy loss was within their control. Thus, any helping professional must choose words and actions carefully, and appropriately intervene if miscommunication has occurred. The potential for further narcissistic injury is always present because of psychological vulnerability.

The therapist must be able to tolerate the unrestrained, affective outpouring of grief – intense sadness, anger, rage, guilt, self-blame, fear of the future, and remorse – while being ever cognizant of his or her own counter-transference to these powerful emotions. If the therapist has experienced a perinatal loss, any self-disclosure should be carefully evaluated as to the appropriateness to the situation at hand and the helpfulness of the content to the patient. Furthermore, if self-disclosure occurs, it is important to process how patients perceive the information, their fantasies, and reactions. This is also true of patient education materials, such as personal stories of pregnancy loss or self-help groups in which members recount their loss. These stories may or may not be helpful, so that processing a patient's interpretation of the information is necessary.

One of the difficulties for couples is that there may be no tangible evidence of their baby's existence that can be mourned. With preimplantation losses and early miscarriages, there are few mementos and rituals that validate the loss. At times, patients enter therapy years after the loss, either consciously aware of unresolved grief or unconscious to other events that ultimately relate to unresolved mourning, such as marital problems, depression, problems with subsequent children, or a pregnancy loss of a family member such as a son or daughter. A task of therapy is, then, to help create mementos and rituals that acknowledge the reality of the lost child.

Therapeutic Goals – Facilitating Grief and Restoring Self-Esteem

Several cognitive-behavioral techniques may be useful in psychotherapy for pregnancy loss and can be presented as options for facilitating grief (see Table 16.2). Couples may want to put together a memory box or album with small things that represent their wished-for child: a sonogram picture, laboratory report, item of clothing or toy that was for the baby, cards and condolences letters received, positive home pregnancy test, and so on. They may also want to consider writing a letter or poem to their baby, in which they name him or her, expressing all their hopes, wishes, and dreams, and then saying goodbye. Keeping a journal of therapy and/or writing a diary of all the events surrounding the loss helps parents find a place to put feelings, so that memories of this special child will never be forgotten. Planning a memorial service, either private or with others, may be helpful even years after the loss. In addition, planting a tree or purchasing a garden statue in their baby's memory may help provide a beautiful, living reflection of their child. Donating money to a special charity, books to a perinatal loss support group, or baby items to a hospital or neonatal intensive care unit may also be a helpful way of recognizing the child. Although these exercises and activities are usually worked on outside the therapy hour, it is often an emotional experience and needs to be processed during the therapy session.

Patients will need assistance in understanding the normalcy of their grief and encouragement for finding ways to express these feelings. Wishes and fantasies will have to be mourned with the realization that the dreams for this special child will never materialize. Where irrational guilt exists, the therapist must carefully explore the origin of the guilt and help patients differentiate between fact and fantasy. At times, patients may need encouragement and assistance in obtaining more medical information to provide the facts. For example, women frequently worry that stress may have been a factor in the loss and need reassurance that there is little evidence that stress causes miscarriages,[56,57] and that babies have been conceived and born under the most horrific of circumstances (i.e., during World Wars and/or natural disasters).

Depression is a common affective response to pregnancy loss.[58–62] A useful intervention may be to tell patients that "depression is often anger turned inwards" and a task of therapy is to help them express what they are angry or unhappy about, while directing the feelings to the source. For example, patients may be feeling very angry at other people, disappointed with their physician, family, or friends who they feel were unsupportive. It can be therapeutic to discuss ways to communicate these feelings to people who have hurt or disappointed them and decide what, if any action, needs to be taken. Do they want to set up an appointment to talk to the doctor or write a letter expressing their concerns? Do they want to speak with their family or write their feelings in a letter that may or may not be mailed? Role-playing in therapy what the patient would like to say can also help reduce angry feelings and model actions. In addition, it provides the opportunity to determine the reality or justifiability of their anger.

It has been said that "a feeling shared is a feeling diminished" and that there is "strength in numbers." Hence, perinatal loss support groups serve as an important therapeutic resource. These groups, available in their community or via the internet, prevent parents from becoming isolated with their grief and help connect them to new relationships that will promote healing. For patients with a history of infertility, the group may help them feel more normal and connected to the fertile world. However, these groups sometimes have the potential to further frighten patients as they may hear stories of perinatal losses they never knew occurred were possible and, in turn, may create more worries about their own future pregnancy. While a support group may not be for everyone, it is suggested that patients need to go about three times before deciding whether or not it is right for them. For many people, a support group or a group of supportive family and friends is all that is needed to heal the grief. For those who are at risk for complicated grief, a perinatal loss support group may stagnate mourning, unless it is used in conjunction with individual and/or couples therapy.

Patients often need the therapist's encouragement and prompting support to take concrete steps toward self-care. In short, grieving people often forget how to take care of themselves. Regular exercise is very important in restoring positive body-image, reducing depression and anxiety, and increasing energy. Other activities enhance a more positive self-image, such as massage therapy, facials, manicures, and so on. Eating planned, nutritionally balanced meals promotes physical healing. Furthermore, patients may need assistance in instituting a schedule and routine in their life that allows for structure to the boundless experience of grief. They also may need permission to involve themselves in activities that are fun and provide relief from the world of grief. These activities assist in restoring self-esteem.

Special Considerations

Multiple Miscarriages

While a miscarriage is considered a somewhat common medical occurrence, the repeated loss of a pregnancy during the first trimester deserves special psychological attention. Early recurrent pregnancy loss (RPL), that is, three or more consecutive spontaneous losses, affects 1–2% of women and is a common presenting problem for treatment at reproductive medical practices.[63] Women with this condition are sometimes referred to as 'habitual aborters,' a medical term that often adds insult to injury. Although a myriad of tests and treatments are available for RPL, the literature is filled with controversy regarding their efficacy.[64,65] Evaluation and management of RPL includes genetic/chromosomal anomalies, endocrine/hormonal factors, immunologic causes, prothrombotic states, anatomical defects, infections, and environmental factors.[31,64] Age is considered a primary risk factor, with one-third of all pregnancies ending in miscarriage after the age of forty, primarily due to chromosomal abnormalities. Despite the debate over evaluations and treatments, some research suggests that the probability of achieving a live birth for an untreated patient after three successive miscarriages may still range as high as 50–70%.[66]

Patients who have experienced repeated miscarriage are usually deeply distressed by the emotional rollercoaster of pregnancy and loss. Gervaize[67] describes these patients as "almost uniformly depressed, overwhelmed, grieving, anxious, ambivalent, angry, and often almost obsessive in the search for a solution to this problem." While medical treatment may vary depending on the causal factors identified or hypothesized, there is an almost universal consensus that psychological support and counseling is a crucial component of care due to the cumulative effect of repeated losses.[58,65,67,68] Patients need thorough information and education on the possible causes of RPL, as well as an understanding that the underlying pathology may never be identified due to the uniqueness of each pregnancy. Counseling and psychotherapy may hold the most hope for improved outcome, although the exact role is still unclear.[67] What is apparent is that psychological support can help to diminish anxiety and depression in subsequent pregnancies.[69,70]

Loss of a Multiple

An often overlooked phenomenon is the loss of a baby in a multiple birth. From early in pregnancy, multiples have a much higher rate of mortality, whether from spontaneous abortion, 'vanishing twin' syndrome (before fourteen weeks' gestation, when a dead fetus is absorbed in-utero), fetal, or infant death.[71] The challenge of bonding with one of more living babies, who may be critically ill, while grieving the loss of another, is often difficult and can be complicated by the mother's own health and well-being following a multiple birth. Frequently, little or no acknowledgment is given to the baby who died, and parents find themselves grieving in isolation, torn between conflicting emotions. Parents need to be encouraged to recognize the loss and mourn as described, while attaching to the surviving child(ren). It is estimated that up to 15% of multiples grow up as singleton survivors and little is known about the long-term implications of this experience.[72] Support groups have formed to serve this special population and are an important resource for their needs.[73]

Elective Termination

Special consideration needs to be given to situations in which couples choose to reduce a multiple pregnancy or terminate a pregnancy after genetic testing reveals an abnormality. The decision to choose to end a pregnancy is never an easy one for people, especially if they have gone to great lengths to achieve it. It is a decision made in an environment of moral, ethical, and social dilemmas that are conflictual. Furthermore, if spontaneous loss is a socially isolating experience, elected loss is in a complete vacuum. Because the issue of pregnancy termination is politically sensitive and highly emotionally charged, there are few resources available to couples for understanding and acceptance. Thus, there is need for education and emotional support for couples faced with these difficult decisions. The therapist needs to be aware of his or her own moral and ethical feelings about these situations, as it is imperative that patients receive counseling in a neutral nonjudgmental environment.

Multifetal pregnancy reduction. Multifetal pregnancy reduction (MPR), an iatrogenic condition, was developed after assisted reproductive technology greatly increased the incidence of pregnancy involving multiple fetuses. Multiple gestation pregnancies pose serious health risks to the mother and children, especially in higher-order pregnancy above twins. The increased risks include loss of the entire pregnancy, premature delivery, preeclampsia, gestational diabetes, and postpartum hemorrhage in the mother, and prematurity, low birth weight, and handicaps in infants. Prematurity can have serious lifelong consequences for children and families and may ultimately result in death after extreme medical intervention has failed. MPR is used to

terminate a preselected number of fetuses in an effort to increase the likelihood of a successful and healthy pregnancy. It is performed at special centers, usually late in the first trimester of pregnancy, and accomplished by means of injection into the cardiac cavities of the selected fetuses, which are eventually absorbed in utero. There have been attempts to address this issue more directly by, regulations in some countries and practice guidelines in others that limit the numbers of embryos transferred. However, this may give a false sense of security as embryos may split in utero and patients may still face reduction decisions.

Because most multiple pregnancies result from infertility treatment, the decision to reduce is a painful irony for couples who so want children. There is intense ambivalence – the risk of morbidity and mortality to the babies, while facing the certainty of loss of some of the babies and risk of loss of the entire pregnancy. Couples do best when they have talked the issues through and are in agreement about whatever decision they make. Despite the concern for psychiatric morbidity, there seem to be few long-term problems for women who resolve their ambivalence and have a successful pregnancy outcome.[22,74]

MPR is a distressing and stressful experience that warrants careful counseling both before and after the procedure. Greenfeld and Walther[75] addressed a plan for assisting couples in which they recommended beginning with pretreatment preparation counseling for women undergoing ovulation induction. Couples need to understand that: (1) multiple pregnancy is a distinct possibility, (2) it carries a significant medical risk to fetuses and mothers, and (3) fetal reduction may be advised. If patients would not consider MPR, they will need to advise the physician before the assisted reproduction procedure and discuss the number of embryos to transfer, or they will need seriously to reconsider participating in this treatment.

If a multifetal pregnancy results, couples need psychoeducational materials to facilitate decision making as well as additional counseling. It is also extremely helpful to have lists of couples who have faced the same decision and are willing to talk to others about their decision to keep the pregnancy or to reduce it. Couples also will need assistance in identifying who they will share their dilemmas and decisions regarding MPR. A recent study indicated that patients can limit the risk of hostile and unsupportive responses and potential stigmatization by selectively sharing their dilemma only with those who are going to be supportive.[76] Counseling should help couples anticipate their emotional responses, be aware of available follow-up, facilitate decision making, and develop a plan for sharing and support.

Pregnancy termination due to genetic birth defect. Prenatal testing has become increasingly available and has led to early detection of genetic defects and fetal anomalies. Preimplantation diagnosis during IVF, CVS during the first trimester of pregnancy, amniocentesis during the second trimester, and high-resolution sonography throughout pregnancy have provided information about a developing baby that a few years ago would not have been known until after birth. However, therapeutic options are limited for many of the problems diagnosed, and parents are faced with the difficult decision: whether to continue or terminate the pregnancy. A painful dilemma is exacerbated when the pregnancy is very much planned and desired. If termination is decided, the procedure is often intrusive and painful, requiring either a D & C in the first trimester or dilation and evacuation, or induction of labor in the second trimester or later.

It seems that women who terminate a pregnancy rarely suffer psychological problems, provided that it occurs in the first trimester and is warranted for genetic, medical, or social reasons.[21] However, psychological sequelae following an elective termination are most often experienced by women who have difficulty arriving at a decision to terminate, have the abortion late in the pregnancy, desired the pregnancy,[75] and were coerced by their partner or others. Even when couples are firm and clear on their decision to terminate for fetal anomalies, grief can be just as intense as it is for those who experience spontaneous loss, as both grieve for their wished-for and wanted baby.[24]

Consequently, intervention after a genetic termination involves similar clinical management to that described for spontaneous loss.[77,78] Patients need to be given the option to participate in all rituals of a perinatal loss as would occur in a normal pregnancy. For example, it is important that they be given the option of seeing and holding the baby, after compassionate preparation of what the baby looks like. Parents' fears and fantasies are often far worse than the reality of any deformities, and spending time with the baby may help bring closure. However, there are several unique issues that need to be recognized in the therapy concerning the *element of choice*, the *perception of loss*, and the *sense of isolation*. First, patients often emotionally struggle with the decision to choose to terminate a pregnancy that was so desired, and yet intellectually know that this is the best for them. They frequently express the wish that the baby had just died versus having to choose to terminate. Second, the narcissistic injury and a perception of defectiveness may be exacerbated due to the fetal anomaly, which may precipitate the discovery of a previously unknown genetic disorder in one or both parents.

In addition, people will experience the loss differently: For some, it will be the loss of a pregnancy, while for others it will be the loss of a baby. Finally, these couples often describe feelings of alienation and shame and may not feel free to discuss the experience with others for fear of rejection or condemnation. In fact, it is important for them to be counseled to choose carefully those people with whom they will talk about the termination. This is a time when they need to surround themselves only with people who they know will be supportive.

Support groups and resources are now available for this special population, offering acceptance and sustenance. While there is currently no international support organization for this population, a number of local/regional groups have formed as well as internet groups, and the physician, genetic counselor, or hospital should be aware of where to locate the support group (see Chapter 15).

FUTURE IMPLICATIONS

As sophisticated and advanced reproductive technologies have become in creating and sustaining life, there will always be reproductive loss. The continuing challenge will be in providing adequate and available resources for psychological support that encourage the positive resolution of grief. More research needs to be done to understand the differences in the way men and women experience the loss; the effect of reproductive technologies on bonding, attachment, and grieving; and investigation of effective interventions that facilitate grieving, especially for those at risk for pathological mourning. Better designed research and the development of grief assessment tools are needed by clinicians. Furthermore, continuing education of the public about the profound nature of perinatal loss will help change social attitudes toward it.

SUMMARY

■ Perinatal death constitutes a major loss for most couples and is a psychically traumatic event.
■ Grieving occurs whether the loss is early or late in the pregnancy, and the intensity is more closely related to psychological attachment than length of gestation.
■ Couples feel intense emotion, often in virtual isolation because of a lack of social support and societal recognition of this significant experience.
■ The narcissistic and object loss occurring at a time of profound developmental change make grieving difficult.

■ The goal of intervention is to facilitate grieving and to restore narcissistic equilibrium.

■ Actions that acknowledge the loss as real and encourage emotional expression help facilitate grief.

■ Multiple miscarriages and loss of a multiple during pregnancy present special psychological challenges.

■ Situations of elected termination of desired pregnancies require psychoeducation, psychological support, and options to follow mourning rituals as in spontaneous loss.

REFERENCES

1. Kirkley-Best E, Kellner KR. Forgotten grief: A review of the literature on the psychology of stillbirth. *Am J Orthopsychiatry* 1982; 52:420–9.

2. Zeanah CH. Adaptation following perinatal loss: A critical review. *J Am Acad Child Adolesc Psychiatry* 1989; 28:467–80.

3. Leon IG. *When a Baby Dies: Psychotherapy for Pregnancy and Newborn Loss.* New Haven: Yale University Press, 1990.

4. Kennell JH, Slyter H, Klaus M. The mourning response of parents to the death of a newborn. *N Engl J Med* 1970; 283:344–9.

5. Lewis E, Page A. Failure to mourn a stillbirth: An overlooked catastrophe. *Br J Med Psychol* 1978; 51:237–41.

6. Stack JM. The psychodynamics of spontaneous abortion. *Am J Orthopsychiatry* 1984; 54:162–7.

7. Bourne S, Lewis E. Pregnancy after stillbirth or neonatal death: Psychological risks and management. *Lancet* 1984; 2:31–3.

8. Herz E. Psychological repercussions of pregnancy loss. *Psychiatr Ann* 1984; 14:454–7.

9. Theut SK, Pedersen FA, Zaslow MJ. Perinatal loss and parental bereavement. *Am J Psychiatry* 1989; 146:635–9.

10. Forrest GC, Standis E, Baum JD. Support after perinatal death: A study of support and counselling after perinatal bereavement. *Br Med J Clin Res* 1982; 285:1475–9.

11. LaRoche C, Lalinec-Michaud M, Engelsmann F, et al. Grief reactions to perinatal death. *Can J Psychiatry* 1984; 29:14–19.

12. Cullenberg J. Mental reactions of women to perinatal death. In: N Morris, ed. *Psychosomatic Medicine in Obstetrics and Gynaecology.* London: Karger, 1972; 326–9.

13. Nicol MT, Tompkins JR, Campbel NA, Syme GJ. Maternal grieving response after perinatal death. *Med J Aust* 1986; 144:287–9.

14. Toedter LJ, Lasker JN, Alhadeff JM. The perinatal grief scale: Development and initial validation. *Am J Orthopsychiatry* 1988; 58:435–49.

15. Kirkley-Best E. Grief in response to prenatal loss: An argument for the earliest maternal attachment. *Dissert Abstr Int* 1981; 42(B):2560.

16. Janssen H, Cuisinier M, Hoogduin K, de Graauw K. Controlled prospective study on the mental health of women following pregnancy loss. *Am J Psychiatry* 1996; 153:226–30.

17. Peppers LG, Knapp RJ. Maternal reactions to involuntary fetal/infant death. *Psychiatry* 1980; 43:155–9.

18. Greenfeld DA, Diamond MP, DeCherney AH. Grief reactions following in-vitro fertilization treatment. *J Psychosom Obstet Gynaecol* 1988; 8:169–74.

19. Farhi J, Ben-Rafael Z, Dicker D. Suicide after ectopic pregnancy. *N Engl J Med* 1994; 330:714.

20. Flam F, Magnusson C, Lundstrom-Lindstedt V, et al. Psychosocial impact of persistent trophoblastic disease. *J Psychosom Obstet Gynaecol* 1993; 14:241–8.

21. Dagg PKB. The psychological sequelae of therapeutic abortion – denied and completed. *Am J Psychiatry* 1991; 148:578–85.

22. Schreiner-Engel P, Walther VN, Mindes J, et al. First-trimester multifetal pregnancy reduction: Acute and persistent psychologic reactions. *Am J Obstet Gynecol* 1995; 172:541–7.

23. Wilson AL, Fenton LF, Stevens DC, Soule DJ. The death of a newborn twin: An analysis of parental bereavement. *Pediatrics* 1982; 70:587–91.

24. Zeanah CH, Dailey JV, Rosenblatt M, Saller DN. Do women grieve after terminating pregnancies because of fetal anomalies? A controlled investigation. *Obstet Gynecol* 1993; 82:270–5.

25. Benfield DG, Leib SA, Vollman JH. Grief response of parents to neonatal death and parent participation in deciding care. *Pediatrics* 1978; 62:171–7.

26. Tudelope DI, Iredell J, Rodgers D, Gunn A. Neonatal death: Grieving families. *Med J Aust* 1986; 144:290–2.

27. Janssen HJ, Cuisinier MC, de Graauw KP, Hoogduin KA. A prospective study of risk factors predicting grief intensity following pregnancy loss. *Arch Gen Psychiatry* 1997; 54:56–61.

28. Neugebauer R, Kline J, Shrout P, et al. Major depressive disorder in the 6 months after miscarriage. *JAMA* 1997; 277:383–8.

29. Hughes P, Turton P, Hopper E, Evans CD. Assessment of guidelines for good practice in psychosocial care of mothers after stillbirth: A cohort study. *Lancet* 2002; 360:114–8.

30. Hughes P, Riches S. Psychological aspects of perinatal loss. *Curr Opin Obstet Gynecol* 2003; 15:107–11.

31. Turton P, Hughes P, Evans CD, Fainman D. Incidence, correlates and predictors of post-traumatic stress disorder in the pregnancy after stillbirth. *Br J Psychiatry* 2001; 178:556–60.

32. Turton P, Hughes P. Post-traumatic stress disorder and management of stillbirth. *Br J Psychiatry* 2002; 180:279.

33. Hughes P, Turton P, Hopper E, McGauley GA, Fonagy P. Disorganised attachment behaviour among infants born subsequent to stillbirth. *J Child Psychol Psychiatry* 2001; 42:791–801.

34. Covington SN, Theut SK. Reactions to perinatal loss: A qualitative analysis of the National Maternal and Infant Health Survey. *Am J Orthopsychiatry* 1993; 63:215–22.

35. Swanson KM. Effects of caring, measurement, and time on miscarriage impact and women's well-being. *Nurs Res* 1999; 48:288–98.

36. Schreiner R, Gresham E, Green M. Physician's responsibility to parents after death of an infant. *Am J Dis Child* 1979; 133:723–6.

37. Leon IG. Psychodynamics of perinatal loss. *Psychiatry* 1986; 49:312–24.

38. Offerman-Zuckerberg J. Psychological and physical warning signals regarding pregnancy. In: B Blum, ed. *Psychological Aspects of Pregnancy, Birthing, and Bonding*. New York: Human Sciences Press, 1980; 151–73.

39. Covington SN. Pregnancy loss. In: *Clinical Management of Psychological Issues in Reproductive Health*. Proceedings of the Twenty-second Annual Postgraduate Course of The American Society for Reproductive Medicine; 1989 Nov 11–12; San Francisco, CA. Birmingham, AL: American Society for Reproductive Medicine, 1989; 19–36.

40. Freud S. *Mourning and Melancholia*. In: J Strachey, ed. and trans. *The Standard Edition of the Complete Psychological Works of Sigmund Freud*, vol 14. London: Hogarth, 1917/1957.

41. Lindemann E. Symptomatology and management of acute grief. *Am J Psychiatry* 1944;101:141–8.

42. Parkes CM. *Bereavement: Studies in Grief in Adult Life*. New York: International Universities Press, 1972.

43. Bowlby J. *Loss*. New York: Basic Books, 1980.

44. Hsu MT, Tseng YF, Banks JM, Kuo LL. Interpretations of stillbirth. *J Adv Nurs* 2004; 47:408–16.

45. Rice PL. When the baby falls!: The cultural construction of miscarriage among Hmong women in Australia. *Women Health* 1999; 30:85–103.

46. Capitulo KL. Perinatal grief online. *MCN Am J Matern Child Nurs* 2004; 29:305–11.

47. Toedter LJ, Lasker JN, Janssen HJ. International comparison of studies using the perinatal grief scale: A decade of research on pregnancy loss. *Death Stud* 2001; 25:205–28.

48. Peppers L, Knapp R. *Motherhood and Mourning: Perinatal Loss*. New York: Praeger, 1980.

49. Cuisiner M, Janssen H, de Graauw C, et al. Pregnancy following miscarriage: Course of grief and some determining factors. *J Psychosom Obstet Gynaecol* 1996; 17: 168–74.

50. Rand CS, Kellner KR, Revak-Lutz R, Massey JK. Parental behavior after perinatal death: Twelve years of observations. *J Psychosom Obstet Gynaecol* 1998; 19:44–8.

51. Shapiro CH. *Infertility and Pregnancy Loss*. San Francisco: Jossey-Bass, 1988.

52. Engelhard IM, van den Hout MA, Arntz A. Posttraumatic stress disorder after pregnancy loss. *Gen Hosp Psychiatry* 2001; 23:62–6.

53. Engelhard IM, van den Hout MA, Vlaeyen JW. The sense of coherence in early pregnancy and crisis support and posttraumatic stress after pregnancy loss: A prospective study. *Behav Med* 2003; 29:80–4.

54. American Psychiatric Association. *Diagnostic and Statistical Manual of Mental Disorders*, 4th ed. Washington, DC: American Psychiatric Association, 1994.

55. Rosenblatt PG, Burns LH. Long-term effects of perinatal loss. *J Fam Issues* 1986; 7:237–53.

56. Milad MP, Klock SC, Moses S, Chatterton R. Stress and anxiety do not result in pregnancy wastage. *Hum Reprod* 1998; 13:2296–300.

57. Nelson DB, Grisso JA, Joffe MM, Brensinger C, Shaw L, Datner E. Does stress influence early pregnancy loss? *Ann Epidemiol* 2003; 13:223–9.

58. Carrera L, Diez-Domingo J, Montanana V, Monleon Sancho J, Minguez J, Monleon J. Depression in women suffering perinatal loss. *Int J Gynaecol Obstet* 1998; 62:149–53.

59. Klier CM, Geller PA, Neugebauer R. Minor depressive disorder in the context of miscarriage. *J Affect Disord* 2000; 59:13–21.

60. Klier CM, Geller PA, Ritsher JB. Affective disorders in the aftermath of miscarriage: A comprehensive review. *Arch Women Ment Health* 2002; 5:129–49.

61. Neugebauer R. Depressive symptoms at two months after miscarriage: Interpreting study findings from an epidemiological versus clinical perspective. *Depress Anxiety* 2003; 17:152–61.

62. Swanson KM. Predicting depressive symptoms after miscarriage: A path analysis based on the Lazarus paradigm. *J Womens Health Gend Based Med* 2000; 9:191–206.

63. Brigham S, Conlon C, Farquharson R. A longitudinal study of pregnancy outcome following idiopathic recurrent miscarriage. *Hum Reprod* 1999; 14:2868–71.

64. Christiansen OB AA, Bosch E, et al. Evidence-based investigations and treatments of recurrent pregnancy loss. *Fertil Steril* 2005; 83:821–39.

65. Swank N. Recurrent pregnancy loss. *Infertility and Reproductive Medicine Clinics of North America* 1996; 7:495–501.

66. Daya S. Habitual abortion. In: LJ Copeland, JF Jarrell, JA McGregor, eds., *Textbook of Gynecology*, 2nd ed. Philadelphia: W. B. Saunders, 2002: 227–71.

67. Gervaize PA. The psychological aspects of recurrent miscarriage. *Infertility and Reproductive Medicine Clinics of North America* 1996; 7:807–23.

68. Li T. Recurrent miscarriage: Principles of management. *Hum Reprod* 1998; 13:478–82.

69. Brier N. Anxiety after miscarriage: A review of the empirical literature and implications for clinical practice. *Birth* 2004; 31:138–42.

70. Cote-Arsenault D, Marshall R. One foot in-one foot out: Weathering the storm of pregnancy after perinatal loss. *Res Nurs Health* 2000; 23:473–85.

71. Bryan E. Loss in higher multiple pregnancy and multifetal pregnancy reduction. *Twin Res* 2002; 5:169–74.

72. Swanson PB, Pearsall-Jones JG, Hay DA. How mothers cope with the death of a twin or higher multiple. *Twin Res* 2002; 5:156–64.

73. Kollantai J. The context and long-term impacts of multiple birth loss: A peer support network perspective. *Twin Res* 2002; 5:165–8.

74. McKinney M, Downey J, Timor-Tritsch I. The psychological effects of multifetal pregnancy reduction. *Fertil Steril* 1995; 64:51–61.

75. Greenfeld DA, Walther VN. Psychological consideration in multifetal pregnancy reduction. *Infertil Reprod Med Clin North Am* 1993; 4:533–43.

76. Britt DW, Evans MI. Multifetal pregnancy reduction: With whom should patients share their situation? *Fertil Steril* 2005; 84:S23.

77. Geerinck-Vercammen CR, Kanhai HH. Coping with termination of pregnancy for fetal abnormality in a supportive environment. *Prenat Diagn* 2003; 23:543–8.

78. Leon IG. Pregnancy termination due to fetal anomaly: Clinical considerations. *Infant Ment Health J* 1995; 16:112–26.

17 Recipient Counseling for Donor Insemination

PETRA THORN

The family the soul wants is a felt network of relationship, an evocation of a certain kind of interconnection that grounds, roots, and nestles.

– Thomas Moore, 1994

Donor insemination (DI) has been shrouded in myth, misinformation and misperceptions, and above all, in secrecy. It has been offered as a 'quick medical fix' for male infertility, with its psychological and social implications ignored. Infertility counselors are increasingly recognizing DI as a family-building alternative and focusing on the short- and long-term implications for recipients, children, and donors. While traditionally DI has been used for heterosexual couples only, more and more lesbian couples as well as single women have been using DI since the 1980s.

During the last decades, the secrecy surrounding DI in some countries has been lifting. Some countries have introduced legislation regulating the rights and responsibilities of those involved in this way of building a family. In other countries, mental health professionals and consumer organizations have spoken out for more awareness for families built by DI. Nevertheless, as a result of different values attached to family, marriage, and the child's well-being, DI remains a morally questionable treatment option in many countries.

In contrast to other types of assisted reproduction, DI is regarded as a 'low-tech' procedure. The female partner is inseminated with the semen of the donor and, depending on her ovulatory status, drugs may be used to induce ovulation. Due to the relative simplicity of the medical treatment, the manifold and complex psychosocial issues involved in DI may be disguised or overlooked. It is not surprising that a growing number of infertility counselors, professional organizations, and government regulatory agencies recommend pretreatment counseling to address:

■ the impact of infertility on the male partner as well as the couple's adjustment to it;

■ the individual's and couple's attitude regarding the use of DI as well as their comfort with social attitudes regarding DI;

■ their management of information sharing.

This chapter

■ gives an historical overview and outlines the current debates regarding DI;

■ addresses legislations and practices in several countries;

■ describes issues and strategies for counseling those using DI to build their family.

HISTORICAL OVERVIEW

Inseminations have been carried out for several centuries. In 1799, Hunter, an English anatomist and surgeon, is said to have achieved the first pregnancy after insemination. In 1885, the French doctor Déhault published a booklet on artificial insemination. One year later, in 1886, the book *Clinical Notes on Uterine Surgery* by the American gynecologist Sims was published and soon translated into several languages and inseminations became increasingly common.[1] The first recorded birth from DI was reported in 1909 in the United States.[2] The actual numbers of individuals and couples who have used DI and the number of children born as a result of it can only be estimated because there are no central registries for births resulting from DI in most countries. In the United States, for example, it is believed that 1,000–7,000 DI treatment cycles were performed annually between 1950 and 1960,[3] with current estimates of at least 40,000 children born yearly.[4] In Great Britain, Mary Barton, one of the pioneers of DI in England, is said to have provided treatment to 899 female recipients between 1940 and 1980.[5] Recently,

Blyth[6] calculated that 15,313 children were born in the period between 1992 and 2000 in Great Britain. For Germany, it is estimated that more than 50,000 children were conceived as a result of DI between 1970 and 2000;[7] a recent survey indicates that at least 500 children are born annually.[8]

Two factors have contributed to the secrecy surrounding the use of DI. Male infertility, in contrast to female infertility, has been a neglected issue in medical research and treatment.[9] Furthermore, male infertility continues to be interwoven with a lack of virility and sexual functioning,[10] both aspects having resulted in stronger stigmatization of male-factor infertility versus female-factor infertility. DI itself has been associated with masturbation and the involvement of a second male has been suggestive of an extramarital affair, both morally questionable exercises. Last, but not least, families built by DI deviate from the common family norm in that DI children conceived by DI are not biologically related to both parents. Although there has been more recognition of other family types based on or including social ties, such as adoptive families, this has not been the case for families built via DI.

In the past, these factors contributed to DI being viewed with suspicion or even as a morally unacceptable treatment. DI was not publicly acknowledged, doctors recommended secrecy, and couples used secrecy to protect themselves and their child.[11] In Great Britain, for example, DI was considered a criminal offense[12] and in Germany it was against the medical code of practice: doctors offering DI services feared losing their license to practice medicine.[13] It was only in the 1980s when these moral objections began to diminish. The advent of in vitro fertilization, oocyte and embryo donation, as well as the increasing practice of cryopreserving semen to decrease infection risks, allowing for more treatment flexibility, resulted in more awareness of DI and greater recognition of the psychological and social implications of this medical treatment. At the same time, these developments highlighted the growing contributions and importance of mental health professionals in helping all parties affected by this form of family-building.

In several countries, the practice of DI has changed considerably over the years, not least because of the introduction of legislation providing legal certainty for the participants involved and symbolically endorsing this way of building a family. Whereas previously, semen providers were granted complete anonymity, many countries, aware of the needs and rights of the offspring to access information about their biological origin, passed laws regarding identification or contact with the donor. In 1986, Sweden[14] was the first country worldwide to grant offspring access to identifiable information about the donor; this was followed by Austria in 1989,[15] Victoria, a state in Australia, in 1995,[16] Switzerland in 2000,[17] and Great Britain in 2005.[18] In 2004, the American Society for Reproductive Medicine published recommendations that encouraged disclosing the use of donated gametes to offspring.[19] In New Zealand, the use of identifiable donors has been practiced for more than ten years and legislation mandating this practice was introduced in 2005.[20] Although there is no agreement within the European Union regarding access to identifiable information about the donor, from 2006 on, all member countries are required to document information about gamete donors for a minimum of thirty years.[21] In addition, consumer organizations[22–25] have been founded in several countries and this consumer movement advocating for increased access to information and disclosure has been instrumental in social policy changes worldwide. Nevertheless, policy changes in other countries have varied. France, several Eastern European countries, Argentina, Israel, and South Africa adhere to anonymity[26] and Italy, where ART legislation was introduced in 2004, banned any treatment using donated gametes.[27]

REVIEW OF LITERATURE

For many years, research in the area of DI was limited to men's feelings about their inability to father a child, couples' experience regarding their use of DI, parental management of information sharing, as well as the evaluation of the children's development. Recently, research has focused on the experiences of children and adults conceived by DI. However, the secrecy and taboo surrounding DI have not only limited the number of these studies but also resulted in small sample sizes and research carried out in the main investigating the wellbeing of young children. Therefore, knowledge resulting from these studies must be seen as preliminary.

Research on Donor Insemination

Traditionally, DI was used only by heterosexual couples who, as a result of male infertility, a previous vasectomy or a hereditary disease transmittable to any offspring, were not able to or decided against achieving pregnancy with the semen of the male partner. Researchers have described several factors as to why these couples may prefer DI to adoption. These include dissatisfaction with the adoption process; the small number of children available for adoption; and the desire to experience pregnancy or the possibility of having a child genetically related to at least one parent 5.[28–31] It has been suggested that couples should not be rushed into treatment to adjust to this different way of building a family,[32–34] and several studies indicate that couples should take from several months to several years between medical diagnosis and the beginning of treatment.[35–37] Both marital and psychological adjustment of couples undergoing treatment has been reported to be within the normal range.[38,39] Once children are born, parental satisfaction has been found to be high.[37,38,40–43]

Earlier investigations also focused on obstetrical outcomes and infant development and reported no increased risks of obstetrical complications or abnormal infant development.[38,44,45] Recently, the development of older children born to heterosexual couples has become a topic of research investigation. One of the most comprehensive studies is the European Study of Assisted Reproduction Families, which included ninety-four families with children conceived by DI up to the age twelve years from Great Britain, The Netherlands, Italy, and Spain.[46] The authors described the psychological and social development of these children to be within normal range and could not detect differences between children conceived by IVF or DI. They concluded that the absence of a genetic link between the father and the child did not interfere with parent–child attachment. Such uneventful developments of younger children were confirmed in a meta-study carried out in 2001[47] and in a recent comparative study of forty-six DI families, forty-eight oocyte donation families, and sixty-nine spontaneous conception families.[48] In all of these studies, only a few parents had informed their children about their biological origins. Apparently, this had not resulted in negative consequences arising from the secrecy for children aged twelve years and younger. Golombok and colleagues,[46] however, stressed that systematic studies of representative samples are necessary to fully understand the long-term consequences of DI for the individuals concerned.

In several countries, among them Australia, United States, Great Britain, The Netherlands, and New Zealand, lesbian couples can now access DI. In other countries such as Germany and several Asian countries, medical guidelines are not favorable toward treating this group, or legislation permits treatment only of married couples.[26] Brewaeys[47] explained that considerable concerns were expressed when treating lesbian couples. Children were feared to develop homosexual tendencies and the absence of a male role model was considered detrimental to child development and the identification process of male children. Nevertheless, a comparison between thirty lesbian families with thirty-eight heterosexual

DI families as well as thirty families with naturally conceived children indicated that there were no differences between the first and the second groups regarding the emotional and behavioral adjustment of children.[49] The nurturing mothers in the lesbian families, however, showed greater interaction with their children than did fathers in the second and third groups. According to the authors, this resulted from the gender difference (men or women) rather than parental sexual orientation. Furthermore, all except one family had told the child about the use of a donor. Similar results were attained in a meta-analysis of six studies carried out between 1994 and 1998.[47] Again, no differences could be determined in the quality of child–parent relations. Despite such positive outcome, Brewaeys and colleagues[50] suggested that these studies should be interpreted with care because the study samples remained small and the children, young.

Only a few studies have investigated the motivations and outcome of single women choosing DI. For many, it was the lack of a male partner, the desire to avoid casual sex, and a strong sense that time was running out reproductively that led them to use DI.[51] Murray and Golombok[52] studied twenty-one solo mother families with a child conceived by DI and compared them with forty-six married DI families. They concluded that maternal satisfaction was high and child development uneventful. Similar to their lesbian counterparts, most mothers in this study intended to disclose the conception to their children but, as a result of the young age of the children, little is known how they will react to the knowledge that they were conceived by an anonymous donor. This is the first study of this group, and again the sample size was small and children were only two years old at the time of the investigation. In conclusion, further research is required to gain a better understanding for this family type.

Research on Disclosure

The nature of information sharing – whether parents talk to their child about their use of DI – has received increasing attention and has been the focus of considerable research. Whereas previously, there was considerable debate among professionals about whether parents should be advised to tell their child about the circumstance of his or her conception, recently legislation and professional guidelines in several countries have supported open information sharing. Writers have claimed that the stigma surrounding infertility, especially male infertility DI, as well as the easy concealability of achieving pregnancy with a donor for heterosexual couples (in contrast to lesbian couples and single mothers) have resulted in most heterosexual parents opting for secrecy.[11,53,54] Studies have confirmed these factors and revealed further parental reasons for nondisclosure[55–58] that include the desire to protect the child from either the distress of finding out that the father is not the genitor or the impossibility of accessing information about the donor; to protect the father from being rejected by the child; the lack of educational material/resources; and lack of support and guidance on how to tell the child.

Both Klock[59] and van Berkel and colleagues[60] found that disclosure rates until 1999 were relatively consistent with only a minority of individuals intending to tell their child about his or her genetic origin. There seems to be some indication that parental attitudes may be changing. In 1999, Rumball and Adair[61] reported that 30% of 181 New Zealand parents had informed their children at a very young age, and of the remaining parents, a further 77% intended to do so at a later stage. However, it should be noted that all of the children in this study were three years and younger. Gottlieb and colleagues[62] studied disclosure attitudes in Sweden and found that 11% of 148 parents in the study had already told their child, while a further 41% intended to do so. In both studies, participants had received pretreatment counseling encouraging information sharing. Daniels and colleagues[63] evaluated pretreatment preparatory/educational seminars for DI in Germany. Ninety percent of the forty-eight couples in these seminars intended to definitely disclose DI to their future children whereas only 42% indicated they would do so prior to the seminar. Two studies conducted in Great Britain in 2004[64] and 2005[65] found that almost half of the parents intended to tell their children about the DI conception. Parents in the latter two studies as well as Rumball and Adair's[61] research also provided reasons for disclosure. They felt that children had a right to this information; parents wanted to avoid the burden of secrecy and the risk of disclosure by somebody else or accidental discovery; and parents believed that technical advances in genetics could result in a genetic mismatch discovered by the offspring, again resulting in 'inadvertent disclosure.' This emerging trend of more openness may reflect legislative and cultural changes as well as impact of counseling and the advent of guidance materials parents can use for talking to their children.

It has been claimed that keeping DI a secret can have a detrimental effect on the development of the children and the families. As a result of the secrecy, research on the experiences of children or adults aware of their DI conception to date is limited. In 2000, Turner and Coyle[66] investigated the experiences of eighteen teenagers and adults conceived by DI. They reported feelings of mistrust, distinctiveness from the rest of the family, abandonment by the donor and professionals who had recommended secrecy, as well as feelings of loss and frustration regarding the unobtainable donor information. They also felt that being denied the right to know their full genetic history posed a threat to their identity. Similar findings were reported by Cordray,[67] conceived by DI himself, who examined the experiences of thirty-six teenagers and adults born as a result of DI. In 2004, Lycett and colleagues[68] compared forty-six families in which parents endorsed openness ($n = 18$) to those who did not ($n = 28$). They reported fewer difficulties among the disclosers than among the nondisclosers. Mothers in the first group reported less frequent and less severe arguments with their children and both parents perceived themselves to be more competent. With respect to the father–child relationship, there was no difference between the two groups. The authors concluded that disclosure could be beneficial to the mother–child relationship. The lack of a negative impact on the father–child relationship may be the result of a more relaxed parenting style in general or the fact that, by chance, the children in the nondisclosing families exhibited more behavioral problems than the children in the other group. Lycett et al.[68] also noted that despite the differences between the two groups, the higher numbers of arguments in the nondisclosing families did not represent dysfunctional relationships but fell within the normal range; instead, the results of the disclosing families reflected particularly positive scores. This study seems to share the same findings of research cited earlier that indicates that younger children who had been told about the DI conception functioned well and had a positive relationship with their parents.

While research suggests that information sharing may have a positive impact on the family, the results of these studies must be interpreted with care. Again, all of them have small sample sizes. In addition, the results of Cordray's[67] survey as well as Turner and Coyle's[66] study may be distorted because respondents were recruited through support networks favoring disclosure and many were informed late in life or under unfavorable circumstances; there may well be a bias toward describing the effect of secrecy negatively or reporting the reactions of such unfavorable disclosure. Therefore, above all, more representative research is needed.

Research on the small number of children born to heterosexual, lesbian couples, and single women in which the children have been aware of their donor conception from an early age, suggests that these children do not show any negative reactions regarding their conception. However, the children do indicate curiosity about the donor and an interest in how they were conceived.

Though some referred to the donor as their 'biological father,' they did not seem to be looking for a father-figure in the donor.[58,61,69,70] Again, research in this area is only beginning and both longitudinal studies as well as investigations with larger number of families and offspring are still to be carried out.

THEORETICAL FRAMEWORKS

No single theoretical framework is universally applicable to the dynamics of using donated sperm to build a family. Family systems theory and the biopsychosocial perspective developed by Engels contribute toward understanding the needs of couples using DI and the dynamics within families built by DI. Identity theory explains the importance of early disclosure for the development of a coherent understanding of oneself. Social stigmatization, which pertains to infertility in general as well as male infertility in particular (see Chapter 3), is also applicable to family-building by DI.

Family Systems Theory

Family systems theory contributes to an understanding of the dynamics within families as well as an understanding of families in their social context. Systems ideas originated in the general systems theory of von Bertalanffy.[71] He proposed that all parts in a system, such as members in the social system of families, are interdependent and relate to each other in a more or less stable and predictable way. Therefore, an intervention at any point in the system will affect the entire system. At the same time, systems display a dynamic balance; they constantly change within, yet retain their structure when moving toward their goals. One of the typical aims of family therapy is to help families achieve a new balance after a developmental crisis or an extraordinary life event, such as infertility, has occurred. The task of all family members is to develop a cognitive as well as affective understanding of this new situation. At the same time, family systems therapists are aware of contextual factors, such as professional recommendations regarding DI; the degree of cultural acceptance of DI; and relevant social policy and legislation regulating DI.

Imber-Black described secrets as systemic phenomena as they impact on the relationships of family members.[72] Therefore, family therapists have extensively addressed the issue of family secrets,[72–74] including the secrecy surrounding infertility and DI.[75–77] Family therapists advise that secrets can result in deception, distortion and mystification, and generate anxieties both for the secret holder and the individual in the family system who is unaware of the secret. This can create barriers between parents and children and result in highly complex situations, particularly in situations in which people outside the nuclear family are aware of the DI, but the child is unaware of the DI conception. Family therapists therefore recommend disclosure of DI in order to avoid distrust and the establishment of rigid, unhealthy barriers in the family system inhibiting communication within and outside the family.

Biopsychosocial Perspective

A biopsychosocial model for understanding the implications of a physical disease was proposed by Engels in 1977.[78] He advocated taking into account human factors when diagnosing and treating patients. Based on a systems understanding, his model recognizes the interrelations between biological symptoms and psychological and social factors in life such as individuals' affective and cognitive reactions, their relationship with their immediate and extended family, as well as any short- and long-term implications of a diseases and its treatment. In the area of family building by DI, Brandon and Warner[79] advocated for more recognition of the psychosocial issues of DI. They spoke out for disclosing DI to the child, providing adequate and age-appropriate information, and developing scripts for sharing DI with children. Recently, several writers have explicitly[80] and implicitly[33,81,82] spoken out for applying a biopsychosocial perspective to family-building by DI. Psychosocial and medical care according to such a model requires an interdisciplinary approach of a variety of professionals and a specific awareness of the implications of the DI conception, not only for the nuclear and extended family, but also regarding the long-term family issues such as information sharing and its impact on child development.

Identity Theory

Theories about identity development suggest that individuals must develop a coherent understanding of themselves.[83] To achieve this personal continuity, a sense of belonging as well as continuity of attitudes and behavioral patterns are vital. Identity does not mean a rigid view of oneself but one continuously renewed and adapted as a result of communication and interaction with others.[83–86] Both subjective and objective personal coherency must be maintained to avoid an identity crisis. Researchers in the area of adoption have found that learning about one's genetic origin late in life or under unfavorable circumstances can be associated with identity disruption and have suspected this to be similar for offspring conceived with the help of DI.[77,87–90] Although children younger than five years are unlikely to be able to cognitively grasp the meaning and some of the implications of adoption,[91] early disclosure has been found important so that children can integrate this knowledge into their development and sense of self which is enhanced when they feel that this is something they have always known about themselves.[92] This suggests that early disclosure about biological origins has the potential to prevent disruption in the identity formation for children conceived by DI.

Stigma Theory

Our understanding of social stigmatization goes back to the work of Goffman,[93] who explained that a stigma is a deeply discrediting attribute marking the bearer as spoiled, and reduces him from a whole and usual person to a tainted, discounted one. As a consequence of this devaluation, so-called normal people justify valuing the stigmatized less. Current researchers in social stigmatization argue that individuals who are unable to cooperate and contribute to the well-being of groups or even threaten successful group functioning run the risk of being stigmatized and excluded.[94,95] Fertility is a vital quality for individuals as it ensures reproduction (and enforces a sense of normalcy, health, and well-being). Therefore, a biocultural perspective helps to explain why individuals suffering from infertility may feel and/or are ostracized. Other writers[96,97] have added that such threats can also be symbolic and often involve deviance from social norms. For the United States, Miall[53] contended that two traditional fertility norms are widely accepted. These are that (1) all married couples should reproduce, and (2) they should want to reproduce. Given that such a pronatalistic attitude is likely to be similar in other Western societies, it is not surprising that infertility is perceived to violate this norm thereby triggering social stigmatization.[55,75,98,99] Furthermore, male infertility has been associated with shame, as it is perceived to be linked to a lack of virility and potency.[100–102] Most societies expect men to be strong, confident, and healthy; men suffering from infertility are typically anxious about being seen to lack masculinity or perceived by others (or themselves) as weak and unhealthy.[10] Finally, despite increasing acceptance for diversity in family composition, sociologists[103] and anthropologists[104–106] have pointed out that family ties based on blood relationships or biological connection continue to be more highly valued cross-culturally than those based on social ties. Families based on or including social ties, such as those built by DI, do not fulfill this norm and run the risk of being stigmatized because of their composition.

CLINICAL ISSUES

Although there is emerging consensus by mental health professionals that pretreatment counseling should be carried out,[107,108] this is not necessarily reflected in legislation and medical guidelines worldwide. In Victoria, Australia, for example, legislation introduced in 1988 requires such pretreatment counseling. For recipients, this legislation delineates the following issues to be addressed in pretreatment counseling:

- information on the legal, psychosocial, and ethical issues involved in DI;
- possible treatment outcome;
- relationship issues for the family such as implications arising from using anonymous versus known donors;
- issues relating to biological siblings born in different families;
- advice that children conceived by DI should be told about their donor origin;
- information that the child has access to information about the donor at age eighteen (in those countries where access is possible).

Such mandatory counseling is perceived to be essential so that couples can make informed decisions.[109,110] Recently, Canada enacted similar legislation.[111] In New Zealand, couples commonly undergo pretreatment counseling, although it is not mandatory.[112] In Great Britain, all clinics must make counseling *available* to couples but only some clinics impose mandatory counseling prior to DI, with research indicating that the majority of couples do not take up counseling even though it is offered.[113] In other countries, individual clinics may require or mandate pretreatment counseling, or this is recommended by medical guidelines.[114] However, because infertility counseling itself remains a fairly new field, there may not be an educated mental health professional available to provide pretreatment counseling; medical professionals may feel capable of providing pretreatment counseling; many medical caregivers may not see the necessity or value of pretreatment counseling;[115] and many recipients remain reluctant to undergo pretreatment counseling for a variety of reasons including stigma about counseling or mental health services in general.

It must also be noted that mandatory counseling, as required by some legislation, has not been universally endorsed. Some couples may perceive this to be an assessment for parental suitability or an unjustified intrusion into their relationship and therefore are reluctant to take part in it. This has led counselors who support mandatory counseling to compare pretreatment counseling to preadoption counseling, which is a universally accepted norm and standard of care. Those opposed to pretreatment counseling suggest that mandating counseling compromises the therapeutic relationship, resulting in clients being less open and forthcoming about issues in counseling.[116] At the same time, there are indications that couples suffering from infertility in general find it difficult to access counseling for a variety of reasons, and mandatory counseling could be seen as an opportunity to make counseling more readily available to everyone.[113,117] It is possible that this is also the case for couples using DI, but currently, there are no data available for this specific subgroup.

One of the challenging issues of mandatory counseling is the issue of when to deny treatment. The lack of exclusion criteria for DI treatment may reflect the difficulty of defining well-substantiated judgments about parental inability to provide adequate childrearing. Although legislation in Great Britain[118] and medical guidelines in some countries[119,120] have argued that the welfare of the child should be taken into account when providing infertility treatment, concrete exclusion criteria have not been defined. The guidelines developed by the Ethics Committee of the American Society for Reproductive Medicine suggest that any exclusion criteria should not discriminate on the basis of disability or other factors pertaining to physical or mental health.[121] They identify the following areas for reasons to deny treatment: uncontrolled psychiatric illness; active substance abuse; ongoing physical and/or emotional abuse; or a history of perpetrating physical or emotional abuse and/or neglect. Furthermore, these guidelines argue that any assessment denying access to treatment should be a group rather than an individual decision and should be transparent for those assessed; for example, by the professionals involved in treatment communicating in writing to the patient and stating the reasons for treatment denial at this particular point in time.

An alternative model to individual or couple counseling is based on the premise that all individuals and couples should be seen by a counselor in a group setting that aims at education and preparation for treatment and parenthood using DI.[33] Thorn and Daniels reported on such preparation seminars in Germany, where counseling is not mandatory.[110] The focus of these seminars was primarily educational with participants receiving comprehensive information on the medical, legal, and psychosocial aspects of DI by experts in their area. The group setting also provided participants the opportunity to meet others interested in DI and to share personal attitudes, concerns, and experiences. Furthermore, during the seminars, a family built by DI talked about their experiences to provide a role model for the group participants. An evaluation of these seminars indicated that all three aspects (information, sharing with others, and exposure to role models) were important factors in reducing feelings of stigmatization and marginalization. Participants felt better informed, better prepared, and more confident about their decision to pursue DI and their ability to discuss their use of DI with significant others and their future child(ren).

THERAPEUTIC INTERVENTIONS

DI is not a treatment for infertility. It does not provide a 'cure' or medical treatment for male-factor infertility. In fact, only the female partner is treated and parenthood is achieved with the sperm of a different male. As this is different from other types of assisted reproduction, writers have pointed out[33,40,109,110] that couples using DI are likely to have specific counseling needs. Counseling should include how the individual partners and the couple are managing the emotional repercussions of the medical diagnosis; grieving the child genetically related to both parents; understanding and exploring medical and social implications of their decision to use DI for family-building; assessing readiness of both partners to proceed with treatment; and addressing information management (disclosure of DI conception) with the child and/or significant others. [see Table 17.1].

Assessing Readiness

Recipient counseling for couples using DI involves different issues to be considered at different stages in the family-building process. Once male infertility has been diagnosed, couples are likely to experience a multitude of emotional reactions including shock, disbelief, and anger. One partner may have more difficulty than the other in accepting and adjusting to the diagnosis. Couples' disagreement about continuation or cessation of treatment using their own gametes is not uncommon, and it is possible that unresolved conflicts of the past reemerge around this issue. Couples are likely to go through a grieving process. For most, the child biologically related to both parents represents a myriad of hopes, dreams, and fantasies. In addition, this process can entail grieving the husband's fertility and the marital equity of each parent's connection to the child they will parent together as well as the couple's autonomous reproductive plans and choices. Couples may also experience shame and isolation resulting from the stigma of infertility as well as depressive reactions, defensiveness, and guilt. Some may want to proceed quickly to DI in continuing their determined

TABLE 17.1. Issues to include in a thorough, structured clinical interview for recipients of donor insemination

Exploring the motivation/reason to use donor insemination

Grieving infertility and the inability to have a child biologically related to both partners

Exploring the pros and cons of adoption (see Table 17.3)

Providing medical and legal information pertaining to the use of donor insemination

Discussing the comfort with using donor insemination (esp. if recipients come from countries where this is illegal)

Determining emotional and financial resources

Deciding on the type of donor to be used (anonymous, known, personal, intrafamilial) and exploring the implications

Exploring the meanings both partners attribute to the donor

Exploring disclosure

Providing information and support for disclosure of DI to the child and significant others

Providing support during pregnancy

Providing support when parents disclose DI to their child

Providing help to establish contact to others using donor insemination, if desired

focus on achieving parenthood at any cost while others wish to proceed quickly to avoid painful feelings or dealing with the psychosocial issues of the male-factor infertility diagnosis. For some couples, it can be helpful to encourage or impose a waiting period (e.g., three to six months) between receiving the diagnosis and commencing DI treatment so that the grieving process can take place and marital and psychosocial adjustment can take place.

To assess readiness for DI (Table 17.2), the couple's reasons (individually and as a couple) for choosing DI can be explored. It is important that both understand the implications of DI in general and take into account the pros and cons of DI versus adoption (Table 17.3). Neither partner should acquiesce to DI because it has been recommended by a professional or because he or she feels coerced by the other partner, family members, societal expectations, or other factors. When 'donor backup' treatment is being considered in conjunction with other treatments, this plan should be carefully explored and considered prior to treatment and should not be a decision by default at the last minute (e.g., after oocyte retrieval during an IVF cycle). Assessing readiness often entails exploring subtle and overt pressures such as the husband who had a vasectomy during a previous marriage and is ambivalent about repeat parenthood, or the wife for whom pregnancy is a paramount requirement of motherhood. For this reason, it is imperative that the couple be in full agreement on the decision to proceed with DI and consider it a positive alternative.

Understanding Disclosure

Another important issue is the question regarding who is informed about DI treatment. For many couples, and especially for women, sharing their fertility difficulties and experiences with significant others is an important means of coping. Given the stigmatizing nature of DI and male-factor infertility, the couple needs to be in agreement about with whom they will share information regarding infertility treatment, diagnosis, and their use of DI. If they do not intend to talk to their future child about his or her DI origin, they must attempt to ensure that their confidants will not disclose this to the child accidentally or not discuss the use of DI with others. When exploring this, couples usually also explore their attitude and beliefs about disclosing the circumstance of their child's conception with the child. Counselors are increasingly supportive of disclosure. However, information sharing will, at least with some couples, not only be an individual decision based on personal preference but also depend on cultural and religious factors such as the degree of acceptance of DI as well as legislation and practices regarding access to donor identity. Acceptance and favorable legislation and/or practices seem to encourage information sharing as parents' fear of stigmatizing is diminished and there is certainty that their children will be able to access this information rather than only learning that an anonymous donor contributed to their conception.[61,62] For many couples, talking to their future children becomes more tangible once they have seen guidance material they can use for disclosure (see Resources List).

Choosing a Donor

In most cases, donors are anonymous. In some countries, it is the doctor who selects the donor according to phenotypological similarities with the male partner, while in other countries, couples choose their

---

TABLE 17.2. Psychological indications for proceeding with donor insemination

Male Partner (or social mother in lesbian relationship)

Ability to manage his (her) inability to be the genitor of the child

For men: Would not see child conceived by DI as a symbol of failure

Views DI and social fatherhood (motherhood) resulting from DI as a positive alternative

For men: Has resolved negative feelings resulting from infertility diagnosis

Female Partner

Continues to see partner in a positive way despite the infertility diagnosis

Couple

Positive couple functioning

Has grieved the loss of a child genetically related to both partners

No coercion to pursue DI by any partner or anybody else

Absence of cognitive functioning or mental incompetence to provide informed consent or to understand long-term implications of choice

The welfare of the child born as a result of treatment or any other child affected by treatment has been taken account of

Ability to manage asymmetrical parenthood and sensitivity toward issues resulting from these differences

Thorough consideration of information-sharing with the child and significant others

Lesbian couples: Agreement which partner is the genetic mother and carries out pregnancy

---

donors from donor profiles that provide nonidentifiable information about the donors such as professional background, hobbies, academic history, nationality, and physical characteristics. Although more common with oocyte donation, the use of an identified, known, or intrafamilial donor is another option for couples. An identified, known, or intrafamilial donor may be a family member (typically the husband's brother), a family friend, or a donor who has been willing to be identified. When an identified, known, or intrafamilial donor is being used, it is important to explore the history of the relationship between the donor and the recipient couple to ensure that there is no coercion or other 'hidden' agendas. Furthermore, the nature of the relationship and boundaries between the child and the donor must be carefully examined and clearly defined for all par-

ties. Should the relationship between the donor and the parents be strained at some time in the future, there is potential for traumatization of the child as well as other family members.[122] In 2003, the American Society for Reproductive Medicine issued an Ethics Committee Report on family members as gamete donors and surrogates.[123] While this report approved of many types of interfamilial gamete donations, it recommended a careful screening to ensure that the decision to donate gametes to a family member protected the autonomy of the donor. It also advised that semen donation should not be carried out in those situations in which the child would result from an incestuous (father-to-daughter donation) or consanguineous union (brother-to-sister donation). Furthermore, it recommended that family members (the extended family of the infertile couple)

TABLE 17.3. Deciding between donor insemination and adoption

Pros of DI	Cons of DI
Wife genetically related to the child and therefore perceived to be closer to a family where child has biological connection to both parents	Asymmetrical parenthood (mother is biological and social mother, father is social father, semen provider is genitor)
Husband and wife can experience pregnancy	Male partner may have difficulty of accepting a child not biologically related to him
Parents can have more genetic information about the child than in adoption	Religious, ethical, or cultural objections to this family composition
Parents can control prenatal environment	More stigmatizing family composition than adoption families
Typically more expeditious and less expensive than adoption	Impossibility to access information about the donor in many countries

must be accepting of the resulting child. Intrafamilial donations that the participants plan to keep secret from the larger family system should be carefully evaluated.

Reproductive Tourists and Immigrant Population

In some countries, such as Italy, all types of gamete donation are prohibited. Couples for whom DI is their only or preferred family-building option often travel to other countries where the treatment they desire is legal and available. This practice has become known as 'reproductive tourism.' Counseling this group is especially challenging for a variety of reasons including language problems, time limitations, cultural differences, financial pressures, and patients' expectations of and investment in treatment success. Counseling must take into account cultural differences: discussing emotional issues about private issues (infertility, sexuality, male-factor diagnosis) during which subtle undertones or nonverbal communications can have very different meanings. Furthermore, counseling must help clients manage their feelings about doing something considered illegal or unacceptable in their home country. It should also help patients address any fears they may have of negative consequences for themselves and the child.[124] It is becoming increasingly common that in many developed countries, the number of foreign inhabitants is rising and clinics are seeing increasing proportions of immigrant patients who are influenced by a religion, culture, and ethnicity. Counselors should create an open atmosphere to allow for addressing cultural issues. Training native speakers in the counseling team can be helpful as it is often difficult to find translator who have a grasp of medical and psychological terms in the second language. At times, one member of the couple may be more proficient in speaking the new language and offer to interpret during the counseling, or translation services may be offered by a family member or friend. However, this is not recommended. It is important to have an impartial translator involved to ensure that each person fully understands the implications of DI and is able to provide informed consent. Information brochures, videos, and internet resources in different languages can also be helpful.[125]

Ending Treatment

During DI treatment, couples require all the support and empathy other couples need when undergoing any other form of ART. They also need to discuss the end of treatment in those cases where conception is not achieved after a reasonable number of treatment cycles and/or when the female partner is of advanced maternal age. A further factor limiting the number of treat-

ment cycles for couples is limited financial resources. In almost all countries, DI is not reimbursed by the national or private health insurance and is therefore an expense of treatment the couple must bear themselves. It is particularly painful for these couples to end treatment for financial reasons because it feels unjust and discriminatory. In these cases, couples may reexplore the possibility of adoption (at least in those countries where adoption is not associated with costs or less costly than DI) or require help to face a life without children.

Achieving Pregnancy

Once pregnancy is achieved, couples are commonly overwhelmed with joy and relief. However, the policy of anonymity in those countries where no or limited information about the donor is available can be challenging for a variety of reasons. Clinical experience indicates that women can experience vivid fantasies about the donor at the beginning of pregnancy, both negative and positive. Such fantasies may be especially strong in those cases where the couple has no information about the donor; after all, these women have become pregnant with the sperm of a man completely unknown to them. In order to validate these affective reactions, it can be important for women to express these fantasies and to normalize them. Typically, these fantasies and fears subside as the pregnancy advances (often helped by modern technology that provides ultrasound pictures of their baby) and usually are quickly overcome once the child is born and is a real person with a unique and separate identity. It can also be helpful to reconsider medical practice and provide at least some nonidentifiable information on donors. Another fear often reexpressed by the male partner at this stage is his anxiety about not being able to bond with the child conceived by DI. This fear may come out of a belief that he would more easily and 'naturally' bond with a child genetically related to him and/or fears that the DI child will look or be remarkably different from him. It can be helpful to educate these men about research that has specifically explored these issues, all of which found the father-child relationship is quite secure.[46–48] This fear may also be indicative that families built by DI are a new family type and our understanding for this family composition is as yet limited. In contrast to traditional adoption, or blended families, families built by DI include both genetic and social relationships but the genitor does not usually have an emotional bond to the child, unless he is a family member or friend. It seems that understanding this and attributing a positive meaning to the donor, yet acknowledging the boundaries between him and the family built with his contribution, is not easy. It is helpful to explore the meanings of fatherhood (reproductive versus social) with both parents and help the father-to-be develop an understanding for his role as father to his child.

Raising a Child

The first years after a child is born are usually associated with the common challenges of adapting to a life with an infant and young child. Couples may seek counseling again once they consider the pragmatics of disclosure. In this phase, counseling can help explore attitudes and provide adequate information as well as guidance on how and when to talk to the child. Educational materials including children's books can be particularly useful (see Resources). Parents in those countries where children cannot access information about the donor may require assurance that even under these circumstances, information sharing can be a positive experience for the family. After all, it prevents the negative consequences of secrecy such as the emotional burden and the corrosive effect of secrets, the perpetuation of a delusion, and deception of the child.

FUTURE IMPLICATIONS

When ICSI was developed in 1993, it was assumed that DI would, by and large, be substituted by this new technology. For a number of reasons, this has not been the case. ICSI is not an effective treatment for many forms of male-factor infertility, or may be financially too expensive, unavailable, or considered too medically invasive. As such, DI remains a financially affordable, easily accessible family-building alternative. Recently, it has been speculated that "artificial" gametes can be developed from embryonic stem cells – animal research has shown that cultured embryonic mouse stem cells can be stimulated to develop sperm formation.[126] It remains to be seen if this technique is successful with human cells.

Although there has been considerable research in the area of DI, there are a number of areas where information is sorely limited. Research is needed addressing more diverse populations, including immigrants, non-middle class families, lesbian and single-mother families; investigation of long-term family adjustment; and comparing the development of families who have chosen openness versus secrecy. To facilitate such research, new avenues for reaching DI families should be investigated.

While DI was shrouded in secrecy in the past, there are some indications that this is changing, albeit at a plodding pace. Government legislation, public policy makers, and consumer organizations are increas-

ingly advocating for openness. Despite the trend to break from a long tradition of secrecy by encouraging or mandating openness about donor gamete conception, there remain a significant number of cultures, religions, countries, societies, and professionals who favor secrecy and nondisclosure regarding donor insemination. However, the move toward openness will probably continue to gain momentum resulting in decreased stigma, greater social acceptance, and more favorable social conditions for these families. There may be many new and unforeseen issues facing these families and the professionals working with them, such as parents with adult children who wish to tell their offspring about their DI conception.[127] As such, mental health professionals will be well served by developing counseling strategies and educational materials to meet these new challenges and dimensions.

SUMMARY

■ Although DI has been occurring for more than 100 years, its acceptance as an alternative family-building option is only occurring. Several countries have, over the last two decades, introduced legislation pertaining to DI.

■ Parental attitudes toward disclosure seem to be changing. Whereas previously, only few parents informed their children of their DI origin, more may intend to do so in the future.

■ Counseling recipients includes grieving the child biologically related to both parents, exploring the pros and cons of DI, assessing readiness, providing support during medical treatment, and helping to manage information sharing. After the birth of a child, it also comprises support and guidance for talking to children about their biological origins.

■ In addition to individual and couple counseling, educational groups providing comprehensive information about family-building by DI and enabling recipients to establish contact with others can be helpful.

ACKNOWLEDGMENT

The author wishes to thank Aline P. Zoldbrod and Sharon N. Covington for the use of their chapter "Recipient Counseling for Donor Insemination" in the first edition of this book as a basis for this chapter.

REFERENCES

1. Semke I. *Künstliche Befruchtung in wissenschafts- und sozialgeschichtlicher Sicht*. Frankfurt: Lang, 1996.
2. Gregoire AT, Mayer RC. The impregnators. *Fertil Steril* 1965; 16:130–4.

3. Zoldbrod AP, Covington SN. Recipient counseling for donor insemination. LH Burns, SN Covington, eds. *Infertility Counseling: A Comprehensive a Handbook for Clinicians*. New York: Parthenon Publishing Group, 1999; 325–44.

4. Orenstein P. Looking for a donor to call dad. *New York Times Magazine* June 18, 1995; 28–51.

5. Snowdon R, Mitchell GD, Snowdon EM. *Artefizielle Reproduktion*. Stuttgart: Ferdinand Enke Verlag, 1985.

6. Blyth E. The UK: Evolution of a statutory regulatory approach. E Blyth, R Landau, eds. *Third Party Assisted Conception Across Cultures. Social, Legal and Ethical Perspectives*. London: Jessica Kingsley Publisher, 2004; 226–245.

7. Schilling G. Kinder nach donogener (heterologer) Insemination in der Einschätzung ihrer Eltern. *Zeitschrift für Psychosomatische. Medizin und Psychotherapie*, 1999; 45:354–71.

8. Thorn P, Daniels K. Die medizinische Praxis der donogenen Insemination in Deutschland. Geburtshilfe und Frauenheilkunde, 2000; 60:630–7.

9. Lee S. *Counselling in Male Infertility*. Oxford: Blackwell Science, 1996.

10. Brähler E, Goldschmidt S, Kupfer J, et al. eds. Mann und Medizin. *Jahrbuch der Medizinischen Psychologie 19*. Göttingen: Hogrefe, 2001; 11–33.

11. Daniels K, Taylor K. Secrecy and openness in donor insemination. *Politics and the Life Sciences* 1993; 12:155–70.

12. Snowdon R, Snowdon E. The gift of a child. *A Guide to Donor Insemination*. Exeter: Allen & Unwin, 1993.

13. Krause W. Vorwort zur deutschen Auflage. Snowdon R, Mitchell GD, Snowdon EM. *Artefizielle Reproduktion*. Stuttgart: Enke Verlag, 1985.

14. Lag om Insemination (1985). Swedish Insemination Act, No. 1140/1984.

15. Fortpflanzungsmedizingesetz – 275. Bundesgesetz, mit dem Regelungen über die medizinisch unterstützte Fortpflanzung getroffen werden, 1992.

16. Szoke H. Australia: Choice and diversity in regulation and record keeping. In: E Blyth, R Landau, eds. Third-party assisted conception across cultures. *Social, Legal and Ethical Perspectives*, 2004; 36–54.

17. Fortpflanzungsmedizingesetz. Über die medizinisch unterstützte Fortpflanzung – Fortpflanzungsmedizingesetz vom 18. Dezember 1998.

18. Human Fertilisation and Embryology Authority (Disclosure of Donor Information Regulations), 2004.

19. American Society for Reproductive Medicine. Ethics Committee Report: Informing offspring of their conception by gamete donation. *Fertil Steril* 2004; 81:527–31.

20. Human Assisted Reproduction Technology Act, 21 November 2004.

21. Richtlinie 2004/23/EG des Europäischen Parlaments und des Rates vom 31. März 2004 zur Festlegung von Qualitäts- und Sicherheitsstandards für die Spende, Beschaffung, Testung, Verarbeitung, Konservierung, Lagerung und Verteilung von menschlichen Geweben und Zellen.

22. Donor Conception Support Group, Australia (http://members.optushome.com.au/dcsg).

23. Donor Conception Network, United Kingdom (http://www.dcnetwork.org).

24. Infertility Network, Canada (http://www.infertility-network.org).

25. Information Donogene Insemination, Germany (http://www.spendersamenkinder.de).

26. Blyth E, Landau R, eds. Third-party assisted conception across cultures. *Social, Legal and Ethical Perspectives*, London: Jessica Kingsley Publisher, 2004.

27. Boggio A. Italy enacts new law on medically assisted reproduction. *Hum Reprod*. Advanced Access publishing, March 24, 2005.

28. Daniels K. Adoption and donor insemination: Factors affecting couples' choices. *Child Welfare*. 1994; 73:1473–80.

29. Czybo JC, Chevret M. Psychological reactions of couples to artificial insemination with donor sperm. *International Journal of Fertility*. 1979; 24:240–5.

30. Baran A, Pannor R. *The Psychology of Donor Insemination*. New York: Amistad, 2nd edition, 1993.

31. Wendland CL, Byrn F, Hill C. Donor insemination: A comparison of lesbian couples, heterosexual couples, and single women. *Fertil Steril* 1996; 65:764–70.

32. Brähler C. Familie, Kinderwunsch, Unfruchtbarkeit. *Motivation und Behandlungsverläufe bei künstlicher Befruchtung*. Opladen: Westdeutscher Verlag, 1990.

33. Mahlstedt P, Greenfeld D. Assisted reproductive technology with donor gametes: The need for patient preparation. *Fertil Steril* 1989; 52:908–14.

34. Goebel P, Lübke F. Katamnestische Untersuchung an 96 Paaren mit heterologer Insemination. *Geburtshilfe und Frauenheilkunde* 1987; 4:636–40.

35. Berger MD. Couples' reactions to male infertility and donor insemination. *Am J Psychiatry* 1980; 137:1047–9.

36. Klock S, Maier D. Psychological factors related to donor insemination. *Fertil Steril* 1991; 56:489–95.

37. Schaible A. Zeugungsunfähigkeit und Kinderwunsch. Akzeptanz und psychische Belastung nach erfolgreicher artifizieller donogener Insemination. Frankfurt: VAS, 1992.

38. Amuzu B, Laxoca R, Shapiro SS. Pregnancy outcome, health of children and family adjustment after donor insemination. *Obstet Gynecol* 1990; 75:899–905.

39. Schover LR, Collins RL, Richards S. Psychological aspects of donor insemination: Evaluation and follow-up of recipient couples. *Fertil Steril* 1992; 57:583–90.

40. Brewaeys A. Review: Donor insemination, the impact on child and family development. *J Psychosom Obstet Gynecol* 1996; 17:1–17.

41. Gillet WR, Daniels K, Herbison G. Feelings of couples who have had a child by donor insemination: The degree of congruence. *J Psychosom Obstet Gynecol* 1996; 17:135–42.

42. Hermann H, Wild T, Schumacher T, Unterberg H. Psychosoziale Situation von Ehepaaren vor der artifiziellen Insemination mit Donorsamen. *Geburtshilfe und Frauenheilkunde* 1984; 44:719–23.

43. Bendvold E, Skjaeraasen J, Moe N, et al. Marital break-up among couples raising families by artificial insemination by donor. *Fertil Steril* 1989; 51:980–3.

44. Milson I, Bergman P. A study of parental attitudes after donor insemination (AID). *Acta Obstet Gynecol Scand* 1982; 61:125–8.

45. Clayton CE, Kovacs CT. AID offspring: Initial follow-up of 50 couples. *Med J Aust* 1982; 1:338–9.

46. Golombok S, Brewaeys A, Giavazzi MT, Guerra D, Mac-Callum F, Rust J. The European study of assisted reproduction families: The transition into adolescence. *Hum Reprod* 2002; 17(3):830–40.

47. Brewaeys A. Review: Parent–child relationships and child development in donor insemination families. *Hum Reprod Update* 2001; 7:38–46.

48. Golombok S, Jadva V, Lycett E, et al. Families created by gamete donation: Follow-up at age 2. *Hum Reprod* 2005; 20:286–93.

49. Brewaeys A, Ponjaert I, Van Hall EV, et al. Donor insemination: Child development and family functioning in lesbian mother families. *Hum Reprod* 1997; 12:1349–59.

50. Brewaeys A, Dufour S, Kentenich H. Sind Bedenken hinsichtlich der Kinderwunschbehandlung lesbischer und alleinstehender Frauen berechtigt? *Reproduktionsmedizin und Endokrinologie* 2005; 1:35–40.

51. Murray C and Golombok S. Going it alone: Solo mothers and their infants conceived by donor insemination. *Am J Orthopsychiatry* 2005; 75:242–53.

52. Murray C, Golombok S. Solo mothers and their donor insemination infants: Follow-up at age 2 years. *Human Reproduction Advance Access Publishing*, February 25, 2005.

53. Miall C. The stigma of involuntary childlessness. *Social Problems* 1986; 4:268–82.

54. Nachtigall RD. Secrecy: An unresolved issue in the practice of donor insemination. *Am J Obstet and Gyn* 1993; 168:1846–51.

55. Schilling G. Zur Problematik familiärer Geheimnisse am Beispiel der heterologen Insemination. *Psychotherapie, Psychosomatik, Medizinische Psychologie* 1995; 45:16–23.

56. Cook R, Golombok S, Bish A, et al. Disclosure of donor insemination: Parental attitudes. *Am J Orthopsychiatry* 1995; 65:549–59.

57. Nachtigall R, Becker G, Szkupinski Quigora S, et al. The disclosure decision: Concerns and issues of parents of children conceived through donor insemination. *Am J Obstet Gynecol* 1998; 178:1165–70.

58. Lindblad F, Gottlieb C, Lalos O. To tell or not to tell – what parents think about telling their children that they were born following donor insemination. *J Psychosom Obstet Gynecol* 2000; 21:193–203.

59. Klock S. To tell or not to tell. The issue of privacy and disclosure. In S Leiblum, ed. *Infertility. Psychological Issues and Counselling Strategies*. New York: Wiley and Sons, 1997; 167–88.

60. van Berkel R, van der Veen L, Kimmel I, et al. Differences in the attitudes of couples whose children were conceived through artificial insemination by donor in 1980 and in 1996. *Fertil Steril* 1999; 71:226–31.

61. Rumball A, Adair A. Telling the story: Parents' scripts for donor offspring. *Hum Reprod* 1999; 14:1392–9.

62. Gottlieb C, Lalos O, Lindblad R. Disclosure of donor insemination to the child: The impact of Swedish legislation on couples' attitudes. *Hum Reprod* 2000; 15:2052–6.

63. Daniels K, Thorn P, Westerbrooke R. Confidence in the use of donor insemination: An evaluation of the impact of participating in a group preparation programme. Submitted *Hum Fertil*, May 2006.

64. Golombok S, Lycett E, MacCallum F, et al. Parenting infants conceived by gamete donation. *J Fam Psychol* 2004; 18:443–52.

65. Lycett E, Daniels K, Curson R, et al. School-aged children of donor insemination: A study of parents' disclosure patterns. *Hum Reprod* advances access publishing 2005; 20(3):810–19.

66. Turner A, Coyle A. What does it mean to be a donor offspring? The identity experiences of adults conceived by donor insemination and the implications for counselling and therapy. *Hum Reprod* 2000; 15:2041–51.

67. Cordray B. An open letter to the HFEA. In: *DC Network Journal* Winter 1999/2000:3–5.

68. Lycett E, Daniels K, Curson R, et al. Offspring created as a result of donor insemination: A study of family relationships, child adjustment, and disclosure. *Fertil Steril* 2004; 82:172–9.

69. Vanfraussen K, Ponjaert-Kristoffersen I, Brewaeys A. An attempt to reconstruct children's donor concept: A comparison between children's and lesbian parents' attitudes towards donor anonymity. *Hum Reprod* 2000; 16:2019–25.

70. Scheib JE, Riordan M, Rubin S. Adolescents with open-identity sperm donors: Reports from 12–17 year olds. *Hum Reprod* 2004; 20:239–52.

71. Bertalanffy L. *General System Theory: Foundations, Development, Application*. New York: George Braziller, 1968.

72. Imber-Black E, ed. *Secrets in Families and Family Therapy*. New York: WW Norton, 1993.

73. Karpel MA. Family secrets: Conceptual and ethical issues in the relational context, ethical and practical considerations in therapeutic management. *Family Process* 1980; 19:295–306.

74. Papp P. Der Wurm in der Knospe; Geheimnisse zwischen Eltern und Kindern. Imber Black, ed. *Geheimnisse und Tabus in Familie und Familientherapie*. Freiburg: Lambertus Verlag, 1995; 85–108.

75. Schaffer J, Diamond R. Infertility: Private pain and secret stigma. In: E Imber-Black, ed. *Secrets in Families and Family Therapy*. WW New York: Norton 1993; 106–20.

76. Bradshaw J. Familiengeheimnisse. *Warum es sich lohnt, ihnen auf die Spur zu kommen*. München: Kösel, 1995.

77. Wiemann I. *Wie viel Wahrheit braucht mein Kind? Von kleinen Lügen, großen Lasten und dem Mut zur Aufrichtigkeit in der Familie*. Hamburg: Rowohlt, 2001.

78. Engels GL. The need for a new medical model: A challenge for biomedicine. *Science* 1977; 196:129–36.

79. Brandon J, Warner J. A.I.D. and adoption: Some comparisons. *Bri J Soc Work* 1977; 7:335–41.

80. Daniels D. Die biopsychosoziale Perspektive. *Orgyn* 2000; 3:11–14.

81. Blyth E. Infertility and assisted conception. *Practice Issues for Counsellors*. Birmingham: British Association for Social Workers, 1995.

82. Thorn P. Familienbildung mit Spendersamen. Eine systemische Innen- und Außenbeobachtung. In: Kontext. *Zeitschrift für systemische Therapie und Familientherapie*, 2001; 4:305–18.

83. Erikson EH. *Lebensgeschichte und historischer Augenblick*. 1. Frankfurt, Auflage, 1977.

84. Krappmann L. *Soziologische Dimensionen der Identität*, 3. Auflage, Stuttgart: Klett Cotta, 1973.

85. Gergen K. *The Saturated Self*. New York: Basic Books, 1991.

86. Giddens A. *Modernity and Self-Identity*. Cambridge: Polity, 1992.

87. Triseliotis J. Donor insemination and the child. *Politics and the Life Sciences* 1973; 12:195–7.

88. McWhinnie AM. Disclosure and development: "Taking the baby home was just the beginning." In: M Singer, M Hunter, eds. *Assisted Human Reproduction. Psychological and Ethical Dilemmas*. London: W. Hurr, 2003:129–53.

89. Feast J. Donor-assisted conception: What can we learn from adoption? In: M Singer, M Hunter, eds. *Assisted Human Reproduction. Psychological and Ethical Dilemmas*. London: W. Hurr, 2003; 76–98.

90. Haimes E, Timms N. *Adoption, Identity and Social Policy*. London: Grower, 1985.

91. Brodzinsky DM. New perspectives on adoption revelation. *Adoption and Fostering* 1984; 29:27–32.

92. Triseliotis J. Identity formation and the adopted person revisited: The dynamics of adoption social and personal perspectives. In: A Treacher, I Katz, eds. *The Dynamics of Adoption. Social and Personal Perspectives*. London: Jessica Kingsley Publisher, 2000; 81–98.

93. Goffman E. Stigma. *Über Techniken der Bewältigung beschädigter Identitäten*. Frankfurt: Suhrkamp 13. Auflage, 1998.

94. Kurzban R, Leary MR. Evolutionary origins of stigmatization: The functions of social exclusion. *Psychological Bulletin* 2001; 127:187–208.

95. Neuberg SL, Smith SM, Asher T. Why people stigmatize: Toward a biocultural framework. In: R Heatherton, R Kleck, M Hebl, F Hull, eds. *The Social Psychology of Stigma*. New York: Guilford Press, 2000; 31–61.

96. Stangor C, Grandall CS. Threat and the social construction of stigma. In: R Heatherton, R Kleck, M Hebl, F Hull, eds. *The Social Psychology of Stigma*. New York: Guilford Press, 2000; 62–87.

97. Pfuhl EH, Henry S. *The Deviance Process, 3rd ed.* New York: Aldine de Gruyter, 1993.

98. Lampman C, Cowling-Guyer S. Attitudes toward voluntary and involuntary childlessness. *Basic and Applied Social Psychology* 1985; 17:213–22.

99. Valentine P. Psychological impact of infertility: Identifying issues and needs. *Social Work and Health Care* 1986; 11:61–9.

100. Mason MC. *Male Infertility – Men Talking*. London, Routledge: 1993.

101. Houghton D, Houghton P. *Coping with Childlessness*. London, Unwin Hyman:1987.

102. Lee S. Male mysteries: Factors in male infertility. In: SE Jennings, ed. *Infertility Counselling*. London: Blackwell Science, 1995; 67–78.

103. Schneider DM. *American Kinship: A Cultural Account*. 2nd ed. Chicago: University of Chicago Press, 1980.

104. Finkler K. The kin in the gene. The medicalisation of family and kinship in American society. *Current Anthropology* 2001; 42:235–63.

105. Strathern M. *Reproducing the Future: Anthropology, Kinship and the New Reproductive Technologies*. New York: Routledge, 1992.

106. Franklin S. Making representations: The Parliamentary Debate on the Human Fertilisation and Embryology Act. In: J Edwards, S Franklin, E Hirsch, F Price, M Strathern, eds. *Technologies of Procreation. Kinship in The Age of Assisted Conception*. New York: Routledge, 1993; 127–65.

107. Burns LH, Covington SN, eds. *Infertility Counselling. A Comprehensive Handbook for Clinicians*. New York: Parthenon, 1999.

108. Boivin J, Kentenich H. *ESHRE Monographs: Guidelines for Counselling in Infertility*. Oxford University Press, 2002.

109. Blood J. Mandatory counselling. *J Fertil Coun* 2004; 11:31–5.

110. Thorn P, Daniels K. A group–work approach in family building by donor insemination: Empowering the marginalized. *Hum Fertil* 2003; 6:46–50.

111. Bill C-6. An Act respecting assisted human reproduction and related research, 2004.

112. Daniels K. New Zealand: From secrecy and shame to openness and acceptance. In: E Blyth, R Landau, eds. Third-party assisted conception across cultures. *Social, Legal and Ethical Perspectives*. London: Jessica Kingsley Publisher, 2004:148–67.

113. Boivin J, Scanlan LC, Walker SM. Why are infertility patients not using psychosocial counselling? *Hum Reprod* 1999; 15:1384–91.

114. American Society for Reproductive Medicine (ASRM). Informing offspring of their conception by gamete donation. *Fertil Steril* 2004; 81(3): 527–31.

115. Kentenich H. The role of the physician in counselling. *ESHRE Monographs: Guidelines for Counselling in Infertility*. Oxford University Press, 2002:11–13.

116. Daniels K. Donor insemination. *ESHRE Monographs: Guidelines for Counselling in Infertility*. Oxford University Press, 2002: 31–2.

117. Kerr J, Brown C, Balen A. The experiences of couples in the United Kingdom who have had infertility treatment – the results of a survey performed in 1997. *Hum Reprod* 1999; 14:934–8.

118. Human Fertilisation and Embryology Act 1990 (c 37).

119. American Society for Reproductive Medicine. Child rearing ability and the provision of fertility services. Ethics Committee Report. *Fertil Steril* 2004; 82:564–7.

120. Richtlinien der Bundesärztekammer: Durchführung der assistierten Reproduktion. *Deutsches Ärzteblatt* 95, Heft 49 (4.12.1998), A-3166.

121. American Society for Reproductive Medicine. Child rearing ability and the provisions for fertility services. Ethics Committee Report. *Fertil Steril* 82:564–7.

122. Nikolettos N, Asimakopoulos B, Hatzissabas I. Intrafamilial sperm donation: Ethical questions and concerns. *Hum Reprod* 2003; 15:933–6.

123. American Society for Reproductive Medicine. Family members as gamete donors and surrogates. Ethics Committee Report. *Fertil Steril* 2003; 80:1124–30.

124. Baetens P. Oocyte donation. *ESHRE Monographs: Guidelines for Counselling in Infertility*. Oxford University Press, 2002; 33–4.

125. Kentenich H. Patients in migration. *ESHRE Monographs: Guidelines for Counselling in Infertility*. Oxford University Press, 2002; 29–30.

126. Newson AJ, Smajdor AC. Artificial gametes: New paths to parenthood? *J Med Ethics* 2005; 31:184–6.

127. Daniels K, Meadows L. Sharing information with adults conceived as a result of donor insemination. *Hum Fertil*. 2006, in press.

18 Recipient Counseling for Oocyte Donation

PATRICIA L. SACHS AND LINDA HAMMER BURNS

> There is only one image in this culture of the "good mother."...She loves her children completely and unambivalently.
>
> – Jane Lazarre

Although the use of donated sperm has been a form of family-building for a century or more, the use of donated oocytes (also known as eggs or ova) did not become a feasible and reliable form of family-building until the 1980s. Oocyte donation (OD) is a direct descendant of the reproductive technology used in in vitro fertilization (IVF) in that oocytes retrieved from one woman are fertilized via IVF, and the resulting embryos transferred to the uterus of another woman. Natural by-products of this technology include the ability to: (1) retrieve mature oocytes for fertilization and (2) create embryos that are not genetically-related to the gestating mother. Just as the use of donor sperm broadened the family-building possibilities for infertile men (e.g., wife's pregnancy) a century ago, donated oocytes have provided new and exciting family-building opportunities for women heretofore unable to conceive. However, currently the biotechnology to cryopreserve oocytes has not been perfected, making the donation of oocytes a far more complicated procedure than sperm donation, because the cycles of the oocyte donor and recipient must be synchronized.

For female-factor infertility, oocyte donation is an applicable treatment for a wide array of conditions including women with premature ovarian failure (POF) or diminished ovarian function; surgically removed ovaries; carriers of genetic diseases; cancer survivors who were treated with chemotherapy and/or radiation; women who have experienced pregnancy loss or recurrent miscarriage; poor oocyte donor and/or embryo quality (particularly when no male factor has been identified as contributing to poor embryo quality); and advanced maternal age. Not only does OD facilitate pregnancy for women with impaired ovarian functioning, but it also improves the possibilities of pregnancy and a healthy fetus, as oocyte donors are typically younger, fertile, and have been medically screened.

Oocyte donation has changed the definition of motherhood – at least in biological and perhaps legal terms – while generating an array of dilemmas including 'stratified reproduction' (the availability of reproductive treatment and potential for exploitation of needy women as donors by the economically advantaged); 'retirement motherhood' (motherhood for women who are well past reproductive age); and 'reproductive tourism' (patients and/or donors traveling across geographic borders because oocyte donation is unavailable, illegal, or cost-prohibitive in their country of residence or citizenship). Furthermore, there are many types of oocyte donation and the terms can sometimes be confusing:

■ *intrafamilial* (e.g., sister-to-sister, cousin-to-cousin);
■ *intergenerational* (e.g., daughter-to-mother, niece-to-aunt);
■ *oocyte-sharing*, whereby an IVF patient donates excess oocytes in exchange for a reduced fee for her own IVF treatment cycle;
■ *split-oocyte donations*, whereby a donor's oocytes are given to two (or more) recipients;
■ *anonymous*, whereby a recipient selects (or is matched with) a paid donor based on nonidentifying information; and
■ *known* (also referred to as identified), whereby a recipient uses oocytes from donor she knows, purportedly not for pay and or unpaid.[1]

In some European centers, recipients choose between donation (i.e., the donor has been recruited by the recipient) or anonymous, so-called personalized anonymity donations (i.e., exchange of the oocytes of a donor recruited by another patient, with those of a donor recruited by a different patient to ensure anonymity between donors and recipients).[2] In the United States, commercial recruitment of oocyte donors has led to escalating fees to oocyte donors and an unregulated growth industry of oocyte donation/surrogacy recruitment agencies contributing to a worldwide phenomenon of reproductive tourists.[3,4] The wide range of oocyte donation possibilities and practices highlights the importance of the role of infertility counselors as integral members of the reproductive treatment team offering OD services in providing psychological preparation, evaluation, and support for women and couples wishing or needing to use donated oocytes to facilitate biological motherhood and family-building.

This chapter describes the psychosocial aspects of family-building through oocyte donation for recipients and their partners. The issues addressed include:

■ an historical overview of recipients using OD, including regulatory approaches of different countries;
■ a review of literature on the motivations, characteristics, donor choices, and selection issues of OD recipients;
■ a theoretical context for understanding OD recipients;
■ identification of clinical issues, regarding psychosocial response to OD, decision making, choosing a donor, and special populations using OD;
■ a framework for the recipient interview, which includes psychoeducation, support, and assessment.

HISTORICAL OVERVIEW

Throughout history, pregnancy, birth, and the ability of women to maintain and nurture the lives of their children have been powerful images reflected across cultures and civilizations in art, literature, and history. Ancient beliefs linked motherhood with divine mythic and mystical powers attributed to a woman's ability to give and sustain life. Images and myths proliferate about the Great Goddess or Earth Mother such as Omikami Amaterasu, mother of the world in Japanese legend; Greek goddess Hera; Hindu goddess Devi, mother of the world – although she had no children; Thrud, the Earth Goddess of Norse mythology married to Thor; or even the Virgin Mary of Christianity – the virgin mother of Jesus. As such, the importance of motherhood as integral to human relationships is well documented across history and civilizations.

Yet, it was not until Dutchman de Graaf's New Treatise on the *Genital Organs of Women* published in 1862 that an ovist (versus two seeds) theory of human reproduction was introduced. Still, even as late as the middle of the eighteenth century, this concept of an oocyte as an integral and equal component to sperm in reproduction was not generally acknowledged in the treatment of infertility.[5] The first successful pregnancy following OD was reported in 1984 by a group from Monash University in Australia.[6] A twenty-five-year-old woman with premature ovarian failure (POF) was the recipient of a single oocyte donated by a twenty-nine-year-old woman undergoing an IVF cycle with a history of bilateral tubal dysfunction: thus, an egg-sharing donation. The pregnancy was without incident until thirty-eight weeks gestation, at which time a Cesarean section was performed for elective reasons. Since that initial success, OD has become increasingly acceptable and an integral part of reproductive medicine practices worldwide and, as such, a common and popular form of family-building. While oocyte donation has provided reproductive hope, particularly for young women whose reproductive life has been sadly shortened by cancer or POF, it has also been used to facilitate motherhood under more questionable circumstances.

According to the Guinness Book of World Records, the oldest woman in the world to give birth was Mrs. Rosanna Dalla Corte of Italy, who was born in 1931 and gave birth to a baby boy on July 18, 1994, when she was sixty-three years old. Her son, conceived via IVF/OD, was her second child – she and her husband had lost their adult son, who was not married and had no children, in a car crash, motivating the couple to become parents again. On November 7, 1996, a sixty-three-year-old, Mrs. Arceli Keh, gave birth to a daughter, becoming the oldest American woman to conceive and give birth following oocyte donation. This was the couple's first and only child and she was conceived after many years of fertility treatment – ultimately achieved because Mrs. Keh lied to caregivers about her actual age. Adriana Iliescu of Romania became the world's oldest mother on January 16, 2005, when she gave birth at age sixty-six to a daughter. Ms. Iliescu, a single woman, used donated oocytes and sperm to achieve the pregnancy that she had regretted not having earlier in her life following more than a decade of infertility treatment. The pregnancy had originally been triplets; however, one triplet was miscarried at ten weeks gestation and the second at thirty-three weeks, triggering a Cesarean delivery at thirty-four weeks. Finally, on November 9, 2004, Aleta St. James, a fifty-six-year-old single American woman, became the oldest woman to give birth to surviving twins, a boy and girl, conceived via donated oocytes and sperm. Each of these pregnancies has made the medical record books but reflect a variety of unique circumstances of this new reproductive frontier. Although pregnancies can be achieved in women of a certain age, they can, and often do, result in complicated pregnancies that endanger the health and well-being of the mothers and their infants.

The practice of oocyte donation, as well as the laws and guidelines regulating it, varies widely across and within countries. This factor dramatically has an impact on the counseling of recipients, particularly regarding donor selection and privacy/disclosure issues.[3] Different approaches include the development of practice guidelines by professional societies (e.g., ASRM, ESHRE), government regulatory agencies (e.g., Great Britain's HFEA, Canada's AHRA, and Australia's RTAC), legislation – typically banning oocyte donation (e.g., Italy) – or benign neglect. Variance across and within countries is due to a variety of factors including religion, culture, and politics. As such, every infertility counselor must be fully aware of the laws and practice standards regarding oocyte donation not only where they practice but also where their patients reside and/or hold citizenship.

A regulatory approach to oocyte donation is exemplified by the United Kingdom's Human Fertilisation and Embryology Authority (HFEA) established in 1991. The HFEA legally mandated anonymity of gamete donors, allowing availability of only limited information about the donor. Originally, the allowable forms of oocyte donation were identified donors (e.g., sisters or friends); recruited altruistic uncompensated donors (identified or anonymous); and egg-sharing by IVF patients (identified or anonymous). However, in April 2005, the HFEA eliminated all donor anonymity and compensation and established a central donor registry so that all donor offspring could access information about their donor upon reaching the age of sixteen. The HFEA's position on the discontinuation of compensation of oocyte donors is in compliance with the European Union Tissue and Cells Directive. The latter promotes 'altruistic donation,' that is, voluntary, unpaid donations, although donors may be reimbursed for expenses and inconveniences related to the donation.[7] The HFEA permits a specific maximum payment amount for reasonable reimbursable expenses to altruistic donors, but prohibits financial remuneration for IVF patients who share or donate their extra oocytes. Accordingly, HFEA regulations specify that counseling be offered to all potential recipients and that it involve information and advice but not screening (i.e., prohibiting or disallowing patients from receiving gametes).[8]

Canada and Australia have similar regulatory approaches. The Infertility Treatment Act was enacted in 1984 in Australia's state of Victoria and was the first to legislatively mandate counseling for all individuals pursuing IVF and/or donor gamete parenthood. Subsequent legislation in 1988 established the Donor Register, which mandates the registration of all donor births and allows all donor offspring at age eighteen access to

identifying information about their donor. Donors have no right of veto. This legislation also established counseling criteria for donors, recipients, and offspring – referred to as donor-linking counseling. Infertility counselors must be licensed and members of ANZICA (Australia/New Zealand Infertility Counseling Association). The Reproductive Technology Accreditation Committee (RTAC), a peer-review accreditation body working in conjunction with the Fertility Society of Australia, accredits all IVF centers in Australia and New Zealand. Currently, three of the five Australian states have legislation regarding reproductive technology (including oocyte donation), with the RTAC overseeing the provision of oocyte donation services including oocyte collection; categories of donors; payment or coercion of donors; matching and exclusion of donors; and information and counseling of donors (*not recipients*). Australia's system is one of combined voluntary regulation and legislative regulation (nationally and across states in the country).[9] In contrast, Canada has the newest regulatory body, the Assisted Human Reproduction Agency, established in 2004. Canadian legislation eliminated donor anonymity; established a central donor registry; prohibited any and all payment to gamete donors (sperm or oocytes); and mandated the provision of counseling services for all individuals participating in assisted reproduction. While HFEA requires that counseling be offered, Canadian legislation mandates that all participants in assisted reproduction participate in pretreatment counseling.

Many countries have legislation specifically directed toward oocyte donation, although the provision of counseling is not addressed. In France oocyte donation became legal in 1994, providing all oocyte donations are voluntary, free, anonymous, and confidential. Clinic staff does anonymous pairing of donors and recipients, under a personalized anonymity system described earlier.[10] Belgium has a similar form of oocyte donation, although known oocyte donations are allowed. Several countries have legally banned any form of oocyte donation, including Germany, Italy, Japan, Kenya, Latvia, The Netherlands, Norway, Portugal, Sierra Leone, Slovenia, Switzerland, and Togo.[11,12] Until 2005, all forms of assisted reproduction were unregulated in Italy,[13] and oocyte donation was banned in Sweden until 2003.[14] It is interesting to note that Sweden was the first country to remove anonymity of sperm donors in 1984, enabling offspring to determine the identity of their sperm donor.

In the United States and Europe, professional organizations have established professional patient care guidelines on oocyte donation, by the Mental Health Professional Group of the American Society of

Reproductive Medicine (MHPG/ASRM) and the Psychological Special Interest Group of the European Society of Human Reproduction and Embryology (PSIG/ESHRE). ASRM professional standards of practice recommend: guidelines for screening and counseling of oocyte donors (1994); guidelines on embryo donation (1996); guidelines for gamete and embryo donation (2002); revised minimum standards offering assisted reproductive technology (2003); ethics committee report on childrearing ability and the provision of fertility services (2004); and ethics committee report on informing offspring of their conception by gamete donation (2004). In 2002, PSIG/ESHRE published the *Guidelines on Counselling in Infertility*, a comprehensive document outlining infertility counseling issues with specific recommendations on oocyte donation.[15] Additionally, ESHRE has a wide array of professional standards of practice issued through Task Force reports including one on gamete donation.[16]

REVIEW OF LITERATURE

Since the initial reports of the first pregnancy achieved via OD, there has been a proliferation of research on the psychosocial aspects of this form of third-party reproduction. A systematic review of published studies from 1983 to 2002 was conducted in an attempt to provide a synthesis of the psychosocial characteristics of OD recipient women.[17] Hersherberg found that multiple research methodologies used were predominantly exploratory, retrospective, and descriptive studies. In the sixteen studies reviewed, 827 OD recipient women participated. This review study identified six areas that were the focus of research: (1) motivation; (2) desired donor characteristics; (3) selection of a known versus an anonymous donor; (4) recipient demographic, educational, and psychosocial profiles; (5) disclosure of the method of conception to family members, friends, and the resulting child; and (6) the relationship between the oocyte recipient and her resulting offspring. Hersherberg noted that the majority of the studies were conducted within the medical and psychological fields (not nursing). Four areas identified are addressed here, as the issues of disclosure to family, friends, and the offspring and the relationship of the recipient to her offspring are addressed in other chapters (see Chapters 26 and 27).

Motivation

Research examining the motivations of OD recipients has generally found that they were motivated to use donated oocytes as a means of conception because they wanted to have offspring; experience pregnancy; nurture an unborn child; have genetically related offspring (e.g., intrafamilial oocyte donation or child genetically related to spouse); and/or as a result of mistrust of the adoption process.[18,19] One study found that the majority (61%) of recipients found the decision to pursue donor oocyte parenthood difficult to some degree while 39% found the decision was not difficult at all.[20]

Desired Donor Characteristics by Recipients

Any analysis or overview of research on OD recipients' preferences or criteria in a potential donor must take into consideration current practices regarding oocyte donation including legislation, regulations, practice guidelines, and infertility patient/consumer movements. Although some description of past preferences may be enlightening, recent developments in legislation in North America and Europe and a growing consumer movement to eliminate donor anonymity may (and probably will) have an impact on desired donor characteristics. As such, research on recipient preferences about specific donor characteristics must be considered within the context of the donation system. In short, recipient preferences (i.e., the ideal donor) may be irrelevant in that the donor is a family member or a fellow IVF patient for whom donor/recipient matching is done by clinic staff and not by the recipient. Recipients more highly invested in specific donor qualities may pursue oocyte donations (e.g., agency donations or internet searches) that are more likely to meet these needs. Unfortunately, this population has not been investigated.

Desired donor characteristics have typically been determined in conjunction with research on other donor/recipient issues. Within this context, research has found that most recipients select oocyte donors on the basis of medical and/or genetic history, race, personality, and intelligence. In a survey of OD recipients in the United States, eighty recipients were asked to generate a wish list of desired traits and physical characteristics they considered important in anonymous oocyte donors. Researchers found that medical history (62%) was the *most important* donor characteristic for recipients, followed by race (49%); smoking/alcohol/narcotics history (44%); intelligence/education (39%); and physical appearance (29%). When recipients' personal demographics were factored in, differences were found in what were rated as important donor characteristics. Intelligence was *most* important to older recipients compared to younger recipients, while physical appearance was more important to younger recipients.[21] A slim majority (52%) of recipients in Finland were interested in knowing the donor's age, profession, physical appearance, hobbies, and place of residence, while fewer (48%) did not want any information regarding the donor.[22]

American researchers Greenfeld and Klock found that the three most important characteristics influencing recipient decisions about their oocyte donors were appearance, intelligence, and personality. Recipients using anonymous donors were significantly more concerned about the donor's medical background and less interested in personality, physical resemblance, and intelligence. Recipients also preferred more information about the donor's family and medical history, and wished to have a photograph of the donor. In contrast, recipients using known donors were satisfied with the information they had about their donor and were more likely to know their donor's religion, number of children, hobbies, profession, and to have a photograph. In both groups, the donor's appearance was valuable because it facilitated recipient/donor matching in terms of resemblance of the women.[20]

In a study that surveyed recipients about their role in the selection of the donor and information recipients desired about the donor, the majority felt that they had little control in choosing the donor, with men feeling they had less control than their wives. Recipients indicated that the most important information in choosing a donor was medical information, talents, and personality characteristics. The researchers concluded that these (American) recipients desired more information about anonymous oocyte donors than known donors and wanted more input in the donor selection process.[23]

Donor Selection Issues – Known versus Anonymous

The various types of oocyte donation (as indicated earlier) offered worldwide can be mind-numbing in variety. Recipient decisions on donor selection are often based more on what is legally or clinically available at the time or place of the donation rather than on the recipients' personal preference. Although there has been considerable research on recipients' decision making and donor selection criteria, in actuality these studies have been conducted on recipients' preferences within specifically defined parameters of donor services available or 'on offer' to the recipient. Thus, no research has examined recipients' preferences when offered all the possibilities of oocyte donation. Rather, this research may be more accurately described as recipients' decisions based on availability of a donor or donation process. As such, recipients' preferences, options, and/or decisions may

be based on pragmatics and practicalities – that is, making the best of what is presented or feasible. This may be supported by research in which recipients reported making donor selection decisions based on what they perceived were their available options.[24]

There has been considerable research on known versus anonymous oocyte donations, often as a backdrop to assessing recipient intentions to disclose the circumstances of their offspring's conception to the child and/or others. However, in considering research on known versus anonymous donations, it must be recognized that definitions of 'known' and 'anonymous' are fluid and evolving. A 'known' donor may be a family member, acquaintance, personally recruited, or a fellow IVF patient 'accidentally' encountered. Anonymous donation may mean secrecy and a sacrosanct commitment to protect the privacy of all parties or a more convoluted arrangement (e.g., 'personalized anonymity'). As such, research on known versus anonymous donations must be considered in terms of these evolving definitions as well as ever-evolving gamete donation laws, policies, and practices.

Researchers in the United States found that the majority of recipients had used anonymous donors because donor anonymity was their preferred choice. When recipients recruited their own donor, their motivations included: dissatisfaction with the treatment program's selection of donors; wanting to meet the donor; and the desire to provide their children with information about the donor. Women using anonymous donors were equally divided between anonymity as their preferred choice and feeling that they had no other option. Among the women who believed they had no other option, some said that they preferred the anonymity anyway, while others reported changing their mind as a result of approaching women they knew (e.g., sisters) who refused or realizing that knowing the donor would be too awkward. Twenty-four percent of the recipients said that anonymity was their preferred choice because they did not want contact with the donor and did not want their children to have contact with the donor. Some feared that the donor would want to participate in parenting or otherwise complicate their relationship with their child.[20]

Despite the popularity of intrafamilial (particularly sister-to-sister) oocyte donation, research has been limited over the two decades it has been practiced. Several very small descriptive studies that investigated identified donations (i.e., sisters or friends) reported an impact on family dynamics. In a study in the United Kingdom researchers found identified donors reported more effects upon the family, particularly regarding secrecy and openness issues.[25] In a study investigating the experiences of donors and recipients in sister-to-sister donations, researchers found that the original self-presentation of donors and recipients changed over time. Sister-to-sister donations appear to be affectively intense experiences with often unanticipated emotional complications for both the recipient and the donor.[26]

In Belgium, where personalized anonymity donations are practiced, Baetens and colleagues found that 69% of recipients chose known oocyte donation over this type of anonymous donation. Even when offered additional financial compensation in the form of free treatment cycles, recipients preferred to use their known donor rather than an anonymous donor. Interestingly, only 28% of the known donors were sisters of the recipient women. Reasons for choosing a known donor included fear of unknown genetic information; personality of the donor; genetic link with the donor (e.g., sister); resemblance between the donor and recipient; pragmatic reasons; preference for known donation; ability to provide information to offspring; and unavailabilty of anonymous donors. An example of pragmatic reasons was the donor's proven fertility because she already had children. Thirty-one percent of the recipients in this study chose personalized anonymity primarily because they desired explicit boundaries between the two families but also because recipients desired independence from the donor (and family); protection of the donor; a wish to minimize the link between the donor and the child; pragmatic reasons (e.g., success rates); and known donation was not possible (e.g., the donor was genetically-related to the husband). Recipient women who had chosen known donations were older than the recipients choosing anonymous donations.[1]

Recipient Characteristics

Few, if any, studies have focused solely on OD recipient characteristics such as demographics, education, age, marital status, and psychological well-being. As such, recipient profiles can be accessed through investigation of other recipient issues (e.g., donor selection or disclosure decisions). A review of research on oocyte donor recipients revealed a profile of the average North American and European recipient as having the following characteristics: married; childless; upper socioeconomic status; and highly educated. The majority were Roman Catholic when religion was identified and the median age in women was forty-one. European and North American studies reported that the vast majority of recipients were Caucasian. Finally, the

majority of recipients used anonymous oocyte donations.[1,18,20,27–29]

In examining emotional well-being and stability among oocyte recipients, one study compared levels of depression in couples pursing OD motherhood on the basis of a diagnosis of primary versus secondary infertility. Beck Depression Inventory scores indicated that women with primary infertility were significantly more depressed than women with secondary infertility. Similarly, husbands with primary infertility were found to be significantly more depressed than husbands with secondary infertility.[30] This research stands out, not because of the reports of higher levels of depression in infertile couples (particularly women), but in that it is the first to document psychiatric symptomatology in recipients. Earlier research on oocyte recipients found that they scored within normal range on psychiatric symptomatology and reported low levels of distress, depression, and other emotional symptoms.[31,32]

THEORETICAL FRAMEWORK

There is no single theoretical framework that is specifically applicable to the use of donated oocytes by infertile women or couples as a family-building option. However, some theoretical perspectives contributing to a better understanding of the psychosocial dimensions of family-building via oocyte donation are specifically: psychoanalytic/feminist theory; stigma theory; attachment and loss theory; and family systems theory.

Psychoanalytic Theory and Feminist Theory

Psychoanalytic theory is based on the work of Freud, on whose thinking psychology and psychiatry evolved as a profession. Historically, a fundamental tenet of psychoanalytic theory was women's envy of men – specifically, penis envy. This approach has been generally debunked or reworked, but it highlights the fundamental importance of reproductive ability in defining an individual's sense of self and the powerful influence of sexuality and reproductive ability in identity formation. Providing a more balanced (less male-dominant) approach, Horney and other feminist psychoanalysts acknowledged the importance of women's unique reproductive capacity in a woman's self-realization and mental health[33] as well as the importance of the desire or need for recreating the mother–child bond as being intimately tied to a woman's identity formation and maturation. According to Horney, reproduction and motherhood are the foundation of women's life and identity and the most powerful factors influencing her self-perception (self-psychology) and, ultimately, her personal fulfillment.

The inability to reproduce for any woman represents a major assault on her identity and a loss of the idealized mother-self.[34] Psychoanalytic theory traditionally viewed childless women as pathological, unable to achieve their functional (and most fulfilling) role in society. This view is often internalized by women, contributing to feelings of inadequacy, defectiveness, or incompetence.

Object-relations theory emphasizes that women's identity formations are significantly impacted by the reality that women are still the primary caretakers of offspring and girls are socialized to form an identity that is intertwined with motherhood and reproduction is a globally universal phenomenon. A woman must form and maintain an identity separate from her mother, which can be a significant challenge for infertile women who are unable to become mothers (unlike their own mothers) and/or are forced to redefine motherhood (via OD) as different but similar to their own mothers. Chodorow[35] emphasized the importance of pregnancy and motherhood in female development, stating that "motherhood begins internally, filled with fantasy" and that "any woman's desire for children, whether immediately fulfilled, fulfilled belatedly, or never fulfilled, contain[s] layers of affect and meaning." There is a self-destruction hidden in the non-reproduction of mothering.[36] Additionally, feminist psychoanalytic theory recognizes the importance of relationships and connections as a basis for women's identity formation and psychological health.[37] Relationship disturbances resulting in disconnections and violations within interpersonal relationships have special significance for women, causing significant psychological distress, even instability.

Feelings of self-reproach, self-blame, and/or guilt are common responses to infertility and clearly impact a woman's sense of self, triggering an array of ego defenses. While achieving motherhood via OD can assuage some of these feelings, replacing self-loathing with self-love, these feelings may not be completely managed even after the child is born. Unresolved feelings about infertility; continued issues with identity and self-esteem; or simply ambivalence about OD may reemerge often during interactions with or decision making about the donor or donation process. Although recipients are typically enormously grateful to the donor for her gift of a life, recipients (often unexpectedly) can also feel jealous, competitive, and threatened (e.g., fantasizing that their husbands will have had an affair with the donor or are attracted to the donor). Fantasies can be undermining forces, sometimes persisting throughout the process of pregnancy and after birth (e.g., the mother's genes will somehow pass from mother to baby through the placenta or breastmilk). Sometimes these are fears and fantasies about which the mother is aware (yet ashamed), but often they are fantasies that are outside the mother's awareness or ability to verbalize. Denial and failure to acknowledge disturbing fantasies can disrupt the donor process and delay self-acceptance and/or maternal/infant bonding. Much of this work is expression of the fantasies; normalizing the experience; and grieving and letting go of the wished-for, deserved, perfect, idealized child and one's self as an ideal, perfect mother.

Oocyte donation enables women to become mothers – reproducing through pregnancy and birth. Although OD mothers make a significant biological contribution toward establishing the life of their child, they do so without a genetic link to their child. Furthermore, although OD motherhood *is* motherhood, it is motherhood achieved with various concomitant losses: loss of health; feelings of normalcy; idealization of motherhood; or the genetically-shared ideal child. These losses can represent a disconnection and alienation for the infertile (recipient) woman, destabilizing her relationships as well as her sense of self and ego mastery. In reality, even normal pregnancy is an odd experience in which a woman shares her body with a separate human being. However, a significant psychological task for OD recipient women is the incorporation of a positive sense of self and a view of the pregnancy and baby as her own child alongside the reality that a foreign body (i.e., the oocyte/embryo) exists physically within her. This is the beginning of feelings of ownership and entitlement to her child as well as the recognition that through pregnancy and birth she will be forever biologically linked to her child (i.e., but for her body, the embryo would not grow into a fetus, and eventually a baby), even though her child is not genetically tied to her in the traditional manner. As such, motherhood achieved via OD can be a profoundly reparative experience. It enables her to achieve motherhood; restore her self-esteem and self-image; and fulfill an important role.

Stigma Theory

Goffman developed stigma theory by explaining that "the stigmatized individual in our society acquires identity standards which he applies to himself in spite of failing to conform to them, it is inevitable that he will feel more ambivalence about his own self."[38] A stigma is a "deeply discrediting attribute marking the bearer as spoiled"[39] which also devalues him or her from the norm to a "tainted" person (outside the norm). Individuals who cannot "contribute to the well-being of their groups"[40] are at risk of alienation and stigmatization. As such, infertile women and couples are vulnerable targets of stigma either due to societal biases against their childlessness or due to their self-perceptions of being different and out-of-sync with their peers. Stigmatizing feelings commonly associated with infertility include feeling damaged, defective, or worthless, and experiencing guilt, despair, isolation, and stress. And while these are feelings that the infertile individual may feel, what is worse is that their feelings of being different and out of sync with their peers enhance feelings of shame, embarrassment, and frustration within the couple's social circle (i.e., family, friends, and community).

Motherhood via OD enables the recipient woman to gain emotional equilibrium through pregnancy and birth and remove the stigma of childlessness by joining the ranks of parenthood. OD enables her to become part of the norm and passing to the outside world, as pregnancy and birth makes her just like anyone else. OD can provide a normalized experience of pregnancy and birth, as it gives formerly infertile men and women the ability to contribute children to their family and society. However, recipients who achieve motherhood via OD may still feel stigmatized because OD is a different form of family-building that breaks some genetic connections and redefines kinship networks along social, not genetic links. For this reason, OD couples may be at risk for stigmatization of themselves and/or their potential child and need to be counseled regarding who they inform of their decision in order to minimize this risk.

Attachment and Loss Theory

Bowlby's theory of attachment is based on the premise that to become a mentally healthy adult the infant and young child must experience a warm, intimate, and continuous relationship with his or her mother in which both parent and child find satisfaction and enjoyment.[41–43] The parent–child feelings are reciprocal, equally loving and intense, and in the process the child becomes an unconditional member of the family. These reciprocal feelings become the foundation for entitlement and claiming, the feelings of attachment in which parents feel that they have a right to their child and they belong to one another. In many respects, bonding, claiming, and entitlement are inextricably intertwined and are fundamental psychological tasks (even challenges) for families created by oocyte donation. It is paramount that the OD mother feels that she is entitled to her child and that they belong to each other despite the lack of genetic linkage. Having achieved motherhood via someone else's oocyte, this can be a signifi-

cant hurdle impeding her bonding and attachment to her pregnancy and, ultimately, her child(ren). Building a healthy attachment and sense of entitlement to her child means acknowledging that OD motherhood is different from traditional biological parenthood, but is still motherhood and parenthood. OD recipient couples must recognize and truly believe that it is the quality of the parent–infant bond that determines healthy development in their child and family system, not genetic ties. Recipient couples may need to be assured that they, in fact, can provide a warm and continuous relationship for their child, despite the lack of genetic links to the mother. They may need to be reassured about the importance of their love and ability to provide a stable, steady, and comforting environment for their child, allowing attachment to happen and setting the foundation for healthy family adjustment.[44]

Bowlby extended his theory of attachment to issues of grief and loss, noting that the levels of attachment determined the grief response – the greater the attachment, the greater the sense of loss and bereavement. Grief reactions to infertility and loss of reproductive ability have been well-documented. Infertile couples must grieve the losses of infertility regardless of how they become parents, relinquishing the ideal child and genetically shared child they deserved and assumed they would have. Grieving is a process and, as such, is typically not completed and resolved before parenthood has been achieved. However, OD recipient couples must, to some extent, come to terms with their feelings of grief and loss in order to truly embrace OD as a positive family-building alternative in their lives.

Family Systems Theory

Family systems theory focuses less on the individual and more on the individual's family as a system of mutually interdependent and interconnected relationships (i.e., emotional attachments). Family systems theory presents developmental stages of family life, noting how nodal events (e.g., births and deaths) can affect the family's development and overall functioning as they cause families to reorganize and adapt. Infertility is an intergenerational family system crisis, impacting not only the infertile couple, but also siblings, parents, and even grandparents – preventing all members within the family system from moving on to the next family life stage. In short, infertility is a crisis within the context of the couple's marriage and within the context of each partner's family-of-origin.

A fundamental principle of family systems theory is the concept of family boundaries, which protect and differentiate the family system. Boundaries are defined not only around the family itself in relation to the outside world, but also within the family through subsystems (e.g., parental subsystem, children subset, and sibling subsystem).[45, p.54] Healthy boundaries are clearly defined (evident) yet permeable, enabling the family to adapt to the movement of family members in and out of the system (e.g., birth and death). Blurred or ambiguous boundaries can make family members uncertain, uneasy, and stressed and impair overall family functioning.[46] Unsure of who is in and who is out of the family system, individuals can become confused by role definitions and responsibilities, further straining family interactions and communications both within and outside of the family. People in general are uncomfortable with ambiguity and uncertainty. Ambiguity causes confused family dynamics, forcing individuals to question their marriage, family, and their own role within these systems.[46,47]

Family systems theory is particularly relevant in intrafamilial (e.g., sister-to-sister) and/or intergenerational (e.g., daughter-to-mother or niece-to-aunt) oocyte donations in that this theory provides a context in which to address the multiple layers of relationships and roles within the family. It allows the assessment of individual, as well as family well-being and functioning of each subsystem within the larger system. Family systems theory has been instrumental in defining the significant negative consequences for individuals and families of boundary violations (e.g., incest or parentified child). It has also been effective in recognizing the power of family relationships to influence individual members of the family, positively or negatively, overtly or covertly. As such, intrafamilial OD/recipient relationships have the potential for threatening family relationships. The whole family system may be put at risk through role confusion, boundary violations, and imbedded decision making; dysfunctional communication patterns; relationship alignments and loyalties; values and belief systems; beliefs about indebtedness and obligation; level of family cohesiveness; and, ultimately, sources of power within the family. Would the OD-sister feel entitled to take a more parental role because she views the offspring as her (biological) child? Would the donor be treated (or expect to be treated) like a special aunt? Will the donor-daughter feel obligated to donate? Will she feel like the child's sister, or another mother? All of these factors can, and do, influence intrafamilial and/or intergenerational OD decisions and should be carefully considered by all participants for these reasons, particularly if there is not a larger cultural or social context that supports these donations.

Finally, the role of secrets in the family can have an impact on the family system and must be carefully considered. Imber-Black[48] described secrets as systemic phenomena that impact relationships of all family members, resulting in deception and generating anxiety for both the secret holder and the unaware. The issue of secrets is particularly important in the context of oocyte donation and must be addressed at the outset to avoid unnecessary injury and damage to the family, recipients, and especially the child. Infertility counselors can use the genogram to outline the family system and assess a variety of family dynamics and values, particularly those regarding kinship beliefs, values, cultural influences, the value and meaning of children, and family functioning over time and across generations (see Chapters 11 and 15). Of particular relevance are the family's beliefs about secrets; how secrets may have been handled or had an impact on the family in the past; and who in the family will know about the donation (and who will not and why not). Recipients and donors should be encouraged to address the issue of disclosure within the family and to the offspring. While these issues are important in all OD families, they are even more relevant in intrafamilial donations. The secrecy about the donation (motivated either by the recipient or the donor) can stress the family system, eventually damaging family relationships and/or threatening the parent–child relationship if the secret is either intentionally or unintentionally revealed – particularly by other family members, not the child's parents. Secrecy about the donation can create an undercurrent of covert communications (positive or negative) between the donor and recipient, straining other family relationships and the overall well-being of the family.

CLINICAL ISSUES

Several clinical issues are relevant in a discussion of OD recipient counseling. These issues concern the psychosocial response to oocyte donations; the process of decision making; selecting a donor whether anonymous or known; and matters related to special populations using OD.

Psychosocial Response and Decision Making about OD

Fundamental to coming to terms with infertility for each couple is defining their goal: reproduction or parenthood. Whether their personal goal is reproduction or parenthood, each partner as well as the couple together must determine which alternatives are acceptable and the direction their future will take. If the goal is reproduction and they have reached the limits of treatments that will allow them to achieve a pregnancy and transmit their own genes, the couple must consider a child-free lifestyle. However, if parenthood is the goal, family-building alternatives such as oocyte donation may be considered.

Women and couples who have been through an array of reproductive treatments over an extended period of time without success often arrive at the threshold of OD from a long and exhausting history of pain, typically involving cyclical episodes of high hopes with a new treatment cycle and hopes dashed when a successful pregnancy is not achieved. Having experienced the vicissitudes of a variety of treatment failures, the recommendation to pursue donor oocyte parenthood may not be particularly surprising, as OD has been part of the long-term treatment care plan or a suspected possibility given the outcomes of previous treatments. This is often the case if the woman is older or has an ovulation-specific infertility diagnosis. For these women, the recommendation of OD may be viewed as a relief and a second chance at biological motherhood. Although OD motherhood means relinquishing a genetic link to the offspring, it does afford women the opportunity to make a "biological contribution to the birth of the child via pregnancy."[15] For other women, OD is an unforeseen treatment recommendation, perhaps made in conjunction with the diagnosis and treatment of a medical condition unrelated to fertility (e.g., cancer), triggering feelings of shock and disbelief. These women may be younger, less mature, and unprepared to consider serious reproductive issues, particularly ones that involve complicated medical treatments and the use of donated oocytes. They typically feel alienated, isolated, and out of sync with their peers, particularly those who have been able to achieve motherhood without problems or challenges. And while OD may offer these women reproductive hope in a real and concrete way, it may feel too overwhelming, given other issues in their lives and their current emotional state.

Whatever the reason for the use of donated oocytes, the necessity of OD represents a variety of losses for most women (and their partners): lost fertility, lost time, lost health, lost youth. As such, the majority of women react with some degree of emotional distress: shock, anger, sadness, anxiety, fear, and/or feelings of being damaged and defective. Whether the woman considering OD has a developing sense of self or a well-established one, the use of oocyte donation to achieve motherhood requires the integration of new, complicated information and feelings about herself, motherhood, and reproduction. At minimum, she must grieve the loss of a child to whom she assumed she would be genetically-linked – a child she and her partner

hoped and dreamed would be genetically shared. She must reconcile dissonant and negative self-perceptions to reestablish a positive self-view before moving forward with this new way of becoming a mother. In short, although OD provides avenues to motherhood, there are a number of psychosocial issues to address and tasks to achieve before OD motherhood can be completely and positively embraced as a family-building option, whether or not it results in the birth of a child.

Partners and spouses of OD recipients often respond with similar feelings of emotional distress in response to the infertility diagnosis and/or the need to use oocyte donation to build a family, although their feelings are typically less intense and/or more likely to be solution-focused. Many recipients fear that the diagnosis and/or OD will impact their partner's feelings about them, while both partners may worry that it will negatively impact their relationship; their future together; and/or their child(ren). There may be concern about how OD will be accepted and treated within their extended families, thereby having an impact on family relationships (i.e., who knows the secret), or in intrafamilial donations concerns about how the relationship between the donor and recipient is affected as well as relationships within the family system. This can become even more problematic in cross-generational intrafamilial donations.

Donor Selection Issues

Choosing a donor is a significant clinical issue, whether the oocyte donation is anonymous or known. Some recipients have virtually no input regarding donor selection criteria or donor anonymity as these decisions and/or alternatives are prescribed by government regulations, standards of practice guidelines, or clinic policies. Others may have a mind-numbing array of choices from clinic recruitment, agencies, the internet, and known situations. As noted earlier, donor anonymity has been eliminated in many countries but remains fundamental to gamete donation in much of the world. Although the removal of donor anonymity enables recipients (and their offspring) to access information about the donor, this does not mean that even in these areas OD recipients have access to extensive information on the donor or are offered a variety (catalog) of potential donors from which they can choose. In actuality, no matter how ooyctes are made available, recipients' choices are typically limited by supply, because oocyte donation remains a medically complicated and physically demanding procedure for women. As such, recipients must be prepared for these realities and limitations: Although oocyte donation does offer them a chance at biological motherhood, it is unlikely to provide them with the ideal, designer perfect and genetically linked child they had anticipated before infertility.

Although the recruitment of oocyte donors either by clinics or recipients is common worldwide using a variety of methods, unique to the United States are paid donors recruited by independent agencies specifically set up for this purpose. With the advent of these brokerage type agencies and internet recruitment resources, recipients have a variety of new opportunities, as well as potential pitfalls, in their search for an oocyte donor. Finally, some recipients turn to a friend or family member as an oocyte donor because these arrangements are more culturally acceptable; psychosocially comfortable; available; and/or accessible. Identified donors may be recruited or volunteer for a variety of reasons (e.g., family ties, compassion, and altruism). However, whatever the circumstances of the donation, recipients and their partners must come to terms with a wide range of issues including their personal beliefs and values about oocyte donation as an acceptable form of family-building; the type of donation; their personal feelings, beliefs, and preferences about donor characteristics; the impact of the form of donation on their marriage, family, and social circle; and disclosure issues.[49]

Research has shown that recipients rank medical and/or genetic history, race, personality, intelligence, and appearance of primary importance.[21,22] The issues of appearance and race can pose significant psychosocial dilemmas, particularly when recipients have no option (e.g., there are no same race or similar appearance donors available at a given time). Of clinical importance is the recipient couple who seeks a donor with specific criteria based on unmet psychological needs, misinformation, or other reasons. An example is recipients choosing a donor of a different race based on a belief that a donor's appearance (i.e., light skin) and, therefore their child, would be more favorably treated by society and gain greater privileges. In this situation, it is important for the infertility councelor to explore the meaning of appearance, race, intelligence, or other donor criteria with the couple to ensure that their decisions are based on emotional stability and health, not narcissistic injury, misconceptions, biases, and/or a belief that they actually can create the perfect child and ensure that their child's future will be perfect in every way. Often recipients have not thought through their own feelings and/or the consequences of these decisions (e.g., how will they handle comments from others about their child's appearance). In fact, the infertility counselor must help recipients consider donor selection issues, particularly a choice that may eventually

highlight their child's lack of genetic connection to the mother. These differences may make the circumstances of the child's conception more obvious and public and (perhaps unintentionally) invade the child's right to privacy about his or her biological origins. As such, the infertility counselor can be instrumental in helping recipients (potential parents) explore their feelings and beliefs about openness about the donation as well as the stigma of infertility; stigma of OD; and potential for their child to experience stigma related to the circumstances of his or her conception. Facilitating open and honest exploration of feelings and communication can ensure that recipient decisions regarding oocyte donation are decisions that will remain comfortable over a lifetime and not reflect a temporary fix of narcissistic wounds.

Whether the donation process is anonymous or known, recipients must consider a variety of issues regarding donor selection. Choosing an oocyte donor is a powerful first step in making their child theirs. However, more often than not, donor selection triggers the reemergence of feelings of grief and loss, as the couple faces the reality of their reproductive situation; searches for the perfect donor (e.g., one that resembles the recipient); and addresses the implications of this assisted reproduction for their marriage, family, and their child. The couple's search for the perfect donor is actually an extension of their search for the perfect child. The role of the infertility counselor in preparing the couple for parenthood is to help them recognize that even if they had a genetically shared child, he or she would not be perfect and might not even resemble them or the child they had imagined. While using donor gametes and selecting a donor may help the couple regain some control over a part of their lives over which they have little control, it should not be viewed as a chance to even up life's score by getting a perfect child that is owed them. Additionally, the infertility counselor can help couples relinquish their attachment to and valuing of biological reproduction and embrace the possibilities of parenthood via oocyte donation. Couples must accept the reality that they will never find a replacement for the wife in any assortment of donor profiles, yet they can find a suitable donor who will help them achieve their goal of a family. Instead, couples should look for something about the donor – for example, hobbies, interests, what she has written about why she wants to donate – that resonates with them and makes them feel connected to her in some way. As such, helping couples to have greater confidence in the selection of a good enough donor can help them come to terms with their ambivalence about OD parenthood and embrace their child as truly theirs – just as he or she is and will be, as a separate individual with their own life.

The shortage or unavailability of oocyte donation as a legally acceptable and viable reproductive alternative has compelled some recipients (and donors) to become reproductive tourists, a phenomenon in which individuals travel across borders to obtain services that are unavailable, regulated, or too costly in their own country of origin.[50,51] While fertility tourism may enable patients to undergo OD, it raises concerns about standards and screening processes for both donors and recipients.[52] Although recipients may be able to obtain the treatment they desire, there are greater risks that the donor (or recipient) may be an unsuitable candidate. Donors may encounter coercion, language barriers, and unavailability of appropriate translators. Additionally, they may be unable to provide informed consent; be enticed by unrealistic promises of financial gain; lack healthcare benefits; or have visitor status visa problems. The same challenges may face recipients seeking treatment in foreign countries. Furthermore, in a single-minded focus on their goal, both donors and recipients may find the medical and psychological assessment for participation in this treatment unfamiliar, unnecessary, and difficult to understand. Language barriers and culture customs may even make it difficult for them to comply with complex treatment protocols and/or provide informed consent. Additional challenges include staff ignorance (or insensitivity) to the cultural and religious issues impacting treatment and the long-term consequences of reproductive tourism in the lives of all parties – donor, recipient, and offspring.[53] The infertility counselor needs to understand the unique cultural issues and reproductive challenges from the patient's country of origin, and may need the assistance of a translator to facilitate counseling.

Anonymous Oocyte Donation

Anonymous oocyte donation involves the matching or selection of a paid donor in which recipients are provided non-identifying information. Information may be extensive or minimal. The recipient couple should be confident that the donor has been appropriately screened[4] medically and psychologically, in accordance with any applicable government regulations and/or professional practice standards, so as to allay any fears about significant psychopathology, health problems, and/or consanguinity. Information may include an extensive self-report profile, which includes a medical family history as well as comments by the potential donor regarding her motivations to donate, and perhaps a photograph of her as an infant, child, or adult. Even so, couples should be aware that the information provided by the donor is often not verified by the treatment facility (or recruiting agency) and is, as such, based on the donor's self-report and veracity. Furthermore, donor anonymity must be respected by recipients and staff alike, despite recipients' sometimes innocent questioning of staff about personal donor information such as personality, appearance, or sense of humor. Repeated questions along these lines may represent other issues for recipients such as lack of emotional readiness for OD parenthood; ambivalence about donor anonymity; lack of partner agreement about OD parenthood; or ineffective or inadequate patient preparation.

Because of the limited supply of donated oocytes, some recipients try to get around the shortfall of donated oocytes through a variety of measures: oocyte donation brokerage-type agencies; the internet; advertising for a donor in university newspapers; or networking through flyers to friends and family.[54–57] Some of these recruitment schemes, fueled by psychological needs for the perfect donor/ perfect baby, offer considerable sums of money for a donor who meets explicit criteria, for example, appearance, intelligence, or specific talents (music or athletics). OD recruitment agencies may be a tempting and appealing solution, however, recipients should carefully consider their claims, as these agencies are not subject to any legal oversight or government regulations. In short, the old adage buyer beware applies. As such, the infertility counselor may be integral in helping recipients become better consumers: aware of any and all current professional and legal standards for appropriate medical and psychological evaluation of potential oocyte donors and be certain that these standards have been applied to any potential donors being considered.

In these situations both recipient and donor are at risk. The donor is at risk of being a commodity coerced to donate body tissue for financial gain, particularly if she is economically disadvantaged or intellectually unable to assess these risks, comply with treatment, or provide informed consent. Recipients are at risk of ending up with an unqualified donor, or one who drops out during treatment because she was poorly prepared. In fact, research shows that, in general, there is a high dropout or rejection rate among first-time potential oocyte donors. Potential donors often opt out once they realize what the donation process actually involves or they may fail to meet medical or psychological criteria for donation (e.g., ongoing medical problem or current chemical abuse/addiction).[58] Although oocyte donation agencies or internet donors may appear to be in more abundant supply, recipients are often disappointed when the dropout rate for these donors is equal to that of other donor recruitment methods, that is,

TABLE 18.1. Reasons for choosing anonymous vs. known oocyte donation

Pros for Using Anonymous:

No potential 'family boundary' issues, as donor is not 'in couple's life'

Easier for couple to maintain privacy

Cons for Using Anonymous:

Feels riskier due to less available information about donor

May be longer wait for donor

Pros for Using Known:

More genetic information about donor; greater comfort level

May be more readily available

May be special person in child's life

Cons for Using Known:

Potential boundary confusion, role blurring

May be too invasive in child's/family's life

Couple may feel 'indebted forever'

significantly high. In fact, one study found that increased compensation to potential oocyte donors did result in a higher percentage of potential donors completing initial questionnaires, but did *not* increase the number of donors who actually donated. The rejection rate (51%) remained the same and comparable to that of other programs and recruitment methods.[59] Infertility counselor and recipients should be aware of current recommended reimbursement amounts governing oocyte donation.

Quasi-known donation situations have increased as couples learn something about the donor, such as a first name, email address, or perhaps have spoken by phone. Although these donations are considered anonymous, it is not uncommon for recipients and donors to figure out or find each other. The concern is that the parties may have begun a relationship that will continue in some form into the future without the safeguards of professional assistance to prepare them for possible future issues and how they plan to handle them. Not only does this represent significantly blurred boundaries but it can also represent hidden agendas, whereby donors and recipients who begin under anonymous circumstances may convert to quasi-known parties, unconsciously wishing to have roles in each other's lives in the future. Such arrangements often move forward with little thought to the long-term well-being of the child. The fact that there is little professional guidance to assist in role clarification and expectations may lead to disappointment or, even worse, damage to the children conceive via this arrangement. As such, both recipients and donors need to be made aware of these issues.

Known Donors

Known oocyte donation is involves a friend, acquaintance, or family member acting as donor. For many recipients, this is a more acceptable means of oocyte donation for cultural and financial reasons. Additionally, the donor may be more accessible and medically reliable, particularly if there is no family history of medical or psychological risk factors (see Table 18.1). The fact that the donor will potentially be known to the child and involved in his or her life is a significant issue in intrafamilial donations. Nevertheless, it cannot be assumed that intrafamilial donations are going to be open. Very often recipients and donors alike wish to keep this arrangement private. If this is the case, all parties must be carefully counseled about the potential negative consequences of this decision (e.g., accidental disclosure and the negative impact of family secrets). Fundamentally, it is critical that the recipient couple and known donor (with spouse/partner) address their desires and expectations regarding the donation; and their future relationship (see Table 18.2); number of planned donations; and implications of negative outcome of treatment and/or conflicts regarding treatment.[60]

Disclosure of donor gamete conception is legally mandated in some countries and recommended by practice guidelines in the United States and Europe. Yet, it remains an area of controversy for recipients and donors – and obviously for offspring. Nevertheless, infertility counselors generally believe that if the child is to know about the means of their conception, it is imperative that he or she hears this information first and foremost from his or her parents, in a manner that is appropriate for them. The primary goal is to avoid emotional damage to the child and ensure the positive integration of this information into his or her identity. Because feelings about the degree of disclosure may change over time, it is also important that the parties agree to communicate; be willing to reassess their positions in the future as needed; and seek the assistance of an infertility counselor if obstacles arise. Discussion, as well as couple and donor agreement about this issue, are integral to pretreatment patient education and preparation (see Chapter 27).

Intrafamilial donations, particularly sister-to-sister donations, can be complex and have significant implications for the family relationship. All the parties (the recipient couple, the donor, and her partner, if any) must agree on who within the extended family is to

TABLE 18.2. Issues to include in a thorough structured clinical interview of OD recipients

Couple's infertility history (CHPI): assessment of how they experienced it and how it was grieved.

How couple decided to do OD and how they feel at present

History of marital relationship; legal difficulties; alcohol/drug use; abuse/neglect

Past traumas and current stressors; coping skills; support network

Assessment of woman's feelings/comfort level with biological inequality attachment concerns

Couple's plans re: openness vs. privacy; known vs. anonymous

Thoughts/fears about donor motivation; information on donor assessment

Cryopreservation/disposition of embryos; prenatal testing, multiples, selective reduction

know and *not know* about the donation. All must be in agreement; have realistic expectations; and an implementation plan. All parties must consider how family members might react to the information and/or subsequently treat the potential child(ren) (i.e., whether the child would experience stigma, discrimination, or special treatment). Particularly in intrafamilial or friend donations, there is the potential for family and relationship boundaries to become blurred, and for confusion to arise around the donor's role in the child's and family's life. The donor may become a special auntie or special friend, with this extra dimension of being potentially enriching for both donor and child. On the other hand, there may be risks of boundary confusion, both on the part of the donor, who may feel entitled to be consulted about parenting or even pregnancy decisions and, on the part of the child, who may wonder who is truly his or her real mother. Either donor or recipient may feel threatened and react by distancing from the sibling relationship or family in general. Roles once clearly defined may be changed (e.g., younger donor sister assuming a more caretaking role) or relationship dynamics may shift – perhaps continuously from comfortable gratitude to uncomfortable indebtedness. Interestingly, one study found discordance over time between sister donors and recipients on the issue of disclosure, with donors wanting more disclosure than recipients.[61]

Special Populations

Women with special medical conditions or circumstances considering OD including younger women with spontaneous premature ovarian failure (POF); older women; women with secondary infertility; and women with complicating medical conditions, face unique issues. These women not only confront unique psychosocial tasks but also have special needs in terms of psychoeducation and support. Additionally, their special circumstances may impact the availability of an oocyte donor or the willingness of a donor to provide oocytes to them (e.g., women over forty-five or with life-limiting conditions).[62]

Younger women with POF face unique psychological challenges. Unlike their older counterparts who may have tried infertility treatment unsuccessfully for years, these women, perhaps in their later twenties or early thirties, are often shocked to be told they simply have little or no ovarian function. They may react with disbelief, anger, sadness, and depression and feel deprived of their chance at a genetic child. The psychological task of the younger POF patient is to reconcile the dissonance of being a young woman with old oocytes, and integrate what has happened to her into her sense of self, so as to be able to view the OD option positively and embrace her potential child. All too often these women are given the diagnosis of POF in one breath and the option of oocyte donation in the next, without thought as to the need to psychologically adjust to this devastating diagnosis before pursuing alternative family-building. Counseling and support allow these women and their partners the time and opportunity to grieve their losses in order to embrace the donor option.

By contrast, the majority of OD recipients are older women in reproductive terms (late thirties and forties) that allow woman of advanced maternal age the opportunity to experience pregnancy, childbirth, nursing, and motherhood when it would have otherwise been impossible. However, pregnancy in older mothers is not without risk – medically and psychosocially – for the mother and her child(ren). Pregnancy and childbirth may be more difficult for older women, and the risks of multiple pregnancy/birth with its associated medical complications from multiple births are increased due to the use of younger, better-quality oocytes. The experience of infertility itself is isolating; becoming a mother at an older age may compound feelings of isolation and abnormality, although it may also go far to repair them. For medical, legal, and ethical reasons, therefore, OD legislation and practice guidelines have established an age cut-off for recipient women, usually in the mid-to-late forties range, although recent studies have also indicated that generally pregnancy outcomes are positive for older mothers.[63–66]

In the case of secondary infertility, where couples already have one biological child, the idea of having a child who is not genetically tied to both the mother and father in the same way can trigger a wide range of emotions and relationship dynamics (often negative). The recipient couple may worry about competition between the children and whether the OD child may experience an inferior or special status within the family or extended family. Donor selection may be driven by a desire to have the child fit into a family look, depending upon how private or open the recipients plan to be. Infertility counselors can help to normalize some of these issues as common concerns all couples have about parenting a second child and, at the same time, explore feelings so that an intelligent decision about whether this is a viable option for their family can be made.

Finally, in the OD recipients with medically complicating or life-threatening illnesses, several issues exist. Long-term, underlying health conditions can and often do affect both the pregnancy and the potential health of the child (i.e., when the woman or man has HIV) as well as the mother's health and lifespan in terms of raising a child. These are important considerations recipients need to address and establish appropriate support resources to assist them in the future.

THERAPEUTIC INTERVENTIONS

Today the consensus, although not necessarily the universal practice, is that all couples considering oocyte donation should have a minimum of one session of pretreatment counseling and that counseling should be made available to them both during and after treatment. Counseling and assessment should be performed by a mental health professional with special training in infertility counseling and reproductive medicine. In intrafamilial and identified situations, separate sessions should be conducted with the recipients and the donor (and her partner/spouse) as well as a joint session with all parties. Although these recommendations have been made by the various professional infertility counseling organizations, in professional practice guidelines; and government agencies/legislation, they are not universally adhered to or applied. Nonetheless, research on oocyte donations has repeatedly found counseling to be integral to the successful preparation of participants and the long-term adaptation of the family cre-

ated via this reproductive technology.[67] Patients and caregivers alike have endorsed the importance of counseling, suggesting that extensive pretreatment counseling should be mandatory, enabling participants to consider the psychosocial ramifications of the procedure, particularly the best interest of the child-to-be.[19,22]

The goal of the recipient couple interview is threefold: psychoeducation, support, and assessment. These three aspects are interwoven throughout the interview and thus are not delineated in the following discussion. The approach to recipient counseling is based upon the assumption that couples are basically normal individuals adjusting to major life crises and decisions.

The Recipient Couple Interview

Prior to the interview, it is helpful for the recipient couple to receive written information about the goals and objectives of the counseling, scheduling, fees for service, and patient education materials. Often patients are anxious and/or suspicious about the reasons for the session and/or why it is required. They may question whether the information provided during the session will be used against them. Having clear, written information in hand before the session helps to minimize or at least clarify some of these concerns. As such, the goals of psychosocial assessment and psychoeducational counseling are to:

- establish a positive relationship where any anticipated or unanticipated problems can be addressed or resolved;
- address issues related to the impact of treatment and the psychosocial implications of third-party reproduction;
- identify any conflicts or issues among the participants;
- evaluate unresolved conflicts or major psychological issues that could be a significant impediment to a positive outcome;
- be available to provide ongoing support and counseling, if desired.

At the beginning of the interview, the infertility counselor and the couple should discuss the purpose of the interview, the infertility counselor's role on the treatment team, and sign any consents and release of information forms. This should cover: (1) who the information discussed in the interview will be shared with (i.e., medical staff treating the patient); (2) where written reports resulting from the interview will be kept (i.e., in a confidential file, separate from the patient's medical records, and/or for internal use only); (3) that

---

TABLE 18.3. Reasons for openness vs. privacy in oocyte donation

Openness:

Honest, trusting relationship between parents and child

Child has right to know its true genetic information

Avoids trauma of finding out at later date when information 'slips' or if medical necessity

Privacy:

No need to tell (unlike adoption) because there is a pregnancy

Avoids possible stigma to child or parents due to unique circumstances of conception

Avoids possible frustration to child of not having access to information or donor

---

impressions, recommendations, and/or any concerns will be shared with the couple during or after the interview; (4) how results of psychological testing, if any, will be handled (i.e., actual testing results will not be released to the couple but will be discussed with them); (5) how decisions regarding treatment will be made (i.e., the medical team); and (6) that parties may wish to seek outside religious and legal counsel.

The clinical interview is comprised of a thorough, step-by-step discussion of the couple's infertility history; how they have experienced and grieved it; how they came to the decision to proceed with OD; and how comfortable they are with it at present. Useful tools for this purpose are the Comprehensive Psychosocial History of Infertility (see CPHI in Appendix 3 and Table 18.2). The first part of the interview consists of a history-taking of the couple's marital relationship, preinfertility sexual functioning, infertility history, and when and how they decided to move ahead with the use of OD. The couple should be asked their thoughts and feelings about the biological inequality with OD, in that their potential child will be genetically related to the husband but not the wife, and what concerns she or he have about her ability to attach to a nongenetic child.

Past and current traumas, disappointments, and stresses should be discussed including how they have coped, both as individuals and as a couple. Significant unresolved infertility issues, including the intensity of the feelings or refusal to deal with them, may indicate that an individual or couple is unprepared at this time for OD parenthood in that they are not ready to emotionally relinquish the genetically shared child they had hoped for and wanted. A prime goal of pretreatment OD recipient counseling is the acknowledgment and restoration of self-esteem diminished by the infertility

diagnosis and treatment. Couples need an opportunity to deal with the issues that emerge as they consider OD parenthood, and address the issues and the implications for the family that they are planning to build.

An important part of the interview concerns a discussion of the couple's view of disclosure regarding OD with family, friends, and, most importantly, a potential child (see Table 18.3). The infertility counselor should ascertain whom the couple has told (if anyone), what reactions they have received, and what kind of family or community support they can expect. Inevitably, couples will not have made up their minds completely on this issue and some ambivalence may persist even after the OD decision has been made. However, they must be encouraged to explore it and not avoid the issue (e.g., we are not even pregnant yet, so we will cross that bridge when we come to it...), thus denying the reality of what they are doing and the future implications of their decisions. This seems to be particularly relevant in intrafamilial donations in which the individual, marital, and family systems dynamics comingle in a multifaceted mix of emotions and issues. The infertility counselor must be prepared not only for avoidant coping but also for a self-presentation that minimizes and/or denies potentially problematic areas in order to qualify for the proposed treatment.

During the interview, the couple should be asked about whether or not they have selected a donor, and if so, based on what characteristics. Their feelings, thoughts, and fantasies about her and her motivation to donate should be explored, and the infertility counselor should offer education, where possible, based on his or her actual knowledge of donors.[15] In identified donations, the importance of a final group session with all parties to address the issues of expectations and hopes regarding future contact, roles, and feelings cannot be overemphasized. How the couple plans to thank the donor should also be addressed, whether financial compensation, or a gift, or memento to show their appreciation. It is important to ascertain whether coercion is involved and also to encourage finding a means to achieve closure, enabling all the parties to effectively move on with their lives and not feel either entitled or indebted to each other forever. Situations in which the donor has offered to donate, perhaps having known about the patient's infertility history for some

TABLE 18.4. Indications and contraindications for the use of oocyte donation[52]

Indications:

Absence of significant psychopathology

Absence of unusual life stressors

Ability to provide informed consent

Ability to comply with medical protocols

Supportive and stable interpersonal relationships

Educational/employment stability

Evidence of positive adaptation to infertility/OD option

Ability to choose donor (assuming availability) with relative ease

Contraindications:

Significant untreated mental illness, substance abuse/addiction

Significant current life stressors impacting compliance with treatment, endanger potential offspring

Inability to provide informed consent

Inability to comply with medical protocols

Marital/relationship instability; lack of social support system; presence of physical abuse; evidence of coercion by partner or other(s)

History of sexual or physical abuse without professional treatment

History of or current legal difficulties

History of perpetrated physical, emotional abuse or neglect

No evidence of having grieved infertility/OD losses

Inability to choose donor (not due to lack of availability)

individual or couple is not prepared to proceed with OD include:

- serious disagreement between partners about the decision to use donated oocytes as evidenced by partner reluctance, coercion, or passivity;
- significant marital conflict and a belief that a baby will repair the marriage or provide a child before a partner exits;
- serious mental health problems that have not been acknowledged and/or treated or impair the individual's ability to comply with treatment or provide informed consent;
- unwillingness to learn about the unique aspects of OD parenting and accept its differences, including acknowledgment of the donor and/or the child's right to information about the donor where this is legally mandated;
- the pursuit of OD parenthood to gain a child who will meet the parent's needs and assuage narcissistic injuries without regard to the child's needs; and/or
- persistent inability to select a donor, not due to lack of availabile oocyte donors.

time, are typically easier for everyone than when the infertile couple has asked for the donation. The ideal donation scenario may be one in which the donor has completed her family and does not wish to have more children, reducing fears and risks that the donor may want to parent the child; may experience infertility herself in the future and regret the donation; or experience medical complications from the donation that may have an impact on her own fertility.

While the position of the infertility counselor is to basically assume that the couple comes to infertility treatment with a history of good mental health, the couple, nonetheless, should be assessed for a history of alcohol and drug use; sexual or child abuse; legal difficulties; past psychiatric issues the individuals may have experienced and how they were addressed; as well as their current level of functioning and use of psychotropic medication. As has been stated, the recipient couple must be made aware at the outset of their interview that there is an assessment component and if problems are identified, they will be discussed during or after the initial interview. Indications that an

The role of the infertility counselor may be to facilitate treatment of the identified problem (e.g., referral to chemical dependency treatment) or to provide referrals to other appropriate caregivers (e.g., marriage counseling, psychotherapy) (see Table 18.4).

In terms of therapeutic management of these situations, the infertility counselor may recommend a *defer, not deny* treatment approach, where patients are urged to seek outside psychotherapy (not with the assessing infertility counselor) for these issues, and return at a later date to be reassessed for their readiness and appropriateness to proceed with OD parenthood. Any decisions to deny treatment are best made by the clinical team (physician, nurse, infertility counselor, etc.). In a study that explored program policies about screening of assisted reproduction participants, researchers found that only 4% of candidates were denied yearly. The majority of programs believed they had a right and responsibility to deny treatment (e.g., evidence of physical abuse), and that decisions were most often based on input from members of the treatment team versus a decision by a single professional.[68]

Integral to the interview (including assessment and care) is the provision of patient education materials such as articles, books, and websites for patients as well as potential children that can help them in their current decision making as well as for future reference. Providing a written resource list or copies of useful articles on the issues discussed is helpful to patients who may hold on to the information for later reference. Of particular interest is a list of storybooks for talking to children about their conception, no matter what the recipient couple's current thoughts on disclosure may be.[69] Research on disclosure indicates that disclosure decisions are less likely to be fixed and more likely to evolve over time and the life of the child.[70–72] In addition, parents' willingness and ability to disclose is often based on the parents' lack of a script or specific instructions or directions on how to tell. As such, patient education materials can be integral in not only giving instruction but also in permission giving: allowing recipients to reconsider the decision over time. Finally, the couple should be informed of any OD support/discussion groups that may be available through the clinic, facilitated by the infertility counselor, or on the internet. These groups provide both educational and emotional support as well as an environment for healing in a safe, nonjudgmental setting with others who are dealing with the same decisions and issues. Of particular importance is providing information on donor registries in the areas in which these are applicable (see Reference list).[73]

FUTURE IMPLICATIONS

Given the scarcity of oocyte donors and the current limitations regarding cryopreservation of oocytes, recent technological developments related to oocytes and ovarian tissue may open new frontiers and treatment possibilities: cryopreservation of oocytes; ovarian transplantation; and ovarian autologous transplantation. Although sperm cryopreservation has been available for decades, the technology for cryopreservation of oocytes is a recent development that, at this time, remains in the research stage. Cases such as the recent one of a young cancer patient who froze her oocytes prior to starting cancer treatment, fertilized the thawed oocytes with her husband's sperm, and then transferred embryos to a gestational carrier who delivered a baby in October 2005,[74] give hope for more successes in the future. Recent studies have shown, respectively, 75% and 90% survival rates of cryopreserved oocytes after thawing, with, respectively, 67% and 82% fertilization rates using ICSI.[75,76] Another

recent development has been case reports of successful donor ovarian-tissue transplant in which a twenty-four-year-old patient received an ovarian tissue donation from her identical twin, resulting in conception and birth of a baby as a result of the donated ovarian tissue (and oocytes).[77] At present, the case appears to have limited applicability because an identical twin was used and thus there was no threat of tissue rejection. Finally, in September 2005, another baby was born when her mother's frozen ovarian tissue was reimplanted into her abdomen following earlier successful cancer treatment for non-Hodgkin's lymphoma. [78] Thus, ovarian autologous reimplantation of preserved ovarian tissue may allow women to have a genetically linked child and for conception to occur traditionally (without IVF). These developments have the potential for expanding the reproductive horizons and possibilities for women of all ages as well as eliminating the need for oocyte donors and/or the synchronization of donor and recipient reproductive cycles. Women may be able to protect or prolong their reproductive lives; prevent the transmission of hereditary diseases; or delay motherhood by cryopreserving their own ovarian tissue in their youth to be used later in life. However, despite the benefits and applications of these technologies, they will no doubt present a unique variety of ethical dilemmas. While we may speculate on how, why, and when these technologies may be used in the future, in reality these new reproductive technologies will probably be applied in ways not yet considered or even imagined.

SUMMARY

■ While sperm donation has been used for more than 100 years, ooycte donation is a more recent family-building alternative of the last twenty years made possible by in vitro fertilization technology.

■ The psychological process of accepting OD as a family-building alternative can be understood by viewing a compilation of theories that involve psycho-analytic and feminist theory, stigma, attachment and loss, and family systems theory.

■ The decision to use donor oocytes has lifelong implications, and recipients need sufficient time to grieve the loss of the shared biological child before they are ready to proceed with treatment.

■ Choosing a donor, whether anonymous or known, is a significant psychological step in the OD process, and each option carries unique issues that must be considered.

■ OD recipients need to be counseled on disclosure issues with regard to family members and friends, as well as the child, and the possible future implications for their child.

■ The clinical interview of the recipient couple by a infertility counselor is crucial in assessing the couple's readiness to proceed, as well as in providing support and psychoeducation.

■ The explosion of new technologies such as oocyte-freezing and ovarian tissue transplant may one day minimize the need for oocyte donors, who are already in short supply.

REFERENCES

1. Baetens P, Devroey P, Camus M, et al. Counselling couples and donors for oocyte donation: The decision to use either known or anonymous oocytes. *Hum Reprod* 2000; 15: 476–84.

2. Ahuja KK, Simons EG, Fiamanya W, et al. Egg-sharing in assisted conception: Ethical and practical considerations. *Hum Reprod* 1996; 11:1126–31.

3. Haase J, Takefman J. *Global Perspectives in Infertility Counselling*. International Infertility Counseling Organization. Postgraduate Course. Montreal, Canada 2004.

4. Kenentich H. Patients in migration. In: J Boivin, H Kentenich, eds, *Guidelines for Counseling in Infertility*. ESHRE Monographs. London: Oxford University Press, 2002.

5. Berriot-Salvadore E. The discourse of medicine and science. In: NZ Davis, A Farge, eds, *A History of Women: Renaissance and Enlightenment Paradoxes*. Cambridge, MA. Harvard University Press, 1993.

6. Lutjen P, Trouson A, Leeton J, et al. The establishment and maintenance of pregnancy using in vitro fertilization and embryo donation in a patient with primary ovarian failure. *Nature* 1984; 307:174–5.

7. Directive 2004/23 E. C. of the European Parliament and the Council (2004) O. J. L102/48 (March 31, 2004).

8. Human Fertilisation and Embryology: The regulation of Donor-Assisted Conception. 9/2004 www.hfea.gov.uk.

9. Cox LW. The role of accreditation committees in oocyte donation. *Reprod Fertil Develop* 1992; 4:731–7.

10. Letur-Konirsch H. Oocyte donation in France and national balance sheet (GEDO). Different European approaches. *Gynecol Obstet Fertil* 2004; 32:108–15.

11. Anderson N, Gianaroli L, Felbergaum R, et al. Assisted reproductive technology in Europe, 2001. Results generated from European registers by ESHRE. *Hum Reprod* 2005; 20:1158–76.

12. Giva-Osagie OF. ART in developing countries with reference to sub-Sahara Africa. In: E Vayne, PS Rowe, PD Griffin, eds. *Current Practices and Controversies in Assisted Reproduction*. Geneva: World Health Organization Report, 2001; 23–30.

13. Boggio A. Italy enacts new law on medically assisted reproduction. *Hum Reprod* 2005; 20:1153–7.

14. Soderstrom-Antilla V, Hovatta O. Oocyte donation to be legalized in Sweden. Excellent results reported from other countries. *Lakartidningen* 2002; 99:3118–21.

15. Baetens P. Oocyte donation. In: J Boivin, H Kentenich, eds, *Guidelines on Infertility Counselling*. ESHRE Monographs. London: Oxford University Press, 2002; 33–4.

16. ESHRE task force on ethics and law. Gamete and embryo donation. *Hum Reprod* 2002; 17:407–8.

17. Hersherberg P. Recipients of oocyte donation: An integrative review. *JOGNN* 2004; 33:610–21.

18. Applegarth L, Goldberg NC, Cholst I, et al. Families created through ovum donation: A preliminary investigation of obstetrical outcome and psychosocial adjustment. *J Assist Reprod Genetics* 1995; 12:574–80.

19. Sewall G, Mason L. Parental acceptance, disclosure, and decision-making amongst recipients in an anonymous donor oocyte program. *Fertil Steril* 1995; 64:S252.

20. Greenfeld DA, Klock SC. Disclosure decisions among known and anonymous oocyte donation recipients. *Fertil Steril* 2004; 81:1565–71.

21. Lindheim SR, Kavi S, Sauer M. Understanding differences in the perception of anonymous parties: A comparison between gamete donors and their recipients. *J Assist Reprod Genetics* 2000; 17:127–30.

22. Soderstrom-Anttila V, Sajaniemi N, Tiitinen A, et al. Health and development of children born after oocyte donation compared with that of those born after in-vitro fertilization, and parents' attitudes regarding secrecy. *Humn Reprod* 1998; 13:2009–15.

23. Heineman-Kuschinksy E, Davis S, Bochard E, et al. Assessment of recipient patient's concerns and feelings associated with anonymous oocyte donation. *Fertil Steril* 1995; 64:S251.

24. Greenfeld DA, Greenfeld DG, Mazure CM, et al. Do attitudes toward disclosure in donor oocyte recipients predict the use of anonymous versus directed donation? *Fertil Steril* 1998; 79:1009–14.

25. Fielding D, Handley S, Duqueno L, et al. Motivation, attitudes and experience of donation: A follow-up of women donating eggs in assisted conception treatment. *J Comm Applied Soc Psych* 1998; 8:273–7.

26. Josephs LS, Grill E, Crone K, et al. Sister ovum donation: Psychological outcomes. *Fertil Steril* 2004; 82:S102.

27. Greenfeld DA, Greenfeld DG, Mazure CM, et al. Social and psychological characteristics of donor oocyte recipients. *Fertil Steril* 1995; 64:S51.

28. Burgos C, et al. Attitudes of patients who underwent oocyte donation: A multicentre study of the Latin American Network of Assisted Reproduction. Presented at the 14th Annual meeting of the European Society of Reproduction and Embryology. Goteborg, Sweden, June 21–24, 1998.

29. Zegers-Hochschild F, Pacheco IM, Fabres C, et al. Psychosocial characteristics of Chilean women participating in an in vitro fertilization program (IVF/ET) with donated oocytes (OD). *Fertil Steril* 1998; 70:S29.

30. Epstein YM, Rosenberg HS. Depression in primary versus secondary infertility egg recipients. *Fertil Steril* 2005; 83:1882–4.

31. Bartlett JA. Psychiatric issues in non-anonymous oocyte donation. *Psychosomatics* 1991; 32:433–7.

32. Golombok S, Murray C, Brinsden P, et al. Social versus biological parenting: Family functioning and the socio-emotional development of children conceived by egg or sperm donation. *J Child Psychol Psychia* 1999; 40:519–27.

33. Ireland MS. *Reconceiving Women: Separating Motherhood from Female Identity*. New York: Guilford Press, 1993.

34. Horney K. *Feminine Psychology*. New York: Norton, 1967/1973.

35. Chodorow NJ. *The Reproduction of Mothering*, 2nd ed. Berkeley: University of California Press, 1978.

36. Chodorow NJ. "Too late": Ambivalence about motherhood, choice and time. *J Amer Psychoanal Assn* 2003; 51:1181–98.

37. Miller JB. Women's psychological development: Connections, disconnections, and violations. In: MM Berger, ed. *Women Beyond Freud: New Concepts of Feminine Psychology*. New York: Brunner/Mazel, 1994; 79–98.

38. Goffman E. *Stigma: Notes on the Management of Spoiled Identity*. Englewood Cliffs, NJ: Prentice Hall, 1963.

39. Kurzban R, Leary MR. Evolutionary origins of stigmatization: The functions of social exclusion. *Psychological Bulletin* 2001; 127:187–208.

40. Neuberg SL, Smith SM, Asher T. Why people stigmatize: Toward a biocultural framework. In: R Heatheton, R Kleck, M Hebl, F Hull, eds. *The Social Psychology of Stigma*. New York: Guilford Press, 2000: 31–61.

41. Bowlby, J. *Maternal Care and Mental Health*. World Health Organization Monograph (Serial No.2), 1951.

42. Bowlby J. *Attachment and Loss: Vol 1 Attachment*. New York: Basic Books, 1969.

43. Bowlby J. *Attachment and Loss: Vol 2 Separation: Anxiety and Anger*. New York: Basic Books, 1973.

44. Cowan PA, Cowan CP. Strengthening couples to improve children's well-being. *Poverty Res News* 2002; 3:18–20.

45. Minuchin S. *Families and Family Therapy*. Cambridge, MA: Harvard University Press, 1974; 54.

46. Burns LH. Infertility as boundary ambiguity: One theoretical perspective. *Fam Process* 1987; 26:359–72.

47. Boss P. *Ambiguous Loss: Learning to Live with Unresolved Grief*. Cambridge, MA: Harvard University Press, 1999.

48. Imber-Black E. *Secrets in Families and Family Therapy*. New York: WW Norton, 1993.

49. American Society for Reproductive Medicine. Guidelines for oocyte donation. *Fertil Steril* 2002; 77:S6–S7.

50. Lee FR. Driven by Costs, Fertility Clients Head Overseas. *New York Times*. 1–25–2005.

51. Pennings G. Legal harmonization and reproductive tourism in Europe. *Hum Reprod* 2004; 19:2689–94.

52. Applegarth LD, Kingsberg SA. The donor as patient: Assessment and support. In: LH Burns, SN Covington, eds. *Infertility Counseling: A Comprehensive Handbook for Clinicians*. New York: Parthenon Publishing, 1999; 369.

53. American Society for Reproductive Medicine Ethics Committee Report. Informing offspring of their conception by gamete donation. *Fertil Steril* 2004; 81:3.

54. Rohr R. Companies offer women $7,000 for donating eggs. *Washington Square News* 1–28–2003.

55. Kolata G. Young women offer to sell their eggs to infertile couples. *New York Times* 11–10–1991.

56. Kolata G. Price of donor eggs soars, setting off a debate on ethics. *New York Times* 2–25–1998.

57. Hoffman J. Egg donations meet a need and raise ethical questions. *New York Times* 1–8–1996.

58. Pennings G. The right to choose your own donor: A step towards commercialization or a step toward empowering the patient? *Hum Reprod* 2000; 15:508–14.

59. German EK, Mukerjee T, Osborne D, Cooperman AB. Does increasing ovum donor compensation lead to differences in donor characteristics? *Fertil Steril* 2001; 78:75–9.

60. Anderson J, Alesi R., Donor issues. In: *Infertility Counsellor's Seminar*, 12 January 1998. Melbourne, Australia.

61. Josephs LS, Grill E, Crone K, et al. Sister ovum donation: Psychological outcomes. *Fertil Steril* 2004; 82:S102.

62. Kump L, Licciardi F, Krey L, et al. An oocyte donor's willingness to donate – does the recipient's lifestyle make a difference? *Fertil Steril* 2003; 80:S140.

63. Porreco RP, Harden L, Gambotto M, Shapiro H. Expectation of pregnancy outcome among mature women. *Am J Obstet Gynecol* 2005; 192:38–41.

64. Callaway LK, Lust K, McIntyre HD. Pregnancy outcomes in women of very advanced maternal age. *Obstet Gynecol Surv* 2005; 60:562–3.

65. Chibber R. Child-bearing beyond age 50: Pregnancy outcome in 59 cases "a concern"? *Arch Gynecol Obstet* 2005; 271(3):189–94. Epub 2004.

66. Paulson RJ, Boostanfar R, Saadat P, et al. Pregnancy in the sixth decade of life: Obstetric outcomes in women of advanced reproductive age. *JAMA* 2002; 288: 2320–3.

67. Tarlatzis BC, Pados G. Oocyte donation: Clinical and practical aspects. *Mol Cell Endocrinol* 2000; 161:99–102.

68. Gurmankin AD, Caplan AL, Braverman AM. Screening practices and beliefs of assisted reproductive technology programs. *Fertil Steril* 2005; 83:61–7.

69. Mahlstedt PP, Greenfeld DA. Assisted reproductive technology for donor gametes: The need for patient preparation. *Fertil Steril* 1989; 52:908–14.

70. Klock SC, Jacob MC, Maier D. A prospective study of donor insemination recipients: Secrecy, privacy, and disclosure. *Fertil Steril* 1994; 62(3):477–84.

71. Nachtigall RD, Pitcher L, Tachann JM, et al. Stigma, disclosure, and family functioning among parents of children conceived through donor insemination. *Fertil Steril* 1997; 68:83–9.

72. Heineman E. Trends of recipient patients concerns and feelings associated with anonymous oocyte donation. *Fertil Steril* 2000; 74:S24.

73. Thorn P, Daniels KR. A group work approach to family-building by donor insemination: Empowering the marginalised. *Hum Fertil* 2003; 6:46–50.

74. www.fertilehope.org.

75. Chen SU, Lien YR, Chen HF, et al. Observational clinical follow-up of oocyte cryopreservation using a slow-freezing method with 1,2-propanediol plus sucrose followed by ICSI. *Hum Reprod* 2005; 20:1975–80.

76. Li XH, Chen SU, Zhang X, et al. Cryopreserved oocytes of infertile couples undergoing assisted reproductive technology could be an important source of oocyte donation: A clinical report of successful pregnancies. *Hum Reprod* 2005; 20:3390–4.

77. Silber SJ, Lenahan KM, Levine DJ, et al. Ovarian transplantation between monozygotic twins discordant for premature ovarian failure. *N Engl J Med* 2005; 353:58–63.

78. Siegel-Itzkovich J. Woman gives birth after receiving transplant of her own ovarian tissue. *BMJ* 2005; 9:70.

19 The Donor as Patient: Assessment and Support

LINDA D. APPLEGARTH AND SHERYL A. KINGSBERG

> *The provision of a gamete is also a life-giving gift that responds to the human needs of others. Yet it is life-giving in a distinctive sense, for it does not keep others alive, but facilitates their ability to create life....*
>
> – Cynthia B. Cohen[1]

The gamete donor plays a unique role in infertility treatment both as a patient and as a provider of reproductive tissue (genetic material). Gamete donation, perhaps as an extension of other forms of medical donations (e.g., blood, tissue, and organs), has in recent decades facilitated thousands of births worldwide. *Donation* refers to a wide range of transactions involving either anonymous or nonanonymous sperm, oocyte, or embryo donors – with the focus of this chapter being the gamete (and not embryo) donor. As such, the physical and emotional well-being as a donor and as a patient is paramount before, during, and after the donation. Ideally, donors should be evaluated both medically and psychologically to ensure that they are physically and emotionally healthy; able to provide informed consent; and capable of tolerating the physical and psychological rigors of the donation process. The work of the infertility counselor is integral in assessing the suitability of the donor, to facilitating the donor's understanding of the implications of donating one's genetic material to another person, and in providing long-term support and education.

Counseling issues and the medical process of gamete donation are unique in that gamete donors are not, according to conventional medicine, 'patients' in need of medical care. Donors are (or at least present with the expectation) that they are physically and psychologically healthy and are not patients either within the medical setting or mental health professional's care. Regardless of this lack of identification as a patient, the donor's psychological well-being and medical needs must always be of critical importance to all caregivers. Despite this caveat, the reality is that worldwide, less attention is given to the psychological assessment, screening, and support of gamete donors than to the stringent medical screenings that are required or recommended. For example, the International Federation of Fertility Societies' Surveillance 2004 Report[2] addresses the issue of gamete donor anonymity versus nonanonymity but does not specifically include psychological assessment or support as part of the general donor work-up.

There is significant variation between countries and within countries regarding gamete donation procedures, policies, and laws as well as differences in the use of donor assessment and counseling.[3,4] Medical evaluation and counseling practice guidelines have been defined by professional societies, such the ASRM and ESHRE; government regulatory agencies, such as Great Britain's HFEA, Canada's AHRA, and Australia's RTAC; and legislation that bans certain forms of gamete donation (e.g., oocyte donation); or, simply by benign neglect. Variance across and within countries has been influenced by a variety of factors including religious laws and beliefs, culture, and politics. As such, every infertility counselor should be aware of the laws and practice standards regarding gamete donation not only where they practice but also where potential donors may reside and/or hold citizenship.

The United Kingdom's Human Fertilisation and Embryology Authority (HFEA) was established in 1991 and exemplified one regulatory approach to gamete donation. The HFEA legally mandated anonymity of gamete donors allowing availability of only limited information about the donor. However, in April 2005 the HFEA eliminated all donor anonymity and compensation and established a central donor registry. Under these regulations, all gamete donors are required to provide identifying information and medical information and be willing to be contacted at some time in the future by any (all) donor offspring. The HFEA's position on the discontinuation of compensation of donors is in compliance with the European Union Tissue and Cells Directive that promotes 'altruistic donation.'

This form of gamete donation is therefore voluntary and unpaid, although donors may be reimbursed for "expenses and inconveniences related to the donation."[5] The HFEA permits a specific maximum financial payment for reasonable reimbursable expenses to altruistic oocyte donors, but prohibits financial remuneration for IVF patients who share or donate their extra oocytes. HFEA regulations specify that counseling be offered to all potential donors although it is not the counselor's responsibility to prohibit or disallow donations; instead they are to provide patient education, facilitate decision making, and address the implications of the donation for the donor[6] (see www.hfea. gov.uk).

Canada and Australia have similar regulatory approaches. The Infertility Treatment Act was enacted in 1984 in Australia's state of Victoria and in 1988 was the first to legislate a donor registry that mandates the registration of all donor births, and allows all donor offspring at age eighteen to access identifying information about their donor. Donors have no right of veto. This legislation also established counseling criteria for donors, recipients, and offspring – referred to as 'donor-linking' counseling. Within this context, infertility counselors, as licensed professionals, receive special training to address the counseling and psychosocial needs of donors as well as offspring and recipients. All fertility clinics in Australia and New Zealand are accredited by the Reproductive Technology Accreditation Committee (RTAC) in conjunction with the Fertility Society of Australia. These regulatory agencies oversee the provision of gamete donation services including gamete collection, categories of donors, payment or coercion of donors, matching and exclusion of donors, and information and counseling of donors. Australia's system is one of combined voluntary regulation and legislative regulation, both national and state[7] (see www.ita.org.au).

In contrast, Canada has the newest regulatory body, the Assisted Human Reproduction Agency, established in 2004. The Canadian legislation eliminated donor anonymity, established a central donor registry, and prohibited all payment to gamete donors (sperm or oocytes). Because of strong opposition to the treatment of gametes as a commodity to be traded for money or other goods, all donor compensation was eliminated.[8] Canadian legislation also mandated the provision of counseling services for all individuals participating in assisted reproduction – including donors. Although U.K. policy requires that counseling be offered, Canadian legislation mandates counseling.

Many countries have legislation specifically directed toward gamete donation, although the provision of counseling is not addressed. According to a report from the International Federation of Fertility Societies (IFFS) in 2004, sperm donation is not allowed in Brazil, Egypt, Iran, Morocco, Saudi Arabia, Tunisia, and Turkey.[2] This legislative position appears to be primarily based on religious beliefs or moral values.

Oocyte donation became legal in France in 1994, provided that all oocyte donations are voluntary, free, anonymous, and confidential. In France, couples are encouraged to bring an oocyte donor who will, in turn, be used anonymously for a different recipient couple. Clinic staff does anonymous pairing of donors and recipients. Referred to as personalized anonymity, recipients recruit a donor (often from family and friends) who subsequently donates their oocytes anonymously to one or more recipients.[9] Belgium has a similar form of oocyte donation although known (identified) oocyte donations are allowed. Several countries have legally banned any form of oocyte donation including Benin, Germany, Italy, Japan, Kenya, Latvia, The Netherlands, Norway, Portugal, Sierra Leone, Slovenia, Switzerland, and Togo.[2] Another form of oocyte donation, referred to as 'egg sharing,' is prevalent in the United States and other parts of the world. It enables fertile women undergoing IVF to donate a portion of their healthy oocytes to other infertile patients – a donation for which they may or may not be compensated.[10] As of 2005, all forms of assisted reproduction are strictly regulated in Italy, and both oocyte and sperm donation are banned.[11] Of interest, Sweden was the first country to remove anonymity of sperm donors in 1984, thus enabling offspring to determine the identity of their sperm donor. Sweden did not pass legislation allowing oocyte donation until 2003.[12]

In the United States, the Mental Health Professional Group of the American Society of Reproductive Medicine (MHPG/ASRM) and in Europe, the Psychological Special Interest Group of the European Society of Human Reproduction and Embryology (PSIG/ESHRE) have established professional practice and patient care guidelines on gamete donation. Within the existing society guidelines, there is a recommendation for psychological counseling for all parties involved in sperm, oocyte, and embryo donation. These guidelines, and those offered by the Mental Health Professional Group of the ASRM,[13] provide a foundation for the practice of donor counseling and assessment that can potentially have legal, psychosocial, and ethical implications (see www.asrm.org).

In 2002, the Psychological Special Interest Group of ESHRE also published the Guidelines for Counselling Infertility, a comprehensive document outlining infertility counseling issues with specific recommendations on sperm and oocyte donation.[14] Additionally, ESHRE has issued a wide array of Task Force reports including one on gamete donation[15] (see www.eshre. com). Included in the ESHRE guidelines are recommendations that the psychological evaluation include an assessment "of the general abilities and intellectual capacity of the donor candidates," along with "minimal information about the donor concerning appearance, education, profession, social background and motivation for donating."[15]

Given the dramatic difference in the laws, regulations, and policies governing gamete donation around the world, a phenomenon known as reproductive tourism has developed. It usually refers to infertile patients traveling across borders to obtain assisted reproductive technologies unavailable or too costly in their home country.[16,17] However, this phenomenon has become increasingly applicable to gamete donors who travel across borders to donate, often commercially recruited and motivated by financial compensation. These donors require special care as they may often have insufficient or inadequate medical and psychological preparation and/or screening and few resources if they change their minds. As such, issues of education, preparation, motivation, and coercion are integral for the proper care of these unique 'donors as patients.'

Counseling gamete donors involves several critical components including evaluation, education, and screening – although this is not a universal recommendation or practice and may present its own set of dilemmas for the mental health professional. Nevertheless, the primary roles of mental health professionals are to protect the emotional well-being of donors; to help them understand as fully as possible the meaning and consequences of their donation; to act as a patient advocate and educator; to access the donor's motivations for donation as well as his or her ability to comply with the medical and/or psychosocial demands of donation; to determine the donor's appropriateness for donation; and finally, if necessary, to address issues relevant to identified donations or directed donations.

This chapter provides a general overview of what is currently known, nationally and internationally, about gamete donation from the donor's perspective, with the purpose of

■ reviewing current literature and research on gamete donors;
■ understanding the theoretical issues involved in the assessment, education, and counseling of gamete donors;

■ defining the clinical issues and therapeutic interventions involved in evaluating, preparing, and counseling gamete donors;
■ providing the psychosocial criteria for acceptance or rejection of donor candidates.

HISTORICAL OVERVIEW

According to historical accounts, artificial insemination was first attempted on Juana, wife of King Henry IV of Castile, in 1677 by Dutch scientist Leeuwenhoek. He had been the first to identify spermatozoa through the newly invented microscope. Subsequent research on sperm identification and manipulation (including cyropreservation) was done on animals. In 1866, Italian physician I. Mantegazza proposed the cryopreservation of sperm and the establishment of human sperm banks to store semen specimens.

The use of donated gametes (specifically by a stranger and not a spouse) is a reproductive phenomenon of the twentieth century. The first cryopreservation of human sperm was reported in 1940 by Shettles, although success was limited by the cryopservation of sperm from only eight donors.[18] The first reported medical use of therapeutic donor insemination was in the United States in 1909,[19] and the first reported pregnancy achieved from cryopreserved sperm was in 1953.[20]

Sperm donation is a noninvasive process requiring relatively little time and physical effort on the part of the donor. It is virtually medically risk-free for the donor as there is no evidence of current or future physical harm from the process of donation. Improved methods of sperm collection were developed in the 1970s and 1980s that led to the development of sperm banks. These banks were typically operated in conjunction with major medical centers offering treatment for infertility. The original practices and policies of these banks (worldwide) protected donor anonymity and maintained a policy of donor privacy and secrecy.[21]

Until the mid-1980s, the work of identifying and screening semen donors was a private and an individual one.[22] In other words, physicians would typically identify medical students, residents, or other graduate-level males, test them for sexually transmitted diseases, and match them accordingly by phenotype. As HIV infection and hepatitis have become more prevalent, semen has been cryopreserved and quarantined for six months. The donor must then retest negative before the frozen semen can be released. With the improved techniques of sperm cryopreservation, there has been a large increase in the number of sperm banks with standardized basic quality assurance.

Until the mid-1980s and despite the availability of cryopreserved donated sperm, many infertile couples continued to use fresh donated sperm because it was believed to be more fertile. However, this practice changed dramatically worldwide with the HIV epidemic of the 1980s during which there were several reported cases of women contracting HIV from freshly donated sperm. Subsequently, much more stringent guidelines for evaluating potential donors (and sperm) were implemented around the world to screen for a variety of infectious diseases, particularly human immunodeficiency virus (HIV) and genetic defects.[23] Today accredited sperm banks offer only cryopreserved semen that has been quarantined six months after which the donor is reassessed for infectious disease status.[24] Sperm is only allowed to be released for donation after this quarantine and reassessment criteria have been met. Still, little attention has been given to sperm donor motivations and/or psychosocial issues (whether short- or long-term). Additionally, counseling has not typically been recommended and/or offered to potential sperm donors.[24]

This situation is in striking contrast to oocyte donors in which recommendations, regulations, and practice standards continue to include psychological assessment, evaluation, and discussion of the donors' feelings and motivations about donation. If and when psychological preparation of sperm donors does occur, it is more likely to be within the context of intrafamilial or identified donation than anonymous donation or within the context of 'donor-linking' in which the donor meets or exchanges information with offspring born as a result of his donation. Furthermore, the change in sperm bank policies regarding the evaluation and screening of donors in the 1980s led to changes in laws and social policies regarding donor anonymity. As noted, Sweden was the first country (of what has now become many) to eliminate donor anonymity in 1984. Additionally, the elimination of donor compensation in some countries may also date back to the tissue storage and social policy changes that occurred in the 1980s.

The first oocyte donation was reported in Australia in 1983 when a twenty-five-year-old woman with premature ovarian failure was the recipient of a single oocyte donated by a twenty-nine-year-old woman undergoing an in vitro fertilization (IVF) cycle due to a history of bilateral tubal dysfunction.[25] Although sperm donation is not medically risky, the same cannot be said for oocyte donation, which is a much more medically complex procedure involving potential medical complications for the donor. Historically, the development of transvaginal ultrasound retrieval has helped increase the availability of oocyte dona-

tion.[26] Oocyte harvesting initially required laparoscopic retrieval, and the necessity for donors to undergo surgery kept the pool of potential donors limited. The main source of donors were women undergoing tubal ligation, or close relatives or friends willing to risk surgery. Another method of retrieval, also developed in the early 1980s, involved artificial insemination of the donor with the recipient male sperm washing the embryos from the uterus for transfer to the recipient female's uterus. This method is no longer used, as it had limited success and numerous problems, including donor infections and retained pregnancies.[27] As cryopreservation of embryos became available, the supply of ova from women going through IVF virtually dried up. Couples chose to fertilize all retrieved oocytes to cryopreserve embryos for their own future use.[28] Fortunately, within a similar time frame, transvaginal ultrasound retrieval was developed, greatly reducing the risk to donors and their recovery time and thus opening up an entirely new potential pool of donors: young anonymous donors, somewhat more analogous to the typical sperm donor. Nevertheless, there is still considerable effort required from the oocyte donor, such as timed injections, blood work, ultrasound examinations, and timing of her cycle with the recipient's.[29]

Unlike sperm donation, the technology for cryopreservation of oocytes remains experimental and is not yet universally applicable. As a result, there are no oocyte 'banks' but instead there exists a labyrinth of oocyte donation possibilities and practices including oocyte-sharing (as in the case of the first oocyte donation), known (most often a sister or friend), or recruited anonymous or identified oocyte donors. The ways and means of oocyte donation are influenced by the laws and standard of practice in the country in which the donation is taking place, and are also influenced by donor recruitment policies. Oocyte donors may potentially be sisters, daughters, or other female relatives of the recipient, friends, or acquaintances. Some donors may wish to be anonymous and have volunteered or been recruited by a medical clinic or a donor oocyte agency, whose sole purpose is to recruit oocyte donors commercially for recipient couples. Donors may also be identified, chosen by recipients from a pool of potential candidates (or the donor may meet the recipients and make a collaborative decision), thus providing donors and recipients more personal control and participation in the donation process.[30] With the entrée of the internet, computerized recruitment is also an increasingly popular means of donor recruitment. Finally, in the United States recently, private recruiting agencies also may offer oocyte donors with a range of levels of identification: photographs and other identifying information, contact with the donor by telephone or electronic mail, and/or a personal, face-to-face meeting with the donor.

REVIEW OF LITERATURE

Psychosocial Status of Donors

Although family-building through the use of sperm donation is used extensively worldwide, there is very little information about the psychosocial impact of this procedure on the donors themselves. Only recently has research begun to look at the psychological effects of sperm donation on donors.[24,31]

The literature is quite limited regarding the emotional and psychosocial status of the gamete donor. Novaes[32] stressed that in general, almost no research is available on the long-term psychological impact of being a gamete donor. There is more information available about the psychosocial issues regarding oocyte donors. These donors, for example, are much more likely to undergo a clinical interview and psychological testing than are their male counterparts. Schover and associates[33] evaluated twenty-six oocyte donor candidates and found that they were significantly more likely than controls to have experienced at least one emotional trauma related to reproduction or at least one family event such as death of a parent, parental divorce, chemical dependency or psychiatric disorder in a relative, or sexual abuse. Oocyte donors themselves had also experienced a significantly greater number of reproductive traumas or family problems than controls. On follow-up,[34] twenty-three women were surveyed with respect to donor satisfaction. Ninety-one percent were moderately to extremely satisfied with the experience; transient adverse psychological symptoms were reported by two donors but resolved with medical or psychological treatment. Although psychological risk factors predicted potential donors' decisions to participate and their compliance, they were not predictive of donor satisfaction on follow-up. Lessor and associates[35] also considered social and psychological characteristics in ninety-five women who volunteered to be oocyte donors and found, on the basis of clinical interviews and psychological test performance, that 73% were acceptable as donors. They noted that the incidence of dysfunction (abandonment, abuse) in family of origin or family of orientation was unremarkable.

Recruitment and Motivation of Donors

Kalfoglou and Gittelsohn[36] conducted a qualitative study of the experiences of thirty-three former oocyte donors. They reported that half of these donors reported that they were motivated primarily by financial compensation. However, some of these women, whose primary motivation was financial, stated that they began to feel more altruistic about the donation as they progressed through the donation process. Other reasons included: the desire to help infertile couples (some knew infertile couples and others had been infertile themselves); the desire to pass on their genes without having to parent themselves; a sense of "genetic pride"; the need to compensate for a previous abortion; and to feel special.[36]

Because many gamete donors are compensated monetarily (e.g., in the United States and Spain), it has been suggested that compensation is an unethical means of obtaining the donor's consent.[37] It has also been recommended that to ensure proper consent to oocyte donation, the infertility counselor should be responsible for exploring these issues with donors so that decisions are made independent of the compensation.[37,38] For example, Lindheim and colleagues[39] found that as the monetary compensation of oocyte donors ($n = 537$) increased ($2,500 to $5,000), the percentage of donors who indicated that their motivation was financial also increased from 39% to 68%. In another study of twenty-five donors, Klock and associates[41] found the lowest levels of satisfaction postretrieval among those donors who indicated they had been motivated by money to donate. Lindheim and colleagues[39] suggest that the "seductive nature" of monetary compensation indicates a need for more attention to the informed consent process and Klock and colleagues[40] also recommend careful screening and counseling of those donors who indicate that financial compensation is a leading motivating factor for the donation.

The issue of recruitment, motivation, and compensation has been a subject of ongoing debate in the United Kingdom. Sauer[41] notes that the United Kingdom and Europe have lagged behind the United States in the number of oocyte donation cycles performed over the past two decades. He believes that this disparity has been largely attributed to governmental restraints that severely limit donor compensation and require donors to be identified eighteen years or more after their participation. Increased compensation, he notes, is unlikely to fix the shortage of donors in the United Kingdom and Europe, and may promote reproductive tourism.

Shenfield[42] echoes this concern by noting that "it is argued that the dangers of inordinate compensation may only increase this possible dearth (of donors) by deterring altruistic donors, and that large payments may be especially prejudicial to the interest and welfare of children born as a result of gamete donation."

Donor Anonymity Issues

In a 1991 report[43] surveying sperm donors themselves, 60% of donors stated that they would agree to some type of personal contact when the offspring reached the age of eighteen. They were also found to be willing to provide in-depth personal, medical, and psychosocial information to recipient families. Recently, however, van den Akker[44] viewed the literature on gamete donors, recipients, and offspring with respect to donor anonymity and disclosure. The author indicates that the importance attached to genetics has led some countries to review the ethics of anonymous gamete donation (e.g., New Zealand) and has led a number of countries (Sweden, Austria, Victoria, Australia, The Netherlands, Canada, and the United Kingdom) to change their laws allowing donor gamete offspring the right to obtain identifying information about their genetic parent. The review points to inconsistencies between and within members of the three groups, regardless of the legislation, and also addresses the importance of testing theoretical models within future research. It argues that there is a need for a better understanding of the underlying problems encountered at a psychosocial level, such as continued preference for anonymity in donors, and the denial in large numbers of recipients of the involvement of a donor in conception. van den Akker[44] adds that the lack of disclosure effectively prevents implementation of legislation because nondisclosure to the offspring means that the child cannot take up the legally available option of finding out identifiable information about the donor.

The use of *known* versus *anonymous* oocyte donors is therefore worthy of discussion. Brill and Levin[45] posited that known oocyte donors often wish to donate their ova because of the close relationship that they share with a sister or good friend. The mental health professional's role is to evaluate and counsel the donor so as to rule out recipient or family coercion, guilt, or the need to 'undo' past reproductive losses. Research[46,47] that has considered donors with past reproductive losses, however, suggests that carefully selected oocyte donors who are counseled about such losses may actually feel at follow-up that donating did console them. In essence, there is very little research addressing the particular psychosocial or emotional needs of the known oocyte donor or the special concerns of the identified oocyte donor. Unlike the known oocyte donor, the identified donor has no familial or social relationship with the recipient couple. Instead, she has been recruited as a donor either by the couple themselves, by a broker or intermediary organization, or by the medical facility. The identified donor then meets with the recipient cou-

ple before the donation occurs and a mutual arrangement is made with respect to the donation. Again, there are no known data regarding this particular population other than anecdotal information with respect to outcomes or satisfaction following the donation. As with other types of oocyte donors, a thorough psychosocial evaluation, including psychological testing, would appear imperative.

Daniels and coworkers[48] extensively studied semen donors in Europe and found that there is a need to take into account the views of donors in forming policies concerning assisted reproduction, as well as a need for the interests of the child to be paramount. In another study, Daniels and colleagues[49] also considered who sperm donors had told about their donation, who they thought should be told, and whether they thought recipient couples should tell the offspring about their conception. These authors thus challenged the dominant view that donor insemination is a practice of medical or legal importance by looking at the attitudes of donors toward both their own family and the family to which they have contributed their genetic material. Swedish donors who were investigated were found to be less likely than donors in other countries to have told people about their involvement in donor insemination, including their partners and their children. Daniels and colleagues[50] also stressed the need for greater social acceptance and endorsement of donor insemination and of the man who would provide his sperm. They suggested that an appropriate goal would be to acknowledge semen donors as men who donate rather than sell their sperm, with the basic motivation of wanting to assist infertile couples. They added that the policies and methods used by clinics and staff play a critical role in the way in which sperm donors are thought of and recruited. In assessing the views and feelings of sperm donors, it was reported that donors perceive DI families as being normal and are very supportive of the autonomy and privacy of these families, but they also have concerns about the needs of the offspring.[48]

Counseling the Gamete Donor

According to Kalfoglou and Geller,[51] there are often ethical challenges created when working with gamete donors. The authors describe an inherent conflict of interest for mental health professionals who may feel pressured by their associated fertility groups to encourage potential donors to proceed. In this case, the authors conclude that this conflict of interest may result in donors not getting sufficient information for consent. However, it may also be the case that a form of checks and balances is present in the case of a psychological screening because mental health professionals often reject potential donors who demonstrate psychosocial instability. Not only is the donor primarily protected, but also the recipients and the fertility program that would be dealing with such a donor are shielded from potential harm. Ultimately, all parties involved can be protected.

Brill and Levin[45] stressed the importance of careful screening and counseling of donors. In addition to a clinical interview, donors should be given the Minnesota Multiphasic Personality Inventory-2 (MMPI-2). They pointed out that although this standardized measure was originally designed to determine psychopathology in a psychiatric population, there is now growing consensus among mental health professionals that the MMPI-2 or similar well-researched measures provide a degree of standardization regarding psychopathology in potential donors. Schover[46] also indicated that the MMPI-2 was useful in identifying oocyte donors with significant psychopathology and noted that profiles suggesting anger and rebelliousness may indicate risk for noncompliance during the medical procedure.

Informed consent on the part of donors also includes an understanding of the potential risks of the procedure. In a study by Gurmankin[52], of the nineteen programs advertising in college newspapers for oocyte donors, Gurmankin found that in an initial telephone call, only 58% of programs volunteered some type of information to donors about the potential risks involved in ooctye donation such as the possibility of infection, PMS-like symptoms, and ovarian hyperstimulation syndrome. There are two major limitations of this study. First, only nineteen programs are represented, and second, it is unclear how many of these programs did eventually provide prospective donors with accurate risk information beyond the first telephone contact. Dear[53], however, suggested that physicians may not be aware of this conflict because they do not necessarily view oocyte donors as patients, but as an instrument to the physician's 'therapeutic capabilities.' The author states that the absence of a medical benefit to oocyte donation would "confound the disclosure process" by not allowing donors to weigh the risks and benefits. That is, from Dear's perspective there is no benefit to oocyte donation, only risk.[53] Of course, an alternate perspective is that gamete donors may experience some benefit particularly if the concept of benefit encompassed financial and psychological benefit and not just medical benefit. However, this study also highlights the importance of the mental health professional's role in assuring informed consent. The evaluation process must include a review of the standard procedures and their potential physical and psychological risks and benefits.

Postdonation Information

With regards to oocyte donors' opinions of their medical treatment, Kalfoglou and Gittelsohn[36] found that the majority of their respondents ($n = 33$) were satisfied with their medical care and believed that the staff at the clinics they used was flexible, supportive, and willing to answer all of their questions. However, not all of those surveyed shared the same opinion of the donation process, including one participant who likened the oocyte donor process to prostitution in that she had no say in what was happening.[36] Some donors indicated that they believed that their health was not the primary concern of the medical staff. Other concerns included donors reporting that the risks of the procedure and the side effects of the fertility drugs were not outlined to them despite repeated requests for this information, that drugs were missing the package insert, that the information was in another language, or that the drugs were from Mexico and illegal to use in the United States. Kalfoglou and Geller[51] also note that several of the donors they surveyed, although generally satisfied with the experience of oocyte donation, believed that it was not the physician's "job to be nice" to them or to act as their advocate, as would be expected from their private physician.[51]

Another study by Kalfoglou and Geller[54] indicated that oocyte donors have a personal interest in receiving information related to the outcome of the IVF procedure that they were involved in. Of twenty-five anonymous donors surveyed, twenty either had received information regarding the outcome of their donation or desired that information. Similarly, Jensen et al.[55] found that a majority of the oocyte donors surveyed indicated that they had a desire to know whether their recipient had become pregnant. The Kalfoglou and Geller[54] study also addressed issues surrounding the consent process to ask donors if they would be willing to have their cryopreserved embryos used for research or shared with another recipient. The authors state that in a review of consent forms used in New York State, there was a lack of information related to what would happen to excess embryos, and that donated embryos would be frozen, used in research, and potentially shared with other women was not made explicit in consent forms.

Klock and colleagues[56] considered factors related to willingness to donate again, and reported that 40% of donors would definitely not donate if there were no compensation. Patrick and associates[57] also followed up with fifty oocyte donors in the United States, and again found that financial remuneration was their primary motivation; however, donors who had children were more likely to indicate a willingness to donate regardless of the compensation being offered. It is evident, based on previous research, that gamete donors have a wide variety of thoughts, feelings, and attitudes about having donated their genetic material to others.

THEORETICAL FRAMEWORK

There are several theoretical frameworks that might be considered regarding gamete donor assessment and support, although, to date, there is no specific theory applicable to gamete donation. Nonetheless, it is important to consider some underlying concepts that may assist mental health professionals in their work with donors.

Exchange Reinforcement Theory and Altruism

Social exchange and reinforcement theory is based on the premise that individuals give to others to obtain certain rewards for themselves. By contrast, *altruism* is defined as "behavior carried out to benefit another without anticipation of external reward."[58] Altruism and exchange and reinforcement theories address the question of what motivates individuals to make major sacrifices to help others: (1) to be helpful; (2 to remove distress for someone else; and/or (3) to gain personal reward or payment.[59] According to psychological egoism, while people may exhibit altruistic *behavior*, purely altruistic *motivations* are impossible. Individuals may very well spend their lives benefiting others without personal material gain. Their most basic motive for doing so, however, is to further their own best interests. The motivation for this form of altruism is that the individual acts to advance his or her own psychological well-being, even when to do so may also benefit others.

In contrast to psychological egoism, the *empathy–altruism hypothesis* contends that individuals experience empathy toward someone in need and are altruistically motivated to help that person. According to this approach to altruism, the individual is primarily concerned about the welfare of another person, not his or her own personal well-being. Within this context, altruism means helping another person without expecting material reward from others. Although the altruistic individual may well experience 'internal' benefit, including good feelings, sense of satisfaction, improved self-esteem, fulfillment of duty, and so on, that benefit is secondary. Some individuals gain substantial emotional satisfaction from acts that they perceive as improving the quality-of-life of others or making the world a better place. In short, the altruistic motivation may be strictly internal given certain circumstances and/or individual personality differences. For others,

what appears to be internally motivated altruism may be a means to an end – the intrinsic internal reward is not improved self-esteem but external rewards (adulation or payment from others) that are more valuable for individuals with this type of personality structure. It should be noted that humans are not exclusively altruistic toward family members, previous co-operators or potential future allies, but, rather, can be altruistic toward people they do not know and/or will never meet.[60,61]

Historically, altruism was the theoretical basis for organ donation (specifically, kidney donation), and the research investigated how the donors experienced organ donations. Simmons and colleagues[59] noted many organ donors found the act of donation a meaningful, altruistic act that was deeply and intrinsically rewarding, primarily from the pleasure of viewing the benefit to the recipient and from the happiness of realizing one's capacity of making a sacrifice to assist another person. However, this research on donors found that donors experienced less positive psychological effects if they were less able to perceive the consequences of the gift or less invested in (attached to) the recipient. Donor decision making was found to be based on moral decision making (with an emphasis on the right thing to do), instantaneous choice (vs. deliberation of alternatives), and postponement (or decision avoidance).[59] Although organ donation was viewed as a positive act that emphasized the resilience of individuals and families, it was also determined that some donors were vulnerable to postdonation distress and there was also potential for family conflict. Research indicated that family donors who reacted more negatively postdonation were more likely to (1) be emotionally less tied to the recipient; (2) experience direct or indirect family pressure to donate; (3) not experience gratitude from the recipient or other family members; (4) feel less obligated to donate (or be helpful); (5) experience high levels of ambivalence about the donation; or (6) have lower self-esteem and overall happiness.

In sum, the theories underlying the notion of organ donation may also be applicable to the gamete donor. Most certainly, many gamete donors have voiced their personal satisfaction gained through helping an infertile couple have a child. Understanding the basis of the individual donor's gratification from the donation can be a useful part of the evaluation and counseling process. In those countries that offer financial compensation to gamete donors, however, acquiring an understanding of the meaning behind the donation can become much more difficult for the mental health clinician.

CLINICAL ISSUES

Several distinct clinical issues are relevant to gamete donation. These include gender differences and attitudes toward donation, the rationale for psychological assessment, and the multiple roles of the mental health professional providing donor counseling and assessment.

Gender Differences and Assessment

Although psychological screening is a necessary component to all forms of gamete donation, there are clear gender differences inherent in the donation process. In contrast to the rigorous medical screening of potential sperm donors, men are rarely evaluated regarding their psychological status, nor are they screened regarding their motivation to donate or their feelings about donation. It is unusual for sperm donor partners to be interviewed or required for informed consent, unless it is a known donor situation. Most oocyte donation programs use a mental health professional for screening purposes and are likely to assess psychological problems, substance abuse, and motivations for donation along with considering psychosocial risks of donation. In addition, some oocyte donation programs require an interview with spouses of donors, who must also provide informed consent. The ASRM guidelines are consistent with this gender difference with their recommendation that psychological counseling be offered to all parties involved in oocyte donation, but not sperm donation. Some explain this gender difference as reflecting the greater medical risk for oocyte donors and the greater likelihood of coercion (in the case of a known donor), given the limited supply of willing oocyte donors.

Psychosocial Assessment: Rationale

Schover[62] pointed out that in the ASRM's 1993 guidelines for gamete donation,[13] there is a suggestion that "psychological counseling be offered to all parties involved in oocyte donation," but no specific recommendation that semen donors undergo psychological screening other than to consider sexual history factors that might increase a man's risk for sexually transmitted diseases.

Regardless of the outcome of an assessment as to the suitability of a potential gamete donor, the mental health professional must also determine that the candidate is able to provide informed consent. Issues of informed consent for gamete donors have been the subject of recent research. A more complicated question in the consent process is whether or not to include a pro-tocol that involves telling donors if there are successful pregnancies and births from their donation as well as other possible dispositions for their donated gametes.

In sum, it is stressed that part of the role of the mental health professional is to assess the overall psychosocial appropriateness of the individual as a gamete donor. The assessment must therefore include an appraisal of the donor's ability to provide informed consent, as well as an evaluation of the mental health and stability of the potential donor.

The Multiple Roles of the Mental Health Professional

In the context of this chapter, the primary roles of the infertility counselor are (1) evaluator/gatekeeper and (2) counselor. The work of the mental health professional is also to ensure true informed consent with regard to the psychological, social, and ethical issues and implications inherent in donation. Both of these responsibilities must be accomplished in a limited period of time, often within a single interview. Following or concurrent with the assessment, the mental health professional may also ultimately engage in psychotherapy either with donors they have evaluated; or, donors referred for therapy from other professionals who conducted the assessment.

The theoretical and clinical bases underlying the need for psychological consultation and evaluation of gamete donors are essentially fivefold. First, as Schover[62] pointed out, psychological screening provides some *protection for the recipient couple*. The clinical interview and standardized psychological testing help rule out major psychiatric disorders believed to have a genetic component such as schizophrenia or bipolar disorder. The evaluation by the mental health professional may reveal significant mental illness in the donor's own history or that of a first-degree relative. The social history and evaluation of the donor's lifestyle can also assist the medical team in determining whether or not a donor may be at risk for HIV infection, other sexually transmitted diseases, or other risk-related behavior.

Second, it is important, particularly in the case of oocyte donors, that they *understand and comply with the medical procedures* required during the donation. Psychological testing and the clinical interview enable the infertility counselor to ascertain more fully the chances that the donor may not follow through with the donation. An unstable family history, sociopathy, and or legal difficulties, an erratic school or work history, or ambivalence about the donation may lead to noncompliance. This situation leads to frustration (and expense) for medical personnel and, more importantly, to great disappointment and upset on the part of the recipient couple.

A third, and very important, rationale behind thorough assessment and counseling of the gamete donor is the *protection of the donor*. As Schover noted, "Donors who are motivated to participate in order to gain restitution for a perceived loss or mistake in the past may be at risk for emotional disappointment or regrets about giving away a potential child."[62] Women and men who donate gametes, fantasizing that the donation gives them a sense of biological immortality or provides them the narcissistic pleasure of having provided the world with an offspring, may have problematic or inappropriate motivations to donate. There is no way that one can predict accurately how a donor will feel about the donation in the months or years to come.

Fourth, there are often questions on the part of recipients about the *matching of donors on the basis of intelligence and/or personality characteristics*. Although the extent to which these traits can be inherited is unclear,[63] it is apparent that some heritability does exist. This is a complex issue and may ultimately put the infertility counselor in a difficult, if not impossible, position with respect to matching gamete donors and recipients. Often, recipients state a preference for donors to be matched to them on intelligence and personality traits rather than on physical characteristics.

Fifth, for recipients using anonymous gamete donors, there is often a desire to have as much *nonidentifying information* as possible about the donor. The infertility counselor can provide recipients additional information regarding a donor's family, education, employment and social history, so as to make the donor more 'real' to them. Having this personal data may also be especially helpful in their efforts to disclose information to their offspring about the donor conception.

An additional role, and responsibility, of the mental health professional when working with gamete donors is that of counselor or psychotherapist. This may occur concurrently with the assessment process or be subsequent to the assessment. Within this context, therapy is conducted in the same manner that the mental health professional would work with other clients. However, there are some particular clinical goals that are often key in this treatment.

First, the potential donor may need to process the impact of donation on his or her current life and in the future. Although the literature review indicates that most donors are satisfied and experience few negative psychological consequences, counseling is essential for the rare situations when a donor experiences psychological distress. There is no research to suggest which particular therapeutic modality (e.g., psychodynamic,

cognitive behavioral, systems, and so forth) is most appropriate to meet the needs of these donors, but the relevant factors to consider are the experience of loss or regret, fantasies regarding the outcome, and/or the impact on current and future relationships with others (partner, offspring, and recipient, particularly if known donation).

Second, another significant need for counseling and support may result when the gamete donor is excluded from a program. If exclusion is for psychological reasons, it may be necessary for the mental health professional to conduct a follow-up interview. The mental health professional will need to explain the reason for exclusion in a way that is protective of the donor's self-esteem. In the role of counselor, therapeutic intervention would further explore the donor's experience of rejection as well as address the issues that led to rejection (e.g., testing that is suggestive of psychopathology, emotional or interpersonal distress, and/or significant unresolved conflict or difficult life circumstances.) It is useful to frame the decision to exclude the prospective donor as "protection rather than rejection" as the first responsibility of all healthcare providers is to "do no harm."

THERAPEUTIC INTERVENTIONS

The clinical interview of the gamete donor is the focus of therapeutic intervention. This interview may involve psychological screening and testing, exploring issues with known gamete donors, assessing donor motivations, psychological implications of medical and genetic screening, and counseling.

Psychological Interview and Screening

Although most programs acknowledge the need for psychological screening of all gamete donors, there is difficulty in determining the factors to be assessed, inclusion and exclusion criteria (see Table 19.1), and variability in the use of standardized psychological testing tools. For example, it has been reported that only 60% of oocyte donor programs have stated psychological criteria for donor rejection and only 59% interview the donor's partner.[64]

The psychological interview is a crucial component in the evaluation of gamete donors. First, it helps screen out individuals with major psychopathology. Second, it permits infertility counselors to address motivation and informed consent issues for the protection of the potential donor; that is, the infertility counselor must assess whether the donor's motivations and expectations are realistic and psychologically healthy.

TABLE 19.1. Psychological indications for acceptance or rejection of a gamete donor	
Positive indicators	**Negative indicators**
Absence of significant psychopathology	Significant DSM-IV axis I or II disorder, including standardized psychological testing score that is two standard deviations above mean
Absence of unusual life stressors	Significant current stress
Use of adaptive coping skills	Chaotic lifestyle, impulsiveness, poor coping skills and judgment
Ability to provide informed consent and understand medical protocols when necessary	Inability to provide informed consent and understand medical protocols when necessary
Supportive and stable interpersonal and/or marital relationships	Marital instability, lack of social support system
Economic stability	Significant economic instability or financial need
Standardized psychological testing within normal limits	Positive history or family history of heritable psychiatric disorders or substance abuse/dependence
Educational/employment stability	Significant history of erratic educational background or employment
	Current use of psychotropic medications
	History of sexual or physical abuse with no professional treatment for donor
	History of legal difficulties/sociopathy
Objection to gamete donation on the part of the donor's partner should be grounds for at least deferment, and probably cancellation, of the donation. The donation should never interfere with or create problems in the relationship between partners or significant relationships.	

Other than altruism as a stated motivation to donate, it is difficult to establish a consensus on psychologically healthy motives. Therefore, it may be easier to rule out unhealthy or unrealistic motivations than to look for the 'correct' list of motivations. Potential gender differences should be considered when motivations to donate are addressed. Men appear to be motivated more by financial compensation, whereas for women the primary reason to donate appears to be altruism.[19] The interviewer must also address any sources of coercion, financial or emotional, and evaluate a potential donor's ability to give informed consent regarding realistic expectations about the medical procedures and to cope with the stress of donation, and the emotional consequences in the near and distant future. Partners of potential donors should also be interviewed and provided with education and information to assist them in giving informed consent to gamete donation. The mental health professional may have only one or two sessions with potential donors; in a limited time, there is need to cover a number of significant issues. The mental health professional should structure the interview and inform the donor of what issues will be addressed at the outset of an interview. The evaluation should include a complete family, psychiatric and reproductive history, and review of psychological testing, discussion of his or her motivations, and psychosocial issues of being a gamete donor. The psychosocial issues will differ depending on whether the donation is sperm, oocytes, or embryos. A more detailed list of content to be covered is listed in Table 19.2.

Sperm Donors: The vast majority of sperm donors are anonymous and present to commercial sperm banks that have their own specific informed consent and screening guidelines and criteria that are often governmentally regulated. In addition, the donation is not medically invasive and of no medical risk to donors. However, anyone conducting a psychological interview with sperm donors must include a discussion of potential future implications of donation. Historically, not only was screening often omitted, but so too was any discussion of what impact donation might have on these typically very young men. It is therefore extremely important for the mental health professional to address this particular issue with men who may not have considered this on their own, prior to their interview. The mental health professional should elicit the donor's perception of the impact of having a genetic child (or several

TABLE 19.2. Issues to include in a thorough, structured clinical interview of oocyte donors [46]

Discussion of donor's motivation

Unrealistic expectations of the psychological benefits of donation

Financial pressures leading to donation out of desperation for money

Past history of reproductive loss and related expectations about donation

Risk for obsessing about unknown outcome for recipients

Risk for grieving the loss of perceived potential offspring

Guilt for past elective abortion or adoption

General coping with emotional losses

Realistic expectations about physical discomfort of shots and side effects, time requirements, discomfort/risk of oocyte retrieval, and hyperstimulation should it occur

History of somatization that might put donor at risk for developing physical symptoms during donation cycle

History of involvement in a lawsuit related to donor's medical care

Significant pressure from family, spouse, partner, or friends regarding donation

Comfort with donation, evidenced by discussion of it with someone close to donor

Assessment of sources of happiness and satisfaction

Assessment of stresses that could impact compliance

Demonstration of stability and goal-directedness

Past history of physical, sexual, or emotional abuse that may make donor vulnerable to feeling victimized

Evidence of stable and happy relationships

Ability to comply with abstinence from sex during ovarian hyperstimulation and oocyte harvesting

Past history or current evidence of major psychopathology or chemical dependency, or first-degree relative with major psychopathology or chemical dependency

children and perhaps from up to ten families) in the present and in the future (particularly for men who do not have children now but plan to parent in the future). Another essential issue for discussion is the limits of anonymity. In the United States, most commercial sperm banks still allow donors to remain 'closed,' that is, offspring will not have access to donors' identities. However, many banks now offer donors the option of being 'open,' that is, offspring will have access to their donors' identities or the donor has the option of choosing to be open if contacted in the future by the sperm bank. In contrast, in the United Kingdom, donors no longer have the right to remain anonymous. According to the Human Fertilization Act, the rights of the offspring outweigh the rights of donors, and offspring have the right to their genetic identities (i.e., the identity of their sperm donors). The impact of this new law on the

number of anonymous donors is yet to be seen. Nevertheless, the implication of this law on the mental health professional's clinical interview is clear: Informed consent must include a discussion of the presumption that anonymity cannot be guaranteed.

Oocyte Donors: Similar to sperm donors, the majority of oocyte donors are anonymous. However, the current necessity to use fresh oocytes increases the likelihood that anonymous donors and recipients may meet, by chance or by design. The clinical interview should include a discussion of this possibility in addition to the informed consent issue that anonymity cannot be guaranteed in the future. Because oocyte retrieval is medically invasive, the interview should ensure that the donor understands the procedures and associated medical and psychological risks. In some fertility clinics, oocyte donors may also be undergoing IVF themselves and donate half their oocytes in a cycle to reduce the cost of the procedure (egg sharing). Additional issues must be addressed with these donors. Obviously, the clinical interview for these donors must include a careful discussion of the emotional ties these women feel to their oocytes and an assessment of motivation versus feeling coerced to donate to reduce the costs of the ART treatment. In some cases, the ability to afford IVF may be tied to their ability to share oocytes. Therefore, the interview must include a discussion of how the donor might feel and what alternate plans she is considering if she is not accepted as a donor. It is important to help these donors identify the factors driving their motivation to donate including financial assistance with IVF, altruism, and empowerment derived from helping other infertile women and couples who are less well-off than them. Finally, the interview must include a discussion of expectations of information regarding outcome. Some IVF programs vary regarding the policy of whether to inform shared donors of the success or not of the recipient's IVF. There must be a discussion of how the donor will cope with the information (both of success and of 'failure') or the lack of any information.

Partners of Gamete Donors: Ideally, the mental health professional's clinical interview should include the partner of the donor if there is one. The partner must also provide informed consent and the interview should include an assessment of the partner's feelings about gamete donation and the potential impact of donation (including future offspring) on the couple.

Embryo Donors: Embryo donors are by definition a couple and should be interviewed as a couple. Unlike sperm and oocyte donors, embryo donors usually come to donate as a result of having excess embryos following their own family building with IVF. Therefore, the psychological interview must include a discussion of all options for embryo disposition including thaw and not use, donation to scientific research, and donation to another infertile couple. The donor couple's feelings regarding their emotional attachment to the embryos should be carefully explored.

Donor couples may feel differently about donating surplus embryos to more than one couple. Although this type of donation is rare, such a donation would require that the donors consider the implications of full genetic siblings being raised in several households.

There are unique considerations for embryo donors who used donated gametes to create the embryo they are considering donating. This situation may trigger a variety of different feelings. Within a couple, differences in desire or motivation to donate embryos may be based on which partner's gametes are being used. Conflict may arise if the partner using his or her gametes feels more entitled to make the decision to donate or not. Resolve, the National Infertility Association in the United States, has published extensive literature that can be helpful to both professionals and patients.[65]

Known Gamete Donor Interview

When known donors are evaluated, the interview must include an additional discussion of this relationship. The use of anonymous versus known donors remains controversial and historically reflects on the significant gender differences in treatment approaches such that sperm donation programs historically used predominantly anonymous donors while oocyte donation began with mostly known donors.[27] Reasons given to justify anonymous sperm donation as preferable to known donation have historically focused on protection of the recipient male; that is, protection of the self-esteem of the recipient and the relationship of the recipient father to the child.[31,66] Little attention was paid to the impact on donors. When the protection of donors was considered, the main concerns were fear of legal liability for resulting offspring, offspring claiming inheritance rights, or donor liability if medical problems developed with offspring. Other concerns included

fear of invasion of future family life by offspring.[67] Although some countries recommend the use of anonymous gametes, ESHRE has proposed a 'double track' system that attempts to address the rights of privacy to the donor (and recipient parents) as well as the right of the offspring to know his or her origins.[15] However, with oocyte donation, the limited number of potential donors initially made the use of known donors the only available option for many couples. Anonymous sperm donation remains the standard, and anonymous oocyte donation is rapidly increasing as more programs expand their attempts at recruiting potential donors. It is interesting to note that the majority of anonymous gamete donors report that if their identity could be revealed to offspring at the age of majority, they would still choose to donate.[24]

With the use of known oocyte donors, there has developed an interest in the impact of known donation on the donor, both male and female. It is extremely important to discuss and assess the following issues surrounding known donation in the counseling of potential donors:

■ How will they feel about any resulting children, since they will most likely have close contact (e.g., many will be donating to siblings)? Are they at risk of perceiving the offspring as their own?

■ How might this donation impact the relationship between donor and recipient? Will it improve the relationship, or is it likely to put a strain on it?

■ What is the plan for disclosure? If disclosure to family and friends is planned, how does the donor think people will react? If disclosure is not planned, can the donor live comfortably with this secret?

■ Does the donor feel coerced or pressured to donate because of the close relationship to the recipient?

Each of these issues should be thoroughly processed in the context of predonation counseling to ensure the donor's ability to give informed consent and to decrease the risk of later regret or relationship difficulties with recipients. Legal consultation should also be advised.

In the process of evaluating known donors, particularly siblings, mental health professionals may be faced with the dilemma of discovering that the donor does not want to donate but because of family pressure, a sense of family duty or loyalty, or a fear of serious family conflict, he or she has agreed to donate. In this case, the mental health professional must not only help the known donor come to his or her own conclusion that donation is not advisable, but also may have to assist the donor by providing a rationale for ceasing the process. This may come in the form of the donor 'failing' the psychosocial screen; or, perhaps preferably, the fertility program informs the recipients that the donor was unsuitable for a more ambiguous or vague 'medical' reason.

Assessing Motivations

The extent to which financial compensation is a motivating factor in providing gametes should be explored. The financial rewards that result from the donation may contribute to the donor's denial about the longer-term implications of the donation. Novaes[32] pointed out that if material reward was not available, the "donor may feel compelled to reflect on the meaning that he (or she) attributes to this altruistic action." She added therefore that financial remuneration could "in the long run be an unethical means of obtaining the donor's consent."

Because a number of studies report that financial compensation is, in fact, a prime motivator, a portion of the evaluation protocol should address this issue. For example, Kalfoglou and Gittelsohn[36] reported that half the donors they interviewed considered the financial compensation to be primary to their decision to donate. Donors who are relying on financial remuneration for survival, that is, to pay rent, buy food, and so on, should be excluded from donation. In such cases, donors are clearly unable to provide informed consent, and are likely to be experiencing difficult life circumstances.

It appears that, for the time being, the policy of financial compensation for gamete donation will be maintained in the United States and in several other countries. As a result, it would seem that it is the responsibility of infertility counselors to help donors understand the meanings and implications of the donation and to protect the donors, as well as recipients, from making inappropriate decisions about gamete donation.

On the other hand, there also appears to be a need for some oocyte donors who have unresolved feelings about past abortions or reproductive losses to compensate in some way for those past experiences by providing oocytes to others. Reproductive trauma should be explored and evaluated by the mental health professional. Assisting donors in working through these issues will enable them to make more informed decisions about their donation.

Medical and Genetic Screening

The medical selection and screening process for sperm and oocyte donors can be rigorous and detailed. Thus, an unanticipated consequence of this process for donors is the discovery of medical or genetic disorders that otherwise would not have been detected until some-

time in the future, if ever. For some, this may be beneficial and protective; for others, such a discovery may cause significant psychological distress. ASRM guidelines are very clear regarding required medical and genetic testing, and ESHRE guidelines allude to the issue of transmittal of genetic disorders. What is much less clear, however, are guidelines regarding genetic counseling for donors, including counseling prior to testing so as to ensure informed consent, counseling that may be necessary depending on the results of the testing, and counseling and requirements regarding future information should offspring have genetic information that would be relevant to donors and their offspring. Clearly, gamete donors' genetic concerns will impact the therapeutic work of the mental health professional.

Psychological Testing

An efficient and effective method of screening potential donors is to use standardized psychological testing and a structured interview by an experienced mental health professional who has extensive knowledge of reproductive issues. Schover[46] developed one of the most comprehensive and useful screening methods for oocyte donors and lists a number of issues that should be assessed by the mental health professional during the interview (see Table 19.2).

In addition, the Mental Health Professional Group of ASRM developed recommendations for screening potential oocyte donors and embryo donors (see Appendixes 5 and 6). There are no equivalent published screening recommendations for sperm donors, but these may be adapted for men. ESHRE guidelines are, at this point, vague with respect to the specific assessment protocol of gamete donors, including the use of standardized psychological testing.

Psychological testing using well-validated objective measures of psychopathology and psychological adjustment is strongly recommended for use in conjunction with the interview. Testing can help identify psychopathology that the interviewer was unable to ascertain, or can validate the results from the interview. It may also provide content areas for further discussion during the evaluation process (see Chapter 5).

Counseling

The mental health professional's counseling intervention is in keeping with the premise that the donor's psychological and medical needs remain paramount. Ultimately, the donor's welfare must be the highest priority during the clinical interview and assessment. With this in mind, the psychological considerations on which one views the gamete donor as patient are based in good part on sound clinical judgment, as well as on potential ethical and legal imperatives. Mental health professionals play an important role in creating an understanding of the nature and meaning of gamete donation for both donors and recipients. Carefully exploring and understanding a donor's motivations for providing gametes may be the single most crucial element in counseling donors with respect to their emotions about the decision to donate. In the case of oocyte donors, it must be stressed that maintaining this as the primary goal for the counselor may create conflict or dissonance with the fertility program that wants or needs more donors and the donor herself who may want to donate even if the counselor deems it not in her best interest. Finally, the structured clinical interview cannot only serve as a vehicle for encouraging donors to consider their feelings about any potential offspring that may be created, particularly when they are donating gametes to a close friend or relative. The interview (as well as psychological testing) also helps provide objective data to support a position that may be in conflict with the wishes of the program or the donor.

FUTURE IMPLICATIONS

As mental health professionals become increasingly involved in reproductive health, it is likely that they will be called upon to provide psychological screening and support to all gamete donors. The growth of third-party reproduction as a parenting alternative has led to the need for increased research into the motivations of donors, as well as an understanding of the short- and long-term implications of donating genetic material for the creation of new life.

The use of gamete donation in family-building also brings with it certain ethical issues that affect not only the decision to donate but also the work of mental health professionals in assessing and counseling gamete donors. Not surprisingly, the very essence of gamete donation begs the question of parenthood: Does parenthood come with the contribution of genetic material, with gestation, or with raising a child?

Similarly, in caring for the psychological well-being of the gamete donor, one must ask what the rights of the donor are. Should the donor be told the outcome of the donation? Is the medical risk taken by young women donors too great? Does a young donor truly comprehend the meaning of the donation if he or she has never had a child? Does the known donor have rights or privileges that are different from those of the anonymous donor? These and other compelling questions will continue to confront mental health professionals, as well as ethicists and healthcare professionals.

As the assessment and counseling of gamete donors becomes more well-defined, it is likely that recipient couples will increasingly request more information about anonymous and identified donors. This need may be based not only on the wish to provide offspring as much information as possible but also on a powerful desire to have the donor matched to the recipient on the basis of personality traits and intelligence, as well as on phenotype. As noted previously, these factors may enable the recipient to feel more emotionally tied to the donor. It may also be an attempt to mitigate the losses inherent in the need for the use of gamete or embryo donation.

Lastly, as the cryopreservation of ova becomes an increasingly successful and utilized technology, it is likely that oocyte donation will also be affected. Donor egg banks may be established similar to sperm banks, and recipients will have more immediate access to donor pools. In that respect, oocyte donors may feel more removed from the process, and less connected to the purpose of the donation. The shift in the technology will, as a result, require the mental health professional to be especially sensitive to the psychosocial needs of donors as well as to issues of informed consent. At the same time, young women who, for a variety of reasons, choose to cryopreserve their oocytes for future use, may therefore be able to use their own oocytes. These women would theoretically no longer require donated gametes to have a child. This concept may have ethical implications, but would also potentially have an impact on the need for donated oocytes.

SUMMARY

■ Historically, the use of gamete donation (sperm) dates back thousands of years.

■ Policies and practices of donation are quite varied across the globe and the number of reproductive tourists is likely to increase as recipients (and donors) travel to countries whose policies support third-party reproduction.

■ Embryo donation has also become a disposition alternative for couples who have excess cryopreserved embryos following IVF cycles.

■ Current research on gamete donors has focused on motivations, the impact of the use of known versus anonymous versus identified donors, and the effects of the donation on the donor's partner and family over the long term.

■ Although there is no specific theoretical framework underlying the need for psychological assessment and support of donors, some of the theory regarding organ donation may be useful in our understanding of gamete donors. The concepts of *altruism* and *exchange and reinforcement* are helpful, but do not fully take into account the donation of genetic material to create a child for another family.

■ The clinical issues of counseling gamete donors reflect the multiple roles of the mental health professional. These roles include gatekeeper, counselor/educator, and, at times, psychotherapist. Paramount in the mental health professional's work is the need to protect the donor.

■ In light of the ethical and psychosocial ramifications of these reproductive procedures, mental health professionals will continue to play a significant role in the area of third- and fourth-party reproduction.

REFERENCES

1. Cohen CB, ed. *New Ways of Making Babies: The Case of Egg Donation*. Commissioned by the National Advisory Board on Ethics in Reproduction (NABER). Indianapolis: Indiana University Press 1996; 94.
2. Donation of gametes. In: Jones HW Jr, J Cohen, eds. IFFS Surveillance '04 *Fertil Steril* 2004: 81:S27, Chapter 6.
3. Blyth E, Landau R. *Third-Party Assisted Conception across Cultures: Social, Legal and Ethical Perspectives*. New York: Jessica Kingsley Publishers, 2004.
4. Haase J, Takefman J. Global perspectives in infertility counseling. International Infertility Counseling Organization, Postgraduate Course. *18th World Congress, International Federation of Fertility Socieities*. Montreal, Canada, May, 2004.
5. Directive 2004/23 E. C. of the European Parliament and the Council (2004) O. J. L102/48 (March 31, 2004).
6. The regulation of Donor-Assisted Conception, *Human Fertilisation & Embryology Authority*, United Kingdom, September, 2004.
7. Cox LW. The Role of Accreditation Committees in Oocyte Donation. *Reprod Fertil Develop* 1992; 4:731–7.
8. Steinbock B. Sperm as property. In: J Harris, S Holm, eds. *The Future of Human Reproduction: Ethics, Choice, and Regulation*. Oxford, England: Clarendon Press, 1998; 160.
9. Letur-Konirsch H. Oocyte donation in France and national balance sheet (GEDO). Different European approaches. *Gynecol Obstet Fertil* 2004; 32:108–15.
10. Anderson N, Gianaroli L, Felbergaum, et al. Assisted reproductive technology in Europe, 2001. Results generated from European registers by ESHRE. *Hum Reprod* 2005; 20:1158–76.
11. Boggio A. Italy enacts new law on medically assisted reproduction. *Hum Reprod* 2005; 20:1153–7.
12. Soderstrom-Antilla V, Hovatta O. Oocyte donation to be legalized in Sweden. Excellent results reported from other countries. *Lakartidningen* 2002; 99:3118–21.
13. Practice Committee of the American Fertility Society. Guidelines for gamete donation: *Fertil Steril* 1993; 59:1S–9S.
14. Baetens P. Oocyte donation. In: J Boivin, H Kentenich, eds. *ESHRE Monographs: Guidelines on Infertility Counselling*. London: Oxford University Press, 2002; 33–4.
15. ESHRE: Task Force on Ethics and Law. Gamete and embryo donation. *Hum Reprod* 2002; 17:1407–8.
16. Pennings G. Reproductive tourism is on the increase in Europe. Presentation at the *21st Annual Conference of the European Society of Human Reproduction and Embryology*. News-Medical. Net, June 20, 2005.
17. Lee FR. Driven by costs, fertility clients head overseas. *New York Times*, January 25, 2005.
18. Shettles LB. The respiration of human spermatozoa and their response to various gases and low temperature. *Am J Physiology* 1940; 128:408–15.
19. Rubin B. Psychological aspects of human artificial insemination. *Arch Gen Psychiatry* 1965; 13:121–32.
20. Sherman JK, Bunge RG. Observations on preservation of human spermatozoa. *Proceedings of the Society of Experimental Biology and Medicine*. 1953; 686–8.
21. Sherman JK. Banks for frozen semen: Current status and prospects. In: E Graham, ed. *The Integrity of Frozen Sperm*. Washington, DC: 1978; 78–91.
22. Daniels KR, Ericsson HL, Burn IP. Families and donor insemination: The views of semen donors. *Scand J Soc Welfare* 1996; 5:229–37.
23. Miller D, Jeffries DJ, Green J, Harris JR, Pinching AJ. HTLV-III: Should testing ever be routine? *Br Med J (Clin Res Ed)* 1986; 292:941–3.
24. Schover LR, Rothmann SA, Collins RL. The personality and motivation of semen donors: A comparison with oocyte donors. *Hum Reprod* 1992; 7:575–9.
25. Lutjen P, Trouson A, Leeton J, Findlay J, Wood C, Renou P. The establishment and maintenance of pregnancy using in vitro fertilization and embryo donation in a patient with ovarian failure. *Nature* 1984; 207:174–6.
26. Sauer MV, Paulson RJ, Lobo RA. Reversing the natural decline in human fertility. *JAMA* 1992; 268:1275–9.
27. Sauer MV, Paulson RJ. Human oocyte and pre-embryo donation: An evolving method for the treatment of infertility. *Am J Obstet Gynecol* 1990; 163:1421–4.
28. Leeton J, Harman J. The donation of oocytes to known recipients. *Aust N Z J Obstet Gynaecol* 1987; 27:248–50.
29. Braverman AM. Oocyte donation: Psychological and counseling issues. *Clin Consult Obstet Gynecol* 1994; 6:143–9.
30. Raoul-Duval A, Letur-Konirsch H, Frydman R. Anonymous ooctye donation: A psychological study of recipients, donors, and children. *Hum Reprod* 1992; 7:51–4.
31. Klock SC, Maier D. Psychological factors related to donor insemination. *Fertil Steril* 1991; 56:489–95.
32. Novaes SB. Giving, receiving, repaying: Gamete donor and donor policies in reproductive medicine. *Int J Technol Assess Health Care* 1989; 5:639–57.
33. Schover LR, Reis J, Collins RL, Blankstein J, Kanoti G, Quigley MM. The psychological evaluation of ovum donors. *J Psychosom Obstet Gynaecol* 1990; 11:299–309.
34. Schover LR, Collins RL, Quigley MM, et al. Psychological follow-up of women evaluated as oocyte donors. *Hum Reprod* 1991; 6:1487–91.
35. Lessor R, Cervamtes M. P'Connor N, Balmaceda J, Asch RH. An analysis of social and psychological characteristics of women volunteering to become oocyte donors. *Fertil Steril* 1993; 59:65–71.

36. Kalfoglou AL, Gittelsohn J. A qualitative follow-up study of women's experiences with oocyte donation. *Human Reprod* 2000; 15:798–805.

37. Kingsberg SA, Applegarth LD, Janata JW. Embryo donation programs and policies in North America: Survey results and implications for health and mental health professionals. *Fertil Steril* 2000; 73:215–20.

38. Gurmankin AD. Extracting eggs: A study of recruitment in oocyte donation. *Am J Bioeth* 2001; Fall; 1:W21.

39. Lindheim SR, Chase J, Sauer MV. Assessing the influence of payment on motivations of women participating as oocyte donors. *Gynecol Obstet Invest* 2001; 52:89–92.

40. Klock SC, Braverman AM, Rausch DT. Predicting anonymous egg donor satisfaction: A preliminary study. *J Womens Health* 1998: 7:229–37.

41. Sauer M. Further HFEA restrictions on egg donation in the UK: Two strikes and you're out! *Reprod Biomed Online* 2005; 10:431–3.

42. Shenfield F. Too late for change, too early to judge, but an oxymoron will not solve the problem. *Reprod Biomed Online* 2005; 10:433–5.

43. Mahlstedt PP, Probasco KA. Sperm donors: Their attitudes toward providing medical and psychosocial information for recipient couples and donor offspring. *Fertil Steril* 1991; 56:747–53.

44. van den Akker OV. A review of family donor constructs: Current research and future directions. *Hum Reprod Update*, September, 2005.

45. Brill M, Levin S. Psychologic counseling and screening for egg donation. In: MM Seibel, SL Crockin, eds. *Family Building Through Egg and Sperm Donation: Medical, Legal, and Ethical Issues*. Sudbury, MA: Jones and Bartlett, 1996; 76–93.

46. Schover LR. Psychological aspects of oocyte donation. *Infertil Reprod Med Clin North Am* 1993; 4:483–502.

47. Bartlett JA. Psychiatric issues in nonanonymous oocyte donation. *Psychosomatics* 1991; 32:433–7.

48. Daniels KR, Curson R, Lewis GM. Families formed as a result of donor insemination: The views of semen donors. *Child Fam Soc Work* 1996; 1:97–106.

49. Daniels KR, Ericsson HL, Burn IP. Families and donor insemination: The views of semen donors. *Scand J Soc Welfare* 1996; 5:229–37.

50. Daniels KR, Curson R, Lewis GM. Semen donor recruitment: A study of donors in two clinics. *Hum Reprod* 1996; 11:746–51.

51. Kalfoglou A, Geller G. Navigating conflict of interest in oocyte donation: An analysis of donors' experiences. *Women's Health Issues* 2000; 10:226–39.

52. Gurmankin AD. Risk information provided to prospective oocyte donors in a preliminary phone call. *Am J Bioeth* 2001; Fall; 1:3–13.

53. Dear JF. Regulating the fiction of informed consent in ART medicine. *Am J Bioeth* 2001; 1:19–20.

54. Kalfogulou AL, Geller G. A follow-up study with oocyte donors exploring their experiences, knowledge, and attitudes about the use of their oocytes and the outcome of the donation. *Fertil Steril* 2000; 74:660–7.

55. Jensen C, Zweifel J, Davidson M, et al. Comparative assessment of pre and post-donation attitudes with respect to potential oocyte and embryo disposition among ovum donors in an egg program. *Fertil Steril* 2004; 82: S304.

56. Klock SC, Stout JE, Davidson M. Psychological characteristics and factors related to willingness to donate again among anonymous oocyte donors. *Fertil Steril* 2003; 79:1312–16.

57. Patrick M, Smith AL, Meyer WR, et al. Anonymous ooctye donation: A follow-up questionnaire. *Fertil Steril* 2001; 75:1034–5.

58. Macaulay J, Berkowitz L, eds. *Altruism and Helping Behavior: Social Psychological Studies of Some Antecedents and Consequences*. New York: Academic Press, 1970.

59. Simmons RG, Klein SD, Simmons RL. *Gift of Life: The Social and Psychological Impact of Organ Transplantation*. New York: Wiley, 1977.

60. Bateson CD. *The Altruism Question*. Hillsdale, NJ: Earlbaum, 1991.

61. Fehr E, Fischbacher U. The nature of human altruism. *Nature* 2003; 425:785–91.

62. Schover LR. Psychological evaluation and counseling of gamete donors. In: Clinical Assessment and Counseling in Third-party Reproduction (XIII). *Proceedings of Annual Postgraduate Course of the American Society for Reproductive Medicine*; Montreal, Quebec, Canada; October, 1993.

63. Plomin R. Environment and genes: Determinants of behavior. *Am Psychol* 1989; 44:105–11.

64. Braverman AM. Survey results on the current practice of ooctye donation. *Fertil Steril* 1993; 59:1216–20.

65. RESOLVE, the National Infertility Association: U.S. Department of Health & Human Services Grant: EAA OP002099, 2002.

66. David A, Avidan D. Artificial insemination by donor: Clinical and psychological aspects. *Fertil Steril* 1976; 27:528–32.

67. Schenker JG. Sperm, oocyte, and pre-embryo donation. *J Assist Reprod Genet* 1995; 12:499–508.

20 Embryo Donation: Counseling Donors and Recipients

LINDA D. APPLEGARTH

For families who benefit, each birth is an epoch event.
– John E. Buster[1]

The use of embryo donation to achieve pregnancy and parenthood is, in terms of human reproduction, a relatively new form of assisted reproduction made possible by in vitro fertilization (IVF). It is estimated that currently there are well over 500,000 cryopreserved embryos in storage around the world. Depending upon embryo stage of cryopreservation, whether or not intracytoplasmic sperm injection (ICSI) procedure was used, the type of thaw technique, and the number of embryos transferred, pregnancy rates from cryopreserved embryos can range as high as 50–70%.[2,3] However, there appears to be no universal standard or measurement to assess the quality of these embryos on a number of parameters including ability to survive thaw, genetic and chromosomal abnormalities, or implantation ability, so more often, pregnancy rates are in the vicinity of 20%. Embryo donation, therefore, may be a psychosocially appealing and medically feasible family-building alternative for both donors and recipients, but it can also be one in which both donors and recipients overestimate the odds of delivering a healthy baby.

The vast majority of embryos for donation are cryopreserved extra or unused embryos from infertility patients who have undergone IVF. Although IVF with fresh embryos is often most successful, there are a number of reasons to create more embryos than will be transferred in a single treatment cycle. Some reasons for creating extra embryos that are cryopreserved for later transfer include: (1) reduced number of ovulation induction cycles for either financial or health reasons; (2) the ability to assess and select the best-quality embryos for transfer; (3) delayed transfer for medical reasons (e.g., ovarian hyperstimulation or cancer treatment); (4) the desire to reduce the risk of multiple pregnancy; and/or (5) to provide another opportunity to achieve pregnancy or enlarge the family without ovulation induction and oocyte retrieval.

Around the world, the practice of cryopreservation and/or donation of embryos may be regulated or monitored by government agencies, legislation, or clinical practice guidelines. In some countries, only a limited number of embryos are allowed for transfer (e.g., United Kingdom). In Latin America, ART procedures are generally not well regulated. Embryo cryopreservation is allowed, but there is no provision for embryo donation. In Italy, the number of embryos transferred is limited and all extra embryos cannot be cryopreserved. As a result, any unused embryos must be donated to another couple and not used for research purposes. Within the applicable parameters, IVF couples with cryopreserved embryos have an array of disposition options: (1) use for one's own family-building; (2) destruction (thawing); (3) donation for research; or (4) donation to another couple for reproduction. Those who choose to donate their excess embryos to another couple may be morally opposed to destroying embryos or to donating them for research. Their sympathy and empathy for the emotional pain of infertility and involuntary childlessness may further contribute to their desire to facilitate parenthood for others who are unable to become parents through procreation or other forms of medical technology. Additionally, some embryo donors may have a sense of moral obligation to use their embryos in a way that is congruent with their personal values or religious beliefs.[4]

Very often embryo donors psychologically view their embryos as having the same potential-child status as their actual children who are alive today, as a result of an IVF procedure during which additionally created embryos were cryopreserved. After all, the embryos donated by post-IVF patients are the potential genetic siblings of the children they already have. Donating their embryos may help a couple feel morally and psychologically comfortable by using their embryos in what they view as a responsible and morally appropriate manner. As such, embryo donors and recipients understandably face a complex array of psychosocial issues involving their personal values, religious beliefs, infertility experiences, beliefs or assumptions about the donation process (including disclosure), and the meaning of parenthood. Additionally, as with other forms of third-party reproduction, counseling donors and recipients must address their motivations, couple consensus, the donation process (e.g., collaborative agreements, legal contracts, and protocols of the treatment facility), and factors influencing the current decision as well as the long-term adjustment of the donors, recipients, and offspring.

Embryo recipient couples often pursue parenthood using donated embryos for medical reasons including repeated treatment failures that result from: (1) idiopathic factors or severe male- and female-factor infertility; (2) multiple pregnancy losses based on issues other than implantation (uterine) factors; (3) transmissible genetic diseases; or (4) absence of or nonfunctional ovaries (with a functional uterus) as well as absent or nonfunctional testes.[5] Additionally, some recipient couples feel that the use of donated embryos is a more equitable reproductive choice when one partner is unable to reproduce, and the use of donated gametes (sperm or oocytes) would create psychological and medical unbalanced genetic ties to their offspring. Finally, some recipients pursue embryo donation for practical reasons because it is a less expensive family-building alternative than oocyte donation or traditional adoption. The process of obtaining donated embryos may also take less time than traditional adoption.

Embryo donation may also be a comfortable parenting alternative for single women or lesbian couples. However, this choice may not be available to these populations in all countries. Certainly, for those women who are suffering from premature ovarian failure (POF) or who are menopausal, the use of existing donated embryos may seem more appropriate than creating new embryos with donor sperm and donor oocytes, especially because gamete donation is not an option in a number of countries. The lack of available embryos or donor oocytes and sperm, however, may lead some individuals and couples to travel to other countries to receive treatments or gametes that may be prohibited in their home countries. This phenomenon, known as reproductive tourism, can impact the work of the mental health professional in that additional education, information, and discussion of the issues and implications may be necessary.

Current practices regarding oocyte donation may also be applicable to embryo donation. Thus, the practice of embryo donation as well as the laws and guidelines regulating it, vary widely across and within countries. These practices dramatically impact the counseling of donors and recipients, particularly regarding psychosocial consultation and evaluation, as well as anonymity and disclosure issues. Some professional societies such as the American Society for Reproductive Medicine (ASRM)[6] and the European Society for Human Reproduction and Embryology (ESHRE)[7] have established practice guidelines for embryo donation. In Latin America ART procedures are not well regulated. Embryo cryopreservation, when allowed, is done without practice guidelines or regulations. In addition, government regulatory agencies (i.e., Great Britain's HFEA, Canada's AHRA, Australia's RTAC) and legislation pertaining to gamete and embryo donation determine practice and policy.

In 1991, the United Kingdom established the Human Fertilisation and Embryology Authority (HFEA) in an effort to regulate assisted reproduction. The HFEA regulations also have an impact on gamete donation, donor anonymity, and counseling of donors and recipients. In April 2005, the HFEA eliminated all donor anonymity and compensation, and established a central donor registry so that all donor offspring can access information about their donor at age eighteen. The HFEA's position on the discontinuation of compensation of gamete donors is in compliance with the European Union Tissue and Cells Directive that promotes altruistic donation, that is, voluntary, unpaid donations although donors may be reimbursed for "expenses and inconveniences related to the donation."[8] Of interest, HFEA regulations require that counseling be offered to all potential donor gamete recipients. However, counseling is defined as information and advice giving but not screening that would prohibit or disallow patients from receiving gametes.[9] It appears that these regulations would also pertain to embryo donors and recipients[9] (see also www.hfea.gov.uk).

Canada and Australia have similar regulatory policies that govern assisted reproduction including embryo donation practices. The Infertility Treatment Act was enacted in 1984 in Australia's state of Victoria and was the first to mandate counseling for all individuals pursing IVF and/or third-party reproduction. In 1988, legislation in Victoria also established counseling criteria for donors, recipients, and offspring – referred to as 'donor-linking' counseling (see www.ita.org.au). Infertility counselors must be licensed and members of ANZICA (Australia/New Zealand Infertility Counseling Association).

Currently, three of the five Australian states have legislation regarding reproductive technology (including oocyte donation) with oversight from the RTAC. Australia's system is one of combined voluntary regulation and legislative regulation (nationally and across states in the country).[10] In contrast, Canada has the newest regulatory body, the Assisted Human Reproduction Agency, established in 2004. The Canadian legislation eliminated donor anonymity, established a central donor registry, prohibited any and all payment to gamete donors (sperm or oocytes), and mandated the provision of counseling services for individuals participating in assisted reproduction. While HFEA requires that counseling be *offered*, Canadian legislation mandates that all participants in assisted reproduction *participate* in pretreatment counseling. Again, it appears that these regulations also apply to embryo donors and recipients.

Many other countries have legislation specifically directed toward gamete donation although the provision of counseling is not addressed. Many allow for some type of known donation, however. More specifically, Plachot[11] reviewed the status of embryo donation in France, Europe, and the United States. The author noted that there is great variability in program procedures and policies in centers in the same country and between countries. Although proposed in a number of ART facilities in the world, embryo donation is more often contemplated than performed. Plachot suggests that this is due to both the absence of information on how to organize this family-building option at a medical clinic, and to legal constraints imposed by law.[11]

In 2005, however, the government of New Zealand published guidelines for embryo donation.[12] Because of psychosocial and ethical issues that embryo donation raises, these guidelines require all applications for embryo donation be submitted for approval. In addition to considering the future welfare of the offspring, the guidelines require donor couples and recipients to undergo counseling so that they are fully informed about psychological, social, and ethical aspects of the process. Both donors and recipients have access to counseling throughout the process, and a joint counseling session between all parties is required. These guidelines were approved by the Minister of Health, and appear to be groundbreaking with respect to the process and implications for embryo donation.

In the United States, Europe, and other countries, professional organizations have established patient care guidelines on psychosocial preparation for embryo donation. The Mental Health Professional Group (MHPG) of ASRM and the Psychology and Counselling Special Interest Group (PCSIG) of ESHRE have published practice guidelines on these issues[6,7] (see also www.asrm.org and www.eshre.com).

This chapter specifically discusses embryo donation as a family-building alternative as it pertains to the emotional and psychosocial preparation of embryo donors and recipients. The terminology used will be that of ASRM and ESHRE, specifically *embryo donation* as opposed to *embryo adoption*. Both terms have been used to refer to this form of assisted reproduction. However, although embryos are accorded more respect than other bodily tissues (e.g., sperm or oocytes), they are not given the rights of persons. Thus, the embryo is not considered a person and the process cannot therefore be viewed as traditional adoption. Nevertheless, there are some parallels between embryo donation and traditional adoption that are compared and contrasted.

This chapter also addresses some theoretical constructs that may underlie the decision to donate embryos or receive them. In addition, there is a discussion of the clinical issues and therapeutic interventions for donors that:

- provides psychosocial assessment and screening;
- assists them in decision making; and
- provides some understanding of the potential implications of these decisions.

Additional issues for recipients of embryo donation include:

- psychosocial preparation and support;
- understanding the implications of the loss of fertility and the loss of genetic connection to the child;
- considering anonymous versus known embryo donation, the nature of the relationship (if any) with the donor couple, as well as related disclosure issues.

HISTORICAL OVERVIEW

The first attempt at in vitro fertilization of mammalian eggs was made in 1878 in Vienna, Austria, although the first successful birth of a human infant conceived via in vitro fertilization did not occur until 1978 in the United Kingdom. In 1984, the first live birth following transfer of a cryopreserved embryo occurred in Australia.[13] Embryo donation, a unique family-building alternative, developed as a direct consequence of assisted reproductive technologies (ART), particularly IVF, emerging at the end of the twentieth century. As such, not much historical context or perspective exists except within the context of human adjustment to the use of reproductive medical technology. Embryo donation is complex, particularly within the context of cultures, religion, national laws, beliefs, and customs. Klock,[14] described embryo disposition studies in various countries and noted that there is wide variation in terms of legislation and/or guidelines that apply to embryo donation. She added that the least common choice of embryo disposition, that is, embryo donation to another couple, is the most complicated of the four options.

REVIEW OF LITERATURE

In general, embryo donation is still a relatively rare occurrence around the world. Hoffman et al.[15] surveyed clinics throughout the United States and found that very few (2%) of the approximate 400,000 cryopreserved embryos are actually designated for donation to other individuals or couples. In Australia, de Lacey[16] found that couples who initially indicated a desire to donate their extra embryos regarded the idea as an idealistic plan rather than a purposeful decision. Their change of mind was attributed to two factors: (1) a change in their standpoint from a childless couple to parents, and (2) a change in the symbolism of the embryo from representing a chance to become pregnant to representing a virtual child in cryostorage. Similarly, Nachtigall and colleagues[17] attempted to ascertain what couples think about their embryos and how they approach making a decision about disposition in light of the significant implications for medical research and embryo donation. The authors concluded that not only is the disposition decision significant and a frequently unresolved issue for couples, but also that couples' deeply personal conceptualizations of their embryos contribute to their ambivalence, uncertainty, and difficulty in reaching a decision.

Lee and Yap[18] also found that embryo donation is currently an uncommon procedure that is associated with many ethical, legal, and psychosocial implications. Their review of the literature, however, supported the notion that it can be a good parenting option for many infertile couples. In 1999, Van Voorhis and colleagues[19] delineated their experiences and provided recommendations for establishing an embryo donation program. They also found that only a small percentage of couples were willing to donate their embryos, even though embryo donation can be a cost-effective treatment of infertility. Nonetheless, Kingsberg and colleagues[20] found that a majority of IVF clinics in the United States indicated that they offer embryo donation to patients; however, as of early 2000, only 37% of programs had actually completed a donation.

Several authors have focused on clinical and administrative aspects of embryo donation including the decisions that couples may face in making disposition determinations.[21,22] Although embryo donation recipients are considered, the articles do not include any specific discussions of counseling. Van Voorhis and colleagues[19] noted that their program provided recipient couples with counseling regarding issues of disclosure to offspring about their embryo donation origin, and addressed the unknown long-term psychosocial consequences of the donation. Soderstrom-Anttila and colleagues[23] evaluated an embryo donation program in Finland, and studied attitudes among donors and recipients. Forty-six couples donated 209 excess frozen embryos, with a clinical pregnancy rate of 28%. These researchers found that significantly more recipients than donors thought the offspring should be informed about the circumstances of conception. However, a higher percentage of donors themselves thought that the child should receive identifying information concerning the donating couple. The researchers emphasized the interest of the offspring, not only regarding knowing his or her genetic origin but also knowing genetic siblings and genetic parents, thus suggesting that these issues should be addressed by embryo donation programs.

Newton and colleagues[24] assessed infertile couples' attitudes toward the procedures of embryo donation in Canada and attempted to identify factors predicting an interest in donation. The authors found that willingness to donate was associated with greater comfort about disclosing personal information, a desire to know the outcome of donation, and willingness to have future contact with a child, but not associated with current family size. They concluded that offering the option of conditional donation could increase the acceptability of embryo donation for some patients. Kovacs and colleagues[25] also considered embryo donation at a large clinic in Australia. They found that of 1,246 couples relinquishing frozen embryos, about 90% opted to discard rather than donate their embryos, with ninety-eight couples on a waiting list to receive donated embryos. The authors concluded that it is important to consider how couples can be encouraged to donate surplus cryopreserved embryos, and they suggested that an education program on relevant legal, social, and clinical issues might facilitate this.

The literature pertaining to counseling donors and recipients of embryo donation is sparse. Data tend to focus primarily on embryo donors and the criteria for donation. Information about how families created from embryo donation are faring is also anecdotal, at best, although it would potentially be helpful information for potential embryo donors and recipients. In the first study worldwide, MacCallum[26] compared families in the United Kingdom with children conceived by embryo donation to those who adopted infants, as well as to those parents who conceived through IVF using their own gametes. The study concluded that embryo donation parents' experience of pregnancy and birth did not seem to result in more positive parenting compared to adoptive parents. Neither did the lack of genetic links between parents and children lead to less positive parenting compared to IVF parents. Despite this limited, but promising data, Belluck[27] found that couples who actually wish to receive donated embryos might have a very difficult time doing so. She noted that many couples who initially said they would donate, later change their minds. Additionally, couples who are willing to donate their excess embryos find that other obstacles arise such as genetic and medical conditions, poor embryo viability, and limited pregnancy success rates.

In 2002 and 2004, Resolve, the National Infertility Association in the United States, received research grants to provide educational materials for infertility patients, professionals, and the general public about issues surrounding embryo donation as a family-building option.[5,28] Initial data gathered from the 2002 project found that 77% of the public believed that the use of cryopreserved embryos should be the personal decision of the couple who created them. Notably, the Resolve data found in a public survey that 75% of those with infertility or a partner with infertility who had considered treatment did not have enough information to make an informed decision about embryo donation. As a result, the organization subsequently published extensive materials related to embryo donation to better educate donating and recipient couples considering embryo donation as a family-building alternative[5,28] (see also www.resolve.org).

THEORETICAL FRAMEWORKS

The theory basis for donor and recipient counseling in embryo donation is generally based on theoretical frameworks that apply to donors and recipients of other forms of third-party reproduction. These include social-exchange theory as well as adoption theory.

Social-Exchange Theory

According to social-exchange theory, individuals seek to maximize rewards and minimize losses in relationship with others. Reciprocity, equity, emotions, motivations, and behaviors all play a part in maintaining a comfortable balance of rewards and losses in interpersonal relationships. Social-exchange theory has been applied to a variety of interpersonal relationships, such as elderly parents cared for by their adult children, and to equity balances in physician–patient satisfaction. Some factors influencing the balance of social-exchange in relationships include power, wealth, morals, justice, communication, and personal relationship, which are intrinsic rewards versus external rewards. This the-

ory suggests that emotions may negatively or positively influence interpersonal relationships, particularly when there is a shared task or goal. Collaboration is most successful when the individuals involved have: (1) the same perception regarding shared responsibility for the success or failure of a task, and (2) find it difficult to distinguish their individual influence or contribution to solving the task. Furthermore, there was greater satisfaction when there was equity in the balance of power within the interpersonal relationship.[29–32]

Social-exchange theory (also referred to as *reciprocal altruism*) has been applied to adoption and may also be a helpful theoretical perspective for considering motivations and decision making in embryo donation for both donors and recipients. There can be a social-exchange relationship, albeit often unconscious, between embryo donors and recipients who must strike an internal balance between rewards and losses. Both recipient couples and donors approach the shared project (embryo donation) motivated to maximize rewards and minimize losses. This appears to occur even if the donation is anonymous. Embryo donation recipient couples may be cognizant of their desire to maximize rewards and minimize losses, and they may also be aware at some level that the donor embryo couple will have similar motivations. The sense of reciprocal altruism seems especially likely because there is financial compensation associated with embryo donation. Most couples who choose to donate their unused frozen embryos do so from moral and religious beliefs as well as from the desire to help another infertile couple and rarely receive or desire financial payment. Viewing their shared task from this perspective can also help both donors and recipients address issues of communication, reciprocity, power, rewards, and losses, particularly when the embryo donation is open and/or the families expect to have some sort of ongoing relationship with one another. In the case of embryo donation, infertility counselors should address the notion of social exchange in these unique, shared goals of giving, receiving, and family-building.

Adoption Theory

Adoption theories can also be a useful theoretical approach for donors and recipients of embryo donation. As in adoption, this form of family-building also involves no genetic relationship between the child and the rearing parents, and the parents must address decisions regarding disclosure about how the child came into the family. Although embryo donation is not as public a form of family-building as traditional adoption, it does involve the possibility of future contact (or a relationship) with the genetic parents and/or genetic siblings.

Freeark and colleagues[33] note the discovery of infertility creates a crisis of normalcy, adequacy, shame, and marginalization, all of which may later impact the couple's experience of becoming adoptive parents. They also add that differences for men and women in emotional reactions have an impact on identity, stigma, coping styles, and opportunities to feel mastery which can set wives and husbands on a different psychological course affecting their efforts to respond as a partnership in adoptive parenthood. In a study in Eastern Europe, Bevc and colleagues[34] found that in dealing with child adoption, the process of coming to terms with infertility and its consequences is an important factor in establishing healthy family relationships and the child's identity within the adoptive family. The authors underscore the need for mental health workers to supply future adoptive parents with a parent preparation program that provides the requisite information and assistance to support the entire family, when the child becomes a member of the family. They report that a fundamental attribute of the program is to offer help to couples in overcoming the traumas resulting from their infertility.

On the other hand, van den Akker[35] found in a retrospective survey that the choice to adopt a child is based on a number of factors, not all associated with infertility resolution. However, the author adds that although it is unlikely that resolution of infertility can be achieved in any population attempting to overcome infertility, the cognitive dissonance identified in this population can, in all likelihood, be generalized to those choosing other options to overcome infertility. Van den Akker[35] states that, "cultural and counseling acknowledgement of postmodern family theory principles is likely to ease cognitive consistency regarding the status of adoptive family hood, and dispel the importance of reproductive options emphasizing a genetic link."

Freeark and colleagues[33] also point out that adoptive parents appear to share the parent–infant interaction more evenly than do biological parents. They concluded that adoptive mothers and fathers have the opportunity for equal participation in the acquisition of their child and more similar experiences (and perhaps more closeness), as they become parents together. This shared experience may increase the woman's satisfaction with the process as it enhances her traditionally prescribed gender role as mother and caretaker, while also stretching the man's prescribed gender role.

The applicability of adoption theory to embryo donation is generally unknown given the lack of research in this area. However, similarities between adoptive parents and embryo donation recipients are evident. Adoptive parents and ED recipients who usually have suffered from long years of infertility and loss, must become comfortable with the reality of rearing a child(ren) who bears no genetic tie to them and must develop positive feelings about their parental role obligations. Couples who choose to donate their embryos may also feel a kinship with birthparents who relinquish their offspring for adoption. In both cases, there are likely to be circumstances that make raising the child themselves very difficult. They are left with their own sense of sorrow or loss while also making the decision (for any number of reasons) to have other people raise and care for their genetic child. Glazer and Sterling thus refer to embryo donors as "high tech birthparents."[36, p. 90]

CLINICAL ISSUES

Because of the intricate and complicated psychological component of embryo donation, it has been recommended that both donor and recipient couples meet with a mental health professional.[6,7] The purpose of these meetings is multifold and generally intended to: (1) explore donors' and recipients' thoughts, feelings, and fantasies regarding undertaking this unique family-building alternative; (2) rule out psychiatric illness and/or psychopathology, substance abuse, marital instability, and other related problems; and (3) provide a forum for a discussion of disclosure issues and/or quality and extent of relationship between donors, recipients, and offspring when applicable. The comfort level of all involved parties must be carefully evaluated before moving forward with embryo donation.

Decision Making and Preparation

In many cases, embryo donors have made the decision regarding the disposition of their unused embryos before meeting with the mental health professional (MHP). Thus, the work of the MHP will be not only to evaluate the psychological status of the donor couple and the appropriateness of this decision, but also to prepare embryo donors for the potential psychosocial effects of the decision. Donating embryos can have an impact not only the donors themselves, but also their children. Exploration and discussion of the donor couple's thoughts and feelings about anonymity/nonanonymity and disclosure will be intrinsic to their sense of psychosocial preparedness and closure. In most countries, embryo donors are not compensated financially for their donation. As a result, motivations to donate for financial gain do not confound embryo donors' decisions.

In countries such as the United Kingdom, Austria, parts of Australia, Canada, Sweden, and Switzerland, ooctye donors are required to provide identifying information to the offspring when he or she reaches age eighteen. Presumably, the same is true for embryo donors. In New Zealand, embryo donor and recipient couples meet together prior to the donation. Although the regulations and guidelines in these countries and others respect the autonomy and privacy of the parties involved, it is likely that the requirement of non-anonymity will deter some embryo donors and/or recipients from following through with this family-building option. Donor anonymity continues to be upheld in France, Belgium, Bulgaria, Czech Republic, Greece, Hong Kong, Israel, Japan, Denmark, Norway, Portugal, South Africa, and Spain. Identifying information is provided, with donor consent, in Iceland, The Netherlands, and the United States.[37]

Recipient couples, as well as single women, considering embryo donation parenthood vary widely in their degree of psychological adaptation to their losses at the time they undertake this parenting option. Mahlstedt and Greenfeld[38] suggested that patient preparation and education are fundamental to all candidates considering assisted reproduction, which is particularly applicable to embryo donation recipients. Pretreatment preparation should emphasize the need for sufficient time to consider this alternative. In short, it should not be a hasty, desperation decision or one based on coercion. Decision making should focus on: (1) identifying and resolving the specific ways in which infertility and infertility treatment have affected individuals and couples; (2) discussing the specific concerns, fears, and fantasies involved in this family-building alternative and developing coping strategies; and (3) assessing and implementing the donation process.

Part of the process of receiving donated embryos will be exploring thoughts, feelings, and fears about parenting a child created by another couple, and who, by pure chance, was a cryopreserved embryo. In all likelihood, the child also will have genetic siblings who are being raised by the genetic parents. This rather surreal situation should be considered by embryo donation recipients as they consider this option, as well as making decisions about disclosure and eventually obtaining identifying donor information.

Grieving the Loss of a Genetic Tie to the Child

For embryo donation recipients, the decision to proceed with a parenting option that does not include having a child who is genetically linked to the parents, involves

loss. The lost dream of having a genetic child can be extremely painful and may be experienced differently by partners. The loss entails mourning each person's biological connection to the child as well as the couple's reproductive hopes and plans. For some couples, these types of losses will have a significant impact on their relationship that, in turn, may require a more ongoing therapeutic counseling intervention as opposed to a supportive one.

We know that men and women respond differently to the stresses and strains of infertility,[39] and it is not surprising that they may also have disparate views and feelings about embryo donation as a parenting possibility. One partner may deny their own fertility prognosis and press to continue treatment long after the other partner has come to terms with the realities presented to them. The anger, sorrow, helplessness, and emotional pain may be such that individual and/or couples therapy is a prerequisite to helping them contemplate and confront the possibility of becoming parents through embryo donation.

The decision to end treatment may come after long, protracted efforts to conceive a biological child who is genetically related to either or both partners. Their sadness may be profound, and for a time, somewhat paralyzing. For other couples, as well as single women, who attempt reproduction later in life, the medical diagnosis and recommendation for third-party assisted reproduction may come quickly, and perhaps compel patients to make decisions about other options earlier in the process. A third group of individuals may make the decision to end treatment based on financial constraints or other limited resources. In any of these cases, there are a multitude of feelings and concerns that warrant careful investigation, input, and support from the infertility counselor.

Grieving the loss of any genetic connection to the child must be given sufficient time to occur before clear decisions can be made about moving forward with embryo donation – or other options. As with the other forms of gamete donation, embryo donation is not a cure or medical treatment for male- or female-factor infertility. If pregnancy is achieved, the etiology and diagnosis of the infertility continues to exist. Ultimately, the therapeutic goal is to assist individuals and couples in integrating their losses into their experience of infertility and make decisions that reach beyond their emotional pain.

Psychosocial Evaluation and Consultation

In many countries, embryo donors and recipients will be referred by the medical practice to the infertility counselor to determine whether or not they are prepared to move forward with the donation. For example, in the United Kingdom, Canada, New Zealand, and Australia, this counseling is either mandatory or must be offered to patients as determined by their respective governments. In some cases, the healthcare staff expects the infertility counselor to evaluate the couple's emotional readiness, define any special circumstances that affect the donors and recipients proceeding with the donation, and thoroughly discuss the many potential psychosocial issues and implications that exist presently or in the future regarding the decision to donate or to parent through embryo donation. The World Health Organization also recommends that adequate counseling should be offered to all couples that undergo embryo donation.[40] It is stressed that, in the case of embryo donation recipients, adequate information should be provided on the limitations and possible outcome of treatment, the likelihood of pregnancy and live birth, the possible side effects of any medication and the risks of treatment (such as multiple birth), the extent to which genetics and infectious screening tests have been performed, and the cost of the treatment.

In some locations, the infertility counselor's evaluation of the recipient couple will determine when, or if, they can move forward with the donation. Additional counseling may also be deemed necessary to assist the recipients in working through their losses in order to deal more effectively with each other, family members, or friends around current or potentially sensitive issues. The extent and impact of the counselor's intervention and/or assessment will vary from country to country. Often, the infertility counselor's input will be one factor in determining whether or not the couple or single woman should move forward with the donation. Ultimately, the decision to proceed may be made by the medical team or by the treating physician.

Some individuals or couples may themselves choose to seek help with complex concerns about embryo donation, or whose relationships may be stressed by long years of infertility and/or differences of opinion about whether or not to donate embryo (donors) or about family-building alternatives (recipients). In such situations, the initial intent is to address and deal with these concerns and differences within a therapeutic context. This will be an opportunity for the infertility counselor to explore not only embryo donation, but also other disposition options (donors) or parenting alternatives (recipients) that may be appropriate to the couple's social and cultural milieu. The individual or couple's issues and concerns can also be addressed within an appropriate timeframe that allows for understanding, resolution, and the development of more effective communication and coping skills.

Anonymous vs. Nonanonymous Embryo Donation

As with other types of third-party reproduction, there are two types of embryo donation: anonymous and known donation. In countries where embryo donation is allowed, some, such as the United States, have no legislation regarding known or anonymous donation and leave the decision up to the clinic and/or the donors and recipients. In clinics that take the responsibility for matching, the donor couple may have limited or no control over the selection process. Efforts may be made to match the recipient couple with the donor couple according to ethnicity, height, weight, and eye and hair color. Because the program is anonymous, it is generally made clear that there will be no ongoing contact with the recipient couple. In addition, the recipient couple must accept the notion that a child born through embryo donation will probably have a genetic sibling(s) being raised in another family. On the other hand, embryo donors may not be told whether a pregnancy and birth occurred.

A number of countries such as the United Kingdom, Canada, and Australia have emphasized the rights and needs of ART children, with the requirement that identifying information on donors should be available to all embryo donation offspring at the age of eighteen or sixteen. There is no requirement, of course, that recipient couples disclose the use of embryo donation to the offspring. Like other forms of third-party reproduction, the idea that donor couples must provide identifying information may impact the decision to donate – both positively and negatively. Most recently, guidelines in New Zealand regarding embryo donation require a face-to-face meeting between donors and recipients prior to the donation, and provide access to counseling services throughout the process.

Disclosure Issues

Some embryo donations are open, that is, donors and recipients have information about one another, have met face-to-face, and/or plan to have some form of ongoing contact; it is also very probable that recipient couples will disclose information about the means of conception to the child(ren). Mental health professionals will often be called upon to assist with this process by clarifying issues, helping to set boundaries, allaying anxieties, and providing the appropriate language for sharing the information.

Donor embryo recipients may choose nondisclosure of the means of conception for several reasons: As opposed to adoption, the couple may wish to keep their infertility secret to hide their shame and protect their

---

TABLE 20.1. Benefits of disclosure and nondisclosure in embryo donation

Benefits of Disclosure

May be in the best interest of the child based on perceived need for medical history and genetic information.

May be in the best interest of the child based on ethical right of child(ren) to know circumstances of conception.

Allows offspring to develop a normative coherent sense of self in relation to genetic origins.

Parents (and others) are not burdened with deception to offspring over a lifetime.

Parents avoid the possibility that child will learn of his or her genetic origins by mistake (e.g., DNA testing or blood testing) or from others outside the family.

Benefits of Nondisclosure

Offspring and parents/family may need to avoid potential stigma in light of specific cultural and religious milieu.

Parents' infertile status remains undisclosed and protected.

Parents may have limited information about embryo donors (if anonymous) and wish to avoid potential confusion and distress on the part of the offspring.

Parents may wish to avoid potential future legal difficulties.

---

self-esteem; they may hope to enhance their sense that the child fully belongs to them; or they may firmly believe that there are no psychosocial benefits to disclosing to the child. Because of the unconventional aspect of embryo donation, the couple may also fear that they or their child will be stigmatized or misunderstood by others. The couple's religious beliefs and cultural background may contribute to stigmatization. In addition, many donor embryo recipient couples may believe that they lack the information and skills necessary to talk with their child(ren) about this complicated issue.

The decision not to disclose (and to maintain secrecy) to the child, or others, may be deeply rooted in sociocultural customs that can lead to reproductive tourism. In countries where reproductive technology is limited or where gamete and embryo donation is not allowed, recipient couples may choose to go to other countries to receive donated embryos. Despite the availability of identifying information regarding the donor couple, these recipients will maintain secrecy, and their offspring will grow up in a different country, perhaps thousands of miles from that of the embryo donors.

Embryo Donation Agencies

There are a number of embryo donation agencies, located in the United States, that provide services to both donors and recipients. These agencies often designate themselves as Christian organizations, but specify that embryo donors and recipients of all faiths can use their services. It appears that a number of embryo donation agencies evolved not only from the wishes of donors to give their unused embryos to other couples, but also

from the social and political climate in the United States that does not condone embryonic stem cell research at this time. These agencies indicate that embryos are available to recipients from all over the world, and delineate the process of donation and adoption of these embryos. Embryo donors are not compensated for their embryos, and the costs of screening, consultation, and shipping of embryos are covered by recipients. In some cases, donors may be reimbursed for storage expenses accrued. Most of these agencies provide for anonymous and nonanonymous donation, and allow donor couples to select the recipient family. Of course, each agency charges a fee for their work in facilitating the donation. Embryo donation agencies handle the required medical and genetic screening, and also perform a home study with each recipient couple. Mental health professionals will often be asked to be involved in this process, particularly if couples need assistance with decision making or if a home study is required.

Known/Anonymous Embryo Donation and Disclosure: Mental Health Professional Bias

Many mental health professionals working in reproductive health and medicine have personal feelings and professional biases that can potentially impact their relationships with patients who pursue embryo donation. Issues of disclosure, secrecy, as well as the possibility of developing a relationship between embryo donors and recipients can be especially difficult for both patients and infertility counselors. Psychotherapists who are experienced in the adoption tradition, especially open adoption, may struggle to maintain neutrality when working with this population. Nonetheless, it is imperative that infertility counselors allow embryo donation recipients the opportunity to explore fully the issues and consequences of choosing this alternative, without the overlay of caregiver personal bias or perspective. As a way of maintaining neutrality, infertility counselors may also choose to provide donors and recipients with a list of pros and cons regarding known or anonymous donation as well as disclosure to the child and others (see Table 20.1), as well as to outline the relevant issues that are pertinent to having a child(ren) through embryo donation (see Chapter 27). Naturally, if the embryo donors and recipients are known to one another, the MHP will need to assess carefully the quality of the relationships, the motivations of all parties to undertake this procedure, and assist both recipients and donors in determining the extent and quality of their future relationships with one another and their children, including how disclosure issues will be managed.

THERAPEUTIC INTERVENTIONS

Therapeutic interventions in counseling for embryo donation may involve several areas, and are globally relevant to those who choose this option. They include:

- evaluating and screening embryo donors regarding the psychosocial and emotional appropriateness of the donation, and counseling embryo donors about the real and potential implications of their decision to donate embryos to another couple;
- assisting the recipient couple or individual in grieving their loss of a genetic tie to the child;
- exploring with recipients the short- and long-term psychosocial implications of accepting donated embryos, including examining their understanding of embryo donation as a parenting option, assessing appropriateness and readiness, providing emotional support, and addressing disclosure issues and/or the relationship (if any) with the donor couple and genetic siblings;
- facilitating exploration of ways of choosing embryos available for donation, such as clinic or agency donation as well as anonymous/nonanonymous embryo donation.

These interventions are also generally consistent with the three separate but related activities suggested in the United Kingdom by the King's Fund Committee Report[41] on infertility counseling that include support, implications, and therapeutic counseling. However, the work of the mental health professional must often go beyond these activities. Specifically, infertility counselors will need to evaluate the psychological and emotional status of embryo donors and recipients. It

may thus be determined that for psychological and/or social reasons, the donation should not proceed. In this respect, the mental health professional may also become a gatekeeper.

Embryo Donors

Couples who are considering donating their unused, cryopreserved embryos to another couple are often confronted with a wide range of thoughts, feelings, and motivations about this decision. A critical role for the mental health professional is to explore the myriad of issues that come up for the donor couple, and assess carefully their psychosocial and marital status. Despite the donor couple's earlier experience of infertility, their desires and feelings about parenting may have changed over time. A thorough discussion of the reasons behind the decision should provide a backdrop for the evaluation. Any ambivalence on the part of one partner, or indications of coercion should be thoroughly evaluated and addressed by the infertility counselor. In the case of divorce or separation, the decision to donate embryos should be a unanimous one for both partners.

The psychological assessment of embryo donors should include a thorough clinical interview(s) with both partners, and may include standardized psychological testing. The goal is to rule out significant psychiatric illness, substance abuse, ambivalence, or coercion regarding the donation, genetic conditions, and indications of marital instability (including domestic abuse) or other factors that may influence the ability to give full informed consent.

An adjunct to screening embryo donors and counseling them about the implications of their decision is the discussion of information about contact with the recipient couple and offspring. For some, the decision to donate may depend on the degree to which they want to predetermine the makeup of the recipient couple. Some couples willingly agree to anonymous donation, although this is no longer an option in some countries (e.g., United Kingdom, New Zealand, Canada, and most parts of Australia). Other couples may want to dictate terms of the donation, desiring recipient couples of a certain socioeconomic level, race, religious orientation, or age bracket.[42]

Embryo Donation Recipients

For most embryo donation recipients, supportive and implications counseling is an integral part of the work performed with the infertility counselor. All three of these approaches, however, are likely to be intertwined with one another as patients are confronted with a myriad of concerns, fears, questions, and

---

TABLE 20.2. Pros and cons of use of donor embryos

Pros of Use of Embryo Donation

Parents are better able to control the health and prenatal environment of the pregnancy.

Parents are able to share the experience pregnancy and childbirth.

May be less costly than adoption or sperm/egg donation.

Parents may be able to hide or protect themselves from stigma of infertility.

Parents may have more social, educational, and genetic information about the embryo donors than in adoption or sperm/embryo donation.

Embryo donation may be a positive alternative for older, single women or lesbian couples who require donor gametes.

Embryo donation provides equity between partners.

Cons of Use of Embryo Donation

The number of healthy embryos available for donation may be limited.

Some parents may be uncomfortable with their country's regulations concerning the use of donated gametes/embryos.

Parents may feel forced to disclose to offspring (and others) and maintain some type of relationship with embryo donors (if known or identified donation).

There may be religious, ethical, or cultural prohibitions to the use of donated embryos.

Parents have no genetic tie to their offspring although their children have genetic non-rearing parents and siblings.

Parents may feel conflicted about disclosure.

The implications of raising a child(ren) created through embryo donation are unknown.

---

uncertainties pertaining to becoming parents through embryo donation.

Part of the counseling work of the mental health professional will be to determine the couple's readiness for embryo donation by exploring their reasons for choosing this family-building option. It is important that both partners have discussed and have a thorough understanding of why embryo donation is the preferred alternative to adoption. Listing the pros and cons of embryo donation may be a useful exercise for both partners as well as for single women (see Table 20.2). An additional task will be to ascertain the psychosocial functioning and mental health of the recipient couple. Despite their potentially long history of failed infertility treatment, disappointments, sadness, and loss, it is important that the couple demonstrate strengths in their relationship with one another, including (but not limited to) good communication skills, the ability to provide caring support and understanding to one another, positive sexual functioning, and no indications of psychiatric illness, substance abuse, or prior history of child abuse or neglect. Signs of a solid, stable relationship would also preclude pressure or coercion on the part of one partner toward another to proceed with embryo donation before he or she is fully prepared. If it is ascertained that the individual or couple is not ready to move forward with embryo donation, they should be encouraged to postpone the donation procedure and address these issues in psychotherapy.

Exploration of Psychosocial and Legal Implications of Donating or Receiving Embryos

As previously discussed, embryo donation is a complicated process. It is one that requires a great deal of effort on the part of all involved parties: the donating couple, the medical team, the recipient couple, and, possibly, the liaison agency that connects donors to recipients. In addition to rigorous medical and genetic screening of donors, as well as recommendations for psychological consultation and assessment, the reality is that few couples choose to donate their excess or unused cryopreserved embryos to other infertile couples.

Resolve, the National Infertility Association, has provided literature to patients and professionals that delineates some of the factors that donor couples need to take into account when donating their embryos.[5] These include:

(1) The knowledge that all rights to the embryos and any offspring resulting from embryo donation will be relinquished;

(2) The likelihood of required psychological counseling before donating embryos;

(3) The possibility that inadvertent damage to an embryo can occur during thaw or transfer;

(4) The right of the clinic or program to refuse to transfer a donated embryo to a recipient who they feel is an inappropriate candidate;

(5) The understanding that if a child is born from the donated embryos, he or she would be a genetically linked sibling to the donor couple's biological children as well as the genetic offspring of the donating couple.

As a result, those who wish to receive donated embryos may have a long wait for embryos that have been legally, medically, and psychologically cleared for donation. This reality can add to an already difficult and painful process for potential recipients

In literature also published by Resolve,[5] it was pointed out that potential recipient couples must be fully informed about the following aspects of embryo donation:

(1) The anticipated fees for medical examination, blood testing, and professional fees that must be assumed for both the donating and recipient couples;
(2) Psychological counseling before and after the transfer process, which is usually mandatory and highly recommended;
(3) The right of a participating practice or clinic to refuse transfer to an inappropriate recipient;
(4) The monitoring regimen and possible risks of medications used during the transfer cycle;
(5) The possible inadvertent damage to an embryo during thaw and transfer;
(6) Clarification of the recipient couple's full responsibility for the embryos and children resulting from the donation, including unknown long-term consequences that could occur in subsequent generations;
(7) Clarification that the donor couple is released from all liability for complications of pregnancy and congenital or genetic malformations in children resulting from the donation.

Appendixes 9–12 provide sample consent forms that embryo donors and recipient couples may be required to sign prior to proceeding with the donation. These consent forms are generally based on policies and procedures in the United States, but could be adapted to a specific country's regulations and/or requirements.

It is within this framework that embryo donors and recipients may have to consider some of the short-term implications of their decision in order to proceed with embryo donation. The availability of acceptable embryos for donation is limited, and the chances of a successful pregnancy may also be limited. Given these realities, it will be important for the infertility counselor to help recipient couples deal with these limitations and responsibilities, and help them cope with another situation that may potentially lead to disappointment, emo-

tional pain, and the loss of a sense of control in their lives.

Counseling and Disclosure

In recent years, many mental health professionals have been helpful to couples that struggle with the disclosure issue. Although they may advocate for openness and against secrecy, believing that a child has a right to know his or her genetic and medical heritage, infertility counselors should only facilitate discussion and consideration of this issue in an unbiased manner. At the same time, embryo donation patients should understand the reasons why nondisclosure may not be realistic or medically or psychologically healthy.

Donor embryo recipients need to feel respected, supported, and allowed to process their fears, fantasies, and concerns about disclosure to their offspring. Greenfeld[43] adds that helpful interventions from clinicians include providing educational materials and resources including what is generally known and what is not known about disclosure. Ultimately, embryo donation recipients must determine for themselves whether or not disclosure is appropriate to their family and cultural milieu. They must also be counseled that they will need to feel comfortable maintaining the secret and understand the inherent risks involved in secrecy, especially in light of the lack of any genetic connection to the child (see Chapter 27).

FUTURE IMPLICATIONS

Although forbidden in some countries, the ability to cryopreserve embryos has given, and will continue to give infertile couples the opportunity to have additional children without undergoing the medical and financial rigors and medications associated with in vitro fertilization. However, many others will have excess frozen embryos that they are unable to use, primarily because they have completed their families. Some of those embryos, as a result, will ultimately be available for donation to another individual or couple.

Embryo donation will, therefore, continue to be a viable family-building option for some people. However, it is important that recipient couples have a realistic view of the actual availability of suitable screened embryos as well as an understanding of pregnancy success rates. Many IVF couples who initially plan to donate excess embryos to other infertile couples, ultimately do not do so. As a result, it is unlikely that embryo donation will take precedence over traditional adoption or other forms of third-party reproduction as a parenting alternative. Nonetheless, the opportunity to have children through embryo donation can lead to much joy and satisfaction in the same way that any other couple does who struggles with infertility, and finally chooses a nongenetic path to parenthood.

The choice to give or receive donor embryos will continue to involve many complex feelings and issues. There will continue to be an ongoing debate about whether and how couples should disclose the use of embryo donation to their child. Certainly, this task will probably be easier for those donor and recipient families who have pursued the option of maintaining some contact or relationship with one another. When the donation is completely anonymous, the waters for all involved parties are murky, and disclosure issues may be more difficult.

With the global community becoming smaller, couples choosing embryo donation may, in fact, be continents and cultures apart from donating couples. MHPs may be challenged to counsel couples from a different country, reproductive tourists, who approach this process in a culturally and/or racially divergent way. Infertility counselors will be called upon to assist in these complex decisions and relationships.

The need for psychological assessment and counseling will continue to be an intrinsic component of the embryo donation process. Men and women, as partners, who choose embryo donation will no doubt grieve the loss of their fertility and genetic connection to the child in different ways and at a different pace. They will also experience different stages of adjustment before, during, and after the donation. Support and input from MHPs will hopefully ease this process for recipients, and, in the long run, enable them to build a healthy and positive future with their child.

It is hoped that as embryo donation continues to be a family-building option, more data will be gained about the impact of this process on donors, recipients, and offspring. Questions regarding how parents may share this difficult (and often confusing) story with their children need to be addressed. The role of the mental health professional in assisting these potential new families cannot be understated. As the science of reproductive technology moves rapidly into the future, it will be critical that continued research be done and information gathered that allows for a greater depth of knowledge about what it means to be an embryo donor, a recipient parent, or a child born of this unique technology.

SUMMARY

■ The notion of donating or receiving human embryos in order to create a child is a complicated psychosocial issue. As a result, it has been recommended (and often mandated) that both embryo donors and recipients meet with a mental health professional in order to more fully comprehend the many aspects and implications of the donation.

■ Although cyropreservation has resulted in hundreds of thousands of excess embryos and IVF couples initially going through treatment may consider donation a viable option, there are, in reality, very limited numbers of embryos available to recipients. Embryo recipients must be counseled about the screening process necessary and relative rates of success of the process.

■ Although embryo donation is an available parenting alternative in a number of countries around the world, data currently are sparse regarding outcomes and the psychosocial consequences of this choice.

■ Theoretical constructs such as altruism and social-exchange theory, grief and loss theory, and adoption theory are useful in understanding how to assist recipients in coping with the inherent losses of infertility and managing alternative forms of parenthood.

■ In general, psychological evaluation and counseling is a critical component of the embryo donation process. For donor couples, it is important that the decision to donate is based on mutual agreement and a clear understanding of future implications. For recipients, it is important to mourn the loss of fertility and to explore thoughts, feelings, fears, and fantasies about embryo donation.

■ To prepare for this family-building option, it is critical to consider issues of embryo donor anonymity/non-anonymity as well as disclosure and secrecy.

■ It is hoped (and expected) that as embryo donation continues to be a parenting option, more research will be obtained about the impact of this alternative on donors, recipients, and especially on offspring.

■ Mental health professionals working in reproductive medicine play an important role in the assessment, preparation, and education of embryo donors and recipients.

REFERENCES

1. Buster J. Historical evolution of oocyte and embryo donation as a treatment for intractable infertility. In MV Sauer, ed, *Principles of Oocyte and Embryo Donation*. New York: Springer-Verlag, 1998; p. 7.
2. Kosasa TS, McNamee PI, Morton C, et al. Pregnancy rates after transfer of cryopreserved blastocysts cultured in a sequential media. *Am J Obstet Gynecol* 2005; 192:2035–9.
3. Ding J, Pry M, Rana N, Dmowski WP. Improved outcome of frozen-trawed blastocyst transfer with Menozo's two-step thawing compared to the stepwise thawing protocol. *J Assist Reprod Genet* 2004; 21:203–10.
4. Appleton TC. Embryo donation. In: J Boivin, H Kenenich, eds, *Guidelines for Counseling in Infertility*. ESHRE Monographs. Oxford University Press, 2002.

5. Resolve, the National Infertility Association: U.S. Department of Health & Human Services Grant: EAA OP002099, 2002.

6. American Society for Reproductive Medicine. Guidelines for gamete and embryo donation. *Fertil Steril* 2004; 82:S8–20.

7. European Society for Human Reproduction & Embryology. Task force on ethics and law: Gamete and embryo donation. *Hum Reprod* 2002; 17:1407–8.

8. European Union Tissue and Cells Directive, 2004/23 E. C. of the European Parliament and the Council (2004) O.J. L102/48 (March 31, 2004).

9. Human Fertilisation and Embryology Authority: The regulation of Donor-Assisted Conception. United Kingdom, September, 2004.

10. Cox LW. The role of accreditation committees in oocyte donation. *Reprod Fertil Develop* 1992; 4:731–7.

11. Plachot M. Embryo donation in France, in Europe and in the United States. *Gynecol Obstet Fertil* 2004; 32:273–9.

12. Ministry of Health. Guidelines for embryo donation for reproductive purposes, National Ethics Committee on Assisted Human Reproduction (NECAHR), New Zealand, 2005.

13. Trounson A, Mohr L. Human pregnancy following cryopreservation, thawing, and transfer of an eight-cell stage human embryo. *Nature* 1983; 305:707–9.

14. Klock S. Embryo disposition: The forgotten "child" of in vitro fertilization. *Int J Fertil Womens Med* 2004; 49:19–23.

15. Hoffman DI, Zellman GL, Fair CC, Mayer JF, et al. Cryopreserved embryos in the United States and their availability for research. *Fertil Steril* 2003; 79:1063–9.

16. De Lacey S. Parent identity and "virtual" children: Why patients discard rather than donate unused embryos. *Hum Reprod* 2005; 20:1065–8.

17. Nachtigall RD, Becker G, Friese C, Butler A, MacDougall K. Parents' conceptualization of their frozen embryos complicates the disposition decision. *Fertil Steril* 2005; 84:431–4.

18. Lee J, Yap C. Embryo donation: A review. *Acta Obstet Gynecol Scan* 2003; 82:991–6.

19. Van Voorhis BJ, Grinstead DM, Sparks AF, Gerard JL, Weir RF. Establishment of a successful donor embryo program: Medical, ethical, and policy issues. *Fertil Steril* 1999; 71:604–8.

20. Kingsberg SA, Applegarth LD, Janata JW. Embryo donation programs and policies in North America: Survey results and implications for health and mental health professionals. *Fertil Steril* 2000; 73:215–20.

21. Beyler SA, Meyer WR, Fritz MA. Disposition of extra embryos. *Fertil Steril* 2000; 74:213–5.

22. Lindheim SR, Sauer MV. Embryo donation: A programmed approach. *Fertil Steril* 1999; 72:940–1.

23. Soderstrom-Anttila V, Foudila T, Ripatti U-R. Embryo donation: Outcome and attitudes among embryo donors and recipients. *Hum Reprod* 2001; 16:1120–8.

24. Newton CR, McDermid A, Tekpetey F, et al. Embryo donation: Attitudes toward donation procedures and factors predicting willingness to donate. *Hum Reprod* 2003; 18:878–84.

25. Kovacs GT, Breheny SA, Dear MJ. Embryo donation at an Australian university in-vitro fertilization clinic: Issues and outcomes. *Med J Aust* 2003; 178:127–9.

26. MacCallum F. Embryo donation families: Psychological implications. *Abstracts of the 20th Annual Meeting of the European Society of Human Reproduction and Embryology*, Berlin, Germany, June, 2004, p. 131.

27. Belluck P. It's not so easy to adopt an embryo. *New York Times*, 1–12–2005.

28. Resolve, the National Infertility Association: U.S. Department of Health and Human Services Grant: 6EAA 0P002102-01-1, 2004.

29. Liang J, Krause NM, Bennett JM. Social exchange and well-being: is giving better than receiving? *Psych Aging* 2001; 16:511–23.

30. Lawler EJ. An affect theory of social exchange. *Am J Soc* 2001; 107:321–52.

31. Koehler, WF, Fottler MD, Swan JE. Physician/patient satisfaction: Equity in the health services encounter. *Medical Care Review* 1992; 49:455–84.

32. Bonacich P. Four kinds of social dilemmas within exchange networks. *Current Research Soc Psych* 1995; 1:1–7.

33. Freeark K, Rosenberg EL, Bornstein J, et al. Gender differences and dynamics shaping the adoption life cycle: Review of the literature and recommendations. *Am J Orthopsych* 2005; 75:86–101.

34. Bevc V, Jerman J, Ovsenk R, et al. Experiencing infertility – social work dilemmas in child adoption procedures. *Coll Antropol* 2003; 27:445–60.

35. van den Akker OB. Adoption in the age of reproductive technology. *J Reprod Infant Psychol* 2001; 19:147–59.

36. Glazer ES, Sterling EW. *Having Your Baby through Egg Donation*. Indianapolis, IN: Perspectives Press, Inc., p. 90, 2005.

37. Boivin J. Worldwide trends in gamete donation: Exploring the changing role of the donor. Paper presented at the Mental Health Professional Group Postgraduate Course: *Children of the ARTs: Psychosocial Challenges to Redefining Family*. Annual Meeting of the American Society for Reproductive Medicine, San Antonio, Texas, October, 2003.

38. Mahlstedt PP, Greenfeld DA. Assisted reproductive technology for donor gametes: The need for patient preparation. *Fertil Steril* 1989; 5:908–14.

39. Hjelmstedt A, Andersson L, Skoog-Svanberg A, et al. Gender differences in psychological reactions to infertility among couples seeking IVF-and ICSI-treatment. *Acta Obstet Gynecol Scand* 1999; 78:42–8.

40. Borrero C. Gamete and embryo donation. In: *Current Practices and Controversies in Assisted Reproduction*: Report on a meeting on Medical, Ethical, and Social Aspects of Assisted Reproduction. Department of Reproductive Health & Research. World Health Organization, Geneva, Switzerland, September, 2001.

41. Kings Fund Centre Counselling Committee. *Report on Counselling for Regulated Infertility Treatments*, United Kingdom, 1991.

42. Mayes G. Frozen in time: Disposition of frozen embryos gives rise to ethical, legal, and yes . . . political considerations. *Medscape Ob/Gyn Women's Health* 2003; 8:1.

43. Greenfeld D. Recipient counseling for oocyte donation. In: LH Burns, SN Covington, eds. *Infertility Counseling: A Comprehensive Handbook for Clinicians*. New York: Parthenon Publishing Group Inc., 1999.

21 Surrogacy and Gestational Carrier Participants

HILARY HANAFIN

The only gift is a portion of thyself.

– Ralph Waldo Emerson

Language and appropriate definitions in the field of third-party family building have been the source of debates among mental health professionals, ethicists, lawyers, and physicians, in a struggle to agree on what words accurately describe and define the roles of the various parties involved. The word *surrogate* was seen as accurate to some because it reflected the intent of the woman as well as her self-perception of her role. To others, *surrogate* was offensive in that the woman was indeed the genetic and birthmother. There has been a tendency by some to eliminate the word *mother* in third-party reproduction (as father has been eliminated from donor insemination third-party reproduction) to reinforce the surrogate's role as a facilitator for intended parent(s). However, others contend that the word *mother* is important so as not to minimize the value and integrity of the woman's role. The choice of terminology became more confusing with the application of in vitro fertilization (IVF), embryo transfer, and gamete and embryo donation. Professional groups around the world and governmental agencies have chosen different terms to describe the woman who gestates another couple's embryo as any of the following: *host surrogate*, *gestational carrier*, and *IVF surrogate*. In this chapter, the term *gestational carrier* (GC) is used to refer to a woman who carries a pregnancy (embryo) conceived by IVF for a contracting couple who are genetically-related as well as the intended parents, or carries any embryos to which she is not genetically related and does not plan to parent herself but, instead, carries the pregnancy for another couple. Infertile couples using a form of surrogacy are most often referred to as *prospective parents*, *intended parents*, or *contracting parents*. In this chapter, the term *intended parents* is used. The traditional term *adoptive parents* has not been widely used in surrogate practices, to differentiate it from traditional adoption of an infant relin-

quished for adoption to an agency or another couple or family. In this chapter, *traditional surrogacy* (TS) refers to a woman who conceives via artificial insemination (AI) using the semen of the husband (male partner) after which the surrogate carries the pregnancy for the intended couple to whom she relinquishes the baby after delivery. In such arrangements, the intended mother may have to proceed with legal adoption of the infant in order to be identified as the baby's legitimate mother although she may have always been the intended mother.

This chapter addresses

■ current practices in psychosocial evaluation and screening of surrogacy participants;
■ the roles of the mental health professional working with surrogates, gestational carriers, and intended parents;
■ common psychosocial problems encountered in surrogacy agreements and procedures;
■ legal and contractual considerations for the mental health professional working in this unique field;
■ the practice of these surrogacy arrangements around the world and the role of the infertility counselor in care and preparation of all participants.

HISTORICAL OVERVIEW

Surrogate parenting has taken place informally throughout time. Although the practice of surrogacy dates back to the Old Testament, it was not practiced in contemporary society formally until the 1970s. In 1977, contractual surrogacy was presented as an option to infertile couples. Traditionally surrogacy was defined as an arrangement in which a woman was or is artificially inseminated with the semen of the husband in an infertile couple, the intended parents, and the resulting baby was or is relinquished by the surrogate (birthmother or genetic mother) to the father and his infertile wife, who, as the intended mother, must legally adopt the child. By 1980, at least three private agencies in the United States were offering services to infertile couples that included the advertisement for and introduction to women who would conceive a child for a contracting couple. By 1986, there were at least six agencies in the United States and one in Europe that arranged for potential surrogate mothers to meet infertile couples. Approximately 500 children were born in the United States as a result of these new and controversial arrangements involving artificial insemination of a surrogate mother. By 2005, the number of agencies in the United States was approximately twenty-three, with a total of 6,000 births by surrogate mothers/gestational carriers occurring in the United States and more than 300 births in Great Britain, according to statistics compiled by the Center for Surrogate Parenting.[1] There is no central reporting of such contractual arrangements, so the actual number is unknown. The majority of these births are the result of the more medically complicated method of conception, IVF gestational carrier surrogacy. While most births occurred in the United States, the medical ability to perform gestational carrier surrogacy is available in first world nations. Gestational surrogacy has been reported in many nations, namely Australia, Canada, Israel, Finland, and Brazil.

This new alternative to childlessness continued despite the public controversy that erupted around it. Public concern about this new form of third-party reproductive parenthood, the industry that developed to facilitate it, and the unique legal and ethical dilemmas surrounding it, became the focus of much debate – and remains so in many parts of the world. The controversies took front page for the public in 1986 when a legal battle ensued between a traditional surrogate named Mary Beth Whitehead and the intended parents. Great Britain began their own public debate in 1985 debate when baby Cotton was born as a result of a traditional surrogate arrangement in which the surrogate agreeably relinquished the infant. A primary concern was the psychological repercussions of surrogacy for the surrogate and for the children involved. Some argued that intentionally creating children who were to be separated physically and legally from their birthmothers and half-siblings was contrary to public and social policy and customs. The commercial nature and fees involved challenged beliefs about maternal attachment and stirred concerns about women's ability to make decisions for themselves. Additionally, curiosity about the enigmatic nature of women who became surrogates was a concern. The media, legal community, and feminist community took an interest in these early volunteer traditional surrogates, while in the psychological community, a small number began to address the complex issues involved in facilitating these parenthood arrangements. To this day, there remains a paucity of psychological research on surrogate mothers and gestational carriers, the infertile couples who contract with them, and the children born as a result of this technology.

As the debates via courtroom and the media continued, the practice of surrogacy grew and broadened in definition. With the technical advances of IVF applied to the practice of surrogacy, in 1987 a gestational surrogate in the United States delivered, via embryo transfer, a baby who was not genetically related to her but was a genetically shared offspring of the intended parents. Also known as gestational carriers, women volunteer to be the host uterus for an infertile couple's genetic embryo. Excitement about this new medical success was accompanied by controversies about the legal and social definitions of mother and motherhood, and parenthood in general. To some, the lack of genetic connection between the baby and carrying mother made a significant difference in defining the relationship and roles of the participating parties, while others found these facts were irrelevant. Another important difference in the pursuit of gestational surrogacy was that IVF clinics and physicians could now offer a new medical procedure to their infertility patients.

Physicians and hospital ethics committees began debating the ethics of participating in the implantation of patients' embryos into gestational carriers. While some IVF centers elected not to provide such a service to their patients, others did so on a case-by-case basis, while a few clinics actually offered the service of finding and matching their patients with carriers or surrogates. The direction IVF clinics took was determined by several factors. There were not laws in most of the United States and in countries worldwide. In the United States, the majority of clinics used professional guidelines and the ethics committees of universities to make decisions. Issues of family law are routinely decided by individual states in the United States. There are laws within some of the states that determine protocols, the enforceability of a contract, and require restrictions of payment to a surrogate. In many countries, national governing bodies took on the task of deciding the fate of this new practice. Commissions were set up to study the impact on public policy, the effect on health services, and the laws determining parentage. The rules determining gestational surrogacy are still evolving. The complexities arise around the finalization of birth certificates and whether the intended mother is ultimately registered as the legal mother in her home country. Furthermore, countries that have strong religious influences in their governing bodies found surrogacy incongruent with the tenets of their religion. For example, countries that are primarily Catholic or Muslim could not support the concept of an outside party involving herself in the creation of a couple's child. Although initially countries struggled with the issues surrounding surrogacy, many developed countries do allow surrogacy as long as the surrogate mother is not financially compensated. For example, surrogacy does occur in Great Britain, South Africa, Canada, Israel, and parts of Australia. Regulations vary and are evolving but most often they include the restriction against financial compensation, restrictions on who is allowed to contract with a surrogate, and mandated involvement by professionals and approval by governing bodies. German governing bodies ruled against surrogacy. It is interesting to note that it was in Germany in the 1980s that an American opened a short-lived commercial surrogacy agency.

REVIEW OF THE LITERATURE

During the 1980s, there was a dramatic increase in the body of literature on surrogate parenting, most of which addressed ethical and social policy issues. The literature and research as they pertain to the dynamics of surrogate mothers, gestational carriers, and the resulting new families were limited. To date, most research has focused on the psychological dynamics and motivations of surrogate mothers and gestational carriers. Franks[2] and Parker,[3] in the first published research in the early 1980s, presented brief articles that explained and described the enigmatic population of surrogate mothers. Parker expanded his work with Reame in 1992, writing a description of forty-four surrogacy pregnancies.[4] In addition, in 1992, the first descriptive study about the new IVF gestational-carrier surrogates was published by Mechanick-Braverman and Corson,[5] while Hanafin[6] and Resnick[7] conducted doctoral dissertations in the 1980s that attempted a broader explanation of the psychological dynamics in third-party reproduction. All researchers were strikingly similar in their conclusions about the motivations and the demographics of surrogate mothers. These studies revealed that surrogate mothers in the United States were motivated by the desire to do something important in their lives, empathy for the childless couple, desire to experience pregnancy again, financial gain, and less often, an opportunity to undo or fix something in their past. Typically the participants were in their late twenties, most often married, and having an average of two children, raised in the Christian/Protestant faith,

and having two years of postsecondary education. Most importantly, none of the research found psychopathology in the participants. Research on surrogate mothers in Great Britain had similar findings. In 1994, Blyth reported on nineteen women serving as surrogates whose motivations and demographics were strikingly similar.[8] In a more interesting study, Resnick[7] compared the psychosocial histories of surrogate mothers and women who were demographic matches. There was no difference between the two groups' childhood histories of attachment and abandonment.

Long-term follow-up studies emerged revealing that over time surrogates/gestational carriers reported minimal remorse about their participation. In 1987, Hanafin[9] reported on thirty-seven surrogates and sixteen new families that had completed a surrogacy program. Ciccarelli[10] conducted a long-term follow-up study of fourteen surrogate mothers. Findings in both studies are similar. In summary, surrogate mothers overall do not regret their involvement, and their satisfaction is positively correlated with a respectful and comfortable relationship with the parents. The respect shown by the parents and the contact with them appears to have significant consequences for the surrogates' long-term comfort and satisfaction with having participated. Recent research published in 2003 in Great Britain by Jadva and colleagues [11] studied thirty-four surrogate mothers who had given birth as a surrogate mother approximately one year earlier. Trained researchers interviewed the women and the data were rated using standardized coding criteria. They found similar results to the earlier research. The surrogate mothers did not appear to experience psychological problems in their relationship with the parents, relinquishing the baby, or in reactions from others. However, two postpartum studies did reveal regrets and struggles for some of the surrogates. Reame and colleagues collected data via interview with ten traditional surrogates in the United States who had given birth between ten and fifteen years earlier.[12] Reame reported that six of the ten felt some degree of remorse, if the parents did not keep their promise to stay in contact. Reame, like Hanafin and Ciccarelli, concluded that the degree of satisfaction with their surrogacy experience correlated with the degree of satisfaction with their relationship with the parents. Blyth's 1994 study of nineteen women in England included nine women who had given birth. Of the nine, one had not relinquished the child and another clearly regretted having become a surrogate. Six of the women were participating for a second time and one for a third time.

Additional research done at the City University in London has provided some insight about the postbirth responses of the intended parents who have become parents via some form of surrogacy. MacCallum and associates in 2003 surveyed, tested, and observed forty-two families with one-year-olds born through surrogacy.[13] They concluded that at this mark, the intended parents generally perceived the surrogacy experience as positive. The relationships with the surrogate had been generally positive with some level of contact maintained after the birth. The parents had told members of their families and friends, and were planning on telling the child. In 2004, the same research team compared these forty-two families created through traditional surrogacy and gestational carrier with fifty-one oocyte donation families and eighty natural conception families.[14] Golombok and colleagues concluded that the parents of children born through surrogacy arrangements indicated greater psychological well-being and adaptation to parenthood than those born by natural-conception parents.

THEORETICAL FRAMEWORK

Women relinquishing children certainly stirs much thought about sociological and psychological issues. Much of the traditional training of mental health professionals would suggest that women who voluntarily relinquish children are flawed people in need of therapy. Furthermore, those who assist women in doing so are colluding with behavior that is unhealthy and against public policy. It is helpful to be aware of theoretical orientations that allow us to look at human behavior in a broader historical and cultural context. Several theoretical frameworks can be used to greater an understanding of surrogacy.

Given the debate of 'altruistic surrogacy' and 'commercial surrogacy,' theories of altruism itself are intriguing. The term altruistic surrogacy is used when the surrogate is receiving no financial compensation beyond reimbursement for expenses. One of the most studied theories about altruism is that of Anna Freud. In her 1936 psychoanalytical writing, *The Ego and the Mechanisms of Defense*, Freud describes some altruistic behaviors as a defense mechanism using projection, identification, or machismo.[15] A person gratifies her own impulses in favor of other people and consequently presents as altruistic. Analyzing altruistic behavior revealed several defense mechanisms against instincts by displacing needs onto others. Anna Freud left unanswered the question as to whether there is genuine altruism, where the gratification of one's own instinct plays no past at all. As mental health professionals, it is worthwhile to look for history and behavior that suggest a surrogate may be sublimating her own needs and projecting them onto the intended parents in a way that may leave her depleted and ungratified. People, especially mothers and pregnant women, need to sublimate and postpone gratification in a healthy way. However, if a surrogate reveals herself to be historically depleted, unsatisfied, and is unaware of her own needs, the concern that surrogacy can be exploitive may be founded.

A more recent discussion of altruism is aptly addressed by Simmons and colleagues. They assessed the impact and the consequences of organ donation in the 1970s.[16] Their conclusions have striking similarity to the conclusions of the small number of studies on surrogates and to the assumptions made by many counselors in the field. For example, Simmons et al. found that donors felt deeply rewarded if they were able to have information about the success and happiness they were able to create by donating. Donors who had more negative responses did not experience gratitude from the recipient. Furthermore, donors who felt coercion, had low self-esteem, ambivalence, or who had less connection to the recipients had more negative reactions. These findings have direct correlation to the evaluation of surrogates/carriers. Surrogates/carriers consistently report that seeing the resulting happiness of their labor and feeling gratitude had a direct correlation on their long-term satisfaction with surrogacy. It is interesting to note that the two early surrogacy programs that began as anonymous programs were short-lived. Even when an act is altruistic, such as a kidney to a relative, there are important clinical issues that mental health professionals can address in hopes of achieving an ethical, satisfactory experience for all participants, minimizing the collusion with pathology and the exploitation.

Beyond the issues of the individual motivation, theoretical frameworks can also be used to understand the context of the individuals. Surrogacy challenges our perceptions of women, maternal attachment, altruism, exploitation, and cultural norms. The practice and the patients need to be viewed in their own historical and cultural context. A sociocultural orientation is helpful when assessing participants and when struggling with clinical issues. Psychologist Jefferson Fish wrote about the importance of relating therapy and assessment to cultural context.[17] Cultural differences exist in infertility, ways of grieving, family relationships, marriage, and the purpose of parenting. Our own assumptions about how women bond to each pregnancy and child are based in culture and history. Beliefs about privacy and the expectations about the duty of extended family are affected by culture. The cultural and social patterns are intrinsic to the understanding of behavior. Fish encourages the vast fields of anthropology and sociology to be included in our understanding of the individual. It is always important for mental health professionals to see participants in these new and evolving practices in a broader cultural context. Other chapters in this book address religious and cultural issues in detail (see Chapter 4).

CLINICAL ISSUES

Legal and Contractual Considerations

Mental health professionals involved in surrogacy/gestational carrier arrangements have several sets of legal paperwork with which they need to be concerned. One is the contract between the couples and the other is the legal documents between the professional and all of the clients.

Mental health professionals (and medical professionals) should refer clients to legal counsel prior to beginning attempts at conception. Being involved in third-party reproduction carries the responsibility of referring clients to other professionals so that they can better protect themselves. With the increase of intended parents and gestational carriers finding each other on the Internet, it is increasingly important that clients be provided with accurate professional guidance. Legal consultation will protect clients from making poorly informed decisions, provide accurate information, and assist in creating a basis for an informed consent argument, if necessary. It is important for clients to know the laws in the place of the birth and in the parents' home. Most surrogate/carrier arrangements involve a contract that outlines the responsibilities and intent of all parties. It also addresses issues of confidentiality, insurance, financial reimbursements (including lack of), termination, misrepresentation, contact, and so on. In addition to being legally significant, the task of reviewing important issues on paper is revealing and can clarify psychological issues.

Like clients, mental health professionals should seek legal counsel and be aware of the standards of care in their country, their mental health profession, and the field of infertility counseling or reproductive health counseling. Japan, Australia, New Zealand, Great Britain, Germany, Canada, and the United States all have professional associations for infertility counselors as do Europe, the Middle East, and South America. In fact, there is now an International Infertility Counseling Organization (see Resource listing). The field of psychological assessment and third-party reproduction is legally complex. Professionals in this field are usually presented with two sets of clients, each with their own agendas, concerns, perspectives, and need for

confidentiality. The control of information – who is entitled to know what – can be tenuous and difficult when such evaluations are provided. It is recommended that professionals address these issues early in the consultations so that they are acting ethically and legally. Their role and purpose need to be explained early on to all participants.

Four documents that mental health professionals may use are a retainer, a psychological informed consent, confidentiality form, and a conflict-of-interest waiver. A *retainer* may include such points as the professional's role, its limitations, the financial remuneration to be paid, and the nature of services to be provided, as well as the manner of action to be taken, if there is a dispute. The *informed consent* outlines the understanding of the clients' roles and the guidelines of the professional's relationship with them. A *confidentiality form* also needs to be considered so that it is clear that the professional does, or does not, have permission to speak to other professionals and to the other client in the arrangement. The other document that is recommended is a *conflict-of-interest waiver*. Third-party reproduction and surrogacy/gestational carrier arrangements, in particular, typically involve the controversial dilemma of one counselor serving two parties. The waiver outlines this very dilemma. It informs the clients that there can be conflicts surrounding what will be withheld and what will be shared with the other party. Additionally, the waiver outlines the possibility that a counselor could give advice that is contrary to the other party's wishes. It is important to define who the client is. These documents do not waive professional liability, which cannot be waived. Finally, before using these documents they should be examined by a legal professional (see Appendixes 8–10 for examples).

Common Problems

Surrogate/carrier arrangements are fraught with the possibility of countless problems, so an important step in minimizing them is taking a *proactive* approach. The planning stage begins after the initial assessment and should address many of the issues already mentioned. However, the most common problems usually fall within three categories: (1) struggles with medical issues, (2) struggles with the relationship, and (3) struggles with logistical surprises.

One of the most trying and disappointing problems for all families is the continual failure of Mother Nature to successfully and safely bring the child into the world, despite everyone's best efforts. Miscarriages, high-risk complicated pregnancies, birth defects, and illness all intrude, despite the best laid plans. A significant psychological issue with this stems from the disparate life experiences that the two couples have had with reproduction. The intended parents and the gestational carrier/surrogate not only have different views of success with fertility and what is 'normal,' but they may also have cultural or religious differences that have an impact on their worldview regarding reproduction. Speaking to these issues directly increases empathy and minimizes painful misunderstandings. The pains of infertility do not end with conception. Where surrogate/carriers tend to feel positive and invincible, the prospective parents may feel anxious, worried, cautious, and hypervigilant. Without understanding the other's perspective, there can be additional strain in the discussion of medical care, prenatal care, and the enthusiasm for exciting but tenuous news.

Beyond these disparate views of Mother Nature, there is the dynamic of 'my body, your baby' or 'my baby, your body.' The prospective parents come to surrogacy having surrendered a great deal already – psychological, socially, even financially. Given that the issues of trust and control are central struggles in surrogacy (as well as infertility), it is inevitable that there will be conflict surrounding prenatal and medical care. The intended parents must decide both when to let a concern go and when to raise it. This discussion sounds simple at first, but can be very taxing to everyone involved. The prospective parents are best served first by having accurate medical information and then choosing their confrontations carefully. As in any relationship, especially one in which trust is a primary component, one needs to make confrontations wisely. A surrogate/carrier and a couple may cause each other significant distress if they are not clear about the other party's limitations and what really matters to them. A mental health professional can be instrumental in deciphering when to let it go and when to make an issue of something. Controversies usually evolve around travel, diet, money, illness, choice of doctor, medication, bed rest, and labor and delivery options.

Assumptions about what type of contact and relationship they will have can be a common source of problems. It is exhausting and hurtful when the two parties have different agendas. Again, providing accurate information and increasing empathy for the other's perspective is usually constructive. It is important that the parties remain on the same team and adversarial positions be avoided. They need each other to make this work, and they need to create a positive legacy for the children. It is a common mistake for couples to mistrust the surrogate/carrier's integrity and consequently offend her. Another common error occurs when a surrogate/carrier misreads a couple's genuine enthusiasm, seeing instead anxiety or aloofness.

Perhaps one of the clearest roles mental health professionals can take is helping these families address issues of closure. Mental health professionals understand the importance of good goodbyes and good endings. Given the understandable awkwardness, exhaustion, and anxieties inherent in surrogacy, it is helpful to clearly plan the birth, hospital stay, and postpartum contact. Giving attention to each family's needs and to simple rituals can be critical in assisting the families leaving whole and happy. Surrogates/carriers, as we all do, need to feel validated, valuable, and trusted. A surrogate/carrier and her family should not feel rushed and pushed aside – dispensable or disposable. Intended parents need to have closure so they feel safe and clear about the psychological dynamics of their child's birthing mother. The postbirth exchange of keepsake or symbolic gifts and thank you letters is helpful. Setting aside time prior to the parent's departure when the carrier/surrogate and her family can visit with the new parents and baby, enjoy the ending, take photographs, and exchange gifts, is recommended. A respectful, warm, and appreciative closure minimizes feelings of exploitation and emptiness for a surrogate/carrier. Attention to closure helps a couple feel secure in the relinquishment and provides a positive story to tell their child. Positive closure is in everyone's best interest.

Surrogacy and the Gay Population

By the late 1980s, gay male couples were contacting commercial surrogate agencies. Initially these cases were rare and were all traditional artificial insemination surrogacy. There is no central reporting of the number of families created for gay couples with the help of a surrogate, but estimations suggest that by 2005 there were several hundred gay men who had become fathers via surrogacy. Some agencies and many countries do not support gay men in this pursuit. However, gay men have become reproductive tourists as well, coming to the United States primarily. The means of conception are both traditional artificial insemination and gestational carrier, with the addition of a donated oocyte. Fertilization of the donated embryos is either by one father or the embryos are divided and half are fertilized by one intended father and the other half fertilized by the other intended father, thus giving both partners the opportunity to potentially parent their own offspring. In some cases, only one partner's embryos are transferred and the remaining embryos are frozen for future children. In other cases, the partners decide to transfer one embryo from each of them into the gestational carrier, potentially resulting in twins who have the same maternal genetics and different paternal genetics.

The mental health professional can be crucial in helping gay couples decide the pros and cons of the various options open to them, while discussing the psychological issues of surrogacy and long-term implications for the children. There are several additional clinical issues involved in surrogacy. The gay male couple is often less versed than their infertile heterosexual counterparts in infertility and pregnancy. They have not been patients and consumers. Consequently, sometimes mental health professionals need to provide more education and support. In this relationship, it is the gestational carrier/surrogate who often knows the most about reproductive technology and therefore needs to be her own advocate. Naivete for any intended parents can cause stress and misunderstandings in the relationship with the surrogate/carrier.

The experience for the surrogate/gestational carrier can be also be different in that there is no woman with whom to share the information and the attention. Some surrogate applicants admittedly prefer helping a gay couple because they do not have to be concerned about the possible control, grief, and loss issues that come with an infertile woman. The surrogate/carriers perceives herself as being free of her fear of impinging on the intended mother. Furthermore, it is important for all to consider that the gestational carrier will not be replaced by a new mother after the birth. The role of the birthing mother may be of more interest to the child in the years to come in that another woman has not replaced her. This dynamic is particularly potent if the surrogate is indeed the genetic birthmother. The matching of surrogates with intended parents is a crucial part to the success of surrogacy. With gay couples creating children via traditional surrogacy, one may give the issues around the long-term relationship special importance.

The culture and beliefs about the gay population certainly play a role in surrogacy. The surrogate/carrier and her family need to be comfortable in helping a gay couple. Furthermore, how she explains the couple to her extended family and community can be a source of stress in that she may be judged more harshly by others. Others' discomfort with gay men becoming parents is an additional issue with which the carrier and her family will contend. However, it is sometimes this very issue that attracts women to helping gay couples. Helping the ones who are least likely to get chosen or about whom society still struggles can, in and of itself, be appealing.

THERAPEUTIC INTERVENTIONS

Historically, psychological screening of surrogates or gestational carrier candidates was considered optional. However, all parties including patients, physicians, and mental health professionals have more legal protection if an evaluation is done. Currently, it is the standard practice of care to provide psychological evaluations of participants in third-party reproduction whether recommended by governmental agencies (e.g., Australia and the United Kingdom), professional societies (e.g., ASRM, ESHRE), or mandated by law (e.g., Canada).[18–20]) The role of the mental health professional in third-party reproduction (as in other areas of infertility treatment) involves assessment and evaluation, patient preparation and education, and occasionally, psychotherapeutic intervention. As such, the clinician observes, assesses, and evaluates participants' behavior and beliefs via a clinical interview that may (and typically does) include psychological testing. Mental health professionals providing evaluations and counseling services for surrogacy and gestational carrier arrangements face a variety of clinical and professional challenges and goals:

■ Determine what is best for all of the parties involved, with particular attention to what is in the best interest of the child (created) as well as any existing children.[21]

■ Apply professional skills according to the professional skills and ethical standards of his or her mental health profession as well as the standards of care in the field of third-party reproduction.

■ Foresee the range of problems that can potentially occur in third-party reproduction and pregnancy and intervene appropriately.

Typically, the mental health professional evaluates potential surrogates or gestational carriers prior to formally contracting with an infertile couple. In these situations, the role of the mental health professional is one of primarily evaluating and preparing the parties and, although ongoing support and assistance may be offered, it is not typically mandatory clinic, agency, professional society, or governmental agency policy. In contrast, in some programs the infertility counselor not only evaluates a potential surrogate/carrier and intended parents, but also provides ongoing individual and group counseling with all parties throughout the process. Whether the role of the mental health professional is ongoing or limited to 'start-up,' mandated by law as in Canada or highly suggested by attorneys, preconception counseling is now considered the standard of care worldwide. As such, infertility counselors must

TABLE 21.1. Contraindications of potential gestational carriers

1. Cognitive or emotional inability to comply or to understand
2. Evidence of financial or emotional coercion
3. Failure to evidence altruistic commitment to become a carrier
4. Psychological testing not within normal limits
5. Unresolved or untreated addiction, child abuse, sexual abuse, physical abuse, depression, eating disorders, or traumatic pregnancy, labor and/or delivery
6. History of major depression, bipolar disorder, psychosis, or diagnosis of a personality disorder
7. Insufficient emotional support from partner/spouse or support system
8. Current marital or relationship instability
9. Excessively stressful family demands, without sufficient support
10. Chaotic lifestyle
11. Inability to maintain respectful and caring relationship with intended parents
12. Evidence of emotional inability to separate from/surrender the baby at birth
13. History of conflict with authority
14. Inability to perceive and understand the perspective of others
15. Motivation to use compensation to solve own infertility
16. Unresolved issues with a previous abortion

American Society for Reproductive Medicine. (2009 pending). Guidelines for Gestational Carriers (see Appendix 7).

have professional knowledge of the field and be prepared to educate consumers (intended parents or gestational carriers/surrogates) about the role, importance, and necessity of preconception counseling.

There has been a significant increase in the number of professional organizations providing outlines for the psychological work involved in third-party family building. Mental health professionals working as infertility counselors should be well-informed about the standards of their own professional practice as well as relevant professional societies, medical associations, and licensing and/or credentialing processes/criteria (see Chapter 31). The European Society of Human Reproduction and Embryology has published Task Force reports on the ethical and the psychological issues involved in surrogacy, including evaluation and assessment of participants in third-party reproduction.[19] Similarly, the American Society for Reproductive Medicine has published guidelines for third-party reproduction. Recommendations and guidelines for working with gestational carriers and surrogates from the Mental Health Professional Group of ASRM are included in Appendix 7.

Assessing Surrogates and Gestational Carriers

The most significant goal of preconception counseling with a potential surrogate or gestational carrier is helping her (and her partner or support system) decide if being a surrogate or gestational carrier will serve a positive, satisfying purpose or a negative, dysfunctional purpose in her life. She needs to be able to provide informed consent, be at peace with the relinquishment of the child, and leave the program whole and unharmed. In an effort to serve both parties, the mental health professional assesses the surrogate/carrier candidate's motivations, her ability to accurately perceive situations, her personality, and her intellectual competency. Table 21.1 provides contraindications for participation as a surrogate or gestational carrier.

For example, it is recommended that a surrogate/gestational carrier have previously given birth, in large part so that she can provide informed consent. If a woman has not given birth and/or has not parented, she is less likely to be able to give informed consent. A woman with no childbirth experience may encounter unknown medical risks and will not be able to fully understand the physical demands that she is undertaking. A woman with no parenting experience may not be as able to predict her own behavior and emotions as they relate to the intended child. Another important criterion is that of financial stability. If a candidate is participating strictly out of acute financial need or pressure, coercion and confounded decision making may be present. Excluding women with risky medical conditions and who have substance abuse histories is also recommended.

Being a surrogate or gestational carrier involves a wide array of ambiguity and potentially emotionally stressful situations. Predicting how a surrogate/carrier will respond to and resolve such issues is key to protecting her and all parties involved. A nonpathological personality that is resilient, adaptable, empathic, and intellectually competent with good ego-strength is ideal. A psychosocial interview is fundamental to assessing her decision-making processes, her social and family relationships, her manner in resolving problems, and her ability to take care of herself and others (e.g., her own children). Special consideration needs to be given to issues of loss and trauma in her history. Table 21.2 lists issues to include in the structured clinical interview.

It is important to use some objective measure to facilitate understanding the potential surrogate/gestational carrier's way of relating to others and responding to

---

TABLE 21.2. **Issues to include in a thorough clinical interview with surrogate/gestational carrier**

Discussion of motivations and her journey to the decision to pursue surrogacy

Expectations about the benefits of serving as a surrogate/gestational carrier

Description of marriage, family life, and support system

Review of current and pending potential stressor or changes

History of pregnancy and postpartum recovery

Reproductive history, including abortions

Childhood family events and traumas

Resolution status of any trauma and loss in adulthood

History of drug/alcohol abuse

History of depression and psychiatric history

Discussion of coping skills when life is difficult

History of lawsuits and difficulty with the law

Discussion of her children and assessment of how she will tell them

History of her own children's lives as it pertains to chaotic life and loss

Expectations about relationship with the intended parents

Expectations about relationship with the potential child

Beliefs about abortion due to birth anomaly

Beliefs about multipregnancy reduction and risk of multiple birth

Fantasies and predictions of her behavior and her needs at time of birth

---

stressful situations. Psychological testing is standardly used to assess potential candidates, both as a means of corroborating the clinical interview and as a method of identifying personality characteristics or lifestyle problems that may impact the candidate's participation. Psychological testing is useful in identifying any number of factors including personality style (e.g., extroversion vs. introversion); psychopathology; and/or potential behavioral problems (e.g., chemical abuse/addiction, hostility toward authority figures, or stress at work). It can also be helpful in identifying the potential candidate's ability to be truthful and forthcoming not only during the clinical interview but also in future dealings with the intended parents and medical caregivers.

Although there is no standard test that is used by every program or one that is universally recommended, the most popular measures are the Minnesota Multiphasic Personality Inventory-2 (MMPI-2) and the Personality Assessment Inventory (PAI). The MMPI-2 is the most universally used psychometric test worldwide because it has been translated into fourteen languages, has been used as a clinical instrument since 1939, and has been researched extensively worldwide. The PAI is also a self-administered test that assess personality and psychopathology. Developed in 1991, it measures twenty-two nonoverlapping scales based on constructs that correlate with the DSM. Research previously sited[3,6] indicates that the surrogate/carrier population typically tries to 'fake good' or look their best on

psychological testing resulting in a repression or outright deception. Surrogate/carriers are often in an application process and are trying to present themselves well. Potential candidates who consistently produce invalid profiles are being deceptive – and although the mental health professional may not be able to determine why or about what they are being deceptive, this fact, in and of itself, is/should be an exclusionary criterion.

Additionally helpful in the evaluation of the assessment is consideration of a candidate's social support system, daily living, resources such as transportation and finances, and immediate family. It is standard to interview a candidate's partner, if she has one. It is anticipated that the partner will make many sacrifices during the process and will be thrust into vague and tenuous circumstances. The strength of the marriage/relationship and his or her motivation for supporting the carrier/surrogate should be assessed. Furthermore, her children are of utmost concern. Discovering how a candidate plans to explain the situation can reveal her own understanding of and empathy for her children's perspective and needs. The mental health professional should consider her participation more carefully if her children have endured considerable loss and/or trauma as the surrogacy/carrier experience may rekindle these issues or the children may not be able to handle an additional stressor. Mental health professionals have a responsibility to protect children psychologically, and proceed more cautiously, with additional counseling or testing, if the interview reveals painful histories for the candidate and/or her children. It is important to weight the ethical and psychosocial complications of reproductive technologies on the children who already exist.[22]

Additionally, the potential candidate's cultural and religious circumstances should be factored into the evaluation and addressed with his or her partner. Cultural and religious beliefs are particularly relevant if the arrangement is intrafamilial. In such cases, the carrier/surrogate may have little social support within her usual community and network and it may be the responsibility of the mental health professional to provide support or connect her with some form of social support that will work for her. The role of the intended parents can be of additional importance if the gestational carrier experiences little support and negativity from her family. Religious and cultural beliefs need to be explored fully around the issues of pregnancy termination and pregnancy reduction. Beyond explaining the medical issues, mental health professional need to understand the candidate's way of thinking as it is tied to her religious and moral decision-making process.

Related to culture is the need to understand how comfortable a carrier is with helping a couple from a different culture, race, or religion. Some carriers are attracted to and comfortable with the differences and can manage the potential miscommunications or ambiguities that occur. Their empathy or their ability to be adaptive is high. Other carriers are best served to work with intended parents from their same sociocultural background. Clarity, communication, and predictability are important for overall satisfaction and minimizing anxiety.

A new form of reproductive tourist is the surrogate/carrier who travels to a different country to conceive and/or deliver a child for intended parents. The logistical variables are important to know and consider prior to contracting. The costs of displacing the surrogate/carrier, restrictions of visas, and potential discomfort for the carrier living and being treated in a foreign land are daunting factors. It is important that the carrier have a support system wherever she is. It is also necessary to have be medical professionals available who speak the same language as the carrier. The intended parents or their associates should not be the interpreters and sole managers of the carrier's medical care. Another consideration is the length of time the carrier must commit to remain in the agreed upon country/state/provence. The surrogate/carrier may be asked to be away from her family or be unable to travel to her family for urgent matters while she is pregnant. Given the rate of high-risk pregnancies, travel can be restricted earlier than expected. Intended parents and surrogate/carriers should proceed with caution and be comfortable with backup plans. If there are plans to relocate the carrier or have her travel in the last month of pregnancy to a new locale, all parties should proceed with caution and have a backup plan in case she cannot be relocated or needs to travel on behalf of her own family.

Mental health professionals might consider doing reference checks and/or criminal background investigations of potential candidates. This may be as simple as an Internet Google search or more formal police background check. If there is a history of prior psychological care, it is advisable to obtain a release of information from the candidate and request a copy of counseling/psychiatric records. It may be helpful to have a conversation with the therapist, particularly if the candidate has currently or recently been in treatment. In addition, history of tobacco usage, chemical dependency/addiction, eating disorders, depression, anxiety, and/or obsessive-compulsive disorder especially related to pregnancy or postpartum should be carefully assessed. It is imperative that a candidate be educated about the protocols and problems that she may encounter. The rate of twins and triplets is well known in the IVF population but gestational carriers need to understand that they may be at increased risk of multiples. As such, they should be encouraged to assess their support system, their own health and well-being, and the impact of confinement on their family.

Providing potential gestational carriers with the opportunity to talk with another carrier can be helpful in two ways. The response to that contact can provide additional assessment information for the mental health professional. Also, speaking with another carrier provides a carrier with additional opportunities for education about the complexities of the process. Providing reading material or websites that describe the IVF process further enhances educational and informed consent. Some of the larger programs in the United States provide gestational carrier support group meetings, usually led by a mental health professional. The carriers attend these meetings from the application process through postpartum recovery.

The focus of the assessment interview may differ depending on which program the woman is considering. Women who are IVF gestational carriers may need to be able to manage a burdensome amount of medical information and logistical inconveniences, as well as give themselves injections for months. Furthermore, beliefs about fetal reduction and perspectives on multiple gestation are very germane. On the other hand, interviews with traditional surrogates typically focus on the feelings and fantasies about the genetic birth child. Many surrogates tend to minimize the genetic link she will have to the infant. However, it is important to explore their feelings and expectations, especially as they relate to their own children, the half-siblings of the child whom the intended parents will raise. Additionally, traditional surrogates typically endure more negative feedback and criticism than gestational carriers, who are genetically unrelated to the baby they carry.

Based on research findings and clinical practice, it appears important that a surrogate/carrier achieve something for herself beyond financial remuneration from the experience. It is appropriate to ask about the amount of financial compensation the carrier is receiving and what role that plays in her motivation. Even if altruistic reasons are cited, it is important to explore what she hopes to obtain for herself and whether it is reasonably obtainable. Pregnancy itself is often cited as a motivation: Many women report an attraction to the pregnancy experience. The opportunity to do something important, unique, and life-affirming is often stated. Most candidates express empathy for childless couples and speak about the joy given to them by their own children. When questioned further, these women typically provide a wide range of examples of their volunteerism or giving (e.g., long-term blood donors) because of the sense of pleasure it gives them and/or a feeling of responsibility to 'make the world a better place.' For some women, empathy for the childless couple/intended parents is increased by having had contact with infertile couples and having witnessed the pain and struggle firsthand. A relatively small percentage of candidates are motivated to be a surrogate/carrier because they view it as an act of healing or redoing some traumatic event or issue in their past. Such attempts to 'undo' or 'redo' a piece of their history is typically related to reproductive losses such as abortion, miscarriage, or relinquishment of a child for adoption. It is important to help the candidate with this motivation realistically assess whether her goals are attainable via being a surrogate or gestational carrier. In fact, the experience of being a GC/TS may create further trigger PTSD and/or actually re-create the same experience of loss and trauma albeit through a different avenue, leaving the woman even more confused and distressed as it was not what she expected from the experience.

Related to motivations and goals are a woman's expectations and concerns about her relationship with the intended parents. It is crucial to explore the surrogate/carrier's hopes for contact and need for openness with the couple. A discussion of her wishes surrounding the relationship with the couple and with the future child will reveal many psychodynamics, as well as ensure that she work with a couple with similar wishes and expectations of the relationship. Unrealistic expectations or even fantasies such as using surrogacy to fill an emotional or social void, issues of mistrust, and a lack of clarity about boundaries in general should be carefully assessed. What the potential surrogate/gestational carrier is looking for in the intended parents and how she sees herself in their lives are important issues to address early on in the process. Her fantasies about her role and attachment to the new family are important to explore. Surrogates/gestational carriers and professionals can mistake the intended parents' physical proximity to the carrier as correlating with the parents' willingness to be involved and generous.

Lastly, questions may vary depending as to whether the gestational carrier is already known to the recipients and as to whether the contract is altruistic surrogacy or fee-based surrogacy. A growing number of countries only permit altruistic surrogacy, resulting in more

known gestational carriers arrangements in which the participants have a preexisting relationship, whether family, friends, or acquaintances. The history of the relationship and the anticipated impact on the relationship should be included in the assessment. Furthermore, exploring the various ways the intended parents can assist the surrogate/carrier and her family despite the prohibition on payment is important. Whether or not financial remuneration is part of the equation, it is recommended that the participants agree upon some form of 'gift' or 'ritual' to formally close the chapter on the event and allow all parties to move on without feelings of obligation and/or ingratitude. Additional questioning of the carrier's husband or partner can be helpful in that there may be less incentive for him to be patient with the demanding process, if he feels that his family is not adequately being compensated for the stress, inconvenience, and potential risk. Even in altruistic surrogacy, when there is a prohibition on fee, the issue of money needs to be addressed. Misunderstandings about lost wages, out-of-pocket expenses such as childcare, travel, clothes, and medical bills need to be clarified prior to conception. Table 21.3 lists psychological indications for acceptance or rejection of gestational carriers.

In intrafamily arrangements the counselor should examine not only the stability of family system but the cultural context in which the reproduction arrangement is taking place. The history of this relationship within the family, and the feelings and beliefs about the arrangements with the extended family. The family system's boundaries (particularly boundary violations such as incest), healthy functioning (e.g., family secrets), communication style, and any signs of coercion should be carefully assessed. Additionally, differences in their power relationship are important to discover. Is the surrogate an employee and having a dual relationship with the parents? Is there family history where one member feels pressured to rescue the infertile couple? Does their culture accept and support a greater degree of secrecy than other cultures? Is there a collusion to keep the genetics of the child or even the pregnancy a secret? Is secrecy normative in their culture or does it reflect unresolved issues? A final issue in intrafamilial and known surrogacy is the control of information. Who tells who, what, and when can be a sensitive topic when the lives of intended parents and surrogates/carriers overlap.

Screening the Intended Parents

Psychological screening of prospective parents attempts to assess their general mental health and

TABLE 21.3. Psychological indications for acceptance or rejection of surrogate/gestational carrier

Positive indicators

History of healthy full-term pregnancy

Experience and competence with motherhood

Motivations that reveal obtainable goals

Motivations that reflect empathy

Spousal support if applicable

Stable lifestyle

No major conflicts or transitions in the next two years

Cognitive ability to provide informed consent and conceptualize risks

Absence of psychopathology

History of making successful decisions for herself

Financial stability

Demonstrates tolerance for ambiguous and unclear situations

Able to express concerns and questions

Negative indicators

Poor pregnancy and medical history

Lack of marital/social support

Acute financial need or coercion

Psychopathology

Unrealistic expectations regarding time involved

Significant current stressors or life transitions

Chaotic lifestyle

Impulsivity or high anxiety

Limited cognitive ability

History of antiauthority behavior and rigidity in thinking

Unresolved or untreated history of child or sexual abuse

History of drug/alcohol addiction/abuse

Unresolved issue concerning prior abortion or reproductive loss issues

Lack of empathy

Inability to communicate in her native language with medical professionals

A potentially useful model for the structured clinical interview is the Comprehensive Psychosocial History for Infertility (CPHI; see Appendix 3). This outlines provides content areas that are relevant to the infertile population. It provides information about the marital stress, level of functioning, history, and social support. The structured interview can help the professional reveal areas of concern.

Often, the tool that is most revealing is a full discussion of the issues surrounding surrogacy. It is important to discuss how they came to this choice. Questions should reveal whether or not it is a joint decision, whether the couple's choice is an informed one, and what each spouse believes surrogacy can realistically provide for them. Education is an important part of the assessment. As with a surrogate or carrier, the motivation to choose surrogacy can be either healthy or unhealthy. Most couples choose surrogacy out of a desire to be connected genetically, to participate in the pregnancy, and to know the child's birthmother. In addition, they often wish to avoid failed adoptions and/or the lack of opportunities to adopt in their country or state.

Revealing information also comes from a couple's perception of the surrogate or carrier and their comfort level with contact with her and her family. The intended parents and the gestational carrier have a relationship that lasts thirteen to eighteen months prior to the birth of the child. It is critical that the intended parents have a reasonable degree of resolution about their infertility. The ambiguous process of choosing a surrogate/carrier, the intense and complicated means of conceiving, the long pregnancy, and the years of parenting all require a couple to be comfortable with the process and with their carrier. The couple's capacity to trust and empathize with the carrier can be predictive of the degree of tranquillity during the process and after birth. Conflicts are less likely to be exacerbated if the couple can contain themselves, appropriately cope, seek assistance, and empathize with the carrier's situation. If the intended parents cannot envision themselves having some contact with the surrogate or carrier, then they should not proceed.

marital stability. For the third-party arrangement to be truly successful, it is important that a couple be empathic, adaptive, and resilient. Participants who are overly intrusive or controlling, who are not comfortable with the concept of surrogacy, or who have personality disorders or active mental health disorders, put the surrogate, the program, and ultimately the child, at risk. The ability to trust, contain anxieties, and be generous in spirit serves couples well. The clinical interview should focus on their histories, decision-making processes, coping abilities and strategies, and marital adjustment. Observing how they treat the professionals and other team members can be revealing and predictive of future behavior.

The evaluation and consultation with the intended parents usually includes a discussion of the future and what they may tell the child, as well as what they anticipate telling family and friends. Often, educating the couple about child development and the myths and realities of adoption research are included. The consultation is typically spent sifting through the feelings about openness and imagining future discussions with the child. Encouraging couples to take the time to create a positive legacy for their child helps empower them to act with integrity and clarity.

The assessment of the couple needs to be culturally sensitive. There are cultural differences in perceptions of privacy, pregnancy, gift giving, family ties, parenting, infertility, and revealing feelings. It is helpful to ask the intended parents directly to educate the counselor about religious and cultural differences and assumptions made due to stereotypes. Discussing intended parents' assumptions about the carrier's culture is a proactive step in minimizing hurt feelings and incorrect assumptions. Also, asking about the traditions and medical care surrounding pregnancy in their culture can prevent simple misunderstandings in the future. A discussion of privacy and secrecy needs to be explored as these pertain to cultural differences. Most importantly, differences that are discovered might be discussed with the gestational carrier so to enhance their relationship and minimize hurt feelings.

It is important for the mental health professional and intended parents to understand any legal issues that may impact this arrangement. The intended parents need to understand the legal consequences of returning to their home with a child born through surrogacy. The logistical and legal issue surrounding being a reproductive tourist are important to explore. Policies vary from country to country and even within countries on such issues as whose name is recorded on the birth certificate, having an impact on the infant's legal status and even issues of privacy (disclosure) about the circumstances of the child's birth. For example, in some countries the carrier's name is on the original birth certificate and that certificate is available to the child in adulthood. Within the United States, some states choose not to honor a legal judgment from a different state and will not amend the original birth certificate. Intended parents who work with gestational carriers in other countries might consult with their consulate in the country of birth and work with a professional who has expertise in the field. The intended parents need to plan to be in the birth country for three weeks to obtain certified birth and passports. Immigration, passports, certified birth certificates, and their home country's regulations about registering children once they return are impor-

tant variables in their psychological comfort. The laws of countries, and even within countries, are often being reevaluated and do change, making it important that the mental health professional remain up-to-date to facilitate informed consent.

Intended parents who are traveling to other countries or far from home also need to be educated about the risks and the unknowns of such a venture. Understanding the medical practices and prenatal care of the carrier's home country is helpful and minimizes misunderstandings. It is common for couples undergoing IVF to be in the clinic's city for two weeks prior to embryo transfer, visit the carrier's country at least once during pregnancy, and remain in that country again for a minimum of two weeks after the birth. If children are born prematurely, new parents can be displaced for months. Having a professional interpreter available is not only a necessity in many circumstances, but also may be legally mandated in some areas. If there is a language barrier, discussions of sensitive medical and psychological and legal issues need to be understood, as thoroughly as possible. For reproductive tourists, it is important that the patients as well as the medical team understand any parameters of their visas that may affect medical treatments. Finally, the issue of payment for medical costs of the newborn child needs to be explored prior to conception. There can be confusion on who is to pay for the pediatrician and hospitalization care when the intended parents are not citizens of the country.

If concerns about the intended parents remain, the counselor may be enlightened by second assessment and/or additional psychological testing by a colleague, interviewing spouses separately, or conducting a follow-up interview. It is advisable to have prospective parents speak with other parents and to do some reading to increase their comfort level and informed consent. Most programs also require documentation regarding medical conditions and marital status. Medical teams and commercial agencies often want to confirm that the intended parents are indeed in need of surrogacy, and are not participating for nonmedical reasons such as convenience. A letter from a doctor about the infertility issue combined with a marriage certificate gives some reassurance to the professional team that the intended parents' presentation is accurate. However, it is not a requirement in all countries that intended parents be married to proceed.

The Joint Session

The meeting between the prospective parents and the surrogate/carrier and her husband or partner, if any,

TABLE 21.4. Issues to review prior to conception in joint session

Pregnancy history of gestational carrier

Infertility history of intended parents

Motivations for participation

Reactions of family and friends

Children of carrier and intended parents existing children, if any

Prenatal care preferences

Prenatal diagnostic testing

Belief and concerns about multipregnancy reduction

Beliefs and concerns about pregnancy termination for fetal anomaly

Contact between the two families during the pregnancy

Contact between the two families after the birth

Preferences regarding delivery and hospital stay

Exploration of religious and cultural differences

Confidentiality concerns

Management of financial issues

Coverage of maternity care costs and for the child's medical care after birth

Legal process for transfer of parentage

Fears about and wishes for their experience with surrogacy

provides a fruitful opportunity to identify any contraindications prior to going forward. It is imperative that the surrogate/carrier candidate and her husband meet both intended parents. Meeting is important both legally and psychologically. Prior to conception, the infertility counselor can facilitate an exchange of information that protects both parties, as well as the counselor. Table 21.4 describes issues to be reviewed in this session. For example, it is helpful to exchange what motivated each participant to pursue surrogacy or become a gestational carrier. It is helpful for the surrogate/carrier to share her motivations, reactions of her children and family, and her concerns about any possible negative effects. The intended parents should share their histories, their families' reactions, and what their day-to-day life is like, so as to build a connection and provide the surrogate/carrier with information for making her decision. The two parties' experience can be enhanced and facilitated when encouraged to educate each other about any cultural differences especially as they relate to privacy, pregnancy, and prenatal care.

Medically, the joint session includes a review of the surrogate/carrier's pregnancy history and general health. It is helpful to provide the opportunity for the participants to discuss concerns about prenatal care (e.g., diet, lifestyle, caffeine, and travel). Even among family members, there are different beliefs about what affects prenatal development and an agreement should

be reached that all parties understand and will abide by. Of particular importance are medical issues such as attending physician, hospital care, prenatal testing, and what to do in the event there are negative pregnancy outcomes (e.g., miscarriage, diagnosis of a fetal anomaly, and multiples). This discussion should include not only 'what do we agree we will do,' but also how the information should be communicated among each other and by medical caregivers. It is not uncommon for intended parents with a history of painful losses to be vigilant (even hypervigilant), especially about medical care. A review of how and with whom both parties should receive medical information is important. The dissemination of information is different during the IVF cycle when the infertile couple is a patient than during the later stages of pregnancy when just the carrier is the patient. Medical insurance issues can be complicated and should be reviewed very carefully. Lastly, a legal contract in which each party is represented by separate legal counsel is paramount. Issues addressed in the contract such as reimbursement arrangements, bed rest, premature labor or delivery, multiples, and miscarriage should be reviewed during the joint sessions, again with an emphasis on communication and agreement on ways of interacting with each other.

The discussion of fetal reduction and pregnancy termination dilemmas is critical as the ethical, moral, and medical dilemmas are weighty. Although not all participants will be able to predict exactly how they will deal with these issues, it is important that the participants consider them and are clear on the decision-making process and have a final agreement. They need to have similar approaches regarding how such difficult decisions will be made.

In surrogacy, almost every issue has a psychological component. A consulting mental health professional needs to raise the topic of finances. Financial issues are important even if the arrangement is altruistic surrogacy or intrafamilial surrogacy. The organizing of financial matters reduces the potential for anger and disappointment. The goal is to minimize discussion of and confusion about money; lost wages, out-of-pocket costs; and so on. Power struggles can be avoided if an objective liaison is used and if each party feels secure in the other's integrity and respect. Again, the intended parents and gestational carrier need to understand the laws regarding financial issues. In many countries and in some parts of the United States, carriers are not allowed to receive any financial compensation, but can receive expense reimbursements.

A joint session should also include a walk-through of the relationship that each participant envisions. As previously discussed, clients' assumptions about the role of openness are ongoing issues. The desire for contact is part of the criteria on which they choose to work together. It is sad, stressful, and hurtful when two families have dramatically different agendas. Surrogate/carriers most often need to see the intended parents responding like parents throughout the pregnancy. Their reward and comfort with relinquishing the baby are significantly increased if they know that the intended parents are eagerly preparing for the baby and are interested in the carrier's well-being as well as her baby's. Achieving some clarity about contact during and after the delivery prevents psychological stress and harm. As discussed earlier, postbirth research on surrogates conclude and Simmon's research on organ donation would support benefit of surrogates seeing and/or hearing about the happiness to which they have contributed. Even within family arrangements, there can be different assumptions about the wish for involvement before and after birth. Contact after the birth has historically been confusing to participants because of the incorrect application of adoption myths. The mental health professional can help by providing structure and definition in the relationship before and after birth. Addressing participants' concerns or assumptions about how the other party feels can help to reduce ambiguities and misinterpretations of the others' behavior. It is advisable for the parties to have professional guidance prior to delivery. Issues related to the transfer of the child, decision making at the hospital, and how to say goodbye, that is, respect for closure and specifics about postbirth contact, should be addressed.

There can be special issues around the relationship when couples seek medical care outside of their own country. With the addition of email to our means of communication, the ability to communicate with other countries has become easier for patients. It is not uncommon for intended parents and gestational carriers/surrogates to email and text-message via mobile telephones frequently so as to maximize the involvement each of the parties feels in the process. The reproductive tourist will need to spend a long period of time in the country of birth that provides opportunities for both parties to share meaningful times, doctor visits, and learn about each other's cultures. Sharing of books

and items unique to each other's countries can enhance the comfort and satisfaction of their experiences. Educating each other and becoming culturally aware and sensitive can actually add to the positive nature of the experience.

Lastly, there needs to be a discussion about the surrogate/carrier's children. Are the intended parents willing to spend time with the surrogate/carrier's children, if that is something the surrogate/carrier and her spouse want? What will her children be told about this unique pregnancy? Does the surrogate/carrier anticipate any difficulties with family members or within her social network? If the intended parents already have a child, it is important to address these same questions. It is commonly recommended that the surrogate's children meet the intended parents, visit with the parents shortly after birth, and participate in some closure so as to minimize any confusion or anxiety about their mother or the new baby.

Guidance should be provided regarding future issues with the intended child, even though the issues may remain ambiguous, evolving, and hard to predict. Will the child be told about the unique circumstances of his or her birth? How will the role of the surrogate/carrier be explained? Will the parents permit contact with the surrogate/carrier if the child desires it? Will the surrogate/carrier allow contact if the child desires it? How will the adults ensure that there is an exchange of medical information as needed? What are each person's fears and concerns about the future? Are there issues regarding contact with extended family, that is, grandparents who wish to meet the carrier? A discussion of possible actions that might minimize long-term issues is useful. These actions may include, for example, writing keepsake letters, assigning an intermediary for contact or emergency issues, and documentation of history. Of course, the critical variable for the child's long-term well-being is likely to be the degree of respect, warmth, and integrity between the two families.

On a final note, in this emotional and pioneering field of infertility counseling, mental health professionals should consider serving only clients with whom they feel comfortable and qualified to assist. It is appropriate and ethical to refer cases to another professional if the decisions to be faced or the personalities involved do not appear to be ones that can be confidentially treated. Furthermore, simply because an individual or couple presents with a reproductive plan that they have developed with or without medical assistance, does not mean that you are required to facilitate this plan – even though this may be the client's expectation. A final means of protection for professionals is to receive consultation on a case and document that they have done so. It is in everyone's best interest to be informed about the legal issues and the profession's code of ethics.

FUTURE IMPLICATIONS

Third-party reproduction, including surrogacy and gestational carrying, is here to stay. The number of surrogate/carrier pregnancies increases each year. The future of third-party reproduction really means the future face of these new blended families. With the increase of options for family-building, there is an increase in the ways in which siblings come to their parents. One family can have children who are homemade, adopted, created by gamete donation, and/or born to a gestational carrier. There are a growing number of families that have three children, each having had a different manner of conception and gestation. These new, blended families will be the source of helpful information, while simultaneously challenging the traditional definition of family and family bonds and, no doubt, presenting new and unique family systems dynamics and challenges.

Related to this issue is the increasing number of children born with four or five adults involved in bringing the child to fruition. Now that physicians can intervene at each step of conception, infertile couples and physicians can find reproductive helpers to serve each separate step. New questions have risen about the process in which an oocyte donor and/or a sperm donor are used and the resulting embryo is implanted into a gestational carrier. The carrier relinquishes the baby to the contracting couple who are the intended parents. The birth of children involving three women – an oocyte donor, a gestational carrier, and the contracting mother – has increased significantly since 1994. Furthermore, some centers report several families having been created by oocyte donor, sperm donor, and gestational carrier, resulting in a child that has no genetic connection to the contracting couple who become the child's parents. Deliberations about these new multidonor conceptions are ongoing and are certain to be taking center stage.

There are also implications and trends given that reproductive technologies are worldwide and access to communities outside of one's own has been made easier by travel, media, and the Internet. For example, it was in 1990 that a British couple had their frozen embryos brought to the United States for transfer into an American gestational carrier with whom they had contracted. Frozen embryos can be created in one country under that country's guidelines and medical costs and then shipped by courier to another country where surrogacy is more abundant. Sometimes this allows an infertile couple to save expenses and pursue a family despite their own country's regulations. The international collaboration for reproductive options has expanded, creating unusual possibilities for blended families. For example, imagine an older Asian couple adopting the remaining frozen embryos of an American couple to implant them into a surrogate who does not speak their language and who grapples with their vast religious differences. Or imagine two gay couples from Europe, who worked with the same oocyte donor and whose surrogate mothers are close friends, have children living in the same community that are genetically related with similar histories. Or imagine a Latin mother and her Asian husband celebrating the birth of their twins with the help of an African American gestational carrier.

One result of the implantation of donor embryos into a gestational carrier is the extension of the possible age of the intended mother. If the intended mother is not donating the oocyte and is not carrying the child, her age becomes a social or legal issue, not a reproductive limitation. The age of parents is an ongoing controversy in clinics and society. Counselors and gestational carriers need to address the concerns they have about more mature parents' health, stability, support system, society's ambivalence, and their own comfort level. Many IVF centers and some countries have guidelines. However, in the United States, it is often left up to the individual physician and attending counselor to provide counsel and consent for parents in their fifties who are contracting with donors and carriers who most often are under thirty-five years.

A correlate to the issue of oocyte donor embryos being implanted into gestational carriers is the increasing concern about multiple gestation. In traditional surrogacy, there is no greater medically significantly risk of multiples than the world of homemade babies. However, with IVF and now IVF with young donor oocytes, there is a significant increase in gestational carriers conceiving twins, triplets, or more. The implication of young mothers conceiving high-risk pregnancies at the hands of IVF clinics on behalf of infertile couples (who may wish an 'instant family') certainly raises concerns of exploitation and poor judgment among participants. The new forms of conception and resulting multiple pregnancy can intensify tensions surrounding prenatal care, decision making, and medical insurance. Regulations concerning the number of embryos that a physician can implant into a patient vary among countries, often affected by the influence of religious beliefs, of socialized medicine, and politics.

Lastly, there are certain to be new legal test cases and an ongoing debate about the definition of *mother* and *father*. As the number of surrogate/carrier arrangements grow with various combinations of gamete donation, it is certain that legislators, judges, and governments will become increasingly involved in defining *family* and family relationships.

SUMMARY POINTS

■ It is important for all participants involved in third-party reproduction to have legal, medical, and psychological consultations.

■ Empathy and integrity are key personality traits in the screening of surrogates, gestational carriers, and intended parents.

■ The positive adjustment of all parties and the tranquility of the case can be increased if the participants are well-matched and invest in preconception discussions.

■ Mental health professionals should encourage participants to clearly define the relationship through legal agreements and counseling sessions. When disagreements arise, they should not expect medical personnel to mediate them, but instead address them with the mental health professional.

■ The paucity of research highlights the need for all professionals to proceed cautiously in this new and ever-changing field.

■ Mental health professionals providing evaluations and counseling services for surrogacy and gestational carrier arrangements tend to play several roles: (1) determining what is best for all of the parties involved, including the existing children; (2) predicting human behavior in a field where the well-being of children and family are at stake; and (3) foreseeing the range of problems that occur in third-party reproduction and pregnancy and to apply these to the unique circumstances of the person's life.

■ The inevitable common problems usually fall within three categories: (1) struggles with Mother Nature, (2) struggles with the relationship, and (3) struggles with logistical surprises.

■ Despite initial hesitation due to religious and cultural concerns, gestational surrogacy has expanded across the globe and is here to stay.

REFERENCES

1. Synesiou K. *Personal conversation*. Encino, CA. 12 February, 2005.
2. Franks D. Psychiatric evaluation of women in a surrogate mother program. *Am J Psychiatry* 1981; 138:1378–9.
3. Parker JP. Motivation of surrogate mothers: Initial findings. *Am J Psychiatry* 1983; 140:117.
4. Reame N, Parker JP. Surrogate parenting: Clinical features of forty-four cases. *Am J Obstet Gynecol* 1990; 162: 1220–5.
5. Mechanick-Braverman A, Corson SL. Characteristics of participants in a gestational carrier program. *J Assist Reprod Genet* 1992; 9:353–7.
6. Hanafin H. *The Surrogate Mother: An Exploratory Study*. Dissertation. Los Angeles, CA: California School of Professional Psychology, 1984.
7. Resnick R. *Surrogate Mothers: Relationship between Early Attachment and the Relinquishment of the Child*. Dissertation. Santa Barbara, CA: Fielding Institute, 1989.
8. Blyth E. I wanted to be interesting. I wanted to be able to say "I've done something interesting with my life": Interviews with surrogate mothers in Britain. *Journal of Reproductive and Infant Psychology* 1994; 12:189.
9. Hanafin H. *Surrogate Parenting: Reassessing Human Bonding*. Paper presented at the American Psychological Association Conference, New York: NY, 1987.
10. Ciccarelli J. *The Surrogate Mother: Post-birth Follow-up*. Dissertation. Los Angeles, CA: California School of Professional Psychology, 1997.
11. Jadva V, Murray C, Lycett E, et al. Surrogacy: The experiences of surrogate mothers. *Hum Reprod* 2003 Oct; 18:2196–204.
12. Reame N, Hanafin H, Kalfoglow A. Unintended consequences and informed consent; lessons from former surrogate mothers. *Hum Reprod* 1999; 14:361–2.
13. MacCullum F, Lycett E, Murray C, et al. Surrogacy: The experience of the commissioning couples. *Hum Reprod* 2003 June; 18:1334–42.
14. Golombok S, Murray C, Jadva V, et al. Families created through surrogacy arrangements: Parent–child relationships in the 1st year of life. *Developmental Psychology* 2004 May; 40:400–11.
15. Freud, A. *The Ego and the Mechanisms of Defense*, Rev. Ed. Madison, CT: International Universities Press, 1936/2000 ed.
16. Simmons RG, Klein SD, Simmons RI. *Gift of Life: The Social and Psychological Impact of Organ Transplantation*. New York: Wiley, 1977.
17. Jefferson F. *Culture and Therapy: An Integrative Approach*. Northvale, NJ: Jason Aronson, 1966; 21–20.
18. Mental Health Professional Group of the American Society for Reproductive Medicine. *Guidelines for the evaluation of gestational carriers*. 2000 [Appendix 7].
19. Shenfield F, Pennings G, Cohen J. et al. ESHRE Task Force on Ethics and Law 10: Surrogacy. *Hum Reprod* 2005; 10:2705–7.
20. Herbert M, Chenier NM, Norris S. Bill C-6: Assisted Human Reproduction Act. Statues of Canada. Library of Parliament, 2004.
21. American Society for Reproductive Medicine. Ethics Committee. Family members as gamete donors and surrogates. *Fertil Steril* 2003; 80:1124–30.
22. American Society for Reproductive Medicine. Ethics Committee. Child-rearing ability and the provision of fertility services. *Fertil Steril* 2004; 82:564–7.

22 Adoption after Infertility

LINDA P. SALZER

I did not plant you, true. But when the season is done –
Then I will hold you high, a shining sheaf above the boughs
and seeds grown wild. Not my planting, but by heaven my
harvest – my own child.

– Carol Lynn Pearson

Adoption is a form of family-building that is a fundamental component of human relationships. At its most basic level, adoption provides children needing parents with homes, while also providing parenting opportunities for adults desiring children. Since antiquity, across continents and cultures, adoption has ensured the survival of at-risk children, improved the quality of life for individuals and couples, created satisfying family relationships, and contributed to societal stability, although often with some measure of psychosocial adjustment, expense, and even sacrifice.

Infertility is a primary motivating factor in the decision to adopt a child.[1,2]. While infertility is universally experienced as a crisis, cultural norms and values have a significant impact on which remedies childless couples consider acceptable to solve involuntary childlessness. Solutions tend to fall into three categories: (1) medical interventions, (2) prayer or spiritual interventions, and (3) realignment of social relationships.[3] However, across all cultures, the realignment of social relationships is often the last or least acceptable alternative. Rosenblatt points out, "... it is 'human' to be concerned about childlessness, that concern with a product of our particular culture and level of technology.... People pray, or take drugs, or cast spells... before they try to change social relationships by adding a spouse, ending a marital relationship or quasimarital relationship, or adopting or fostering."[3, p. 2] Adoption is a means of realigning relationships, whatever form it involves, including intrafamilial, domestic, international, and/or transracial. Because the realignment of social relationships comes at great psychosocial cost, there is now a greater awareness of the emotional effects of adoption on birthparents, adoptive parents, and adoptees. It is emotionally and socially difficult for humans to create new attachments, sever old ties, and move outside traditional social norms or customs. Whereas many forms of adoption have historically been cloaked in secrecy and shame (particularly for birthparents), adoption practices now encourage a more collaborative arrangement among the participants, further acknowledging the challenges of social realignment.

This chapter addresses adoption from the perspective of infertility and the role of the infertility counselor in helping couples and individuals with this process. As such, some forms of adoption that are less frequently motivated by infertility (e.g., intergenerational and/or intrafamilial adoption) will be discussed only as they pertain to infertility. This chapter includes:

■ an historical overview of adoption;
■ a theoretical understanding of adoption, changing psychological perspectives, and the developmental tasks of adoptive families;
■ the different types of adoption options available today and the growing complexity of adoption;
■ common fears and psychological concerns regarding adoption among infertile couples, including the need to address unresolved infertility issues;
■ therapeutic stages that infertile couples undergo in considering adoption as an option and how infertility counselors can assist prospective adoptive parents in making decisions.

HISTORICAL OVERVIEW

Prehistoric and primitive people knew little about reproduction and, as a result, children were valued as part of the kinship group, offering potential labor, caregiving of elders, and survival of the tribe. With the onset of monogamous heterosexual relationships, the role and importance of children became complex as they became valued as progeny, property (particularly in patriarchal societies), or for spiritual purposes. Historically, children were adopted because they were orphaned or relinquished by their birthparents because of age, marital status, illness, and/or poverty. Adoptive parents were motivated by involuntary childlessness, social savior desires, or the need for children as laborers or religious legacies. Nevertheless, adoption was often equated with significant social stigma. It represented public shame and embarrassment related to sexuality, exemplified by a failure to fulfill proper social roles, and was generally different from the norm. Birthparents were viewed as sexually promiscuous or irresponsible, while infertile couples were considered to be reproductive failures. Adoptees were often viewed as a second choice by their adoptive parents (or the community) or seen as the embodiment of their birthparents' sexual misbehavior, bearing the shame of illegitimacy and/or abandonment. While attitudes toward adoption have dramatically changed, particularly in the nineteenth and twentieth centuries, the social stigma of adoption remains in many cultures and countries to varying degrees even today.[4,5]

During the nineteenth century, adoption was affected by extraordinary migrations from Europe, particularly to North America and Australia, often leaving large numbers of orphaned children. Poverty and disease added to this orphaned population. Homeless children or those residing in poorhouses were often taken advantage of by being pushed into child labor situations. This was frequently done with the belief that these children were being rescued from their unfortunate lives. In Australia, aboriginal children were taken from their families in an attempt to be saved by giving them training to become house servants. A similar practice occurred in the United States where American Indian children were placed in orphanages and forced to speak English in a concerted social effort to eliminate their traditional culture and adopt Western ways.

During the twentieth century, a variety of global wars triggered waves of international adoptions. Most notably were the initial transracial adoptions of Chinese infants, spearheaded by American author Pearl S. Buck and others who were determined advocates for homeless children in China and other Asian countries. Buck founded Welcome Home, the first international transracial adoption agency in the United States, arguing persuasively that race should not be a factor in finding homes for children.[6] A dramatic increase in international adoptions began after World War II, primarily as a North American philanthropic response to the plight of thousands of orphaned European children left homeless by the war. Although these were international adoptions, they were not, for the most part, transracial adoptions. The transracial international adoption movement became more extensive after the Korean War (1950–53) and the Vietnam War (1964–75), which precipitated an increase in international adoptions throughout the world.[7] In addition, pervasive poverty and social chaos led to greater numbers of children being adopted from the former Soviet Union, Latin America, and Eastern Europe at the end of the twentieth century.[8]

The adoption policies of every country are determined by its history, culture, governmental policy, socioeconomic status, and changing politics. China is a prime example. When China instituted its one-child-per-family policy, its goal was to lessen population growth. One result, however, has been the abandonment of baby girls who were considered less desirable than male heirs. With the overcrowding of orphanages, the Chinese government began to facilitate the adoption of these children beginning in 1992. Another example is Romania, which attempted to increase its population through measures that banned abortion and promoted pregnancy. This country also found a growing number of abandoned babies who could not be cared for due to poverty and inadequate social and medical resources. These children were increasingly institutionalized.[9] In Guatemala, where more than half of the population is rural and relies on subsistence farming, the fertility rate ranks near the top of all Latin American countries. As a result, birthmothers often place their infants for adoption shortly after birth for both social and economic reasons.[10]

Adoption laws were established in North America, Australia, and Great Britain during the 1920s (nationally or by states or provinces) with the goal of establishing adoption as a legitimate social practice; developing specific clear regulations; and preventing the abuse of children and protecting their rights. The basis for these laws was a belief that removing a child from a poverty-stricken environment or negative social surroundings and giving him or her a position in proper society was an act of salvation. At that time, attitudes toward sexuality, especially involving young unwed mothers, were harsh and moralistic. Birthmothers rarely had the opportunity to keep their child and abortion was virtually impossible. More emphasis was placed on the rights of the adoptive parents than on the best interests of the child during this time.[11] In recent years, there has been a shift to a stronger child welfare focus in most Western countries.

Over time, what began primarily as a philanthropic movement to adopt internationally shifted to more personal reasons for such adoptions. This was motivated, in large part, by the needs of childless couples as the availability of children for domestic adoption declined. While kinship (including step-parent and skipped-generation adoptions), independent, and agency adoptions previously accounted for the vast majority of adoption placements in the United States, international adoption became more popular – and more feasible. Fewer children were available for domestic adoption (particularly in developed countries) due to lower fertility rates, access to legalized birth control and abortion, decisions to delay marriage and conception, increased independence and autonomy for women, and a growing social acceptance of single parenthood – all contributing to an increase in international adoption.[12] Furthermore, some prospective adoptive parents (e.g., older, single, or homosexual) found it difficult to adopt in their home country and others were uncomfortable with the increasing preference by birthparents, particularly in the United States, for open adoption placements.[4]

In addition to historical changes in the process and types of adoption, there have been significant changes in the attitudes toward adoption, particularly in Western or developed countries. The 1950s saw the beginnings of a movement away from adoption as a social stigma, where issues were handled in shame and secrecy, toward a more open, accepting attitude. This coincided with a greater awareness and understanding of the psychosocial needs of birthparents, adoptive parents, and adoptees. Adoption, which traditionally involved the domestic adoption of infants at birth, typically had been anonymous, closed placements with little exchange of information between birthparents and adoptive parents – often leaving adoptees uninformed of their adopted status. Birthmothers were expected to forget the birth of their child and move on with their lives, while adoptive parents were similarly encouraged to forget their infertility. Adoptive parents were often unaware of the significance of birthparents in their children's lives or reluctant to acknowledge their impact. Adoption, for all parties, frequently became a family secret with the potential for psychologically traumatic consequences.

Although, historically, social stigma was a motivation for secrecy, many believed that these practices were truly in the best interests of the child, adoptive parents, and/or birthparents. Early works by Paton in the 1950s and Triseliotis in the 1970s emphasized the psychosocial importance for adult adoptees of information on their biological origins.[11] These works significantly affected legal reform in several countries, offering open access to birth certificates for adult adoptees, and set

a precedent for legislation in Australia, Canada, and some states in the United States. As a result, there is greater awareness in many Western countries that adoption is a process in which the needs and interests of all participants must be acknowledged and balanced. Today, birthparents are increasingly viewed as interested and relevant parties in the adoption process, and are more likely to be active participants in the adoption plan. Adoptive parents have become more aware of the importance of information about their child's heritage and are more interested in meeting with or communicating with birthparents. Adoptees are less likely to experience adoption as a socially stigmatizing part of their heritage and are more likely to benefit from greater social acceptance and access to information about their birthparents and heritage. Although there are many levels of openness in adoption today, adoption is more likely to be seen as a positive collaborative family-building process.[13]

Greater world attention to adoption issues and the rights of children is also evidenced by The Hague Convention of May 29, 1993, on the Protection of Children and Cooperation in Respect of Intercountry Adoption.[14] This convention was based on the United Nations Convention of 1989 on the Rights of the Child that resulted in the establishment of the UNICEF International Child Development Centre in 1999. The UN Convention established definitions and categories of adoption: *domestic* (also referred to as in-country or national), *intercountry*, and *international*. Domestic adoption involves a child and adoptive parents of the same nationality and the same country of residence. *Intercountry* adoption involves a change in the child's country of residence (birth country), regardless of the adoptive parents' nationality. *International* adoption involves parents whose nationality differs from the adopted child, regardless of the parents' country of residence. The purpose of The Hague Convention was to: (1) prevent abuse, such as abduction or sale of children; (2) regulate standards for legal consent of an adoption; (3) set standards for a child's move to a new country; and (4) establish the status of the adopted child in the country of placement. It notes that intercountry/international adoption may be considered only if there is no suitable alternative for the child in his or her country of origin. Furthermore, by setting principles, providing standards and safeguards, and creating a network of cooperating institutions, it has provided the impetus for looking at adoption (particularly intercountry/international adoption) in new ways. For simplicity, in this chapter, the term *domestic adoption* will be used to refer to in-country or national adoption and the term *international adoption* will describe issues related to both intercountry and international adoptions.[14]

REVIEW OF LITERATURE

There is extensive research on multifaceted aspects of adoption. For the purposes of this review, literature has been grouped into four areas: adoptive parent adjustment, adoptee adjustment, openness in adoption, and issues related to transracial and international adoption.

Adjustment to Adoptive Parenthood by Infertile Couples

Recognizing that the transition to parenthood is markedly different for adoptive and biological parents, several authors have investigated the unique challenges, stresses, and potential conflicts that can impact the path to adoption.[15–17] In that most adoptive parents have been infertile with a history of significant loss, various factors have been identified as potentially influential in their adjustment to adoptive parenthood. These factors include years of medical treatment, psychological disappointments, narcissistic injury, and marital conflict, as well as unresolved feelings about these issues, all of which can have an impact on adoptive parenting skills and, by extension, the development of the adopted child.[15–20] It has been suggested that the adjustment of infertile couples to adoptive parenthood may be influenced by both negative factors (stigma; ignorance; racism; or cultural kinship beliefs) and positive factors (purposeful and positive attitudes toward parenthood; more extensive education and preparation; greater maturity and economic resources; or marital stability).[16,17,21,22] Researchers have speculated that additional factors affecting this transition to adoption include the time elapsed between diagnosis of infertility and the adoption of a child; the coping mechanisms used by adoptive parents during infertility; and feelings of deprivation – defined as the adoptive parents' sense of loss owing to their infertility.[15,18,20] Although these are valid considerations in understanding the effects of infertility upon adoption, much of this work involved theoretical constructs based on clinical experience, not research-based evidence.

In a short-term longitudinal study that investigated the transition to parenthood, Levy-Shiff and colleagues explored preadoption/prenatal parental expectations and postadoption/postnatal parental experiences in 104 Israeli couples who were first-time adoptive and biological parents. The researchers used questionnaires and interviews to investigate the extent to which individual and contextual antecedents in the expectancy period predicted parental experiences when the infants were four months old. The researchers found that the transition to parenthood in biological and adoptive families differed markedly. Adoptive parents expressed more positive expectations about parenthood and reported more satisfying experiences in their transition to parenthood than did biological parents. Predictors of parental experiences were found to be: (1) parental expectations and depressive mood for both groups; (2) ego-strength for the biological parents group; and (3) feelings of deprivation, social support, and self-concept for the adoptive parents. These researchers found that the high level of adjustment in the adoptive parents to their parental role did not support the view that difficulties surrounding the adoption process handicap adoptive parents' experiences. They suggest that preparenthood deprivations may increase the rewards and gratifications associated with parenthood. The increased age (and thereby maturity) of the adoptive parents may also make them more resourceful and better equipped to adapt to the stresses of parenthood.[17]

Psychosocial Adjustment of Adoptees

The long-term psychological adjustment of adoptees is an area that is increasingly receiving research attention. Most early studies were not longitudinal and generally focused on confidential (also known as closed) adoptions, that is, no contact between birth and adoptive families and no identifying information. Research in recent years has broadened to include more emphasis on open adoptions, the study of children's development over time, and the effects of early deprivation, loss, or maltreatment. A 1994 study[23] involving 715 adoptive families found that adolescents adopted in infancy were no more likely to suffer from mental health or identity problems than nonadopted teenagers. Many others, however, have found that adopted children are overrepresented in the mental health system.[24–27] In a review of the research literature, Brodzinsky reported that, in general, adoptees are at an increased risk for various behavioral, psychological, and academic problems compared with a nonadopted population. Despite these risk factors, however, most adoptees do exhibit normal adjustment.[25] Brodzinsky notes that adoption has a lifelong impact and that it will be a factor at every point of the child's development.[26] A number of studies have indicated that "as the placement age increases, so does the risk for psychological problems, substance abuse and behavioral/educational problems. . . . Children who have spent years in orphanages, who have experienced early deprivation, lack of stimulation, multiple/inconsistent caretakers, and separation from siblings are at risk.... Prenatal exposure to drugs or alcohol, as well as poor maternal care, are often critical challenges to the long-term outcomes for adoptees."[27, p. 41]

A longitudinal study of 190 adopted families in the United States, from 1987–2000, found that compatibility within the family was a key factor in the psychosocial adjustment of adoptees.[28] The researchers found that "when the study children were in middle childhood, the strongest predictor of problematic adjustment outcomes (internalizing and externalizing) was the parent's perception of the child's incompatibility with the family" and that "the higher degrees of perceived compatibility maintained from middle childhood to adolescence were associated with higher degrees of psychosocial engagement (defined as adolescents' active use of inner resources to interact positively with others in family, peer, and community contexts) and attachment to parents and lower problem behavior."[28]

Recent studies indicate that adopted children are at increased risk for learning and attentional problems. In a 1991 study of 7,194 special education students in the United States who had been classified as being neurologically impaired, perceptually impaired, or emotionally disturbed, it was found that adoptees were overrepresented in these groups. They accounted for three to four times the number that one would expect given the percentage of adoptees in the general population.[29] Brodzinsky notes that "since the rate of learning disabilities is roughly 5–15% of the school-aged population, adoptees may be at a rather high risk of running into some sort of a problem in school."[26] The Attention Deficit Disorder/Attention Deficit Hyperactivity Disorder (ADD/ADHD) rate in the general school population is estimated at 3–7%, while rates for adopted children are reported at approximately 20%.[30] All of these learning/attentional difficulties may be due to hereditary factors, poor prenatal care (including prenatal maternal drug or alcohol use), complications during pregnancy or delivery, or adverse conditions during infancy and early childhood. Recent research indicates that, for all children, early trauma and deprivation will affect brain development. This research implies that environment has a more significant influence on the development of a child's brain than was previously thought.[31]

Openness in Adoption

Some of the earliest research on adult adoptees was completed by Paton, who found that adoptees are in need of information regarding their biological past

and recommended the use of contact registries and legislative reform regarding openness.[32] A later study explored the long-term effects of adoption by means of extensive interviews with all members of the adoption triad. The findings suggested the need to open records for adult adoptees and recommended that agencies reevaluate their practice of sealing birth records.[33]

A significant project in this field has been a longitudinal study investigating the long-term effects of openness for all members of the adoption triad. The study, originally conducted from 1987–1992, involved 190 adoptive fathers, 190 adoptive mothers, 171 adopted children, and 169 birthmothers. It investigated four sets of issues, including variations in openness; the relationships between birth and adoptive parents; the relationship between the children's participation in openness and their adjustment to and understanding of adoption; and the adjustment of birthmothers, as affected by level of openness. Results included the following: (1) in those families with fully disclosed adoptions, there seemed to be no fear on the part of the adoptive parents that birthparents would try to reclaim their child or interfere with their family; (2) openness did not affect the adoptive parents' ability to establish a sense of entitlement; and (3) openness did not guarantee that birthmothers would successfully resolve their grief.[34]

Subsequently, a summary of this research on open adoption reported generally positive outcome for adoptees, adoptive parents, and birthparents. It was noted that children who remained in contact with their birthparents had a better understanding of adoption and showed more positive socioemotional development. In this summary, it was also concluded that birthmothers in open adoption were better able to resolve their loss than those having no contact with the adopted family.[35] Based on this ongoing study, the researchers noted recently that there is no single form of adoptive arrangement that is the best for everyone and that levels of openness can change over time. As a result, an important task of the counselor is to educate all members of the triad to expect and prepare for change throughout the adoption experience.[36]

Transracial and International Adoption

With the dramatic increase in international adoptions, greater attention has been devoted to how adopted children come to terms with issues related to transracial and/or international adoption and how they develop a cohesive personal identity. An overrepresentation of adopted children in mental health treatment has been attributed to a number of factors including: the trauma of adoption; maltreatment or neglect prior to adoption; preexisting medical conditions (e.g., fetal alcohol syndrome); attachment disorders; and learning disabilities due to institutionalization and/or prenatal conditions.[26,37–41]

Many studies have noted the effects of early adverse experiences on the later adjustment of the adopted child. In a study of eighty children adopted in The Netherlands from Romania, researchers found that 20% of the adoptees met the criteria for post-traumatic stress disorder (PTSD–Type I and II). Type I PTSD was attributed to the adoption process itself, in that the child was separated from his or her biological mother or family. This trauma has been referred to as adopted child pathology[42] or adoption syndrome and cumulative adoption trauma.[43] Type II PTSD was attributed to violence; physical, sexual, and/or emotional abuse; or malnutrition, all of which may contribute to constant feelings of fear, insecurity, hypervigilance, and abandonment. This has been referred to as a postinstitutionalized syndrome.[44] Hoksbergen and colleagues found that the two groups did not differ with respect to gender, age, or health on arrival, physical development, family composition, and length of stay in the placement country (The Netherlands). They concluded that whether the adoptees suffered from Type I or II PTSD, they required immediate postplacement aftercare by professional counselors for an extended period of time. Although these researchers specifically investigated children coming from Romanian institutions, their observations suggest immediate assessment at time of placement for all children arriving from institutions and the offer of professional counseling to adoptive parents and their children.[45]

A Dutch longitudinal adoption study, initially completed in 1986–1987 and 1990, investigated the prevalence and developmental course of problem behaviors in a sample of 1,538 adopted and nonadopted adolescents. Results showed a higher rate of problem behaviors for adoptees than nonadopted children, as determined by both parent and self-reports. There were a substantial number of children who became increasingly maladjusted over the three-year study and it was noted that adolescence may be a time of increased vulnerability for adoptees. Despite these problems, the study concluded that the majority of adopted children were functioning well as adolescents.[46] This study was later extended to an investigation of young international adult adoptees (72.5% of the original sample) and nonadopted young adults (78.1% of the original sample). Results showed that the adoptees were 1.52 times as likely to exhibit an anxiety disorder as the nonadopted young adults, 2.05 times as likely to have

a problem with substance abuse or dependence, and, for adopted males, 3.76 times as likely to have a mood disorder.[47]

A 1992 study in The Netherlands investigated 2,148 international adoptees (aged 10–15 years) to assess the impact of early adverse experiences on later adjustment. It was found that early neglect, abuse, and a history of multiple caretakers increased the risk of later maladjustment. These researchers found that the age of a child at time of placement for adoption was not significant, in and of itself. However, the older a child was at the time of placement, the greater the likelihood that he or she had experienced trauma or adversity prior to adoptive placement.[48]

A 2005 meta-analysis in The Netherlands addressed just these issues by comparing international with domestic adoptions, as well as a control group of nonadoptees, to determine the effects of international adoption on behavioral problems and mental health referrals. Researchers examined adoption studies dating from 1950 to 2005 throughout the world (not limited to English-language publications). As in previous research, they found that adoptees were generally overrepresented in mental health services, although international adoptees had fewer behavioral problems and were less often referred to mental health services than domestic adoptees. The researchers concluded that most international adoptees were well-adjusted but were more likely to be given mental health referrals than nonadopted controls. Overall, preadoption trauma and/or deprivation were found to influence adoptee emotional well-being and long-term adjustment whether it was an international or domestic adoption.[49]

In one study, researchers used qualitative measures (interviews and children's kinetic family drawings) to assess bicultural identification in internationally adopted children and their parents. Although the researchers reported good psychosocial adjustment and strong family attachment, most of the children struggled with a sense of being different and some experienced feelings of loss and sadness. Children's understanding of their own cultural identity appeared to follow a pattern of development similar to theories of their understanding of adoption. Additionally, parents differed (with other adoptive parents and even with their spouses) on how to incorporate their child's birth culture into the family's identity. Some of the parental approaches to their children's biculturalism included: avoiding discussions of race/ethnicity and the use of labels; pointing out to their children that other people in the family had been immigrants or were adopted; and confronting other children (or their parents) who had made derogatory comments. Some parents felt at a loss to prepare their children for prejudice and discrimination. Others were concerned about scaring their children or making them defensive.[50]

THEORETICAL FRAMEWORK

Attachment and Loss Theory

Attachment and loss theory (based on Bowlby's[51] work) is built on the premise that the infant's attachment to the mother or a primary caregiver provides the security necessary for the child to explore his or her environment. It provides an understanding of affectional bonds and their meaning. Failure to form a primary attachment in early childhood can be related to an inability to develop close personal relationships in adulthood. Attachment is a reciprocal process between adults and children (with a parent responding to a child and a child responding to a parent) and, as such, is influenced by the losses and/or traumas that each has experienced. For the infertile individual or couple, some of the losses affecting attachment might include: a biological child, dreams of a fantasy child, parental roles, ties to one's spouse and extended family, and personal identity. For the adopted child, there can also be a multitude of losses and/or traumas, including: lack of or loss of secure, responsive care in infancy; loss of a caregiver(s) or multiple changes in caregivers during childhood; abuse and/or neglect; and loss of a familiar environment, including language, sounds, foods, and/or culture. The personality and resiliency of the child can also have a significant effect on attachment. Full attachment occurs when both parents and child feel that the other is an irreplaceable part of their lives. Factors in attachment that are particularly important concepts in adoptive parenting include: bonding (the process of attachment), claiming, and entitlement. Claiming refers to the mutual process by which an adoptive family and an adoptee come to feel that they *belong* to each other. Entitlement refers to the adopted parents' sense that they have both a legal and emotional right to be parents to their child. In many respects bonding, claiming, and entitlement are inextricably intertwined processes in the adoptive family.

Building a sense of entitlement means acknowledging that adoption is different from traditional biological parenthood. However, biological and adoptive parenthood share more similarities than differences. When a child has been adopted, the parents have the same responsibilities as any parent in caring for and guiding that child. The parent–child feelings are equally loving and intense, and the child becomes an unconditional member of the family. A basic question to be considered by all adoptive parents and their children, however, is "Who are the *real* parents of this child?" Adoptive parents must develop a sense of security in their role as the *real* parents both for their own sake and for the comfort and security of the child. Developing this sense of *entitlement* means that they believe that a child is really theirs and that they are really the parents.

Bowlby extended his theory of attachment to issues of grief and loss, which are significant factors in infertility and adoption in that the level of attachment defines the level of grief and loss. In this respect, it is attachment to the child that the infertile couple imagined and expected they would have. The infertile couple has to grieve this loss no matter how they become parents because the extended anticipation stage of parenthood has often produced an ideal child or expectations of themselves as an ideal parent. Grieving is the ability to let go of unfulfilled dreams and replace them with a comfortable reality. Not all grieving will occur before an adoption is completed, but couples should have resolved many of these feelings and be able to embrace adoption as a positive choice in their lives. For most couples, adoption is a second (or even third) choice toward parenthood, and the losses from infertility must be emotionally resolved. When this fails to happen, problems will often develop in the adoptive family.

Identity Formation

Identify formation is an individual's core sense of self, self-worth, and identifiable boundaries. According to Erickson's psychosocial theory (based on Freud's psychoanalytic theory), personality develops according to steps predetermined by individual readiness to be driven toward, to be aware of, and to interact with a widening social world, a world that begins with a dim image of mother and ends with an image of humankind. Erickson contended that development consists of the progressive resolution of conflicts between a child's needs and social demands. At each of the eight stages of development, conflicts must be resolved, at least partially, before progress can be made on the next stage. The failure to resolve problems at any given stage can result in psychological issues that can have an impact on an individual over a lifetime. As such, identity formation begins in childhood, develops within the context of the family, and is consciously shaped in adolescence.

The developmental stages from childhood to adulthood (stages 1 through 6) include trust versus mistrust; autonomy versus shame; initiative versus guilt; industry versus inferiority; identity versus diffusion; and intimacy versus isolation. Adolescence triggers an identity crisis in which the young person must successfully form an identity, separating and individuating from his or her parents, while establishing life goals and a sense of self in the larger world.[28]

Adopted children may have more difficulty with identity formation because they have incomplete or inaccurate information about their birth family history or they do not feel they have full membership in the adoptive family. Also, as they establish their personal boundaries, they must cope with the ultimate attack on self-worth – abandonment by their birth families. Adoptive parents must recognize the particular issues of identity formation for their children, as well as their own issues of identity formation as the parents of adopted children, which may involve children of different races, cultures, assisted reproductive technologies, or other unique qualities that set them apart. Within this context, adoptive parents cannot rely on traditional means of identifying with their children or with other parents.

Family Systems and Developmental Tasks of Adoptive Families

Family systems theory focuses on the family as a collection of individuals who are interconnected and have mutually interdependent relationships (i.e., emotional attachments) with one another. A primary premise of this theory is that the behavior of any one person in the family is directed or influenced by others in the family and must be understood in the context of the whole unit. Family systems theory provides the ability to recognize how events in the family – nodal happenings – can affect the family's development. Family transitions and other nodal events such as marriage and parenthood require families to reorganize and adapt. Infertility typically occurs at a junction between developmental stages, that of a newly married couple and of a family with young children. It becomes an obstacle that challenges the completion of life goals and developmental tasks, resulting in stress and requiring adaptation or reorganization on a number of levels.

Every adoption occurs within the framework of the family system of those involved. It involves the creation of a new kinship network that forever links two families together through the child, who is shared by both. As in marriage, the new family created through adoption does not signal the absolute end of one family and the beginning of another, nor does it sever the psychological ties of the earlier family. Instead, it expands the family boundaries of all those involved.[52] Use of the genogram to identify extended family history will often reveal issues that affect feelings about adoption and aid in assessment of the couple's family system (see Chapters 4 and 15). How do family members view adoption? What significance does genetic continuity have in the extended family? How do the relationships with one's parents and the parenting that one received as a child affect the desire for a biological child? These are just a few of the many questions raised by exploration of family history and family system dynamics.

In family systems theory, the developmental tasks of the adoptive family are (1) resolving feelings about infertility; (2) recognizing and accepting the differences that adoption brings; and (3) learning to deal with society's negative views of adoption (including being able to handle the many questions and comments that accompany adoption). Kirk[15] was the first to present a theoretical framework of adoption that did not involve a psychoanalytic approach. He contended that an adoptive family is exposed to different developmental tasks and challenges that must be resolved for satisfactory adjustment of both the family system and its members. Adaptive adjustment in adoptive families involves two different forms of acknowledging difference: *acceptance of difference* and *rejection of difference*.[15] Kirk contended that adoptive parents who are able to strike a balance in their behavior are generally the healthiest. They accept the difference by not trying to pretend that adoption is just the same as biological parenthood. However, at the same time, they do not dwell on the differences; they recognize that adoption and biological parenthood are more alike than different. In addition, Kirk was one of the first in the field to promote greater openness in the adoptive parent–child relationship, especially in the telling process, and greater openness and honesty in the placement process.

Another category of behavior in adoptive families, identified by Brodzinsky, is *insistence of difference*.[52] Typical of this category are people who continuously raise the topic of adoption with others, constantly dwell on it, and always identify themselves and/or their child in terms of adoption. Such behavior generally indicates a sense of insecurity and difficulty with a sense of entitlement.

Learning to deal with adoption within the context of society is a third important step in reaching a sense of entitlement and family adaptation. Those who are secretive and continue to feel uncomfortable or embarrassed about being an adoptive family are exhibiting problems in this area. They may see adoption as second best or are fearful of being viewed differently or negatively as an adoptive parent. Negative societal views do exist, and the public is naturally curious about adoption or assisted reproductive technologies as different forms of family-building. Adoptive parents have a responsibility to act as educators and to dispel inaccurate or prejudicial information.

Complex Adoption Theory

The definition of family has increasingly broadened to include a wide variety of adoptive placements, including international adoptions, foster care adoptions, skipped generation/kinship placements, and open adoption. As adoption has become more complex, a broader conceptual framework for understanding these placements has become necessary. Shapiro, Shapiro, and Paret[9] developed an integrated conceptual approach to adoption that provides a better understanding of the complex factors that influence all family members in these new adoptive structures. Their theoretical approach to adoption addresses three influential perspectives: (1) developmental, (2) ecological, and (3) ethnographic.

From the developmental perspective, the most significant factors influencing an adopted child's healthy development are the child's age at the time of placement and the quality of care provided prior to adoption. Developmentally, the important factors that need to be assessed in an adopted child's development are:[9]

■ the impact of diverse sociocultural contexts on children;
■ the concept of developmental lines and the assessment of delayed development;
■ the history and effects of primary attachment relationships;
■ the history and trauma of disruption and loss;
■ special issues in identity formation in adoptive families structures;
■ interactive environmental and biological risk factors, such as prenatal exposure to alcohol and drugs;
■ the nature of infant temperament and other biological factors.

The ecological perspective includes cultural, social, demographic, and familial factors that surround an adopted child and affect his or her growth and development. For example, this includes the negative effects of prejudice on a child in a transracial adoption as well as the effects of poverty, lack of social support, and/or the mental and physical problems of a caregiver.[9]

The ethnographic approach is based on ethnographic theory that "suggests that parents and children are the 'experts' in the subjective experience of their own painful family histories."[9] Each family's and individual's experience is unique and personal, yet may not be openly shared and expressed. Typically, adoptive family members come together with histories of loss, discontinuity, and difference. The ethnographic approach allows family members to tell "this part of the story while receiving the empathy of the listener" and "is helpful in mourning the past losses that were often invisible to others, and in constructing a more positive personal identity."[9] This approach allows for the adopted child's expression of feelings and personal identity development, while supporting familial attachment and the development of a family identity.

CLINICAL ISSUES

Infertility and adoption counselors offer many kinds of clinical guidance in preparing individuals and couples for adoption. Educating prospective adoptive parents in the wide range of choices available is an important aspect of adoption counseling. Before any decisions are made, infertility counselors can help patients explore their fears and expectations about adoption, as well as resolve lingering concerns related to infertility. It is crucial to address these issues before embarking on an adoption path. Once this decision has been made, counselors can also help individuals or couples deal with the issues of birthparents and the relationship they wish to have once adoption has occurred.

Patient Education: Adoption Options

The numerous options available for adoption today can be confusing and overwhelming. However, this range of choice does allow prospective adoptive parents to determine what best suits their needs and their family values. Each has advantages and disadvantages that need to be carefully considered. As noted earlier, adoptions can be either domestic or international. Included in these categories are agency, transracial, identified, or independent (private) adoption arrangements – all of which have their own set of complex circumstances and psychosocial issues.

Domestic Agency Adoption
Domestic adoption (also known as in-country or national adoption) involves a child and adoptive parents in the same country of residence. Agency adoptions represent a wide variety of possibilities and vary

according to country. Some examples are a government agency (e.g., involving children for whom parental rights have been terminated and are, as a result, wards of the state), a social service agency (e.g., having a religious affiliation such as Catholic Charities), or a private firm that facilitates adoptions. In traditional agency adoptions, the birthmother (or birthparents) places the child with an agency, which then selects (matches) the adoptive parents from the agency's list of prospective parents. These individuals or couples have undergone preadoption screening and preparation through a home study. The prospective parents may express their particular desires or needs, but the agency determines the match. In many cases, the birthparents and adoptive parents remain anonymous to each other, although nonidentifying information is generally exchanged. In recent years, an increasing number of traditional agencies have begun to offer birthparents and adoptive parents more choices about contact and information exchange. In addition, some agencies operate a portfolio system, in which prospective adoptive parents complete a portfolio that includes a statement about themselves, photos, and sometimes a video presentation. Birthparents are then shown numerous portfolios and given the opportunity to select an individual or couple for possible placement of their child. A meeting with the adoptive parents usually, but not always, follows the birthparent's selection before the final decision is made. Depending on agency guidelines and the preferences of the birth and adoptive parents, this may be a single meeting or one of many typically but not always.

Agencies generally establish rules for their placements, and these can be interpreted in a positive or negative light, depending on one's needs and/or preferences. For example, many agencies place a baby in foster care prior to making an adoption placement to ensure that the birthparents have relinquished their parental rights before the placement occurs. This may be the agency's choice to protect adoptive parents from the worry of bringing a child home and subsequently having the birthmother change her mind. Or, it may be a legally mandated practice. This practice may be viewed as a drawback by adoptive parents who wish to care for their child immediately from birth or a positive safeguard. In addition, agencies may have restrictions (again, either agency policy or legal mandate) regarding age, religion, marital status, length of marriage, criminal background, sexual orientation, and medical or mental health history. On occasion, an agency might also stipulate that one parent stay home on a full-time basis or that the couple complete medical treatment for infertility before pursuing adoption. Counseling is pro-

vided to both adoptive and birth parents when working with an agency. Although counseling can also be arranged in an independent placement, it occurs more routinely in an agency adoption.

In recent years, many nontraditional private agencies have emerged with innovative approaches to placement. Some, for example, encourage open placements, facilitating meetings between adoptive parents and birthparents, offering extensive exchange of history and identifying information, and establishing plans for future communication or visitation. These changes have been encouraged by consumers (birthparents and adoptive parents) who prefer or expect such arrangements based on the experience of others who have adopted or various adoption support organizations worldwide. Many adopted children now often receive mementos from a birthmother – a letter, pictures, or special gift – in hopes of facilitating their child's emotional growth and adjustment and/or ameliorating feelings of abandonment. Such mementos may help some adoptees with identity formation, comfort birthparents with relinquishment issues, and assist the adoptive parents with incorporating the child into their family system.

Some infertile individuals or couples who are seeking to adopt a healthy newborn may be deterred by lengthy waiting lists or restrictions of an agency. Others may feel that they can meet the challenges of a child with more complex issues. As a result, they choose to investigate government and social service agencies for the possibility of adopting special-needs children who have significant emotional, physical, and/or mental disabilities. Also included in the special-needs category are sibling groups and older children, who often have a history of abuse or neglect with concomitant physical and psychological problems. In recent years, there has been a trend toward deinstitutionalization of children with the goal of permanent placement for special needs and older children. As a result, such children are readily available but require exceptional parents who are flexible people willing to commit a tremendous amount of time, money, and effort to their child. Extra resources, including counseling, academic assistance, and medical care, are often necessary and can be costly and time-consuming. It should be noted that, in the United States, the 1997 Adoption and Safe Families Act provided health coverage for all adopted special-needs children.[53] Although the rewards are potentially great for both parent and child in these families, it is clear that care for a special-needs child can be stressful and emotionally draining. Children with special needs typically arrive at their adoptive homes with an array of physical and emotional scars, needing immediate intervention by qualified professionals. This history can interfere with healthy attachment to adoptive parents, as well as causing behavioral and/or emotional problems in adoptees. A stable, loving home, in and of itself, may not be enough to cure such tragic histories and/or traumatic problems. As such, prospective adoptive parents should have an accurate understanding of their child's special circumstances and realistic expectations of what can be achieved. Perhaps more than other parents, these individuals must have considerable energy, patience, courage, hope, commitment, and resources.

Domestic Independent Adoption

Independent adoption (also referred to as private adoption) occurs when an individual or couple locates a birthmother and makes an independent arrangement for placement of the baby without the assistance of an agency. Sometimes the birthparent/intended parent contact is made through a facilitator or an intermediary (friend, physician, or attorney). In other situations, the prospective adoptive parents advertise in a magazine or newspaper, or they network in a variety of ways to locate a birthmother. Networking might include: (1) talking to friends, relatives, colleagues, and professionals; (2) sending out resumes, letters, or brochures; (3) obtaining contacts through the Internet; or (4) posting calling cards or announcements on bulletin boards and in other community areas. Most often, independent adoption arrangements are domestic, but they have become increasingly international with the birthmother traveling to the adoptive parents' residence to give birth and/or relinquish her baby (or vice versa).

There is a wide range in cost for independent adoptions, depending on the extent of medical, legal, and other pregnancy-related expenses. A birthmother is generally reimbursed for the expenses involved with pregnancy and delivery. If she has insurance for her medical care and the legal costs are contained, an independent adoption can be relatively inexpensive. However, when she requests payment for living costs (e.g., rent, clothing, and transportation) during the pregnancy, as well as extensive medical and legal fees, the cost can be significant. It is illegal in most countries to pay specifically for a baby, a policy that has been further enforced by The Hague Convention.

Although prospective adoptive parents often look to independent adoption as a means of taking control of their childlessness and achieving parenthood with fewer obstacles (e.g., agency policies) or delays (e.g., agency wait-list), in actuality there is a wide variation in waiting time for independent adoptions. It is possible for an independent placement to occur quickly, but

some couples advertise or network for long periods of time, even years, without locating a birthmother or finding one with whom they can make an acceptable collaborative agreement. While luck frequently plays a role, there can be any number of extenuating circumstances. Due to the unpredictability of such adoptions, prospective adoptive parents should not embark on an independent placement without being emotionally, physically, and financially prepared for the unexpected: whether that is sudden parenthood when they receive a child within months of starting the process or the disappointment of numerous false starts in which the birthmother/parents change their decision regarding placement. Although preplacement counseling (e.g., home study) may not be required in independent adoptions, both adoptive and birth parents should seek counseling to facilitate coping and adaptation.

Potential adoptive parents and birthparents may prefer independent adoption for a variety of reasons. One advantage is that many feel that independent adoption provides a greater sense of control than an agency adoption. As they are actively participating in the location of or placement of their child, they typically feel more involved in the decision-making process. Although this feeling of increased control may be unrealistic because so many aspects of the process remain unpredictable, many still find it preferable to the passive waiting list process in agency adoptions. Another reason many prefer independent placements is that it enables intended parents and/or birthparents to avoid restrictions imposed by other methods of adoption. This might be true for individuals who are remarried, older, chronically ill, single, wealthy, homosexual, and/or have legal problems (e.g., illegal immigrant or convicted felon). Finally, many prefer this form of adoption because it provides prospective adoptive parents with the opportunity to adopt their infant immediately after birth and/or to be present at the delivery. Although some independent placements are completely anonymous, the majority of birthparents and prospective adoptive parents pursue this option because they prefer greater involvement between parties and increased information sharing. Adoptive parents and birthparents decide together the parameters of contact and communication (if any) during the adoption process and in the future.

Despite a variety of advantages, independent adoption also has significant disadvantages. Emotional and financial risks are significantly higher in an independent placement than in a placement through a reputable agency and the process is less predictable. The greatest risk is that, until parental rights are legally terminated, birthparents can reclaim the child. Laws regarding the relinquishment of parental rights vary widely for both international and domestic placements, so it is very important to know the specific laws applicable where the adoption will occur. Although most adoptions proceed smoothly one after a baby has gone home with the adoptive parents, there is significant risk of a birthparent reconsidering placement and/or even reneging at the time of birth or shortly thereafter. It is not uncommon for an adoption plan to fall through at any point during the time of pregnancy, delivery, or postplacement, and prospective parents need to be prepared for this reality. Another disadvantage of independent adoption is the unpredictability of the financial costs that can leave many unsuspecting couples financially or emotionally devastated. Hidden costs might include high advertising fees, telephone costs, a search that takes an extended period of time, travel expenses to meet prospective birthparents, attorney's fees, and medical or living expenses for the birthmother. The final costs for medical and legal services are often unclear until the delivery and placement are completed, making it almost impossible to estimate what the total expenditures will be (e.g., long hospitalization due to pregnancy complications). Furthermore, any expenses paid to a birthmother are not refundable should she change her mind regarding the placement. Therefore, it is extremely important to encourage couples adopting independently to carefully watch expenditures prior to placement and to get advice from a reputable attorney as well as a qualified mental health professional. Although most birthmothers are legitimate, well-meaning individuals, there have been unfortunate scams in which dishonest people have taken advantage of desperate and/or naïve infertile couples.

Another form of domestic adoption, which combines both independent and agency elements, is *identified adoption*. This is an adoption in which an individual or couple locates a birthmother (or vice versa) through independent efforts and an adoption agency subsequently oversees or facilitates the placement. This may be an interfamilial adoption or it may be strangers who have encountered each other via some form of networking. This form of adoption is most prevalent in states or countries that do not allow independent placements. All or parts of the agency services are provided to the parties involved.

International Adoption

As with domestic adoption, international placements can be completed through an agency in the country of origin; an agency or orphanage in a foreign country; or an adoption attorney/intermediary (i.e., independently). It should be noted, though, that The Hague Convention ensures adherence to standard regulatory process in all international adoptions. The countries that originally signed The Hague Convention 2000 were equally divided between countries of origin and receiving countries. Among countries of origin, South and Central American countries were strongly represented, with less of a showing from Eastern European countries. As in the past, Africa remains largely outside the global framework of international adoption. Asian representation is patchy with noticeable absentees such as India, China, and Korea.[54] The major receiving country worldwide is the United States, which currently takes in approximately 17,000 children per year through international adoption (comprising almost half of all the children subject to international adoption globally). In 2003, the five countries accounting for the greatest number of international adoptions in the United States were China (6,859), Russia (5,209), Guatemala (2,328), South Korea (1,790), and Kazakhstan (825).[55]

International adoptions are not without a variety of unique challenges, advantages, and disadvantages. Fees for international adoptions are typically comparable with a domestic placement, with waiting times varying from 6–18 months, which may be shorter than for a domestic agency adoption. Travel requirements vary from country to country but generally require, at minimum, a passport. Some countries and agencies have restrictions on age, marital status and length of marriage, number of biological children presently in the family, criminal history, health factors (including obesity), and/or work status (e.g., requiring one parent to be at home full-time). While international placements require considerable paperwork and may involve extensive red tape, prospective adoptive parents can typically follow the steps to placement without much difficulty when given guidance from an agency, attorney, mental health professional, and/or support organization.

The children most often available for international adoption are six months of age and older. The age at which a child is adopted can be a significant factor, especially if the child is receiving poor or inadequate institutional care and/or has preexisting health problems (e.g., prematurity).[9] All too often, there is insufficient information available, and the pediatric history of the child's early months may be limited. It is not unusual for children to arrive with health problems that were previously unnoted – and, as such, a surprise to adoptive parents. One important factor influencing a child's health and well-being at the time of placement is the quality of care the child received in his or her country of origin from birth until placement.[9] Some countries have a well-established foster care system (e.g., Korea), while others have a private, religious orphanage system (e.g., South America) or a governmental orphanage system (e.g., Eastern European countries). Still other countries have a combination of private and government-run orphanages (e.g., China).

Understandably, the economic and political atmosphere of a country can influence the level of physical, medical, and emotional care provided to children available for adoption. Therefore, it is important for prospective parents to remain up-to-date about adoption policies in their own country, as well as the country of origin of their awaited child. Changes often occur due to political events, government policy, natural disasters, and/or issues related to the adoption process. It is not unusual for countries to suddenly terminate placements, providing little information about when/if adoptions will be reinstated or placements will be completed. Therefore, it is important for prospective adoptive parents to deal with a reputable agency, intermediary, or orphanage and to obtain as much information as possible before placement and/or accepting a referral. Adoptive parents must also be certain that appropriate healthcare can be obtained in their own community. They may be particularly interested in making contact, before placement, with a clinic that specializes in international and/or adoptive medicine. Very often, it is helpful for preadoptive parents to consult with a pediatrician or pediatric psychologist to review the information they have received about their child, both to evaluate the appropriateness of the referral and in preparation for care, if the child is placed.

Many infertile couples who turn to international adoption are attracted by the availability of children for placement and the relatively low risk related to birthparents. It is unlikely that birthparents (if living) will want a collaborative placement agreement in an international situation. In fact, in the majority of international placements, birthparents are anonymous and there is little information available about them medically or psychosocially. For couples who worry about a birthmother changing her mind or later appearing in the child's life, international adoption often is more appealing than other forms of adoption.

Nonetheless, parents who adopt internationally are not simply adopting a child – they are also adopting their child's culture, heritage, and ethnicity. Infertility counselors must help clients assess their ability to deal with these differences. Couples need to determine how they feel about parenting a child who will probably not resemble them and who may differ in other ways. They also need to consider how a child will look not only as an infant but also when fully grown. Those who adopt internationally must be willing to help their child identify with the culture in which he or she is being raised, as well as the child's country of origin. As couples assess their own feelings, they will also need to consider how their extended family, friends, and community will respond to their child being different. Societal challenges may be a prominent factor in an international adoption, with the possibility of rude, ignorant, or intrusive questioning, staring, discrimination, and greater attention from the public, whether positive or negative. The possibility does exist for international adoptees to experience some measure of racial discrimination and prejudice. However, Bartholet[56] found no evidence to suggest that the experiences of international adoptees are any worse than others who experience racism and discrimination. A greater risk factor may be that internationally or transracially adopted children may lose some of their unique ethnocultural heritage and identity. This can be worsened when it is partially reinforced by parents who are innocent and caring, but inept in their expectations.[12] Those who successfully adopt from another country generally view the racial or ethnic diversity of their family as an enriching experience, particularly if the family works to incorporate the background differences of the child into the family system and family identity.

Transracial Adoption

During the past thirty years, there has been considerable controversy over the adoption of children of color by Caucasian individuals or couples. In 1972, the National Association of Black Social Workers in the United States presented opposition to transracial adoptions and, as a result, the majority of states and agencies in the United States instituted policies that favored domestic same-race adoption placements. A similar stance was taken for Native American children with recommendations for same-race placements. Unfortunately, there were an inadequate number of African American or minority adoptive families available for same-race placements, leading to a growing number of children remaining in institutional or foster care. As a result, in 1994, the Multiethnic Placement Act (MEPA) was passed in the United States. The primary objective of this legislation was to decrease the time spent by children in foster care placement and open up more avenues to permanent placement, which included transracial placements. Prospective adoptive parents could no longer be denied the ability to adopt on the basis of race, color, or nationality. Still, many agencies and prospective adoptive parents remain cognizant of the long-held opposition to transracial adoptions and have been less open to adopting transracially within the United States. Consequently, Canadians and Europeans are adopting an increasing number of minority American children, while Americans continue to adopt children from other countries, transracially, at the highest rate of any country in the world. One study estimated that approximately 65% of all international adoptions in North America involve children and parents of different racial backgrounds.[57] Predominant arguments against transracial adoption include: (1) loss of heritage or connection to ethnic-racial identity experienced by adoptees; (2) exploitation of people living in weak, poverty-stricken countries by those in richer, more powerful nations; and (3) the inability or unwillingness of adoptive parents to support their adopted children's original culture and heritage.[1]

Despite the concerns of mental health professionals regarding the psychosocial well-being of children raised in transracial homes, there is little evidence that these placements are problematic. Research has indicated that "adopted children placed transracially do just as well, in all respects, as children placed in same-race homes"[58] and that, "long-term studies show consistently encouraging outcomes over time."[9] Based on the results of their almost thirty-year investigation of transracial adoption, Simon and Alstein[59] concluded that transracial adoptees show no special problems. However, Bartholet[60] contended that children who are assigned minority status must understand how others view them to protect themselves physically and emotionally from racism. Adoptive parents do need to respect and encourage the racial and ethnic identity of their child, as well as help him or her deal with discrimination in the community. It is important to assist children in developing supportive peer relationships, including friends of the same race/ethnicity, and to provide the opportunity to live in a racially integrated community where difference is accepted.

Programs such as EuroAdopt[61] (begun in Sweden) suggest ways to support transracial adoptees through: (1) get-together facilities (e.g., children's camps); (2) establishment of special-interest groups; (3) homeland tours; (4) summer camps in the country of origin; (5) programs that help families explore the child's roots; and (6) reports from the countries of origin. Post-placement services, typically offered by adoption agencies or consumer support organizations, can be a beneficial means of supporting transracial adoptees and their parents.

Home Studies

Throughout the world, anyone who wishes to adopt must complete a home study or assessment. The process of the home study varies considerably, depending on the agency and/or professional completing it, but it generally involves some or all of the following components: (1) assessment of the prospective adoptive parent(s) and their motivation for adoption, (2) financial statement, (3) medical screening and history, (4) fingerprinting/ legal background check, (5) personal references, (6) psychological screening, and (7) verification of identity. Individuals and couples may be asked to complete lengthy questionnaires or an autobiographical statement for use in the assessment. A variety of documents are also typically required such as birth certificates, marriage licenses and divorce decrees (if applicable), letters of employment, and so on. The traditional idea of a home study was of an intimidating white glove approach to evaluating a couple and their home for potential parenthood. In recent years, the home study has generally been restructured into a preparation process, providing opportunities for parent education about the unique nature of adoption and facilitating the transition to adoptive parenthood. In addition, prospective adoptive parents are encouraged to increase self-awareness, explore concerns about adoption, and gain psychosocial support as waiting parents. Many agencies now provide, in addition to interviews and home visits, waiting parent groups, meetings with birthparents (to gain greater understanding of their perspective), support resources, and workshops on parenting skills.

Regardless of the home study format and the degree of compassion shown by the social worker, most prospective adoptive parents expect it to be a threatening experience. This, again, represents a loss of control for the couple because they are not able to move toward parenthood without the approval or intervention of others. Many prospective adoptive parents feel resentful, recognizing that the rest of the world does not need to be evaluated for parenthood. Frustration and a sense of powerlessness can reemerge, as well as resentment toward the invasion of privacy, issues often reminiscent of infertility. It is important that adoption professionals understand these reactions and not establish an adversarial relationship with those wishing to adopt. Traditionally, adoption counselors have been advocates for the child and, while this remains a significant role, their support of adoptive and birthparents is an equally important role. When couples feel a supportive, positive relationship with the social worker or infertility counselor, they are typically more willing to communicate openly, discuss their anxieties, educate themselves regarding the unique aspects of adoptive parenthood, and ask for help when needed. Although some view the home study as unfair, it can and should be a beneficial process for adoptive parents.

Expectations and Fears about Adoption

For most infertile people, the decision to adopt does not occur quickly or easily. More often it represents an evolution of feelings and a process that includes grieving, information gathering, decision making, implementation of the decision, and, ultimately, adapting to adoptive parenthood. During early medical treatment, when couples are hopeful of success, any mention of adoption can produce panic, that is, fear that they might not succeed in their quest for a biological child. Anger can also occur, as others insensitively and simplistically remark, "Well, you can always adopt" or "If you adopt, you'll probably get pregnant." The general public fails to understand the complex emotional issues, the time required to make this decision, the financial expense, and the myriad of other emotional, social, and physical challenges involved in becoming adoptive parents.

A common fear for many infertile individuals and couples is whether or not one can love an adopted child to the same degree as a biological child. Although parent–child attachment is not determined by biological links, many people continue to believe that a blood/genetic connection is necessary for close, committed parent–child relationships. This may be a previously unrecognized or unexplored assumption which preadoptive parents must emotionally and intellectually face. Expressing and examining these fears will not only make preadoptive parents more comfortable with and prepared for adoption, but it can also make them better parents. Furthermore, exploring these fears also involves acknowledging their fantasies. Although fantasies of an ideal biological child are common, infertile couples must put these dreams to rest and accept that there is no perfect child (either biological or adopted), nor is it possible to be perfect parents. Accepting a child for who he or she is, with his or her unique characteristics, is in large part what makes adoption (and parenthood) successful.

Very often couples considering adoption fear that an adopted child will ultimately reject them in favor of their birthparents. Opportunities to search for biological parents are becoming more available through mutual disclosure registries, private investigations, and opening of birth records. However, motivations and experiences vary widely when adoptees search. Some adoptees (perhaps with idealized or unrealistic expectations) are disappointed when the contact, reunion, and/or relationship falls short of what they had anticipated. For other adoptees, meeting birthparents is a positive experience that enhances their life, as well as the relationships with their adoptive family. Motivations for searches are varied and are influenced by the circumstances of the adoption, as well as the adoptee's own life stage and experiences. Adoptees may seek contact to obtain information about their heritage, to learn more specific details about their placement, or to acquire medical history that adoptive parents cannot provide. Other adoptees are motivated by psychological needs, such as identity issues – a search for self in one's biological or genetic heritage. Adoptive parents must be reassured that a search does not imply inadequacy on their part as parents or as an adoptive family. In fact, current research indicates that the decision to search is an idiosyncratic one that is not based on any definable reasons (e.g., unhappiness with adoptive parents; unmet psychological needs; or need for medical information). Search factors are not predictable and appear to relate more often to the adoptive person's personality and personal experiences than to a set of definable factors.[62]

Another concern for prospective adoptive parents is whether an adopted child will be at risk for increased psychological and/or medical difficulties. As reported earlier, adopted children have been found to be overrepresented in the mental health system. This overrepresentation may be due to the willingness of adoptive parents (versus biological parents) to acknowledge even minor problems and enlist professional assistance. Or it may be due to preexisting conditions in the child, such as the circumstances of the adoption; prenatal factors; age of the child at the time of placement; a history of abuse or neglect; and/or medical or mental health conditions. Adopted children, in general, may experience periods of anger or depression in dealing with their loss and yet successfully resolve these issues.[30] Ultimately, if one or both preadoptive parents is expecting or is psychologically invested in a problem-free parenting experience, this may be an indication that they are uneducated and/or illequipped for adoptive parenting and the unique challenges (and rewards) it offers. Unmatched or unrealistic expectations of adoption may represent unresolved grief and/or inadequate preparation for adoptive parenthood (see Chapter 26).

Resolving Feelings about Infertility

The experience of infertility involves many losses, perhaps most significantly the basic assumption of fertility.

This includes a genetically shared love child that is traditionally conceived as well as the experience of pregnancy, a psychosocial event for both the couple and their extended family. Further affected by the experience of infertility are one's life goals and expectations, social status, self-esteem, control of personal destiny, belief in a predictable world, genetic continuity, and expectations about parenthood (e.g., breast-feeding). For infertile couples, these losses typically occur following a series of failed treatments, disappointments, and sobering realities before the final acknowledgment that parenthood cannot be achieved via traditional conception, pregnancy, and birth. As such, infertile couples considering adoption must mourn these losses and gain a healthy perspective on these experiences (e.g., recognizing that all feasible medical efforts were made and that their primary goal is truly to become parents). When individuals have not faced and resolved these feelings, they may have difficulties with attachment, forming an identity as an adoptive family, or being effective parents (e.g., helping their child deal with his or her own issues of loss).

In resolving infertility, a couple must recognize the potential for tremendous happiness and fulfillment as parents, despite their inability to produce a biological child. Parenthood is not reproduction but, rather, the day-to-day guidance, love, and caregiving of devoted mothers and fathers. In preparation for adoption, counselors must help individuals and couples come to terms with their infertility issues, recognizing that resolution is a process and not an event. As a result, even after adoptive parenthood has occurred, feelings about infertility may linger, although the majority of issues should be largely resolved before placement. Indications of unresolved infertility might include:

■ intense feelings of sadness and anger, perhaps manifested in avoidance of pregnant women;
■ refusal to acknowledge grief or disappointment about infertility;
■ continuing resentment of infertility and a sense of feeling cheated;
■ inability to spend time around the children of others;
■ strong fear that an adopted child will fall short of family standards or expectations;
■ ongoing fantasies about the perfect biological or genetically shared child;
■ discomfort with or refusal to discuss adoption issues;
■ decision to keep adoption secret from others and/or the child due to shame or embarrassment.

When there is evidence of significant unresolved infertility issues, including the intensity of feelings or refusal to deal with them, it may indicate that an individual or couple is unprepared for adoption at this time. Ultimately, this may impact their ability to provide an emotionally healthy family environment and promote the psychological well-being of a child. The bottom line is *adoption is not a solution for infertility and is not the right choice for everyone*. Indications for infertility and adoption counselors that an individual or couple should not proceed with adoption include:

■ serious disagreement between partners about the decision to adopt, evidenced by partner reluctance, coercion, or acquiescence;
■ belief that adoption is a temporary solution for infertility, as indicated by the assumption that it is only a matter of time before returning to medical treatment and the possibility of a biological child;
■ significant marital conflict and a belief that a baby will repair the marriage or provide a child before a partner exits;
■ serious mental health problems that have not been acknowledged and/or treated;
■ unwillingness to learn about the unique aspects of adoption and accept how it differs from biological parenthood;
■ pursuit of an adopted child who will meet the parent's needs, assuaging narcissistic injuries, and not to meet the needs of the child.

Relationships with Birthparents

All prospective adoptive parents must accept the reality of their child's birthparents and the significance of birthparents in their child's life. For some couples, the idea of a birthmother/father relinquishing their child for adoption is incomprehensible. They may be unable to differentiate between their own special circumstances (ready and willing to have a baby but unable to) and those of the birthparents (physically able to have a child but unprepared or unable to parent for a variety of reasons). It is not unusual for women experiencing infertility to feel anger at others who get pregnant easily, unexpectedly, or unintentionally. Some prospective adoptive parents may continue to feel anger and resentment toward a birthmother who was able to conceive, yet never wished to have a child or be a parent. Being happy that a birthmother has decided to place her baby is not the same as being able to empathize with her predicament and the difficulty of her decision. Often, when adoptive parents meet the birthmother and/or father, they can better understand their unique predicament and recognize them as real people with real problems and feelings. Particularly in open adoptions, negative attitudes about birthparents can interfere with the ability to establish a collaborative agreement, develop a healthy sense of entitlement to their adopted child, and later discuss adoption comfortably with their child. Feelings of competition with the birthparents and/or fears of the birthparents reemerging to reclaim (physically and/or emotionally) their child can also be problematic. These are normal and sometimes valid concerns for prospective adoptive parents and, as such, need to be fully addressed early on.

In open or collaborative adoptions, prospective adoptive parents must determine what kind of relationship, if any, they wish to have with the birthparents. These arrangements occur more often in domestic adoptions, but have become more common in international adoptions as well. Prospective adoptive parents must assess their preference and level of comfort with the various forms of adoption available today: anonymous, semi-open, or fully open placements. A fully open relationship typically involves ongoing communication and physical contact (e.g., visits on holidays) among all parties: birthparent(s), adoptive parents, and child. The terms of the placement, including the degree of openness and extent of future contact, need to be clarified before the adoption occurs and should be explicitly stated, preferably in a written legal agreement. This can prevent much confusion, misunderstanding, and ill-will in the future. Those approaching adoption for the first time are often wary of contact with the birthmother, feeling threatened by or uneasy with her presence. Despite such fears, it is important that prospective adoptive parents obtain as much information as possible about the birthparents at the time of placement – whether the placement is anonymous, semi-open, or fully open. This might include talking to or meeting the birthparents or extended family, exchanging extensive information, sending letters and/or pictures on an ongoing basis, or maintaining contact through visits, telephone calls, or email. Many couples find that, as they feel more secure in their parental role, their fears dissipate and they may later regret not taking the opportunity to meet the birthmother and/or obtain additional information. Meeting face-to-face with birthparents, gathering information, taking pictures, and asking a birthmother for a letter to her child at the time of birth can be invaluable in future years, when a child is interested in learning more about his or her origins. Furthermore, when adoptive parents can demonstrate their understanding of the child's emotional needs by providing this information, it can enhance their child's trust in them.

THERAPEUTIC INTERVENTIONS

There are several kinds of professionals that prospective adoptive individuals and couples may encounter in their quest to adopt. Adoption intermediaries are those who bring together birthparents and prospective adopters, and may sometimes serve in a counseling role, although they are not typically trained mental health professionals. Attorneys, independently or through an agency, facilitate the legal transfer of parental rights to the child. Finally, infertility or adoption counselors help individuals or couples explore whether adoption is the right path for them; assist them in examining the many options available for adoption; educate them regarding the unique nature of adoptive parenthood; make appropriate referrals for additional guidance; provide emotional support during the transition to adoptive parenthood; and explore feelings about infertility and adoption. These various professionals and their roles often overlap and, ideally, work in concert to facilitate the adoption and the healthy adjustment of the new family.

Most people who consider adoption will travel through numerous emotional stages before making this decision. Counselors can assist individuals and couples with these various stages, including: (1) initial consideration of adoption as a family-building option; (2) helping couples grieve; (3) gathering information; (4) forming a decision as a couple; and (5) facilitating the transition to adoptive parenthood. These stages do not occur in a structured, straightforward manner and are not mutually exclusive. Rather, they are pieces of the complicated emotional journey toward reaching parenthood.

Considering Adoption as a Family-Building Option

Couples generally move from infertility treatment to adoption in one of two ways. Some feel the need to complete every medical option available before they can begin to consider adoption. They want to determine and feel that biological parenthood is definitely beyond their grasp. Unfortunately, this approach is difficult because the field of infertility treatment is constantly changing and expanding, with new treatment options available at an increasingly rapid pace. Even when a couple is told that their situation is hopeless and that no further medical treatment can be offered, it can be very difficult for them to accept in this era of ever-evolving assisted reproductive technologies. This makes it very difficult to end treatment and pursue adoption strictly from a medical point of view (see Chapter 24).

A confounding factor is that patients are often offered medical treatments that are actually forms of adoption (e.g., donor insemination, oocyte donation, or embryo donation) and may fail to consider the psychosocial issues of adoption in their decision making (e.g., relinquishing and grieving the genetically shared child). Other couples begin to consider adoption while in the midst of infertility treatment. They may be frustrated with treatment failures and experiencing diminished hope, but have not yet reached the end of medical options. Some couples will have realistic expectations about treatment success, recognizing that time or medical success rates are not in their favor, while other couples are panicked about the *possibility* of unsuccessful medical treatments. Whatever the case, many infertile couples approach adoption as a means of considering their future choices, knowing that they eventually want to become parents.

As partners begin to consider adoption, they must allow time to privately do some soul-searching, examining their own personal beliefs, needs, and fears. Each individual should determine how the losses of infertility have affected him or her personally. Individuals will need to consider which losses are most significant to each of them, and which of these losses could be addressed by making a decision to adopt. Each must assess his or her needs and be able to separate the experience of pregnancy from that of becoming a parent. Although most people desire both the pregnancy and parenting experience, many have a primary focus. Most couples who ultimately choose adoption find that their desire for parenthood is more important than a desire to reproduce. If the need for genetic continuity and/or a longing to experience pregnancy are the most significant factors, adoption will not fulfill these needs and the couple must honestly accept that this is how they feel, at least for the present. Sometimes these feelings will change over time but, until that occurs, adoption should not be pursued.

Those considering adoption must carefully assess their views on the role of genetic factors versus the environment in affecting the development of a child. Genetic inheritance will not only influence physical characteristics but also personality traits, intelligence, and interests. Environment clearly plays a role in a person's development, but all children will display specific inherited characteristics. These traits may be significantly different from those produced in one's biological child, but not necessarily worse. This is another challenge for adoptive parents: incorporating the child's differences into the family system and family identity in a positive manner that enhances and supports both unity and individuality.

Should couples pursue adoption before ending their medical treatment? It is advantageous for couples to discuss the possibility of adoption while still in treatment and to begin exploring this vast field. The prospect of adoption can be overwhelming because of its complexity and the diverse avenues available. It often takes considerable time to evaluate all the alternatives and forms of adoption. Not only will this accelerate the process if a couple later pursues adoption wholeheartedly, but many find that it also relieves the stress of medical treatment by assuring them that parenthood is ultimately possible. It also provides them with a sense of control lost during infertility treatment, as they can take action to learn more about alternative family-building. In the meantime, if medical treatment is successful, a couple has simply educated themselves about adoption.

Because some agency adoptions involve lengthy waiting lists, it can be beneficial for couples to begin the adoption option while still in medical treatment. However, if a couple is planning to pursue independent adoption, they should be nearing the end of treatment. Independent placement can occur quickly, and couples must be emotionally and physically prepared for this possibility. This also applies when an agency with a shorter waiting list or with a portfolio service is used. *Actively pursuing both independent adoption and infertility treatment is not recommended, unless an individual or couple is fully emotionally prepared for a child to result in either or both cases.* Couples must allow time to educate themselves about adoption, such as birthparent issues, talking to children about adoption, handling social situations, resolving lingering feelings about infertility, and understanding the psychological impact of being an adoptive parent and an adopted child. Couples must also prepare physically and emotionally for the arrival of a child, as well as getting themselves ready for their new role as parents. Understandably, they may be apprehensive about making purchases for a baby or preparing a nursery, but these early joys should not be missed and are an important part of the transition to parenthood and attachment to their adopted child. Those who continue with treatment may not be able to invest their time and emotions in anticipation of a child's arrival or the important psychological tasks of preparing for adoptive parenthood. An unwillingness to stop treatment can be a significant indicator of a failure to resolve infertility issues; an inability to accept adoption as a joyful and fulfilling path to parenthood; a reliance on others (e.g., physician) for life's decisions;

or ambivalence about adoptive parenthood. It may also indicate that the couple has an unequal investment in adoptive parenthood, with failure to reach a committed joint decision.

Helping Couples Grieve

Often, infertile couples become stuck in their inability to grieve and cannot move comfortably toward adoption. Infertility counselors can help individuals and couples identify their reasons for their failure to grieve:

- *extreme anger*: inability to accept that infertility is a situation over which they have no control;
- *unresolved guilt*: a view that they are bad people deserving of their infertility or that they have contributed to their diagnosis of infertility through some negative actions;
- *shame and embarrassment*: a belief that infertility is too personal, shameful, or embarrassing to admit to others;
- *fear*: a need to remain in control, due to fear that grief will be devastating;
- *denial*: inability to admit that severe infertility exists, an unwillingness to accept a negative prognosis from multiple specialists, or unrelenting and unrealistic pursuit of assisted reproduction.

In addition, some people are unable to grieve because the losses of infertility are too many or too intangible. In such cases, couples may develop a ceremony for mourning, in which they mark the end of their treatment efforts and embark in a new direction. Helping couples (and even their extended family) plan and execute a ritual can be a helpful therapeutic intervention.

Many couples become fixated on the idea of their biological and genetically shared child because they have idealized and become attached to the fantasy of what that child would be. They imagine their own best qualities (and their partner's) and believe that their offspring will have a composite of all their respective positive characteristics. It is important to address the unlikelihood of this perfect outcome, perhaps by having the couple list the worst characteristics of themselves and their family, and then imagining their biological child as a composite of those traits. This scenario may help couples recognize that children come as they are and not as they are wished-for or imagined. Furthermore, while ideal children are not real children, ideal parents are equally unrealistic and impossible.

For individuals who have been unable to grieve, infertility counselors can encourage their exploration of these issues by helping them picture their fantasy biological child. Who would he or she look like? What color hair and eyes would the child have? What would they name him or her? The infertility counselor can suggest that they imagine different parenting experiences and ask them to consider how their life would be different if infertility had not been an issue. If individuals are experiencing difficulty with verbalizing these thoughts, they may find it easier to express themselves in writing or in an artistic endeavor. The therapist might ask clients to write a letter to their unborn, hoped-for child. Sometimes, feelings will also emerge through dreams. Interpretation of these dreams can be helpful in addressing previously unspoken feelings.

One of the most important aspects of grieving and ultimately resolving infertility is revealing oneself to others, that is, being able to communicate openly about infertility with one's partner, close friends, and family. Infertility counselors should encourage clients to join an infertility support organization or a preadoption group. For those who have been secretive about infertility, a group normalizes their experience, giving them the opportunity to share feelings with others who intimately understand the infertility crisis and to learn how others have handled this experience. Isolation can lead to enhanced feelings of being damaged or unworthy. Participating in a group can help the infertile person view this crisis in a more constructive manner with less self-blame, anger, and isolation. For those who find a group logistically or emotionally impossible, the Internet is another means of connecting with others, as well as gaining information (see Resource list).

Gathering Information

When first considering adoption, many individuals and couples are overwhelmed by the scope of the field – the various forms of adoption, the extensive psychological issues, the logistics, paperwork, and financial considerations. Most have just emerged from the frustration and devastation of infertility, having educated themselves in the complexities of the medical world, only to find that adoption brings an equally great challenge, another maze, and an additional financial hurdle. Often, infertile couples are often shocked and overwhelmed when the reality of adoption sets in: It can be as complex and frustrating as infertility and its medical treatment. Early on, the quest of adoption for many couples seems to raise more questions than answers.

One of the most important stages in the adoption process is information gathering. Couples need to understand the many options available and the psychological issues of adoption before they can proceed further. Infertility counselors should recommend that couples read extensively on all aspects of adoption, for example, how-to-adopt guides, books from the perspective of the birthparents, books about life as an adoptive parent, and literature geared to children. Adoption is often a difficult and challenging process and, as such, prospective adoptive parents need to avail themselves of all educational opportunities. They should attend adoption conferences, join an adoption support organization, network with friends, relatives, and professionals, and openly share their goals. An adoption support group is a valuable resource for meeting others who have adopted, becoming familiar with issues in adoption, and obtaining information on the how-to options (e.g., referrals to agencies, attorneys, or knowledgeable professionals). This is especially true if they are adopting internationally or transracially. Most support organizations offer monthly informational meetings, newsletters, videotapes, annual conferences, referral services, informal peer or professionally led support groups, internet websites, and library services.

Increasingly, access to the Internet is having a significant effect upon all aspects of adoption because of the richness of its resources. On the positive side, it provides more visibility for children in foster care and those with special needs who are in need of permanent placement (e.g., photo listings of waiting children). It also offers the general public greater opportunity for adoption education and awareness. In addition, it provides adoptive parents, birthparents, and adoptees access to the many pre- and post-placement adoption resources available, as well as a community of support. On the negative side, it must be noted that not all information on the internet is accurate and there is the possibility of illegal business being conducted or illegitimate claims being made.

Although the Internet is a highly efficient, rapid, far-reaching source of information for those interested in adoption, material obtained online must be verified, cross-checked, and generally approached with caution. Individuals must take personal responsibility for assessing the value of the information found on the Internet. In general, those sites that are clearly structured, up-to-date, and well-maintained will indicate a higher standard of quality.

Forming a Decision as a Couple

Partners often begin to consider adoption at different points in their infertility treatment and they may initially disagree about the decision to adopt. It is normal for partners to view this option differently. Couples often panic when they express dissimilar points of view, and this fear can impede further communication. Partners need to share their fears and skepticism with one another in an honest and open fashion. Adoption does require a leap of faith and can be both an exciting and frightening proposition. Often, the differences that partners express are not as disparate as they initially seem. For example, couples may agree on the next step in their decision-making process (e.g., going to an informational meeting about adoption) but be at odds on the timing of the decision (e.g., pursuing adoption immediately or waiting until after the next course of medical treatment). In addition, individuals often do not accurately express what they feel. For example, a partner might state, "I could never adopt," when actually what he or she means is, "I'm not ready to stop treatment" or "I'm not ready to consider adoption *now*." Infertility counselors can assist couples explore their opinions and listen carefully to one another in order to better understand the feelings behind differing points of view.

Often, conflict between partners develops because each has an internal conflict or ambivalence that is not being honestly acknowledged and/or expressed. The infertility counselor can serve as an objective and supportive third party, helping the couple to unravel these issues. During early discussions, couples often try to balance each other's point of view, consciously or unconsciously. One may take a strong proadoption stance with no expression of anxiety or ambivalence, while the other counteracts with a firm negative standpoint. Counseling can help couples identify points of agreement – similar fears, desires, objectives, or needs – that are often present. They can be given the task of making individual lists of pros and cons regarding adoption and then comparing these lists with one another. This is often helpful in clarifying differences and similarities. Infertility counselors should emphasize that talking about adoption is not a decision to pursue it. However, exploring adoption and other family-building alternatives is an important component in coming to terms with the infertility experience. The process itself (like infertility) can strengthen relationships and increase individual self-knowledge and self-confidence.

When couples hit an impasse, it may be necessary to retreat from the conflict and to agree on a future date for further discussion. This may be several weeks or even months later. Placing the issue on hold, with the purpose of exploring individual feelings and gaining greater knowledge, often brings a change in perspective and more openness in future talks. Couples should be told that opinions about adoption often change over time as individuals deal with their feelings, reassess their situation, or learn more about adoption. It is not unusual for a person to adamantly oppose adoption at one point and later successfully adopt.

Facilitating the Transition to Adoptive Parenthood

Couples should communicate with friends and family about their adoption journey, garnering support as expectant parents. Although some will feel most comfortable on an agency list awaiting a baby, they should also continue to share their goals with others. Networking can be exceedingly important because adoption leads might come unexpectedly from any source. Very often couples agree to equalize the infertility experience through adoption: The partner undergoing the least medical treatment takes the responsibility for investigating and/or implementing the adoption decision. This strategy can be helpful when spirits lag, especially for couples investigating adoption while completing medical treatment.

Although many adoptions proceed quickly and smoothly, the adoption process is most often frustrating and time-consuming. Babies and children *are* available for adoption, but couples need to be creative and patient in their efforts. Most who persevere will successfully adopt, but there may be disappointments and dead ends along the way. Infertility counselors can be helpful in offering much needed encouragement and support during the course of adoption. For those couples who experience disappointment and may be on the verge of abandoning their plans, it is important to emphasize that persistence will generally succeed. Many begin to feel persecuted – first by their reproductive problems and failed infertility treatment, and then by their lack of success in adoption. Helping couples understand that such disappointments are common in the adoption process can help normalize their experience and bolster sagging spirits.

Infertility counselors working with prospective adoptive couples need to understand that once a child has been identified, the waiting period can be extremely stressful. For all would-be parents, the anticipatory stage of parenting is ambiguous and stressful, filled with worries about what to expect, what the child will be like, and how life will change with parenthood. Adoptive parents face the same feelings as all prospective parents, but there are also concerns that are unique to the adoption process. Will the adoption plan succeed and, if so, when and how? Will the birthparents change their mind? If international travel is required, adoptive parents often face a number of logistical concerns. How long will they have to stay in the country? Where will they stay? What about their jobs and other responsibilities? Will the political situation of the country remain stable and will the adoption follow an established, predictable process? Feelings of failure and pessimism during infertility (particularly if unresolved) can be exacerbated or reemerge during the adoption process. While all prospective parents need tremendous amounts of support and encouragement, this is an even greater necessity during adoption.

Infertility counselors can be instrumental in helping preadoptive couples with the transition to parenthood. Because this is both an exciting and stressful period, couples should be encouraged to recognize the stressors unique to their situation and develop a coping plan. This may include setting constructive goals, identifying stress reduction strategies, and developing a plan for handling the adoption process. Some ideas for remaining busy with constructive goals include preparing their home for children, learning more about adoption or parenthood, meeting with other adoptive parents, and attending baby care classes. Stress reduction strategies may include focusing on enjoyable couple activities, individual hobbies, and using their social support network. Couples should be encouraged to spend positive time together, renewing areas in which their relationship might have been eroded by infertility – particularly their intimate relationship. In addition, they should be encouraged to see themselves as parents, communicating about how they plan to be a parenting team. Counselors can assist couples to develop an adoption implementation strategy in which they spell out their plans for problem-solving about the adoption, communicating with the agency or adoption facilitator, and managing the unexpected happenings that are certain to occur during the waiting period. Finally, couples should enlist the support of friends and family prior to placement that may involve educating them about adoption issues, the adoption process, or their child's unique heritage.

FUTURE IMPLICATIONS

Infertility and involuntary childlessness will always be important elements of the human condition. Realigning social relationships, by creating families via adoption, is a psychosocially stressful process for all participants in the adoption triad: parents unable to care for their birth children, infertile couples, and children in need of families. Research that identifies the effects of adoption on all members of the triad, but especially adoptees, will need to continue in future years, offering clinicians an increased understanding of the needs and feelings of each group. Much of the existing research has focused on the immediate process of forming adoptive families and the short-term effects on members of the triad. More extensive research is needed on the long-term implications for adopted children and their families, especially as international and transracial adoptions increase and adoptive family-building becomes more complex. In the future, it is hoped that adoption will be increasingly viewed as a positive family-building alternative, providing parenting opportunities for the infertile and offering permanent families for children in need. Adoption, like infertility, is becoming more visible to the community and, as such, less shameful for all members of the adoption triad. This visibility should help destroy misconceptions and better educate the general public about adoption as a positive family pattern.

SUMMARY

■ The world of adoption has substantially changed in recent years. As the domestic adoption of healthy infants has become more difficult, the number of international and transracial adoptions has risen. The implementation of The Hague Convention has provided standards and safeguards throughout the world for international placements.

■ Adoption is becoming increasingly complex, with a multitude of genetic, biological, social, psychological, and environmental factors affecting the development of a child and the adjustment of the adoptive family. Although most adoptees are psychosocially well-adjusted, they are at greater risk for a variety of difficulties (e.g., behavioral, emotional, educational, and neurological). The need for thorough preadoption counseling to understand and prepare for these issues is essential, as well as the necessity for postadoption services to help families handle the many challenges of adoption.

■ Most individuals and couples succeed with adoptive placement, but they often must persevere longer in their efforts to adopt. Disappointments with failed placements are common, with high emotional and financial risks.

■ In many countries, the traditional secrecy in adoption is giving way to greater openness among members of the adoption triad at the time of placement and in postplacement years. Research indicates the importance for adoptees of having knowledge regarding their genetic and birth history.

■ Those who move from infertility to adoption need to grieve their many losses and resolve the issues of infertility in order to successfully move on. They must also accept that there are differences between adoptive and biological parenthood. The infertility counselor may be crucial in helping prospective adoptive parents face these significant issues.

■ Although adoption has become less socially stigmatizing, negative stereotypes of adoption remain. As a result, adoptive parents have the responsibility of educating others, as well as advocating for themselves and their children.

REFERENCES

1. Rojewski J, Rojewski J. *Intercountry Adoption from China*. Westport, CT: Bergin & Garvey, 2001.
2. Tessler R, Gamache G, Liu L. *West Meets East: Americans Adopt Chinese Children*. Westport, CT: Bergin and Garvey, 1999.
3. Rosenblatt PC, Peterson P, Portner J, et al. A cross-cultural study of responses to childlessness. *Behav Sci Notes* 1973; 8:221–31.
4. Bharadwaj A. Why adoption is not an option in India: The visibility of infertility, the secrecy of donor insemination, and other cultural complexities. *Soc Sci Med* 2003; 56:1867–80.
5. Ezugwu F, Obi S, Onah H. The knowledge, attitude and practice of child adoption among infertile Nigerian women. *J Obstet Gynaecol* 2002; 22:211–6.
6. Evans K. *The Lost Daughters of China*. New York: Tarcher/Putnam, 2000, p. 135.
7. Selman, P. Intercountry adoption in Europe after The Hague Convention. In: R Sykes, P Alcock, eds, *Developments in European Social Policy: Convergence and Diversity*. Bristol: Policy Press, 1998.
8. Evan B. Donaldson Adoption Institute. *International Adoption Facts*, 2001 (www.adoptioninstitute.org).
9. Shapiro V, Shapiro J, Paret I. *Complex Adoption and Assisted Reproductive Technologies*. New York: Guilford Press, 2001.
10. Howard C. Domestic or international: Choosing an adoption path. *Adoptive Families Magazine* 2003 (www.adoptivefamilies.com).
11. Winkler R, Brown D, van Keppel, et al., eds. *Clinical Practice in Adoption*. Elmsford, New York: Pergamon Press, 1988.
12. Kim WJ. International adoption: A case review of Korean children. *Child Psychiatry and Human Development* 1995; 25:141–54.
13. Van den Akker O. Adoption in the age of reproductive technology. *J Reprod Infant Psychol* 2001; 19:147–59.
14. Child Welfare League of America–National Data Analysis System. *International Adoption: Trends and Issues*, 2003 (ndas.cwla.org).
15. Kirk HD. *Shared Fate: A Theory and Method of Adoptive Relationships*, 2nd ed. Port Angeles, WA: Ben-Simon Publications, 1984.
16. Brodzinsky D, Huffman L. Transition to adoptive parenthood. *Marriage and Family Review* 1988; 12:267–86.

17. Brodzinsky D. A stress and coping model of adoption adjustment. In: D Brodzinsky, M. Schechter, eds, *The Psychology of Adoption*. New York: Oxford University Press, 1990; 3–24.

18. Matthews R, Matthews AM. Infertility and involuntary childlessness: The transition to nonparenthood. *J Marriage Fam* 1986; 48:641–9.

19. Schechter M. About adoptive parents. In: E Anthony, T Benedek, eds. *Parenthood: Its Psychology and Psychopathology*. Boston: Little, Brown, 1970; 353–71.

20. Humphrey M. The effect of children upon the marriage relationship. *Br J Med Psychol* 1975; 48:273–9.

21. Humphrey M, Kirkwood R. Marital relationship among adopters. *Adoption Fostering* 1982; 6:44–8.

22. Levy-Shiff R, Goldschmidt I, Har-Even D. Transition to parenthood in adoptive families. *Develop Psych* 1991; 27:131–40.

23. Bower B. Adapting to adoption: Adopted kids generate scientific optimism and clinical caution. *Science News* 1994; 146:104–5.

24. Miller B, Fan X, Grotevant H, et al. Adopted adolescents' overrepresentation in mental health counseling: Adoptees' problems or parents' lower threshold for referral? *J Am Acad Child Adol Psychiatry* 2000; 39: 1504–11.

25. Brodzinsky D.Long-term outcomes in adoption. *Future of Children* 1993; 3:153–66.

26. Brodzinsky D, Schechter M, Marantz Henig R. *Being Adopted: The Lifelong Search for Self*. New York: Random House, 1993.

27. Riley D, Singer E. The dynamics of adoption. *Family Therapy Magazine*, January–February 2003; 37–43.

28. Grotevant H. *Adoptive Families: Longitudinal Outcomes for Adolescents*. (Final Report), 2001 (www.fsos2.che.umn.edu/mtarp).

29. Brodzinsky D, Steiger C. Prevalence of adoptees among special education populations. *J Learn Disabil* 1991; 24:484–9.

30. Gray D. *Attaching in Adoption*. Indianapolis, IN: Perspectives Press, 2002.

31. National Clearinghouse on Child Abuse and Neglect Information. In: *Focus: Understanding the Effects of Maltreatment on Early Brain Development*, 2001.

32. Paton J. *Adoptees Break Silence*. Action, CA: Life History Study Center, 1954.

33. Sorosky A, Baran A, Pannor R. *The Adoption Triangle*. New York: Anchor Books, 1978.

34. Grotevant H. McRoy R. The Minnesota/Texas adoption research project: Implications of openness in adoption for development and relationships. *Applied Devel Sci* 1997; 1:168–86.

35. Grotevant H. What works in open adoption? In: M Kluger, G Alexander, P Curtis, eds, *What Works in Child Welfare*. Washington, DC: CWLA Press, 2000.

36. Grotevant H, Perry Y, McRoy R. Openness in adoption: Outcomes for adolescents within their adoptive kinship networks. In: D Brodzinsky, J Palacios, eds, *Psychological Issues in Adoption: Research and Practice*. Westport, CT: Praeger Publishers, 2005.

37. Borders L, Black L, Pasley B. Are adopted children and their parents at greater risk for negative outcomes? *Family Relations* 1998; 47:237–41.

38. Sharma A, McGue M, Bensen P. The emotional and behavioral adjustment of United States adopted adolescents: Part I. *Children and Youth Services Review* 1998, 18:83–100.

39. Friedlander M. Ethnic identity development of internationally adopted children and adolescents: Implications for family therapists. *J Mar Fam Ther* 1999; 25:43–60.

40. Lindblad F, Hjern A, Vinnerljung B. Intercountry adopted children as young adults – a Swedish cohort study. *Am J Orthopsychiatry* 2003; 73:190–202.

41. Burrow AL, Finley GE. Transracial, same-race adoptions, and the need for multiple measures of adolescent adjustment. *Am J Orthopsychiatry* 2004; 74:577–83.

42. Feder L. Adoption trauma: Oedipus myth, clinical reality. *International Journal of Psycho-Analysis* 1974; 55: 491–3.

43. Lifton BJ. *Journey of the Adopted Self*. New York: Basic Books, 1994.

44. Cline FW, Helding C. *Can This Child be Saved? Solutions for Adoptive and Foster Families*. Milwaukee, WI: World Enterprises, 1999.

45. Hoksbergen R, ter Laak J, van Dijkum C, et al. Posttraumatic stress disorder in adopted children from Romania. *Am J Orthopsychiatry* 2003; 73:255–65.

46. Versluis-den Bieman H, Verhulst F. Self-reported and parent reported problems in adolescent international adoptees. *J Child Psychology & Psychiatry* 1995; 36:1411–28.

47. Tieman W, van der Ende J, Verhulst F. Psychiatric disorders in young adult intercountry adoptees: An epidemiological study. *Am J Psychiatry* 2005; 162: 592–8.

48. Verhulst F, Althaus M, Versluis-den Bieman H. Damaging backgrounds: Later adjustment of international adoptees. *J Am Acad Child Adol Psychiatry* 2000; 39:1504–11.

49. Juffer F, van IJzendoorn MH. Behavioral problems and mental health referrals of international adoptees: A meta analysis. *JAMA*. May 2005; 293:2501–15.

50. Friedlander ML, Larney LC, Skau M, et al. Bicultural identification experiences of internationally adopted children and their parents. *J Couns Psych* 2000; 2:197–8.

51. Bowlby J. *Attachment and Loss: Attachment*. New York: Basic Books, 1969.

52. Brokzinsky DM, Schechter MD, eds. *The Psychology of Adoption*. New York: Oxford University Press, 1990.

53. Evan B. *Donaldson Adoption Institute: Foster Care Facts / Fact Overview*, 2002 (www.adoptioninstitute.org).

54. Duncan W. The Hague Convention on protection of children and co-operation in respect of intercountry adoption. In P Selman, ed, *Intercountry Adoption: Developments, Trends, and Perspectives*. London: British Agencies for Adoptions and Fostering, 2000; 40–52.

55. US Department of State, *International Adoption Trends*, 2003; (www.adoptivefamilies.com).

56. Bartholet E. Adoption among nations. In: *Family Bonds: Adoption and the Politics of Parenting* Boston: Houghton Mifflin, 1993; 118–63.

57. Reitz M. Groundswell change in adoption requires anchoring by research. *Child Adol Soc Work J* 1999; 16:327–54.

58. Alexander-Roberts C. *The Essential Adoption Handbook*. Dallas, TX: Taylor Publishing, 1993.

59. Simon R, Alstein H, Melli M. *The Case for Transracial Adoption*. Washington, DC: American University, 1994.

60. Bartholet E. *Nobody's Children: Abuse and Neglect, Foster Drift, and the Adoption Alternative*. Boston: Beacon Press, 1999.

61. Sterky K. Maintaining standards: The role of EurAdopt. In: Selman, ed, *Intercountry Adoption: Developments, Trends and Perspectives*. London: British Agencies for Adoption and Fostering, 2000; 389–404.

62. Wrobel G, Grotevant H, McRoy R. Adolescent search for birthparents: Who moves forward? *J Adol Research* 2004; 19:132–215.

23 Involuntary Childlessness

GRETCHEN SEWALL AND LINDA HAMMER BURNS

Farewell dear child, thou ne'er shall come to me.
— Anne Bradstreet

While the reasons for wanting children vary across time and across cultures, the personal desire for children falls into three categories: (1) *normalcy desires*, or the equation of normal adult personhood with marriage and parenting; (2) *immortality desires*, or the conviction that personal perpetuity can be achieved through children, who serve as extensions of self; and (3) *quality of life desires*, or the existential equation of happiness and life-meaning with having children.[1] Although having children is both desired and expected in all cultures, the meanings attached to children and parenthood; perceptions of infertility; sexuality; and medicine, and the nature of communication about these issues vary widely from culture to culture.[2] Children are valued for a variety of reasons including: (1) *social security desires* (i.e., children ensure their parents' survival); (2) *social power desires* (i.e., children serve as a valuable economic resource in a patriarchal social structure); and (3) *social perpetuity desires* (i.e., children continue group structures into future generations).[3]

In a cross-cultural study of childlessness, Rosenblatt and colleagues[4] found that infertility was considered a crisis across all cultures and solutions to infertility fell into three categories: (1) medical interventions; (2) prayer or spiritual interventions; and (3) realignment of social relationships. Infertile couples have used all three measures – social, spiritual, and medical – as remedies for involuntary childlessness throughout history and across cultures. Most challenging is when every culturally acceptable and feasible remedy for childlessness has been pursued and, yet, the couple (and/or individual) remains childless. For these couples, coming to terms individually, as a couple, and within their social community can be excruciatingly painful and immensely challenging. As such, childlessness and the inability to become a parent is an experience of profound loss and suffering for both men and women, hav-

ing an impact on their individual emotional well-being; marital stability; relationships with extended family; social standing; and religious faith. Furthermore, factors impacting the acceptance of childlessness following infertility include the burden of medical treatment that is primarily borne by women (even with male-factor diagnosis); the acceptability of other roles for women; the social stigma of childlessness within the couple's culture; the degree of negative consequences of childlessness; the availability/acceptability of medical treatment or adoption as remedies for childlessness; and religious traditions.

While some may decide to be childless as an acceptable personal or marital choice, the focus of this chapter will be involuntary childlessness following infertility. This chapter addresses:

- historical and cultural roots of childlessness;
- incidence and pathways to childlessness following infertility;
- etiological differences in causes, consequences, and rates of childlessness in developed and developing countries across the globe;
- clinical issues of childlessness including grief and loss; decision making; gender differences; pronatal societal and economic pressures; and cross-cultural issues;
- adaptation for couples (particularly women) when childlessness is the only alternative;
- childlessness as a lifestyle alternative.

HISTORICAL OVERVIEW

In ancient Greece, a wife did not enter definitively into her husband's family until she produced a child. Romans, like the Hebrews and Greeks before them, thought the purpose of marriage was to give a man legitimate children – preferably sons.[5] Roman citizens

411

were encouraged to procreate as part of their civic duty following the first legislation enacted to stimulate marriage and offspring introduced by Augustus (Roman emperor from 27 BCE–13 CE), who even offered rewards for those couples who produced many children. Interestingly, the first Roman divorce, that of Spurius Carvilius, surnamed Ruga, in 230 or 231 BCE, was the result of his wife's childlessness.

Early Judaism taught that marriage was an obligation as well as a divine commandment and blessing and, as such, the only sanctioned way that a couple could fulfill their obligation to reproduce. However, a man (without input from his wife) could divorce his wife for 'shameful' behavior (Deut. 24:1), which included barrenness. There are a variety of examples of childlessness in the Torah (also known as the Old Testament Bible), notably Sarah and Rachel, who 'resolved' or 'endured' childlessness, depending on one's perspective. Still, the tradition remains within Orthodox Judaism that a husband may divorce his wife (although not vice versa) if the marriage is childless.

Within Islam, the purpose of marriage was/is also to produce children. According to Islamic law, if a marriage was/is childless for seven years, the husband can/could divorce his wife (with or without her knowledge) and/or take another (usually younger) wife.[6,7] Within a social and religious system in which motherhood was/is a woman's only acceptable role/job, childlessness is a problem of significant proportions and consequences. Fatherhood bestows social stature, generativity, and economic value while providing a means of transmitting property. Historically (and even today), childless Islamic women have had few choices: Either their husbands could return them to their natal families or they could remain with their husband, raising his children from other wives.

Early Christian teachers, such as Saint Augustine, declared that married couples should engage in sex only to beget children. In medieval Europe, the Christian church introduced the concept of marriage as a holy sacrament through which the participants obtained God's grace and, as such, was irrevocable. With marriage being an 'insoluble sacrament,' solutions to childlessness were limited for infertile couples. Motherhood was considered the fulfillment of a woman's God-given role and children a blessing for economic, social, religious, and emotional reasons. With the ideal marriage ranking below virginity and widowhood, it was not uncommon for the medieval childless wife to seek shelter in a religious community (convent) and fulfill her nurturing roles through religious life. With the advent of romantic love during the medieval period in Europe, the meaning and purpose of marriage expanded to include companionate marriage. As such, children were not only an important means of fulfilling economic, individual, and social roles, but they also became a reflection of the parents' love and affection for each other. Childlessness or barrenness was socially stigmatizing and often considered the fault of the woman herself. Infertile women or those who had suffered miscarriage or stillbirth were often accused of witchcraft, a belief system that lasted well into the modern era and continues today in some parts of the world. Barrenness for the Christian was considered a test of faith and religious leaders advised barren women to strengthen their faith and find other ways to lead a more godly life. "Rather she should be more fruitful in all the good works of Piety and Charity."[8]

In Latin America, following colonization by European countries, the Roman Catholic Church and the beliefs of the indigenous peoples influenced both attitudes and traditions regarding family, reproduction, and sexuality. Gender roles were proscribed. *Machismo*, literally translated as maleness and virility, is a cultural belief that men are responsible for the honor, welfare, and economic well-being of their family. Influencing the behavior of women is *marianismo*, based on the cult of the Virgin Mary, which contends women are spiritually superior to men and therefore capable of enduring suffering, particularly that inflicted by men. Within this context, childless women are expected to be self-sacrificing and to persevere; accept their fate; pray; or pursue religious solutions (e.g., light candles and make pilgrimages to shrines) – a tradition that continues in many Hispanic cultures.[9]

Historically, ancestor worship is the oldest and most pervasive Asian religion, based on the ability of the living to communicate directly with the dead and the ability of the dead to influence current events in this world. In most Asian cultures, the family unit is multigenerational (preserving the continuity of generations) and patriarchal. A woman is absorbed into her husband's family through marriage and holds a position of status beneath her father-in-law, mother-in-law, and husband. Within this rigid family structure, sons are more valued than daughters because they provide family continuity and contribute to the economic success of the family. As such, children exist for the well-being of their parents and extended family. In a study of a Chinese farm family, Wolf[10] described the importance of a child as evidence of an unbroken chain of men: "Every new bride brings hope of at least one more link in the chain of descent; every birth brings certainty." Childlessness, particularly for women, is a tragedy of multidimensional proportions, interrupting the ancestral line, displacing a woman as the primary wife, and precipitating her loss of social power or even a home, particularly if her childlessness requires that she return to her natal family. A significant impact of the Cultural Revolution during twentieth-century China was the deconstruction of an ancient feudal system and the implementation of the communist government's one-child-per-family policy. As a consequence, childlessness produced a new set of psychosocial issues, most predominantly the use of reproductive technologies to ensure the birth of the single revered son and/or the abandonment or relinquishment for adoption of baby girls.

In some Asian countries such as Vietnam, it is widely believed that although the purpose of marriage is to have children, few couples can attain a special and coveted form of marital sentiment with each other without the birth of children.[11] This viewpoint seems to be more prevalent in countries in which the nuclear family is primary (versus the multigenerational family unit common in China and India). It is believed that giving birth and raising children creates a special bond between husband and wife that helps make the conjugal relationship flow more smoothly. As a result, childlessness prevents a couple from achieving that special happiness, a focal point for their relationship that cannot be achieved any other way.

In Africa as in South America, the role of women; the meaning of children; and beliefs about reproduction are influenced by tribal beliefs and religion (most predominantly Islam and Christianity). Although some African cultures are matriarchal, the majority are patriarchal societies in which women are considered the property and/or responsibility of the male family members (e.g., her father, brothers, and/or husband). While female reproduction is highly valued in some cultures, others value female virginity because of beliefs, myths, and/or superstitions (e.g., sexual intercourse with a virgin will cure or immunize her male partner from disease). Infabulation or female circumcision is a cultural practice that supported the importance of female virginity. The practice is considered the number one health hazard to African women by the World Health Organization. Ironically, female circumcision is a significant causal factor in female infertility (e.g., infection and pelvic inflammatory disease), yet a woman's infertility is often attributed to evil spirits or superstitious beliefs about her. In contrast, in many African cultures male-factor infertility is so socially stigmatizing it is denied and/or concealed. Childless couples face not only significant social stigma but also few positive remedial alternatives. Husbands, forced to deny male-factor infertility, often divorce their current wife and/or take an additional, typically younger wife who can pro-

vide children. Women seek covert impregnation from another man (adultery); may be physically harmed or killed by their husband or his family; or are forced into poverty when divorced and/or returned to their natal family.[1,12,13] Today in many African cultures, infertility is a dilemma because of the social factors that contribute to its increased incidence, including a sexual system that emphasizes fertility over female virginity; polygamy (helpful in producing extra work units and based on a belief in a man's biological need for numerous partners and sexual encounters); and limited access to reproductive medicine services. Childless women are treated so badly that they are frequently less fearful of being caught in adultery or undergoing any number of medical treatments than they are of remaining childless.[14]

Although the value and reasons for having children may have changed as the world moved away from agrarian, tribal or feudal social structures to urbanization and industrialization, children remain fundamentally important. In the past, children may have been valued for primarily economic reasons (e.g., labor value to the family), but with the Industrial Revolution in eighteenth-century Europe, the family home became a private retreat from the challenges of the world.[8] Reproduction and procreation shifted from a matter of survival to a source of personal happiness, resulting in smaller families and a focus on parent/child relationships. As children became more valuable as a source of personal happiness, childlessness took on new psychosocial dimensions. Dally[15] contended that, prior to the Industrial Revolution, motherhood was never a psychologically significant role for women – and, in fact, many women interpreted motherhood and childbirth as burdensome to their own health and well-being. Fewer workers were needed after the Industrial Revolution, so motherhood became an important and worthy occupation for women, taking women out of the workplace and thereby, providing more jobs for men. As a result, motherhood became an idealized and glorified occupation – and gave women something to do. Childless women were viewed as maladjusted and unable (or unwilling) to conform to appropriate gender roles – a viewpoint influenced by the burgeoning science of psychiatry and an earlier feminist movement in which women demanded the right to vote in democracies around the world.

Pronatalism, or actions that encourage childbearing for religious or political reasons, has a long history that continues even today around much of the world. However, newer pronatalistic forces as a psychosocial response swept the globe at the end of World War II, putting increasing pressure on women to have children and many of them. Women who were not mothers were considered selfish, deficient, or worse – defiant or deviant. Furthermore, it was believed that education and a career could hinder a woman's reproductive potential.[8] Intentional childlessness during these years was so stigmatized that demographers assumed it was practically nonexistent.[16] During the rebirth of the feminist movement in the 1960s and early 1970s in North America, economic forces, legalization of abortion, and advances in technology and medicine (e.g., reliable contraception and ARTs) released many women from reproductive obligation. In developed countries education, expanded career choices, reliable and effective birth control, and delayed childbearing combined with divorce and cohabitation contributed to expanded roles and life goals for women. As such, birth control and reproductive technology had an impact on women's reproductive behavior and decisions,[17,18] allowing women to move out of the home and away from reproduction as her sole identity and profession. In contrast, some countries used these technologies for other purposes (e.g., China's one-child-per-family policy or the practice in India of using reproductive technology to ensure the birth of a male child).

Still, increased reproductive freedom has not been globally universal nor has it been without cost to women worldwide. Postponement of childbearing has resulted in increasing numbers of women seeking medical treatment for reproduction failure due to advanced maternal age. These women are childless not by choice but by chance or circumstance, often misled by the advances in reproductive medicine and birth control to believe their reproductive life is limitless and self-determined. Another consequence of industrialization, globalization, and increased availability of ARTs is the stratification of reproduction. In short, many men and women around the world remain childless because they cannot access medical treatment for infertility; it is economically beyond their means; or unavailable in their area. Childlessness all too often is an uncomfortably imposed fate because medical treatment or adoption are alternatives financially or socially feasible for the select few: financially well-off, educated, mobile couples living in developed or developing countries.

REVIEW OF THE LITERATURE

Both a human and global phenomenon, the World Health Organization defines infertility as a worldwide health disease afflicting an estimated 60 million to 80 million couples across the globe.[19] Infertility carries with it social and personal stigma and can be misidentified as voluntary, circumstantial, or simply

delayed childbearing. These difficulties most likely contribute to underreporting of a hidden or concealed disease and/or social circumstances.

Causes and Incidence of Childlessness

The numbers of combined voluntary and involuntary childless women has increased in most industrialized countries since the late nineteenth century. As previously stated, education, career choices, birth control, and delayed childbearing along with divorce and cohabitation have contributed to this phenomenon. Most recently, a growing and more visible population of American and European men and women recognize 'child-free' as a desirable life choice. This trend started in the early 1980s and continues today. Prior to this period, rates of childlessness in America varied. The lowest rate reported by the U.S. National Center for Health Statistics occurred in 1975, when 9% of women between the ages of twenty and forty-four were childless. In 1993, this percentage had risen to 16% and by the year 2000, at least 20% in this age group were childless. The only other time such a high rate of childlessness occurred was during the Depression years (1929 to 1934), when 22% of American women remained childless, statistics that may be representative of all developed countries.[20]

Consequences of Involuntary Childlessness

An exception to the rise of voluntary childlessness in developed countries is within the Jewish population of Israel. Voluntary childlessness is still virtually nonexistent within this group.[21] Israeli society is family oriented and emphatically pronatal. A number of factors including Jewish religious tradition; demographic competition with Arab neighbors; fear of death due to military conflict; and child-centered everyday culture have sustained a relatively high fertility level among Israeli Jews. Married Jewish women in Israel have an average of 5–8 children.[21] Within this pronatalistic society, childlessness (including involuntary) can be thought of as a form of social deviance. Childlessness deprives a woman of her gender identity and expected personal achievement.[22,23] Public and healthcare policies clearly reflect the high social value of fertility in Israel[24] as couples are provided, at no cost, whatever treatment is necessary to produce two children.[21] As a result, Israeli women may be 'relentless' in their pursuit of pregnancy and medical treatment to achieve it. Remennick's study of twenty-six infertile Jewish women in Israel[21] indicated that not one subject in her study saw childlessness as a life option.

In Egypt as in many Islamic cultures, women engage in prolonged treatment rather than face the societal, religious, and personal identity crises of childlessness.[3] For Hispanic childless women, the price of maintaining this social façade can be particularly painful. Emotional privacy and stoicism in both men and women are valued to protect the comfort of others. Solutions and peace are found by turning to one's faith. Devotion to God, trust in divine intervention, and prayer will bring a sense of tranquility and normalcy to believers. It is thought that once this is achieved, the miracle of life is possible,[9] highlighting how childlessness is *not* acceptable.

In a study of Chinese infertile men and women, parental expectation was the leading source of stress for men, while women found being unable to meet societal childbearing role expectations as the most stressful.[25] In a similar study, men report grieving the discontinuation of the family heritage as a significant stressor.[26] The pressure to have children is multifaceted and includes personal desires to maintain ancestral ties; preserve family continuity; prevent loss of face; and elevate a woman's status within her own home and community by producing a son. Belief systems about family, ancestor cults, illness, and cure are all important factors influencing feelings about childlessness and infertility treatment.

Worldwide, infertility affects at least 14% of the reproductive population. However, only a very small proportion is able to acquire suitable treatment.[27] Regional differences impact the incidence, causes, and availability of treatment as well as societal and psychological interpretation and response.[16,19,20] In resource-poor countries, children are an economic necessity as well as highly valued for cultural and personal reasons. Voluntary childlessness is not considered a reasonable option. A young woman who does not procreate faces enormous interpersonal and societal problems and also substantial risk. Studies in Bangladesh, Nigeria, Mexico, and Zimbabwe indicate women have legitimate fears of the consequences of infertility. Maltreatment by her spouse and in-laws (e.g., divorce, expulsion from her husband's house, emotional and/or physical abuse, and murder) are common consequences of the inability to conceive and/or bear children.[1,19,28–30] Once removed from the home, the childless woman is often reduced to poverty and social isolation (e.g., prostitution). As such, childlessness is a major factor in the spread of STIs in many parts of Africa.[19,31]

In Nigeria, where women are the husband's property, the wife is typically blamed for infertility and then neglected or forced into the role of extended family slave.[19] The estimated number of infertile persons in Nigeria is 12 million, yet actual figures are probably higher. Primary causes are tubal factor, severe oligospermia, and azoospermia.[12] This significant and growing number of life- and population-threatening sterility in Nigeria was treated by less than 600 total ART treatment cycles in Nigeria in 2000.[12] During this same period, 99,639 ART cycles were performed in the United States.[32] Governments, policy makers, and influential research institutions must face stark realities and ensuing long-term impacts of the inequities of available prevention and treatment of infertility in countries where people and populations are in danger. This 'stratified reproduction' results in some being able to achieve their reproductive desire while others (e.g., poor women of color) are disempowered and despised as reproducers.

Daar and Merali state, "The central difficulty associated with infertility in developing countries is that infertility transforms from an acute, private agony into a harsh, public stigma with complex and devastating consequences. Infertility has the potential to disrupt peace, exacerbate poverty, and devastate communities. The harms caused by infertility are pervasive, socially embedded and serious, precisely because infertility interacts with a complex network of social relationships, social expectations and social needs."[13] It is becoming evident that infertility is far more dangerous for women in resource-poor countries than for those of the developed world.

Women often verbalize a fear about childlessness leading to loneliness and regret in old age. Also of concern is the loss of connection with the next generation. Studies have shown, however, that older childless women in developed countries have other goals and interests to give their lives meaning. Interestingly, having children has been found to contribute neither to happiness nor to overall satisfaction in later life.[16] Gerontologists describe the effects of being childless in later life as 'benign.'[33]

In some countries, aging provides women with enhanced power and prestige in which they attain the role of respected elder with venerated social status. However, childlessness for women in these cultures may represent aging in a negative manner. For example, childless women in West Africa are referred to by a word that implies 'agelessness,' implying unnatural, abnormal, and negative supernatural power. As a result, she is avoided and stigmatized.[6] In many indigenous cultures infertility continues to be attributed to witches, spirits, jealous co-wives, adultery, or an unclean womb – all factors that attribute blame to the infertile woman herself and rarely to her male partner. The family – which typically includes the larger extended family network of husband, wife(s), sons, daughters-in-law, and grandchildren – is valued above the well-being of the individual. The principle of extended genealogical groupings persists in the thinking of people, and tribal pedigree is considered fundamental in determining and justifying traditional authority and political power. For this reason, infertile men may have multiple wives or be pressured by family members to take another wife if their marriage is childless – although only 4–5% of Islamic men actually practice polygamy.[34] In a study of infertile women in Pakistan, the primary reasons for seeking infertility treatment were: having someone to carry on the family name; feeling alone; *akharat par maan bap bun kar uthna* (getting up as a parent on judgment day); not having a male heir; social pressure; coercion by in-laws; and/or social isolation.[35]

THEORETICAL FRAMEWORK

Family Systems Theory

According to family systems theory, the family life cycle framework defines a series of stages with expectable timelines that most people imagine as their predictable life course.[36] Successful passage through family life cycle stages depends on the effectiveness of developmentally appropriate negotiations of tasks and stressors. Carter and McGoldrick[37] delineated six stages of the American family life cycle, a model that acknowledges the confluence of situational, developmental, and family-of-origin (historical) stressors. The stages and their tasks are:

1. *Unattached young adult*, during which tasks include separation and individuation; development of close relationships; and establishment of an identity linked to educational, job, or career goals;
2. *Married couple*, during which the marital dyad is established and relationships with family-of-origin and social support network are realigned;
3. *Family with young children*, during which the marital bond adjusts to include children, incorporates parenting roles, and redefines relationships with extended family (including grandparents);
4. *Family with adolescents*, during which parents flexibly support their adolescent's drive for autonomy and self-definition while redirecting their attention to their own personal and professional development and taking care of older family members;
5. *Parents launching children*, during which parents support their children's physical separation from the family while renegotiating their marital relationship to a more intimate dyad (downsizing). Parents develop an egalitarian relationship with adult children; reorganize the family system to include others (e.g., in-laws, and grandchildren); and cope with the failing health or death of their own parents;
6. *Family in later life* is a stage in which couples explore new family and social roles; address loss and mortality issues; and adjust to the role of honored family elder.

To decide to have children and to implement that decision is an implicit part of most marital contracts and is an expectation of men and women entering marriages worldwide and across all cultures. Childless couples are indefinitely stuck in the 'couple stage' of family development, imposed on them by reproductive failure, making it more difficult for them to define boundaries between themselves (the couple) and their families-of-origin. Ambiguous boundaries (who is in the system and who is not) create emotional discomfort for the childless couple and their extended family, as well as their social community. As a result, childless couples may respond with rigid boundaries between themselves and their families-of-origin in an attempt to protect themselves against emotional intrusion; shame about infertility; or offers of 'what to do.' Alternatively, childlessness may precipitate the loss of necessary, healthy boundaries by sharing private emotions or information with others or allowing outsiders to influence couple dynamics (e.g., decision making). In-law relationships can also become strained when a couple experiences childlessness (whether it is a decision to accept one's fate or embrace childlessness when treatment has been unsuccessful). For many couples – and across many cultures – the privileges and responsibilities of adulthood are often withheld until the adult couple has produced children. As such, involuntary childlessness is an intergenerational family crisis. Parenthood enables couples to move into the next stage of the family life cycle while at the same time enabling their own parents to move into the next developmental stage of *their* family life cycle. Or put another way, childlessness stops the whole family system from moving forward through the predictable stages of the family life cycle. The importance of the transition to parenthood is particularly true in patriarchal societies or cultures in which ancestors are highly valued and/or worshipped. In short, childless couples trapped in the 'couple stage' of the family life cycle can feel lost in a painful 'no man's land' of quasi-adulthood, on the fringe of family dynamics, where individual, couple, and family roles are ill-defined and/or uncomfortable while at the same time feeling responsible for preventing other family members and/or the family system from moving forward.

Involuntary childlessness is a crisis in which all members of the family system must adapt and adjust as they rework family boundaries; redefine the meaning of family; and determine how the family system will move forward through the family life cycle when a couple (and grandparents) is without children. Couples must alter their life, goals, and personal identities. R. Matthews and A. Matthews[38] contend "nonparenthood is likely to have as significant an impact on family and personal identity as parenthood itself." They conclude that the transition to *nonparenthood* is as important and demanding a transition for families and individuals as the more traditional transition to parenthood. The childless couple must redefine the meaning of family to include a marital dyad without children. These are challenging tasks for individuals, couples, and families and, as with any transitions, adjustments, and redefinitions, the ability to make these changes in a healthy fashion will depend on the stability and well-being of the individual, marital dyad, and family system prior to the crisis of infertility and involuntary childlessness.

Psychoanalytic Theory

Fundamental to psychoanalytic theory are three fundamental tenets: *self psychology*, or the cohesion and fulfillment of the self as an individual's primary aim; *ego psychology*, or the focus on defensive and coping devices used to deal with distressing feelings; and *object relations theory*, which focuses on the mental representation of objects; "the relationship of the self to one's world of inner objects; and the repetitive reenactment of this internal world in the context of ongoing interpersonal relationships."[39] Historically, a fundamental tenet of psychoanalytic theory was women's envy of men – particularly the power that was symbolized through the male reproductive organ (i.e., penis envy). This approach has been generally debunked or reworked, but it highlights the fundamental importance of reproductive ability (and healthy organs) in defining an individual's sense of self and the powerful influence of sexuality and reproductive ability in identity formation.

Psychoanalytic theory traditionally viewed childless women as pathological, unable to achieve their functional (and most fulfilling) role in society. This view, still held in a variety of cultures, limits women's roles to their reproductive abilities as well as the way in which women think of themselves. Object-relations theory emphasized that women have had the primary caretaker role for both female and male offspring, which significantly impacted identity formations as girls have the challenge of formation and maintenance of an identity separate from their mothers. In terms of developing an individual sense of self, Erickson[40] identified eight stages of life critical in human psychosocial development. While they parallel family development, the focus of Erickson's stages is on individual development and tasks that balance the negative and positives in each developmental stage. The stages most pertinent to involuntarily childless men and women are:

- *young adulthood*: Intimacy versus isolation;
- *adulthood*: Generativity versus self-absorption;
- *senescence*: Integrity versus disgust.

Successful achievement of developmental tasks contributes to happiness and success in later tasks. Developmental tasks are based on physical maturation; cultural pressures; and privileges and include the aspirations and values of the individual. Erickson's generative task of midlife is an excellent example of how the successful accomplishment of a developmental task need not be restricted to reproduction (as is very often the socially and culturally defined norm). Generativity can also expand beyond childbearing to include a multitude of creative endeavors; mentoring possibilities; and nurturing opportunities allowing the mature adult to guide and influence the next generation. As Erickson pointed out, failure to move through this developmental stage leads to a "pervading sense of stagnation and interpersonal impoverishment" potentially impacting healthy adjustment later in life.

Feminist Theory

Feminist theory, jumping off from psychoanalytic theory, has considered women's identity apart from sexual reproduction and cultural context that defines families in which children are not present. In recent decades, particularly in industrialized countries, remaining childless emerged as a trend within the broader context of changes in women's political, economic, and social status.[41] The second wave of feminism in North America late in the twentieth century championed changes in women's status, even though cultural and religious expectations of women continued to be based on sexual reproduction.[41] As such, feminist theory continued, to a large extent, to regard childless women as dysfunctional despite a movement among feminists to subvert women's association with sexual reproduction and extend the notion of families to include individuals without children.

Ireland[42] suggested a variation of object-relations and Lacanian[43] theory to better understand the woman who is not a mother. "Unlike the male, who must reject his early identification with mother and shift his identification to father, the daughter's identity evolves through a path of continual relatedness; she will never have to completely relinquish her earliest maternal identification."[44] Consequently, the desire or need for recreating the mother–child bond is intimately tied to a woman's identity formation and maturation. Unfortunately, because the childless woman identifies with her mother, it is difficult for her to see herself in roles of competency and independence beyond the role of motherhood. Simply put: All mothers are women, but not all women are mothers. The mother who models a multifaceted personality extending beyond her 'good' or 'bad' mothering offers her daughter more opportunity to identify with and be influenced by her mother's personality and creative expression of identity. Motherhood is no longer the one and only defining component of a woman. Ireland[42] contended that personal identity based on an expanded view of femaleness better enables a woman to develop to her full potential.

Lacan[45] emphasized human subjectivity in the way in which language structures identity and formation of gender roles. Lacan perceived the father as facilitating the shift from the fused unit of the mother–infant bond to two separate beings. According to Lacan, acquisition of language is key to assuming a separate identity, as it opens a reflective space between one's self and one's immediate experience. Language based on a patriarchal society does not fully represent the female experience (i.e., being given her father's name followed by her husband's). As such, particularly in patriarchal societies, it is the father who is in the position to assist his daughter by supporting a new voice and language in society, particularly in the developed world.

Social Psychology and Stigma Theory

Social psychology is the study of how individuals influence and are influenced by the thoughts, feelings, and behaviors of other people. Attitudes, social cognition, and social interactions all contribute to social behavior and interactions. Individual attitudes and beliefs about infertility, reproductive failure, and childlessness are experienced by the individual within a social context – whether that of marriage, family, community, society, or as part of humankind. Failure to comply with

individual developmental tasks or societal expectations often results in feelings of embarrassment, abnormality, shame, and isolation. As summarized by Greil,[46] "the essence of infertility's burden has to do with the inability to proceed with one's life according to life course norms that are both reinforced by others and accepted as valid by the affected individual." Infertile men and women feel that they have a personal defect and are damaged or worry that they are being perceived this way by others. Goffman explained this as stigma: "Given that the stigmatized individual in our society acquires identity standards which he applies to himself in spite of failing to conform to them, it is inevitable that he will feel more ambivalence about his own self."[47] Feelings of ambivalence about him or herself are enhanced by feelings commonly associated with infertility, such as being damaged, defective, or worthless, as are strong feelings of guilt, despair, isolation, and disstress. Stigma is enhanced by a sense that one is not operating within the social norm even when one wishes to do so. According to stigma theory, childless men and women deviate from the 'ordinary and natural' life course and are, as such, deeply discredited by their community and within their own self-concept. They may not reveal their childless status, or selectively disclose, in an attempt to avoid experiencing social stigma.

Stigma is a common occurrence for individuals and couples experiencing involuntary childlessness. In a Canadian study that explored attitudes toward voluntary versus involuntary childlessness among the general public, the researchers found that, although there was some stigma regarding voluntary childlessness, involuntary childlessness was not universally stigmatizing and may actually lead to some positive attributions.[48] Despite a trend toward increasingly more voluntary childlessness or acceptance of childlessness following failed medical treatment, numerous studies have shown that childless women continue to feel or be stigmatized.[49] Generally, these childless individuals, regardless of cause, are characterized as being selfish, moody, and emotionally maladjusted. An investigation of childlessness in Bulgaria found that women, when given the opportunity, protested the stigma and mistreatment through voicing their anger and appealing to social change through organized action.[50] It is often presumed that childless individuals will be miserable and lonely in old age, although research indicates that both men and women actually benefit from their child-free status. A study by Connidis and McMullin[51] on geriatric childless women suggested no significant difference in subjective well-being between older child-free women and older mothers. Women reported better health, greater feelings of well-being, and greater marital satisfaction[52,53] in studies on geriatric populations.[54,55]

The stigma of childless women may be better understood within the social context of childlessness. In a study examining childlessness among Arab women, researchers found that childlessness resulted in significant social stigmatization for infertile women and placed them at risk of serious social and emotional consequences.[56] By contrast, childless women in south India found it impossible to pass or selectively disclose the 'invisible' attribute despite serious efforts to destigmatize themselves.[57] In Arab countries, poor village women of childbearing age were devalued in ways affluent and professional women were more able to avoid. However, researchers also found that south India women were able to create spaces for childless marriages within the margins of families and culturally prevalent definitions of womanhood.

In short, having children and building a family are universal norms infertile couples face worldwide. Childlessness, whether voluntary or involuntary, represents a nonnormative experience, exposing the childless man or woman to a variety of stigmatizing experiences and feelings and triggering an array of destigmatizing behaviors that may or may not be successful.

CLINICAL ISSUES

Central to the clinical issues of childlessness is the cultural and societal context in which it is experienced. As clinical treatment and client populations are becoming more international, practitioners must widen their clinical lens and expand their understanding and management of childlessness. Reproductive tourism[58] is bringing highly varied cultures and new clinical experiences and dilemmas into infertility clinics around the world. The infertile woman who travels across international borders may have done so because continued childlessness is not safe or realistic for her. This means the healthcare provider/counselor must consider unfamiliar or atypical reproductive options or family-building alternatives. For example, the husband may take a second wife (sometimes a younger female relative) while the first, infertile wife remains in the home as caretaker, or she may show respect for the husband by emphasizing the need for IVF rather than the need for donar insemination (DI).

The danger of childlessness due to voluntary delay, or ongoing but unsuccessful medical treatment, lies in the possibility of never making the decision to live without children. Endless treatment options can keep the wound open and delay healing. Year after year, grief persists and festers. Fulfillment and happiness become as elusive as parenthood. The focus of a man or woman's identity becomes a sense of not having, not belonging, and not sharing. The cost of unresolved grief can be the additional losses of relationships, marriage, jobs, career, and other life plans. There is also a substantial risk of depression, anxiety, and other mental and physical health difficulties.[59–64]

Paths to Childlessness

Defining and understanding a client's pathway to childlessness is the first step to a therapeutic working relationship. Ireland[42] found that women who had not given up and had spent years in infertility treatment, were more traditional in their values than those who sought little or no medical treatment. These 'traditional women' identified with a feminine sex role and planned to devote a major part of their adult life to motherhood. Career was more often secondary to the primary role of motherhood. For these women, the central issue had become one of mourning: "The mourning process is necessary if the traditional woman is to be able to view herself and others like her in positive, rather than damaged terms."[42] Infertility treatment can create an extended period of denial as each month involves hopes of motherhood, when it is perhaps more appropriate to face the reality of infertility, and, as such, childlessness.

The cause of infertility, ages of partners at the time of diagnosis, treatment options, and financial resources all influence the couple's attitudes about childlessness and their willingness or the necessity of considering the possibility of never having children. A growing number of women in developed countries enter the fourth and fifth decades of their lives without having experienced motherhood. According to Ireland, "At some point, all are awakened by an internal voice or external event that calls their attention to the timeline of their lives; [and] they realize that motherhood is not going to happen."[42] This can precipitate feelings of panic, fear, and a sense of loss of control which may be brief or continue for years.

These 'transitional' women, according to Ireland, want a career and family. For some, the delay is caused by marrying later in life or marrying a partner who does not want children, is not ready for children, or already has children. Single women may suffer from involuntary childlessness, as well as the absence of marriage or a committed life partner. Many of these women are admittedly ambivalent about motherhood. Without actively seeking motherhood, a woman can drift into her middle and later years without children. As she waits, she misses her opportunity to fully realize her creative and nurturing self as a mother. By not making a conscious choice and recognizing her own responsibility in creating in her circumstances and fate, she may struggle to maintain a positive and coherent sense of self.

THERAPEUTIC INTERVENTIONS

The life crisis of infertility has many faces around the world, each within a cultural and religious context and within a family system with its own stories and solutions. The professional equipped with an international perspective and understanding of infertility can more fully appreciate and focus on a client's place and experience of infertility. Within this framework, universal truths of healing and meaningful human connection are made between the therapist and client(s). Once achieved, hope accompanied by culturally realistic and safe solutions to reproductive problems is made possible.

The global causes and solutions to increasing rates of sterility lie outside the therapeutic relationship between infertility counselor and client. Clearly, social, economic, and health policy reforms are needed to address these growing world problems. Improved availability and access to preventive and medical treatment will better serve women in countries in Africa than simply building more IVF clinics. Childless women living within male dominant cultures, with little educational and economic opportunity, will continue to be at risk. Action taken by politicians, social scientists, anthropologists,[1] medical caregivers, the media, mental health professionals, and organizations (e.g., World Health Organization) have exposed the world to the harsh and dangerous realities faced by childless women around the world. With awareness and knowledge, for these women, new possibilities may emerge.

Facilitating Grief and Loss: The First Step

Those who could someday join the large cohort of happy and fulfilled child-free adults would benefit from limited or extended grief work. Letting go of the possibility of giving birth and having children involves an unfocused grieving of many losses. It is a mourning of the loss of an experience rather than an actual death even with a history of perinatal loss. One must face the loss of the dreamed-of child; the loss of whatever part of one's identity was wrapped up in those dreams; and the loss of a destiny that one always assumed would be achieved. It also includes the abstract loss of hope

and a sense of control in life.[8] This grieving is lonely and isolating, because childlessness brings to the surface losses that are largely unrecognized by others. Also called 'disenfranchised grief,' the infertile couple once again find themselves outside of the world of treatment and the world of parenthood.[65] Generally, the longer the pursuit of pregnancy and parenthood, the longer the mourning period. Denial, avoidance, or minimization of this pain can easily result in emotional paralysis and the inability to make concrete changes and develop new goals. Psychological health and well-being can be restored as the mourning process is completed.[8]

Viorst,[66] in a review of loss across the lifespan, states that loss is part of adult life. We must all develop the skill to accept loss to allow for growth and to regain control over our lives:

Throughout our life we grow by giving up our deepest attachments...[and] certain cherished parts of ourselves. We must confront, in the dreams we dream, as well in our intimate relationships, all that we never will have and never will be.

Shapiro[67] contended that: "Couples can't rein in control over their emotions and private lives until they cease their quest for a baby." With the many treatment options available today, deciding to stop treatment can be more difficult than staying on the treatment treadmill. Medical intervention locks the couple into a cycle of hope, followed by the crushing despair of failure. They often feel they cannot give up and think that if they keep trying, eventually something will work. Only the honest and realistic acceptance of their circumstances allows their hope and energy to return.

When there is little choice associated with a couple's situation or there has been ambivalence about parenthood, the transition to a child-free existence can occur without an emotional upheaval or crisis. This was often the case in previous generations, when treatment options were limited and generally unsuccessful. Now, with the array of ARTs and third-party reproduction, treatment options can extend into the fifth and sixth decades of both men and women. For couples seeking treatment today, the decision to end the medical quest for pregnancy is more difficult and is often more emotionally traumatic (see Chapter 24).

To be effective, infertility counselors must understand the clients' personal experience of loss within their societal, cultural, and religious context. With this knowledge, infertility counselors can help individuals and couples process their losses and then, in time, guide decision making and assist their transformation of identity in pursuit of new life meaning. Ultimately, the goal

---

TABLE 23.1. Client exercises

Exercises to access feeling and acknowledge losses

What is it about parenting that drives you?

What is your dream of parenthood?

Describe your infertility crisis beyond your diagnosis and treatment.

What are some stereotypes of childless people?

Compare yourself to these stereotypes. Do they fit?

What makes it difficult for you to consider living child-free?

What do you grieve the most?

What is the difference between not having children and not being a parent?

Exercises to end treatment and say goodbye to the dream child

What do you need to do to finish treatment?

How have your feelings about treatment changed over time?

Could your desire to parent be met in other ways?

Develop a ritual or ceremony to say goodbye to your dream child.

Develop a plan and vocabulary for explaining to others why you do not have children.

Look at how your life is set up. What changes have you already made and what changes do you need to make to accommodate a child-free life (e.g., house, career, pleasure activities)?

What opportunities lie ahead of you?

---

is to help the client consciously accept and find fulfillment and safety in their new and unexpected life journey.

Facilitating Decision Making

Carter and Carter[68] wrote: "Choosing to be childfree after infertility is not giving up hope, it is finding hope of a good life again, only this time without children." *Child-free* is a hopeful word used to describe the positive potential in life.[68] A conscious, deliberate decision to live child-free does not mean resigning oneself to a life without children. Rather than drifting into lifelong childlessness, one can believe that for every loss there is a potential gain. This decision allows for new growth and new goals and the ability to invest renewed energies into work, family, and hobbies. To live child-free is a choice requiring clarity of thoughts, feelings, and communication before becoming acceptable to both partners. This reengineering of self and family is an active process in which living child-free is a way to fulfill the goals of parenthood in other positive, constructive ways.[55,69,70] People with the desire to nurture and love should be encouraged to find ways to do this without having children. The move to a child-free life is a creative adaptation from sorrow, pain, and loss.[8]

Difficulties in making decisions about options for family-building, or conflicts over these options, are common presenting problems for clients seen in clinical practice. Either of these problems can lead to the decision to remain child-free. Couple counseling is recommended if the couple has not been able to come to an agreement on being child-free. Each person needs an opportunity to verbalize and have his or her feelings acknowledged. Compromise is always the goal but may not be possible if one partner is determined to be a parent and the other partner is equally invested in *not* being a parent or if childlessness is culturally unacceptable. By helping the couple appreciate each other's views and by renewing their commitment to each other, possible solutions can emerge. Generally, client(s) and infertility counselor agree to a time-limited contract with clearly defined goals. Typically, goals will be met within two to ten sessions.

After years of dashed hopes and recurrent disappointments, denial of or the inability to feel and identify feelings is common. This emotional whitewash has the potential of leading to clinical depression. Using solution-focused therapy or a cognitive-behavioral framework, infertility counselors can help clients reconnect with their feelings in a safe and supportive environment. It is suggested that sessions end with homework assignments and/or exercises that can be used during or between sessions (Table 23.1). For clients suffering from long-standing depression or dysthymia, a thorough assessment may lead to a referral and further evaluation for pharmacological intervention in conjunction with longer-term, insight-focused and interpersonal psychotherapy. As the depressive symptomatology recedes, work in therapy typically returns to active decision making within an outcome-focused framework.

As stated earlier, confronting loss is the first step in deciding to remain child-free. Telling one's story offers an opportunity to identify losses. Verbalizing personal motivations to parent is also valuable. Work outside the session can be as simple as listing losses or as elaborate as creating a ritual or ceremony to say 'good-bye' to the dream child. For some, creative expression such as drawing, painting, poetry, or collage can be helpful in facilitating bereavement and moving on.

Basic strategies for decision making involve taking control of one's life; developing a positive identity; and reasserting goals and priorities.[68] Rubin[28] offers a very useful model for helping clients with decision making. Assessment starts with looking for and identifying possible 'decision blocks': (1) resignation or holding on to pain; (2) believing there is only one correct decision; (3) holding on to all possible options rather than choosing any one path; (4) procrastination; and (5) guilt over previous decisions. The work in therapy is to identify the individual or couple's particular obstacles and, through the use of therapeutic interventions, overcome these blocks to allow the process of decision making to unfold.

According to Rubin's[28] model, the next task is to establish a foundation for decision making based on personal values. When consumed by the blindfold of infertility, the perception and definition of self become myopic. It is suggested that either during or between sessions, the clients take the time to create a list of priorities. Possible items on the list might be health, quality of life, religion, education, culture, family influence, and security. As clients develop a list, they see themselves as full human beings with the ability to alter their behavior to match their values and create or follow other life plans not involving parenthood.[68]

The final task entails committing to the decision. This means operationalizing the decision to stop treatment and moving from being childless or the state of having less to the position of choosing a child-free life. For most couples, it is a gradual process that happens over time. They may find it takes months or even years before being child-free feels right or comfortable. Rarely do partners move through this process in the same way and with the same timeline. Allowances should be made for individual and gender-specific differences. Eventually, everything begins to fall into place, and concrete evidence of moving on appears. Perhaps a house is purchased without a large family room and four bedrooms, or an application to graduate school is completed or a career move is made. For others, it might be new hobbies; meaningful volunteer work; new friends; or a renewed focus and commitment to their marriage. Realistically, for some couples moving on may be doing so separately because the meaning and purpose of marriage (to have children) has been nullified by childlessness. In these instances, the infertility counselor's work may involve facilitating an amicable marital dissolution; helping both or either partner grieve the lost spouse as well as child; and helping to explore other life goals at possibilities.

Addressing Pressures of Pronatalism

Despite the commonly held perception of global overpopulation, statistics show increased rates of infertility and childlessness in many countries.[1] The right to reproductive function and health are a matter of public policy and population survival. Women in many developing countries often do not have the individual position in society or the personal choice to not have children even when their marriage is infertile. They suffer tremendously and are often powerless to change their circumstances. For these women, the personal experience of infertility in a pronatalist culture, religion, and/or society is brutal. Children secure family survival through labor contributions and, later, by supporting aging parents. Children also serve to sustain political position as well as ethnic and religious identity.[1] A macro-sociopolitical approach supporting significant global changes in health policies, resource distribution, and allocation is needed to address these far-reaching problems. In the developed world, pronatalistic pressures felt by infertile women are often more personal in nature. Gradually, more women are facing this pressure and fighting back. Over the last decade, evidence in developed societies suggests it has become somewhat easier and more acceptable to not have children. Still, the pressure from parents, friends, casual acquaintances, religion, and society is still present. Stereotypes persist, the most common being that the childless couple or woman is self-centered. Strangely, those who choose to remain childless are often called upon to justify their decision, while prospective parents are rarely asked why they want a baby or parents why they have children. Some women without children have said that their lives symbolize a threat to people whose daily lives are largely mandated by their role as parents. Interestingly, wanting to have children could be considered a selfish desire, while parenting as a job demands daily acts of selflessness. A significant clinical issue to explore with involuntarily childless couples is the reasons they originally and currently wish to be have children: to please parents; cement a marriage; fulfill traditional roles; prove youthfulness by reproducing; have someone to love and be loved by; and have someone to care for them in their old age. Although having children may satisfy many of these desires, children actually require years of endless responsibility, hard work, and money and can actually threaten a couple's relationship. Marital satisfaction studies done on Western populations tend to follow a U-shaped curve, with marital happiness starting out high, dropping when children are young, and climbing again after children leave home.[29] One must consider whether motives for having children are not perhaps narcissistic and self-serving. It is ironic that these are often the adjectives used to describe childless individuals, particularly in the developed world.

As women and men age, general societal tension may ease in that people stop asking and waiting for the couple to have children. Lang[16] found that the older women she interviewed expressed very little concern about stigma and stereotypes and did not feel devalued for not having children. Several studies, such as Grimmig and associates'[71] study on older German childless men, found benefits such as husbands presenting themselves with more self-confidence and seeing themselves as more attractive than their peers who were fathers. In the United States, Dalphonse[72] found that nonparents enjoy having more leisure time and money to spend on themselves.

Carter and Carter[68] described being child-free as a 'closet choice' in that even today, many infertile couples are reluctant to discuss their choice because they find it threatening and distressing to disappoint parents and friends will not or do not understand. Typically, couples must find their own support and thus experience solace through their own resolution.[16] It is likely that over time, others will accept their choice as they see the peace and renewed energy in the couple's life. Women at an infertility support group spoke of the peace and relief they experienced as the transition to a child-free life was made.[73] They felt they were once again masters of their own destiny and had moved beyond tragedy to acceptance and opportunity. Wardell[74] suggests, "All lives are filled with compromises, one of which can be to become childfree." Child-free was never a goal or desire, but it can become a very reasonable compromise for many couples stuck on the treadmill of infertility.[29,74]

For some, the use of birth control or surgical sterilization helps to avoid dissonance and help the couple feel greater control of their reproductive lives – addressing overwhelming feelings of loss of control often triggered by infertility. Sterilization ensures that the door to parenthood is, indeed, closed and hopes and plans for the future are directed elsewhere. Furthermore, birth control prevents an unexpected (and often advanced maternal or paternal age) pregnancy after a couple has made new life plans without children. As friends' children grow up and leave home (moving into family life stages that are again focused on the marital dyad), childlessness often becomes less of an issue. Choosing to be child-free does not mean permanent liberation from feelings of loss. It does, however, mean

becoming healthy enough to embrace both loss and gain, and exercising the human ability to adapt to life's circumstances.[75]

Addressing Impact on Relationships

A necessary and distinctive characteristic of the child-free life is the possible presence of new and meaningful relationships. As a couple works through the decision to stop treatment and accept a child-free life, they are forced to reexamine the choices, goals, and dreams that they made together. The partners' new hopes and aspirations may be different from one another. One person may even decide to continue with the quest to have children in his or her life, while the other is pleased to have new opportunities and experiences without children. Clinical experience suggests that couples staying together tend to recommit to each other and direct their nurturing and creative energy toward themselves, marriage, and each other rather than toward treatment and children.

Snarey[76] found that men coped with infertility in three different ways: (1) substitution of a nonhuman object; (2) taking part in activities with other people's children; (3) and self-centeredness. He found that the coping mechanism a man used had an impact on his long-term adjustment in a positive or negative way, in that men who coped by investing in themselves were more satisfied with childlessness and a child-free lifestyle. These men were also more likely to divorce than remain married.

A difficult aspect of childlessness can be the realignment of relationships in the extended family – particularly with the would-be grandparents. How does an adult progress to the role and developmental stage of 'grandparent' when their offspring is child-free? Even adult children feel pressure and work to please their parents and gain parental approval, particularly in cultures in which the well-being of the family or community is considered more important than individual happiness (see Chapter 4). In Lang's[16] study, several women described tension in their relationships with their mothers, who interpreted their daughters' rejection of motherhood as 'a spitting in their face.' Not until daughters and sons move beyond the childbearing years and into middle age will most older parents let go of their expectation and dreams of being a grandparent, and pressure (unspoken or verbalized) from the family subsides. Infertility counselors can be helpful in setting realistic expectations.

Today, divorce of a 'barren' spouse and/or polygamy remain common consequences of childlessness for women from many developing countries.[1,11,14] Husbands and family members are often the primary source of physical danger, harm, and even murder. The small minority of women who have the resources and means to travel to infertility treatment centers that provide forms of third-party reproduction unavailable to them may not be able to return to their community without a pregnancy and/or a child.

FUTURE IMPLICATIONS

The World Health Organization defines access to basic healthcare as a fundamental human right. Today, large populations of people around the globe are not able to exercise this right, in terms of human fertility. Millions of people today do not have access to basic reproductive education or treatment for prevention of rapidly growing rates of permanent sterility. The economic and social stratification of world societies has reinforced equal stratification of reproductive health treatment and service. A just and decent world gives opportunity for all men an women, regardless of race, culture or economic position, the right to seek and receive safe and effective infertility treatment. Conversely, women and men around the globe whose procreative health provides economic security and a place and role in society and the family, deserve the right to openly accept their loss of reproductive function, knowing their family system, community, culture, and religion would realign to accommodate their circumstances. Ultimately, our goal as healthcare providers must extend beyond the narrow view of a medical cure for the select and privileged few. Rather, as infertility counselors and researchers committed to our field and those we serve, our work and goal is to promote and protect the welfare of those who seek, need, and deserve our help, everywhere.

As the incidence of voluntary childlessness and delayed childbearing increases, men and women will have more opportunities for fulfilling and satisfying lives without children. Infertility counselors will be called upon to help these clients to accept their childlessness with courage and find culturally and economically appropriate solutions to their childlessness. We will aid in their discovery of new ways to nurture and develop meaningful and creative ways to contribute and engage in life – without giving birth and becoming parents. This also includes helping patients take responsibility for their decisions for or against children, rather than deciding through avoidance or a decisional drift of repeated treatment trials and failures.

Individuals and institutions of today's industrial world need to continue to challenge prevailing pronatalist norms and values, and to encourage envisioning new possibilities for individuals and society. More and more women are now valuing themselves and others as complete, mature, and feminine women without the once required rite of passage of childbirth. At the same time, growing awareness of the serious reproductive and human rights problems in developing countries will hopefully lead to changes in world health policies and improved healthcare for women and the reduction of the spread of STIs (e.g., HIV, AIDS) due to childlessness. This may stimulate changes in the cultural stigma and economic realities of childlessness in many developing countries. Religious institutions may be enlisted to increase tolerance and embrace families who do not or cannot have children.

In this new world of global travel and trade as well as growing economic interdependence and limited resources, it is up to infertility counselors as leaders in the field of reproductive health and technology, to help build and reinforce a new definition of 'family values.' This is a value for families that we can support through action and the demand for change that truly nurtures and improves the family of humankind in this twenty-first century. This has become our work, our opportunity, and our mission.

SUMMARY

■ While it is estimated that 14% of the world's population suffers from involuntary infertility and sterility, recent evidence suggests this estimate is inaccurate due to underreporting because of social stigma, personal risk, and misidentification.

■ Infertility counselors as leaders, researchers, educators and effective clinicians in reproductive health face increasing demands to address issues of reproductive tourism and global inequalities of reproductive health treatment.

■ The global stratification of reproductive treatment is, on a humanist level, a violation of basic human rights. Solutions to this growing and far-reaching problem are complex, requiring macrosociopolitical as well as grassroots and individual innovation and change.

■ In developing countries, the acute private agony of infertility is transformed to harsh public stigma with complex and devastating consequences.

■ Within most patriarchal societies and in developing countries, cultural traditions, economic realities, religious beliefs, and the power differences between genders all preclude voluntary childlessness for women and even involuntary childlessness.

■ Family system, psychoanalytic, feminist, and stigma theory as well as social psychology all contribute to a better understanding of the theoretical foundations for counseling interventions for involuntarily childless individuals and couples.

■ An individual's and couple's pathway to childlessness sets the stage for the grief process, decision making, and the transition to a child-free life. Culture, religion, and ethnicity contribute to the infertility counselor's development of an appropriate treatment plan as road maps for the therapist.

■ Women living in societies that accept childlessness need help from the infertility counselor to recognize, acknowledge, and ultimately accept losses so as to realistically and honestly transform negatives into positives.

■ Culture and religion, gender and role definition, and identity are all closely tied to the desire to have children. A child-free life requires redefining one's identity and life goals within these contexts.

■ Women and men deciding on a child-free life will need anywhere from several days to several years to make the transformation. The steps include: identifying and overcoming decision blockers; clarifying priorities; and committing and investing in the decision.

■ Historical and present-day societal pressure to procreate is based on pronatalism, a force required for the continuation of the species, and may be motivated by cultural, religious, and political agendas.

■ A child-free life includes reevaluating and committing to significant relationships. Communication and nurturing are core elements in a meaningful and satisfying life.

■ In developed countries, the increasing number and greater visibility of women who choose not to give birth and raise children are helping to encourage a broader definition and expression of meaningful, creative, and successful lives for men and women.

REFERENCES

1. Inhorn MC, Van Balen F, eds. *Infertility Around the Globe: New Thinking on Childlessness, Gender and Reproductive Technologies*. San Francisco and Berkeley, CA: University of California Press, 2002.

2. Chun K, Balls Organista P, Marin G, eds. *Acculturation: Advances in Theory, Measurement, and Applied Research*. Washington, D.C.: American Psychological Association, 2003.

3. Inhorn MC. *Infertility and Patriarchy: The Cultural Politics of Gender and Family Life in Egypt*. Philadelphia, PA: University of Pennsylvania Press, 1996.

4. Rosenblatt PC, Peterson P, Portner J, et al. A cross-cultural study of responses to childlessness. *Behavior Science Notes*, 1973; 8:221–231.

5. Yalom M. *A History of the Wife*. New York: Harper Collins, 2001.

6. Bledsoe CH. *Contingent Lives: Fertility, Time and Aging in West Africa*. Chicago, IL: University of Chicago Press, 2002.

7. Goodwin J. *Price of Honor: Muslim Women Lift the Veil of Silence on the Islamic World*. New York: Little Brown & Co., 1994.

8. Tyler EM. *Barren in the Promised Land*. New York: Basic Books, 1995.

9. Jenkins GL. Childlessness, adoption and milagros de dios in Costa Rica. In: MC Inhorn, F Van Balen, eds. *Infertility Around the Globe: New Thinking on Childlessness, Gender and Reproductive Technologies*. San Francisco and Berkeley, CA: University of California Press, 2002.

10. Wolf M. *The House of Lim: A Study of a Chinese Farm Family*. Englewood Cliffs, NJ: Prentice-Hall, 1968.

11. Pashigan MJ. Conceiving the happy family: Infertility and marital politics in northern Vietnam. In: MC Inhorn, F Van Balen, eds. *Infertility Around the Globe: New Thinking on Childlessness, Gender and Reproductive Technologies*. San Francisco and Berkeley, CA: University of California Press, 2002.

12. Giwa-Osagie O. ART in developing countries with particular reference to sub-Saharan Africa. *Current Practices and Controversies in Assisted Reproduction: Report of a Meeting on Medical, Ethical and Social Aspects of Assisted Reproduction*. World Health Organization. 2001 Sept.; 17–21:22–7. Available at: http://www.who/int/reproductive-health/infertility/27.pdf. Accessed 3/22/2005.

13. Daar A, Merali Z. Infertility and social suffering: The case of ART in developing countries. *Current Practices and Controversies in Assisted Reproduction: Report of a Meeting on Medical, Ethical and Social Aspects of Assisted Reproduction*. World Health Organization. 2001 Sept.; 17–21:14–21. Available at: http://www.who/int/reproductive-health/infertility/27.pdf. Accessed 3/22/2005.

14. Gerrits T. Infertility and matrilineality: The exceptional case of the Macua of Mozambique. In: Mc Inhorn, F Van Balen, eds. *Infertility Around the Globe: New Thinking on Childlessness, Gender and Reproductive Technologies*. San Francisco and Berkeley, CA: University of California Press, 2002.

15. Dally A. *Inventing Motherhood: The Consequences of an Ideal*. New York: Schocken Boos, 1982.

16. Lang SS. *Women Without Children: The Reasons, the Rewards, the Regrets*. New York: Pharos Books, 1991.

17. Jamison PH, Franzini LR, Kaplan RM. Some assumed characteristics of voluntarily childfree women and men. *Psychology of Women Quarterly* 1979; 4:267–73.

18. Shields S, Cooper PE. Stereotypes of traditional and nontraditional childbearing roles. *Sex Roles* 1983; 9:363–76.

19. Boonmongkon P. Family networks and support to infertile people. *Current Practices and Controversies in Assisted Reproduction: Report of a Meeting on Medical, Ethical and Social Aspects of Assisted Reproduction*. World Health Organization. 2001 Sept.; 17–21:281–6. Available at: http://www.who/int/reproductive-health/infertility/27.pdf. Accessed 2/14/2005.

20. Hastings DW, Gregory RJ. Incidences of childlessness for United States women, cohorts born 1891–1945. *Soc Biology* 1914; 21:178–84.

21. Remennick L. Childless in the land of imperative motherhood: Stigma and coping among infertile Israeli women. *Sex Roles: A Journal of Research* December 2000:1–16. Available at: http://www.findarticles.com/p/articles/mi_m2294/is_2000_Dec/ai_75959829/. Accessed 2/14/2005.

22. Stanworth M, ed. *Reproductive Technologies: Gender, Motherhood and Medicine*. Cambridge, UK: Polity Press, 1987.

23. Whiteford LM, Gonzales L. Stigma: The hidden burden of infertility. *Social Science & Medicine* 1995; 40:27–36.

24. Peritz E, Baras M. *Studies in the Fertility of Israel*. Jerusalem: Hebrew University, 1992.

25. Lee T-Y, Chu T-Y. The Chinese experience of male infertility. *Western J Nursing Res* 2001; 23:39–48.

26. Lee S. *Counselling in Male Infertility*. London: Blackwell Science, 1996.

27. Bentley G, Mascie-Taylor CG, ed. *Infertility in the Modern World*. Cambridge, UK: Cambridge University Press, 2000.

28. Rubin TI. *Overcoming Indecisiveness: The Eight Stages of Effective Decisionmaking*. New York: Harper and Row, 1985.

29. Renne KS. Childlessness, health and marital satisfaction. *Soc Bio* 1976; 23:183–97.

30. Strauss B. *Involuntary Childlessness: Psychological Assessment, Counseling and Psychotherapy*. Seattle, WA: Hogrefe and Huber, 2002.

31. Caldwell JC, Orubuloye IO, Caldwell P. Fertility decline in Africa: A new type of transition? *Population and Development Review* 1992b; 18:211–42.

32. www.cdc.gov/reproductivehealth/ART00/nation.htm. Accessed 2/14/2005.

33. Alexander BB, Rubinstein RL, Goodman M, Luborsky M. A path not taken: A cultural analysis of regrets and childlessness in the lives of older women. *The Gerontologist* 1992; 32:618–26.

34. Khayata GM, Rizk DE, Hasan MY, et al. Factors influencing the quality of life of infertile women in United Arab Emirates. *International Journal of Gynecology and Obstetrics* 2003 Feb; 80:183–8.

35. Bhatti LI, Fikree FF, Khan A. The quest of infertile women in squatter settlements of Karachi Pakistan: A qualitative study. *Soc Sci Med* 1999; 49:637–49.

36. Carter B, McGoldrick M. *The Family Life Cycle: A Framework for Family Therapy*. New York: Gardner, 1980.

37. Carter B, McGoldrick M. *The Changing Family Life Cycle: A Framework for Family Therapy*. Boston: Allyn & Bacon, 1988.

38. Matthews R, Matthews AM. Infertility and involuntary childlessness: The transition to nonparenthood. *J Mar Fam* 1986; 48:641–9.

39. Barron JW, Eagle MN, Wolitsky DL, eds. *Interface of Psychoanalysis and Psychology*. Washington, DC: American Psychological Association, 1992.

40. Erickson E. *Identity and the Life Cycle*. New York: Norton, 1980.

41. Hird MJ, Abshoff K. Women without children: A contradiction in terms? *Canadian Journal of Comparative Family Studies* 2000; 31:347–66.

42. Ireland M. *Reconceiving Women: Separating Motherhood from Female Identity*. New York: Guilford Press, 1993.

43. Lacan J. *Four Fundamental Concepts of Psychoanalysis*. New York: Norton, 1978.

44. Klein M. Early stages of the oedipus complex. *Int J Psychoanalysis* 1928; 9:167–80.

45. Lacan J. *Feminine Sexuality*. New York: Norton, 1985.

46. Greil AL. *Not Yet Pregnant: Infertile Couples in Contemporary America*. New Brunswick NJ: Rutgers University Press, 1991.

47. Goffman E. *Stigma: Notes on the Management of a Spoiled Identity*. Englewood Cliffs, NJ: Prentice-Hall, 1963.

48. Lampman C, Dowling-Guyer S. Attitudes toward voluntary and involuntary childlessness. *Basic and Applied Social Psychology* 1995; 17:213–22.

49. Mueller KA, Yoder JD. Stigmatization of non-normative family size status-statistical data included. *Sex Roles: A Journal of Research*. December 1999:1–15. Available at: http://www.findarticles.com/p/articles/mi_m2294/is1999_Dec/ai_61892280/. Accessed 2/24/2005.

50. Todorova I, Kotzeva T. Social discourses, women's resistive voices: Facing involuntary childlessness in Bulgaria. *Women's Studies International Forum* 2003; 26:139–51.

51. Connidis IA, McMullin JA. To have or not to have: Parent status and the subjective well-being of older men and women. *Gerontologist* 1993; 33:630–6.

52. Houseknecht SK. Childlessness and marital adjustment. *Journal of Marriage and the Family* 1979; 41:259–65.

53. Renne KS. Childlessness, health, and marital satisfaction. *Social Biology* 1977; 23:183–97.

54. Zhang Z, Hayward MD. Childlessness and the psychological well-being of older persons. *The Journal of Gerontology* 2001; 56B:S311–S320.

55. Lafayette L. *Why Don't You Have Kids? Living a Full Life Without Parenthood*. New York: Kensington Books, 1995.

56. Fido A, Zahid M. Coping with infertility among Kuwaiti women: Cultural perspectives. *International Journal of Social Psychiatry* 2004; 50(4):294–300.

57. Riessman CK. Positioning gender identity in narratives of infertility: South Indian women's lives in context. In: MC Inhorn, F Van Balen, eds. *Infertility Around the Globe: New Thinking on Childlessness, Gender and Reproductive Technologies*. San Francisco and Berkeley, CA: University of California Press, 2002.

58. Fathalla M. Current challenges in assisted reproduction. *Current Practices and Controversies in Assisted Reproduction: Report of a Meeting on Medical, Ethical and Social Aspects of Assisted Reproduction*. World Health Organization. 2001 Sept.; 17–21:1–12. Available at: http://www.who/int/reproductive-health/infertility/27.pdf. Accessed 3/22/2005.

59. Newton CR, Hearn MT, Yuzpee AA, Houle M. Motives for parenthood and response to failed in vitro fertilization: Implications for counseling. *J Asst Reprod Technol Genet* 1992; 9:24–31.

60. Berg BJ, Wilson JF, Weingartner PJ. Psychological sequelae of infertility treatment: The role of gender and sex-role identification. *Soc Sci Med* 1991; 33:1071–80.

61. Boivin J, Takefman JE, Tulandi T, Brender W. Reactions to infertility based on extent of treatment failure. *Fertil Steril* 1995; 63:801–7.

62. Edemann RJ, Connolly KJ. Psychological aspects of infertility. *Br J Med Psychol* 1986; 59:209–19.

63. Domar A, Seibel M, Benson H. The mind/body program for infertility: A new behavioral treatment approach for women with infertility. *Fertil Steril* 1990; 53(2):246–9.

64. Greenfeld D, Mazure C, Haseltine F, DeCherney A. The role of the social worker in the in-vitro fertilization program. *Social Work in Health Care* 1984; 10(2):71–9.

65. Doka KJ, ed. *Disenfranchised Grief: New Directions, Challenges, and Strategies for Practice*, Champaign, IL: Research Press, 2002.

66. Viorst J. *Necessary Losses*. New York: Ballantine, 1986.

67. Shapiro C. *Infertility and Pregnancy Loss: A Guide for the Helping Professionals*. San Francisco, CA: Jossey-Bass Publishers, 1988.

68. Carter JW, Carter M. *Sweet Grapes. How to Stop Being Infertile and Start Living Again*. Indianapolis, IN: Perspectives Press, 1989.

69. Wardell H. The childfree lifestyle. *Aribella: The Magazine for Today's Woman* [On-line Journal]. 4 January 2002. Available at: http://www.aribella.com/childfree.htm. Accessed 2/14/2005.

70. Cain M. *The Childless Revolution*. New York: Perseus Publishing, 2001.

71. Grimmig RE, Jaiser F, Pfrunder D. Self concept and body image in involuntary sterility. *Psychother Psychosom Med Psychol* 1992 Jul; 42(7):253–9.

72. Dalphonse S. Choosing to be childfree. *ZPG Report*. 1997 May–Jun; 29(3):1, 6. Available at: http://www.ncbi.nlm.nih.gov/entrez/query.fcgi?cmd=Retrieve&db=pubmed. Accessed 7/18/2005.

73. Resolve, Aronson S. *Resolving Infertility: Understanding the Options and Choosing Solutions When You Want to Have a Baby*. New York: Harper Resource, 1999.

74. Wardell H. *Childfree After Infertility: Moving From Childlessness to a Joyous Life*. Lincoln, NE: iUniverse, 2003.

75. Anton HL. *Never to be a Mother: A Guide for All Women Who Didn't – or Couldn't – Have Children*. San Francisco, CA: Harper, 1992.

76. Snarey J. Men without children. *Psychology Today* 1988 Mar; 22(3):61–2.

24 Ending Treatment

JANET E. TAKEFMAN

The line between failure and success is so fine that we scarcely know when we pass it: so fine that we are often on the line and do not know it.

– Elbert Hubbard, 1927

A question frequently posed within the context of the infertility clinic is when to stop treatment, or when to advise patients that 'enough is enough.' This question poses a number of problems when trying to establish evidenced-based answers. First, there is no clear end point for cessation of unsuccessful fertility treatment as there is always some probability of success inherent in further attempts. Furthermore, unlike other treatments, there is no continuum of benefits of infertility treatment, with the only satisfactory outcome being a live birth. Finally, the decision to continue or end treatment is often based on a different set of criteria depending on whether it is physician- or patient-initiated, which may present a conflict of interest situation. The physician bases the decision to end treatment on medical probabilities of success; the patient, on personal costs and rationalizations. However, only limited information is available about this decision-making process because only a few studies have been specifically designed to address why, when, and how people end treatment. Considering the experience of infertility treatment for the majority of individuals is failure rather than success, given the less than 50% overall success rate of IVF treatment, this is a conspicuous lapse. However, we can understand this end of treatment process better by extrapolating from related areas of study.[1] Such studies include, but are not limited to, research on patients who drop out of treatment, and qualitative studies of patients' experiences following failed treatment cycles. It is based on these studies that clinical recommendations can be suggested.

Despite the paucity of direct studies, it is well-accepted that ending treatment is a difficult and complex psychological process for both physician and patient.

This chapter

■ appraises current research related to factors that impact the decision to end treatment;
■ describes the psychological process that patients navigate in abandoning treatment;
■ applies theoretical frameworks to comprehend this stage of ending treatment;
■ provides guidelines for health professionals to assist both physicians and patients in improving ending treatment consultations.

HISTORICAL OVERVIEW

Research and clinical efforts within the discipline of health psychology have traditionally focused attention on two main aspects of medical interventions. Treatment perseverance and the stresses associated with a prolonged treatment process have received the most attention, followed by difficulties relating to post-treatment adjustment. The theoretical evolution of this research was promoted by such groundbreaking works as Benson's mind–body model of illness and health,[2] which recognized the interplay of biological, psychological and social influences on the treatment of disease, and by Lazarus and Folkman's model of stress and coping,[3] which was developed to provide a framework to understand adjustment to health-related problems.

The field of psychological aspects of infertility and its treatment has followed this same convention and evolution. Thus, a substantial amount of research exists on the process of participating in infertility treatments with its accompanying social, interpersonal, and emotional difficulties (see Part III of this book) and examination of the process of decision making regarding alternatives to biological parenting, once treatment has failed (see Parts VI and VII of this book). What has been neglected in the clinical literature is examination of the psychological processes that must take place when patients transition from actively pursuing treatment in the hope of having a child to accepting that it will not yield their desired result – the process of ending treatment. It was not until the late 1980s when a few studies were published that this aspect of infertility treatment was recognized as an important area of study.[4–6]

REVIEW OF LITERATURE

The review of literature will examine factors that have an impact on the end of treatment. They include: sociodemographic, interpersonal, emotional, and fear factors.

Sociodemographic Factors

Parity is a significant predictor of withdrawal from treatment. Callan and colleagues found that 50% of women who intended to stop IVF were more likely to have children already, compared with only 25% of those with no children who were considering ending treatment.[5] Daniluk and Mitchell found that family size was a significant factor in couples' decisions regarding continuing IVF.[7] For the 34% of the sample who had achieved multiple births, most were not intending to pursue further treatment. Conversely, having only one child was a reason to continue with treatment. Interestingly, Throsby[8] also found that one of the important motivators of why couples try IVF is to produce a sibling for an existing child. However, she elaborated that concern about the possible loneliness of an only child was balanced against concern that getting involved in IVF would negatively affect that child in terms of parent absences, resources, and emotional availability. Thus, paradoxically, while having an only child is one of the determinants of why couples seek out treatment; it is also a reason why they withdraw from treatment before accomplishing their goal. Another study showed that if the female partner of the couple had a child, ending treatment was more likely than if the male partner had a child.[9]

Finally, people who are more open-minded about alternative ways of forming a family are likely to react more favorably to ending treatment. van Balen and colleagues in The Netherlands found that life-satisfaction scores after the end of treatment were higher for infertile couples who were exploring other options to natural conception.[10] Similarly, planning to adopt was the main factor discriminating distress scores for those

couples who experienced treatment failure with those intending to adopt being less distressed,[11] and a Norwegian study found that the psychological crisis of treatment failure could be resolved through adoption.[12]

Age of the woman, per se, does not seem to be a predictor of voluntarily dropping out of treatment except when actively recommended by her doctor.[13] However, a few studies have found that male age is a predictor of treatment dropout, with women married to older partners less likely to continue with treatment.[14]

Gender is critical to decision making about further treatments. First, it has been well-established that women, compared to men, are more likely to initiate treatment, want to try new treatments, and want to continue on with treatment.[15] Blenner[6] in her theory of stages through infertility treatment found that men were more likely to disengage or let go of treatment before women. This greater interest in pursuing treatment in women has been attributed to the notion that parenthood is a more valued developmental goal for women.[16] This hypothesis has been supported by different studies that demonstrate, for example, that childbearing is rated as a more vital life goal by women than men,[17] that the value of life without children is rated as poorer in women compared to men,[18] and that women appear to benefit more from having children after infertility than do men.[19] For a more comprehensive review of these gender differences, read Chapter 3.

Finances have long been presumed to be an important factor in determining whether couples persist with medical treatment for infertility, especially IVF and other costly assessments or treatments. Furthermore, it is likely that a certain number of people do not even begin treatment due to poor financial resources and turn immediately to more affordable alternatives such as adoption or foster care. However, recent studies have shown the impact of economic concerns on deciding to end treatment may have been overestimated in developed countries. This evidence mainly comes from international studies that were carried out in countries where IVF treatment is subsidized by the state. In two Dutch studies (a country where three IVF cycles are covered by public health insurance), one reported a cumulative dropout rate of 62.4%, in which only 13.9% was due to physician recommendation,[20] and the other had a 30% dropout rate before the third cycle.[13] In Australia, couples who ended treatment had undertaken only two and a half of the six subsidized treatment cycles available to them.[21] In Sweden, couples participated in an average of one and a half of three cycles allowable.[22] In all these studies, psychological factors played a more central role in ending treatment than economics.

In summary, on the basis of these sociodemographic findings, health professionals should be aware that childless women who are not open to alternatives to natural conception will likely persist longer with treatment compared with their male counterparts, regardless of age or economic status and, perhaps consequently, react more negatively to the suggestion to end treatment.

Interpersonal Factors

Although earlier research[23–25] suggested that the stress associated with infertility had damaging effects on most marriages, it has since been well-established that for the majority of couples marital satisfaction and commitment tend to be strengthened as couples face the onslaught of the infertility experience together.[26] Specifically pertaining to treatment dropout, one recent study reported that only 2.3% of 500 couples had ended treatment because of marital discord,[27] and another reported only 1.3% of couples dropped out of treatment because of separation or divorce.[28] Slightly higher statistics were recently reported in a study from Sweden, which found that 15% of 242 couples reported ceasing treatment without achieving a birth because of divorce or marital problems.[22]

For most couples, the choice to marry is synonymous with the decision to eventually form a family. Therefore, it is not surprising that relationship issues have been identified as one of the significant predictors of treatment persistence or abandonment. Daniluk and Mitchell found that people who felt that infertility had had a negative impact on their marriages were less likely to want to try IVF for a second time.[7] Conversely, Stauss and colleagues found that couples who felt their union would be threatened by not having a family were those who most persisted with treatment and were reluctant to end it.[18] This was supported in Daniluk's longitudinal, qualitative analysis of thirty-seven couples who were going through the transition to biological childlessness.[29] Participants expressed a sense of uncertainly and foreboding about the future of their relationships if they accepted the reality that treatment would not yield a child. Moreover, she reported that eventually 10% of these couples ended treatment because of the strain it had on the partnership. An interesting finding with important clinical implications was that couples who ended treatment without consensus continued to have feelings of emotional distress years later compared with couples who were in agreement about discontinuing at the time they ended treatment.

Thus, on the basis of these findings, the recommendation to end treatment may elicit a wide range of reactions; from relief that the marriage will not have to endure this pressure any longer, to fears that it will trigger the demise of the relationship. Congruence between spouses would be an important outcome to elicit from couples to ensure long-term relationship stability and satisfaction.

Emotional Factors

Optimism, or patients overestimating their chances of success, is one of the most reliable findings in studies that have profiled the infertility patient.[18] Theoretically, this optimistic bias is considered an important variable in determining adjustment to threatening events.[30] The magnitude of the optimistic bias in IVF has led some to examine its effect on emotional reactions if treatment fails. However, no link was found between pretreatment optimism and reactions to treatment failure,[31] nor was optimism during treatment found to compound negative reactions when treatment was unsuccessful.[32] This is important to note for clinical purposes as there exists among mental health professionals and patients alike a misconception that the lower a patient's expectations are, the less emotionally distraught they will be following a treatment failure. These data cited suggest otherwise. Conversely, a common recommendation that medical staff make to patients during treatment is to 'think positively,' as this will improve participation. This concept too has no empirical basis.

However, optimism does appear to play a role in decision making about initiating treatment[9] and in ending treatment.[18] Callan and colleagues found that patients who continued with treatment perceived the psychological burden of treatment no differently from those who discontinued, but the former group continued because they were more optimistic about the chances of success with further attempts.[5] Similarly, it has been demonstrated that patients' beliefs about the likelihood of success are based more on their own optimistic bias than physicians' estimations of their chances.[22,27] However, physician optimism can, and often does, influence a woman to continue IVF treatment when she is ambivalent.[5]

Based on these findings regarding optimism as a trait, we could predict that optimistic patients may have a harder time accepting the end of treatment and will be less impressed and/or influenced in their decision-making process by the physician's opinion of their chances.

Psychological distress is another factor that has been studied with respect to treatment persistence. However, the literature is murky because of the lack of precision in terminology. A number of vague terms have been used to describe this psychological variable in studies that looked at ending treatment. These include: 'psychologically too stressful,'[28] 'psychological burden,'[22] 'psychological reasons,'[13] 'emotional costs,'[21] 'emotional stress,'[33] 'reached limit,'[34] and 'emotional exhaustion.'[29] Such terms are, obviously, too broad and difficult to operationalize. To illustrate this point, when Olivius and colleagues[22] categorized the spontaneous comments made by 143 couples who had discontinued IVF, the most common reason given for discontinuing treatment prior to completing three, free IVF cycles was 'psychological burden,' attributed to 26% of the sample. However, this psychological burden category included earlier failed treatments, late pregnancy miscarriage and abortion due to chromosomal abnormalities, as well as feeling social pressure to quit and too many doctor appointments.

In one of the few studies that used standardized measures of distress, it was shown that pretreatment levels of distress were predictive of early dropout rate.[13] This Dutch study consisted of a sample of 380 women entering their first IVF cycle who were given a battery of psychological questionnaires before and after treatment. It was shown that subjects who dropped out of treatment of their own volition had significantly higher pretreatment anxiety and depression scores than subjects who continued on with treatment. Thus, it was reasonable to conclude that the most common reason for ending treatment was emotional distress, in that the more anxious or depressed a woman was prior to IVF treatment, the more likely she was to end treatment prematurely.

It is noteworthy that despite the psychological ordeal of treatment, many couples do not regret having tried. The Australian follow-up study of 211 patients who had their last appointment some three years prior to the start of data collection, indicated that almost all were satisfied that they had tried the medical options available, even though 60–70% perceived treatment to be a significant stressor.[21] Similarly, in two different qualitative studies, one from Canada,[29] the other from the United States,[6] all participants recalled their attempts at treatment as essential to reaching closure and precluding any regrets later on. All women stated they would do nothing differently if they had it to do over again, in spite of the fact they never achieved pregnancy.

In contrast to the above paragraph, some evidence also exists suggestive of a continued negative impact of childlessness. For example, two studies demonstrated that even though life satisfaction scores were in the high range, scores for childless women were lower than the scores of those who became parents through other means.[19,35] Furthermore, studies have shown that many years after treatment women still report intrusive thoughts about infertility,[12] still consider infertility an emotional issue,[21] still report fertility-related stress,[19] and still yearn for a biological child.[34] It would seem therefore that although global quality-of-life is fairly good among couples who remain childless, there can be some continuing, negative residual effects.

Fear Factors

Fear plays a significant role in understanding couples' reluctance to end treatment. There are three existential-type fears that individuals must grapple with and confront in the process of ending treatment.[1] The first is the fear of not being able to cope with the emotional ramifications of ending treatment. Daniluk[29] proposed that one of the main factors preventing couples from ending treatment is the fear that reactions would be unbearable and impossible to cope with. A second fear is that life without children will be comparatively deficient and remarkably unfulfilling. In other words, many couples persist with treatment because they cannot imagine a satisfying future life without genetically-conceived children. For them, being told that treatment is over is tantamount to being told they have no future. Finally, many couples fear their relationship will not survive without children. As mentioned earlier, for many couples (and according to many religions and cultures) the basis of a committed relationship is the formation of a larger family. Thus, ending treatment would be synonymous to the destruction of the core couple either from within, due to a couple's own beliefs, or from external social or religious pressures.

As mental health professionals, our goal is to help infertile couples overcome these fears. It is a basic counseling tenet that any decision made in fear is the wrong decision. Thus, we must empower and fortify couples with factual information about ending treatment so that their decision making is not prejudiced by fears, but rather based on objective and relevant evidence.

In conclusion, it seems clear that how an individual reacts to advice about ending treatment will differ according to a variety of social, demographic, interpersonal, emotional, and psychological factors. As infertility counselors, it is our responsibility to be cognizant of these factors so that we can advise physicians how best to approach the topic of ending treatment with patients in order to offer optimal counseling to clients who are facing these situations and dilemmas.

THEORETICAL FRAMEWORK

To date, most theories on coping with tragic life events have focused on psychopathology (e.g., depression) rather than successful adaptation (e.g., renewed energy). However, most studies on the consequences of tragic life events find that the majority of people manage to cope in impressively resilient ways to even the most adverse setbacks in their lives.[36] These findings are echoed in the following experiential models that have been proposed to explain how an infertile individual deals with withdrawing from treatment. Three paradigms have been postulated in three separate studies to explain the long and complex process required for infertile individuals to transition from 'not yet pregnant' to 'not going to be pregnant,' to use Throsby's terminology.[8] This process is seen as a necessary rite of passage for the infertile individual to ultimately accept and come to terms with letting go of the dream of a genetically-conceived child. All three theories were based on qualitative analyses because this type of methodology is better suited to track adaptation over time than quantitative research designs.

Infertility-Stage Theories

Blenner's stage theory[6] was based on the reports of twenty-five infertile married couples as they moved from pretreatment to posttreatment. The theory is based on three concepts: engagement, immersion, and disengagement and includes eight stages within these concepts. *Disengagement* marked the beginning of the process of ending treatment. The three stages of disengagement were 'letting go,' 'quitting and moving out,' and 'shifting the focus.' Blenner described the stage of letting go as a turning point when couples and individuals began to entertain the notion that treatment would not work and, therefore, should not continue. Cognitively, couples started to question the fairness of life and the investment of further energy in treatment. It was a time when they began to reexamine their options. Emotionally, individuals felt less pain and more in control of their lives. They found peace in the belief that they had done all they could do to reach their reproductive goals. In the next stage of quitting and moving out, individuals ceased treatment. Couples felt relief at not being ruled by the demands of treatment. The stage of moving out occurred in many directions, from pursuing adoption to remaining childless. Shifting the focus, the final stage, was described as a peaceful resignation with a new focus on the future. Although pangs of grief recurred, usually precipitated by specific events such as a friend's pregnancy, individuals were able for the most part to cope with their biological childlessness.

In Daniluk's three-year longitudinal, qualitative study[29] a sample of thirty-seven couples, was asked the question: "How do couples make sense of their infertility and reconstruct their lives when faced with the permanence of biological childlessness?" She developed a four-stage model based on a continuum of themes that included: 'hitting the wall,' 'reworking the past,' 'turning toward the future,' and 'renewal and regeneration.' In comparing these two models, Daniluk basically magnified Blenner's disengagement stage by providing more details and adding time frames to the stages. In Daniluk's analysis, the first ten months after abandoning efforts to conceive were experienced as a time of hitting the wall. The couples came face-to-face with their worst fears and the undeniable reality that their infertility was permanent. This was a stage of profound sadness and grief. Couples experienced the next ten months as an attempt to make sense of their years of trying to conceive, which was characterized by reworking the past. During this stage, anger and frustration were expressed and couples questioned the viability of their marriages. It is a stage defined by instability. The third ten-month period, referred to as turning toward the future, was a time when couples demonstrated a willingness to consider future life scenarios other than biological parenthood. Emotionally, this period was described as a time of stability and personal control. The final stage, renewal and regeneration, was a ten-month period in which couples regained a sense of who they once were, while taking comfort in knowing they had survived great adversity. By this point, most of the couples were able to identify some greater purpose to their infertility.

Finally, Throsby[8] drew her model from in-depth interviews with fifteen infertile women and thirteen couples, all of whom came from IVF programs without having achieved a live birth. However, she makes the point that even when IVF is successful, the end of treatment is still not clearly marked because the successful cycle may provide the motivation to return to treatment to try for a second child (or more) to complete the family. Thus, the point at which treatment ends is really always subjective, based on a myriad of personal and medical factors. Her study identified seven key rationalizations or discourses that participants used to help them come to terms with having abandoned treatment. These included (1) doing everything possible, (2) desperation, (3) resistance, (4) benevolence, (5) the sensible consumer, (6) fertility, and (7) fitness to parent. These discourses were not considered mutually exclusive and frequently overlapped within individual accounts. These discourses allowed participants to make sense of their biological childlessness while still feeling they conformed to society's norms and expectations regarding their role as women. Throsby drew heavily on the understanding of motherhood as stemming from a social and cultural rather than biological imperative, and that gaining closure required conforming to this ideology regardless of one's actual capacity to reproduce.

Cognitive Adaptation Model

In comparison to the stage theories that were developed specifically observing infertile subjects, the cognitive adaptation model was developed primarily from work with women diagnosed with breast cancer. It contends that individuals who successfully adapt to a personal tragedy address three basic themes in coming to terms with the event.[30] First is to try to find meaning in what happened. This task was also posited by both Blenner's and Daniluk's models. A second task is to gain mastery over the threatening event and regain control over one's life. Daniluk showed that for those who do not achieve pregnancies, the restoration of personal control is one of the greater challenges.[29] Some achieve control by making decisions about careers, education and other significant pursuits,[29,34] whereas, others do so by rejecting further treatment even when a possibility of success exists.[6] Third, people coping with tragic events try to enhance the self. Tragic events often make survivors feel badly about themselves regardless of whether they had any control over the occurrence of the event. The profound negative effect of infertility on women's self-esteem is well-established. Infertile women have been shown to have poorer self-esteem, especially body esteem, compared with women who have never been infertile.[37] Similar decrements in self-esteem have also been reported for men, especially when the cause of infertility is male-factor.[38]

This limited analysis, based on the few theoretical studies addressing the topic of adaptation to biological childlessness or disease, offers some interesting perspective on coping with the end of treatment. Clearly, the sadness of infertility never wholly remits, but individuals do seem to attain a fair level of contentment and happiness in life. Those unable to achieve a healthy level of adjustment are those who are likely unable to find a way of valuing a life without children or to perceive any positive value from their experience with infertility.

CLINICAL ISSUES

Medical training encourages treating a patient until the medical problem is resolved. Unfortunately, infertility treatment does not always resolve the problem in favor of a pregnancy or live birth. Consequently, many couples continue treatment even in the face of futility. Wischmann pointed out that deciding to stop treatment is often more difficult than continuing.[39] Furthermore, physicians who have not been trained to abandon treatment efforts, encounter regularly the need to counsel a patient that they have exhausted all reasonable means to conceive a genetic child and it is time to discontinue treatment. This section will discuss some of the clinical issues mental healthcare providers must consider in counseling both the physician and patient on ending treatment.

Physician-Recommended Dropout

The Ethics Committee of the American Society for Reproductive Medicine made recommendations in 2004 for doctors treating infertility patients when treatment would not likely be successful.[40] Basically, it was concluded that physicians have a right to refuse to initiate a treatment which they regard as futile or with very poor prognosis, as long as they have made a reasonable medical judgment and have fully informed the patient. An important clinical issue that arose from this discussion is the conflict of interest between patient and physician. On the one hand, patients have an interest to do anything they can to have a child while on the other hand, physicians have an interest in minimizing harm to patients by not offering treatment that will not be helpful, and may, in fact, impair a patient's physical health or jeopardize emotional well-being. It was made clear that this is a delicate consult in which frustration and misunderstanding can erupt, if not handled correctly. Because of this, the Ethics Committee further suggested that physician-recommended treatment termination should include a referral to a psychological counselor. A final recommendation was that this end of treatment consultation would be an appropriate time when physicians could broach the topic of alternative family-building options with patients.

Further support for the role of counseling in this type of situation came from a recent Dutch study that compared the psychological sequelae for patients who were denied further treatment by physicians (actively censored), compared with those who discontinued treatment voluntarily (passively censored).[13] It found that although at pretreatment levels of depression and anxiety did not differ, at posttreatment the actively censored patients reported higher levels of depression and anxiety than those who self-terminated. It was concluded that this group of patients was therefore most in need of psychological support.

Thus, because physicians are being encouraged to end treatment when appropriate and discuss options to biological parenting with patients, and because the evidence suggests that patients will have severe reactions to such recommendations even when warranted, infertility counselors must be prepared to offer their expertise and skills to both parties.

Delivering Bad News

Ending treatment, whether patient- or physician-initiated, is not considered good news, thus, we must find a way to approach this topic so as not to compound difficulties. Boivin and colleagues showed that mood alternates during an IVF cycle among elation–sadness, confidence–worry, and frustration–relief, depending on negative or positive feedback.[41] Thus, when counseling patients on end of treatment decisions and adaptation, the mental health professional must be conscientious about presenting the information in the most positive light possible. For example, telling a patient she did everything she was supposed to do in following her treatment regimen is more positive than pointing out that her case is hopeless. In a related study, Groff and colleagues studied how women responded to the bad news of receiving the diagnosis of premature ovarian failure (POF).[42] Of 100 women, 71% were unsatisfied with the manner in which the physician informed them about their POF status and 89% reported experiencing significant emotional distress at the time of diagnosis. Most importantly, the degree of emotional distress was significantly correlated with the degree of dissatisfaction with the manner in which the women were told of the diagnosis. In this study, most women felt the bad news consult could have been handled more effectively by the physician if they had been allotted more time, been given more thorough information, and felt the physician was sensitive to their emotional needs. The article also provided a model for the physician when delivering bad news.

Staff–Patient Communication

Studies have shown that patient dissatisfaction with IVF programs is influenced by total quality of care management, which inherently involves staff–patient communication.[33] Common patient complaints include: insufficient time to talk about concerns and questions;

insufficient information provided; poor understanding of medical advice; and lack of empathy expressed by medical staff. Patient-centered communications are a simple and basic remedy for these complaints. These involve more open-ended questions with greater scope for patients to raise their own concerns. Patient-centered communications support an emotionally focused approach, which has been shown to be particularly helpful in medical situations that are uncontrollable and unpredictable such as ending treatment.[1] Schmidt and colleagues showed that practicing patient-centered communication in IVF clinics was associated with treatment satisfaction when treatment ended.[44] Thus, infertility counselors can serve an important role to medical staff by educating them on improving staff–patient communication around the delicate issue of ending treatment will better meet overall psychosocial needs of their clientele.[45]

Weinman, in his review of effective doctor–patient communication, listed its benefits. Short-term benefits include better adherence to advice, increased patient recall, greater comprehension, more confidence in advice, more positive appraisal of quality of service, and reduced emotional reactivity. Long-term benefits include better coping, better decision making, improved patient self-management, quicker emotional recovery, and increased patient satisfaction.[43]

Mandatory Counseling

Certain countries such as Canada and Australia mandate precounseling for IVF patients, while other countries, such as the United Kingdom, mandate the offering of counseling. Hammarberg and colleagues found that after a mandated session, about 60% of couples felt it had helped them understand the emotional issues of IVF. However, only 16% agreed that the session was useful in helping them decide whether to continue with treatment.[21] Eighty percent of couples stated they would want to receive counseling about the option of ceasing treatment. Therefore, one clinical question is: Should counseling be mandated for the end of treatment given the complexity of psychosocial issues involved in making the decision and adjusting to it?

Couple Consensus

As presented in the literature review, individuals resolved their biological childlessness with more ease if, at the time of discontinuing treatment, there was agreement between the spouses to proceed in this manner.[29] It is essential that infertility counselors are aware of this finding and offer couple counseling to achieve consensus before couples actively cease treatment. This is an important point for medical caregivers as well, who may not be in the position to assess couple agreement when they make a recommendation to discontinue treatment and therefore should strongly recommend that the couple be seen for counseling to ensure healthy adjustment following their consultation.

In conclusion, the mental health professional can be a significant asset to both the patient and physician by being well informed of the clinical issues around this final phase of treatment. The counselor should be an effective communicator and be prepared to educate, counsel, or advise at any point during the end of treatment process.

THERAPEUTIC INTERVENTIONS

Counseling the Physician

The infertility counselor is often in a position to assist the physician in an end-of-treatment consult with the patient. As experts in emotional concerns, the best evidence-based advice mental health professionals can give physicians includes:

1. At the end of each unsuccessful treatment, on an ongoing basis, the physician and other caregivers should be reevaluating the probabilities of success with the patient and appraising the patient's/couple's limits of endurance and level of adjustment.
2. The physician should let the patient set the agenda, once the advice to end treatment has been conveyed and digested.
3. The physician should give the patient permission to express concerns and feelings, listen with empathy, and be prepared to deal with intense emotional responses.
4. The physician should help the couple reflect on all they have done to achieve a pregnancy so that they will not blame themselves, but rather accept that they have done all they could reasonably do.
5. The physician can point out the positive aspects of ending treatment, such as relief from constant pressure, privacy reintroduced into the relationship, opportunity to focus on other life pursuits, redirecting emotional and financial resources toward different goals, and so on.
6. The physician should ensure that the information is presented with a positive slant and that any hopeful information is offered along with the disappointing.

7. The physician should reassure patients of continued attention and care so they will not feel abandoned.
8. The physician should broach the subject of alternative options to natural conception to be discussed at a second meeting, if the couple appears overwhelmed. Suggestions of reading materials or resources regarding alternatives are useful to prepare the patient for the next meeting.
9. The physician should try to resolve any differences between the spouses in how they assess the situation.
10. The physicians should refer the patient to an infertility counselor to help them transition in an adaptive manner from 'not yet pregnant' to 'not going to be pregnant.' The physician should reduce the stigma of this referral by assuring them that at this stage, it is a good idea for all patients to consult a counselor.

Counseling the Patient

Various therapeutic interventions within the field of infertility counseling are covered elsewhere in this book. However, it may be helpful to review some guiding principles to be considered when counseling patients on ending treatment.

1. Before helping clients manage and adjust to the end of treatment, it is important to help them reach the decision to end treatment. Thus, within a counseling framework, first encourage patients to explore whether emotionally they have reached the end of their tether. Help them do a cost–benefit analysis of continuing treatment versus ending it. Costs should include not only the obvious financial costs that many clients immediately consider but also the costs to the relationship, to keeping their lives on hold, to their emotional well-being, to their careers, to relationships with family and friends, and so on. They should be encouraged to be equally candid with themselves about the benefits of continuing treatment, some of which they may have not expressed or even considered, such as continued relationships with infertile friends or clinic staff. Although it is clear that the answer to the question "when is enough, enough?" is highly personal and individual, it is a question that the infertility counselor is uniquely prepared to help patients investigate.
2. If the circumstances involve a couple, the mental health professional must be sure to include both partners and impress upon them how important

couple consensus is for the future health of their relationship. Within the couple framework, it is important to help them work through this process together with mutual empathy and understanding.

3. As highlighted by the various theoretical frameworks reviewed, it is critical that patients be given the opportunity and place to review their infertility experience emotionally and cognitively, as this is a necessary prerequisite to putting the dream of a genetically-conceived child to rest and moving forward. It is equally important for the counselor to bear witness to their client's grief and loss.

4. Help clients find meaning in all they have endured and to feel proud of themselves that they have simply survived the crisis of infertility.

5. Following that, patients need to be helped in creating a new reality for themselves with a redefined sense of self and purpose, which includes renewed life goals and immediate future plans, for both the individual and couple.

6. Impress on the patient that there is no timeframe for this transition process. For some it may take weeks, for others, months or years (although Daniluk[29] postulated about 3.6 years from beginning to end).

7. Reassure patients that clinical experience and research findings are very convincing that the pain of infertility does subside and that a fulfilling and contented life is attainable. Furthermore, if they are determined to be parents, this can be accomplished, albeit through other means of family-building.

8. To offer optimal care, be aware of all the contributing factors reviewed previously (e.g., optimism and anxiety) that will facilitate better or poor adjustment for any given individual and intervene accordingly.

9. Above all, whether offering psychodynamic, cognitive-behavioral or supportive counseling, it is incumbent upon the infertility counselor to do so in a nonjudgmental and compassionate manner with respect for this challenging period.

FUTURE IMPLICATIONS

As assisted reproductive technologies become more successful and expectations from both consumers and caregivers rise for better outcome results, patients' hopes for their wished-for genetic child will be more feasible. Thus, the challenge to mental health professionals will be to monitor the toll these expectations take on the emotional, interpersonal, and social well-

being of clients and to intervene on their behalf so that the choices they make regarding continuing or ending treatment are in their true best interests. Despite previously unimaginable reproductive successes, treatment failures are inevitable and continued treatment is not feasible or realistic for all patients. As such, the role of the mental health professional is integral for both patients and caregivers. Infertility counselors can, and should, use their expertise to judiciously advise medical staff regarding the end of treatment care plans and decisions, using language they understand and evidence-based recommendations, while advocating for the emotional well-being of the patient.

Furthermore, there is no doubt that third-party or collaborative reproduction procedures are on the rise and viewed as a panacea to childlessness. In their zeal to help, treatment providers may be too quick to encourage patients to give up on their dream of a genetic child. An ever-increasing role for infertility counselors will be to ensure that patients are ready to move in this direction. Counselors must establish that patients are not feeling coerced by either partner, family, or doctor to end treatment, and that they have had an opportunity to grieve for their biological childlessness.

Finally, to maintain credibility within the treatment team, counselors must be cognizant of the latest research findings and, if possible, participate in research opportunities.

SUMMARY

■ Not until recently has research examined the psychological ramifications and implications regarding that point in time when an infertility patient transitions from 'not yet pregnant' to 'not going to be pregnant.'

■ Despite the paucity of studies, the empirical literature is definitive that ending treatment involves a long, complex, and difficult mental process for the patient.

■ How an individual reacts to ending treatment will be dependent on a number of social, demographic, interpersonal, emotional, and psychological factors.

■ Different clinical issues exist between physician-recommended and patient-initiated end of treatment.

■ A patient-centered, emotionally focused approach is the optimal communication format for the end of treatment consult.

■ The mental health professional is in the best position to assist both the physician and the patient in managing the multifaceted aspects associated with ending treatment.

■ The role of the infertility counselor is to help patients make the decision to end treatment, to bear witness to their grief, to encourage them to deconstruct and make sense of their infertility experience and find meaning in it, to assist them in redefining life goals, and to promote long-term adjustment.

REFERENCES

1. Boivin J, Takefman J, Braverman A. Giving bad news: 'It is time to stop.' In: N Macklon, ed. *Assisted Reproduction in the Complicated Patient*. London: Taylor & Francis Books, 2005; 233–40.

2. Benson H. *The Mind/Body Effect: How Behavioral Medicine Can Show You The Way To Better Health*. New York: Simon & Schuster, 1979.

3. Lazarus RS, Folkman S. *Stress, Appraisal and Coping*. New York: Springer Publishing, 1984.

4. Leiblum S, Kemmann E, Colburn D, et al. Unsuccessful in vitro fertilization: A follow-up study. *J IVF & ET* 1987a; 4: 46–50.

5. Callan VJ, Kloske B, Kashima Y, et al. Toward understanding women's decisions to continue or stop in vitro fertilization: The role of social, psychological and background factors. *J IVF & ET* 1988; 5:363–9.

6. Blenner JL. Passage through infertility treatment: A stage theory. *IMAGE* 1990; 22:153–8.

7. Daniluk JC, Mitchell J. Response to parenthood following in vitro fertilization. *J Soc Ob/gyn Canada* 1993; March Supplement: 47–57.

8. Throsby K. No-one will ever call me Mummy: Making sense of the end of IVF treatment. *New Working Paper Series* Issue 5, November: London School of Economics: Gender Institute, 2001.

9. Fortier C, Wright J, Sabourin S. Soutien social et abandon de la consultation médicale en clinique de fertilité. *Journal International de Psychologie* 1992; 27:33–48.

10. van Balen F, Trimbos-Kemper TCM. Long-term infertile couples: A study of their well being. *J Psychosomatic Ob/gyn* 1993; 14:53–60.

11. Bryson CA, Sykes DH, Traub AI. In vitro fertilization: A long-term follow-up after treatment failure. *Hum Fertil* 2000; 3:214–20.

12. Sundby JS. Long-term psychological consequences of infertility: A follow-up study of former patients. *J Women's Health* 1992; 1:209–17.

13. Smeenk MJ, Verhaak CM, Stolwijk AM, et al. Reasons for dropout in an in vitro fertilization/intracytoplasmic sperm injection program. *Fertil Steril* 2004; 81:262–8.

14. Goldfarb J, Austin C, Lisbona H, et al. Factors influencing patients' decision not to repeat IVF. *J Asst Reprod Gen* 1997; 14:381–4.

15. Stanton A, Tennen H, Affleck G, et al. Cognitive appraisal and adjustment to infertility. *Women Health* 1991; 17: 1–15.

16. Berg BJ, Wilson JF, Weingartner PJ. Psychological sequelae of infertility treatment: The role of gender and sex role identification. *Soc Sci Med* 1991; 22:1071–80.

17. Collins A, Freeman EW, Boxer AS, et al. Perceptions of infertility and treatment stress in females as compared with males entering in vitro fertilization treatment. *Fertil Steril* 1992; 57:350–6.

18. Strauss B, Hepp U, Staeding G, et al. Psychological characteristics of infertile couples: Can they predict pregnancy and treatment persistence? *J Comm Appl Soc Psych* 1998; 8:289–301.

19. Abbey A, Andrews FM, Halman LJ. Infertility and parenthood: Does becoming a parent increase well-being? *J Consult Clinic Psych* 1994; 62:398–403.

20. Land JA, Courtar DA, Evers JLH. Patient dropout in an assisted reproductive technology program: Implications for pregnancy rates. *Fertil Steril* 1997; 68:278–81.

21. Hammarberg K, Astbury J, Baker HWG. Women's experience of IVF: A follow-up study. *Hum Reprod* 2001; 16:374–83.

22. Olivius C, Friden B, Borg G, et al. Why do couples discontinue in vitro fertilization treatment? A cohort study. *Fertil Steril* 2004; 81:258–61.

23. Daniluk JC. Infertility: Intrapersonal and interpersonal impact. *Fertil Steril* 1988; 49:982–90.

24. Hirsch AM, Hirsch SM. The effect of infertility on marriage and self-concept. *JObNN* 1989; 18:13–20.

25. Newton CR, Hearn MT, Yuzpe AA. Psychological assessment and follow up after in vitro fertilization assessing the impact of failure. *Fertil Steril* 1990; 54:879–86.

26. Greil AL. Infertility and psychological distress: A critical review of the literature. *Soc Sci Med* 1997; 45:1679–704.

27. Malcolm CE, Cumming DC. Follow-up of infertile couples who dropped out of a specialist fertility clinic. *Fertil Steril* 2004; 81:269–70.

28. Osmanagaoglu K, Tournaye H, Camus M, et al. Cumulative delivery rates after intracytoplasmic sperm injection: 5 year follow-up of 498 patients. *Hum Reprod* 1999; 14:2651–5.

29. Daniluk JC. Reconstructing their lives: A longitudinal, qualitative analysis of the transition to biological childlessness for infertile couples. *J Counsel Develop* 2001; 79:439–49.

30. Taylor SE. Adjustment to threatening events: A theory of cognitive adaptation. *Am Psychol* 1983; 38: 1161–73.

31. Boivin J, Takefman J. Stress level across stages of in vitro fertilization in subsequently pregnant and nonpregnant women. *Fertil Steril* 1995; 64:802–11.

32. Boivin J, Takefman J. The impact of the IVF-ET process on emotional, physical and relational variables. *Hum Reprod* 1996; 903–7.

33. Domar AD. Impact of psychological factors on dropout rates in insured infertility patients. *Fertil Steril* 2004; 81:271–3.

34. Brew T. Benefit finding in women's lives following unsuccessful infertility treatment. *Dissertation, Cardiff University*, Cardiff, Wales; 2002.

35. Leiblum SR, Aviv A, Hamer R. Life after infertility treatment: A long-term investigation of marital and sexual function. *Hum Reprod* 1998; 13:3569–74.

36. Ickovics JR, Park CL, eds. Thriving [Special edition]. *J Social Issues* 1998; 54:2.

37. Wright J, Duchesne C, Sabourin S, et al. Psychological distress and infertility: Men and women respond differently. *Fertil Steril* 1991; 55:100–8.

38. Nachtigall RD, Becker G, Wozny M. The effects of gender-specific diagnosis on men's and women's response to infertility. *Fertil Steril* 1992; 57:113–21.

39. Wischmann T. Facing the end of treatment. In: J Boivin, H Kentenick, eds. *Guidelines for Counselling in Infertility*. ESHRE Monographs: Oxford University Press; 2002: 25–6.

40. The Ethics Committee of ASRM. Fertility treatment when the prognosis is very poor or futile. *Fertil Steril* 2004; 82:806–10.

41. Boivin J, Scanlan LC, Walker SM. Why are infertile patients not using psychosocial counseling? *Hum Reprod* 1999;14:1384–91.

42. Groff A, Covington S, Halverson L, et al. Assessing the emotional needs of women with spontaneous premature ovarian failure. *Fertil Steril* 2005; 83:1734–41.

43. Weinman J. Doctor–patient communication. In: A Baum, S Newman, J Weinman, et al., eds, *Cambridge Handbook of Psychology, Health and Medicine*. Cambridge: Cambridge University Press, 1997:282–7.

44. Schmidt L, Holstein B, Boivin J, et al. High ratings of satisfaction with fertility treatment are common: Findings from the Copenhagen Multi-Centre Psychosocial Infertility (COMPI) Research Programme. *Hum Reprod* 2003; 18: 2638–46.

45. Boivin J, Kentenick H, eds. *Guidelines for Counselling in Infertility*. ESHRE Monographs: Oxford University Press 2002:25–6.

25 Pregnancy after Infertility

SHARON N. COVINGTON AND LINDA HAMMER BURNS

If I could only feel the child! I imagine the moment of its quickening as a sudden awakening of my own being which has never before had life. I want to live with the child, and I am as heavy as a stone.

– Evelyn Scott

The pregnancy following infertility treatment is a premium pregnancy: precious, priceless, and precarious. It is also a high-stakes pregnancy, usually representing a considerable investment of time, emotion, energy, money, and medical treatment. Furthermore, the pregnancy after infertility may be the result of medical treatments facilitating conception, such as in vitro fertilization (IVF), donated gametes, or pregnancy in a gestational carrier or surrogate. The postinfertility pregnancy may be affected by the side effects of assisted reproductive technologies (ARTs), such as complicated multiple gestation, multifetal reduction, high-risk pregnancies/deliveries, and the ultimate risk – loss of the whole pregnancy. Pregnancy after infertility is more than a planned pregnancy: It is a deliberate pregnancy. Once achieved, it can be a distressing realization that it involves a myriad of new challenges and perils demanding considerable psychological and physical adjustments.

This chapter addresses the unique aspects of pregnancy after infertility and:

■ defines how the pregnancy after infertility is different from other pregnancies;
■ outlines the psychological tasks of the postinfertility pregnancy;
■ addresses issues of psychopathology and psychiatric treatment in the postinfertility pregnancy;
■ delineates the unique characteristics of the postinfertility pregnancy, including multiples, third-party reproduction, and pregnancy in the older mother;
■ specifies therapeutic interventions for helping the previously infertile couple manage the typically precious and highly valued postinfertility pregnancy.

HISTORICAL OVERVIEW

Although pregnancy is a universal experience, how it has been experienced by men and women has varied dramatically over the centuries and across cultures. While pregnancy has typically been considered a uniquely female experience, there are accounts of the couvade experience in which men either mimic or display culturally determined pregnancy-related behaviors. During his thirteenth-century trip to China, Marco Polo described the custom in China of fathers taking to bed with their new baby for forty days while friends and kinsmen visited – a custom based on the belief that the mother had done her share, so should not have to endure more.[1] Similarly, according to tradition in an Amazonian tribe, men prepared for delivery by restricting their diet and after birth were confined to hammocks unable to work, smoke, or handle weapons for several weeks during which the mother returned to her work in the forest and cared for her husband and new baby.[1] It is thought that the couvade experience is a means of supporting the importance of the father in the child's life and facilitating father–child attachment, although there is some thought that it may be yet another reflection of how men were more valued and even in childbirth warranted center stage. In fact, from prehistoric times until the twentieth century, women's lives were shorter than men primarily due to the risks of childbirth. Maternal deaths were primarily the result of puerperal infection but also caused by toxemia, hemorrhage, and other factors such as underlying conditions (e.g., malnutrition or gestational diabetes) and circumstances (e.g., abortion). In fact, until the twentieth century the majority of women worldwide did not live to experience menopause, dying before the age of forty due to complications of childbirth. However, with the industrial revolution, the role of women and the experience of childbearing changed dramatically.

Simkin[2] reviewed how childbearing has evolved during the twentieth century and how social changes have influenced the experience of pregnancy for women. At the turn of the century, women rebelled against the Victorian custom of confinement during pregnancy and entered society, bringing about the introduction of maternity clothes and bottle-feeding. By the 1920s, in a further attempt to gain control of their reproductive lives, women in developed countries were attempting to limit pregnancies through the widespread use of birth control. By the 1950s, natural childbirth and childbirth education became popular in North America, Australia, and Europe due to the work of British obstetrician Grantly Dick-Read, who suggested that the primary cause of labor pain was fear and tension.[1] He introduced the idea of 'childbirth without fear' upon which French obstetrician Ferdinand Lamaze based his controlled breathing techniques (the Lamaze method) for coping with labor pain.[1] By the 1970s, fathers had entered the delivery room and maternal–infant bonding was advocated – particularly by French obstetrician Frederick LeBoyer,[1] who suggested that birth should take place in a calm, quiet, dimly light environment to facilitate mother–infant attachment. This was also a time of burgeoning medical technology, including the development of ultrasound, amniocentesis, genetic counseling, neonatology as a new medical specialty, and the first baby conceived by IVF. The 1980s continued the trend of delayed and controlled childbearing, with increasing emphasis on the perfect baby.

The decade of the 1980s also saw a number of firsts in reproductive technology: the first child conceived by a donated oocyte, the first pregnancy carried in a gestational carrier, the first surrogate pregnancy, and the first conception using intracytoplasmic sperm injection (ICSI). By the end of the twentieth century, parenthood and pregnancy could involve deceased parents (pregnancy maintained in a brain-dead mother or pregnancy achieved by sperm harvested from a deceased father); cloning of embryos; the birth of twins several months apart; and genetic testing of embryos before implantation. At the beginning of the twentieth century, women were attempting to reject reproductive destiny by gaining greater control of their reproductive lives. Now, as the twenty-first century unfolds, women are attempting to gain even greater control of reproduction by extending their childbearing lives through the use of frozen oocytes, donated gametes, and volunteer carriers. And while historically, primitive culture did not understand

the contribution of the male to human reproduction (e.g., the attribution of pregnancy to spirits by Trobriand Islanders), women of the twenty-first century have the freedom to reproduce without traditional procreation or the participation of a husband or man.

In this new century, the meanings of pregnancy, conception, motherhood, and parenthood have been forever changed and altered, yet continue to exist within a cultural context that defines these experiences. Traditionally, there has not been a distinction between biological or genetic parenthood and psychological or social parenthood. However, conception and pregnancy now entail various forms of prenatal adoption, donated gametes or embryos, surrogacy, and gestational carrier, as well as intentional versus biological parenthood and conception after death. Traditional means of determining parenthood, such as genetics, bloodlines, or physical pregnancy, have given way to 'parenthood by intention,'[3,4] altering the experience of pregnancy and, ultimately, the experience of parenthood. Thus, while pregnancy after infertility has much in common with normal pregnancies, there is also much about it that sets it apart.

REVIEW OF LITERATURE

While the psychology of infertility has received considerable research attention, investigation of psychological factors in pregnancy after infertility has been limited. Research has traditionally focused on obstetrical outcomes, especially following particular fertility treatments such as donor insemination conceptions and assisted reproductive technologies (ARTs). Pregnancies following ARTs have consistently been found to be at greater risk for pregnancy complications and problem deliveries, including increased incidence of preterm labor and delivery; low birth rate; multiple gestations; preeclampsia; and Cesarean deliveries.[5] Huber and Ludwig[5] reviewed multiple studies on ART obstetrical outcome and concluded that while higher rate multiple pregnancies following ART were a critical factor (sevenfold), singleton pregnancies were also at higher risk.[6] The risk factors associated with pregnancy and delivery problems may be the result of the initial infertility diagnosis, multiple gestations, advanced maternal age, prenatal testing, multifetal reduction, or conception via IVF/ICSI.[7] Pregnancies conceived with cryopreserved embryos do not appear to have any additional risk to the pregnancy or fetus.[5] The risk factors disappear when a surrogate mother, rather than an infertile mother, carries the pregnancy. Huber and Ludwig conclude, "that it seems certain types of infertility per se do contribute to the risk of pregnancy complications, but not the ART procedure used to induce the pregnancy. This has to be included in the counselling of these patients"[5, p. 68] (see Table 27.1 for a review of outcome studies).

Several studies have examined external stress factors and the impact on pregnancy outcomes. Klonoff-Cohen and Natarajan examined specific concerns about IVF/GIFT (i.e., side effects, surgery, anesthesia, not enough information, pain, recovery, finances, missing work, and delivery) in 151 women undergoing treatment to determine the association (if any) on reproductive outcome.[8] They found that women who were very concerned about the finances associated with IVF had a very high risk (odds ratio = 11.62) of *not* achieving a successful live birth delivery. Other studies have looked at the impact of catastrophic events (September 11th in New York City and earthquakes) on pregnancy outcome and found a significant decrease in the delivery rate for IVF patients[9] as well as preterm delivery dates.[10] Thus, pregnancy outcome after infertility may not only be influenced by a concomitant of medical issues, but also by a variety of factors including daily hassles or major life stresses.

Increased anxiety and cautious attachment to the postinfertility pregnancy have been a frequent research finding. Garner[11] noted that reactions to pregnancy after infertility fell between two extremes: *denial/avoidance* (women who denied pregnancy and failed to seek appropriate prenatal care for several months) and *hypervigilance* (women who repeatedly called the clinic with exaggerated fears over even normal/minor pregnancy symptoms). Anxiety has been described as a 'waiting to lose' period, when previously infertile pregnant women are constantly alert to signs of impending miscarriage and have little confidence that a baby actually will be born.[12] In addition, a prior reproductive loss has been identified as significantly increasing anxiety for both partners, resulting in difficulty in coping as they anticipated a negative outcome and withdrew emotional investment in the pregnancy.[13–15] One study[16] reported that previously infertile pregnant women avoided preparing for their baby and attempted to control every aspect of the pregnancy in an effort to distance normal feelings of trepidation, ambivalence, and fear of the unknown. Previously infertile pregnant women were also found to have elevated depression scores compared to never-infertile women.

Several studies have found no differences in mood or adjustment post partum of women who became pregnant following infertility compared to controls.[17–19] However, a recent study from Australia found a significant increase of early parenting difficulties, including mild to moderate maternal depression and anxiety as

well as infant sleeping and eating problems, with mothers who had conceived through ART.[20] The authors conclude that postpartum mood disturbance may be affected by multiple factors associated with ART, such as multiple birth and Cesarean surgery. Furthermore, a recent systematic review concluded that past infertility and assisted conception may constitute risk factors for postpartum mood disorders.[21]

Research also indicates that previously infertile women have difficulty letting go of the rituals of infertility; separating from the infertility team; developing a new support network; and investing in a pregnancy that they might yet lose.[22] Relinquishing infertility "involved efforts to let go of the negative identity, feelings, and thought patterns developed over the course of the struggle to conceive."[22] Previously infertile women also reported a higher incidence of guilt and shame that they associated with their formerly infertile status.[23] These women continued to harbor feelings of failure and malformation about their reproductive ability or, if the baby was conceived by donor gametes or surrogacy, embarrassment about the circumstances of the child's conception. Guilt was associated with their relationships with their friends who remained infertile. Glaser and Strauss[24] found that previously infertile women struggled with three issues during pregnancy: (1) *selflessness*, defined as the belief that all their energy and effort should be devoted and directed toward the baby; (2) *lack of entitlement*, defined as having no right to complain or expect more because they had what they wanted – a baby; and (3) *vulnerability*, defined as their feeling that they were more medically at risk than they had ever been and perceived their baby to be at greater risk as well.

Little is known about men's responses to pregnancy after infertility. In one study[25] of previously infertile husbands' responses to pregnancy in their wives, the men experienced couvade symptoms consistent with the incidence in the general population. Nevertheless, a husband's responses to pregnancy may be influenced by the circumstances of conception; the demands of pregnancy such as bedrest or hospitalization; the emotional stability of the expectant mother; and his own psychological well-being.

THEORETICAL FRAMEWORK

Although early literature focused on the psychoanalytic interpretation of the symbolic meaning and experience of pregnancy,[26,27] pregnancy is now considered a normal developmental process signaling arrival into adulthood and acceptance of adult roles. Pregnancy and parenthood represent a bridge between generations central to the human experience and to a woman's sense of self, gender identity, and self-esteem.[28] Physical, intrapsychic, and interpersonal adaptations are needed to successfully adjust to pregnancy, delivery, and, ultimately, parenthood.

Pregnancy is a time when profound physical and emotional changes occur within a short period of time. During pregnancy, a woman faces monumental issues: the sharing of her body with another; changes in her body image; changes in her relationship with others; attachment to the baby she is carrying while at the same time preparing to separate from it; as well as feelings about motherhood in general, herself as a mother, and the mothering she received as a child.[29] The physical demands and emotional stresses of pregnancy can have an impact on a woman's coping ability and style, her relationship with significant others (especially her spouse/partner) and her own psychological adjustment, including her individuation, ego development, and consolidation of self.

Even when a pregnancy is wanted, some ambivalence is normal and probably universal. During pregnancy, women often feel a sense of accomplishment; heightened self-esteem; increased feelings of femininity; and comradeship with other women. At the same time, there may be feelings of resentment and even hostility about the changes taking place that are beyond a woman's control both physically and psychosocially. When things go well, pregnancy can be a narcissistically rewarding period – a gratification of the body's performance – or, if there is a problem, a narcissistically wounding period – anxiety and distress about the body's competence during pregnancy and delivery. Feelings of ambivalence, anxiety, or fear may increase self-doubt and lower self-confidence, thereby complicating adjustment to pregnancy and parenthood. Furthermore, adjustment to pregnancy is affected by a number of factors in a woman's life, including previous life experiences; prior psychological adjustment; the meaning of this pregnancy in her life; her dependency needs; and her relationship with her partner and others.[29] Physical and emotional dependence on her partner may clash with a woman's own desire for independence and self-sufficiency during pregnancy. These issues may arise when the pregnancy is complicated by bedrest or other medical restrictions.

The meaning of the pregnancy after infertility varies and is highly individual. It may represent hopes, dreams, miracles, expense, overinvestment, success, fulfillment, or even a burden or hindrance. Following years of infertility, the developmental transition to parenthood can be difficult and stressful for a couple. The postinfertility pregnancy may involve its own unique challenges: fears of pregnancy loss; the strains of a medically complicated pregnancy; and attachment to a nongenetically related baby or a baby being carried by someone else. Fundamentally, the tasks of pregnancy are influenced by the experience of infertility in general and the previously infertile pregnant woman's experience of *this* pregnancy. Ultimately, not only do previously infertile couples arrive at pregnancy differently, but their experience of pregnancy is also significantly different.

Psychological Tasks of Pregnancy after Infertility

The abrupt transition from long-standing infertility to potential parenthood is a psychological challenge requiring a rapid revision of identity and internal reconfiguration.[30] Olshansky[31] described the identity shift in the formerly infertile woman as a confusing psychological state in which the expectant mother with a history of infertility and/or reproductive loss simultaneously straddles the two worlds of infertility and pregnancy. She has difficulty seeing herself as a normal pregnant woman and feels that her experiences with infertility, medical treatment, and childlessness set her apart from other pregnant women. She may feel that she has no right to complain about the physical demands of pregnancy because either her support network is tired of hearing about her not being pregnant or she herself feels that she should feel only gratitude for this pregnancy. Some women pregnant after infertility are unable to relate to the 'whining' about the discomforts of pregnancy from women who have had no problems with conception; or they may feel that they are not entitled to whine as they worked so hard to achieve this pregnancy and fear others will be critical of them.

Furthermore, Olshansky[32] contends that difficulty in letting go of the infertility experience contributes to the paradoxes of pregnancy after infertility: simultaneous feelings of contradictory emotions. The paradoxes involve the 'embrace of contraries,' such as happiness about pregnancy and fear of loss or perception of self as defective due to infertility. The normalization of pregnancy for the previously infertile woman consists of a complex identity shift from an infertile and childless identity to one of pregnancy and, ultimately, motherhood. It involves the ability to experience pregnancy as a normal developmental process that is gratifying and involves its own set of tasks, responsibilities, and goals.

Unique to the pregnancy after infertility are donated gametes, surrogate mothers, or gestational carriers, resulting in confused physical and psychological boundaries. Here one is circumventing rather than overcoming infertility, for although pregnancy may be achieved, the original infertility diagnosis or problem is not cured.[23]

The developmental tasks of normal pregnancy that are made more difficult by infertility include:[33]

■ *validation of pregnancy*: This is difficult after infertility because confirmation and affirmation of the pregnancy are less an event than a process, often involving repeated pregnancy tests, ultrasounds, and examinations. Acceptance and assimilation of the reality of the pregnancy may be more tentative and difficult, especially if the process involves a significant period of time;
■ *fetal embodiment*: The expectant mother's incorporating the fetus into her body image may be especially difficult if she perceives her body to be defective or unreliable after the experience of infertility or prior problem pregnancies. Recognizing the baby as part of her body may be threatening, which is reinforced if there are complications during the pregnancy or conception achieved by donated gametes or embryos;
■ *fetal distinction*: Recognition of the fetus as a separate entity is actually the beginning of parental bonding, attachment, and acknowledgment of the baby's individuality and separateness. Sometimes fetal distinction is delayed or suspended until the final status of the pregnancy has been determined, as in cases of threatened miscarriage, possible fetal reduction, or waiting for results of prenatal testing;
■ *role transition*: This involves redefinition of the self as a parent and integration of the baby as a separate person within the family. This may be a formidable task when a couple has been defined as childless in a child-filled world. The wounds from infertility may make it difficult to bond with the miracle baby or deal with the infant's many needs.

According to Colman and Colman,[34] the psychological tasks of the childbearing years are defined in terms of pregnancy as a developmental stage that inaugurates a much longer one: parenthood. The six tasks of pregnancy are: (1) accepting the pregnancy; (2) accepting the reality of the fetus; (3) reevaluating the older generation of parents; (4) reevaluating the relationship between the two partners; (5) accepting the baby as a separate person; and (6) integrating the parental identity. Each of these tasks can have special meaning and challenges to the previously infertile couple who may have difficulty acknowledging the reality of the pregnancy or baby; have experienced long-term marital adjustment problems; or have unrealistic expectations of self as a parent or of their child.

The pregnancy after infertility has its own unique challenges and tasks. Glazer[35] defined the tasks of pregnancy after infertility in terms of how it differs from normal pregnancy: (1) fear of loss of the pregnancy, (2) fear of having a baby with defects, (3) difficulty in becoming an obstetrical patient (as opposed to an infertility patient), (4) feeling neither fertile nor infertile ('in a no-person's land'), and (5) fear of having a high-risk pregnancy. She further defined the issues of the postinfertility pregnancy as:[36]

■ *ambiguity*: the process versus the event of pregnancy confirmation in normal pregnancies, although it can apply to other forms of ambiguity in the postinfertility pregnancy, such as the ambiguity of genetic ties to the pregnancy (e.g., donor gametes);
■ *isolation*: feelings of alienation and not belonging to either the fertile or infertile worlds;
■ *fear or anxiety about the pregnancy*: including fears about pregnancy outcome and parenthood but possibly also anxiety about one's ability to manage the pregnancy or delivery or fear of the response of others, should they discover the circumstances of conception;
■ *loss* (fundamental to infertility) *involves*: the multiple losses of pregnancy after infertility, including the potential for pregnancy loss, the necessity of fetal reduction, the loss of a 'normal' pregnancy experience, and/or the loss of a support network, such as friends left behind in the world of infertility after pregnancy is achieved;
■ *technological bewilderment*: the myriad medical technologies that contribute to creation and/or maintenance of the postinfertility pregnancy.

CLINICAL ISSUES

Psychopathology during Pregnancy after infertility

Early investigations[37] into the incidence of psychiatric hospitalizations during pregnancy found a decrease, supporting the belief that normal pregnancy was a time of relative calm, providing protection from psychiatric illness. However, subsequent research has shown either a small decrease or an unchanged incidence of major psychiatric illness during pregnancy.[29] The most significant factor predictive of psychiatric illness during pregnancy is prior history of mental illness.[29] The significance of psychiatric illness during pregnancy primarily involves its potential effect on obstetrical outcome (prematurity, low birth weight, and subsequent child morbidity); disturbances of mother–infant relationship; and inability to comply with medical care or appropriately care for oneself or the pregnancy.[38,39]

Mood, Anxiety, and Personality Disorders

Although a first episode of major depression is unlikely to erupt during pregnancy, *reoccurrence* of major depression during pregnancy is a possibility both patients and caregivers must always consider. Apart from a history of a prior major depressive episode, additional risk factors include presence or absence of prior children; instrumental support during pregnancy; prior pregnancy loss; disturbed marital relationship; stressful life circumstances; and medically high-risk pregnancy.[29] Furthermore, depression during pregnancy may be more common than previously thought. In a recent review of studies involving more than 19,000 women in Canada, researchers found that depression during pregnancy is relatively high, around 7.4% of women in the first trimester and rising to over 12% in the second and third trimesters.[40] Because a history of major depression is such a significant predictor of depression during pregnancy and postpartum, it has been suggested that women with a history of depression should be carefully screened before conception, as well as during pregnancy and postpartum.[41] In addition, preparing women by educating them about risk factors, symptoms, and treatment options can provide understanding and preventive care.

Depression during pregnancy can be particularly painful for a previously infertile pregnant woman who may have (mistakenly) believed that the long-awaited pregnancy would be a time of happiness and health. Furthermore, depression can be surprising and distressing to the women's spouse, family, and caregivers. However, patients and caregivers can be reassured by the availability of a variety of treatment options that have been found to be successful, including interpersonal therapy, cognitive-behavioral therapy, and medications.[42] In addition, research has shown that some antidepressant medications appear to have no detrimental impact on the fetus and can be a relatively safe, effective treatment approach.[43,44] However, the U.S. Food and Drug Administration recently issued an alert stating that exposure to paroxetine (Paxil) in the first trimester of pregnancy may increase the risk of congenital malformations, particularly cardiac malformations,[45] so patients should seek appropriate medical consultation (e.g., psychiatrist specializing in women's health) regarding any medication taken during pregnancy. Whether treatment involves psychotherapy and/or medication, patients need to understand that there is evidence that untreated depression, as well as other psychiatric conditions, may affect their baby (i.e., fetoplacenatal integrity and fetal central nervous system development).[46] In short, depression needs to be assessed, either through history taking, screening tools, and/or questioning so that, when identified, these pregnant women receive appropriate support and treatment.

Although pregnancy does not appear to increase the risk of depression during pregnancy, several studies found that depression during pregnancy is a significant predictor of postpartum depression.[47,48] Other predictive factors for postpartum depression include lack of social support; stress in terms of increased daily hassles; unstable relationship with the baby's father; family history of depression and/or alcoholism; and more difficult pregnancy, labor, or delivery.[49–51] One study found the strongest risk was sick leave during pregnancy and a high number of visits to the antenatal care clinic, often related to complications during pregnancy (hyperemesis, premature contractions, and psychiatric conditions), as predictive of postpartum depression.[52] The experience of infertility combined with stressors such as high-risk pregnancy; loss of social support postinfertility; relationship problems; and the effects of ovulation-inducing medications may increase vulnerability for depression in previously infertile pregnant women.[20,21] In addition, research has indicated higher rates of depression in women following miscarriage (11% versus 4% of community women), indicating another potential risk factor.[53]

As with depression, women with prior anxiety disorders are not protected from anxiety, phobias, or panic disorders during pregnancy[54] and may be at increased risk for triggering or worsening of anxiety disorders postpartum, for example, obsessive-compulsive disorder.[55–57] Although some anxiety during pregnancy is typical, especially if the focus is on the fetus rather than the woman herself, overwhelming anxiety that impairs functioning is not. For postinfertility pregnant women, certain levels of anxiety are common and predictable,[17] although a comprehensive psychiatric history or objective measures with attention to prior episodes of panic and anxiety attacks may be the best diagnostic tool.

The impact of personality disorders during pregnancy has not been investigated, but the developmental tasks of pregnancy may be profoundly influenced by characterological disturbances which include: difficulty with assumption of adult roles; revival of unresolved developmental or childhood conflicts; ambivalence toward the fetus; changes in internal boundaries and body image; reactivation of separation and individuation struggles; and resurgence of mother–daughter conflicts.[58] Personality disorders involve a pervasive, persistent, and maladaptive pattern of perceiving one's environment and behaving. As such, these disturbances can significantly affect patient behavior and care, especially during a stressful postinfertility pregnancy.[59] Overdependence, violence, grandiosity, hypervigilance, emotionality, self-aggrandizement, wariness, and sociopathy are common presenting features in women with personality disorders. The risks of these problems involve a patient's vulnerability to overwhelming feelings of despair, hopelessness, and anxiety; reduced functioning; and/or increased pathological behavior that may endanger the pregnancy or her ability to receive appropriate care as a result of her disturbing behavior.[59]

Eating Disorders and Hyperemesis Gravidarum

Eating disorders, contrary to popular belief, do not diminish in intensity during pregnancy. Pregnancy may, in fact, trigger more intense risky eating behaviors, endangering the infant's life, maternal health, and intrauterine growth, reducing infant birth weight, and increasing congenital anomalies.[29,60,61] When symptoms of disordered eating diminish as the pregnancy progresses, they frequently resurface postpartum.[62] One study[63] found that compared with women whose eating disorders were in remission, women with an active eating disorder during pregnancy gained less weight and encountered more pregnancy complications.

Although not a psychiatric disorder, hyperemesis gravidarum is a rare condition of intractable vomiting resulting in dehydration, ketonuria, weight loss, and/or electrolyte imbalance and may require hospitalization. It is common for women to be so debilitated that they are unable to function normally, even when vomiting does not require hospitalization. Furthermore, the severe emotional and physical distress of hyperemesis gravidarum can be demoralizing to the point of precipitating a major depressive episode. Psychological management usually includes supportive counseling, psychoeducation, progressive relaxation, visualization, hypnosis, accupuncture, accupressure, relief of guilt, identifying and lessening exacerbating factors, and assisting patients with self-assertion to limit contact with food, experiences, and individuals who worsen symptoms.[64] Occasionally, psychotropic medication is also appropriate in addition to medical managment of the condition.

Interestingly, one study[65] of patients with hyperemesis gravidarum found a history of an eating disorder in 50% of women who had presented to an infertility clinic for ovulation-induction treatment and had failed to disclose to their caregivers that they suffered from an eating disorder. Given the high prevalence of disordered eating in the infertility population and the impact of weight on treatment outcome, it has been suggested

that all infertility caregivers address the issue of eating disorders and dieting behavior before proceeding with treatment.[65,66]

Pseudocyeses and Pregnancy Denial

Pseudocyesis (false pregnancy) is a syndrome in which an otherwise nonpsychotic woman firmly believes that she is pregnant and develops physical signs of pregnancy when she is not pregnant. Although there are no firm psychological or physical explanations for pseudocyesis, it has been postulated that cultural pressures to have children, an inordinately strong desire to be pregnant, and the strain of infertility may be causative factors.[29,67]

Denial of pregnancy is characterized by refusal to accept the pregnant state, failure to affiliate with the fetus, and no evidence of preparatory behavior (e.g., wearing maternity clothes and acquiring things for baby).[68] Denial may range from subtle failure to adjust one's lifestyle to pregnancy to frank psychotic denial of pregnancy in the face of physical evidence. For previously infertile pregnant women, some denial of pregnancy or delayed acceptance of the pregnancy is normative, often the result of an ambiguous pregnancy confirmation process that contributes to disbelief or unreality. Attainment of certain landmarks of pregnancy such as a certain number of weeks of gestation, confirmation of fetal heartbeat, or fetal movement may help validate the reality of the pregnancy for a previously infertile couple. Often, women are consciously aware of denying or avoiding the pregnancy as a means of self-protection against pregnancy loss, even though they remain involved in caring for the pregnancy. In more serious situations, women may avoid or refuse medical care or directly jeopardize the pregnancy through risky behaviors while professing a desire for a child, indicating significant internal conflicts and psychological disturbance.[69] This phenomenon may be more common in patients who thought to try ARTs one last time but did not expect it to be successful. Thus, having emotionally adjusted to childlessness or a single-child family, shifting to acceptance of the new child may be more challenging than it would appear.

Complicated Pregnancy after Infertility

Although most pregnancies after infertility are uneventful, many are not. A woman who becomes pregnant after infertility is at a one-third greater risk than the general population of experiencing pregnancy complications and loss.[70] Complications may be due to pre-existing conditions or to factors unique to this pregnancy. The original infertility diagnosis (e.g., uterine fibroids, luteal phase disorder, or cervical problems) may contribute to pregnancy complications, or complications may be related to conception (e.g., multiple gestation). Other problems of pregnancy include complications of advanced maternal age, gestational diabetes, toxemia, hyperemesis gravidarum, hypertension, or preexisting medical problems, such as multiple sclerosis, arthritis, or obesity. All of these complications increase the risk of pregnancy loss and vulnerability of both mothers and infants, and highlight how the pregnancy following infertility is not normal.

When pregnancy complications arise, psychological distress in both mother and father is common. The mother-to-be may have to relinquish or reduce her work responsibilities, restrict her activity, abdicate the care of her other children, and submit to varying degrees of medical intervention, while experiencing anxiety about the baby and her own health. Wohlreich[71] described how obstetrical complications shatter previous plans and hopes for the pregnancy while exposing the mother to a confusing array of medical information, tests, and treatments. Women who become pregnant after infertility often feel cheated of a normal pregnancy and delivery, an experience that many feel is owed to them after the trials and tribulations of infertility. They often experience pregnancy complications as another blow to self-esteem and confidence in their ability to perform basic life tasks or their body's ability to function in a normal fashion. Ruminating about the cause of the pregnancy problems, many women blame themselves for real or imagined wrongdoing, such as failure to comply with minor medical instructions (e.g., missing a daily prenatal vitamin), sexual intercourse, or temporary ambivalence about the pregnancy.

Nausea and Vomiting

Nausea and vomiting occur in the majority (50–90%) of pregnancies and are at best nuisances that dispel some of the magic of the precious pregnancy.[29] Occasionally, nausea and vomiting continue episodically or continuously throughout the pregnancy, although not severe enough to be considered hyperemesis gravidarum. Nevertheless, feeling unsettled and sick is distressing for a previously infertile expectant mother, often increasing her anxiety about her baby, dampening her enjoyment of the pregnancy, and potentially contributing to pregnancy complications by retarding maternal weight gain and fetal growth. Furthermore, although nausea and vomiting are common and normal in early pregnancy, these symptoms may trigger a recurrence of anorexia or bulimia in women with a history of an eating disorder. And while food aversions and cravings are typical and normal in pregnancy,

they too may trigger the reemergence of disorder eating.[64] Women experiencing difficulty in eating during pregnancy due to nausea, vomiting, food aversions, or cravings may find it helpful to consult a nutritionist for guidance. Ginger has also been found to be effective in relieving the severity of nausea and vomiting for some women,[72] as well as acupuncture and some vitamin therapies.[73] Of course, these treatments should be adopted with the approval and collaboration of her physician/obstetrician.

Pregnancy Bedrest

Bedrest, a common prescription for the problem pregnancy, can be physically and psychologically demanding. Restriction of activity and limited social interaction can contribute to emotional distress, including regression, anxiety, resentment, vulnerability, and feelings of sadness and helplessness. Loss of control, one of the issues of particular significance during infertility, often reemerges during a pregnancy that requires bedrest and/or hospitalization. Boredom, although usually unidentified and underestimated, can be a true nemesis of the bedrest pregnancy, affecting compliance with medical care and the emotional well-being of the mother-to-be. Financial problems; dependence on the care of others (often parents and in-laws); relinquishment of roles (e.g., employee and parent); and loss of social network at the workplace are additional stressors. Furthermore, husbands may become restless, resentful, or overwhelmed, further stressing the marital relationship, especially when the demands of caring for other children or assuming the wife's relinquished duties may impair the husband's own well-being. Creative ways of coping with the demands of the bedrest pregnancy include telephone networking with other bedrest mothers; reading materials; college courses on television or on the internet; visits from home healthcare providers; and computers for work or networking with others.[74]

Whether pregnancy complications require surgery, bedrest, extended hospitalization, or simply activity restrictions, an expectant mother may experience a myriad of negative emotions, further spoiling her pregnancy and robbing her of the normal pregnancy experience she expected or felt she deserved. Extended hospitalization may increase the mother's ambivalence about the pregnancy or the baby, especially if she feels or is even treated by caregiving like a 'living intensive care incubator' in which the baby's well-being is a higher priority than her own. Failure to bond or delayed bonding to the baby may result from the mother's fears about her own well-being, ability to carry the pregnancy, or losing the pregnancy. In contrast, hospitalization with the constant availability of medical care may give some women a false sense of security and confidence about the outcome of the pregnancy. They may find the hospital environment so reassuring that they react with profound disbelief and despair if the pregnancy outcome is negative.

Some women are better able to handle the psychological stressors of the complicated pregnancy, whereas others find it beyond their ability to cope, precipitating extreme psychological or marital crisis. Some women willingly tolerate the discomforts and restrictions of a bedrest pregnancy, while others consider the rigors of the complicated pregnancy punishment or simply intolerable. Some expectant mothers experience the sacrifices of a bedrest pregnancy as a means of being a good mother, psychologically facilitating the transition to motherhood. For other women, high levels of anxiety, depression, guilt, ambivalence, or conflicts about dependency needs result in noncompliance with care, increased conflict with caregivers or loved ones, or decreased confidence in herself as a mother.

A history of infertility may place a pregnant woman at risk for psychological problems that may be further exacerbated by a complicated pregnancy. Obstetrical risk factors for depression during and after pregnancy include toxemia, hyperemesis, fetal malpresentation, hydramnios, placental defects, and multiple gestations.[75] Whether the complications of pregnancy after infertility are physical or psychological, they take a toll on the woman, her partner, her relationship with her baby, and her caregivers. Pregnancy complications stress marital relationships; compromise and even endanger the expectant mother's health; threaten the well-being of the pregnancy; and impede the developmental tasks of pregnancy, including attachment to the infant and transition to motherhood. Furthermore, pregnancy complications after infertility highlight the qualities of isolation, ambiguity, loss, fear, and technological bewilderment unique to the pregnancy after infertility. While conflicted and ambivalent feelings about the demands of a complicated pregnancy are normal for women pregnant after infertility, these women and their partners require a great deal of support and understanding from family, friends, and caregivers to successfully navigate this challenging experience.

Multiple Pregnancy

Pregnancies following infertility are frequently the result of ovulation-enhancing medications and/or assisted reproductive technologies, in which multiple gestation is a common consequence. Multiples are, in effect, 'too much of a good thing,' contributing to

preterm labor and delivery; fetal growth restriction and low birth weight; obstetrical complications such as toxemia, preeclampsia, anemia, gestational diabetes, and cervical incompetence, resulting in extended bedrest or long-term hospitalization; and neonatal disabilities or mortality as well as maternal mortality.[76] Multiple gestations following assisted reproduction have increased by at least 200% since the early 1970s, placing a heavy burden on obstetrical care and neonatology units.[77] One study[78] comparing international outcomes in assisted reproduction found the incidence of twins to be 20–25%, triplets 2–5%, and quadruplets 2.8% and reported that multiple gestation was the major factor contributing to high perinatal mortality rates.

The risk of the multiple or 'super-twin' pregnancies is, unfortunately, often beyond comprehension for infertile couples, even when they have been informed of the possibility. Patients may significantly underestimate the risks associated with multiple births in their decisions regarding how many embryos to transfer[79] and respond to the news of a multiple pregnancy with delight and without apprehension, even though the reality is that these pregnancies are risky for both mother and babies. In fact, in a study[80] of attitudes regarding multiple births, previously infertile women were significantly more positive about having multiple gestations than the infertile control group. However, the previously infertile woman expecting multiples expressed greater worry about losing the pregnancy and more concern about potential consequences to her health, attractiveness, and marital relationship.

Couples facing a multiple pregnancy need assistance in understanding the risks; consideration of pregnancy options; preparation for the birth; and, ultimately, education about the issues and demands of raising multiples. One of the remedies for multiple gestation is multifetal pregnancy reduction (MPR).[81] It involves the termination of one or more fetuses usually with reduction to triplets or twins, in order to increase the possibility for a successful pregnancy. However, MPR is not a procedure without risk, as the entire pregnancy may be lost and there is an increased risk of preterm delivery and fetal growth restriction.[82]

For many previously infertile couples, the concept of terminating a much-longed-for pregnancy is particularly offensive and disturbing. Marital conflict and frustration are understandable, as are individual responses of distress and sadness in addition to ethical or religious dilemmas, cultural factors, and extended family issues. Feelings of panic and dismay are also common as couples consider challenging decisions regarding the pregnancy and termination. Some couples choose to reduce a twin pregnancy to a singleton because they had not anticipated the possibility of multiples or because of economic or social reasons – often to the shock and dismay of caregivers. Other couples reluctantly accept a procedure that is in opposition to their personal wishes and/or moral beliefs. Some women experience MPR as the loss of another child, not unlike miscarriage, stillbirth, or a chemical pregnancy following IVF. Furthermore, it is a loss that usually occurs in isolation, without the support or knowledge of family and friends, within a social context of stigma and censure regarding pregnancy termination. Still others refuse MPR, choosing to take their chances – hoping to beat the odds with the pregnancy they have.

Despite the obvious emotional side effects of MPR, research[83,84] has shown that women who have undergone the procedure handle it fairly well without long-term feeling of guilt, remorse, or regrets. Ideally, all couples pursuing assisted reproduction should be educated early on, preferably before conception, about the possibility of a multiple pregnancy and the option of MPR, so that they can consider and prepare for decision making about this possibility (see Chapter 16).

Although women may not be at greater risk of psychiatric illness following MPR, its impact should not be minimized or maximized, but should be avoided whenever possible with proper prepregnancy educational counseling and appropriate medical treatment. It cannot be overlooked that the 'super-twin' pregnancy is an iatrogenic condition. Professional societies (e.g., ASRM and ESHRE) have established practice guidelines on the number of embryos to transfer to minimize the possibility of multiple gestation, while some countries have government agencies (e.g., HFEA) or laws (e.g., Italy) to regulate this practice. The economic, social, psychological, and health costs of multiple pregnancies are great and prevention is the most important means of decreasing multiple gestations.[76]

Pregnancy and Third-Party Reproduction

An issue of pregnancy after infertility that is unique to the previously infertile is third-party reproduction, which includes pregnancies conceived using donated sperm, oocytes, or embryos and pregnancies in a surrogate or gestational carrier. Although studies of obstetrical outcome following donor insemination conception have revealed no increased obstetrical risk of problematic outcomes, this has not been the case for other forms of third-party reproductive technologies. While the advent of oocyte donation has provided a means for women without ovarian function to experience pregnancy and delivery, there is some evidence that pregnancies conceived via oocyte donation, especially in women

with ovarian failure, should be considered obstetrically high-risk because of the higher incidence of pregnancy complications and multiples.[85] There is considerable evidence of increased cardiac risk for Turner's syndrome patients during pregnancy following oocyte donation and it is recommended that they be adequately screened with echocardiography before treatment.[86]

Third-party reproduction involves physical and psychological complexities that can complicate a pregnancy and the transition to parenthood as well as strain the well-being of the partners and the marriage.[87] If the pregnancy is the result of donated gametes or embryos, the psychological tasks include attachment to an infant to whom one or both parents are not genetically related, genealogical bewilderment, resolution of issues regarding secrecy versus disclosure, and psychological adjustment to feelings of ambivalence, anxiety, resentment, confusion, and apprehension.[88–90] If the third-party pregnancy is carried by a gestational carrier or surrogate, the psychological tasks for the intended parents include attachment to the fetus; establishment of appropriate boundaries with the gestational carrier or surrogate; management of fear and anxiety regarding the pregnancy and its outcome; and management of social attitudes.[91]

Pregnancy in the surrogate or gestational carrier involves a complex array of unique psychological tasks. Preliminary research on the psychological adjustment to surrogate pregnancy has shown a strong prenatal attachment between the surrogate/carrier and the fetus.[92] In addition, some surrogate mothers may experience grief responses at the time of relinquishment, resulting in feelings of loss or abandonment after the birth or resentment at no longer being the center of attention[91] (see Chapter 21).

For the intended parents, surrogate/carrier pregnancies may enhance feelings of powerlessness, lack of social support, and uncertainty about parenthood. Running parallel with the desire and need to attach to the expected child are the parents' fears that the surrogate/carrier may change her mind, not surrender the child, or not take proper care of herself, thereby endangering the pregnancy or baby. Research[93] has indicated that intended (versus carrier) mothers have a high need for affection and may need to feel that the surrogate/carrier cares about them and their husband. Furthermore, the intended mother may attempt to shape and nurture her child by forming a positive relationship with the surrogate/carrier.

Infertility counselors can provide assistance to intended parents and the surrogate/carrier by defining and facilitating the tasks of pregnancy and by supporting the individuals as they move through them.

These tasks include preserving the autonomy of the carrier/surrogate; protecting the rights and responsibilities of all parties; preventing any adverse maternal outcomes for the carrier/surrogate; avoiding psychosocial traumatization of all parties, particularly the disadvantaged carrier/surrogate; facilitating attachment between the intended parents and the baby; and providing ongoing counseling for all parties, especially the carrier/surrogate, for at least six weeks postpartum.[94] It is a delicate balance for infertility counselors between preventing exploitation and protecting autonomy for the carrier/surrogate, while protecting the rights and responsibilities of the genetic or intended parents.[95]

The pregnancy achieved through donated gametes involves unique tasks of pregnancy. Before conception, the infertile couple must assimilate complex medical information, cope with one parent's loss of genetic contribution, as well as the loss for both partners of the genetically-shared pregnancy, and undergo varying levels of medical treatment. During pregnancy, the expectant mother must come to terms with carrying a fetus that is not genetically related either to her, her husband or her other children, often harboring secret fears about the baby's appearance or normalcy. Just after the birth, new parents may experience heightened anxiety attributable to fears that the baby's physical characteristics will be distinctively different from the parents, somehow publicizing the circumstances of the conception.[92]

Secrecy about the means of conception is a unique feature of the donor gamete pregnancy, because this pregnancy is not visibly different from any other pregnancy. This factor can be both a positive, in that it enables the normalization of pregnancy and parenthood, and a negative, in that it makes it easier to avoid the difference of this pregnancy. Hence, decisions about disclosure that began before conception will continue to be revisited during the pregnancy and long afterward.

The issues of the postinfertility pregnancy – ambiguity, isolation, fear, loss, and technological bewilderment – are most apparent in third-party reproduction. The ambiguity of these pregnancies involve ambiguous bloodlines, loyalties, and relationships, as well as new definitions of parenthood, kinship, and family roles. Intended parents may not share the circumstances of the conception or pregnancy with family and/or friends, leading to increased isolation and/or feelings of stigma. The fears of this pregnancy are more complex: Will the carrier or surrogate relinquish the child? Will the donor be of the same race? Could there be a laboratory mixup of gametes or embryos? Will the use of donor gametes become an issue for a spouse, the child, or the family in the future? The losses of the third-party pregnancy

are also unique, including loss of control of the prenatal environment, loss of predictability, and even loss of the pregnancy experience.

Finally, technological bewilderment is fundamental to third-party pregnancies – donated gametes, donated embryos, gestational carrier, surrogacy – resulting in a myriad of complexities for both parents and children, boundary violations, and confusion between the fetus, surrogate/carrier, and intended parents.[96] Although reproductive technologies provide family-building opportunities previously unimaginable, they are not without dilemmas, ethical challenges, and confusion about parental roles, definitions, and kinship ties. Not surprisingly, parents-to-be in third-party reproduction often feel ill-prepared for the challenges of these pregnancies or the stresses of parenting under such unique circumstances. Although there has been an increasing demand from both infertility patients and mental health professionals to improve patient education and preparation, provide appropriate psychological support and evaluation, and better equip patients for these unique pregnancies, the majority of women and their partners remain ill-prepared for their third-party pregnancies.[97]

Pregnancy in the Older Mother

There is a growing trend toward pregnancy in older mothers, especially in the infertile population. Medically termed *elderly gravida*, it encompasses pregnant women over the age of thirty-five. However, with the advent of donated oocytes, women have given birth after age sixty, a practice not generally recommended or condoned for social, ethical, and medical reasons. There is growing evidence that increasing maternal age is associated with specific adverse pregnancy outcomes including miscarriage, congenital abnormalities, gestational diabetes, preeclampsia, gestational diabetes, toxemia, hypertension, macrosomia, placental abruption, preterm delivery, low-birth rate, and perinatal mortality.[98] Nonetheless, although maternal and fetal outcome may be threatened, pregnancies in women over age forty may be considered relatively safe as the occurrence of perinatal death is still relatively rare.[99] Nevertheless, it is generally accepted that women over the age of forty have a consultation with a perinatologist to rule out any underlying health concerns (e.g., obesity, hypertension) that may impact their ability to successfully carry a pregnancy.

If the pregnancy in an older mother involves her own gametes, the fetus is at increased risk of a variety of problems related to increased maternal age, such as chromosomal abnormalities, molar gestations, and monozygotic twining (see Chapter 15). Consequently, prenatal testing is seriously recommended for these older mothers, which can often affect their feelings about the pregnancy and/or attachment to the fetus (see Table 25.1). Some prenatal testing, such as serum alpha-fetoprotein testing, involves a simple blood test and is less invasive. Other genetic tests such as amniocentesis, chorionic villus sampling, fetoscopy, and percutaneous umbilical blood sampling are more invasive and involve some risk of losing the pregnancy.

The whole issue of the 'less than perfect' baby is another consideration of these pregnancies and can be a significant psychological hurdle. Terminating a much-longed-for pregnancy is never easy but can be even more challenging if it represents the end of one's childbearing possibilities or ending a pregnancy achieved after considerable investment of time, treatment, finances, and emotional energy. Equally difficult or challenging can be the care of a disabled or handicapped child after years of infertility when one or both parents are well into middle age. In one study[100] of previously infertile couples, undergoing amniocentesis and prenatal testing contributed to feelings of adversity, uncertainty, and hope that reprised elements of the infertility experience and affected the pregnancy experience in a negative way. Interestingly, the majority of the infertile women under age thirty-five in this study refused amniocentesis, reflecting, in the researcher's opinion, a greater sense of the value of the pregnancy and baby.

Older first-time mothers typically represent a last chance at biological parenthood, frequently following a quest for a 'baby at any price.' They often willingly risk their own health and well-being for the longed-for pregnancy and baby, reasoning that, if the baby is healthy, then complications or risks to their own health are acceptable.[101] Apart from the medical considerations, the complex social situation of older primigravidae – remarriage, stepchildren, adult children from previous marriages, older or younger spouse, aged parents – frequently complicates their adjustment to parenthood and parental satisfaction.[102–104]

Pregnancy Following Secondary Infertility

Pregnancy in the secondarily infertile couple has not been investigated but has its own set of experiences and issues. Secondary infertility may follow a period of prior infertility, complicated pregnancy, or pregnancy loss, so that additional infertility treatment was anticipated. By contrast, previous conceptions and pregnancies may have been uneventful, while the subsequent pregnancy was achieved after considerable medical intervention. If a woman's other children are younger and still require

considerable care, this precious pregnancy may be more difficult to safeguard and manage – especially if bedrest is required. On the other hand, the comfort of a child may ameliorate feelings of anxiety, distress, and worry about this pregnancy.[105]

Of special consideration in the postsecondary-infertility pregnancy is the conception achieved via donated gametes or carried by a surrogate/gestational carrier, while previous conceptions were genetically-shared pregnancies. The postinfertility third-party pregnancy highlights 'the new blended family,' composed of children each with a unique reproductive beginning. But it can be a mixed blessing: Although it provides a longed-for child, it presents parenting family and relationship challenges. The third-party postsecondary-infertility pregnancy involves ambiguous genetic ties, more complicated pregnancy management, and a redefinition of family and kinship meanings. Furthermore, the postsecondary-infertility mother-to-be may be unable to interact with her social support system in the same manner in which she did during prior pregnancies, and obstetrical care may be based on inaccurate assumptions from her prior pregnancy history, enhancing her feelings of ambiguity, isolation, and technological bewilderment.

THERAPEUTIC INTERVENTIONS

A pregnancy after infertility is an exciting, terrifying, delightful, and frightful time for couples. Infertility counselors can play a special role in assisting patients in moving from infertility through the transition to becoming expectant parents to eventually, new mothers and fathers. There are six areas in which infertility counselors can facilitate and support the adaptation to pregnancy and the preparation for parenthood: (1) facilitating the adjustment to pregnancy; (2) assisting in decision making about prenatal care and testing; (3) developing and strengthening coping skills; (4) assessing for potential psychopathology and intervening; (5) identifying and providing support resources; and (6) advocating with caregivers.

Facilitating the Adjustment to Pregnancy

Moving from the identity of an infertile person to that of an expectant parent, and finally to the long-awaited identity as mother or father occurs in rapid succession once pregnancy is established. Couples often need help from infertility counselors in making the transition. The psychological tasks of pregnancy – validation, fetal embodiment, fetal distinction, and role transition – occur in a maturational process that infertility counselors can help to facilitate through education, support, and discussion. Understanding the unique aspects of pregnancy after infertility will also help in the adjustment. Mothers have to be able to take in their developing baby as part of themselves before they can separate from the infant during the birth process and see it as an individual.

Recognizing that there are unique challenges in pregnancy after infertility, couples also need encouragement to find as many opportunities as possible to normalize the pregnancy experience for both partners. One area that will need to be addressed is a couple's sexual relationship, which often is negatively affected by years of infertility. Renewing sexual intimacy encourages closeness, pleasure, and communication on which new parents can draw. However, couples may have many fears about sex during pregnancy and will need reassurance and concrete information that an orgasm does not precipitate labor or premature rupture of membranes in nonproblematic pregnancies. In addition, minimal spotting after intercourse is usually not harmful or troublesome.[106] Beginning to reestablish sexual intimacy is an important component in infertility healing and essential in assisting toward marital stability as child(ren) grow. Through education and support, infertility counselors can dispel myths and fears such as this, which can, and often do, interrupt healthy adjustment to pregnancy and parenthood.

Facilitating Decision Making

Once pregnancy is established, the formerly infertile couple often faces a new set of medical experiences and decisions. Some of the many decisions they must consider during pregnancy are diagnostic and/or prenatal testing; other medical interventions; the use of a midwife, obstetrician, or perinatologist; hospital or birthing facility; and birthing plan or preferences. Making the shift from the infertility practice, where the couple may have been involved for years, to an unknown obstetrical practice is often difficult for patients. It becomes yet another loss, as they leave behind caregivers who have shared in some of the most intimate aspects of their lives and may have become part of their primary emotional support system. There may be concerns that the new caregivers will not appreciate the preciousness of their pregnancy, be as invested in their care, or accommodate their medical and/or psychological special needs. A pregnancy support group sponsored by the reproductive medical practice is an ideal method for assisting infertility patients in these transitions by providing an understanding environment of the unique issues specific to this pregnancy, as well as continuing a con-

nection to the infertility clinic. In effect, a pregnancy support group acts as a bridge between the two medical practices (reproductive and obstetric) and two psychological experiences (infertility and pregnancy) (see Chapter 10).

The pregnant couple may also be faced with decisions about prenatal screening and/or testing, requiring support and understanding about their feelings and values, which are often conflicted and ambivalent (see Chapter 15). In addition, couples will have to explore and examine the risks of the procedures compared with potential benefits of the information obtained from them. For example, if a couple knows that they would not terminate the pregnancy of a genetically affected fetus, it may not be worth the risk of having procedures that may jeopardize the pregnancy by precipitating a miscarriage. With any of these decisions, it is always better that couples be educated, informed, and prepared for the possibilities well before having to make the choices. Infertility counselors can provide additional support as a familiar anchor, aware of their personal situation and knowledgeable of who they are, apart from this crisis. Table 25.1 describes decisions regarding obstetrical and genetic testing and how these decisions may alter the psychological adaptation to pregnancy.

Strengthening Coping Skills

Pregnancy after infertility could well be called the definition of the anxious pregnancy. Couples often need assistance in identifying and strengthening coping mechanisms during this anxious and challenging period. Nine months often feels like nine years to the previously infertile pregnant couple. Thus, one of the first tasks may be to help them adopt the 12-step program motto of 'one day at a time' because looking too far down the road and anticipating all the 'what ifs' can be, and is, overwhelming. For some, it may mean breaking the pregnancy period into even smaller components (one hour at a time) as a means of managing anxiety and trepidation. Breaking the pregnancy into a more manageable time frame, such as trimesters, may help to compartmentalize worries and fears, adjusting to the current demands versus the potential ones. Other cognitive-behavioral techniques may be useful, such as breathing exercises (e.g., yoga breathing, graduated breaths, and counting breaths); being mindful (e.g., staying in the moment or mindful meditation); cognitive restructuring (e.g., challenging negative thoughts – "Is this true? Is this helping me right now? Is there another way of looking at this?"); and writing index cards with positive, reality-based messages to refer to when anxiety increases (e.g., "I am doing all I can to

TABLE 25.1. Altered adaptation to pregnancy with amniocentesis[113]

Event	Adaptive response
First trimester	
1. Confirmation of pregnancy	Acceptance of pregnancy
Early second trimester	
2. Preamniocentesis counseling	Insulation from hurt due to potential subsequent loss leads to delayed acceptance of pregnancy and even anticipatory grief
Awareness of procedure-related miscarriage risk	
Risk of fetal abnormality(ies) assessed	Tentative pregnancy phenomenon
Early to mid-second trimester	
3. Sonography performed	Pregnancy suddenly equals baby and becomes a reality, especially for father
Baby looks normal	Enforces dream of healthy baby
Abnormality detected	Point of loss
4. The wait (about 2 weeks)	Continued detachment, delayed acceptance, guarded emotional investment in pregnancy – all in anticipation of potential loss
Mid- to late second trimester	
5. The results	
Abnormal	Decision making
	Grieving process
Normal	Equating normal results on one of two specific tests with normal baby, resulting in greater letdown if baby is born with problems undetectable by amniocentesis
Sex of baby	Reconciliation of fantasies of not 'wished for' sex, naming of baby, elaboration of fantasies, intensified bonding
6. Birth (after abnormal results)	Potentially enhanced coping due to opportunity to prepare for event/loss
7. Birth (after normal results)	
Good outcome	Reconciliation of fantasies regarding idealized child (normal process)
Unexpected outcome	
Death	Grieving process
Birth defect	Grief, adjustment – feeling of betrayal if test results normal

ensure a healthy pregnancy. All indications so far are that my pregnancy and baby are fine."').

Increased anxiety and vigilance are common in the pregnancy after infertility, perhaps representing a long-standing dependency on medical technology or a need to maintain contact with caregivers who have become a primary source of support and reassurance. Hypervigilant coping is often represented by repeated requests or demands for verbal reassurance or repetition of medical tests or by difficulty in relinquishing the infertility treatment team for more appropriate obstetrical care. The result of hypervigilant coping may be an overreaction to the common and normal symptoms and physiological changes of pregnancy such as nausea, heartburn, or backache and misinterpreting them as signs of problems with the pregnancy or the baby. Hypervigilance often includes requests for weekly physician visits, repeated ultrasound examinations, special medications, self-imposed bedrest, weekly psychotherapy visits, or sexual abstinence. Cognitive-behavioral interventions, including stress relaxation techniques, increased social support, and keeping a journal, may be useful in managing this acute anxiety and worry.

It may be that couples with a history of infertility are more aware of what can go wrong with a pregnancy.[107] Hence, they seek out ways of ensuring the safety of the pregnancy, even when there is no evidence that it is endangered. Other couples use avoidant coping to handle their numerous fears. Coping through avoidance may include not telling friends and family about the pregnancy; delaying or refusing to use maternity clothing; resisting transfer to obstetrical care from the infertility clinic; not following medical advice; and consciously resisting bonding with the baby. Furthermore, avoidant coping impedes problem solving and mastery of the tasks of pregnancy, further diminishing self-esteem and self-confidence as an effective parent. While hypervigilance and avoidance may be normal coping responses to the pregnancy after infertility, they are effective only in the short term and become problematic (i.e, a defense) when they become the primary way a woman deals with her feelings. Infertility counselors need to be able to assess when any coping mechanism begins to impede normal adaptation to pregnancy, relationships with others, and/or psychological functioning.

Assessing Emotional Distress

Infertility counselors may be called on to assess and intervene with emotional problems, which may be preexisting or precipitated by this pregnancy. Women with a history of depression, anxiety or panic disorder, eating disorders, or other psychological problems may need to be followed more closely during pregnancy and postpartum. In addition, these women (and their families) need to be educated early in the pregnancy about risk factors, treatment options, warning signs, and action plans to minimize the effects of their mental illness on their own well-being as well as that of the pregnancy and baby. Furthermore, marital problems may surface after the years of infertility and will need to be addressed as couples prepare for the transition to parenthood, the next great marital stressor.

Sometimes women who become pregnant after infertility react with feelings of bitterness toward the pregnancy or the baby. They may feel that they have 'paid their dues' during infertility treatment and are 'owed' an effortless pregnancy or delivery. Resentment about the additional physical demands and psychological stresses of pregnancy or even resentment of the baby itself may surface, much to the alarm of the woman, her partner, and caregivers. In extreme situations, newly pregnant infertility patients may be so overwhelmed and disturbed by the experience that they demand an abortion or act out their distress in equally alarming ways. Careful and immediate assessment and intervention are needed to understand the basis for this extreme reaction and provide appropriate diagnosis, treatment, and support.

Because depression and anxiety are common concerns in the pregnancy after infertility, several tools have been developed for assessing depression during pregnancy as a means of predicting postpartum depression: These include: the Antepartum Questionnaire,[108] the Antenatal Questionnaire,[109] and the Edinburgh Postpartum Depression Scale.[110] However, standardized measurements for depression and anxiety (e.g., Beck Depression Inventory, Beck Anxiety Inventory) may be just as effective in assessing psychological disturbance, especially if administered repeatedly during the pregnancy. Most women who develop postpartum depression (PPD) acquire the condition by six weeks after birth although it may emerge up to eighteen months after delivery.[111] As such, infertility counselors may need continued involvement postpartum with patients at risk of developing PPD.

Providing Resources

Many postinfertility pregnancy patients need assistance in accessing and using pregnancy resources, which often feels like unfamiliar and foreign territory. It is important that couples be encouraged to normalize the pregnancy as much as possible and become involved with the same support resources available to pregnant women or couples who conceived procreatively the fertile pregnant group – childbirth classes, pregnancy exercise programs, support groups, preparation for parenthood classes, and parents of multiples organizations. Couples also need access to information and reading materials on pregnancy, prenatal testing, or normal obstetrical care, as well as any special problems or circumstances of this unique pregnancy. The internet has become a powerful source of information for many issues related to infertility as well as pregnancy, helping to lessen feelings of loneliness and isolation that follow infertility and prepare for parenthood as well as normalize the pregnancy experience. However, caution must be used, as information received on the internet may not be accurate. As such, infertility counselors can be a useful resource in guiding patients to appropriate websites (see Resources).

Advocating with Caregivers

The history of a woman pregnant after infertility may include physical and emotional losses following failed medical treatments, marital disruption, sexual dysfunction, and/or even serious psychiatric illnesses such as depression, anxiety, eating disorders, or obsessive-compulsive disorder. She may have idealized pregnancy as a state of bliss and fulfillment or fantasized that her baby would be perfect in every way or that she would be the perfect all-knowing, all-caring mother. Furthermore, a woman's own stage of life may influence her adjustment to pregnancy. For example, the first-time mother in her late twenties will experience pregnancy differently from the woman who is pregnant in her forties after an extended period of secondary infertility. As a consequence, women may need assistance from infertility counselors in navigating and negotiating the pregnancy path. This may mean advocating for patients, when they are unable, with physicians, other caregivers, employers, or family members. For example, an infertility counselor may want to be in contact with the obstetrician to coordinate care and help the physician better understand the patient and her past infertility experience. Often, infertility counselors are bridges between the worlds of infertility and obstetrical caregivers and, as such, are able to explain or discriminate normal and abnormal responses to pregnancy in a previously infertile patient.[112] Working with caregivers toward the best interest of a woman pregnant after infertility, is a further extension of the collaborative reproductive healthcare approach advocated throughout this text.

FUTURE ISSUES

Although pregnancy is as old as mankind, the way conception is achieved has changed drastically in the last few years. However, the future may hold more changes in the ways in which babies are carried to term. Third-party reproduction with gestational carriers and surrogates has already been an example of some of these changes. The next century may see babies gestated in vitro rather than in vivo, in a manner not unlike that envisioned in Aldous Huxley's *Brave New World*. Continued research is needed to understand the psychological adaptation to pregnancy after high-stakes infertility treatment. Olshansky[23] outlined three possible future directions for research on pregnancy after infertility:

■ delineation of the differences in experiences of infertility and correlation of those different experiences with subsequent experiences of pregnancy;
■ more diverse sampling in research on those pregnant after infertility, including the various reproductive technologies, cultural perspectives, economic factors, and pregnancy experiences;
■ gender differences in responses to pregnancy after infertility.

Other resources need to be developed to assist this special population (targeting the special needs of the previously infertile pregnancy). Educational materials are needed on normal pregnancy, pregnancy complications, delivery, and parenting. Support resources, especially pregnancy support groups, childbirth education classes, and preparation for parenthood classes for the previously infertile pregnant couple are sorely needed. There must also be education and training of obstetrical staff about the special circumstances, needs, and

unique characteristics of a women who are pregnant after infertility.

SUMMARY

■ The pregnancy after infertility is a premium pregnancy with additional potential medical and psychological challenges before a successful outcome (i.e., birth of healthy infant) is achieved.
■ The psychological tasks of pregnancy – validation, fetal embodiment, fetal distinction, and role transition – are challenged and complicated by the infertility experience.
■ The psychological tasks of pregnancy after infertility involve addressing the issues of ambiguity, isolation, fear, loss, and technological bewilderment.[36]
■ The pregnancy after infertility is at higher risk for complications, including multiple gestation, problems related to advanced maternal age, premature delivery, low birth weight, and perinatal loss. Additionally, potential complications for the mother include problems related to the infertility diagnosis (e.g., PCOS or incompetent cervix) or problems related to the pregnancy (e.g., hypertension, gestational diabetes, and toxemia).
■ The postinfertility pregnancy is often marked by high anxiety, hypervigilance, or denial as typical coping mechanisms. In addition, there may be an increased risk of depression, anxiety, obsessive-compulsive disorder, eating disorders, and other psychiatric illness in the postinfertility pregnancy.
■ There are six areas in which infertility counselors may assist pregnant couples: (1) facilitating in adjustment to the pregnancy, (2) assisting in obstetrical decision making, (3) strengthening coping mechanisms, (4) assessing and treating maladaptive responses, (5) providing additional resources, and (6) advocating for patients.

REFERENCES

1. Rothman BK. *Encyclopedia of Childbearing: Critical Perspectives*. Phoenix, AZ: The Oryx Press, 1993.
2. Simkin P. Childbearing in a social context. *Women Health* 1989; 15:5–21.
3. Gordon ER. Blended families: Adopted, ART, and natural children. In: *Postgraduate Course XII: ART Parents and Children*. American Society for Reproductive Medicine; Seattle, WA, October 7–8, 1995; 78–83.
4. Macklin R. Artificial means of reproduction and our understanding of the family. *Hastings Cent Rep* 1991; 21:5–11.
5. Huber G, Ludwig M. Obstetric outcome of pregnancies after assisted reproduction. In: M Ludwig, ed. *Pregnancy and Birth After Assisted Reproductive Technologies*. Berlin: Springer-Verlag, 2002; 56–68.

6. Koudstaal J, Braat DDM, Bruinse HW, et al. Obstetrical outcome of singleton pregnancies after IVF: A matched control study in four Dutch university hospitals. *Human Reprod* 2000;15:1819–25.

7. Wennerholm UB, Bergh D, Hamberger L, et al. Obstetric outcome of pregnancies following ICSI, classified according to sperm origin and quality. *Human Reprod* 2000; 15:1189–94.

8. Klonoff-Cohen H, Natarajan L. The concerns during assisted reproductive technologies (CART) scale and pregnancy outcomes. *Fertil and Steril* 2004; 81: 982–8.

9. Spandorfer SD, Grill E, Davis O, Fasouliotis SJ, et al. September 11th in New York City (NYC): The effect of a catastrophe on IVF outcome in a New York City based program. *Fertil and Steril* 2003; 80:51.

10. Glynn LM, Wadhwa PD, Dunkel-Schetter C, et al. When stress happens matters: Effects of earthquake timing on stress responsivity in pregnancy. *Am J Obstet Gynecol* 2001; 184:637–42.

11. Garner CH. Pregnancy after infertility. *J Obstet Gynecol Neonatal Nurs* 1985; 14(suppl):58–62.

12. Harris BG, Sandelowski M, Holditch-Davis D. Infertility and new interpretations of pregnancy loss. *J Matern Child Nurs* 1991; 16:217–20.

13. Phipps S. The subsequent pregnancy after stillbirth: Anticipatory parenthood in the face of uncertainty. *Int J Psychiatry Med* 1985; 15:243–64.

14. Cuisinier M, Janssen H, de Graauw C, et al. Pregnancy following miscarriage: Course of grief and some determining factors. *J Psychosom Obstet Gynaecol* 1996; 17:168–74.

15. Bernstein J, Lewis J, Seibel M. Effect of previous infertility on maternal-infant attachment, coping styles, and self-concept during pregnancy. *J Women's Health* 1994; 3:125–33.

16. Bernstein J, Mattox JH, Kellner R. Psychological status of previously infertile couples after a successful pregnancy. *J Obstet Gynecol Neonatal Nurs* 1988; 164(suppl):404–8.

17. McMahon C, Ungerer J, Tennant C, et al. Psychosocial adjustment and the mother–baby relationship for IVF mothers. *Symposia of the Mental Health Professional Group*, American Society for Reproductive Medicine, Boston, MA; November, 1996.

18. Klock SC, Greenfeld DA. Psychological status of in vitro fertilization patients during pregnancy: A longitudinal study. *Fertil and Steril* 2000; 73:1159–64.

19. Halman LJ, Oakley, D, Lederman R. Adaptation to pregnancy and motherhood among subfecund and fecund primiparous women. *J Maternal-Child Nursing* 1995; 23:90–100.

20. Fisher JR HK, Baker HWG. Assisted conception is a risk factor for postnatal mood disturbance and early parenting difficulties. *Fertil Steril* 2005; 84:426–30.

21. Scottish Intercollegiate Guidelines Network. *Postnatal depression and puerperal psychosis. A national clinical guideline.* Edinburgh: SIGN Executive, 2002.

22. Sandelowski M, Pollock C. Women's experiences of infertility. *Image J Nurs Sch* 1986; 18:140–4.

23. Olshansky EF. Identity of self as infertile: An example of theory-generating research. *Adv Nurs Sci* 1987; 9: 54–63.

24. Glaser BG, Strauss AL. *The Discovery of Grounded Theory.* Chicago: Aldine Press, 1967.

25. Holditch-Davis D, Black BP, Harris BG, et al. Beyond couvade: Pregnancy symptoms in couples with a history of infertility. *Health Care Women Int* 1994; 15:537–48.

26. Benedek T. Parenthood as a developmental phase. *J Am Psychoanal Assoc* 1959; 7:379–417.

27. Deutsch H. *The Psychology of Women*, Vol 1, New York: Grune & Stratton, 1944.

28. Notman MR, Lester EP. Pregnancy: Theoretical considerations. *Psychoanal Inq* 1988; 8:139–59.

29. Miller LJ. Psychiatric disorders during pregnancy. In: DE Stewart, NL Stotland, eds, *Psychological Aspects of Women's Health Care*. Washington DC: American Psychiatric Press, 1993; 55–70.

30. Raphael-Leff J. *Pregnancy: The Inside Story*. London: Jason Aronson, 1995.

31. Olshansky EF. Psychosocial implications of pregnancy after infertility. *NAACOG Clin Issues Perinat Womens Health Nurs* 1990; 1:342–7.

32. Olshansky EF. Pregnancy after infertility: An overview of the research. Course XII: ART Parents and Children. American Society for Reproductive Medicine; Seattle, WA, October 7–8, 1995; 5–13.

33. Clark AL, D Affonso, eds. *Childbearing: A Nursing Perspective*. Philadelphia: FA Davis, 1976.

34. Colman LL, Colman AD. *Pregnancy: The Psychological Experience*. New York: Noonday Press, 1991.

35. Glazer E. *The Long-Awaited Stork*. New York: Lexington Books, 1990.

36. Glazer E. Parenting after infertility. In: MM Seibel, AA Kiessling, J Bernstein, et al., eds. *Infertility and Technology: Clinical Psychological, Legal, and Ethical Aspects*. New York: Springer-Verlag, 1993; 365–72.

37. Pugh TF, Jerath BK, Schmidt WM, et al. Rates of mental disease related to child-bearing. *N Engl J Med* 1963; 268:1224–8.

38. Gise LH. Psychiatric implications of pregnancy. In: SH Cherry, R Barques, N Kale, eds, *Rovinksy and Gutmacher's Medical, Surgical, and Gynecologic Complications of Pregnancy*, 3rd ed. Baltimore, MD: Williams & Wilkins, 1985; 614–54.

39. Callahan EJ, Desiderato L. Disorders of pregnancy. In: EA Blechman, KD Brownell, eds, *Handbook of Behavioral Medicine for Women*. New York: Pergamon Press, 1988; 103–15.

40. Bennett HA, Einarson A, Taddio A, Koren G, Einarson TR. Prevalence of depression during pregnancy: Systematic review. *Am J Obstet Gynecol* 2004; 103:698–709.

41. Lusskin SI. Mood disorders during pregnancy and the postpartum period. *Obstet Gynecol Board Review Manual* 1999; 5:15–23.

42. O'Hara MW, Rehm LP, Campbell SB. Predicting depressive symptomology: Cognitive-behavioral models and postpartum depression. *J Abnorm Psychol* 1982; 91:457–61.

43. Chambers CD, Johnson KA, Dick LM, et al. Birth outcomes in pregnant women taking fluoxetine. *N Engl J Med* 1996; 335:1010–15.

44. Altshuler LL, Cohen L, Szuba MP, et al. Pharmacologic management of psychiatric illness during pregnancy: Dilemmas and guidelines. *Am J Psychiatry* 1996; 153:592–606.

45. http://www.fda.gov/medwatch/safety/2005/safety05.htm#Paxil. Accessed 11/01/05.

46. Cohen LS, Rosenbaum JF. Psychotropic drug use during pregnancy: Weighing the risks. *J Clin Psychiatry* 1998; 59:18–28.

47. O'Hara M, Zekoski E, Phillips L, et al. Controlled prospective study of postpartum mood disorders: Comparisons of child-bearing and nonchildrearing women. *J Abnorm Psychol* 1990; 99:3–12.

48. O'Hara MW. Social support, life events, and depression during pregnancy and the puerperium. *Arch Gen Psychiatry* 1986; 43:569–73.

49. Powell S, Drotar D. Postpartum depressed mood: The impact of daily hassles. *J Psychosom Obstet Gynaecol* 1992; 13:255–63.

50. O'Hara M, Rehm L, Campbell S. Postpartum depression: A role for social network and life stress variables. *J Nerv Ment Dis* 1983; 171:336–41.

51. O'Hara MW, Zekoski EM. Postpartum depression: A comprehensive review. In: R Kumar, IF Brockington, eds. *Motherhood and Mental Illness*. London: Butterworth, 1988.

52. Josefsson A, Angelsioo L, Berg G, et al. Obstetric, somatic, and demographic risk factors for postpartum depressive symptoms. *Am J Obstet Gynecol* 2002; 99:223–8.

53. Neugebauer R, Kline J, Shrout P, et al. Major depressive disorder in the 6 months after miscarriage. *JAMA* 1997; 277:383–8.

54. Villeponteaux VA, Lydiard RB, Laraia MT, et al. The effects of pregnancy on preexisting panic disorder. *J Clin Psychiatry* 1992; 53:201–3.

55. Neziroglu F, Anemone R, Yaryura-Tobias JA. Onset of obsessive-compulsive disorder in pregnancy. *Am J Psychiatry* 1992; 149:947–50.

56. Brandt KR, Mackenzie TB. Obsessive-compulsive disorder exacerbated during pregnancy: A case report. *Int J Psychiatry Med* 1987; 17:361–6.

57. Cowley DS, Roy-Byrne RP. Panic disorder during pregnancy. *J Psychosom Obstet Gynaecol* 1989; 10:193–210.

58. Notman MT. Reproduction and pregnancy: A psychodynamic developmental perspective. In: NL Stotland, ed, *Psychiatric Aspects of Reproductive Technology*. Washington DC: American Psychiatric Press, 1990; 13–24.

59. Stotland NL. Personality disorders. *Prim Care Update Ob/Gynecol* 1997; 4:57–60.

60. Abrams BF, Laros RK. Pregnancy weight, weight gain and birth weight. *Am J Obstet Gynecol* 1986; 154:503–9.

61. Hollifield J, Hobdy J. The course of pregnancy complicated by bulimia. *Psychotherapy* 1990; 27:249–55.

62. Lacey JH, Smith G. Bulimia nervosa: The impact of pregnancy on mother and baby. *Br J Psychiatry* 1987; 150:777–81.

63. Stewart DE, McDonald OL. Hyperemesis gravidarum and eating disorders in pregnancy. In: S Abraham, D Llewellyn-Jones, eds. *Eating Disorders and Disordered Eating*. Sydney, Australia: Ashwood House, 1987; 52–5.

64. Downey J, Whitaker A. Nausea and vomiting of pregnancy: Behavioral aspects of diagnosis and management. *Clin Consult Obstet Gynecol* 1994; 6:258–64.

65. Stewart DE, Robinson GE, Goldbloom DS, et al. Infertility and eating disorders. *Am J Obstet Gynecol* 1990; 163:1196–9.

66. Abraham S, Mira M, Llewellyn-Jones D. Should ovulation be induced in women recovering from an eating disorder or who are compulsive exercisers? *Fertil Steril* 1990; 52:566–8.

67. Ladipo OA. Pseudocyesis in infertile patients. *Int J Gynaecol Obstet* 1979; 16:427–9.

68. Brezinka C, Huter O, Biebl W, Kinzl J. Denial of pregnancy: Obstetrical aspects. *J Psychosom Obstet Gynaecol* 1996; 15:1–8.

69. Miller LJ. Psychotic denial of pregnancy: Phenomenology and clinical management. *Hosp Community Psychiatry* 1990; 41:1233–7.

70. Bernstein J. Pregnancy after infertility. *Serono Reprod Med Infertil Nurses* 1986; Sept 27–28:68–81.

71. Wohlreich MM. Psychiatric aspects of high-risk pregnancy. *Psychiatr Clin North Am* 1986; 10:53–68.

72. Vutyavanich T, Kraisarin T, Ruangsri RA. Ginger for nausea and vomiting in pregnancy: Randomized, double-masked, placebo-controlled trail. *Obstet Gynecol* 2001; 97:577–82.

73. ACOG Practice Bulletin. Nausea and vomiting of pregnancy. *Obstet Gynecol* 2004; 103:803–14.

74. Johnson SH, Kraut DA. *Pregnancy Bedrest: A Guide for the Pregnant Woman and Her Family*. New York: Henry Holt, 1990.

75. Nadelson CC. 'Normal' and 'special' aspects of pregnancy: A psychological approach. In: CC Nadelson, MT Notman, eds., *The Woman Patient, Medical and Psychological Interfaces, vol. 1: Sexual and Reproductive Aspects of Women's Health Care*. New York: Plenum, 1978; 279.

76. The ESHRE Capri Workshop. Multiple gestation pregnancy. *Hum Reprod* 2000; 15:1856–64.

77. Callahan TL, Hall JE, Ettner SL, et al. The economic impact of multiple gestation pregnancies and the contribution of assisted reproductive techniques to their incidence. *N Engl J Med* 1994; 331:244–9.

78. Lancaster PA. International comparisons of assisted reproduction. *Assist Reprod Rev* 1992; 2:212–21.

79. Newton D, McBride J. Single Embryo Transfer (SET): Factors affecting patient attitudes and decision-making. *Fertil Steril* 2005; 84:S3.

80. Leiblum SR, Kemmann E, Taska L. Attitudes toward multiple births and pregnancy concerns in infertile and non-infertile women. *J Psychosom Obstet Gynaecol* 1990; 11:197–210.

81. Greenfeld DA, Walther VN. Psychological consideration in multifetal reduction. *Infertil Reprod Med Clin North Am* 1993; 4:533–43.

82. Silver RK, Ragin A, Helfand BT, et al. Multifetal reduction increases the risk of preterm delivery and fetal growth restriction in twins: A case-control study. *Fertil Steril* 1997; 67:30–3.

83. McKinney M, Downey J, Timor-Tritsch I. The psychological effects of multifetal pregnancy reduction. *Fertil Steril* 1995; 64:51–61.

84. Schreiner-Engel P, Walther VN, Mindes J, et al. First trimester multifetal pregnancy reduction: Acute and persistent psychological reactions. *Am J Obstet Gynecol* 1995; l72:541–7.

85. Seelig AS, Ludwig M. Oocyte Donation. In: M Ludwig, ed, *Pregnancy and Birth After Assisted Reproductive Technologies*. Berlin: Springer-Verlag, 2002, 69–84.

86. Karnis MF, Zimon AE, Lalwani SI, et al. Risk of death in pregnancy achieved through oocyte donation in patients with Turner syndrome: A national survey. *Fertil and Steril* 2003; 80:498–501.

87. Bertrand-Servais M, Letur-Konirsch H, Raoul-Duval A, et al. Psychological considerations of anonymous oocyte donation. *Hum Reprod* 1993; 8:874–9.

88. Pados G, Camus M, Van Steirteghem A, et al. The evolution and outcome of pregnancies from oocyte donation. *Hum Reprod* 1994; 9:538–42.

89. Braverman AM. Oocyte donation: Psychological and counseling issues. *Clin Consult Obstet Gynecol* 1994; 6:143–9.

90. Schover LR. Psychological aspects of oocyte donation. *Infertil Reprod Med Clin North Am* 1993; 4:483–502.

91. Parker PJ. Motivation of surrogate mothers: Initial findings. *Am J Psychiatry* 1983; 140:117–18.

92. Braverman AM, Corson SL. Characteristics of participants in a gestational carrier program. *J Assist Reprod Genet* 1992; 9:353–7.

93. Braverman AM. Surrogacy and gestational carrier: Psychological issues. *Infertil Reprod Med Clin North Am* 1993; 4:517–33.

94. Reame NE. The surrogate mother as a high-risk obstetrical patient. *Jacobs Inst Women's Health* 1991; 1:151–4.

95. Reame NE, Parker PJ. Surrogate pregnancy: Clinical features in 44 cases. *Am J Obstet Gynecol* 1990; 162:1220–5.

96. Lester EP. Surrogate carries a fertilised ovum: Multiple crossings in ego boundaries. *Int J Psychoanal* 1995; 76:325–34.

97. Mahlstedt PP, Greenfeld DA. Assisted reproductive technology with donor gametes: The need for patient preparation. *Fertil Steril* 1989; 52:908–14.

98. Goldman JC, Malone FD, Vidaver J, et al. Impact of maternal age on obstetric outcome. *Obstet Gynecol* 2005; 105:983–90.

99. Jacobsson B, Lafors L, Milsom I. Advanced maternal age and adverse perinatal outcome. *Obstet Gynecol* 2004; 104:727–40.

100. Sandelowski M, Harris BG, Holditch-Davis D. Amniocentesis in the context of infertility. *Health Care Women Int* 1991; 12:167–78.

101. James C. Impact the psyche of the cycle: Pregnancy after forty. In: *Postgraduate Course XI: American Society for Reproductive Medicine*; Seattle, WA, October 7–8, 1995, p 135.

102. Windridge KC, Berryman JC. Maternal adjustment and maternal attitudes during pregnancy and early motherhood in women of 35 and over. *J Reprod Infant Psychol* 1996; 14:45–55.

103. Berryman JC, Windridge KC. Pregnancy after 35 and attachment to the fetus. *J Reprod Infant Psychol* 1996; 14:133–43.

104. Frankel SA, Wise MJ. A view of delayed parenting: Some implications for a new trend. *Psychiatry* 1982; 45: 220–5.

105. Rosenblatt PA, Burns LH. Long-term effects of perinatal loss. *J Fam Issues* 1986; 7:237–53.

106. Shapiro CH. Is pregnancy after infertility a dubious joy? *Soc Casework J Contemp Soc Work* 1986; 67:306–13.

107. Reamy KJ. Sexuality in pregnancy: An update. *Clin Consult Obstet Gynecol* 1994; 6:265–73.

108. Posner NA, Unterman RR, Williams KN, et al. *Antepartum Questionnaire: APQ*. Albany, NY: Department of Obstetrics & Gynecology, Albany Medical Center, 1996.

109. Cooper PJ, Murray L, Hooper R, et al. The Development and validation of a predictive index for postpartum depression. *Psychol Med* 1996; 26:627–34.

110. Cox JL, Holden JM Sagovsky R. Detection of postnatal depresseion: Development of the 10-item Edinburgh Postnatal Depression Scale. *Br J Psychiatry* 1987; 150:782–6.

111. Stowe ZN, Nemeroff CB. Women at risk for postpartum-onset major depression. *Am J Obstet Gynecol* 1995; 173:639–45.

112. Burns LH. Pregnancy after infertility. *Infertil Reprod Med Clin North Am* 1996; 7:503–20.

113. Benkendorf J, Corson V, Allen JF, et al. Perinatal bereavement counseling in genetics. In: *Strategies in Genetic Counseling: Reproductive Genetics and New Technologies*. White Plains, NY: March of Dimes Defects Foundation, 1990; 136–48.

26 Parenting after Infertility

LINDA HAMMER BURNS

Your children are not your children. They are the sons and daughters of life's longing for itself…you may strive to be like them, but seek not to make them like you.

– Kahil Gibran

The legacy of infertility extends beyond the children and families created through medical treatment and reproductive technologies: The impact may be experienced in the long-term adjustment and psychosocial development of the family system and its individuals. The legacy of infertility often includes multiple losses; prolonged yearning for a child; intrusive reproductive technologies; possibly third-party reproduction; a tenuous, highly anxious pregnancy; and/or an exorbitant investment of time, energy, and money to have children. Exceptionally determined and purposeful, previously infertile parents may be aware of their reasons for wanting to be parents, but less cognizant of the potential challenges and actual joys of parenthood. Once parenthood is achieved, these parents are often equally determined about parenthood as they were about infertility. Their goal is often to be the world's best parents and they are not satisfied with being simply good enough parents. Furthermore, most previously infertile parents believe that parenthood is worth it: They value their children; take the responsibilities of parenthood seriously; savor the pleasures of their children; and do their best to act in the best interests of their children. Nevertheless, many previously infertile couples refer to their history of infertility as the shadow, a legacy that resurfaces long after parenthood is achieved and emerges in various ways long after the maelstrom of infertility has passed.

The role of the infertility counselor has always involved not simply supporting individuals and couples pursuing infertiltiy treatment, but providing care over the long term to families with a history of infertility. The issue of parenting after infertility treatment has become even more relevant with a recent American Society of Reproductive Medicine Ethics Committee[1] report recommending that fertility programs withhold services when there are reasonable grounds for thinking that patients will be unable to provide adequate child-rearing to offspring and/or may endanger the child. This report further recommends that decisions to deny treatment should be made jointly among members of the treatment team with input from the mental health professional as part of the treatment team. Examples of factors that may be considered reason for refusal or postponement of treatment are uncontrolled psychiatric illness; substance abuse; ongoing physical or emotional abuse; or a history of perpetrating physical or emotional abuse. As this chapter reviews how the experience of infertility impacts families created via infertility treatment and the parenting experience (particularly in special circumstances), the best interests of the child and the welfare of the family and its members are important considerations about which the mental health professional should always be cognizant. While adoptive parenting (see Chapter 22) and children conceived via assisted reproduction (see Chapter 27) are addressed elsewhere, this chapter addresses:

■ the unique psychosocial issues of and the transition to parenthood after infertility;
■ special parenting situations, including the older parent; parenting after secondary infertility; parenting multiples; parenting after third-party reproduction; remarriage parenting issues; solo parenting; gay/lesbian parenthood;
■ the role of the infertility counselor in facitating post-infertility family adjustment.

HISTORICAL OVERVIEW

Historically, children were valued by primitive and pre-historic peoples for their ability to contribute to the kinship (tribe) through their labor (e.g., food gathering and caregiving of elders). With the evolution of civilization and the advent of monogamous relationships that were

459

legally sanctioned by society and/or religious tenets, the role and importance of children became more complex. Children were valued as validation of the marital relationship or a woman's role (function) in society, as progeny and property.[2]

By the seventeenth century, children in agrarian societies were valued for their labor, while urban children were economically useless, especially orphans or children from large, poor, or disadvantaged homes. In colonized areas (e.g., America, Canada, Australia, Africa, South America, and Southeast Asia) children were necessary for propagation of the colonies (particularly by the colonists) and, most importantly, for economic survival of the colonials. Furthermore, childlessness was thought to be the result of a woman's sinful ways, and the very idea of attempting to alleviate infertility was viewed as defiance of God's will, particularly in Puritan America.[3,4] Cultural shifts during the eighteenth century in industrialized countries affected family life and patterns of family formation, moving families away from a communal society to a society founded on single-family units of married couples and their offspring.[4] Before the industrial revolution of the nineteenth century, children were valued or devalued primarily for their economic utility. With the industrial revolution, women and children were removed from the workforce and moved to the home. Child labor laws in the early twentieth century created monumental social change worldwide: Children came to be valued for their affectional ties, companionship, and stimulation and childrearing as a job for women (motherhood). Thus, children became *functionally worthless*, *economically useless*, but *emotionally priceless* companions.[5]

It has been suggested that this shift in values may explain differences in the meaning of children to men and women.[6] Historically, men invested in having children (especially sons) out of a need to have a material and spiritual heir; children (like wives) were the chattel property of men. With the industrial revolution, children became less valuable as *economic* investments providing economic return although they remained valuable as economic heirs (e.g., estates, titles, fiefdoms, and businesses). Nevertheless, children, particularly in the developed world, became more valuable as *emotional* investments providing emotional warmth and affection, especially for women. This value shift is thought to account for the decline in men's investment in children,[6] while at the same time contributing to the increase of women's investment in children. To make motherhood a career for women, motherhood became an ideal, a role for women, encouraged by economic necessities, psychological theories, and cultural values.[7] Whether the result of the industrial

revolution or patriarchal culture, women have historically and continue to be, primarily valued for their reproductive and childrearing capacities. Across cultures motherhood was/is a primary role and sole vocation, and, as such, women expect (and/or were expected) to obtain all of their emotional, intellectual, and personal gratification from motherhood similar to the rewards men receive from their work. As such, infertility leaves women unemployed and emotionally unfulfilled at a very fundamental level even when they have a career or other generativity measures in their lives.

By the beginning of the twentieth century, reproduction had become less a matter of having children than of having the *right* children: Only worthy parents were fit to bear and rear worthy children. This cultural shift, termed the *privatization of happiness*, represented a shift in the developed world from the community as a source of emotional investment and reward to a society in which the nuclear family was the ideological center of happiness.[3] It can be argued that this became the basis for the eugenics movement of the twentieth century and other attempts to create the *ideal* child and/or family (e.g., Nazi Germany). In this view, the current high value of children – 'a child at any price' – is the result of a cultural shift in which public life appears bankrupt and alienating, so that couples with or without children continue their pursuit of happiness in the private areas of their lives with children remaining the focus of this private drive for happiness.[3] It has also contributed to the 'medicalizing of motherhood' in which pregnancy, childbirth, and infertility became a female disability. Medicalizing motherhood began with the movement of childbirth away from the home and midwives to direct management of maternity care by physicians at hospitals and/or medical centers. Childbirth became a medical event, and infertility became not simply a social and/or marital crisis but a medical crisis involving increasingly complex and invasive treatments to facilitate conception and birth in hopes of creating the perfect nuclear family.[8]

REVIEW OF LITERATURE

Although interest in postinfertility families has grown among reproductive health professionals, it has yet to capture the curiosity of the broader community of mental health professionals and researchers, although families created via assisted reproductive technologies have gained considerable attention in recent years. However, there continues to be a significant lack of research in such areas as: the impact of infertility's legacy from the child's perpective (e.g., the child's perception of parenting or family dynamics); the impact on family developmental transitions on older children, adolescent, or adult offspring; family dynamics and adjustment; parental attitudes or behaviors; and comparisons of expectations before and after parenthood.

Part of the problem is the tendency of postinfertility parents to blend with the larger population of parents, so that other professionals are unaware of the legacy of infertility and the difficult issues faced by these parents and families. In addition, infertility has been treated as a medical, not a psychosocial or family system issue and, as such, has received more attention from the medical community and less within the mental health community. For these reasons, it has been difficult to formulate a research agenda or define research questions that address the long-term adjustment of family members or family systems, especially because the goal of medical treatment has been achieved and, consequently, medical professionals and patients alike anticipate no further problems.

Investigations historically have focused on medical treatments facilitating parenthood and less on actual parenting and/or the child. An inordinate amount of research has focused on parenthood achieved by third-party reproduction (e.g., donated gametes or gestational carrier) and other forms of assisted reproduction [e.g., in vitro fertilization (IVF) or intracytoplasmic sperm injection (ICSI)], particularly disclosure decisions. Recently, a few studies have addressed the psychological adjustment of previously infertile parents and investigating factors influencing posttreatment parental adaptation and child development.

Motivations for Parenthood

Hoffman and Hoffman[9] in a conceptualization of motivations for parenthood in a normal population enumerated nine reasons: adult status and social identity; expansion of self; moral values; group ties and affection; stimulation and fun; achievement and creativity; power and influence; social comparison; and economic utility. A study of motives for having children in involuntarily childless couples[10] found that the desire for children was very strong, especially among women, even after a lengthy (8.6 years) period of infertility. For both men and women, the primary motive for wanting children was happiness and well-being, while social control and continuity were unimportant to both men and women.[11] Assessed motives for parenthood of infertile women and men participating in an IVF program, reported that women placed greatest emphasis on fulfilling gender-role requirements, while men were more likely to stress a desire for marital completion as motivation. Although the long period of infertility treatment appears to stimulate the process of thinking and rethinking the reasons for having children, most couples do not abandon the desire for a family. Furthermore, this process may help infertile men and women develop a more realistic perception of the demands and rewards of children.

Postinfertility Adjustment to Parenthood

Historically, against this backdrop, it was thought that previously infertile parents would be more appreciative and conscientious parents – reinterpreted as more overprotective and overinvested parents. In 1943, a study of overprotective mothers concluded, "Mothers who suffer the trials of prolonged anticipation of the first born, long periods of relative sterility, or spontaneous miscarriages or stillbirths, are rendered obviously more apprehensive and protective in their attitude toward the offspring than if childbirth occurred without these circumstances."[12, p. 401] By contrast, it was speculated that a history of infertility resulted in parents who were more hostile, abusive, or neglectful of their children – perhaps acting on lingering feelings of shame, self-reproach, frustration, or long-standing marital conflict about infertility. One case report[13] went so far as to conclude that child abuse and abortion were manifestations of parental hostility toward children resulting from prior infertility and reproductive failure. Finally, it was theorized that a history of parental infertility could produce disturbances in children and the family system. In a 1971 investigation of child-centered family systems, Bradt and Moynihan[14] concluded that prematurity and adoption (as evidence of reproductive failure) increased the risk of a child's becoming disturbed and the emotional focus of a family, as evidenced by a child's acting out to escape the pressure and responsibility of the family's happiness. However, none of these theories or speculations ever produced conclusive research evidence that families with a history of infertility were at greater risk for psychological disturbance in the children, the family system, or problem parenting.

Maternal identity after infertility has also been the focus of investigation. Dunington and Glazer[15] found no significant difference in prenatal maternal identity between previously infertile mothers and noninfertile mothers. However, previously infertile mothers lacked self-confidence in their ability to perform mothering tasks; sought more reassurance about the normalcy of their baby; and showed more identity confusion between career and maternal identities. In a preliminary evaluation from a study of children born by anonymously donated oocytes, Olshansky[16] found that previously infertile mothers were more likely to report feelings of guilt and shame, which they associated with their formerly infertile status. These women continued to harbor feelings of failure and malformation about their reproductive ability and felt embarrassed about the circumstances of the child's conception. Research indicates that previously infertile parents are satisfied with their parental roles but have more difficulty adjusting to parenthood. In a comparison study of infertile couples, Abbey and colleagues[17] found that previously infertile mothers experienced greater global well-being, while previously infertile fathers (but not mothers) experienced greater home-life stress.

In a study evaluating perceptions of parenthood in previously infertile parents who had become parents via infertility treatment or adoption, but not assisted reproductive technologies (ARTs),[18] no significant differences were found between adoptive or procreation parents. However, in comparison to a control group, the previously infertile parents were more likely to be satisfied with their marital relationship than with their parenting ability. The majority (50%) of procreation parents considered their parenting conscientious/secure while only 20% of previously infertile rated their parenting in this way. Thirty percent of the procreation parents versus 25% of previously infertile parents rated themselves as overprotective/child-centered, while 20% of both procreation parents and previously infertile parents rated themselves as abusive/neglectful. While none of the procreation parents rated themselves as *both* overprotective and abusive, 35% of the previously infertile parents did. In addition, the previously infertile parents were more likely to report problems in bonding to their child and were more likely to nominate or identify psychological problems in their children. This early study was helpful in identifying how the experience of infertility is not a transient event in the lives of the individuals and couples who experience it, but one that can have ongoing consequences impacting long-term family and individual functioning.

In a recent study,[19] researchers developed the Parenting after Infertility Survey (PAI), a sixty-four-item questionnaire consisting of eight theoretically and empirically derived subscales that measure postinfertility parental adjustment. It is not a unitary scale but multifactorial and, as such, is not intended to measure a distinct construct. The eight subscales are: being a perfect parent; disclosure of children's origins; emotional aspects of infertility; expectations for children; expectations for self; effects on family relationships; effects of infertility treatment; and overprotection of children. Although the majority of respondents (67%) indicated that parenthood erased most of the unhappiness experienced during infertility, 16% disagreed with

this statement. In addition, 39% stated that infertility had left a permanent scar on their life; 34% felt they were overprotective in their parenting due to their experience with infertility; and 16% stated that some family members disapproved of the way in which they had achieved parenthood. The four subscales with the highest internal consistency were: being a perfect parent; disclosure of children's origins; emotional aspects of infertility; and overprotection of children.

ARTs Treatment and Adjustment to Parenthood

Recent research has focused considerable attention on parenthood achieved via IVF with attention to family functioning, marital satisfaction, and parent–child relationships. Greenfeld and colleagues[20] found, in a survey study of parents who had conceived following IVF, that half of the mothers felt the IVF process had created special feelings of attachment to their child, causing some difficulty in initial parent–child separation. Mushin and colleagues,[21] in a study of post-IVF children, found no cases of child neglect, abuse, or severe disturbance in the child, although three of fifty-two couples felt that IVF had altered their perceptions of their child. Another study[22] compared IVF parents to procreation parents and found no differences between the two groups in emotional health of parents and children or marital adjustment. However, the IVF parents gave higher positive ratings for feelings about their babies and their personal freedom, while more also reported feeling overprotective toward them.

In a longitudinal study in Australia of mothers and their infants conceived by IVF, McMahon and colleagues[23] investigated psychosocial adjustment, child behavior, and the quality of the mother–child attachment during pregnancy and postpartum. They found no significant differences between the IVF mothers and procreation mothers on satisfaction with motherhood or marriage. However, during pregnancy, the IVF mothers expected their babies to be more difficult; talked less to their babies in utero; and delayed preparation for the baby. At four months postpartum, IVF mothers reported lower self-esteem and diminished self-confidence in their ability to care for their infants. In the second part of this study, the researchers[24] assessed mothers and infants at twelve months and found that IVF mothers of first-born singleton babies and procreation mothers reported comparable levels of parenting stress, anxiety, and depression, as well as similar attachment to their child. However, even though IVF mothers reported more difficult behavior and reactivity in their children, no observable behavioral differences were found between IVF infants and procreation infants. When the first child was five years old, researchers found that IVF mothers reported a more external locus of control than did procreation mothers, but there were no notable differences on other measures. Within the IVF group, higher levels of treatment predicted lower parenting stress. While this long-term study has confirmed a growing body of research indicating overall positive adjustment in IVF parents, it noted that individual differences among IVF mothers should be considered particularly in terms of treatment experience (e.g., repeated IVF cycles or complicated pregnancy).[25]

For previously infertile parents, the transition and adjustment to parenthood are often more challenging and complex than for noninfertile parents. In two studies of young children (age range: fifteen months to eight years), researchers compared parents via ARTs to procreation parents. Golombok and colleagues[26] compared children conceived via IVF and children conceived via donor insemination to two control groups: procreation children and adopted children. Researchers found that on the issues of warmth, emotional involvement with the child, and parent–child interaction, the quality of parenting was superior in the IVF and DI parents in the first cohort of children conceived by IVF to reach adolescence. In a subsequent study that assessed IVF families, adoptive families, and procreation families, the few differences in parent–child relationships that were identified appeared to be associated with the experience of infertility rather than with IVF per se. The IVF children were found to be functioning well and did not differ from the adoptive or procreation children on any of the assessments of social or emotional adjustment.[27]

Similar findings were reported in a comparison study of IVF parents compared to procreation couples. Interestingly, the procreation parents experienced decreased marital satisfaction in the first year postpartum, whereas the IVF couples did not. Additionally, the children in the IVF group were assessed by their parents as being more regular/habitual, sensitive, and manageable.[28] In a multicenter study in which IVF/ICSI and IVF-conceived children were compared to procreation children from five European countries: Belgium, Denmark, Greece, Sweden, and the United Kingdom, very few differences were found between the IVF/ICSI, IVF, and procreation families. The only significant differences were that mothers in the IVF/ICSI-conceived families reported fewer hostile or aggressive feelings toward the child and higher levels of commitment to parenting than the procreation mothers.[29] In a similar study in Taiwan, IVF mother–child pairs and procreation mother–child pairs were compared in terms of quality of parenting; family functioning; and emo-

tional and behavioral adjustment of children aged three to seven years. Teachers rated IVF mothers as displaying greater warmth but not overprotective or intrusive in their parenting behaviors toward their children and IVF children as having fewer behavioral problems than procreation children. In contrast, IVF mothers reported less satisfaction with family functioning. A significant mediating factor was family composition: IVF mothers with only one child experienced less parenting stress than did procreation mothers with only one child.[30]

Parenting after Third-Party Reproduction

Recently, research has focused on issues of third-party reproduction (donor gametes, gestational carrier, and surrogacy) and the impact of this form of family-building on family functioning and/or parent–child relationships. Although major issues of postinfertility parenthood achieved through third-party reproduction involve disclosure versus secrecy: to tell or not to tell the child about the circumstances of his or her conception and/or birth and the well-being of the child (those issues are addressed in Chapter 27). However, several studies have compared different forms of family-building to asssess any impact on the family and/or marital relationships.

In 1997, a study compared family functioning and the social and emotional development of children in families created via ARTs in Western Europe with families created via ARTs in an Eastern European country (Bulgaria), where there was a history of specific pronatalist interventions. Researchers found greater difficulties in parental adjustment and child behavior in ARTs families in Eastern Europe. The researchers concluded that although the outcomes of ARTs for family functioning and child development appear to be independent, to some extent at least, the social context in which these treatments are carried out may influence long-term family adjustment.[31]

In a European study (conducted in the United Kingdom, Italy, Spain, and The Netherlands), family relationships and the social and emotional development of children in families created as a result of the two most widely used ARTs (i.e., IVF and DI) were compared to procreation and adoptive families. Mothers of children conceived by ARTs expressed greater warmth; were more emotionally involved; and interacted more with their child. Additionally, they reported less stress associated with parenting than mothers of procreation children. Similarly, ARTs fathers interacted more with their child and contributed more to parenting than fathers with a procreation child.[32] Findings from the second phase of this longitudinal study found that the

ARTs families were similar to adoptive and procreation families in terms of the quality of parent–child relationships. There was more positive functioning among the ARTs families, with the possible exception of over-involvement with their children in a small proportion of ARTs mothers and fathers. Overall, ARTs children were functioning well and did not differ from the adoptive or procreation children on any of the measures of psychological adjustment, leading the researchers to conclude that IVF and DI families with an early adolescent child were well-functioning.[33]

Golombok and associates[34] also compared parents who had conceived via DI and oocyte donation (OD) with parents who had procreation children on dimensions of psychological well-being of the parents; the quality of parent–child relationships; and infant temperament. Differences identified indicated more positive parent–child relationships among the OD than the procreation parents as well as greater emotional involvement with the child. It was concluded that parents with OD or DI conceived infants did not appear to be at risk for parenting difficulties. In addition, Golomok and associates compared families created through surrogacy arrangements with OD and procreation families on psychological well-being of the parents; the quality of parent–child relationships; and infant temperament. Differences identified between the surrogacy families and the other family types indicated greater psychological well-being and adaptation to parenthood by mothers and fathers of children born through surrogacy arrangements than by the procreation parents.[35] Similarly, families created via OD, DI, adoption, and IVF were assessed in terms of parents' emotional well-being; the quality of parenting; and children's socioemotional development in families with a child who is genetically unrelated to the mother or the father. Differences were found to exist between families according to the presence or absence of genetic ties between parents and their children in that there was greater psychological well-being among mothers and fathers in families where there was no genetic link between the mother and the child. Families did not differ with respect to the quality of parenting or the psychological adjustment of the child.[36] More positive parent–child relationships and greater emotional involvement with the child were found among gamete donation parents than procreation parents. Infants conceived by OD or DI were found to be at no greater risk for parenting difficulties.[36]

In summary, based on longitudinal, multicentered studies comparing adjustment to parenthood achieved through various avenues (e.g., ARTs, adoption, or surrogacy) it would appear that, in general, the vast majority of the marriages, children, family systems, and parent–child relationships are stable and well-functioning. Although some variation can be expected, particularly when the individual's unique circumstances are taken into consideration (e.g., culture or pregnancy circumstances), overall it is reassuring to know that families created through ARTs are happy, resilient, and well-adjusted. Of course, these studies have focused on families in developed or developing countries (e.g., Europe, Eastern Europe, North America, and Australia). As such, it cannot be assumed that the levels of adjustments or issues of stigma; societal acceptance; family identity; and/or the legacy of infertility or ARTs will have the same universally positive adjustment. It is an area that warrants greater research attention, particularly in light of the lack of universal access to treatment (stratification of treatment); reproductive tourism; and the lack of consistency of care (medically and psychologically) across treatment centers worldwide. However, it is a helpful starting point to know that, to date, within the geographic areas defined, research has indicated that postinfertility parents felt they appreciated their children more and did not consider the means by which they had achieved parenthood a significantly negative factor in parent–child relationships or long-term family adjustment.[37]

THEORETICAL FRAMEWORKS

The Tasks of Parenthood

Parenthood is recognized as a major developmental milestone in the lives of men and women, often marking a symbolic entry into adulthood. Parenthood implies a certain stability, maturity, and willingness to assume adult roles and responsibilities. Physical, interpersonal, and relational adaptations are required to successfully adjust to pregnancy, delivery, and parenthood. While some well-adjusted previously infertile couples anticipate and adapt to the demands of parenthood quite well, others arrive at parenthood with unrealistic expectations, utopian fantasies, or idealized perceptions of their child or themselves as parents. In short, adjustment to parenthood after infertility involves all of the regular tasks of parenthood, in addition to the unique tasks of postinfertility parenthood.

Fundamentally, parenthood involves the physical and psychological care of a child ensuring his or her well-being, growth, and development from infancy to adulthood. It involves setting behavioral standards for the child and providing for the child a culture of the values of family and society. The six stages of parenthood according to Galinsky[38] are:

- image-making stage
- nurturing stage
- authority stage
- interpretive stage
- interdependent stage
- departure stage

The *image-making stage*, beginning in pregnancy or preadoption, involves fantasizing about the child who is to arrive and envisioning oneself as a parent. The *nurturing stage*, lasting from birth until the child learns to say 'no,' involves cementing attachment to the child and reconciling the real infant with the imagined infant. During the *authority stage*, as the child enlarges his or her environment, primary parental responsibilities are to keep the child out of danger while allowing the child sufficient freedom and independence to safely explore the world. An important issue for parents is how to enforce limits and manage conflict with the child; avoid battles of wills; and adapt to changes in the child. During the *interpretive stage* (latency age), parental tasks involve explaining the culture and physical world to the child so that he or she absorbs parental values. An additional parental task is keeping up with the child's physical, emotional, and intellectual growth. The *interdependent stage* begins just before puberty and, for parents, involves reconciling two images: their self-image as parents of a maturing child and their image of their child versus the child's self-image. During this stage, discipline and communication must adapt to the child's increased autonomy and maturity. The *departure stage* is marked by the child's leaving home and taking personal responsibility for his or her life, during which parental tasks are letting go and accepting the child's separation and individuation. During this stage, parents often have the mistaken belief that "this is it; we're done," not realizing that departure is often a coming and going process that can evolve over several years and involve repeated relaunching of adult children.

Some issues of parenthood are often more challenging for previously infertile parents, especially those regarding their child's autonomy, separation, and individuation; parental acceptance of the child's identity, independence, and maturity; and parental authority, discipline, and enforcement of age-appropriate limits. Each stage of the child's development represents specific challenges for previously infertile parents, highlighting how infertility presents difficulties to parents long after the reproductive crisis has passed.

Tasks of Parenthood for Previously Infertile Parents

The process of the transition to parenthood for previously infertile parents involves, according to Sandelowski and colleagues,[39] four different tasks:

- *facing infertility*: the process of revealing, concealing, and accommodating the consequences and meaning of infertility;
- *mazing*: the recursive, iterative, and capital-intensive process of the pursuit of parenthood;
- *relinquishing infertility*: involves a couple's efforts to divest themselves of the infertility identity, thoughts, feelings, and behavior patterns;
- *reconstructing infertility*: the process in which a couple seeks to understand and gain interpretive control of their infertility experience.

All of these tasks are fundamental to adaptation not only to the infertility experience but also to parenthood as the couple incorporates infertility into their couple and family history and relinquishes it in preparation for parenthood.

Glazer[40] presents another theoretical model on the tasks and transition to parenthood for previously infertile parents. She defined the tasks as:

- giving up of the fantasized child;
- developing a realistic approach to bonding;
- accepting ambivalence;
- redefining and realigning the family.

Accordingly, previously infertile parents must surrender the child they had anticipated or felt that they deserved in preparation for acceptance of the child they will actually parent. A form of *relinquishing infertility*, giving up the fantasy child involves grieving the child whom the infertile couple dreamed of having, often an idealized child who is perfect in every way. *Developing a realistic approach to bonding* involves recognizing that bonding is not a love at first sight event but an attachment process that takes on average eighteen months.

While all new parents experience some ambivalence, previously infertile parents are often frightened or distressed by their doubts about parenthood; themselves as parents; or their child. During infertility, many women and men make a private bargain to be perfect parents if they are just given the opportunity to become parents, only to discover, once they actually *are* parents, that they have made an impossible bargain. Glazer[40] suggested that this bargain is an example of magical thinking in that parents must relinquish the ideal in order to experience the real feelings of parenthood – ambivalence, disappointment, discouragement, and confusion – along with its joys.

Finally, *redefining and realigning* the family, similar to Sandelowski and colleagues reconstructing infertility, involves postinfertility parents recognizing how their family and children may be different than traditional definitions of family. The postinfertility family may be the result of ARTs and/or third-party reproduction (e.g., OD, DI, surrogacy, gestational carrier, or adoption). These family-building alternatives challenge traditional definitions of kinship and relatedness – defined by Gordon[41] as the new blended family. In the new blended family, each child may enter the family via a unique reproductive beginning or adoptive process that differs from other siblings' origins and even the parents' reproductive beginning. Still, despite the fact that these families have complex biogenetic origins, their social and experiential relationships are more like those of traditional nuclear families than of stepfamilies.

CLINICAL ISSUES

After years of anticipating parenthood, postinfertility parents may have unrealistic, even idealized expectations of themselves as parents and/or their children. Previously infertile parents may simply look to parenthood as a pancea, termed by Burns[18] the 'baby as the eraser' syndrome in which the arrival of the longed-for child will remove all previous emotional distress, particularly infertility-specific distress. Failing to address any residual feelings or intrapsychic conflicts regarding infertility, postinfertility parents may view their children as a cure or balm for the psychological wounds caused by infertility. Or even more compelling, they may expect their children to provide (albeit emotional) compensation (or payback) for the trials and tribulations of infertility. Expecting an ideal child with special talents or abilities who will realize the parents' unmet needs or unfilled dreams is a formula for more disappointment and emotional distress, putting undue pressure on the child and the family system. Furthermore, parents may pressure themselves to be perfect parents (versus good enough parents), often to the exclusion of other roles (e.g., spouse/partner, friend, or son/daughter). Issues of separation and individuation, parental overprotection, and enmeshed or child-centered family systems are potential problems, particularly as these parents (and even their caregivers) often refer to these children created through ARTs as special, precious, priceless, and miracle babies.[42,43]

Special Parenting Issues after Infertility

Parenting after infertility presents some special clinical issues for older parents, the only child after secondary infertility, postinfertility parents of multiples, and parenthood achieved via third-party reproduction. Furthermore, questions regarding disclosure to a child born through donor gametes, surrogacy, or gestational carrier are a major concern to parents as are parenting adopted children.

Older Parenthood

Older parenthood has received increasing attention, particularly in the developed world, in which ARTs can and does facilitate pregnancy for men and women with age-related diminished fertility. Older parenthood has medically and traditionally been defined as first-time motherhood after age thirty-five, although ARTs has pushed this parameter to motherhood after age fifty-five or fatherhood after age seventy-five. These older parents are often more likely to receive public attention due to media coverage, an unfortunate circumstance as it gives the general public the impression that older parenthood is: (1) the norm; (2) easily attainable; (3) occurs naturally without ARTs; and (4) has no negative consequences for the parents and/or child(ren). Motivations for older parenthood may be lack of opportunity earlier in life; repeat parenthood in a subsequent marriage; replacement of a child lost to death; assuagement of a new (childless) partner; or an attempt to maintain youth and postpone aging. Older parenthood is often experienced within the context of numerous life responsibilities and demands concurrent with other midlife events such as aging parents; high work demands; peers' adjusting to empty nests; age-related health issues in one or both parents; and other major life crises.[44]

A major issue for older parents and their children is the parents' health and life expectancy. An elderly parent may not survive to see or participate in the important milestones of his or her child's life, requiring the younger spouse to assume primary parenting responsibilities if the older spouse becomes ill or aged, or dies. A younger surviving spouse may face the emotional, financial, and physical challenges of single parenthood that are enhanced by the financial drain of earlier medical treatments for infertility; children from previous marriages or relationships; or the care of the older or infirm spouse and/or parents. Retirement may not be possible, employment must continue, and/or the family's standard of living may decline due to a lost income or increase due to inheritance or death benefits.

The impact of older or elderly parenthood on children has rarely been investigated, especially when related to infertility. Furthermore, issues of age and impact on children are often met with resistance and even hostility by potential older parents. One study[45] found that older parents exhibited increased anxiety about all decisions relating to their children and had a tendency to overemphasize all aspects of the parent–child relationship. In an interview study[46] of adult last-chance children raised by older parents, adult children spoke about the pros (parents with greater patience and more life experiences) and cons (parents unable to participate in physical activities) of having older parents. In summary, older parenthood after infertility entails a number of significant issues and challenges that are often minimized or ignored by the potential parents.[47]

Parenting the Only Child after Secondary Infertility

Secondary infertility may come as a surprise to parents or may be expected after persistent infertility treatment. However, couples experiencing secondary infertility are not expecting to be parents of only children and often have difficulty relinquishing the family of their dreams. This is particularly true in cultures in which single-child families or an only child of the wrong sex is unacceptable or stigmatizing. Although a child at home may ameliorate some of the pain of infertility, he or she may also exacerbate it by reminding parents of the joys and possibilities of parenthood. Additionally, having a single child may be a significant motivation for another child – providing a sibling for an only. The challenges of parenting an only child while undergoing infertility treatment involve distinguishing the parents' wish for another child from the child's wish for a sibling; addressing the child's feelings (pro and con) about being an only child; coping with the grief of not having another child or the ideal family size; managing societal pressure for a larger family; educating oneself about the advantages of an only-child family; guarding against overindulgence or overinvestment in the only child; closing the family boundaries and moving on; and managing the feelings of vulnerability regarding an only child.[44]

One of the challenges of secondary infertility for parents is protecting their child from internalized parental longing and grief for the wished-for baby. Parental conversations about another child, medical treatments, doctor visits, medications, and infertility treatments may be misinterpreted by the child. If younger than two years, he or she may not be aware of or affected by infertility treatments. However, older children may be acutely aware of what is happening in the family and feel distressed by it.[48] Young children may interpret their mother's constant medical care as evidence that mother is very ill and respond with fears of losing the mother (e.g., her death) or being abandoned (e.g., adopted child's fear of being removed in favor of the preferred biological child).[48] Children may experience parental distraction and emotional distance as dissatisfaction with them. Furthermore, they may believe that something is wrong with them or feel responsible for the parents' inattentiveness. Children feeling "Am I not enough?" or "What's wrong with me?" may respond with overcompliance, hypervigilance of the parent, or rebellious uncooperativeness and acting-out in a bid for attention and affirmation.[49]

Historically, having an only child has been considered a negative family constellation producing self-centered and socially impaired children. However, current research does not support this belief. Only children have been found to have more social skills than children with siblings, especially later-born children, and to be psychologically very stable.[50] Research on only children as adults has consistently found few significant differences in behavioral outcomes between them and children raised with siblings. In addition, only children are more likely to be more educated than non-only children.[50]

Parenting Multiples

Twins, triplets, and other multiples have become increasingly common after infertility treatment and are usually considered a blessing, albeit mixed, by many previously infertile parents. After a lengthy period of childlessness, many infertility patients prefer a multiple birth as their treatment outcome and may even actively pursue or encourage this outcome unaware of the challenges (even dangers) that multiples pose to the pregnant mother and/or the children.[51] Some of the significant challenges include management of limited resources (time, money, energy, and attention) and the well-being of all family members, especially other siblings who are not included in the aura of specialness. As such, the complexity and challenges of parenthood broaden with multiple births with the potential for precipitating psychological distress (particularly in mothers). In a matched comparison study of parents of preschool twins conceived spontaneously, with infertility treatment, or via IVF, Monro and colleagues[52] found that the IVF parents, especially the mothers, reported more difficulty in social relationships following multiple pregnancy and parenthood. However, a similar study found no difference in families with twins naturally conceived and families with twins conceived following infertility treatment.[53] In a study evaluating psychological well-being in mothers of multiples following IVF, Garel and Blondel[54] reported that, at one year, the majority of mothers experienced considerable fatigue, stress, social isolation, and strained marital relationship. In addition, they felt their relationship with their children was often disturbed and that it was difficult to give adequate attention to each child. Other researchers found that each increase in multiplicity was associated with increased risks of maternal depression.[55] Researchers have found that women who conceived multiples after infertility treatment were more delighted when informed of a multiple pregnancy than those who conceived spontaneously.[56,57] Factors associated with poorer maternal adjustment were triplets or more; physical health problems in the children; higher rates of maternal depression; and overall poorer parent–infant synchrony and infant–mother adjustment. Additionally, the exclusivity of the parent–infant relationship was compromised.[58]

By contrast, previously infertile parents often find caring for an instant family an enjoyable immersion experience in which both parents are actively and energetically involved.[59] They enjoy the special attention that their family and children receive, as well as the additional involvement of their own parents, family members, and friends despite the challenges if posed by prematurity; special needs and disabilities in the children; financial burdens (e.g., loss of the mother's income); the mother's loss of her social network at the workplace; public invasions of the family's privacy; breast-feeding and childcare challenges; unanticipated family configuration; separate individuals versus packaging multiples as a group; absence of a one-to-one relationship with each child; adequate childcare help; and household arrangements to accommodate multiples.[44] Despite the challenges of health problems in the children; unmet family needs; maternal and/or paternal depression; and parental stress, one study found increased marital solidification as parents coped with the inordinate stresses of multiple births.[60]

Unique issues for parenting multiples include establishing each child's unique individuality, managing the issues of separation and independence not only from the parents but also from each child; twin talk; and the special twin (or multiple) bond.[61] Despite these distinctive factors, research indicates that multiples are at no increased risk of more difficulty with issues of individuality, separation, and independence than singletons, even when the multiples have been conceived following infertility treatment.[61,62]

Parenthood after Third-Party Reproduction

Parenthood after third-party reproduction – donated gametes, embryos, gestational carrier, or surrogacy – is unique, as it separates biological (genetic) parenthood from psychosocial (rearing) parenthood. A baby may be genetically related to both psychosocial parents yet carried by another woman (gestational carrier) or genetically related to the psychosocial father and carrying mother but not the psychosocial mother (traditional surrogacy). Or a child may not be genetically related to either psychosocial parent yet be carried by the psychosocial mother (donated embryo). A child may be genetically related to the father but not to either the psychosocial or the carrying mother (donated oocyte) or genetically related to the carrying mother but not to the psychosocial father (donor sperm). The inequity of the biological or genetic contribution of each psychosocial parent can contribute to marital conflict; differing feelings of ownership or investment in the child; and divergent opinions on disclosure, affecting family dynamics and kinship definitions. All of these variations of biological and psychosocial parenthood make third-party reproduction more psychologically complex and can create confusion regarding definition of family boundaries and dilemmas for how families adapt and manage the dynamics and definition of these complex family systems over time. Infertile couples often choose donated gametes (sperm or oocyte) as a family-building option because, in comparison to adoption, it is expeditious; typically more economical; less socially obvious; allows control of the prenatal environment; and offers genetic or biological connection to one partner. Parenthood achieved by donated gametes (sometimes referred to as prenatal adoption or complex adoption) is psychologically similar to traditional adoption in that couples must relinquish the genetically shared child they had hoped for and expected. Infertile couples often choose parenthood via third-party reproduction to avoid some of the perceived negatives of adoption, such as involvement or relationship with the relinquishing parents. However, increasingly, intended parents using third-party reproduction do so through an open, identified, and collaborative process. [63,64]

Furthermore, in many parts of Europe and North America, Australia, and New Zealand, donor anonymity has been eliminated and donor registries have been established either voluntarily or through legislation. Consequently, an important task for these parents involves defining appropriate boundaries and relationship parameters for ongoing interactions between them, their child, and the gamete donor and/or surrogate/gestational carrier.[44,64] One of the most significant challenges of parenthood via surrogacy or gestational carrier is how it affects the legal definition of motherhood. While it is banned in several countries, where it is practiced, genetic or intended mothers are often legally required to adopt the child born to a gestational carrier or surrogate. Gestational carriers and surrogates may be a previously unknown woman hired to carry a pregnancy or may be a compassionate friend or family member volunteering to be a surrogate or gestator. Dual relationship in third-party reproduction, including family members who donate gametes, may increase the psychological perplexities within the family and contribute to potential problems for parents, child, and the nuclear and/or extended family later in life. A pregnancy carried by someone else can delay maternal bonding; contribute to lingering feelings of loss; and enhance feelings of insecurity, anxiety, and loss of control. [63,65]

Fundamentally, the more complex the method of achieving pregnancy and the more participants involved in the conception/birth, the more complex the psychological implications and emotional reverberations are for all participants: childrearing parents, reproductive helper and children.[64,66] Families must decide how they will integrate these relationships into their life, often within a social context of stigma, secrecy, ambiguity, and laws and/or practice guidelines in which donor anonymity has been eliminated and donor registries established. Thus, third-party parents must come to terms with feelings of isolation and difference and with the lack of societal, familial, or social support.[65] They must also address the potential and actual psychological impact on their child of his or her unique biological beginning and, as such, infertility counselors can be an important ongoing resource as the family matures and develops.

Finally, a major parenting issue for third-party reproduction parents is the issue of whether or not to tell their child about the unique circumstances of his or her conception and birth. Various factors influence this decision including the family's unique situation, culture, religion, values, country of residency, and infertility history as well as the family's structure: nuclear two-parent family, solo mother, gay or lesbian couple, or step-parent family. For some couples, circumstances determine the decision such as the existence of older siblings from whom a surrogacy pregnancy cannot be hidden or solo parents and/or homosexual couples who have little motivation to hide circumstances of their child's conception. In contrast, nondisclosure (privacy or even secrecy) about the circumstances of the child's conception/birth may be the only acceptable alternative – even when anonymity has been legally mandated or the reproductive helper (i.e., gamete donor/gestational carrier) is a family member. Personal preference or cultural norms may be motivations for privacy or parents may wish to minimize

stigmatization of the child and/or family. Parents must be prepared for their child learning about their beginnings in an unplanned and/or hurtful manner that is more damaging than an open discussion in which the information comes from loving parents.[67] Whether or not parents decide to tell or not tell, research indicates that all parents base their decisions on the same principle: what they believe to be in the best interests of *their* child and *their* family.

For many parents, the issue is not about *whether* to tell, but more about *how* and *when* to tell (see Chapter 27). As such, infertility counselors can provide a neutral environment for facilitating decision making and examination of thoughts and feelings, as well as providing support, educational materials, and resources.[67–70] Parents should be reminded that disclosure decisions at the time of treatment need not be final, permanent decisions. Instead they should be prepared for a lifetime of conversations about parenting their child whose unique reproductive history involves its own sets of parenting challenges. Disclosure is not an event but a process. As such, parents should consider these discussions an opportunity to educate their child and facilitate the integration of this information into the child's (and family's) identity. Infertility counselors serve as an ongoing resource in this process and are frequently asked by parents for assistance, sometimes years or decades after the initial consult and/or parenthood has been achieved.

Solo, Gay, and Lesbian Parenthood

While solo parenting was, in the past, a phenomenon of life circumstances (i.e., divorce, widowhood, and unplanned pregnancy), solo, gay, and lesbian parenthood via ARTs became increasingly popular by the end of the twentieth century. Although the use of assisted reproduction by single and homosexual men and women is not universally available worldwide, since the 1980s it has been a popular means of achieving parenthood for many Europeans, North Americans, and Australians.

Research comparing the quality of parent–child relationship and socioemotional and gender development of seven-year-old children in lesbian, heterosexual families, and solo-mother families found positive mother–child relationships and well-adjusted children in all the families.[71] A literature search of studies that had assessed the psychological well-being of children and the quality of parenting after infertility treatment found that in lesbian families, the psychosocial development of children (median age 6.1 years) and the quality of parenting were not different from those in heterosexual two-parent families after infertility treatment or natural conception.[72]

Although solo mothers via DI have not been found to be at greater risk for psychiatric or social problems, the lack of a co-parent may be a risk factor for social stigma, social isolation, and financial challenges.[73] As such, the infertility counselor may be helpful in identifying social support networks and potentially unhealthy parent–child relationships such as enmeshment and/or maternal expectation that the child will meet the parent's emotional (and social) needs (and not vice versa).

Overall, there is considerable evidence that children raised in lesbian couple families are stable and well-functioning despite the risk of social stigma due to having two moms. However, these parents are more likely to be financially and socially stable. Infertility counselors may be helpful in addressing issues of stigma, social development, and healthy family functioning. Additionally, effective pretreatment counseling is optimum in addressing any issues that may impact parenting (e.g., relationship problems; legal issues for same-sex partners; unrealistic expectations; and ongoing mental health problems).

THERAPEUTIC INTERVENTIONS

The transition to parenthood, loosely defined as the period from pregnancy through the first year of the life of a first-born, is always a period of change and stress as the parents, marriage, and new infant adjust to one another. This transition for previously infertile parents may involve a number of risk factors and challenges during both pregnancy and parenthood. Previously infertile parents may arrive at parenthood with exhausted coping abilities; diminished marital satisfaction; and depression or psychological distress.[74] The elongated anticipation of parenthood may have contributed to overidealization of the child or parenthood, resulting in unrealistic expectations of one's self or spouse as a parent, or misperceptions of normal infant behavior.[74–77] By contrast, previously infertile parents may be buffeted from normal decreases in marital satisfaction following parenthood because they are typically older, better educated, married longer, and less likely to define their marriage solely in romantic terms.[21,74,76,77] Furthermore, the experience of infertility may have enabled the couple to acquire more egalitarian relationship patterns; effective problem-solving skills; and healthier communication allowing them to discuss sensitive topics and feelings.[74,78] Previously infertile new mothers, although lacking self-confidence, may be more comfortable turning to their husbands for support and encouragement and establishing a team approach to parenthood that fosters skills attainment in both partners.[17,22,75,79]

The infertility counselor can be particularly helpful in addressing parenting issues in families with a history of infertility by normalizing parenthood; faciltating adaptation to parenthood; assessing mental health and family functioning; and collaborating with other professionals.

Normalizing Parenthood for Previously Infertile Parents

For the infertility counselor, the most important intervention in facilitating the adjustment to parenthood for previously infertile men and women is *normalizing* parenthood and the parenting experience. Moving from the identity of an infertile person to that of competent parent can be challenging, but one that can be normalized by highlighting how family life stages and the psychological tasks of parenthood occur in a maturational process that is the same regardless of how a parent has achieved the parental role. Infertility counselors can ease the transition by providing educational materials, resources, and referrals to support groups that emphasize the acquisition of parenting skills (for both men and women) and deemphasize how they are different parents.

Another way in which previously infertile parents feel different can be the way in which they have achieved parenthood (e.g., third-party reproduction or adoption). For previously infertile parents, integrating the manner in which they achieved parenthood into their personal and family identity is a process – one that is more challenging for some individuals than for others. Nevertheless, it is an important task for parents as their ability to successfully integrate this information will set the tone for their family and for their children. However, this is not to minimize the challenges of being different or how psychologically painful stigma can be.

Previously infertile parents should be encouraged to continue to view themselves as a couple even though they may prefer, even delight in being able to view themselves as a real family and as parents. Early on, they should be encouraged to strike a balance between their marital relationship and their roles as parents such as investing in their partner and partnership as much as they emotionally invest in their child(ren). Whether enchanted or overwhelmed with their roles as parents, previously infertile parents should be encouraged to maintain a healthy sexual relationship; social life; good communication; and shared activities that they, as a couple, have always found enjoyable.

Part of normalizing the parenting experience is acknowledging it is and can be stressful. Regardless of how gratifying it is to have finally achieved parenthood, parenting stress can and does occur on a regular basis and is no reflection of the parents' competency or skill. However, many previously infertile parents feel they do not deserve to complain; ask for assistance; or feel entitled to support and comfort. Expecting themselves to be ideal parents, they may feel ill-equipped to handle or even acknowledge parenting stresses. However, identifying the healthy coping mechanisms they used during infertility and highlighting their resiliency in managing the crisis of infertility can help them recognize their capacity for managing this new role as well. Infertility counselors can help parents set a healthy balance between appropriate parental concerns and hypervigilant, controlling parenting. Having spent years in the medical world of infertility, previously infertile parents may pathologize normal behavior and minor childhood illnesses (e.g., low-grade fever following vaccinations). This anxious coping is not only detrimental to the parents but also potentially detrimental to the child and the parent–child relationship.

Facilitating Adaptation to Parenthood after Infertility

Adapting Galinsky's[38] stages of parenthood, infertility counselors can assist previously infertile couples in their transition to parenthood. During the *image-making stage* of parenthood, previously infertile parents must relinquish their fantasy child and their infertile identity, thoughts, feelings, and behavior patterns. Lack of social support during pregnancy and/or parenthood; stigma (especially if parenthood was achieved through third-party reproduction) and altered self-concept involving feelings of incompetence or inadequacy are frequent and familiar feelings for previously infertile parents. In addition, relinquishing infertility may include letting go of important relationships – medical staff at the infertility clinic; friends from infertility support organizations; or enjoyable activities such as get-togethers with childless friends. Bernstein[76] suggested that disturbances of parenting after infertility may be related not only to psychosocial distress during infertility treatment (see Table 26.1) but also to the lack of appropriate role models for parenting after infertility; delayed attachment to the baby, especially during pregnancy; and cognitive dissonance, a disparity between what was imagined about parenthood/the baby and the actual experience.

During the *nurturing stage*, previously infertile parents must establish a comfortable means of bonding

---

TABLE 26.1. Potential impact of infertility[76]

Transition to parenthood

Increased anxiety levels during pregnancy and/or adoption period

Lack of role models

Possibility of delayed bonding

Cognitive dissonance: gap between ideal and real self and between fantasy and real child

Ethical and emotional issues related to means of achieving parenthood

Factors affecting parenting

Decreased self-esteem and self-efficacy

Altered body image and self-concept

Impaired marital communication

Isolation from family and friends

Grieving over losses associated with infertility: anxiety, depression, and anger management issues

---

to their child, through baby massage, bedtime rituals, and special lullabies. In addition, parents need to come to terms with and understand the normalcy of their ambivalence about parenthood (e.g., fatigue or no time to oneself) and their baby (e.g., colicky and unlikeable characteristics). Previously infertile parents may become overprotective – enmeshed; excessively involved; infantilizing their child; preventing independent behavior; and stunting the child's emotional growth.[4] Often, the child does not view their parents' overprotection as an indication of their parents' insecurity and self-protection, but as a justifiable lack of confidence in the child's ability to manage in his or her life or to venture into the world.

For previously infertile parents, the *authority stage* can be particularly challenging as parents recognize the need to set limits; agree and collaborate on discipline; and define their roles as authority figures for their children. Some of the potential problems for previously infertile parents include overprotective parenting; difficulty with appropriate discipline; and unrealistic expectations of parenting or the child.[18,40,76,77] They may become hypervigilant or overindulgent, while attempts at discipline are half-hearted and inconsistent. They may manage their feelings of loss and grief about infertility by holding the child too close or by limiting the child's attempts at increased self-sufficiency and self-reliance.

Discipline problems in postinfertility families often represent two extremes: rigid, strict control of the child or the inability to set appropriate behavioral limits. Previously infertile parents may be hesitant to become angry with their child out of a mistaken belief that it is inappropriate; may feel guilty about their angry feelings at their longed-for child; may fear that negative feelings will damage their child or the parent–child relationship; or may misperceive anger as an unacceptable emotion. Some parents may recognize that their anger is disproportionate to the situation but have little insight into the factors influencing this response, such as unrealistic expectations of the child; inappropriate behavior in the child; or disappointment that the child or parenting is not more emotionally rewarding. These parents often need assistance in learning how to set appropriate limits and boundaries with their children and recognizing and managing their feelings.

During the *interpretive stage*, parents of children born as a result of third-party reproduction face issues of disclosure and interpreting the culture of reproductive technology for their child. Questions of whether the child has a moral right to know and privacy as a primary family value must be considered; agreed upon by both parents; and interpreted for the child. For previously infertile parents and their children, the interpretation of reproductive technology (even IVF) or family-building options (e.g., gamete donation and adoption) may mean realignment of the family. These families must adapt to new definitions of kinship and relatedness; normalize parent–child relationships; and acknowledge the child's unique origins and circumstances in the family. Just as important, families with a history of infertility must recognize the ways not only in which they are unique and different but also in which they are much the same as all families.

Adolescence, or the *interdependent stage* of parenthood, is often a challenging time for both parents and children. It involves the reconciling of two images: the parents' self-image and their image of the child as he or she is. During this stage, discipline and communication must adapt to the child's increased autonomy and maturity. Reemergence of common psychological responses to infertility may occur at this time including grief, anxiety, depression, feelings of isolation, and diminished self-esteem as the child challenges the parents' values, belief systems, and limits. Previously infertile parents may have difficulty allowing or acknowledging their child's increased independence and may actively or unconsciously infantilize (prevent appropriate movement toward adulthood) the young person's separation by impeding individuation, autonomy, and independence.

Frequently, parental impediments to a child's maturation involve the issues of the child's sexual development, sexual behavior, and/or reproductive ability. For previously infertile parents, their child's sexual devel-opment can be a bitter reminder of infertility and their own reproductive losses. They may respond to the child's developing sexuality by avoiding the topic – failing to prepare the child for menstruation or failing to provide sex education or birth control information – perhaps covertly fulfilling their own reproductive hopes and dreams. Additionally, after infertility, family meanings about sex and reproduction may overemphasize procreation and ignore the other meanings of sex, such as commitment, caring, sharing, or play.

Finally, the *departure stage* is marked by the young adult's leaving home either temporarily (e.g., going to college) or permanently (e.g., marriage). For many previously infertile parents who devoted extensive time and money to having child(ren), departure may entail a reexamination of these prior decisions: Was it worth it? What will their own financial stability be in retirement or old age? What are their obligations or responsibilities to the child after a certain age? Departure represents an acknowledgment of the discrepancy between what they hoped their family/child would be and who their child has actually become, for better or worse.

Unrealistic expectations place an undue burden on parents and pressure children to be perfect, grateful, successful, and emotionally rewarding – an impossible feat. Danger signs of disturbed parenting after infertility are overemphasis on excellence or exceptionality in the child or self as a parent; inability to see the child in realistic or objective terms; belief that the child is perfect and flawless; inappropriate expectations of the parent–child relationship to meet the parents' emotional needs; imposition of the parents' hopes and dreams onto the child; splitting of parents; parent-child enmeshment; parental inability to allow age-appropriate or peer-appropriate behavior; infantalizing the child; refusal to allow or train the child in age-appropriate problem-solving; extreme conflicts with the child regarding separation and individuation; inadequate or inappropriate discipline; parental rejection; neglect or abuse; and repeated boundary violations.

Perhaps more than any other topic in infertility counseling, parenting after infertility demands a family therapy approach even if only one family member (e.g., one parent or the child/young adult) is being seen. A family with a legacy of infertility and/or reproductive losses has a unique legacy and with it, its own unique history of experiences, decisions, losses, and circumstances. Each person in the family system always has his or her unique perspective, a tenet that is even more relevant in these families created under special circumstances, through often extraordinary special treatment, and with distinctive consequences and requirements. As such, the infertiltiy counselor (as well as any other professional) working with these families and family members must be prepared to address the unique legacy of infertility, addressing problems and psychosocial issues from the perspective of each family member.

Assessing for Mental Health and Family Functioning

Worldwide, the estimated incidence risk of postpartum depression in the eighteen months following the arrival of a child (whether via adoption, birth, and/or gestational pregnancy) is 10–15%.[80] Furthermore, the rate of maternal depression is twice as high in mothers with disabled children via a multiple pregnancy conceived via infertility treatment than in mothers of multiples conceived via procreation.[56] Risk factors for developing post-partum depression and/or anxiety in the general population are: (1) stressful life events, (2) poor marital relationship, (3) inadequate social support, (4) personal and family history of psychopathology, and (5) combined effects of vulnerability factors and stressful events.[81] When the risk factors for postpartum depression in the general population are combined with risk factors related to a history of infertility; infertility treatment; complex reproduction and/or adoption; and the transition to parenthood after infertility, it is clear that previously infertile parents may be especially vulnerable to developing postparenthood mental health problems. It is therefore helpful for the infertility counselor (as well as other caregivers) to educate postinfertility parents about the signs and symptoms of anxiety and depression; symptom levels that are normal and those that are problematic; and how to access support and treatment, if needed. These parents should be encouraged to seek help and not interpret the development of these problems as a personal flaw or failure either as an individual or parent. Postparenthood depression and anxiety in either parent is painful and can be a significant mental health crisis for the individual and the family, robbing the parent(s) of the joys of parenthood and their child; impairing individual functioning (e.g., work) and physical health; interfering with relationships (including marriages); and interrupting parent–child bonding. Parental depression has the potential for harming the parent, but it can and does harm the well-being of the child(ren). As such, patient education and expeditious interventions are warranted and made easier by educated patients and caregivers.

Part of the transition to parenthood is the evolution of the family system from a couple unit to a family with children. Healthy family adjustment involves maintaining a healthy couple identity while incorporating the child into the family as a unique and separate individual who belongs within the family. Helping couples identify the qualities of a healthy family system can be another important role for the infertility counselor. In addition, the infertility counselor is useful in identifying dysfunctional patterns, particularly those related to marriage and parenting including poor couple communication and team building; dysfunctional family system patterns (e.g., child-centered, enmeshed, laissez faire, overprotective, abusive, or neglectful); and/or dysfunctional parenting behaviors (e.g., abuse, neglect, and boundary violations). By helping couples identify and correct these patterns and problems early on, infertility counselors facilitate healthy adjustment to parenthood as well as long-term family health and well-being of all family members.

Collaborating with Other Caregivers

As addressed earlier, pretreatment counseling can provide education and support as well as increase informed patient decision making, particularly with regard to ARTs by facilitating discussion of risks (e.g., multiples); identifying potential mental health (e.g., depression screening); and/or relationship problems; and by encouraging patients to look beyond the goal of pregnancy to parenthood.[55] By helping patients recognize that the infertility experience can have a lasting impact even after parenthood has been achieved, infertility counselors can aid the transition to parenthood. Specifically, infertility counselors can help infertile couples make pretreatment reproductive decisions within the context of the parents they will be and the families they are creating, rather than from the simplistic standpoint of pregnancy at any price *now*.[60,82]

Finally, infertility counselors often collaborate with other professionals working with parents after infertility, acting as a bridge between infertility and parenthood, two very different worlds. Infertility counselors often educate pediatricians, pediatric mental health professionals, family physicians, and family therapists about the legacy of infertility; the implications of third-party reproduction; and normalizing for these professionals postinfertility parenting issues and behaviors. This is yet another application of the collaborative reproductive healthcare approach and the role of the infertility counselor advocated throughout this book.

FUTURE IMPLICATIONS

Today, parenthood after infertility involves a variety of meanings, challenges, and responsibilities. In the twenty-first century, how postinfertility families and children adjust to the unique legacy of infertility and assisted reproductive technologies remains to be seen. Although there appear to be indications of risk factors and vulnerabilities in postinfertility families, there is also plenty of evidence that these families adapt and adjust in a healthy and positive fashion. Infertility counselors are in an excellent position to prepare postinfertility families for the challenges of adjustment, as well as conduct research on these parents, families, and children.

Previously infertile parents may present soon after conception or birth, requesting assistance with adjustment to parenthood or at a later point in the child's or family's life – most often at points in the life cycle that involve separation, individuation, and autonomy. When problems occur, these parents are most likely to present for help to school psychologists, social workers at child mental health centers, family physicians, pediatricians, pastors, or mental health workers within the legal system. Unfortunately, these professionals are often unaware of the family's history of infertility, reproductive losses, and use of assisted reproductive technologies and therefore are often less likely to understand the child's unique legacy. Consequently, it is important to review with infertility patients, when appropriate, the unique issues of transition to parenthood and family adaptation. The role of infertility counselors may increasingly entail assisting parents, children, and families with the consequences of reproductive choices that facilitated their longed-for miracle babies but with lifelong ramifications.

SUMMARY

■ Parenthood after infertility is full of joys, challenges, and, at times, complications due to the circumstances of the conception/birth.
■ Research indicates that, despite the protracted nature of infertility treatment, infertile families are no more vulnerable to psychological disturbance than noninfertile families. Furthermore, previously infertile couples evidence stronger marital satisfaction; have more egalitarian relationships; and are more emotionally expressive than their procreative counterparts.
■ The developmental stages of parenthood, applicable to all couples, are image-making, nurturing, authority, interpretative, interdependent, and departure.
■ Previously infertile parents face unique psychological tasks in their transition to parenthood: giving up the fantasy child; realistic bonding; accepting ambivalence; and redefining the meaning of kinship and family.

■ Special issues include: parents who are older; parenting multiples; secondary infertility; solo, homosexual, and/or adoptive parenthood; and/or third-party reproduction parenthood. Any or all of these issues may isolate parents who lack a social support system; may be exhausted physically, emotionally, and financially; and experience greater social stigma and shame regarding the means through which they achieved parenthood.

REFERENCES

1. American Society of Reproductive Medicine. Ethics Committee. Child-rearing ability and the provision of fertility services. *Fertil Steril* 2004; 82:3. www.asrm.org.
2. Leduc C. Marriage in ancient Greece. In: G Duby, M Perrot, eds, *A History of Women: From Ancient Goddesses to Christian Saints*. Cambridge, MA: Harvard University Press, 1992.
3. May ET. *Barren in the Promised Land: Childless Americans and the Pursuit of Happiness*. New York: Basic Books, 1995.
4. Marsh M, Ronner W. *The Empty Cradle: Infertility in America from Colonial Times to the Present*. Baltimore: Johns Hopkins University Press, 1996.
5. Zelizer V. *Pricing the Priceless Child: The Changing Social Value of Children*. Princeton, NJ: Princeton University Press, 1994.
6. Griel AL. *Not Yet Pregnant: Infertile Couples in Contemporary America*. New Brunswick, NJ: Rutgers University Press, 1991.
7. Dally A. *Inventing Motherhood: The Consequences of an Ideal*. New York: Schocken, 1993.
8. Rothman BK. *Recreating Motherhood*. New Brunswick, NJ: Rutgers University Press, 2000.
9. Hoffman LW, Hoffman M. The value of children to parents. In: JT Fawcett, ed, *Psychological Perspectives on Population*. New York: Basic Books, 1973; 19–73.
10. van Balen F, Trimbos-Kemper TCM. Involuntary childless couples: Their desire to have children and their motives. *J Psychosom Obstet Gynaecol* 1995; 16:137–44.
11. Newton CR, Hearn MT, Yuzpe AA, et al. Motives for parenthood and response to failed in vitro fertilization: Implications for counseling. *J Assist Reprod Technol Genet* 1992; 9:24–31.
12. Levy DM. The concept of maternal overprotection. In: EJ Anthony, T Benedek, eds, *Parenthood: Its Psychology and Psychopathology*. New York: Little, Brown, 1970; 387–409.
13. Calef V. Hostility of parents to children: Some notes on infertility, child abuse, and abortion. *Int J Psychoanal Psychother* 1972; 10:76–96.
14. Bradt JO, Moynihan CJ. Opening the safe: A study of child-focused families. In: JO Bradt, CJ Moynihan, eds, *Systems Therapy: Selected Papers: Theory, Technique, Research*. Washington, DC: Groome Center, 1971.
15. Dunington R, Glazer G. Maternal identity and early mother behavior in previously infertile and never infertile women. *J Obstet Gynecol Neonatal Nurs* 1991; 20:309–17.
16. Olshansky EF. Parenting after infertility. In: *ART Parents and Children*. American Society of Reproductive Medicine, Seattle, WA, October 7–8, 1995; 59–65.

17. Abbey A, Andrews FM, Halman LJ. Infertility and parenthood: Does becoming a parent increase well-being? *J Consult Clin Psychol* 1994; 62:398–403.

18. Burns LH. An exploratory study of perceptions of parenting after infertility. *Fam Syst Med* 1990; 8:177–89.

19. Frances-Fischer JE, Lightsey OR. Parenthood after primary infertility. *J Counsel Therap Coup* 2003; 11:117–28.

20. Greenfeld DA, Ort SI, Greenfeld DG, et al. Attitudes of IVF parents about the IVF experience and their children. *J Assist Reprod Genet* 1996; 13:266–74.

21. Mushin DN, Barreda-Hanson MC, Spensley JC. In vitro fertilization children: Early psychosocial development. *J In Vitro Fertil Embryo Transf* 1986; 3:247–52.

22. Weaver SM, Clifford E, Gordon AG, et al. A follow-up study of 'successful' IVF/GIFT couples: Social-emotional well-being and adjustment to parenthood. *J Psychosom Obstet Gynaecol* 1990; 14:5–16.

23. McMahon C, Ungerer J, Tennant C, et al. Psychosocial adjustment and the quality of the mother–child relationship at four months postpartum after conception by in vitro fertilization. *Fertil Steril*. 1997; 68:492–500.

24. Gibson FL, Ungerer JA, Leslie GI, et al. *Psychosocial adjustment, child behavior and quality of attachment relationship at one year postpartum for mothers conceiving through IVF.* Presented at the American Society for Reproductive Medicine, Boston, MA, November, 1996.

25. McMahon CA, Gibson F, Leslie G, et al. Parents of 5-year-old in vitro fertilization children: Psychological adjustment, parenting stress, and the influence of subsequent in vitro fertilization treatment. *J Fam Psychol* 2003; 17:361–9.

26. Golombok S, Cook R, Bish A, et al. Families created by the new reproductive technologies: Quality of parenting and social and emotional health of the children. *Child Develop* 1995; 66:285–98.

27. Golombok S, MacCallum F, Goodman E. The "test-tube" generation: Parent–child relationships and the psychological well-being of in vitro fertilization children at adolescence. *Child Dev* 2001; 72:599–608.

28. Sydsjö G, Wadsby M, Kjellberg S, et al. Relationships and parenthood in couples after assisted reproduction and in spontaneous primiparous couples: A prospective long-term follow-up study. *Hum Reprod* 2002; 17:3242–50.

29. Barnes J, Sutcliffe AG, Kristoffersen I, et al. The influence of assisted reproduction on family functioning and children's socio-emotional development: Results from a European study. *Hum Reprod* 2004; 19:1480–7.

30. Hahn C, DiPietro JA. In vitro fertilization and the family: Quality of parenting, family functioning, and child psychosocial adjustment. *Develop Psychol* 2001; 37:37–48.

31. Cook R, Vatev I, Michova Z, et al. The European study of assisted reproduction families: A comparison of family functioning and child development between Eastern and Western Europe. *J Psychosom Obstet Gynaecol* 1997; 18:203–12.

32. Golombok S, Brewaeys A, Cook R, et al. The European study of assisted reproduction families: Family functioning and child development. *Hum Reprod* 1996; 11:2324–31.

33. Golombok S, Brewaeys A, Giavazzi MT, et al. The European study of assisted reproduction families: The transition to adolescence. *Hum Reprod* 2002; 17:830–40.

34. Golombok S, Lycett E, MacCallum F, et al. Parenting infants conceived by gamete donation. *J Fam Psychol* 2004; 18:443–52.

35. Golombok S, Murray C, Jadva V, et al. Families created through surrogacy arrangements: Parent–child relationships in the 1st year of life. *Develop Psychol* 2004; 40:400–11.

36. Golombok S, Murray C, Brinsden P, Abdalla H. Social versus biological parenting: Family functioning and the socioemotional development of children conceived by egg or sperm donation. *J Child Psychol Psychiatry* 1999; 40:519–27.

37. Adamson D, Baker V. Multiple births from assisted reproductive technologies: A challenge that must be met. *Fertil Steril* 2004; 81:517–22.

38. Galinsky E. *Between Generations: The Six Stages of Parenthood.* New York: Times Books, 1981.

39. Sandelowski M, Harris BG, Black BP. Pregnant moments: The process of conception in infertile couples. *Qualitat Health Res* 1992; 2:273–82.

40. Glazer E. Parenting after infertility. In: M Seibel, AA Kiessling, J Bernstein, SR Levin, eds, *Technology and Infertility: Clinical, Psychosocial, Legal, and Ethical Aspects.* New York: Springer-Verlag, 1993; 399–402.

41. Gordon ER. Blended families: Adopted, ART, and natural children. In: *ART Parents and Children.* American Society of Reproductive Medicine, Seattle, WA, October 7–8, 1995:78–83.

42. Colpin, H. Parents and children of reproductive technology: Chances and risks for their well-being. *Intern J Fam Care* 1994; 6:49–71.

43. Golombok S, MacCallum F. Practitioner review: Outcomes for parents and children following non-traditional conception: What do clinicians need to know? *J Child Psychol Psychiatry* 2003; 44:303–15.

44. Glazer ES. *The Long-Awaited Stork: A Guide to Parenting After Infertility.* New York: Lexington Books, 1990; 3.

45. Frankel SA, Wise MJ. A view of delayed parenting: Some implications for a new trend. *Psychiatry* 1982; 45:220–5.

46. Morris M. *Last Chance Children: Growing Up with Older Parents.* New York: Columbia University Press, 1988.

47. Rosenthal, MB, Kingsberg SA. The older infertile patient. In: LH Burns, SN Covington, eds, *Infertility Counseling: A Comprehensive Handbook for Clinicians.* New York: Parthenon Press, 1999; 283–97.

48. Clapp D. Secondary infertility. In: M Seibel, AA Kiessling, J Bernstein, SR Levin, eds, *Technology and Infertility: Clinical, Psychosocial, Legal, and Ethical Aspects.* New York: Springer-Verlag, 1993; 313–17.

49. Simons, HF. Secondary infertility. In: Burns LH, Covington SN, eds, *Infertility Counseling: A Comprehensive Handbook for Clinicians.* New York: Parthenon Press, 1999; 313–24.

50. Falbo T. Only children: A review. In: T Falbo, ed, *The Single-Child Family.* New York: Guilford Press, 1984; 1–24.

51. Ryan GL, Zhang SH, Dokras A, et al. The desire of infertile patients for multiple births. *Fertil Steril* 2004; 81:500–4.

52. Monro JM, Ironside W, Smith GC. Successful parents of in vitro fertilization (IVF): The social repercussions. *J Assist Reprod Genet* 1992; 9:170–6.

53. Tully LA, Moffitt TE, Caspi A. Maternal adjustment, parenting and child behaviour in families of school-aged twins conceived after IVF and ovulation induction. *J Child Psychol Psychiat* 2003; 44:316–25.

54. Garel M, Blondel B. Assessment at 1 year of the psychological consequences of having triplets. *Hum Reprod* 1992; 7:729–32.

55. Ellison MA, Hotamisligil S, Lee H, et al. Psychosocial risks associated with multiple births resulting from assisted reproduction. *Fertil Steril* 2005; 83:1422–8.

56. Yokoyama Y. Comparison of child-rearing problems between mothers with multiple children who conceived after infertility treatment and mothers with multiple children who conceived spontaneously *Twin Research* 2003; 6:89–96.

57. Cook R, Bradley S, Golombok S. A preliminary study of parental stress and child behaviour in families with twins conceived by in-vitro fertilization. *Hum Reprod* 1998; 13:3244–6.

58. Feldman R, Eidelman AI. Parent–infant synchrony and the social-emotional development of triplets. *Develop Psychol* 2004; 40:1133–47.

59. Leiblum SR, Kemmann E, Taska L. Attitudes toward multiple births and pregnancy concerns in infertile and non-infertile women. *J Psychosom Obstet Gynaecol* 1990; 11:197–210.

60. Ellison MA, Hall JE. Social stigma and compounded losses: Quality-of-life issues for multiple-birth families. *Fertil Steril* 2003; 80:405–14.

61. Bryan EM. *Twins, Triplets and More*. New York: St. Martin's Press, 1992.

62. Noble E. *Having Twins*. Boston: Houghton Mifflin, 1991.

63. Cooper SL, Glazer ES. *Beyond Infertility: The New Paths to Parenthood*. New York: Lexington Books, 1994.

64. Braverman AM. Oocyte donation: Psychological and coounseling issues. *Clin Consult Obstet Gynecol* 1994; 6:143–9.

65. Braverman AM. Surrogacy and gestational carrier: Psychological issues. *Infertil Reprod Med Clin North Am* 1993; 4:517–33.

66. Sorosky AD. Lessons from the adoption experience: Anticipating times of developmental conflict for the ART child. In: *ART Parents and Children*. American Society of Reproductive Medicine, Seattle, WA, October 7–8, 1995: 137–61.

67. Nachtigall RD, Quiroga SS, Tschann JM, et al. Stigma, disclosure, and family functioning among parents of children conceived through donor insemination, *Fertil Steril* 1997; 68:1–7.

68. McWhinnie AM. Outcome for families created by assisted conception programmes. *J Assist Reprod Genet* 1996; 13: 363–5.

69. Klock SC, Maier D. Psychological factors related to donor insemination. *Fertil Steril* 1991; 56:489–95.

70. Mahlstedt PP, Greenfeld DA. Assisted reproductive technology with donor gametes: The need for patient preparation. *Fertil Steril* 1989; 52:908–14.

71. Golombok S, Perry B, Burston A, et al. Children with lesbian parents: A community study. *Develop Psychol* 2003; 39:20–33.

72. Hunfeld JAM, Fauser BCJM, de Beaufort ID, et al. Child development and quality of parenting in lesbian families: No psychosocial indications for a-priori withholding of infertility treatment. A systematic review. *Hum Reprod* 2002; 8:579–90.

73. Jacob MS. Lesbian couples and single women. In: LH Burns, SN Covington, eds, *Infertility Counseling: A Comprehensive Handbook for Clinicians*. New York: Parthenon Press, 1999, 267–81.

74. Klock SC. The transition to parenthood among fertile couples: A review of the psychological literature. In: *ART Parents and Children*. American Society of Reproductive Medicine, Seattle, WA, October 7–8, 1995; 17–35.

75. Applegarth L, Goldberg NC, Cholst I, et al. Families created through ovum donation: A preliminary investigation of obstetrical outcome and psychosocial adjustment. *J Assist Reprod Genet* 1995; 12:574–80.

76. Bernstein J. Parenting after infertility. *J Perinat Neonatal Nurs* 1990; 4:11–23.

77. Bernstein J, Mattox JH, Kellner R. Psychological status of previously infertile couples after a successful pregnancy. *J Obstet Gynecol Neonatal Nurs* 1988; 17:404–8.

78. Benezon N, Wright J, Sabourin S. Stress, sexual satisfaction and marital adjustment in infertile couples. *J Sex Marital Ther* 1992; 18:273–84.

79. Raoul-Duval A, Bertrand-Servais M, Frydman R. Comparative prospective study of the psychological development of children born by in vitro fertilization and their mothers. *J Psychosom Obstet Gynaecol* 1993; 14:117–26.

80. Foli KJ, Thompson JR. *The Post-Adoption Blues: Overcoming the Unforeseen Challenges of Adoption*. New York: St. Martin's Press, 2005.

81. O'Hara M. *Psychological Aspects of Women's Reproductive Health*. New York: Springer Publishing, 1995.

82. Glazebrook C, Sheard C, Cox S, et al. Parenting stress in first-time mothers of twins and triplets conceived after in vitro fertilization. *Fertil Steril* 2004; 81: 505–11.

27 Assisted Reproductive Technology and the Impact on Children

DOROTHY A. GREENFELD AND SUSAN CARUSO KLOCK

Children are the living messages we send to a time we will not see.

– Neil Postman, 1982

The miraculous birth of Louise Brown, the first baby conceived through in vitro fertilization (IVF), raised the hopes of infertile couples everywhere. Since her birth in 1978, more than 100,000 babies worldwide have been conceived through IVF and other assisted reproductive technologies (ARTs).[1] Women infertile as a result of tubal problems were the first patients, but in a very short time IVF became the treatment of choice for a host of reproductive disorders in men and women alike. ART innovations such as oocyte donation, embryo cryopreservation, gestational surrogacy, and intra-cytoplasmic sperm injection (ICSI) have made parenthood possible to an entirely new cohort of patients, such as women without ovarian function, women without a uterus, and men who are quadriplegic or otherwise unable to ejaculate. These innovations have, in turn, introduced and redefined the family in a new way.

Infertility treatment centers throughout the world initially focused on the infertile couple with little regard to the possible long-term impact of treatment on the children they were helping to create. Historically, the goal of treatment was pregnancy and the focus was on the medical and psychological aspects of the treatment itself. Mental health practitioners working in the field focused on the 'roller coaster' of euphoria and dysphoria associated with infertility and its treatment, particularly on the emotional impact of treatment failure.[2–4] As the technology has advanced with increasing numbers of children resulting from these complex reproductive technologies, greater attention has been given to the overall medical and psychological well-being of the families that were created. Integral to the current information available about children born as a result of ART, is the question of what children *themselves* know and understand about the process of their conception and/or birth via ARTs.

The impact of ART on children so conceived is the focus of this chapter. The chapter includes:

■ a history of the scientific innovations that have led to complex ART family possibilities;
■ an examination of medical and psychological research on how ART families are faring, in particular the children;
■ the significance of disclosure to ART offspring about their conception and birth;
■ a discussion of therapeutic interventions to assist parents raising children conceived through ART.

HISTORICAL OVERVIEW

The birth of Louise Brown, while certainly a milestone, which meant that "reproductive medicine would never be the same,"[5] was achieved after years, indeed centuries, of scientific research. Much of the research then, as it is now, was accomplished with animals. For example, Lazzaro Spallazani in 1779 achieved the first artificial insemination using frog semen that he had collected and mixed with unfertilized frog oocytes. He repeated the process in 1782 by successfully artificially inseminating a cocker spaniel.[6] John Hunter, a Scottish physician, achieved the first human pregnancy as a result of artificial insemination in 1870. He directed a man infertile as a result of hypospadia to collect semen in a 'warm cup' and inject it into his wife's vagina using a syringe.[7] In 1891, the first mammalian embryo transfer was accomplished by Walter Heape, who demonstrated that fertilized ova could be flushed from a rabbit's fallopian tubes and transferred to a surrogate mother.[7] After mating two angora rabbits, he transferred the embryos to a Belgian hare. Thus, the Belgian hare "represents the first mammal ever to have given birth to offspring not genetically her own."[8]

Patrick Steptoe and Robert Edwards, the so-called 'fathers of IVF,' began their collaboration in 1968 in England. Edwards, a biologist, and Steptoe, a gynecologist, had each been influenced early in their careers by the emotional devastation of infertility among their patients. Early in his career, Edwards artificially inseminated mice and studied mouse embryos, which ultimately led him to work on the maturation of human embryos in vitro. Steptoe perfected the use of the laparoscope. The two began their collaboration late in their careers and achieved the first IVF pregnancy some ten years later.[9]

Animal research resulted in the successful freezing and thawing of mouse embryos in 1971.[10] The first baby born as a result of cryopreserved human embryos was Zoe Leyland in Australia in 1984.[11] Prior to that achievement, clinics either transferred all the embryos to their patients' uteri or discarded them. While the advantages of embryo cryopreservation are many, the process has ultimately led to problems of embryo disposition, with tanks around the world full of 'abandoned embryos.'[12] The abandoned embryo phenomena has led to a maelstrom of ethical and social policy discussions as well as a burgeoning industry in the United States of 'embryo adoption' agencies.

In Australia in 1983 a twenty-nine-year-old woman going through IVF donated one of her oocytes to a twenty-five-year-old woman with premature ovarian failure, thus resulting in the first birth through oocyte donation.[13] While the treatment was initially developed and used for women with missing or surgically removed ovaries or without ovarian function, in a short time oocyte donation became a treatment for women with recurring pregnancy loss, genetic disorders, and even advanced maternal age.[14] Although surrogacy has been occurring since biblical times, the first documented case of contractual surrogacy in the United States in 1976 involved the use of artificial insemination of a *traditional* surrogate by the intended father.[15] In 1985, the first baby born as a result of IVF and embryo transfer to a *gestational* surrogate was reported in California.[1] Currently, surrogacy and oocyte donation have become common and have facilitated many uniquely constructed families. For example, gay male couples may now start a family through the use of oocyte donation and surrogacy using the sperm of one of the male partners. Lesbian couples may choose to have a baby with one partner donating oocytes to the other so that one woman is the genetic mother of the child, while the other woman is the birth mother.

Assisted reproductive technologies, that began twenty-five years ago as a way to help infertile couples realize their dream of having a child, have been used to create families through a wide array of applications of these medical technologies. There are today tens of thousands of children in families worldwide conceived and born as a result of these technologies. These children, and their families, are now being systematically investigated in terms of their physical health and emotional well-being.

REVIEW OF THE LITERATURE

Studies of Physical Well-Being

Studies of the physical health of ART (IVF, GIFT, ICSI) children have primarily come from Europe, where ART and birth registries are established and accessible. One of the first studies assessing the health of IVF children was from the United Kingdom.[16] In the early 1980s, shortly after IVF became an effective treatment for infertility, the Medical Research Council in the United Kingdom set up a Working Party on children conceived by IVF. This group developed a voluntary registry of births from IVF beginning in 1983 from all clinics licensed under the Voluntary Licensing Authority (the precursor to the Human Fertilization and Embryo Authority; HFEA). In this study, the authors assessed preterm deliveries, low birth weight, multiple gestations, and birth defects from 1978–1987. The IVF data were compared to national statistics and adjusted for maternal age and multiplicity of gestation. The average age of the mothers and fathers was thirty-four and thirty-six years, respectively. Nineteen percent of the deliveries were twins, and 4% were triplets or higher order pregnancies. Twenty-four percent of the deliveries were preterm compared to 6% in the national average. Thirty-two percent of the babies were of low birth weight (LBW) compared to 7% in the national average. When multiples were excluded, the IVF singletons had a 12% rate of LBW, which was still higher than the national average. The rate of stillbirths and neonatal death was about twice the national average for IVF babies: 11.7 per 1,000 for singletons and 39.7 per 1,000 for twins. The rate of congenital malformations among the IVF children was 2.9%, which was in keeping with the national average. The authors speculated that the high rates of preterm births and LBW were due to maternal factors or infertility-related problems. The higher rate of perinatal mortality was seen to be due to the higher rate of multiple pregnancy. The authors were cautious in their conclusions related to the congenital malformation rates because of the lack of statistical power due to small sample size. They acknowledged that a sample of at least 10,000 children was necessary to adequately determine if there is a higher rate of congenital abnormality among IVF children because the base rate for congenital abnormalities is so low.

A similar French study reported the results of 7,024 clinical pregnancies from IVF resulting in 5,371 births (24% miscarriage rate) from 1986–1990.[17] These data were collected from the voluntary French birth registry managed by the French National Institute for Health and Medical Research (INSERM). In this sample, 34% of infants were from twin pregnancies and 10% were from triplet pregnancies compared with a multiple pregnancy rate of 2.3% in naturally conceived pregnancies in the French general population. Twenty-nine percent of all the infants were premature: 9% of singletons; 43% of twins, and 90% of triplets. The prematurity rates for IVF singletons were double that of naturally conceived singletons. The perinatal mortality rate was 27 per 1,000 and was significantly higher for multiple pregnancies. In terms of congenital malformations, 2.8% of all children were born with one or more major or minor malformations. When terminated pregnancies were included, the rate of malformations rose to 3.3%. However, the rate of malformations was not higher than that in the general population. A limitation of the study was that the data were not inclusive because participation in the registry was voluntary. The registry data for obstetric outcome and child health represented only 55% of all pregnancies because most ART centers did not continue to care for the patient through pregnancy to delivery. Despite these shortcomings, the authors concluded that prematurity, morbidity, and perinatal mortality are more frequent in ART than natural conception and that multiple pregnancy is not the only explanation for this finding.

In 1999, Bergh and colleagues reported on the health of children born after IVF in Sweden from 1982–1995.[18] A strength of this study was that the researchers compared the health of 5,856 IVF babies with over 1.5 million naturally conceived babies in the general population. IVF mothers were significantly older, were less likely to smoke, and had lower parity than mothers in the general population. Twenty-seven percent of deliveries were multiple births (23.9% twins, 2.8% triplets, and 0.2% quadruplets). Of the 3,305 singletons from IVF, 11.2% were born before thirty-seven weeks gestational age compared with 5.4% in the general population. 2.6% of the IVF babies weighed less than 1,500g at birth (very low birth weight; VLBW) and 9% weighed less than 2,500g (LBW). This was a fourfold increase in these events compared to the data from the naturally conceived babies. Perinatal mortality (8.2/1,000) was slightly higher in the IVF group. In terms of congenital malformation, 316 of the 5,856

IVF infants were identified with a malformation (5.4%) according to ICD–9 classification. The comparable figure for the naturally conceived babies was 3.9%. The authors then excluded babies with 'minor' malformations, at which point the rates more closely approximated that of the general population. The strengths of this study are that it included the entire population of IVF babies in Sweden for a thirteen-year period. It had a control group and had high birth follow-up data. The authors attributed the increased risk of medical complications at delivery and birth defects to the five-year average age difference in IVF mothers, their lower parity, and the 27% rate of multiple pregnancy in the IVF group. They acknowledged, however, that the IVF singletons were at a higher rate of prematurity (11.2%) than their naturally conceived counterparts. In a related study by Wennerholm et al. using the same birth registry information, the authors found a rate of 7.9% of congenital malformations in 1,139 infants conceived with ICSI/IVF,[19] again a rate higher than the general population.

Similar studies on IVF and ICSI children's health have been reported from Denmark,[20] The Netherlands,[21,22] Finland,[23] and Belgium[24] (see Table 27.1). All of these studies were able to track large numbers of IVF and naturally conceived children through the use of birth registries in their country. In general, IVF pregnancies had 25% and 30% multiple pregnancy rates. When compared to naturally conceived controls, IVF infants tended to weigh less and be delivered earlier, but this effect disappeared when a control group was matched to the IVF group on maternal age, parity, and plurality of pregnancy. However, in one study using only singleton pregnancies, a significantly lower overall birth weight was found for IVF infants compared to infants from matched control mothers.[25] The rates of perinatal death were between 17 and 22 per 1,000 births, although differences in definition across studies make it difficult to compare these rates.[18,21] The rates of congenital abnormality among IVF births among these European studies ranged from 2.3% to 6.6% depending on the classification system used, the percentage of entire sample assessed, and length of follow-up. Due to the low base rates of congenital abnormalities in the general population, very large samples are needed to have enough statistical power to determine if IVF children have a statistically significant higher rate of congenital abnormalities. Pooling data from several countries registries may be needed to meaningfully answer this question.

In a highly publicized study, Hansen and colleagues investigated the incidence of birth defects after ICSI

TABLE 27.1. Summary of studies of infant outcome

Study	Perinatal Death				Congenital Abnormalities (per 1,000)
	% Twins	% Triplets	% LBW	% Preterm	
MRC, 1988 11.7 n = 1,388	19	4	32	24	2.9%
FIVNAT, 1995 27 n = 5,371	34	10	–	29	2.8%
Bergh et al., 1999 8.2 n = 5,856	24	2.8	9*	11*	5.4%
Wennerholm et al., 2000 n = 1,139	17	<1	–	–	7.9%
Westergaard et al., 1999 21.8 n = 2,245	24.3	1.8	23 7*	24 7*	4.8%
Koudstaal et al., 2000 17 n = 307 singletons only	–	–	–	–	2.3%
Anthony et al., 2002 n = 422	–	–	–	–	3.2%
Koivurova et al., 2002 n = 304	–	–	–	–	6.6%
Bonduelle et al., 2002 23.3 n = 2,955	42	4.0	26.5 7.8*	29.3 9.0*	4.6%
SART/ASRM, 2002 n = 16,175	32	4.7	–	–	–
Schieve et al., 2002 n = 42,463	43	12	13.2*		
Hansen et al., 2002 n = 837	37 (all multiples)		22	32	9.0%

* singletons only

and IVF in a sample of Australian infants.[26] Using data from three birth registries, the researchers evaluated the rate of birth defects in infants born via ART from 1993 to 1997. In Australia, the Human Reproductive Technology Act of 1991 established the Reproductive Technology Register, which has recorded all births from ART since 1993. The researchers compared births from the ART registry to those in the general birth registry and cross-referenced it with data from the Western Australia Birth Defects Registry. Birth defects were classified using the ICD–9 classification system and were later defined as 'major' or 'minor' according to CDC (U.S. Centers for Disease Control) definition. The prevalence of major birth defects for IVF, ICSI, and naturally conceived infants up to one year in age were calculated. Odds ratios of the relative risk for each group were calculated. Maternal age, parity, and infant sex were also used to calculate relative risk. The sample included 301 infants conceived with ICSI, 837 with IVF,

and 4,000 who were naturally conceived. Mothers of the ART infants were older, less likely to have a previous child, and more likely to be white and married. ART infants were more likely to be born via Cesarean section, preterm birth, and low birth weight. The rates of birth defects for the groups were as follows: 8.6% ICSI (n = 26); 9.0% IVF (n = 75); and 4.2% naturally conceived (n =168). There were no significant differences in rates of birth defects across clinics. The results were similar and remained significant when only singletons were considered, when analyses were restricted to only singletons born at term, and when analyses were adjusted for maternal age and parity. In this study, two-thirds of the birth defects were diagnosed in the first week of life, and more than 90% were diagnosed by six months of age. When pregnancies that were terminated because of fetal abnormalities were included, the rates of major birth defects increased to 8.6% in the ICSI group, 9.4% in the IVF group, and 4.5% in the naturally conceived group. The authors postulated that possible causes for these findings were the advanced maternal age of ART mothers, the underlying cause of the infertility, the medications used during ovulation induction or to maintain the pregnancy, and factors associated with the procedures themselves such as freezing and thawing of embryos or delayed fertilization of the oocyte.

The data in the United States regarding the health of IVF/ICSI children are limited. The national ASRM/SART registry tracks procedure- and pregnancy-related ART data but it does not include data on infants' health. In a recent summary describing the data from the United States in 2000, there were 99,989 IVF cycles initiated and 73,406 transfers among 383 reporting programs. There was a delivery rate of 29.9% per retrieval and a 16.7% pregnancy loss rate. Sixty-four percent of the deliveries were singletons, 31% were twins, 4% were triplets, and 0.2% were higher order multiples.[27] The absence of an ART birth registry is a major drawback with the U.S. infertility treatment industry.

A recent study used the SART/CDC data from 1996–1997 to look at LBW and VLBW among ART infants.[25] The authors analyzed the birth weights of the 42,463 infants (excluding stillbirths) born as a result of ART. Infants were classified on the basis of maternal age, parity, plurality of pregnancy, and type of procedure (fresh versus frozen embryo transfer). The data from the ART infants were compared to the expected numbers from the birth data in the United States in 1997 matched for maternal age. In this study, 43% of the ART infants, were singletons, 43% were twins, 12% were triplets, and 1% were quadruplets. The percent of LBW (2,500 g or less) was 13.2% among singletons to 100% from quadruplets. The rate of VLBW (1,500 g or less) for singletons was 2.6% and up to 66.9% for quadruplets. The authors concluded that the use of the ARTs accounts for a disproportionate number of LBW and VLBW infants in the United States, in part because of the increased rates of multiple gestations but also, in part, due to use of assisted reproductive technology; the rates of LBW and VLBW were seen in singletons as well.

Very few studies have assessed infant health when the infant was born via previously cryopreserved embryos. Two such studies from England have been published. Wada et al.[28] found that mean gestational age and birth weight were not significantly different in infants born from fresh versus cryopreserved embryos. There were no differences in perinatal mortality rates and a lower incidence of major congenital abnormalities in the cryopreserved group. Sutcliffe and colleagues[29] reported on the health of ninety-one cryopreserved embryo children and a group of naturally conceived children. They found the cryopreserved embryo group children had significantly lower birth weight and prematurity than the naturally conceived children. There were no significant differences between groups in the rates of minor and major congenital abnormalities. Among the cryopreserved embryo group, the major congenital abnormalities that were noted were one child with Down's syndrome, one with Beckwith-Wiedemann syndrome (BWS), and one with hypophosphatemic rickets.

Finally, DeBaun and associates have reported the first evidence that ART is associated with large offspring syndrome in humans.[30] In this study, the authors monitored the birth defect registry for BWS. BWS is a congenital disorder that involves the overgrowth of several organs and a high incidence of neoplasia. The primary features are macrosomia, macroglossia, midline abdominal wall defects, and a predisposition for cancer. It has recently been determined that it is caused by epigenetic, as opposed to genetic, changes, which the authors described as "stable alterations in DNA as opposed to changes in the DNA sequence itself." The sites of the alterations for BWS are in the loss of imprinting in the H19 and LIT1 gene. The loss of imprinting can change the methylation of the gene that in turn changes the growth instructions in the developing embryo. The authors established a BWS registry in 1994 and found that seven children with BWS were born after IVF. The prevalence of ART was 4.6% among BWS patients but in the United States, ART accounts for only 0.76% of all live births, leading the authors to conclude that ART infants are overrepresented in the BWS registry and that there is a sixfold increase in BWS in children born after ART. Genomic DNA samples were collected from six of the seven children with BWS born after IVF. Five of the six children had abnormal imprinting of the LIT1 with hypomethylation. One child showed abnormal imprinting at the H19 site. The authors concluded that the relatively high rate of ART conception among BWS children demonstrates a relationship between the two. The biological data from these children support the occurrence of imprinting changes and altered methylation of the gene known to be associated with BWS.

A series of articles discussing the possible explanations to altered genetic expression among embryos created in vitro was published recently. Khosla and colleagues[31] reviewed the literature on culture media on embryonic development, particularly in reference to gene expression and phenotype. DeRyke and associates reviewed the data related to epigenetic risks related to embryos and offspring from IVF.[32] The epigenetic modifications they discuss are methylation and imprinting. Thompson and colleagues extended these discussions and suggested that the epigenetic modifications seen in in vitro-produced embryos may be more subtle than originally thought and that cellular stress induced by in vitro procedures may alter embryonic gene expression and contribute to phenotypic abnormalities after ART.[33]

These recent articles are thought-provoking and highly complex. They are based in some part on data from the animal literature where various pregnancy and offspring abnormalities have been observed at higher rates than in humans. The general findings in the human literature on birth defects and malformations after ART (except for those of Hansen et al.) continue to show rates of births defects among ART infants similar to or only slightly higher than naturally conceived infants. The exception to this is Hansen et al.'s data, in which maternal age, parity, multiplicity, and birth weight were controlled for and rates of birth defects were still roughly twice as high among ART offspring.

Sutcliffe [34, p. 29] provides important commentary regarding the interpretation of the data from outcome studies of ART children. He points out that the following methodological difficulties in the studies may limit their validity:

(1) matching criteria for the study and control groups need to be rigorous to limit factors that may also be affecting the outcome variable of interest, for example, socioeconomic status as it may affect intellectual development;

(2) follow-up rates need to be at least 80% of the sample of interest to provide reasonable confidence in the generalizability of the findings;

(3) statistical power calculations should be completed in studies using standardized measures to ensure that the sample is large enough to answer the question at hand;

(4) longer follow-up of children is needed to determine if a congenital abnormality is present;

(5) consistent definitions of congenital malformations across studies are needed to aid comparisons.

With all infant outcome studies, it should be kept in mind that large numbers of infants need to be studied because the base rate of birth defects remains low. It is unclear if the information from these studies warrants a change in our preconception counseling of patients regarding the risks of birth defects after ART. However, in light of these ART data, the establishment of an ART birth registry in the United States, the international pooling of data, and international collaboration research is warranted to accurately document and assess facts about ART children's health and to enable future research with large enough numbers to generate reliable and valid results.

Studies of Psychosocial Health

In addition to physical health, the psychological health and development of ART children has been of interest. Two studies in the mid-1980s assessed the development of IVF infants between twelve and thirty-seven months and found no evidence of abnormal development.[35,36] Since 2000, there have been several studies of pregnancy and early infancy comparing IVF versus naturally conceived infants.[37–41] Most of these studies have used small samples and self-report measures of infant temperament, but they provide the first available data on the psychosocial development of ART children.

A study from Greece looked at the impact of fertility treatment and IVF on communication between mothers and their infants. Researchers videotaped infants at four, seven, thirteen, and twenty-one weeks of age and their mothers from two groups: naturally conceived infants conceived through fertility treatment other than IVF, and IVF-conceived infants. Results showed that infants from fertility treatment and IVF were developing no differently than naturally conceived infants, but their mothers seemed to be more attentive and the babies seemed to be more playful. The authors felt that differences were related to the success of the treatment after infertility and not to stressors associated with IVF.[37]

A study of IVF children in Australia compared the development, behavior, and temperament of sixty-five IVF singletons with a matched group of sixty-three naturally conceived controls at one year of age. A methodological strength of this study was the administration of the Bayley Scales of Infant Development instead of reliance on self-report data about the infant from the parent. The investigators also used measures of receptive and expressive language, social development, and maternal assessment of behavioral problems. The results indicated that there were no significant differences between the IVF and control infants on any measures except the receptive language measure, in which IVF infants scored lower but still within the normal range. Additionally, a significantly higher percentage of IVF mothers rated their one-year-old as 'behaviorally difficult' than control mothers, 35% versus 16%, respectively. The authors concluded that the differences in maternal perception of infant behavior may be an extension of the IVF mothers' lower level of self-efficacy in caring for their infants at four months postpartum than was found by their colleagues in an earlier part of this study.[38,39]

A group from The Netherlands studied twenty-seven IVF families and twenty-three matched families with naturally conceived children at nine years of age. Parenting behavior, parenting stress, and the child's psychological development were assessed by parent questionnaires, and teachers' behavioral ratings were obtained for the majority of children. Parents were also asked if they had informed their child of their IVF origin. Results indicated that parenting behavior and parenting stress scores did not differ between groups. All the child behavior measures were within the normal range for both groups. Twenty-six percent of the IVF parents had informed their child about their IVF origin, 59% said they intended to tell, and 11% did not know if they would tell, while one couple was certain they would not tell. Parents who had informed their child had done so between the ages of four and eight years. Parenthetically, children who were informed had significantly higher problem behavior scores as reported by their mother and father compared to IVF children who had not been informed. The scores were still within the normal range and are based on small numbers of children and parents. The authors concluded that in general there are very few behavioral and psychological differences between IVF and naturally conceived children at nine years of age.[42]

Hahn and DiPietro[43] reported the results of a study of IVF and matched control families from Taiwan whose children were between the ages of three and seven. In this study, the researchers found that parents of IVF children were more similar than dissimilar to parents of naturally conceived children. There were some specific differences found, with IVF mothers reporting more feelings of protectiveness toward their children and greater separation anxiety as their child grew older. IVF mothers with one child reported less parenting stress than their control group counterparts and with other mothers with more than one child.

The aforementioned studies demonstrated that the psychosocial development of IVF children is generally good. There may be specific differences in parenting related to a past infertility history, but these differences do not appear to be significant over the long term. Another aspect of the impact of ART on child development is third-party reproduction that has generated ongoing research and discussion, particularly regarding issues of privacy and disclosure attitudes among donor gamete families.

Studies Addressing the Issue of Disclosure

Golombok and colleagues reported the outcome of a European study of IVF, DI, adopted, and naturally conceived children in the United Kingdom, Italy, Spain and The Netherlands.[44,45] In this longitudinal study, the researchers followed 116 IVF families, 111 DI families, 115 adoptive families, and 120 families with naturally conceived children for twelve years. Children with birth defects or who were from a multiple pregnancy were excluded. The researchers assessed parental marital adjustment and individual anxiety and depressive symptomatology in the parents. Interview data ascertained the quality of parenting and observational ratings of the mother–child interaction in the home. The Parenting Stress Index (PSI) was also administered. In addition, the child's mother and teacher assessed children's emotions, behavior, and relationships. Results indicated lower anxiety and depression levels in mothers of assisted reproduction children compared with mothers of naturally conceived children. ART mothers also provided significantly higher levels of warmth and emotional involvement to their children than the naturally conceiving mothers. The ART group and adoption groups were similar on these two dimensions of parenting. No significant differences were found in the children's behavior or emotional problems or with the children's feelings toward their mother or father. None of the DI children in this study had been told about their origin. Seventy-five percent of DI parents stated that they were definitely not going to tell their child about the circumstances of his or her conception, 13% were undecided, and 12% planned to tell. Still, more than half (56%) had told friends or family about the circumstances of their child's conception.

In the second phase of this study, 102 IVF, 94 DI, 102 adoptive, and 102 families with naturally conceived children were assessed from the original sample.[45] Measures of parental depression, anxiety, and parental stress were included as well as interviews with both parents and the child to ascertain relationship quality. Children's behavior was assessed by parent and teacher rating scales. Results indicated no differences in general measures of parental depression, anxiety, or marital satisfaction. Some specific differences were noted, with ART mothers reporting greater enjoyment of motherhood and greater emotional involvement with their children than naturally conceiving mothers. ART mothers were also more likely to be rated as overconcerned or overprotective of their child. ART fathers were rated as displaying more warmth toward their child than the natural conception or adoptive fathers.

An additional finding by these researchers was that only 8.6% of the parents in the sample had told their child that he or she had been conceived by DI. Ten percent planned to tell in the future, 12% were undecided, and 70% had decided against it. Half of the IVF parents and 95% of the adoptive parents had told their children about the circumstances of their origin. The most common reason given for not telling was to protect the child, which involved concern about the impact of telling on family relationships, particularly the child's relationship to the father. Two-thirds of couples believed there was no need to tell the child. No differences were found between the IVF and DI families on any of the variables related to parenting or psychological adjustment of the child. The researchers speculated that the absence of a genetic link between the father and the child did not interfere with the development of a positive relationship between them. DI fathers were as warm and involved with their children as IVF fathers. Potential biases in the study were that interviewers could not be blind to the type of family they were interviewing. The study also included only healthy, singleton children, and therefore outcomes of ART families with multiples or children who have special needs cannot be assumed to be the same.

In a recent study, Golombok and colleagues[46] studied forty-eight families with a child conceived with oocyte donation, forty-six with a child via donor insemination, and sixty-eight families with a naturally conceived child. At the time the child was one year old, the intention to tell was assessed: 46% of donor insemination families and 56% of oocyte donation parents intended to tell their child. When the child was two years of age, the investigators interviewed and administered self-report questionnaires to the parents and children. The investigators found that gamete donation mothers viewed their children as more vulnerable than natural conception mothers. No other differences were noted on the questionnaire measures. From the interview data, the investigators found that gamete donation mothers reported higher levels of joy and pleasure from parenting. For the oocyte donation mothers, no differences in parental variables were found between the 27% of the women who used a known donor compared to the 73% who used an anonymous donor. It was also noted that mothers of donor insemination children had higher levels of overprotectiveness than oocyte donation mothers. No such differences were noted among fathers. In terms of the children's development, no differences on developmental measures were noted between groups. Comparisons were then made to determine if there was any difference in child outcomes based on intention to tell the child of their gamete donation origin, and no

differences were found. In the discussion, Golombok and colleagues noted that the nature and quality of fathers' relationships with their donor sperm and donor oocyte children were no different. Based on this research, previously noted concerns regarding hostility or distance in donor sperm fathers may be less salient than previously thought.

In another English study, Lycett and colleagues[47] in a similar study investigated the impact of disclosure and privacy on the development of forty-six donor insemination offspring between the ages of four and eight years of age. Twenty-eight (60%) families did not plan to disclose (nondisclosers); eighteen (40%) had or planned to disclose to the child donor origin (disclosers). At the time of the study, 15% of the marriages had separated or divorced (no difference between disclosers and nondisclosers). In terms of the parent–child relationship, nondisclosing mothers reported that the child was more of a 'strain' than disclosing mothers and disclosing mothers reported fewer and less severe arguments than nondisclosing mothers. There were no differences for fathers between disclosers and nondisclosers on parent–child variables. Interestingly, the researchers point out that the hypothesized difficulties in father–child relationships in donor insemination families were not found in this study. Instead, difficulties, when they were found, were in the mother–child interactions, indicating that nondisclosure may have a greater impact on mothers than fathers. This is similar to the earlier observations that male infertility and donor insemination treatment has a significant impact on the female partners of the male infertility patient.[48] In addition, the researchers reiterated that disclosure did not necessarily produce more positive family functioning because both groups scored in the normal range on assessment measures.

Researchers in the United States studied mothers and fathers of oocyte donation offspring who had used anonymous and known donors. Parents from five centers across the country were queried about the amount of information they had about the donor, their relationship (if any) to the donor, and their disclosure decisions. The authors found no differences in plans to inform the child based on the use of a known or anonymous donor. Eighty percent of both groups had told others about using a donor to conceive, but two-thirds reported that they would tell no one if they had it to do over again. Regarding telling the child, there were no significant differences between couples using a known or anonymous donor: Approximately 10% had told the child, 49% planned to tell, 31% did not plan to tell, and 10% were unsure. For men, the amount of information known about the donor was significantly related to intention to tell the child, with men who knew more about the donor being more likely to tell the child. This relationship between disclosure to the child and information known about the donor was not found for the recipient mothers.[49,50]

In a unique scenario in which donor offspring from a California sperm bank could obtain identifying information about their donor (an 'identity-release' donor) upon reaching age eighteen, Scheib, Riordan, and Rubin[51] reported on the disclosure status of twenty-nine adolescents between the ages of twelve and seventeen who had been conceived using identity release donors. Forty-one percent of the youths were in lesbian couple families, 38% in single-woman families, and 21% heterosexual couple families. These adolescents were told of their donor sperm origin at a median age of seven years. Most reported feeling neutral or positive about their donor origin and felt that it was, 'a fact taken for granted' in their development and that they felt 'very loved and wanted by their family.' When asked about feelings about their donor, almost half (48%) reported feeling 'somewhat to very positive' about the donor, 86% reported 'curiosity' about the donor, and 51% reported being 'appreciative.' When asked what information they would like about the donor, the following were identified: a photograph (96%), current circumstances (89%), feelings about being contacted (79%), donor's health (69%), and family history (65%). In terms of seeking the donor's identity, 86% reported that they were 'moderate' to 'likely' to request identity release, with youths from single-women households more interested than lesbian households. Almost two-thirds of youths thought they would want a relationship with the donor.

These findings highlight the psychological complexity of disclosure among gamete donation families and provide the best estimate of actual parent disclosure behavior. However, the research findings may be biased due to low participation rates (particularly among those less likely to disclose, thus possibly overestimating the percentage of disclosers) and assessment of intention rather than actual disclosure. But given these limitations, there is a growing trend toward more openness in gamete donation families and it appears likely that at least half of sperm and oocyte donation parents are telling others and telling the child about their donor gamete origin.

An International Perspective on Disclosure

While studies of the health and psychological well-being of ART children cross international borders and apply to all children conceived via assisted technologies, stud-ies of disclosure may indeed be influenced by differences between countries and cultures, given that laws and customs very greatly among nations. However, a trend toward openness appears to be worldwide and is increasingly evident in international policies regarding disclosure regarding circumstances of conception and birth to offspring. For example, Australia, Austria, Canada, Germany, The Netherlands, New Zealand, Sweden, and Switzerland have moved toward providing offspring with access to identifying information about their donor.[52,53] Interestingly, Sweden was the first to enact legislation that ends donor anonymity when the child reaches a certain age, and Austria enacted the same laws shortly thereafter, in 1992. However, in both cases these laws apply only to sperm donors because neither country allows oocyte donation. In Iceland, the choice between anonymity and disclosure is made by the donors themselves. If the donor chooses to be anonymous, no identifying information is provided to recipients or offspring. If the donor chooses to be identified, the clinic maintains a file on the donor that may be reviewed by the (adult) offspring.

In the United Kingdom, the Human Fertilization and Embryology Authority (HFEA) was established in 1990. As part of its larger regulatory role, the HFEA maintains a confidential record of all gamete donors and all recipients of gamete donation. Although the identity of the gamete donor is not revealed to the recipients or their offspring, the identity is known to the authorities and is maintained to trace the donor and prevent further donation if the offspring are found to have a hereditary disorder and to prevent marriage between the offspring of the same donor.[54] Furthermore, HFEA mandates counseling be offered for all infertility patients, including those using donor gametes. In 2005, the HFEA changed the law ensuring donor anonymity providing offspring with the possibility of obtaining their donor's identity.

In the United States, there is no single consistent policy regarding choices between anonymity and openness. Some clinics require the use of anonymous donors only, whereas others are open to choices of known donors, intrafamilial donors, or donors recruited by agencies. The Ethics Committee of the ASRM released a statement in 2004 recommending "while ultimately the choice of recipient parents, disclosure to offspring of the use of donor gametes is encouraged." The committee also suggested that programs and sperm banks keep careful records with the anticipation that offspring would one day contact them for more information.[55] The ASRM Practice Guidelines suggest that all participants in third-party reproduction be counseled prior to treatment.

THEORETICAL FRAMEWORK

There are several theoretical frameworks regarding child development and family functioning that can frame ART child development issues. From an object relations perspective, Ainsworth[56,57] and Bowlby [58,59] have written extensively about the importance of the child's attachment and relationship to the mother as it relates to child development. This concept has also been extended by Lamb and others[60–62] to include the importance of the child's relationship with the father. From this perspective, the quality of the parent–child relationship is believed to affect the child's interactions with others and how the child reacts in novel or challenging situations. To the extent that the experience of infertility alters the ability of the parents to form appropriate relationships with their children (i.e., increasing the likelihood of overprotectiveness or detachment), attachment theory would predict that the children of previously infertile parents would be at greater risk for developmental difficulty.[63] Thus far, there has been little research supporting this view. In terms of donor offspring, attachment theory would predict that the more secure the relationship to the parents, the better the donor sperm or donor oocyte child would respond to the disclosure of their gamete donation origin. This supposition would be based on the primary importance of the relational aspects of parenting as opposed to the genetic component of parenting. Two studies that have investigated this supposition have found mixed results.[47,64]

Another important theoretical perspective to be considered when working with ART families is the family systems approach.[65–67] Within this model, the family is viewed as a system that is made up of different components but is connected and interdependent and that each part is related to the other in a stable manner over time. The family is made up of a series of triangular relationships, for example, mother, father, and child, that are the foundation of the family. When there is disequilibrium between two people, a third person enters to restore equilibrium. Troubling behaviors can be viewed as a way for gaining closeness or distance between the people in the dyad. In the context of donor children, the donor can be viewed as the 'third person' to restore equilibrium to the infertile couple. After the child is born, maintaining privacy about the donor child's origin can be viewed as a way to maintain equilibrium for the parent–child triad or it could be conceptualized that the 'secret' is the event that creates imbalance which is then seen in acting out in the parents or child. Understanding the couple's history and relationship dynamic becomes important in predicting how the family unit will function with the addition of a donor child. This would seem to be particularly important in the subgroup of couples who disagree with one another regarding the disclosure decision because the discordance could be acted out in a way that would be damaging to the child.

CLINICAL ISSUES

The mental health professional working with ARTs is constantly challenged by new treatment options and new cohorts of patients presenting novel family configurations. Each new group presents intriguing issues that are often ethically, socially, and psychologically complex. The clinician's mixed role of gatekeeper, therapist, counselor, and educator can often be difficult as the treatment evolves and patients' needs and concerns rapidly change.

Mental health professionals working in ART are also aware that their time with patients is usually quite limited. In most cases, the counselor may be afforded only one or two meetings with stressed and troubled potential parents. These patients often have long histories of infertility, and they may have a very difficult time imagining the reality of rearing one or more infants – let alone imagining this child's needs as an adolescent or adult. These may avoid difficult subjects in a defensive, even superstitious attempt to 'not jinx their chances' of pregnancy. Clinicians often are adept at helping patients cope with the sorrow associated with infertility, with the possibility of treatment failure and the experience of anticipatory grief. Inevitably, there is less time to deal with the prospect of success, of dealing with the emotional turmoil associated with a complicated pregnancy and the transition to parenthood.

Furthermore, the complexities of the treatments often lead to new issues relatively unfamiliar to the therapist, such as the new family configurations made possible by donor gametes – hence the ART cliché that a child can have five 'parents': the intended father, the intended mother, the sperm donor, the oocyte donor, and the surrogate. ART has created such novel family possibilities as single women having a child with donor sperm and donor oocyte, or donated embryo, children created with posthumous sperm, and children created by same-sex couples, each presenting the clinician with new and complex challenges that must be addressed, if at all, within a very limited time frame. As the mental health professional works with infertile individuals and couples, two central issues emerge specifically relevant to children: (1) the transition to first-time parenting among previously infertile couples, and (2) the role of the mental health professional in helping

---

TABLE 27.2. Issues to address regarding disclosure and privacy[70]

What role do you believe genetics plays in a person's personality, sense of humor, values, goals, etc.?

Are secrets necessarily lethal or detrimental?

Is there information that parents have a right to keep private?

Do you feel that a child has an inalienable right to know about his/her genetic origins?

Are there any dangers in telling your child about his/her donor conception?

Would you want to know if your parents used a gamete donor?

Can you live with a secret?

When are the parents' right to privacy superseded by a child's right to know?

Are feelings about disclosure or privacy entangled with the husband's or wife recipient's feelings of shame or discomfort about their fertility?

How will the child's family and community react to the use of donor?

How would you feel if your child 'discovered' the donor circumstances of his/her conception at some time in the future?

How important is it to you to manage or control the means of disclosure? Given your situation, how feasible is it to maintain secrecy and for how long?

How will you/would you feel if family or community knew about the child's donor conception?

Can you imagine any circumstances in which donor conception as a secret could be used in a negative manner by your partner?

If the laws regarding donor gametes change, how comfortable would you be with your child having access to information about the donor?

How would you feel about a central donor registry?

---

couples discuss and develop their plan regarding disclosure of the circumstances of their child(ren)'s conception and/or birth.

THERAPEUTIC INTERVENTIONS

Talking to Prospective Parents about Disclosure

Consultation with a mental health professional (MHP) is often required or suggested for couples seeking donor sperm or oocytes to conceive. The consultation includes a discussion of the logistics of donor selection, treatment time frame, and an exploration of treatment expectations and attitudes regarding disclosure. Surprisingly, the disclosure discussion is often the couple's introduction to the subject despite medical treatment plans developed with medical caregivers. Thus, the discussion can be pivotal, so long as it is both instructive and reassuring. In approaching the discussion of disclosure, mental health professionals may find themselves torn between maintaining 'therapeutic neutrality' and the impulse to advocate for a particular stance regarding disclosure. We believe that initially it is important for the mental health professional to allow the couple to express their thoughts and feelings about the issue before any recommendations are made, and that the primary role of the MHP is to help the couple come

to a decision that works best for them.[68] In allowing the couple to consider and express their perspective, the MHP is also learning about this particular couple's unique circumstances influencing their lives and that of their prospective children. For example, do they think the gamete donation origin of their child will make a significant difference in the day-to-day parenting of a child or in the child's future development and, if so, in what ways? This information is often best explored through a discussion of the couple's opinions of the 'nature versus nurture' aspect of parenting. This type of discussion can help the parents understand each other's perspective and help determine how great an impact they anticipate from the gamete donation process (see Table 27.2).

Factors that will influence disclosure to the child include: religion, culture, the existence of other children in the family, extended family functioning, and the community in which the couple will raise their child(ren). Treatment-related factors that may influence disclosure to the child include: recipient age, knowledge about the donor, and relationship to the donor. For example, in the United States couples using a recruited donor generally do not have access to the donor's identifying information. Couples should consider how they will store the information they do have about the donor and how will they respond to the child's questions about the donor. During the mental health consultation, there is an opportunity for the couple to hear about the experiences of other donor gamete families and to learn about current studies of disclosure. Not surprisingly, if this is the couple's introduction to the issue of disclosure, they are typically unaware of current trends toward more openness so may have never considered the topic, individually or as a couple. Additionally, the MHP may find that one partner may be inclined to be open about the process while the other may prefer to keep it private. When the disagreements are extreme (e.g., each rigidly adhering to opposite viewpoints), it may signify that the couple is not ready to proceed,[69] but for the most part, these disagreements are a healthy part of the give and take between couples with a strong relationship. Sometimes these differences relate to which individual is the infertile partner or they may reflect common gender differences (women typically are more open about infertility than are men). In cases of sperm donation, for example, men typically plan to maintain privacy, while most women plan to disclose.[68] This difference can provide the basis for a discussion of their individual concerns and reasoning. Often, the discussion leads directly to a recounting of which friends and family already have been informed about the couple's plans. The couple can then be helped to understand the impact of their decision and actions by tying together the issues of disclosure to others with the issue of disclosure to the child. For example, it is common for women to have told their best friend, sister, and/or mother, and for the husband to have told no one. When one partner becomes aware that the other has already disclosed to others, both partners quickly understand that the situation has changed in that the child may now be a risk to inadvertently learn from someone else. Clearly, the more people who know about the donation, the less control the couple has over keeping this information private. Providing the couple with a safe environment to openly discuss the topic, educational materials, as well as encouragement to return at a later date – even after the child is born or has grown older – may be the best interventions the MHP can provide in certain circumstances (see Table 27.3).

Telling the Child

Many couples who are seen for a pretreatment consultation are so intently focused on the difficulties involved in getting pregnant that it is difficult for them to imagine that they may in fact be successful and end up with a baby. Even if they can imagine a baby, it is often hard for them to imagine anything beyond the infancy of their potential child. When they do imagine a disclosure discussion with a potential child, they often believe that this will be a one-time telling and that there is one best age for it. Generally, they think of it as a discussion for a comparatively grown child. In fact, the discussion is ongoing and frequently repeated, evolving as the child grows and matures. The mental health professional can help make this process comprehensible by providing scenarios for when the child is a preschooler, a preadolescent, and a teenager, describing how the donor gamete information may affect the child at each phase. Also, some children may be very curious about the donor, whereas others may not. The differences in the child's interest level must be taken into consideration in the disclosure scenario. Conceptualizing the discussion of the disclosure over an eighteen-year time frame can help the couple understand that the disclosure decision is a lifelong process and is fundamentally about the child, not the parents (see Table 27.4).

When thinking about talking to children, most couples have not found the exact words and the mental health professional can help by suggesting approaches that are appropriate for the developmental stage of the child. The toddler and preschooler can be told that their parents worked hard to bring them into the family, that a doctor helped them, or that they were special and wanted very much. As the child grows and learns about reproduction and as issues come up in the family (e.g., of family trait similarities and differences), the parents may use those topics as an opening to tell the child about their gamete donation origin. Children vary greatly in their readiness for disclosure, and information must be tailored to the needs of each child. Parents should be encouraged to remember that they know their child better than anyone else and that their knowledge can guide them in the timing and the extent of the disclosure.

When a child is told, the parents may also want to discuss who else, if anyone, knows about the child's gamete donation origin. In addition, the child's disclosure to his or her friends may also be discussed, usually in the context of a discussion of other information-sharing patterns within the family and outside the family. For some families, gamete donation will be considered very private, to be discussed only within the nuclear family. For other families, it may be discussed in the wider social circle.

If a couple plans to maintain privacy, it is also helpful to discuss with them the consequences of this choice. At the very least, a decision to maintain privacy usually requires nondisclosure with all others to prevent inadvertent discovery by the child that can, understandably, be hurtful and traumatize the child and the parent–child relationship. Similarly, a decision to maintain privacy requires awareness of possible future scenarios, both

---

TABLE 27.3. Pros and cons of disclosure to children regarding third-party reproduction[71]

For disclosure

Child has a fundamental right and need to know about biological genetic origins

Medical information is critical, and nondisclosure may limit the information received and/or may lead to wrong information being given about the recipient's genetic history

Secrets are lethal and may permanently hurt the family and/or the child

Children born using assisted reproduction will sense that there is something different, and this difference will affect their sense of self and their relationship with their families

Parents are able to control and manage the disclosure and prevent unintended disclosure

Manner in which child is told or discovers will impact child's relationship with parent more than disclosure itself

Parents agree that openness is a family value

Genetic and biological information are fundamental to an individual's sense of self and personal identity

Believe it is best for child

For privacy

Telling will undermine parental role and parental connection to child

Disclosure has potential of making parents' infertility public

May jeopardize parents' connection with the child

Beliefs and ideas regarding disclosure may change over time

Believe it is best for child

Individuals do not have a fundamental right to know about their genetic origins

Medical information can be incorporated into the child's and family's medical history to ensure accurate information

All families have secrets, and we do not know that this is a 'lethal' secret

Children born through donor gametes will not sense anything different when raised in a home where the parents are loving and unconflicted about the use of a donor gamete

Sperm donation has been commercially available for decades, and less formally for centuries, under the restrictions of privacy and these families appear to have managed well. In short, privacy seems to have worked for these families

---

medical and social, in which the child's genetic information might require disclosure. It is also important to note that a couple's feelings regarding privacy may change over time and they need to retain information that they may want to share later if they change their minds. Understanding that raising children is an ongoing process and that beliefs often evolve through time and circumstance is reassuring to couples, encouraging them to continue their discussions together and to always factor in the unique characteristics and personality of their own child and his or her needs.

Fortunately for mental health professionals and the potential parents they counsel regarding gamete donation and talking to children, there are a number of useful resources. It is also important that MHPs inform couples of their availability to assist them long after treatment has ended and their families have been created.

FUTURE IMPLICATIONS

As this chapter has described, we know a great deal about the impact of ART on its participants and we are learning more and more about the health and well-being of ART offspring. However, we have little first-hand knowledge about ART offspring entering adulthood and their unique experiences growing up. As we approach the end of the third decade following the birth of Louise Brown, we can anticipate that thousands of ART offspring around the world will be entering their reproductive years and many will be making their own transition to parenthood.

We have yet to know what if any impact the ART treatment itself may have on the fertility of offspring so conceived. For example, will the large doses of progesterone taken by their mothers in order to have them affect their daughters' ability to conceive? Will ICSI conceived

TABLE 27.4. Discussing third-party reproduction with children[72]

Early years

Assure child of parent's unconditional love, how much he/she was wanted, happiness of parents when he/she was born

Assess child's readiness for information about sexuality, reproduction, own story

Explain simple facts of reproduction, various ways families are made

Tell child the story of his/her own arrival in family

Emphasize the nongenetic parent's role as parent

Middle years

Reassure child of unconditional love of both parents

Explain that child's place in family was something both parents wanted, that child would not be here if both parents had not made the decision together

Build on basic facts of reproduction to explain difference in child's conception

Reassure child that he/she was carried in mother's uterus, born like everyone else

Reassure child about donor: good person wanting to help other people have children

Later years

Reassure child of unconditional love of both parents and parents' shared wish for him/her

Explain why parents choose this option to have children (because of infertility)

Share information about how conception occurred (e.g., clinic, physicians, process, presence of father at insemination, reaction to pregnancy as part of child's own family story)

Explain various reasons why donors decide to assist individuals to become parents

Share available genetic history and information about the donor

Normalize experience for child: there are many others who have been conceived in this fashion

Recognize that the feelings of confusion, sadness, and pain are appropriate – may even reassure by explaining that parents had same feelings as child now has

Explain that sharing this information with others is his/her choice; it may be difficult and not everyone will understand. Help child process who he/she would like to tell and why. Support child if he/she wishes to keep it private

Offer child help in talking to others (e.g., therapist, pediatrician) if he/she wishes

sons have their own sperm problems? As mental health professionals in the past have counseled DES daughters about their loss of fertility because of the drugs their mothers took in order to have them, mental health professionals in the future may be counseling ART offspring about their own loss of fertility.

Certainly, mental health professionals can anticipate that as donor offspring reach adulthood, some of them may feel the need to explore the details of their conception and to learn more about the donors who participated in it. It may well be that these young men and women will turn to mental health professionals to provide counsel and guidance to assist them in their search and facilitate their adjustment to the situation. Indeed, as these individuals come to terms with their ancestry and history, their experiences may change and expand our understanding of the nature of personal identity, attachment, and family structure. As MPHs learn how to help and guide this new generation, they may also have the opportunity to expand their knowledge of how people come to understand who and what they are.

SUMMARY

■ ARTs have helped thousands of couples worldwide achieve their dream of having a child.

■ Studies of physical health of ART children indicate higher rates of multiple births, prematurity, and low birth weight. It is unclear if these are due to the technology itself or related to the underlying infertility problem within the couple.

■ Studies of congenital abnormalities of ART children demonstrate slightly higher levels of abnormalities, but methodological problems make these results difficult to interpret.

■ Studies of the psychosocial development of ART children show no differences from naturally conceived children.

■ Disclosure to children about the nature of their conception is a challenging concern for many ART parents. Mental health professionals can play a pivotal role in helping couples come to resolution around this issue.

■ Future issues within ART include PGD for sex selection and treating gay male couples.

REFERENCES

1. Trounson A, DK Gardner, eds. *Handbook of in Vitro Fertilization*. 2nd ed. New York: CRC Press, 2000.

2. Mahlstedt PP. The psychological component of infertility. *Fertil Steril* 1985; 43:335.

3. Mazure CM, Greenfeld DA. Psychological studies in in-vitro fertilization/embryo transfer patients. *J In Vit Emb Trans* 1989; 6:242.

4. Berg BJ, Wilson JF. Psychological functioning across stages of treatment for infertility. *J Behav Medicine* 1991; 14:11.

5. Duka WE, DeCherney AH. *From the Beginning: A History of the American Fertility Society 1944–1994*. American Fertility Society, 1994.

6. Betteridge K. An historical look at embryo transfer. *J Reprod Fertil* 1981; 62:1–13.

7. Gosden R. *Designing Babies: The Brave New World of Reproductive Technology*. New York: Freeman, 1999.

8. Silver L. *Remaking Eden: Cloning and Beyond in a Brave New World*. New York: Avon Books, 1997.

9. Edwards R, Steptoe P. *A Matter of Life*. London: Sphere, 1982.

10. Wilmut I, Rowson L. The successful low temperature preservation of mouse and cow embryos. *J Reprod Fert* 1973; 33:352–3.

11. Trounson A, Mohr L. Human pregnancy following cryopreservation, thawing and transfer of an eight cell stage human embryo. *Nature* 1983; 305:707–9.

12. Klock S, Sheinin S, Kazer R. The disposition of unused frozen embryos. *N Engl J Medicine* 2001; 365:68–9.

13. Lutjen P, Trounson A, Leeton J, et al. The establishment and maintenance of pregnancy using in vitro fertilization and embryo donation in a patient with primary ovarian failure. *Nature* 1984; 307:174.

14. Sauer MV, Paulson RJ, Lobo RA. Reversing the natural decline in human fertility. An extended clinical trial of oocyte donation to women of advanced reproductive age. *JAMA* 1992; 268:1275–9.

15. Walters L. Ethics and new reproductive technologies. In: *Current Therapy of Infertility -3*. CR Garcia, L Mastroianni, RD Amelar, L Dubin, eds. Philadelphia: BC Decker, 1988.

16. MRC working party on children conceived by in vitro fertilization. Births in Great Britain resulting from assisted reproduction, 1978–1987. *BMJ* 1990; 300:1229–33.

17. FIVNAT. Pregnancies and births resulting from in vitro fertilization. French national registry analysis of data 1986–1990. *Fertil Steril* 1995; 64:746–56.

18. Bergh T, Ericson A, Hillensjo T, et al. Deliveries and children born after in vitro fertilization in Sweden 1982–95: A retrospective cohort study. *Lancet* 1999; 354:1579–83.

19. Wennerholm U, Bergh C, Hamberger L, et al. Incidence of congenital malformations in children born after ICSI. *Hum Reprod* 2000; 15:944–8.

20. Westergaard H, Johanson A, Erb K, et al. Danish National in vitro fertilization registry 1994 and 1995: A controlled study of births, malformations and cytogenetic findings. *Hum Reprod* 1999; 14:1896–902.

21. Koudstaal J, Braat D, Bruinse H, et al. Obstetric outcome of singleton pregnancies after IVF: A matched control study in four Dutch university hospitals. *Hum Reprod* 2000; 15:1819–25.

22. Anthony S, Buitendijk S, Dorrepaal C, et al. Congenital malformations in 4,224 children conceived after IVF. *Hum Reprod* 2002; 17:2089–95.

23. Koivurova S, Hartikainen A, Gissler M, et al. Neonatal outcome and congenital malformations in children born after in vitro fertilization. *Hum Reprod* 2002; 17:1391–98.

24. Bonduelle M, Liebaers I, Deketelaere V, et al. Neonatal data on a cohort of 2,889 infants born after ICSI (1991–1999) and of 2,995 infants born after IVF (1983–1999). *Hum Reprod* 2002; 17:671–94.

25. Schieve L, Meikle S, Ferre C, et al. Low and very low birth weight in infants conceived with use of assisted reproductive technology. *NEJM* 2002; 346:731–37.

26. Hansen M, Kurinczuk J, Bower C, et al. The risk of major birth defects after intracytoplasmic sperm injection and in vitro fertilization. *NEJM* 2002; 346:725–30.

27. SART and ASRM. Assisted reproductive technology in the United States: 2000 results generated from the American Society for Reproductive Medicine/Society for Assisted Reproductive Technology Registry. *Fertil Steril* 2004; 81:1207–20.

28. Wada I, Macnamee C, Wick K, et al. Birth characteristics and perinatal outcome of babies conceived from cryopreserved embryos. *Hum Reprod*. 1994, 9:543–6.

29. Sutcliffe A, DeSouza S, Cadman J, et al. Outcome in children from cryopreserved embryos. *Arch Dis Child* 1995, 72:290–3.

30. DeBaun MR. Niemitz EL. Feinberg AP. Association of in vitro fertilization with Beckwith-Wiedemann syndrome and epigenetic alterations of LIT1 and H19. *American Journal of Human Genetics* 2003 Jan; 72:156–60.

31. Khosla S, Dean W, Reik W, et al. Epigenetic and experimental modifications in early mammalian development: Part II. Culture of preimplantation embryos and its long-term effects on gene expression and phenotype. *Hum Reprod Update* 2001: 7:419–27.

32. DeRyke M, Liebars I, Van Steirteghem A. Epigenetic risks related to assisted reproductive technologies. *Hum Reprod* 2002; 17:2487–94.

33. Thompson JG, Kind KL, Roberts C, et al. Epigenetic risks related to assisted reproductive technologies: Short- and long-term consequences for the health of children conceived through assisted reproduction technology: More reason for caution? *Hum Reprod* 2002; 17:2783–86.

34. Sutcliffe A. *IVF Children The First Generation: Assisted Reproduction and Child Development*. London, UK: Parthenon Publishing Group, 2002.

35. Mushkin DN, Barreda-Hanson MC, Spensley JC. In vitro fertilization children: Early psychosocial development. *J In Vitro Fertil Embryo Transf* 1986; 3:247–52.

36. Yovitch J, Parry T, French N, et al. Developmental assessment of twenty in-vitro fertilization (IVF) infants on their first birthday. *J In Vitro Fert and Embryo Transfer* 1986; 3:253–7.

37. Papiligoura Z, Trevarthen C. Mother–infant communication can be enhanced after conception by invitro fertilization. *Infant Mental Health Journal* 2001; 22:591–610.

38. MacMahon C, Ungerer J, Tennant C, et al. Psychosocial adjustment and the mother–baby relationship for IVF mothers from pregnancy to 4 months postpartum. *Fertil Steril* 1997; 68:492–500.

39. Gibson FL, Ungerer JA, Tennant C, et al. Parental adjustment and attitudes toward parenting after in vitro fertilization. *Fertil Steril* 2000; 73:565–74.

40. Klock SC, Greenfeld DA. The psychological status of in vitro fertilization (IVF) patients during pregnancy: A longitudinal study. *Fertil Steril* 2000; 73:1159–64.

41. Greenfeld DA, Klock SC. Transition to parenthood among in vitro fertilization patients at 2 and 9 months postpartum. *Fertil Steril* 2001; 76:626–7.

42. Colpin H, Soenen S. Parenting and psychosocial development of IVF children: A follow-up study. *Hum Reprod* 2002; 17:1116–23.

43. Hahn CS, DiPietro J. In vitro fertilization and the family: Quality of parenting, family functioning and child psychosocial adjustment. Develop Psychol 2001; 37: 37–48.

44. Golombok S, Brewaeys A, Cook R, et al. The European study of assisted reproduction families: Family functioning and child development. *Hum Reprod* 1996; 11:2324–31.

45. Golombok S, Brewaeys A, Giavazzi MT, et al. The European study of assisted reproduction families: The transition to adolescence. *Hum Reprod* 2002; 17:830–40.

46. Golombok S, Jadva V, Lycett E, et al. Families created by gamete donation: Follow-up at age 2. *Hum Reprod* 2004; 20:286–93.

47. Lycett E, Daniels K, Curson R, et al. Offspring created as a results of donor insemination: A study of family relationships, child adjustment and disclosure. *Fertil Steril* 2004; 82:172–9.

48. Klock SC. Psychological aspects of donor insemination and male infertility. *Infertl Reprod Clinics N America* 1993; 4:455–69.

49. Greenfeld DA, Klock SC. Disclosure decisions among known and anonymous oocyte recipients. *Fertil Steril* 2004; 81:1565–71.

50. Klock SC, Greenfeld DA. Parents' knowledge about the donor and their attitudes toward disclosure in oocyte donation. *Hum Reprod* 2004; 19:1575–9.

51. Scheib J, Riordan M, Rubin S. Adolescents with open-identity sperm donors: Reports from 12–17 year olds. *Hum Reprod* 2004; 20:239–52.

52. Gottlieb C, Lalos O, Lindbald F. Disclosure of donor insemination to the child: The impact of Swedish legislation on couples' attitudes. *Hum Reprod* 2000; 15:2052–6.

53. Pennings G. The 'double track' policy for donor anonymity. *Hum Reprod* 1997; 12:2839–44.

54. Firth L. Gamete donation and anonymity: The ethical and legal debate. *Hum Reprod* 2001; 16:818–24.

55. The Ethics Committee of the American Society for Reproductive Medicine. Informing offspring of their conception by gamete donation. *Fertil Steril* 2004; 82(Suppl 1):S212–S216.

56. Ainsworth M. Attachment as related to mother–infant interaction. In: JS Rosenblatt, RA Hinde, C Beer, M Busnel, eds. *Advances in The Study of Behavior*. New York: Academic Press, 1979; 9:1–51.

57. Ainsworth M, Blehar MC, Waters E, et al. *Patterns of Attachment*. Hillsdale, NJ: Erlbaum, 1978.

58. Bowlby J. *Attachment and Loss: Vol 1 Attachment*. New York: Basic Books, 1969.

59. Bowlby J. *Attachment and Loss: Vol 2 Separation: Anxiety and Anger*. New York: Basic Books, 1973.

60. Lamb ME. The development of father–infant relationships. In: ME Lamb, ed. *The Role of the Father in Child Development*. New York: Wiley, 1997, 3rd edition, pp. 104–20.

61. Pleck JH. Paternal involvement: Levels, sources and consequences. In: ME Lamb, ed. *The Role of the Father in Child Development*. New York: Wiley, 1997, 3rd edition, pp. 66–103.

62. Lamb ME. Attachments, social networks and developmental contexts. *Human Develop* 2005; 48:108–12.

63. Burns LH. An exploratory study of parenting after infertility. *Fam Systems Medicine* 1987; 8:177–89.

64. Chan R, Raboy B, Patterson C. Psychosocial adjustment among children conceived via donor insemination by lesbian and heterosexual mothers. *Child Development* 1998; 69:443–57.

65. Foley V. Family Therapy. In: R Corsini, ed. *Current Psychotherapies* Itasca, IL: FE Peacock, 1979, 2nd ed. pp. 460–99.

66. Bowen M. The use of family therapy in clinical practice. In: J Haley, ed. *Changing Families*. New York: Grune & Stratton, 1971.

67. Satir V. *Conjoint Family Therapy*. Palo Alto, CA: Science and Behavior Books, 1983.

68. Klock SC, Jacob MC, Maier D. A prospective study of donor insemination recipients: Secrecy, privacy, and disclosure. *Fertil Steril* 1994; 77–84.

69. Vercollone CF, Moss H, Moss R. *Helping the Stork: The Choices and Challenges of Donor Insemination*. New York: Macmillan, 1997.

70. Braverman M. Oocyte donation: Psychological and counseling issues. *Clinical Consult Obstet Gynecol* 1994; 6: 143–9.

71. Braverman AM. Issues in privacy and disclosure in donor gametes. Presented at the Eighth National Conference for IVF Nurse Coordinators and Support Personnel, Serono Symposia, Boston, MA, M28–30, 1995; 63–8.

72. Probasco KA. Discussion with children about their donor conception. Insights into infertility. Serono Symposia, Longwell, MA: Summer 1992; 5, 10.

28 Infertility Counseling in Practice: A Collaborative Reproductive Healthcare Model

SHARON N. COVINGTON

Where no counsel is, the people fall: but in the multitude of counsellors there is safety.

– Proverbs 11:14

Infertility counseling is a specialty that combines the fields of reproductive health psychology and reproductive medicine. Counseling, in its purest form, means giving advice or guidance, and often includes consoling or giving comfort to those in need. All infertility healthcare providers, from physicians and nurses to laboratory technicians and administrative assistants, have the opportunity to counsel and console patients going through reproductive medical diagnosis and treatment. In this sense, psychosocial care is the responsibility of *all* members of the treatment team as it entails 'treating the patient, not the disease.' Nonetheless, increasing specialization and collaboration in all fields of healthcare practice have brought the need for psychological services to the reproductive medical practice. While there is no clear international agreement of who can or should provide infertility counseling services, there is an increasing awareness and growing consensus that it needs to be a mental health professional and that services are integral to the optimum care of the infertile patient. Mental health professionals have become increasingly important in reproductive healthcare. This has been the result of technological advances in reproductive medicine and the recognition of the complex psychosocial issues and demands facing infertile patients. The role of infertility counselors in reproductive medicine extends beyond advising and comforting: It requires specialized skill, knowledge, and training in the interrelation of the medical and psychological aspects of infertility to appropriately evaluate and treat the emotional consequences of impaired fertility. Infertility counseling includes psychological assessment, psychotherapeutic intervention, and psychoeducational support of individuals and couples experiencing fertility problems. The focus of patient care for infertility counselors is the psychological care and treatment of the individual and/or couple within the context of the medical condition and infertility treatment.

This chapter

- gives a historical overview of infertility counseling practice;
- presents a theoretical framework for the provision of infertility counseling services based upon collaborative reproductive healthcare models;
- discusses clinical issues facing infertility counselors in establishing a collaborative practice with patients, medical staff, colleagues, and professional and consumer organizations;
- identifies the process for integrating infertility counseling into clinical settings through practice models, role identification, practice management, and helpful tips;
- reflects on issues for the future of infertility counseling practice.

HISTORICAL OVERVIEW

While the psychological sequelae of infertility has been addressed in the literature for more than fifty years,[1,2] it has only been within the last twenty-five years that infertility counseling has emerged as a recognized profession and a specialization within the mental health professions. Traditionally, the role of the mental health professional was to cure the neurosis that was thought to be the cause of a patient's (usually a woman's) infertility. However, as this approach fell into disfavor, counselors working in infertility clinics began increasingly to provide psychological support, crisis intervention, and education to ameliorate the stress of infertility and enhance quality-of-life.[3]

Historically, the integration of infertility counseling in medical treatment of infertility has focused on patient symptomatology, using a more traditional medical model. In this situation, counseling is provided on an as-needed basis when the patient expresses or the caregiver identifies distress, or crisis intervention is provided when symptomatology has impaired patient functioning, particularly with compliance in medical treatment. However, over time a shift has occurred with provision of infertility counseling required or recommended for specific treatments or certain populations (e.g., IVF, donor insemination, oocyte donation, and single women).[4–6] Here, infertility counseling is specific to the situation and reflects a concern for patient preparation and education, understanding of the implications, and assessment of psychological readiness for treatment. While remediation of symptomatology continues to be a function of infertility counseling, the shift to these preventative aspects of care is essential in service provision.

The importance of including infertility counseling as part of reproductive medical treatment became clearer in many countries in the early 1980s as a consequence of an enormous technological leap: the first successful birth following in vitro fertilization (IVF) in 1978 (see Chapter 31). Additional advances in assisted reproductive technology (ART) changed the image of parenthood through surrogacy, gestational carrier, oocyte and embryo donation, furthering the need for specialized counseling services for families being created through these extraordinary measures. Issues regarding the relationships between third-party participants, disclosure to offspring of their genetic heritage, and the eventual ban in some countries of anonymous gamete donation including donor linkage counseling (i.e., meetings between donors and recipients facilitated by infertility counselors) added more impetus to the field. The role of the infertility counselor expanded to meet the psychological challenges of assisted reproductive technologies and third-party reproduction through psychosocial assessment, support, treatment, education, research, and consultation.[7]

Today, infertility counselors serve as an integral part of the reproductive medical team. Public awareness and consumer demand, legislation and regulatory bodies, as well as professional guidelines have moved infertility counseling from the background to the forefront of patient care in reproductive medicine. Infertility counseling is no longer considered an elective adjunct service available to a minority of needy infertility patients. Nor do the services or skills of mental health professionals providing infertility counseling need to be further justified or defended. Infertility counseling is now recognized as a separate body of knowledge and professional services integral to reproductive medicine and patient care.

REVIEW OF LITERATURE

Early work in the area of the psychology of infertility and the role of mental health professionals focused on the psychosomatic basis of infertility and sterility.[1,2,8–10] Historically, gender bias regarding the woman as the cause of infertility was evident: Treatment was provided by psychiatrists (primarily male) who employed a psychoanalytic orientation, and the focus of treatment was on patients (almost exclusively women) who were seen as having unresolved, hostile feelings about motherhood or their relationships with their own mothers. Thus, if infertility could not be identified in medical terms, it was viewed as a psychosomatic reaction requiring extended psychoanalytic treatment of the woman to cure her neurotic response to her childlessness.

Gradually, a change occurred in the literature as the emotional distress of infertility was seen as a *consequence* rather than a *cause* of infertility. With this change came a growing recognition of the need for supportive counseling services for couples undergoing infertility treatment. One of the earliest articles, by Berger,[11] discussed the role of psychiatrists consulting in an infertility clinic as both helping couples deal with the outcome of infertility treatment and identifying psychological factors as possible causative agents of infertility, particularly related to sexual function. Other articles[12–14] described counseling services provided at reproductive medical clinics by mental health professionals, involving assessment of emotional symptomatology associated with infertility and enhancement of quality-of-life for patients. Thus, there was an increasing recognition of the psychological sequelae of infertility as a consequence of the emotionally intrusive and protracted nature of the medical treatment process.[15,16] As this recognition has increased, so too has the awareness of the need for skilled mental health professionals to provide these services.[17]

The development of IVF and other assisted reproductive technologies (ARTs) facilitated the involvement of mental health professionals as part of the medical treatment team.[18–21] A number of authors have recommended the inclusion of psychological services for the evaluation and treatment of participants in the more involved fertility therapies.[4,5,22,23] Recommendations have been suggested for provision of counseling services for patients undergoing assisted reproductive technologies including IVF; sperm, oocyte, or embryo donation; and surrogacy or gestational carrier participants. Other recommendations for counseling have been based on concern about marital or psychological functioning, the best interest of the child, inability to provide informed consent, or partner coercion. The role of the mental health professional as part of the treatment team[24] and coordinator of third-party services[25] continues to expand.

With more mental health professionals being drawn to infertility counseling, some studies have looked at personal reproductive history as an issue for counselors. Covington and Marosek[26] surveyed the personal reproductive histories of nurses and mental health professions working in the field of reproductive medicine and found that 52% of respondents ($n = 100$) had been diagnosed with infertility and 67% received medical treatment for infertility at the same clinic where they were employed. Of the infertile respondents, 71% began working in reproductive medicine *after* the diagnosis. In a similar study of genetic counselors, Martin and Walker[27] found that 36% of survey respondents ($n = 522$) identified themselves as personally affected in some way by a genetic disorder or reproductive difficulties. A majority (88%) of the genetic counselors could identify ways in which their personal history was helpful and beneficial in counseling, while fewer (23%) were able to identify ways in which it presented challenges. Interestingly, 49% of the genetic counselors reported disclosing their personal reproductive or genetic history to a client at least once. Both of these studies address the issue of how personal reproductive history and related counter-transference may influence the professional's work and patient care in the field of reproductive medicine, in both positive and negative ways.

THEORETICAL FRAMEWORK

Collaborative Reproductive Healthcare

This chapter focuses on the emerging role of the infertility counselor as part of the medical treatment team. The model of practice has a basis in a biopsychosocial approach, described throughout this book, where the diagnosis and treatment of medical conditions are considered in terms of a variety of aspects impacting an individual's experience of the illness and treatment: physiological, psychosocial, experiential, interpersonal, familial, and societal. According to this approach, influential factors include the context in which the individual experiences the diagnosis, illness, and treatment (e.g., individual's overall health, functional status, and emotional well-being). This approach emphasizes the importance of the healthcare provider and patient as collaborators in the diagnosis, treatment, and health maintenance to achieve optimum results.

The collaborative family healthcare model expanded on the biopsychosocial model to emphasize and encourage two changes in the provision of healthcare: (1) the integration of mental health professionals (behavioral healthcare) as integrated members of a multidisciplinary treatment team; and (2) a redefinition of the patient from an individual to an interpersonal system (e.g., couple, parent–child, and family). It emphasizes a cohesive partnership among the primary provider, the patient, the patient's family, and other providers, particularly mental health professionals. This practice style integrates biomedical and psychosocial factors, and overcomes the mind and body split of the traditional medical model. It recommends a seamless collaboration between psychosocial, biomedical, nursing, and other healthcare professionals, all taking into consideration the patient within the context of his or her interpersonal relationships (e.g., marriage, family, and community). Healthcare professionals and patients (couples) are equal participants in the healthcare process. It is suggested that the collaborative family healthcare model improves the quality of health care delivery and may also improve cost-effectiveness of treatment.[28]

The collaborative family healthcare model has its roots in the United States in family practice (general practice) at the end of the twentieth century. However, within the same timeframe, reproductive medicine around the world was moving toward a more integrated and collaborative approach to the treatment of infertile couples by recognizing the importance of all members of the multidisciplinary team: reproductive endocrinologists, urologist, nurses, mental health professionals, genetic counselors, embryologists, and other professionals working in the field as consultants (e.g., perinatologists). This holistic approach minimizes rigid distinctions between fields (but not expertise), allowing all members of the team to provide psychological support or counseling and expecting mental health professionals to be educated and trained about the medical diagnosis and treatment of infertility. It has even been suggested that multidisciplinary collaborative approach provides a creative and integrating force by improving patient care, providing an arena for evidence-based research as well as system-based curriculum for professional development (physician, nursing, and mental health training).[29,30] The following represents two theoretical models for collaborative reproductive healthcare.

The Ten-Step Circular Process Model

This integrative model focuses on different critical points during the infertility diagnosis and treatment process to maximize effective collaboration between patient and team members. It was developed by Swiss physician Johannes Bitzer and serves as a framework for integrating patient counseling within the medical

TABLE 28.1. Ten-step circular process[23]

Step 1: Introduction and initiation of a working alliance

Step 2: Problem assessment and monitoring

Step 3: Clarification about problem definition and negotiation about objectives and priorities

Step 4: Exchange of hypotheses and decision making concerning diagnostic procedures

Step 5: Investigations, diagnostic procedures

Step 6: Information giving about results

Step 7: Elaboration of options to resolve infertility problem

Step 8: Decision making about specific options

Step 9: Treatment procedures

Step 10: Evaluation of outcome

environment proposed by the European Society of Human Reproduction & Embryology (ESHRE) *Guidelines for Counselling in Infertility*[23] (see Table 28.1). The model involves a ten-step medical cycle whereby psychosocial needs and counseling are identified and addressed in terms of purpose (i.e., why it is necessary); objective (i.e., what is to be achieved); typical issues (i.e., potential problem areas); and communication skills (i.e., attitude and knowledge needed for success). It is a fluid model in which the cycle may restart at different points or terminate at any step. *Step 1* is the *introduction and initiation of a working alliance* and provides a basis for the helping relationship. *Step 2* involves *problem assessment and monitoring* where information is gathered about the patients' psychosocial experience and history with infertility. In *Step 3*, there is *clarification about problem definition and negotiation about objectives and priorities* when the patient's problems are summarized and possible limitations to treatment are discussed. During *Step 4*, an *exchange of hypotheses and decision making concerning diagnostic procedures* takes place regarding possible causes of and diagnostic plans for impaired fertility. *Step 5* concerns *investigations and diagnostic procedures* that allow for more patient information and for the patient and caregiver to elaborate a problem-solution plan. *Information giving about results* is *Step 6*, when the team informs the patients about results and their implications. In *Step 7*, the *elaboration of options to resolve infertility problem* is presented and processed with the patient based on the diagnosis. During *Step 8*, the team and patients discuss *decision making about specific options* including advantages, disadvantages, and possible outcomes. *Treatment procedures* occur during *Step 9*, when patients and team take action with diagnostic tests and/or treatments. *Step 10*

completes the cycle with *evaluation of outcome* with the team and patient accessing the results of previous steps, and may eventually mean that the cycle may be reentered at a previous step. This model presents a biopsychosocial approach that underscores the responsibility of all members of the treatment team to address psychosocial needs of the patient.

The Six Phases of Infertility Treatment Model

The conceptualization of integrating infertility counseling into clinical practice may be viewed along a continuum of medical treatment. Covington[31] and Feldman[32] developed a theoretical framework for examination of counseling issues and provision of services within a six-phase model of infertility treatment. This model also underscores the importance of integrating medical and psychological services throughout the infertility treatment process, normalizing the counseling experience and preventing problems in later phases by providing services and interventions early on (see Table 28.2). In *Phase I, seeking help*, the mental health professional, typically on a limited basis, provides support and psycho-education, normalizing the feelings and experiences of infertility as well as what to expect with medical evaluation. During *Phase II, medical evaluation*, the infertility counselor's role broadens to include increased understanding of a couple's psychosocial functioning in relation to their infertility diagnosis and treatment. Services may involve assessment, education, or psychotherapeutic interventions to promote effective coping and/or more adaptive behavior. In *Phase III, beginning treatment*, patients characteristically have a renewed sense of hope about the success of treatment plans, as well as increased stress as treatment begins or becomes more intense. Continued support and education are provided by the infertility counselor and involve managing treatment demands, enhancing coping strategies, and preparing for realistic expectations of treatment success. *Phase IV, further treatment*, may continue over several years, often dominated by feelings of frustration and failure or obsessive determination. During this phase, the infertility counselor helps patients deal with the consequences and chronicity of infertility, express or manage the myriad of negative feelings, and begin preparing for consideration of childlessness and/or other family-building alternatives. Patients often enter *Phase V, third-party reproduction*, psychologically depleted, only to face complex decisions about assisted reproductive technology or third-party reproduction. Counseling is vital to assess psychological readiness, explore implications of decisions, and prepare for the outcome of treatment. Finally, in *Phase VI, ending treatment*, the infertility counselor helps patients reach a decision about ending treatment,

TABLE 28.2. Six phases of infertility treatment and counseling tasks

Phase[32]	Task[31]
I. Acknowledging a fertility problem: seeking help	Support education, information, and resources
II. Undergoing medical evaluation	Psychosocial assessment and support education Preparation for treatment
III. Treating infertility problems	Support and education Identifying coping mechanisms Stress management Emotional and therapeutic counseling Preparing for outcome
IV. Further treatments: investigating and treating additional diagnosis	Stress management and coping strategy Emotional and therapeutic counseling Exploring alternatives
V. Attempting noncoital conception: donor gametes and assisted reproductive technologies	Emotional and therapeutic counseling Implications counseling Psychosocial assessment and support Facilitating decision making Exploring alternatives preparing for outcome
VI. Deciding to end treatment and redefine family: adoption and childlessness	Grief and therapeutic counseling Pursuing alternative family-building Preparing for outcome
Any stage: adjustment to pregnancy and parenthood	Support and education Redefining self/couple as parents Emotional and therapeutic counseling

grieving the losses, and redefining family so that resolution and closure can occur. By giving meaning to the infertility and integrating it into the sense of self and the marital history, patients are able to let go of infertility and move on without impairment or damage. During any phase of treatment, if pregnancy or the decision to adopt occurs, the counselor's role is to assist in the adjustment to pregnancy and/or parenthood, which is influenced by the infertility experience.

CLINICAL ISSUES

Taking a collaborative approach to infertility counseling practice involves working in a meaningful, respectful manner toward a mutual goal of quality care and support. To meet this goal, infertility counselors form a variety of collaborative relationships involving their patients, medical staff, other mental health professionals, and professional and consumer organizations. Each of these relationships presents unique opportunities and challenges.

Patient Collaboration

Undoubtedly, the most important collaborative relationship an infertility counselor establishes is with the infertility patient. This book is devoted to assisting the MHP in creating a foundation of knowledge and understanding to form a productive working relationship with patients experiencing a variety of reproductive health issues. However, it has been noted that one of the reasons MHPs (as well as other healthcare providers) are drawn to this work is out of their own personal experience with reproductive loss.[26,33] From the intimate exposure to their own pathos with infertility, many counselors (and other medical caregivers) learn about the needs and issues with which infertility patients struggle. Some may enter the field as a consequence of their infertility, perhaps wanting to use the experience to heal their own wounds or to make something positive come from it, while others may be established mental health professionals wanting to grow professionally and personally from the experience with an infertility counseling practice. Whatever the reason or motivation, having a personal experience with reproductive loss presents the counselor with unique perspectives as well as challenges.

A normal part of the therapeutic process is transference and counter-transference, a projection of thoughts, reactions, and feelings that occur naturally in all relationships. It is the unconscious transferring of experiences from a past interpersonal situation to another in the present that helps the therapist understand the patient and deepen the relationship. The resulting conscious and unconscious reactions and feelings that may be triggered in the therapist (counter-transference) also have the potential to facilitate the interpersonal work or, if not understood, complicate it. When the MHP has a lived experience with reproductive loss, it becomes crucially important that they have worked through and come to some resolution with their own feelings before entering the journey with their infertile patients.

All members of the treatment team, including infertility counselors, are at risk for compassion fatigue, a cumulative state of stress and tension from helping (or wanting to help) a traumatized or suffering individual, and which may occur suddenly. Compassion fatigue is different from burnout, an extreme state of dissatisfaction on many levels with one's work (often work environmental factors) that emerges slowly over time. It is a consequence of the deep caring, empathy, and sympathy for another's suffering or misfortune, an experience made more difficult if the caring professional has also suffered the same misfortune.[34]

Figley[34] contends that mental health professionals are vulnerable or susceptible to compassion fatigue due to a complex set of circumstances. First, compassion fatigue may be a natural by-product of the therapeutic relationship in that no matter how hard one tries, the therapist may not be able to be protected from the intensity of a patient's trauma. Second, empathy is a major resource and integral part of the therapeutic relationship, yet empathy can be a key factor in the induction of traumatic material from the primary to the secondary victim (i.e., the therapist). Consequently, the therapist as helper may be traumatized as well. Third, many trauma workers have experienced some traumatic event in their lives and a danger may arise from the therapist overgeneralizing his or her experiences and methods of coping and overpromoting these as helpful methods for the patient. Fourth, unresolved trauma for the therapist will typically be activated by reports of similar trauma in clients. Thus, infertility counselors with a similar reproductive history as their patients must be conscious of their counter-transference reactions and level of compassion fatigue so that they seek appropriate support, supervision, consultation, and/or psychotherapy for issues that occur in their practice.

Medical Staff Collaboration

Forming a strong, trusting, respectful relationship with physicians, nurses, genetic counselors, laboratory, and administrative personnel provides the foundation for infertility counselors in the collaborative reproductive healthcare model. Mental health professionals working in reproductive medicine often spend a great deal of time educating the medical team about what they do and how best to use their services, especially when first establishing a collaborative relationship. Role negotiation and clarification seem to remain an important and fundamental task of infertility counselors, a mission that is usually ongoing.[35,36] As in any relationship, it may take years to form a cohesive, collegial association and the process of working side-by-side in patient care may provide the best avenue toward the medical staff's understanding of what infertility counselors do. And like any relationship, there continues to be renegotiation and reshaping over time, as it is a fluid process.

The decision of when infertility counseling is essential and when it is optional may be left to the discretion of each medical practice or may be mandated by the government. The medical treatment team may look to the infertility counselor for assistance in defining when counseling should be required or recommended. Or the medical practice may have its own ideas about the necessity or applicability of counseling – which may conflict with the counselor's opinions, institutional recommendations, country regulations, or professional guidelines.

Inevitably, there are times in working with the medical team when an infertility counselor feels their role, skills, and services are undervalued and diminished, at best, or simply disregarded, dismissed, disrespected, and ignored, at worst. For example, the physician may make psychosocial decisions without the counselor's input or disregard suggestions the counselor has made in patient care. In some situations, the medical practice may refer a patient for counseling or assessment as a formality and have no intention of using the recommendations from the infertility counselor. As a result, infertility counselors may find themselves in an ethical dilemma of contracting with and accepting payment from a client for a service that they know is not really being provided. By the same token, the medical practice may not use a MHP at all, except when the patient is in a crisis, often during or following a treatment cycle. The MHP's role as a patient caregiver may be clear to the MHP and patient, yet the collaborative role with the medical team may be more complicated and complex. While there are no easy or simple answers to working through blocks to an effective collaborative relationship, being able to rely on the support and assistance of others working in the field is crucial.

Colleague Collaboration

Infertility counseling, like infertility, can be very challenging work and, at times, may be very isolating. As counselors struggle with difficult cases, ethical challenges, feeling unsupported by the medical team, family demands, and/or other taxing situations, having the support of other MHPs, particularly other infertility counselors, is critical. To begin, anyone doing infertility counseling should join both the reproductive medical society of their country or region as an allied health professional and, if available, the related psychosocial group (see Chapter 31). These infertility counseling organizations offer, among other things, continuing education, collaborative research, professional representation, and networking opportunities. With the advent of the internet and telecommunication, members are able to communicate with each other via listserves and email groups. These internet groups have become a lifeline for many infertility counselors, offering the ability to consult and exchange information and resources across continents.

Supervision and mentoring are another aspect of colleague collaboration. While it is ideal to have clinical supervision with a MHP who has infertility counseling experience, it is important that there be some appropriate place and person for the counselor to discuss their clinical work. If no one is available in the counselor's community, supervision or consultation could be arranged over the telephone or by email with an experienced infertility counselor. Peer supervision groups with others doing infertility counseling also are very useful. Mentoring may be offered through professional organizations (e.g., MHPG) and provide a means for helping an infertility counselor establish his or her practice; however, it is not a substitute for good clinical supervision.

Consumer Advocacy Organization Collaboration

The influence of infertility consumer advocacy groups in the growth and development of infertility counseling cannot be overlooked and, as such, is important to recognize as another collaborative relationship. Barbara Eck Menning, a nurse who was experiencing infertility, founded the first consumer advocacy group, Resolve, in 1974. Similar organizations quickly sprang up around the world and, today, infertility patients have a global forum of consumer groups through the International Federation of Infertility Patient Associations (IFIPA), a consortium of twenty member groups representing fifteen countries. These groups have been instrumental in educating the public about the emotional toll infertility plays in people's lives. They have been activists in medical organizations, with legislators, and the media to promote awareness and provide quality resources to infertility patients. As a result of the efforts of these organizations, infertility patients have become a powerful and influential group. Most importantly, consumer groups universally support the availability of infertility counseling to patients by qualified and skilled mental health professionals.[37]

In some ways, the founding of infertility patient organizations may be the single most influential event in the growth of infertility counseling. Mental health professionals often play an active role in these consumer organizations, serving on the executive boards of the institutions, facilitating support groups, helping to develop and write patient education materials, speaking, mediating internet programs, and engaging in consumer advocacy on local and international levels. Having infertility counselors actively involved in these organizations is mutually beneficial and can serve as a means of building both practice and support organization.

THERAPEUTIC INTERVENTIONS

This section clarifies areas involved in establishing an infertility counseling practice. It describes models for provision of services; roles of the infertility counselor; practice management issues; and practical tips for collaborative reproductive healthcare practice.

Models for Practice

Infertility counseling may be integrated into clinical practice in three ways, with the infertility counselor providing services as an independent private practitioner, independent consultant to the program, or employee of the reproductive medical practice. These practice frameworks are on a continuum from complete independence from the medical practice to complete integration into it as an employee. In each area, there are advantages and disadvantages for infertility counselors, patients, and the medical practice.

Independent Clinical Practice

Mental health professionals involved in their own independent private or group practice may serve as an outside referral source to a reproductive medical practice or physician. Patients are seen in the office of the counselor, which is separate and apart from the medical clinic where they receive care. Infertility counseling may be a small percentage of a general counseling and psychotherapy practice or the entire focus of the mental health professional's practice. In the independent clinical practice approach, the counselor operates completely independent of the referring physician or medical clinic, and communication between the counselor and medical team is limited and structured by traditional parameters of information exchange. Fee-for-service arrangements are handled between the therapist and patient, and patients must sign appropriate authorization for release of information. Thus, the therapist's primary responsibility is to the patient, not the referral source. Boundaries of the relationship are clearly defined and separate, an understanding that is underscored by the separate facilities.

Because the therapist operates completely independently of the medical practice, there is little potential for therapist coercion or conflict of interest – a distinct advantage of this arrangement. Patients often find this arrangement more comfortable: They feel freer to express negative feelings about care, objectively assess medical treatment alternatives, and discuss issues that they worry will impact the availability of care or alter the physician's positive feelings toward them. Disadvantages of this arrangement range from minor logistical problems to major impediments to care when patients refuse to sign an authorization for release of information or allow the therapist to share information with the medical staff that clearly has an impact on medical care or patient compliance.

Independent Practice Consultant

In this arrangement, the mental health professional is a consultant who works as an independent contractor to the medical practice. This arrangement represents a middle ground between the completely independent, off-site infertility counselor and the infertility counselor who is an on-site, practice employee. The infertility counselor usually sees patients at the medical practice, either renting office space from the medical practice or making some other arrangements for the use of office space. The counselor usually bills the patient on a fee-for-service basis, independently and separately from the medical practice. However, the infertility counselor may bill the medical practice for specific services that the clinic provides to patients, such as the initial counseling session, preparation for IVF, evaluation of oocyte donors or gestational carriers, or clinic support groups. The infertility counselor operates as an independent consultant and receives no benefits that an employee of the practice would normally receive.

The advantages of this arrangement include convenience for the patient, facilitation of crisis intervention, and continuity of care because of therapist proximity. Because services are integrated as an accepted part of treatment, the counseling experience is normalized. Being on the premises can also help the infertility counselor better understand the particular clinic's procedures and policies, which can facilitate patient education and preparation. In addition, the members of the treatment team may feel more comfortable consulting or discussing treatment problems with a counselor who is readily accessible. Infertility counselors often find the informal, curbside consultation one of the keystones of educating medical staff about the psychology of infertility.

A further advantage is that there is minimal expense to the practice for providing infertility counseling services. Because fee-for-service is handled independently of the medical clinic, the issues of coercion and job security are less relevant, although the counselor is still dependent on the medical practice for referrals. This arrangement allows greater integration of care, as the therapist operates and interacts more as a staff member, while maintaining professional and financial independence. However, the therapist positioned as a member of the treatment team may be advantageous in some situations (e.g., when a united front is required) or detrimental in other situations (e.g., when the counselor disagrees with medical treatment decisions).

The drawbacks of this arrangement often involve role misunderstandings, unclear boundaries, and boundary violations, particularly regarding confidentiality. Patients viewing the therapist as affiliated or associated with the practice may have more difficulty disclosing or establishing a therapeutic alliance, especially if they have disagreements with the medical practice or patients may expect or assume the MHP will share delicate information with the treatment team that the patient has been unable or reluctant to do. Boundaries of the relationships between the infertility counselor, staff, and the patient must be more clearly defined, discussed, and addressed early in counseling, so that issues of confidentiality and the therapist's role are clearly understood by all parties. This can be emphasized by the signing of appropriate release forms or written information that explicitly defines the counselor's relationship with the medical clinic. Nevertheless, the potential for confusion and misunderstanding is always there when counseling services are provided on the same premises as the medical clinic. When the therapist is on the premises, communication between the treatment team and infertility counselor is often less formal and may unwittingly involve unauthorized discussions or sharing of information.

Practice Employee

The third practice approach involves the mental health professional as a salaried employee of the medical practice and, as such, a formal member of the treatment team. This approach enables the integration of medical and psychological care with close collaboration between the members of the treatment team and the patient. Fees for counseling are billed by and paid to the medical practice, and the infertility counselor receives a predetermined salary. Because the counselor is a salaried staff member and consequently dependent on the practice for employment, there may be ethical concerns that the counselor's judgment is vulnerable to coercion or undue influence from the employing medical clinic and may be susceptible to bias or lack of objectivity. The infertility counselor may feel that her or his job may be jeopardized by recommendations that are unfavorable to the practice, such as rejection of an oocytes donor or disagreement with physicians. However, these concerns may not be as significant as they may seem at first in that the mental health professional has ethical standards and legal requirements of licensure that supersede employment responsibilities. Although the infertility counselor is part of the treatment, professional standards of confidentiality and relationship boundaries remain and should be clearly understood by all parties, including patients.

An advantage of this approach is that the infertility counselor is perceived and operates as an integral and equal member of the treatment team, attending patient care conferences and participating, when appropriate, in treatment decisions. Patient care may be more comprehensive, as the counselor is in the clinic, readily available, and patients are encouraged to access this service. Additionally, the MHP may have an active role in establishing clinic policies or as a member of the ethics committee. It is also thought that this approach legitimizes the importance of the psychological aspects of infertility, making it okay for patients to accept or take advantage of referrals for counseling. However, the disadvantages of this approach are similar to those described earlier, including boundary violations, conflicts of interest, and role confusion.

Roles in Practice

Infertility counselors serve as a resource to patients and staff by providing psychological services that support and enhance quality care. They can provide a variety of services including:[7]

■ assessment of patients' functioning in relation to their infertility;
■ evaluation of psychological readiness of participants for medical procedures, including recipients, gamete donors, surrogates, or carriers;
■ support, intervention, and treatment for the consequences of infertility or for underlying mental disturbances that could affect medical treatment;
■ education about psychological sequelae of infertility affecting individuals and families, and ways to deal with them;
■ research on reproductive psychology and on families created through advanced technology;
■ consultation with and support of the medical staff.

The role of the mental health professional involves both counseling and assessment. Counseling in its purest form entails advising and guiding patients about their options and treatments. Ideas and feelings are expressed in an atmosphere of mutual respect, trust, and safety. In addition, counseling involves knowledge of human behavior, interpersonal relationships, and family dynamics. With the knowledge of people and of reproductive medical treatment, infertility counselors can educate and assist patients with their choices and the possible consequences of their decisions.[37] Silman[38] delineated three areas of fertility counseling:

■ helping clients determine what it is they desire or seek;
■ exploring the implications of the desire, both physical and emotional, that might be overlooked in the 'excitement of the chase' for a baby;
■ supporting the decision with realistic information.

In assessment, infertility counselors offer psychological screening of participants in various assisted reproductive technologies and third-party reproduction. When the mental health professional is in this role, she or he may be seen as a gatekeeper recommending inclusion or exclusion of patient participation in treatment. Clearly, infertility counselors must be explicit with patients at the outset as to their role – counseling or assessment. If a decision is made to withhold or postpone treatment, the infertility counselor has a responsibility to inform the patient as to the reason for denial or deferral, and refer the individual or couple for follow-up counseling apart from the medical clinic.[39] Helping the patient understand the reasons for deferral and the need for more counseling may help to engage them in a postponement decision. Furthermore, a slippery slope exists for the mental health professional who is seeing an infertility patient in ongoing therapy and is asked to provide clearance for their patient needing treatment (i.e., donor gamete or IVF). Changing roles from counselor to evaluator raise serious ethical issues (e.g., dual relationships) and may threaten the therapeutic alliance. Keeping therapeutic boundaries completely clear and separate is usually in everyone's best interest (MHP and patient), and a referral to an independent infertility counselor for assessment or clearance is optimal.

If a recommendation to withhold or postpone treatment is made by the infertility counselor, a team consensus for exclusion is preferable and recommended by professional guidelines. In this sense, the counselor is not the gatekeeper; rather, the multidisciplinary team is sharing responsibility for inclusion and exclusion. It is important for the team to have developed written protocols and guidelines for denial or deferment of treatment that they include under what circumstances treatment may be denied (i.e., active substance abuse, untreated mental illness, or serious marital discord) and how it will be handled (i.e., letter to patient, phone call, or appointment with staff member). However, there may be situations in which the infertility counselor makes a recommendation for denial or deferral of treatment with which the team disagrees, or the team decides to overrule the counselor's recommendation. In these situations, the mental health professional should clearly document the reason for exclusion or postponement, including supporting information and evidence of notification to the treatment team for recommendations. Denying or deferring treatment is never easy for the mental health professional or medical staff. Thus, it may be helpful to look upon these recommendations as *protection* of the parties involved rather than *rejection*, because it is the first responsibility of medicine and all helping professionals *to do no harm*.

The role of evaluator and/or exclusion decisions are often difficult, and some infertility counselors find them objectionable and against their ethical beliefs. Some counselors refuse to make clear recommendations and instead provide a patient profile leaving the decision for inclusion or exclusion to the medical team or attending physician. However, this can be particularly problematic when the medical team, unable or unwilling to assess complex psychosocial issues, expects or depends on the expertise of the mental health professional. Ultimately, if the infertility counselor is uncomfortable or opposed to screening or evaluation, she or he should not accept these referrals and should notify medical practitioners accordingly.

Practice Management

It bears repeating that patients need to be made aware, at the beginning of any interview required or recommended by the medical clinic, of the counselor's role as part of the treatment team and, specifically, how it pertains to this interview. Issues of confidentiality and sharing of information with the medical team should be discussed, and signed consent to share information (when appropriate) should be obtained. Fees and billing arrangements should be in writing and discussed, especially in cases of third-party reproduction, in which the contracting parents may be financially responsible for evaluations. Counseling records and notes should be kept separate from medical records and under the therapist's (not clinic's) control. If a report is to be written, shared with the medical team, and/or made a part of the medical record, the patient must be made aware of this. Finally, the results of psychological testing should be reviewed with the patient in a manner that is understandable to her or him. If there are clinic policies regarding testing, such as requirements that patients

TABLE 28.3. Health and behavior assessment and intervention CPT codes[40]

CPT Code	Service*
96150	Assessment – initial
96151	Reassessment
96152	Intervention – individual
96153	Intervention – group
96154	Intervention – family w/ patient
96155	Intervention – family w/o patient

* Charge is in "units" – 15 minutes = 1 unit

score within a certain range, the patient should be made aware of this policy.

It is helpful to have patient information on the infertility counselor and the psychosocial services offered available in written materials, such as a practice brochure or handout. If counseling is required, such as for third-party participants, it is important to have clear, written information outlining why patients are being counseled or assessed, the goals to be achieved, how to make appointments, fees, billing and cancellation policy, testing information (if appropriate), and other relevant information. It is also helpful for the infertility counselor to have files of articles and resource information available to give patients as a psycho-educational part of the counseling session.

As MHPs have increased their involvement in treating patients with medical conditions, an important shift has occurred in the United States regarding coding for billing of services that allows for reimbursement. Previously, the Current Procedural Terminology (CPT) coding system required psychotherapy intervention codes and a mental health diagnosis, such as those in the Diagnostic and Statistical Manual of Mental Disorders, Fourth Edition (DSM-IV), for infertility patients to be eligible for insurance reimbursement.[40] However, in 2002, the coding system was changed to allow mental health professionals to apply health and behavioral assessment and intervention services for the prevention, treatment, and management of physical health problems (see Table 28.3). When a physician has made a physical health diagnosis (i.e., infertility), usually an International Classification of Diseases, Ninth Edition (ICD-9) code, services for assessment and intervention (i.e., donor oocyte recipient counseling) related to the diagnosis may be used for billing. However, these health and behavioral codes cannot be used for psychotherapy services, addressing the patient's mental health diagnosis, or on the same day as a psychiatric CPT code.[40]

This change reflects the growing role of mental health professionals in physical healthcare and a move away from the pathologizing the psychosocial experience of infertility and other medical conditions. Consequently, it is important that infertility counselors use these procedural codes when appropriate.

Practical Tips

As MHPs transition into the model of an infertility counselor doing collaborative reproductive healthcare, they must consider changes in the way they approach their practice. Recognizing the challenges this presents for clinicians, Haley and associates developed ten practical tips for psychologists working in primary healthcare.[41] These ten tips are good advice and easily adapted to MHPs working in reproductive medicine.

1. Do not wait for your patients to come to you. In traditional practice models, MHPs depend on direct referrals from the physician or other mental/healthcare provider. This practice has inherent flaws – physicians may not pick up issues that warrant a mental health referral and, when a referral is made, up to 50% of patients never follow through.[42] In addition, patients may hear this recommendation as a message that it is all in their heads, which further complicates follow-up for psychosocial services.

Normalization, location, and accessibility to infertility counseling services is a critical component to service delivery. When these services are viewed as a part of total reproductive healthcare and integrated into practice, patients view it as a normal aspect of their care. Physical proximity helps to ensure patient follow-through, as well as provides the opportunity for informal consultation between medical staff and infertility counselor regarding patient care. Infertility counselors also have the opportunity to reach out to patients through informal meetings and support groups, and medical staff are frequently reminded of this referral option by the physical presence of the MHP.

2. Many of your patients really are sick (i.e., infertile). Infertility counselors need to obtain full information about a patient's infertility and general health history as part of their overall assessment. The patient's subjective view of infertility is particularly important and understanding the ways they have responded to it, within the context of their family and culture. One of the most helpful aspects for infertility counselors of practicing within the medical setting is the ability to consult easily with the physician and nurse about the likely impact of a medical condition on psychological functioning. For example, a woman diagnosed with premature ovarian failure (POF) is dealing with a number of symptoms related to decreased estrogen (hot flashes, bone loss, and dry eyes, etc.) which affect her functioning as well as impair her fertility. Physical functioning affects individual and family dynamics, and vice versa, much more than is acknowledged in traditional psychological theory.[43] Thus, information about the medical management of the infertility (i.e., diagnosis and treatment), prognosis, and its effect on daily functioning need to be a part of the infertility counselor's treatment plan, as well as necessitating active collaboration.

3. No more 'Lone Ranger' – Join the 'posse.' Full collaboration with the reproductive medical team allows for comprehensive infertility services to be provided without distinction between physical and mental health. Haley and associates point out, "Successful collaboration involves . . . developing a collegial relationship with the referring provider, eliciting his or her explanation about the patient's problems, clarifying any questions, and securing his or her support for the psychological treatment."[41, p. 241] It also involves a strong working alliance with all members of the staff, knowledge and a respect for each of their areas of expertise. Physical proximity not only allows for better integration of psychosocial services but also for ability to introduce a patient to services through a joint session or meeting with the doctor or nurse. Communication between the infertility counselor and the physician or nurse regarding the patient's care (and vice versa) is fundamental in achieving effective teamwork. In short, infertility counselors cannot work in isolation and must see themselves as one part of the whole.

4. Psychotherapy is not enough. As has been discussed throughout this chapter, the role of the infertility counselor extends beyond traditional psychotherapy to a broad base of skills and services. Although infertility counseling is a specialized field, it involves a generalized skill set that demonstrates personal and professional flexibility. MHPs working in this field need to be able to provide a broad base of clinical services (such as psychotherapy, crisis intervention, and stress management), consultation and education services, research, as well as working with community, professional, and policy organizations. Collaborative reproductive healthcare means that infertility counselors cannot limit themselves to only clinical services but must look to the larger picture (and skill set) for practice.

5. Patients do not know why they are seeing you unless you tell them. Although infertility patients are often aware of the emotional responses to this condition (i.e., depression, anxiety, stress, and marital conflict), they frequently want their medical providers to be able to treat these problems. Patients may perceive a referral to a MHP as the physician thinks they are crazy, does not want to be bothered by them, or wants to get rid of them. Even in the most Westernized of cultures, a referral to a MHP may be looked upon as stigmatizing, further exacerbating these feelings in infertile people. When the MHP is involved in the referral, such as during a joint meeting with the patient and physician, there is the opportunity to model for the physician how to make a recommendation for counseling that is well-received by the patient.

One tactic is to help patients understand the multidisciplinary approach to infertility treatment and the specialized care that each member brings to the treatment team. To begin, it is important to clarify the patient's understanding of why they were referred to the infertility counselor and to address any misconceptions as to role and purpose of counseling. Clarifying confidentiality issues is crucial in defining communication with the physician/treatment team, even if it is only in acknowledging the referral. Physicians expect some communication about their patients with consulting healthcare providers, usually a brief description of diagnosis and treatment recommendations. Patients need to understand how this communication and collaboration is directed toward their best care, and be in agreement with the sharing of information.

6. Hurry up. Physicians and MHPs have very different practice styles, both in the time they see patients (i.e., fifteen-minute increments versus fifty-minute session) and approach (i.e., concrete solutions versus method and process). Reproductive medical practices operate at a rapid pace and outcomes of the interaction are expected quickly, which is in contrast to traditional psychotherapy practice. Communication with physicians needs to be clear, precise, and problem-focused. Referral questions need to be clarified so that solutions, or the need for further exploration and consultation, may be identified. In effect, infertility counselors need to take a problem-focused approach and learn how to communicate in the same language and style as physicians.

What is most important is timely and concise communication between physician/team and infertility counselor. Written reports to the medical team need to be completed quickly (ideally within a day) and should be summarized with essential findings and specific recommendations. If a report is longer than a page, a summary section of the most critical information with bullet points should be included because physicians rarely have the time to read a full report. Similarly (when applicable), notes in medical records should be brief, specific, and not speculatative. A follow-up phone call or email to the nurse or physician briefly describing the consultation and recommendations is essential, if a written report will not be available promptly.

7. Do not give any tests you cannot carry in a briefcase. While psychologists may be well-versed in administering a number of psychological tests, the acceptability and time required to complete these tests (as well as the fact they must be scored and interpreted only by those trained in the testing, usually psychologists) may limit usefulness in general infertility practices. Brief screening instruments that enhance the identification of patients who might benefit from seeing the infertility counselor are most useful to the medical team. These include the Primary Care Evaluation of Mental Disorders Brief Patient Health Questionnaire (PRIME-MD Brief PHQ), the Beck Depression Inventory (BDI), and the Beck Anxiety Inventory (BAI) to detect mood disorders, and the Fertility Problem Inventory (FPI) to determine the level of psychological stress with infertility. These validated tests can be easily administered and scored by any member of the treatment team to assess psychological distress, facilitate referral, or measure improvement over time for infertility-specific test (see Appendix 4).

8. Stand up for what you know, and ask about what you do not know. All MHPs working in reproductive medicine must demonstrate their expertise to the treatment team. They must be able to give decisive opinions on behavioral issues in patient care and be well-versed in current research on psychological aspects of infertility. Physicians are trained to challenge each other on evidence-based medicine, and infertility counselors should be prepared to operate in a similar manner (see Chapter 7). Infertility counselors need to be able to communicate their knowledge devoid of psychological jargon, which others may not understand or find distancing and condescending. While training in infertility counseling includes a broad knowledge of reproductive medicine, there will be times when the counselor is unfamiliar or unaware of new procedures or terminology. He or she must be comfortable and willing to ask questions to acquire the knowledge, as well as be involved in continuing education activities that involve both the medical and psychosocial aspects of reproductive healthcare. Mutual respect of the knowledge and skills each member of the treatment team brings to the practice is fundamental to effective collaboration.

9. No specialists allowed – be prepared for anything and everything. Infertility counseling is a specialized area of practice and yet patients bring a history to the experience beyond their impaired fertility. Patients may be dealing with a variety of situations and life experiences that impact their care – other medically complicating conditions, such as cancer, HIV, or genetic disorders; remarriage and step-families; gay or lesbian couples; single people; older couples; and experiences from different cultures – to name a few. MHPs need to be prepared for a diverse range of problems and be able to generalize their skills to the patient's special needs.

10. Refer out when necessary. The infertility counselor will not have the time, or necessarily the training, to see all patients of the practice with a wider spectrum of issues. He or she must be prepared to assess relatively quickly what type of care is needed and identify appropriate referral sources. For example, patients may request infertility treatment as a result of long-standing sexual dysfunction and a referral to sex therapist may be most appropriate. Or a substance abuse problem may be discovered in the course of evaluation, and a referral to a drug and alcohol treatment program is in order. In most cases, the infertility counselor will assess the situation and decide if the problems can be addressed within the context of the reproductive medical practice environment. With more complex cases where specialized or extensive intervention is needed, patients will be referred elsewhere for treatment. Consequently, it is important for the infertility counselor to have established a referral base of subspecialty mental health professionals and caregivers (i.e., acupuncturists, spiritual advisors, or psychopharmacology). In these situations, the infertility counselor may then serve as a bridge between physician and the outside referral source, to provide continuity of care. This is another aspect of collaborative care, the MHP collaborating with other mental health caregivers to improve and/or maximize patient well-being.

FUTURE IMPLICATIONS

Reproductive medicine will continue to change as advancing technology presents increasingly complex options and choices for patients. As clinical practice has become more specialized, so too has the need for more specialization of the staff members who make up the infertility treatment team. Infertility counselors provide psychological assessment, insight, and judgment that can assist the medical team in making increasingly difficult ethical and clinical decisions, as well as improving patient care.

To accomplish this task, infertility counselors must be highly skilled therapists who are knowledgeable about the medical and emotional aspects of reproductive medicine. There is an increasing need for training programs, practicums, and continuing education workshops on infertility counseling, especially its application within the specific mental health professions. International collaboration with other mental health professionals working in the field of reproductive health psychology will be crucial to achieve these objectives

Credentialing and the need to establish defined standards of care in infertility counseling is a more immediate goal. Qualification guidelines have been established in the two largest professional organizations, ASRM/MHPG and ESHRE/PSIG. Nonetheless, they are just that: *guidelines*. Furthermore, while a number of countries have mandated the provision of infertility counseling (Great Britain, Australia, and Canada), it is less clear who is considered qualified to provide these services.

Increasingly, mental health professionals working in reproductive medicine have indicated the belief that specialty status or credentialing is necessary for infertility counseling. How it should be accomplished is a greater question. The British Infertility Counseling Association (BICA) has developed the Infertility Counseling Award, a specialty status system based upon resume and case review. However, its usefulness may be in questions as, to date, only a very small number of counselors have actually applied and even fewer have actually met the requirements to obtain this credentialing. Infertility nurses in the ASRM experienced a similar difficulty when attempts were made to establish certification in reproductive endocrinology nursing that was later abandoned due to lack of participation and problems in administering the examinations. On a parallel note, Burns and Figlerski surveyed members of ASRM/MHPG in 1999 and 2002 to assess members' interest in credentialing and specialty status. Although the majority in both studies believed there should be special credentialing in infertility counseling, they were reluctant to participate in the process.[44] All of the respondents considered themselves expert in the field, yet were increasingly unwilling to pursue credentialing/specialty status, the more rigorous the requirements. Respondents were willing to: obtain continuing education credits (74%); make an application (70%); attend postgraduate courses (66%); take a certification exam (34%); undergo skills/knowledge evaluation to maintain certification (31%); pursue Diplomate status (30%); submit cases for review by a board (20%); and complete an internship, mentorship, or fellowship (10%). The establishment of meaningful credentials in infertility counseling that are accepted by practitioners and recognized by the reproductive medical team remains a challenge.

It is becoming increasingly important for infertility counselors to be involved in scientific research about the psychological aspects of infertility, the impact of reproductive technology, and the efficacy of various psychological interventions. Possibly the most important area of research is the long-range impact on offspring and families created by advancing reproductive technologies. Families are being created today through technologies that just a few years ago were thought to be fiction, not unlike Aldous Huxley's *Brave New World*. As much as infertility counselors may advise patients about the implications of these technologies, no one can predict how someone will feel tomorrow about his or her decisions, let alone ten years from now. Age, experience, unexpected life events, and societal changes are only a few factors influencing feelings as time goes on. Thus, it is crucial for infertility counselors to be involved in and aware of research and clinical practice in ways that provide a greater understanding of families affected by a legacy of infertility and/or created through assisted reproductive technologies.

SUMMARY

■ Although all members of the reproductive medical team counsel and console patients, infertility counselors are mental health professionals who provide specialized services of psychological assessment, psychotherapeutic intervention, psychoeducational support, psychological research, and staff consultation.

■ The collaborative reproductive healthcare model is based on biopsychosocial theory and emphasizes a seamless collaboration between all members of the reproductive medical team, including infertility counselors, and the patient to provide optimum care.

■ In this model, infertility counseling is viewed along a continuum of the medical process, where the medical and psychosocial aspects of infertility treatment are integrated.

■ Effective collaboration in infertility counseling involves patients, medical staff, other mental health professionals, and community and consumer organizations.

■ Infertility counseling services may be incorporated into clinical practice in three ways: (1) referral to an independent, private practitioner who is outside the medical practice; (2) use of an independent contract consultant, who is affiliated with the practice; or (3) hiring of an employee, who is an infertility counselor and a staff member.

■ Infertility counselors must explicitly define their roles and responsibilities to patients and staff.

■ Credentialing and/or specialty status of infertility counselors is necessary to help ensure quality standard of care.

■ Infertility counselors must be involved in research on the psychological aspects of infertility, the impact of reproductive technologies, and the efficacy of psychological interventions.

REFERENCES

1. Marsch EM, Vollmer AM. Possible psychogenic aspects of infertility. *Fertil Steril* 1951; 2:70–9.
2. Rubenstein BB. Emotional factors in infertility: A psychosomatic approach.*Fertil Steril* 1951; 2:80–6.
3. Bresnick E, Taymor ML. The role of counseling in infertility. *Fertil Steril* 1979; 32:154–6.
4. Klock SC, Maier D. Guidelines for the provision of psychological evaluations for infertile patients at the University of Connecticut Health Center. *Fertil Steril* 1991; 56:680–5.
5. Covington SN. Preparing the patient for in vitro fertilization: Psychological considerations. *Clin Consider Obstet Gynecol* 1994; 6:131–7.
6. Daniels KR. Management of psychosocial aspects of infertility. *Aust N Z J Obstet Gynaecol* 1992; 32:57–63.
7. Covington SN. The role of the mental health professional in reproductive medicine. *Fertil Steril* 1995; 64:895–7.
8. Benedek T. Infertility as a psychosomatic defense. *Fertil Steril* 1952; 3:527–41.
9. Fischer IC. Psychogenic aspects of sterility. *Fertil Steril* 1953; 4:466–7l.
10. Ford ESC, Forman I, Willson JB, et al. A psychodynamic approach to the study of infertility. *Fertil Steril* 1953; 4:456–65.
11. Berger DM. The role of the psychiatrist in a reproductive biology clinic. *Fertil Steril* 1977; 28:141–5.
12. Rosenfeld DL, Mitchell E. Treating the emotional aspects of infertility: Counseling services in an infertility clinic. *Am J Obstet Gynecol* 1979; 135:177–80.
13. Sarrel PM, DeCherney AH. Psychotherapeutic intervention for treatment of couples with secondary infertility. *Fertil Steril* 1985; 43:897–900.
14. Covington SN. Psychosocial evaluation of the infertile couple: Implications for social work practice. In: D Valentine, ed, *Infertility and Adoption: A Guide for Social Work Practice*. New York: Haworth Press, 1988; 21–36.
15. Menning BE. The emotional needs of infertile couples. *Fertil Steril* 1980; 34:313–9.
16. Mahlstedt P. The psychological component of infertility. *Fertil Steril* 1985; 43:335–46.
17. Monach J. Counselling – Its role in the infertility team. *Hum Fertil* 2003; 6:S17–21.
18. Greenfeld D, Mazure C, Haseltine F, et al. The role of the social worker in the in-vitro fertilization program. *Soc Work Health Care* 1984; 10:71–9.
19. Freeman EW, Boxer AS, Rickels K, et al. Psychological evaluation and support in a program of in vitro fertilization and embryo transfer. *Fertil Steril* 1985; 43:48–53.
20. Stotland NL. Contemporary issues in obstetrics and gynecology for the consultation-liaison psychiatrist. *Hosp Community Psychiatry* 1985; 36:1102–8.
21. Paulson RJ, Sauer MV. Counseling the infertile couple: When enough is enough. *Obstet Gynecol* 1991; 78:462–4.

22. Braverman AM. Ovum Donor Task Force of the Psychological Special Interest Group of the American Fertility Society. Survey results of the current practice of ovum donation. *Fertil Steril* 1993; 59:1216–20.

23. Boivin J, Kenenich H, eds. *Guidelines for Counseling in Infertility*. ESHRE Monographs. Oxford University Press, 2002.

24. Kainz K. The role of the psychologist in the evaluation and treatment of infertility. *Womens Health Issues* 2001; 11:481–5.

25. Gagin RM, Cohen M, Greenblatt L, et al. Developing the role of the social worker as coordinator of services at the surrogate parenting center. *Soc Work Health Care* 2004; 40:1–14.

26. Covington SN, Marosek KR. Personal infertility experience among nurses and mental health professionals working in reproductive medicine. *Fertil Steril* 1999; 72:S129.

27. Martin MS, Walker ME. Exploring the impact on the genetic counseling process when the counselor has a significant genetic or reproductive history. *J Genet Couns* 1995; 4:327–32.

28. Doherty WJ. The why's and levels of collaborative family health care. *Fam Sys Med* 1995; 13:275–81.

29. Bitzer J. Quality assessment and quality in psychosomatic obstetrics and gynecology: Old wine in new bottles? *J Psychosom Obstet Gynecol* 2001; 22:67–8.

30. Watkins KJ, Baldo TD. The infertility experience: Biopsychosocial effects and suggestions for counselors. *J Counsel Develop* 2004; 82:394–420.

31. Covington SN. The psychosocial evaluation of the infertile couple within the medical context. In: *Counseling the Infertile Couple (IX)*. Proceedings of Twenty-third Annual Postgraduate Course; 1990 Oct 13–14; Washington, DC. Birmingham, AL: American Society for Reproductive Medicine (formerly the American Fertility Society), 1990; 26–48.

32. Feldman PR. Infertility: A view of its medical and emotional aspects. In: *Counseling the Infertile Couple (IX)*. Proceedings of Twenty-third Annual Postgraduate Course; 1990 Oct 13–14; Washington, DC. Birmingham, AL: American Society for Reproductive Medicine (formerly the American Fertility Society), 1990; 2–23.

33. Rosen A, Rosen J. eds. *Frozen Dreams: Psychodynamic dimensions of Infertility and Assisted Reproduction*. New York: Analytic Press, 2005.

34. Figley CR, ed. *Compassion Fatigue: Coping with Secondary Traumatic Stress Disorder in Those Who Treat the Traumatized*. New York: Brunner/Mazel, 1999.

35. Applegarth LD. The role of the mental health professional: What are the boundaries of our responsibilities? In: *ART Parents and Children: An Integration of Clinical Experience and Psychosocial Research to Counsel the Next Generation (XII)*. Proceedings of Twenty-eighth Annual Postgraduate Course of the American Society for Reproductive Medicine; 1995 Oct 7–8; Seattle, WA. Birmingham, AL: American Society for Reproductive Medicine, 1995; 175–82.

36. Covington SN. Historical Overview of Infertility Counseling and Models of Service. In: *Infertility Counseling: An Emphasis on Therapeutic Interventions*. Proceedings of the Thirty-second Annual Postgraduate Course of the American Society of Reproductive Medicine; 1999 Oct 25–6; Toronto, Canada. Birmingham, AL: ASRM, 1999; 1–11.

37. Covington SN. Reproductive medicine and mental health professionals: The need for collaboration in a brave new world. *Orgyn* 1997; 3:19–21.

38. Silman R. What is fertility counseling? In: SE Jennings, ed., *Infertility Counselling*. Oxford: Blackwell Science, 1995; 205–13.

39. Covington SN. Ethical issues in infertility counseling. In: National Advisory Board on Ethics in Reproduction. Washington, DC. *NABER Report* 1996; 2:4–6.

40. American Psychological Association Practice Directorate and Interdivisional Healthcare Committee. *Health and Behaviour CPT Coding System*. 2002.

41. Haley WE, McDaniel SH, Bray JH, et al. Psychological practice in primary care settings: Practical tips for clinicians. *Prof Psychol Res Prac* 1998; 29:237–44.

42. Callahan CM, Hendrie HC, Dittus RS, et al. Improving treatment of late-life depression in primary care: A randomized clinical trial. *J Am Ger Soc* 1994; 42:839–46.

43. McDaniel SH, Hepworth J, Doherty WJ. *Medical Family Therapy: A Biopsychosocial Approach for Families with Health Problems*. New York: Basic Books, 1992.

44. Burns LH, Figlerski L. Task Force on Credentialing Report 1999, 2002, 2005. www.asrm.org, MHPG website. Retrieved 11/1/2005.

29 Ethical Aspects of Infertility Counseling

NANCY STOWE KADER AND DOROTHY A. GREENFELD

Knowledge not based on ethics cannot . . . bring real honor or profit to its master.

– Marie de Jars

Since the beginning of in vitro fertilization (IVF) and the advent of assisted reproductive technology (ART) more than twenty-five years ago, mental health professionals (MHPs) working in the field of reproductive medicine have counseled couples struggling with complex ethical decisions resulting from the very treatment that promises such hope. The overlap between ethical dilemmas for patients and how they psychologically experience these issues is an ongoing part of the work between the MHP and the infertile couple. Indeed, as clinicians strive to understand and assist patients in dealing with unprecedented ART developments, the interface between psychological and ethical issues has steadily shaped and defined the role of the MHP in the ART milieu.

This chapter

■ addresses ethical issues and challenges as they relate to mental health professionals and infertility;
■ reviews literature produced by ethics committees and mental health professionals;
■ describes ethical principles and the role of an ethics committee;
■ identifies ethically complex clinical issues for programs, such as requests for posthumous reproduction;
■ provides a model for establishing an ethics committee in the practice;
■ suggests implications for future counseling dilemmas in fertility programs.

HISTORICAL OVERVIEW

Since the time of the ancient Greeks, healthcare professionals have accepted special moral obligations governing their practices. The injunction 'first, do no harm,' loosely derived from the Hippocratic oath, is held by physicians (and by extension, all healthcare profession-

als) to be the foundation of their professional ethic. Over time, each of the various healthcare professions has adopted a code of conduct to guide them as they carry out their specific responsibilities.

Despite the acceptance of ethical codes of behavior, the medical profession has historically conducted research and experimentation upon human subjects, sometimes offering benefits to their patients, but at times causing harm. A need for broader and more internationally based rules of conduct was realized after World War II when the Nuremberg trials disclosed the medical atrocities inflicted by German physicians upon their prisoners. In 1947, the Nuremberg Code was accepted as international law, asserting the principle of voluntary and informed consent along with other safeguards on human experimentation. The postwar ethical ferment also led to the formation of the World Medical Association, a national body which produced, in 1954, "Principles for Those in Research and Experimentation." These principles became the precursor to the adoption of the Helsinki Declaration in 1964 (last amended in 1989), wherein most of today's familiar rules on voluntary consent and the protection of the autonomy of the human subject were firmly established.[1]

Physicians in the United States were not faultless during this era. It was not until 1972 that the infamous Tuskegee Study was halted amid acrimony and outrage. News reports disclosed that hundreds of poor black men in Tuskegee, Alabama, had been monitored since the 1930s to learn the long-term effects of syphilis without being told they were part of a study; and even worse, they were not given treatment even after penicillin proved to be effective. The outrage over this immoral violation of human rights led to the congressional creation of the National Commission for the Protection of Human Subjects of Biomedical and

Behavioral Research. The regulations drawn up by this body form the basis for our current ethical requirements over human experimentation today. Furthermore, this tumult instigated new interest in ethical behavior in medicine leading to a new field of inquiry, which we know today as bioethics.[2,3]

By the 1970s, a new discipline emerged from the interaction of two fields of study, ethics and the biological sciences, coining a new term: bioethics.[4] Ethics is the philosophical study of morality, where one task is to provide a systematic means of evaluating moral problems. Bioethics takes on a more specific mission, that of *applying* ethical insights to real problems in biomedicine, especially those arising out of actual practice situations. These are not theoretical problems to be studied in the abstract, but real problems affecting real people, so it is important that the answers put forward in the field achieve something more than moral correctness. They must also be clinically useful, practical, and reasonably acceptable to those affected by them. Historically, philosophers and legal scholars typically addressed these matters. However, mental health professionals quickly became directly involved in bioethical concerns because "many ethical questions raise psychological issues."[5]

Because of the particular vulnerability of their patients, mental health professionals (including those working in infertility clinics) have developed extensive and complex guidelines regarding their ethical obligations to their patients. However, the cascade of rapid technological advances in the treatment of infertility in the mid-twentieth century has introduced a steadily increasing number of complex, new health-related moral problems in the infertility clinic, issues that could not be easily resolved by simply referring to a professional code of ethics.

ART and Ethics

Reproductive medicine has been at the forefront in producing technological challenges to traditional moral thinking beginning with the 1978 announcement of the first IVF birth of Louise Brown in Great Britain, an announcement that raised moral anxieties around the world. The ethical issues engendered by subsequent advances in ART treatment (such as oocyte donation, embryo cryopreservation, intracytoplasmic sperm injection (ICSI), pre-implantation genetic diaqnosis (PGD), and the potential for harvesting stem cells from embryos) have led to a robust and increasingly urgent ongoing ethical debate. This is equally true of ARTs treatments that are only potentially feasible at this time (e.g., cloning).

Since the early days of IVF, as programs were formed and treatment teams were put together, mental health professionals at once became vital members of the team. As members of the treatment team, they were asked to participate in institutional ethics committees where crucial decisions were made about ART treatment. The role of the mental health professional in ART is in itself a focus of ethical debate. For example, is it appropriate for the MHP to be a gatekeeper – helping to determine whether a specific treatment is appropriate for a specific individual or couple? Does the MHP's role include an obligation to assess patients for their suitability to take on the role of parent?

ART organizations worldwide have formed ethics committees to address issues arising as a result of these new technologies. The American Society for Reproductive Medicine (ASRM) established an Ethics Committee in 1985 that initially consisted of four obstetrician/gynecologists, an attorney, an attorney/ethicist, a reproductive biologist, and an endocrinologist.[6] The Committee held a news conference to announce its first report in 1986 entitled "Ethical Considerations of the New Reproductive Technologies."[7] In subsequent years, the membership has changed and in 1999, for the first time, the Committee included a mental health professional.

Another ART professional organization began at a meeting in Helsinki in the early 1980s when fellow scientists R. G. Edwards of the United Kingdom and J. Cohen of France conceived the idea for a European organization that would meet to stimulate research and study in reproductive medicine. In 1985, the European Society of Human Reproduction and Embryology (ESHRE) held its first meeting in Bonn, Germany. ESHRE currently has more than 4,000 members representing 101 countries. In 1990, ESHRE formed a special task force on Ethics and Law. The group has addressed such issues as postmortem reproduction, cloning, surrogacy, and sex selection. All members of the task force are members of ESHRE and are generally either physicians or mental health professionals. In any case, MHPs have valuable input.[8]

The Ethics Committees for both ASRM and ESHRE publish papers that are recommendations and guidelines for practitioners working in the field of ART. That is quite different from organizations established as a result of laws passed governing ART treatment. For example, following passage of the Human Fertilisation and Embryology Act of 1990, the Human Fertilisation and Embryology Authority (HFEA) was established in the United Kingdom. This licensing organization included a code of practice guidelines for all licensed infertility clinics that outlined the proper specific treatment procedures and activities. The HFEA also developed and maintained a formal register of "information about donors, treatments and children born as a result of those treatments."[9] In 2003, the HFEA established a Law and Ethics Committee to address ethical dilemmas (e.g., stem cell research, advances in PGD). Members of that committee, as are all members of HFEA, are appointed by health ministers of the United Kingdom and require that the Chair, Deputy Chair, and at least half the members are neither doctors nor scientists involved in ART. They are often members of the clergy, philosophers, and lawyers.[9]

REVIEW OF THE LITERATURE

Literature from Ethics Committees

The aforementioned organizations and their Ethics Committees have published literature addressing the ongoing ethical concerns of MHPs, ART treatment teams, and patient participation in these treatments. For example, the sixth edition of the HFEA Code of Practice manual published in 2004 includes sections on surrogacy, oocyte donation, embryo storage, and oocyte sharing with an emphasis on the welfare of the child so conceived. There is also a section on various aspects of counseling, including 'implications counseling,' that is, making sure that the person being counseled understands the treatment; 'support counseling' – emotional support offered during times of particular stress, such as treatment failure; and 'therapeutic counseling' – providing coping strategies for participants.[9] An important issue regarding counseling under HFEA is the provision that counseling be *offered*, not necessarily taken up. Furthermore, although HFEA provides specifics on what the counseling should include, it does not specifically address who is qualified to provide this counseling.

The ESHRE Task Force on Law and Ethics has published a number of papers resulting from committee discussions of current ethical concerns. This committee faces unique challenges in that it is not a governing body but a professional organization representing 101 countries. As such, their recommendations on policy must take into consideration very diverse cultural, religious, and ethical approaches, as well as government laws regarding infertility treatments and family-building options. For example, several papers concern aspects of oocyte donation such as disclosure to donor offspring and payment to oocyte donors.[10–15] Because in some countries payments to oocyte donors are illegal, some of the ESHRE recommendations

have addressed the ethical and practical applications of oocyte-sharing and other unique donor recruitment policies and practices between IVF patients and recipients.[16–19] Several papers from the task force have addressed ethical issues in posthumous reproduction[20–24] and concluded that it was generally acceptable and supported by most centers, but that "each case should be discussed and authorized by a multidisciplinary committee that includes physicians, clergy, psychiatrists, psychologists, sociologists and other appropriate parties."[21] Other papers looked at the issue of legitimizing surrogacy in Israel[25] and in the United Kingdom.[26–28] Ethical and social concerns of prenatal sex selection (also called gender selection or family balancing) were addressed,[29–34] including a survey of geneticists from thirty-seven nations where 46% approved of performing sex selection for family balancing.[32]

The Ethics Committee of the ASRM has published statements that address current issues in ART programs and go to the heart of clinical concerns for MHPs working in the field of reproductive medicine. For example, a common clinical concern is acceptance or rejection of a specific individual or couple for a specific treatment based on their potential to be good parents. A recent paper addressed this issue and recommended that programs should not discriminate against persons with disabilities, yet identified reasons to reject potential treatment candidates including uncontrolled psychiatric problems, substance abuse, and a history of perpetrating physical and/or emotional abuse or neglect. The committee recommended that rejection decisions should be made by the various members of the treatment team, which may include assessments by the MHP[35] and should, ideally, be based on the clinic's (preferably predetermined) policy and/or treatment protocol. In a recent report, regarding disclosure to offspring about their donor gamete conception, the committee recommended that "while ultimately the choice of the recipient parents, disclosure should be encouraged," counseling and informed consent should be required for donors as well as recipients.[36] Intergenerational gamete donation, using family members as donors and surrogates, is another common clinical concern that was addressed in a recent report. The Committee concluded that while the use of sibling donation (brother to brother, sister to sister) is generally acceptable, intergenerational gamete donation and surrogacy arrangements are 'especially challenging' and require special attention such as monitoring for undue influence of a relative and the appearance of incest.[37] Two statements addressed the issue of sex selection.[38,39]

In 1999, in a statement on sex selection and PGD[39] the Committee found that IVF with PGD solely for sex selection should be discouraged because of the risk for gender bias, social harm, and the diversion of medical resources from genuine medical need.[39] Another statement in 2001 addressed the use of sperm selection techniques for nonmedical gender selection. The Committee recommended that if such techniques prove to be safe and effective, physicians should be free to offer these services for sex selection for 'gender variety' as long as couples understand the risk of failure and would agree to accept the child of opposite sex if the treatment should fail.[38] A statement regarding financial incentives for oocyte donors recommended that donors not be compensated more than $10,000.[40]

Literature from Mental Health Professionals

The interface between psychological issues and ethical dilemmas associated with ART has been addressed in the mental health literature. Considerable literature has addressed ethical dilemmas faced by MHPs themselves in their complex roles as educators, counselors, and gatekeepers.[41,42] Covington described the role of the MHP in the infertility practice as encompassing five primary functions: assessment and evaluation; intervention and treatment; education; research; and consultation.[43] She pointed out the importance of working with an ethics committee and provided a model for establishing an ethics committee in the infertility practice,[44] as well as a model when working independently, inspired by research by Chally and Loriz.[45] Gordon and Barrow describe ethical, legal, and moral issues that have become "part and parcel of the infertility counselor's domain," such as fetal reduction, posthumous reproduction, and sex selection.[42]

Other research described the overlap between psychological and ethical issues associated with ART and how the role of the MHP has extended to counseling in such complex areas as preimplantation genetic diagnosis with its potential for sex selection, posthumous reproduction, and disposition of unwanted embryos.[5] Rosenthal described ethical and psychological aspects of oocyte donation and the problem of "counseling donors in the abstract." By that, the author means envisioning future scenarios where, for example, a donor may find herself infertile.[46]

An unsettled and often contentious debate among MHPs working in ART is whether assessment includes the role of program 'gatekeeper.' Some clinicians feel that part of their role is that of gatekeeper, assessing if, when, how, or whether an individual and/or couple can

or should proceed with a specific treatment. From this perspective the role of the MHP is one that takes into consideration the best interest of the potential child, the ability of the participants to provide informed consent, and/or comply with the medical treatment plan. Others feel that the role of the MHP is to provide support, education, and preparation but not to determine which patients are psychologically eligible for treatment, asserting "no one monitors the fertile world." Still others try to take a middle of the road approach, which encompasses aspects of both roles, recognizing that as educated professionals, the MHP has an ethical duty and professional responsibility to provide some measure of assessment as well as education, preparation, and support.[5,42]

THEORETICAL FRAMEWORK

IVF programs and members of ART treatment teams (including MHPs) have two resources to turn to when they are grappling with ethically difficult treatment decisions: an institutional review board (IRB) and an ethics advisory committee. While the IRB is particularly useful to scientific research and ethical issues regarding the development of *new* treatments and technologies, ethics committees are particularly helpful for discussion of the moral and ethical impact of *established* treatments and technologies.[47]

The purpose of the IRB is to review biomedical research to be clear about the rights of study subjects and to make sure that investigators follow the principles of the Helsinki Declaration. Those principles are that research should be conducted by scientifically qualified and competent researchers; that research should be properly designed; that the confidentiality of subjects should be maintained; and that subjects should be able to give informed consent. The institutional review board is generally regulated by the state or the government.[47]

Unlike IRBs, ethics committees are not governed by the state or government regulation and were created to address moral dilemmas resulting from particular medical technology. The first ethics committee was established in the United States in 1962 after the development of the arteriovenous shunt and canula, which made dialysis possible. The marvel of the technology meant that the demand exceeded the availability, and a small group met, whose initial role was to determine who was an appropriate candidate for dialysis.[47] The role of the ethics advisory committee includes case review, education, and policy review. However, Elias and Annas point out that "the far more important role of the ethics committee is the protection of the dignity of the patients."[48]

While there is no overarching single ethical theory per se, bioethics has turned to a special set of principles as key to helping clarify the basic moral issues. These principles are autonomy, beneficence, nonmaleficence, and justice. They were originally introduced by Beauchamp and Childress in an early textbook in bioethics and are now so well accepted that their use has earned a term: principlism.[49] Each principle provides an important point of view in assessing moral problems and can be used to remind the clinician of the important moral values at stake.

Autonomy

This principle holds that people have the right to determine their own actions based upon their personal values and beliefs.[49] It is the principle that forms the basis of informed consent and respect for privacy. In an ART setting, autonomy refers to an individual's reproductive rights and choices. It includes the individual's right to medical information about the treatment being considered and the individual's right to make decisions about which treatment to accept (if any) or reject (e.g., refuse treatment).[4] However, since assisted reproduction depends on the cooperation of more than one individual, the autonomous choices of each participant can conflict, causing a need for mediation.

Beneficence

This principle represents an obligation to promote the well-being of patients, protecting them from harm while promoting and encouraging the greater good. It is closely aligned with the principal of nonmaleficence, balancing actions between good and potential harm. There may be overlap between the principles of beneficence and nonmaleficence when, for example, a patient with a medical disorder that would be exacerbated by pregnancy requests IVF treatment, or HIV incongruent couples request husband inseminations which could increase risk of disease transmission to the uninfected spouse.

Nonmaleficence

This principle identifies the obligation to 'do no harm,' and may at times conflict with the principal of autonomy or other principles. Illustrative is a physician's refusal to treat in order to refrain from harming the patient, although the refusal may compromise the patient's autonomy.[4] The physician who recommends transferring no more than two embryos while the couple requests transferring multiple embryos is another good example. Because this principle is at the core of

the Hippocratic oath, it may take precedence in decision making.

Justice

This principle concerns fairness and equity, specifically with regard to sharing the burden (costs) and in the distribution of resources (benefits) to all members of the community. With the exception of countries where there is uniform health insurance that covers infertility treatment, much of the world does not meet this standard. Lack of insurance coverage, variations in covered services, and the frequent determination by insurance companies that infertility is not as a disease, often make infertility treatment unavailable to patients with low income. This is particularly true with third-party reproduction (oocyte donation and surrogacy), where generally only wealthy couples can afford these reproductive services, even in countries with mandated health coverage. This phenomenon has been referred to as 'stratified reproduction' to describe transnational inequalities whereby some people are able to achieve their reproductive desires, often through recourse to globalizing technologies, while others – usually poor women of color around the globe – are disempowered (and even despised) as reproducers.[49] A further consequence of stratified reproduction is 'reproductive tourism,' in which infertile individuals or couples with financial means travel across borders to access ARTs that are not available for legal, religious, or cultural reasons in their own country.

CLINICAL ISSUES

Decisions that may be a routine part of treatment can be ethically and morally troubling for many couples. Some couples may be troubled about the disposition of embryos. Other couples may struggle with the dilemma of selective reduction of a multiple pregnancy. For other couples, the quandary may be about whether or not to use a family member or a friend as a gamete donor or whether to disclose the donor conception to the child, friends, or family. A dilemma for some couples may be whether or not to pursue parenthood using medical treatments that are opposed by their religion, culture, or family. Additionally, couples may present for treatment in various states of psychosocial distress potentially impairing functioning and/or ability to comply with treatment or there can be disagreement about treatment involving coercion of one partner by the other. These are just a small sample of the sorts of issues that arise continually in a reproductive medicine clinic.

Mental health professionals and their treatment teams experience their own ethical dilemmas and may find themselves uncomfortable with some treatment decisions. Issues that inevitably arise include requests for infertility treatment from patients with a concomitant illness such as HIV/AIDS, women of advanced maternal age, intergenerational gamete donation, same-sex couples, and patients requesting posthumous reproduction. This underscores the value of having access to an ethics committee (or the importance of developing such a committee) for the practice.

Treating Patients with Concomitant Illness

Some prospective mothers face concerns about embarking on fertility treatment because of a history of a serious preexisting illness such as a heart condition, cancer, or HIV infection. The question at stake is whether a pregnancy will exacerbate the illness or whether the severity of illness might necessitate the use of a donor or surrogate. In either case, the ethical question can be settled by assessing known scientific data, considering how similar cases have been handled, and evaluating the likelihood that ovulatory stimulation or pregnancy could cause a recurrence of symptoms or a risk to the patient's/offspring's health or life. Often such risks can be quantified, allowing participants to be given the right to choose their own options with a clear understanding of the degree of risk involved. However, sometimes these risks cannot be quantified or the patient may choose to proceed with treatment against medical advice.

Initially, pregnancy was contraindicated in patients with established HIV infections, but recent research introduced methods that decrease the possibility of transmitting the virus to others, making it safer to attempt fertilization and pregnancy. Nevertheless, the potential for transmission, not only to the child but also to a noninfected partner, necessitates careful consideration of each case.[50] An instance where a healthy person assumes an unnecessary risk for a potential goal (versus a necessary risk to save a life) adds a difficult moral dimension to the problem. In some cases, the assessment of the emotional stability of the participants by the infertility counselors might be the deciding factor for guiding the process. Furthermore, the infertility counselor may be in the best position to provide appropriate education, support, and therapeutic assistance, enabling individuals and couples to come to terms with the psychosocial and medical realities of their situation.

Treating Women of Advanced Maternal Age

ART treatment teams are increasingly faced with requests from women of advanced reproductive age seeking medical assistance to become pregnant. Oocyte donation has afforded older women the opportunity to give birth well beyond menopause, and many are taking advantage of this opportunity. In this situation, clinicians must struggle with questions such as whether the life expectancy of the prospective mother should be a consideration in determining whether to proceed. How should clinicians weigh the risks of pregnancy against the rights of a woman to choose such treatment? And what about the children? Should programs be concerned about the children raised by mothers who will presumably have a lifespan considerably shorter than women who bear children before menopause?

At present, guidelines regarding the ethical propriety of this extension of the normal reproductive age vary greatly. For example, ESHRE, the Canadian Fertility and Andrology Society (CFAS), and the ASRM have *not* issued clear guidelines on this issue and have not addressed the most pressing question, 'What is the appropriate age limit for acceptance of women into treatment?' The exception is the HFEA, which determined that recipients of donor oocytes should not be older than the age of forty-five, based on the view that it is in the best interest of the child to be parented into young adulthood.

In the United States, there is great disparity among programs accepting postmenopausal women into treatment. For example, Practice Guidelines from the ASRM recommend that all recipients of oocyte donation over the age of forty-five undergo thorough medical evaluation including cardiovascular testing and a high-risk obstetrical consultation before treatment. The guidelines do not specify recommendations for age restrictions, however.[51] A statement from the ASRM Ethics Committee asserted that oocyte donation to postmenopausal women "should be discouraged" and that programs should determine eligibility for proceeding with treatment on a 'case by case' basis in which a woman's health, medical and genetic risks, and provision for childrearing are considered.[52]

Concerns about these patients and their potential children include health risks of pregnancy in older mothers, the potential of pregnancy triggering ongoing health problems (e.g., gestational diabetes becomes Type 2 diabetes) that may impact the woman's lifespan, and lack of energy and stamina in older women impairing their ability to raise young children. Furthermore, the children themselves may be at risk physically (e.g., pregnancy-related complications that impair the mother's and baby's health) or psychosocially (e.g., increased likelihood of losing their mothers in childhood or young adulthood). In a paper presented at the annual meeting of the ESHRE in 2005, De Swiet described the increase in the number of first-time mothers over the age of thirty-five. In the United Kingdom, in 2000–2002, 10% of women in their first pregnancy were older than thirty-five compared with 3% in 1988–1990. De Swiet argued that because pregnancy in older women is associated with a range of medical and social issues, "someone else rather than doctors should legislate or make policy statements regarding these issues."[53]

Intergenerational Gamete Donation

In terms of gamete donor identity, rules, regulations, and guidelines vary greatly around the world. For example, in some countries donor anonymity is encouraged and even protected, whereas in others donor identity is the law (see Chapters 17 and 18). In countries where familial donation is acceptable, *intragenerational* gamete donation, such as sister to sister oocyte donation and brother to brother sperm donation, is, generally speaking, much less ethically and psychologically complex than *intergenerational* gamete such as daughters donating oocytes to mothers, and fathers donating sperm to fathers, and vice versa.[54]

The ASRM Ethics Committee addressed the subject in a recent statement and underscored two reasons that the counseling is challenging for MHPs working with families seeking intergenerational gamete donation: concerns about undue influence and the perception of incest.[37] A good example is when the mother remarries and wants to use her daughter as the donor. The daughter may be financially or otherwise dependent on her mother and stepfather and may therefore feel obligated (if not coerced). At the same time, she may be troubled by the idea of creating a baby with her stepfather even though conception would take place in the Petri dish. Finally, she may have some conflicting feelings about being both biological mother and sister to this child.

Treating Gay Male Couples

Because fertility treatment centers offering ART routinely accept lesbian couples for treatment, they inevitably must address the issue of whether they also should treat gay male couples. In recent years, gay males, as well as lesbian women, have become more open about their homosexuality, their relationships, and their determination to become parents.[55,56] Yet while papers from many different countries have appeared in the literature about lesbians seeking assisted reproduction to have children, the issue of gay men seeking treatment has only been addressed in the United States. The ESHRE "Guidelines for Counseling and Infertility" includes a section on reproductive services for lesbian couples, but no mention of gay males seeking such service.[57] In a joint policy statement published in 1999, the CFAS discussed the increasing number of lesbians seeking treatment but made no recommendations about gay men who were not included.[58] HFEA has not addressed the issue of gay men and ART and in fact has little to say about treatment of lesbians other than in their publication on "Patients' Guide to DI."

A recent survey of ART programs in the Unites States makes clear that programs are more likely to reject gay males than they are lesbians.[59] Some common questions about gay fathers include: Can men (and, in particular, gay men) be sufficiently nurturing if they raise a child without a woman in the household? Will children raised by gay fathers face more difficulty with their own sexual maturation? Others may question whether it is ethically acceptable for programs to accept lesbians for assisted reproduction while refusing to treat gay males.

A growing body of research supports the notion that children being reared in homosexual homes are not harmed and are not more likely to become homosexuals themselves.[60] These factors have led more ART programs to consider treating same-sex couples of both genders. Gay males give the same reasons for parenthood than heterosexual males do, that is, the desire to nurture children, to have the constancy of children in their lives, and to achieve a sense of family that children provide.[61,62] Parental motivation was considered in a study comparing attitudes toward parenting of heterosexual and gay fathers. Gay fathers were more likely to express "the higher status accorded to parents as compared to non-parents" as a motivation for parenting. The authors also asked subjects to describe their interaction with their children. They found no reported differences in terms of intimacy or involvement with the children, although gay fathers reported greater warmth and responsiveness and more limit setting.[63,64]

It appears that same-sex couples, including gay male couples, are increasingly determined to become parents and many are seeking infertility programs to assist them. Programs need to develop appropriate policies if they are to serve these couples with a focus on the specific needs and concerns they bring to the treatment. There is also a need for continuing studies of treatment outcome for gay couples to help improve the quality of care.

Posthumous Reproduction

The ability to retrieve and preserve sperm from a newly deceased male to be used for later fertilization is called posthumous sperm procurement (PHSP.)[65] While not a routine issue for ART programs, there has been a noted increased demand in many countries. However, the procedure has been banned in many countries including Canada, Denmark, Egypt, France, Germany, Korea, Norway, Spain, Sweden, and The Netherlands. [65] In contrast, it is performed in the United States, although not universally. For example, a 1997 survey of ART programs in the United States reported that twenty-five requests for PHSP were honored by fourteen facilities nationwide although none of these facilities had policies in place for the procedure at the time of the request.[66] By 2002, another study determined that forty-two requests for PHSP were honored and that twenty-one programs reported that they had established protocols for the procedure.[67] One such program described the development of their guidelines regarding this issue. The program recommends a one-year waiting period following the death before proceeding with using the posthumous sperm, both for time to grieve and because survivors' feelings often change over time.[68]

The possibility of fathering a child after death clearly creates a number of ethical, legal, and psychological issues for ART programs, the surviving family, and, especially, the potential children. Issues that PHSP raises include the idea that the shock of losing a loved one might propel the living partner to act hastily to create a new family, perhaps making a commitment which is impulsive or motivated primarily by the grieving process.[69] Furthermore, the status of the child, who may come into existence years after the parental death, can be controversial in terms of legal recognition and inheritance rights, especially when there are competing siblings or other stakeholders in estates or other legal matters. For these reasons, the well-being of the resulting child should be the overriding concern, not the comfort of the surviving partner.

Posthumous reproduction has been conditionally accepted in some countries, most notably The Netherlands and the United Kingdom; however, it may occur privately in other countries when it is not specifically banned. It has been more readily accepted in situations where the death of a partner interrupts the parenting plans of a couple in a committed relationship. It is more difficult when no prior planning has been done before death and when no consent has been given, especially if new partners become involved after the death.[68] The parents of the deceased, for example, might balk at the possibility of a new spouse raising their grandchild.

In rare cases, cryopreserved embryos are left behind when both genetic parents have died. It is not clear what the legal status of the resulting children would be, although one state court has ruled that such children should not be able to inherit the parent's estate, while another state has offered the opposite opinion in a similar case.[69]

In general, the practice of posthumous reproduction raises a classic conflict between the principle of autonomy for the prospective parent and the principle of beneficence with regard to the future of the prospective child. The important moral issue at stake should be to adequately protect the future dignity and legal status of the child.

Now that we are seeing improved survival rates in cancer patients as well as greater awareness on the part of patients and their oncologists regarding the importance of fertility preservation before treatment, men and women are increasingly preserving their gametes before undergoing chemotherapy and radiation. In a statement on fertility preservation and cancer treatment, the ASRM Ethics Committee recommended that posthumous reproduction be allowed only when the "deceased has specifically provided an advance directive and the surviving spouse or other designee agrees that it is a sound one." The report underscored the importance of informing these patients of their options for gamete disposition in the case of their death.[70]

THERAPEUTIC INTERVENTIONS

There are two therapeutic interventions regarding ethical decision making for infertility counselors. The first involves establishing an ethics committee, when one does not exist or when one does not have access to such a body in a reproductive medical practice. The other approach concerns MHPs who practice independently of a clinic and provide a framework for autonomous decision making.

Establishing an Ethics Committee in the Infertility Practice

When a core group of clinicians begins to recognize the value of interdisciplinary dialogue and joins together to shape the clinic's goals and practices, the first step toward the formation of an ethics committee has been taken. To fully engage in ethical review, the next step is to deliberate about specific cases and their implications for the policies of the program. It is not obligatory that a formal ethics committee be run by a trained ethicist, but it is important that leadership is assumed by an interested clinician who takes on the responsibility for gathering information, acquainting the group with ethical codes and professional practice guidelines, and introducing styles of reasoning (ethical principles) that meet with the program's needs and keep the focus of discussion within acceptable boundaries.

A reasonable goal for membership would be the inclusion of representatives from major facets of the practice: physicians, nurses, laboratory scientists, mental health professionals, and administrative staff. Better decisions are usually made when more diversity in representation is included and when more variety in opinions and ideas are obtained for consideration. Some committees add experts from the outside public, perhaps inviting representatives from religious or educational institutions, or from local hospitals, although this can be problematic for two reasons. Some of these participants may be lacking in the necessary medical and scientific knowledge base required by the practice, so that their ideas and suggestions are not as practical or useful as those of clinicians working in the field. However, it is just this lack of information and personal agenda that may make their opinions valuable to the committee, as they may reflect the greater society who is also 'unknowledgeable.' Confidentiality is more likely to be breached by an increase in public participation, especially in a small community. Good decisions are apt to arise when details and contexts are fully considered, and yet these discussions can impinge on the privacy of the individuals involved and their families. Despite this concern, diversity in points of view and standpoints is a necessary component of the ethics committee to ensure that decisions do not arise from local custom or prejudice alone, or for the sole benefit of the practice, and to incorporate the widest array of ethical ideas and points of view.[71] Ethics committees can be run in a variety of ways, although most popular is the advisory body that attempts to educate one another to elevate the deliberative process working toward consensus. Some important factors that should be considered when setting up an ethics committee are listed here.

Important Components of an Ethics Committee
■ *Clear Goals:* Will the committee create policies for the practice or act in an advisory role only?
■ *Who Are the Stakeholders:* Does the committee act to protect the patient's interests, but also work to protect the clinic from bad publicity and from litigation?
■ *Membership:* Are all facets of the practice represented? Should outside members be incorporated? Is some special expertise in ethics or in medical knowledge required?
■ *Decision-Making Process:* Will decisions be made by majority vote or by consensus? How will deliberations proceed when conflicts arise?
■ *Confidentiality:* Fewer members might lessen the risk of violating confidentiality but heighten the risk of poor decision making. Signed statements of confidentiality might serve to remind members of the importance of their project.
■ *Setting the Agenda:* How are cases brought to the committee, how do employees suggest issues for discussion, and how are they framed for group deliberation? Can patients bring issues to the group?
■ *Historical Record Keeping:* Who keeps track of the membership, the minutes of the meetings, and makes files for future reference of decisions?

Role of Ethics Committees in the Infertility Practice
The ethics committee can serve at least three functions by helping: (1) protect clinics and practitioners from legal liability; (2) protect patients and clients against moral or ethical lapses in their treatment; and (3) prevent the possibility that public controversy or internal dissent can upset the stability of the practice itself. The committee can add confidence to decision makers in several ways: by developing internal guidelines and policies; by reasoning toward the best ways to proceed in the more unusual or new types of cases; by considering the moral ramifications of various treatments; and by weighing reasons for rejecting an applicant if a case cannot be reconciled with the clinic's overall mission or ethical goals, or would be harmful to the patient and/or potential offspring.

The ethics committee's goal is usually to find specific solutions, not to rethink or reargue moral issues that are already fixed or have become commonplace. As time goes on, many formerly controversial moral problems are settled and time is wasted rehashing issues because certain treatments have become standard of care. It would not make sense, for instance, to reengage in a discussion about the validity of using in vitro fertilization (IVF), using surrogates to carry pregnancies, using oocyte and sperm donors, and so on, every time one of these services is required as part of a treatment plan. Furthermore, it is important that the ethics committee be prepared to clarify ethical issues in more detail, even though they seem to be settled practice. For example, some patients present at the clinic with a preexisting goal or treatment plan and are upset when their wishes are not carried out. The committee may need to help the patient reassess their goals, or they may need to reassess their own practice commitments to make allowance for unusual situations.

An important role of the ethics committee is to develop treatment protocols for the practice and then to consider how or when cases fit into them. One of the first steps of the committee might be to develop mid-level principles to cover the more common procedures and activities, therefore narrowing with more specificity the types of cases that ought to be examined in more detail.

TABLE 29.1. Atonomous ethical decision making[45]

1. **Clarify the ethical dilemma.** Whose problem is it, and who should make the decision? Who is affected by the decision? What ethical principles are related to the problem?

2. **Gather additional data.** Having as much information as possible about the situation helps in decision making. Speak to other professionals working with the patient or collaborate with other colleagues regarding similar situations. It is important to be up-to-date on laws or regulations related to the issues, any legal cases related to the ethical questions, as well as ethic statements by reproductive medical organizations that may be applicable.

3. **Identify options.** If feasible, brainstorm with others to identify as many alternatives as possible. The more options identified, the more likely that an acceptable solution will be found.

4. **Make a decision.** Think through the options identified; some will be more feasible than others. Determine which option is most acceptable.

5. **Act.** Carry out the decision. It may be necessary to collaborate with others to implement the decision as well as to identify options.

6. **Evaluate.** After acting on a decision, evaluate its impact. In retrospect, was the best course of action made, or would an alternative have been better?

Mid-level principles might include, for example, general policies on appropriate age boundaries or restrictions on the number of cycles to be allowed for oocyte donors or surrogates; or they might include more specific rules like the establishment of 'gatekeeping' standards: the principles for determining acceptability and suitability of specific candidates for specific treatment. When these sorts of mid-level principles, based in ethical reasoning, are adopted, overall deliberations can be abbreviated and more time spent on the difficult and unusual situations that develop.

Exceptions to the policies will always occur because of special needs or circumstances, and the ethics committee can be an invaluable resource in determining when these exceptions are valid. In every clinic, some applicants for assisted reproduction will be turned away for various reasons; a situation that is painful both to the applicant and to the clinicians, who generally feel a morally based impulse to treat all who exhibit need. They are professionally trained to provide help and assistance. Even though the denial of treatment might be well-considered, clinicians worry that the applicant will look elsewhere, perhaps to a less scrupulous place, to address their reproductive desires. This is a good reason to make the ethics committee the appropriate forum for examining difficult cases, determining their grounding, and ensuring that caution and prudence have not outweighed morality, before rejection is final.[72]

Autonomous Ethical Decision Making

The lack of an organized ethics committee does not exempt clinical staff members from the requirement to engage in moral reasoning. Of course, every professional is required to be aware of and practice according to the ethical standards unique to their profession, but infertility counseling and reproductive medicine, in general, often presents unique and unforeseen ethical dilemmas for the caregiver, patient, and the treatment team. No healthcare professional can ever be immune from the necessity to forward her or his ethical concerns to the appropriate decision makers so that they can be given due weight in the actual implementation of treatment. The role of ethical emissary is often embodied by the MHP who may be called on to inform the clinic's leadership when ethical issues arise, and also to translate ethical guidelines to the patient and partners in treatment. In lieu of an organized ethics committee, the lone clinician may assist in the identification of important moral issues, the development of policies and protocols to cover daily routines, the promotion of the consistent application of moral values by the employees, and the setting up of procedures that allow for the expression of misgivings by staff members, so that moral qualms can be adequately addressed.

Many MHPs providing infertility counseling services practice independent of a clinic, yet regularly face situations that test their moral and/or ethical views. Covington[44] adapted a theoretical framework for decision making by infertility counselors with ethically challenging situations, based upon the work of nurses Chally and Loriz, aptly referred to as "ethics in the trenches."[45] The framework involves six steps for MHPs to use to help determine a course of action when working alone or without the benefit of an ethics committee, and is viewed in Table 29.1.

FUTURE IMPLICATIONS

The past two decades have introduced remarkable transformation to the world of ART. Infertility counselors working in early IVF programs would have been hard put to predict a future that would have included the possibility that a child from IVF could have had five parents: the intended mother, the intended father, the sperm donor, the oocyte donor, and the gestational carrier. The idea that a woman over fifty would routinely give birth through oocyte donation, or that a dead man could father a child, or that a homosexual male couple could have a child through oocyte donation and surrogacy would have been truly hard to imagine. Now we know we are working in a rapidly evolving discipline and that we can expect the unexpected, that we will have to try to understand each new development and work to define guidelines for whatever challenges the future brings.

ART for the treatment of the infertile may very well become ART for the fertile. For example, now that we are on the verge of perfecting oocyte freezing, infertility counselors in future may very well find themselves counseling healthy young women who want to pursue a career and preserve their oocytes for future use. One can imagine an ethically challenging scenario where these healthy young women may be offered a discount on their freezing fees if they elect to 'donate' some of their oocytes to another woman.

The future is already here in the sense that fertile couples persist in their quest for sex selection with PGD in order to achieve 'family balancing' or 'gender variety,' two inadequate terms. What about the couple who feels that their family would be 'balanced' with one child, and that child should be a girl? Or a boy? As the horizons of reproductive technology continue to expand exemplified by cloning being visible in the distance, infertility counselors will be increasingly called upon to address the issue: Simply because something can be done, does not mean it necessarily should be done. In short, while the application of bioethical principles and the use of ethics committee may make decision making a bit more comfortable, ethical dilemmas and conundrums in reproductive medicine will continue to expand in exponentially unpredictable ways.

SUMMARY

■ The interface between psychological and ethical issues has defined the role of the mental health professional in the field of ART.

■ The mental health professional is often in a singular position to identify ethical concerns, to lead ethics discussions, and to promote the application of ethical values.

■ Mental health professionals have addressed the ethical and psychological impact of ART in the literature.

■ An ethics committee as part of the ART team enhances communication of moral concerns, and the delivery of sound guidelines and program policies.

■ The principles of autonomy, beneficence, non-maleficence, and justice are basic values in medicine and are necessary requirements for moral deliberation.

REFERENCES

1. Jonsen AR, Veatch RM, Walters L. *Source Book in Bioethics: A Documentary History*. Washington, DC: Georgetown University Press, 1998.
2. Caplan A. Twenty years after: The legacy of the Tuskegee Syphilis Study. *Hastings Ctr Report* 1992; 22:29–32.
3. Gamble VN. Under the shadow of the Tuskegee: African Americans and health care. *Am J Public Health* 1997; 87:1773–8.
4. Holm S. Not just autonomy: The principles of American biomedical ethics. *J Med Ethics* 1995; 21:332–8.
5. Cooper S. Ethical issues associated with the new reproductive technologies. In SR Leiblum, ed., *Infertility: Psychological Issues and Counseling Strategies*. New York: John Wiley and Sons, 1997.
6. Duka WE, DeCherney AH. From the beginning: A history of the American Fertility Society, 1944–1994. Birmingham: The American Fertility Society, 1994.
7. The Ethics Committee of the ASRM. Ethical considerations of the new reproductive technologies. *Fertil Steril* 1990; 53:S2.
8. ESHRE: www.eshre.com.
9. Code of Practice, Sixth Edition, *Human Fertilisation and Embryology Authority*. London: HFEA, 2003.
10. Ahuja KK, Simons EG, Edwards RG. Money, morals and medical risks: Conflicting notions underlying the recruitment of egg donors. *Hum Reprod* 1999; 14:279–84.
11. Ahuja KK, Simons EG, Mostyn BJ, Bowen-Simpkins P. An assessment of the motives and morals of egg share donor: Policy of "payments" to egg donor requires a fair review. *Hum Reprod* 1998; 13:2672–78.
12. Kan AKS, Abdalla HI, Ogunyemi BO, et al. A survey of anonymous oocyte donors: Demographics. *Hum Reprod* 1998; 13:2762–6.
13. Lindheim SR, Frumovitz M, Sauer MV. Recruitment and screening policies and procedures used to establish a paid donor oocyte registry. *Hum Reprod* 1998; 13:2020–4.
14. Abdalla H, Shenfield F, Latarche E. Statutory information for the children born of oocyte donation in the UK: What will they be told in 2008? *Hum Reprod* 1998; 13:1106–9.
15. Ahuja KK, Simons EG. Cancer of the colon in an egg donor: Organizational selection and assessment of women entering a surrogacy agreement in the UK. *Hum Reprod* 1999; 14:262–6.
16. Ahuja KK, Mostyn BJ, Simons EG. Egg sharing and egg donation: Attitudes of British egg donors and recipients. *Hum Reprod* 1997; 12:2845–52.

17. Englert Y. Oocyte donation: Ethics of oocyte donation is challenged by the health care system. *Hum Reprod* 1996; 11:2353–7.

18. Englert Y, Rodesch C, Van den Bergh M, et al. Oocyte shortage for donation may be overcome in a programme with anonymous permutation of realed donors. *Hum Reprod* 1996; 11:2425–8.

19. Ahuja KK, Simons EG, Fiamanya W, et al. Egg-sharing in assisted conception: Ethical and practical considerations. *Hum Reprod* 1996; 11:1126–31.

20. Blood D. Responses to the consultation document of Professor S. McLean. *Hum Reprod* 1998; 13:2654–6.

21. Benshushan A, Schenker JG. The right to an heir in the era of assisted reproduction. *Hum Reprod* 1998; 13:1407–10.

22. Ahuja KK, Mamiso J, Emmerson G, et al. Pregnancy following intracytoplasmic sperm injection treatment with husband's spermatozoa: Ethical and policy considerations. *Hum Reprod* 1997; 12:1360–3.

23. Bahadur G. Posthumous assisted reproduction (PAR): Cancer patients, potential counselling and consent. *Hum Reprod* 1996; 11:2573–5.

24. Hervey TV. Buy baby: The European Union and regulation of human reproduction. *Oxford J of Legal Studies* 1998; 18:207–34.

25. Benshushan A, Schenker JG. Legitimizing surrogacy in Israel. *Hum Reprod* 1997; 12:1832–4.

26. McGee G. Trials and tribulations of surrogacy: Legislating gestation. *Hum Reprod* 1997; 12:407–11.

27. Brazier M, Golombok S, Campbell A. Symposium: Reference documents on the ethics and laws of human reproduction. Surrogacy: Review for the UK health ministers of current arrangements for payments and regulation. *Hum Reprod* Update 1997; 3:623–8.

28. Shenfield F, Pennings G, Devrocy P, et al. ESHRE Task Force on Ethics and Law ID: Surrogacy. *Hum Reprod* 2005; 20:2705–7.

29. Sureau C. Gender selection. Gender selection: A crime against humanity or a fundamental right? *Hum Reprod* 1999; 14:867–8.

30. Benagiano G, Bianchi P. Gender selection. Sex preselection: An aid to couples or a threat to humanity? *Hum Reprod* 1999; 14:868–70.

31. Simpson JL, Carson SA. Gender selection. The reproductive option for sex selection. *Hum Reprod* 1999; 14:870–2.

32. Wertz DC, Fletcher JC. Ethical and social issues in prenatal sex selection: A survey of geneticists in 37 nations. *Soc Science Med* 1998; 46:255–73.

33. Dawson K, Trounson A. Ethics of sex selection for family balancing. Why balance families? *Hum Reprod* 1996; 11:2577–8.

34. Pennings G. Ethics of sex selection for family balancing. Family balancing as an acceptable application of sex selection. *Hum Reprod* 1996; 11:2339–46.

35. ASRM Ethics Committee. Child-rearing ability and the provision of fertility services. *Fertil Steril* 2004; 82:564–7.

36. ASRM Ethics Committee. Informing offspring of their conception by gamete donation. *Fertil Steril* 2004; 81:1124–30.

37. ASRM Ethics Committee. Family members as gamete donors and surrogates. *Fertil Steril* 2003; 80:1124–30.

38. ASRM Ethics Committee. Preconception gender selection for nonmedical reasons. *Fertil Steril* 2001; 75:861–4.

39. ASRM Ethics Committee. Sex selection and preimplantation genetic diagnosis. *Fertil Steril* 1999; 72:595–8.

40. ASRM Ethics Committee. Financial incentives in recruitment of oocyte donors. *Fertil Steril* 2000; 74:216–20.

41. Covington SN. Establishing an ethics committee in your private practice. Serono *Insights into Infertility Newsletter*; 1996.

42. Gordon ER, Barrow RG. Legal and ethical aspects of infertility counseling. In: LH Burns, SN Covington, eds. *Infertility Counseling: A Comprehensive Handbook for Clinicians*. New York: Parthenon, 1999.

43. Covington SN. The role of the mental health professional in reproductive medicine. *Fertil Steril* 1995; 64:895–6.

44. Covington SN. Confronting and dealing with ethical dilemmas in infertility counseling. In post-graduate course: *Infertility Counseling: Survival Skills for the New Millennium*. American Society for Reproductive Medicine Annual Meeting. San Diego, CA. October 21–22, 2000.

45. Chally PS, Loriz L. Ethics in the trenches: Decision making in practice. *AJN* 1998; 98(6):17–20.

46. Rosenthal JL. Psychological aspects of care. In: MV Sauer, ed, *Principles of Ooctye and Embryo Donation*. New York: Springer, 1998.

47. Hindle PA. Charting uncharted waters: The role of the ethics advisory committee. In: MM Seibel, SL Crockin, eds, *Family Building Through Egg and Sperm Donation: Medical, Legal, and Ethical Issues*. Boston: Kluwer Academic Publishers, 1994.

48. Elias S, Annas GJ. *Reproductive Genetics and the Law*. Chicago: Year Book Medical Publishers, Inc., 1987.

49. Beauchamp TL, Childress JF. *Principles of Biomedical Ethics: 5th Edition*. Oxford: Oxford University Press, 2001.

50. ASRM Ethics Committee. Human immunological virus and infertility treatment. *Fertil Steril* 2002; 74:218–22.

51. ASRM: Guidelines for oocyte donation. *Fertil Steril* 2002; 77(Suppl):S6–S8.

52. ASRM: Ethical considerations of assisted reproductive technologies. *Fertil Steril* 1997; 67(Suppl):25–35.

53. De Swiet M. Pregnancy and advanced maternal age. *Hum Reprod* 2005; 20:Suppl 1, p. 49.

54. Marshall LA. Intergenerational gamete donation: Ethical and societal implications. *Am J Obstet Gynecol* 1998; 178:1171–6.

55. Patterson CJ. Family relationships of lesbians and gay men. *J of Marriage and Family* 2002; 62:1052–69.

56. Johnson SM, O'Connor E. *The Gay Baby Boom: The Psychology of Gay Parenthood*. New York: New York University Press, 2002.

57. ESHRE: Guidelines for counselling and infertility. *Hum Reprod* 2001; 16:1301–4.

58. CFAS Joint Policy Statement: Ethical issues in assisted reproduction. *SOGC* 1999; 21:21–1.

59. Gurmankin AD, Caplan AL, Braverman AM. Screening practices and beliefs of assisted reproductive technology programs. *Fertil Steril* 2005; 83:61–7.

60. Wainwright JL, Russell ST, Patterson CJ. Psychosocial adjustment, school outcomes, and romantic relationships of adolescents with same-sex parents. *Child Dev* 2004; 75:1886–98.

61. Bigner JJ, Jacobsen RB. Parenting behaviors of homosexual and heterosexual fathers. *Journal of Homosexuality* 1989; 18:163–72.

62. Bigner JJ. Raising our sons: Gay men as fathers. *Journal of Gay and Lesbian Social Services* 1999; 10:61–8.

63. Miller B. Gay fathers and their children. *Fam Coord* 1979; 28:544–52.

64. Mallon GP. *Gay Men Choosing Parenthood*. New York: Columbia University Press; 2004.

65. Hurwitz JM, Batzer FR. Posthumous sperm procurement: Demand and concerns. *Obstet Gynecol* 2004; 59:806–8.

66. Kerr SM, Caplan A, Polin G, et al. Postmortem sperm procurement. *J Urol* 1997; 157:2154–8.

67. Hurwitz JM, Macdonald JA, Lifshiz LV, et al. Posthumous sperm procurement: An update. *Fertil Steril* 2002; 78:1001:S242.

68. Tash JA, Applegarth LD, Kerr SM, Fins JJ, Rosenwaks Z, Schegel PN. Postmortem sperm retrieval: The effect of instituting guidelines. *J Urol* 2003; 170: 1172–5.

69. Batzer FR, Hurwitz JM, Caplan A. Postmortem parenthood and the need for protocol with posthumous sperm procurement. *Fertil Steril* 2003; 6:1263–9.

70. ASRM Ethics Committee. Fertility preservation and reproduction in cancer patients. *Fertil Steril* 2005; 83:1622–8.

71. Kuhse H. New reproductive technologies: Ethical conflict and the principle of consensus. In: K Bayertz, ed, *The Concept of Moral Consensus*. Boston: Kluwer Academic Publishing, 1994.

72. Fletcher JC. Ethics committee and due process. *Law Med Hlthcare* 1992; 4:291–3.

30 Legal Issues in Infertility Counseling

MARGARET E. SWAIN

The science of legislation is like that of medicine in one respect: that it is far more easy to point out what will do harm than what will do good.

– Charles Caleb Colton, 1825

The mental health professional occupies a unique and diverse position in the arena of infertility intervention. The infertility counselor may be viewed variously as a patient advocate, gatekeeper, counselor, confidante, and liaison. Whatever the role, within the boundaries of acceptable practice, the infertility counselor is subject to the laws, standards and regulations governing this profession. These include ethics codes, practice guidelines, case law, legislation, and facility procedure. The application of these standards to infertility practice sometimes strains the intentions and the practical dimension of these guidelines, which, in turn, invites uncertainty in their day-to-day use. As rapid advances in fertility treatments pose unprecedented and ever-increasing moral and ethical dilemmas, the mental health practitioner is often called upon to be the arbiter of ethical behavior.

The construct of the family has fundamentally changed since the development of assisted conception and the introduction of third-party reproductive collaborators. Basic questions regarding medical intervention, intrusion into the marital relationship, suitable candidates for treatment, and allocation of treatment resources have no easy answers. The evolving view of the nuclear family carries with it uncertainty and misunderstanding. What, and who, constitutes this basic societal group is no longer a simple concept. Confounding the question are widely varying cultural and religious mores. Furthermore, the legal status of children, parents, and reproductive collaborators continues to be debated. Rights are resolved on a case-by-case basis, but no uniform approach to these complex issues currently exists. These factors combine to create an uneven landscape for the infertility counselor. Beginning with Freud, psychotherapy historically concentrated primarily on the individual, yet, clearly, the infertility client does not exist, nor is he or she treated, in a vacuum.

Patients' choices are affected by conditions and occurrences in the local community, as well as in the larger global society.

This chapter:

■ gives a brief historical review of reproductive events and the law;
■ reviews the status and practice standards of the mental health professional, especially as they apply to infertility counseling;
■ identifies legal dilemmas posed by practice in the area of infertility; and
■ discusses legal aspects of assisted conception, both domestically and internationally, with a view toward their impact on counseling.

The terms 'mental health professional' (MHP), 'counselor,' 'therapist,' or 'mental health provider' may be used interchangeably throughout this chapter to identify a psychologist, social worker, psychiatrist, marriage and family therapist, or psychiatric nurse.

HISTORICAL OVERVIEW

Reproductive law has paralleled reproductive technology, by striving to resolve a new set of complex moral and social questions never before contemplated. Reproductive rights were considered and upheld for the first time in the United States' landmark case of *Skinner v. Oklahoma*.[1] There, the Supreme Court ruled that a 1935 law permitting forced sterilization of a population of criminals was unconstitutional. Thereafter, news of medical and social developments in the area of reproduction periodically appeared in both professional and lay publications. Donor insemination was highlighted in 1945, when the *British Medical Journal* reported its use. A subsequent report by the Archbishop of Canterbury recommended criminalizing the process, but concerns of resultant underground activity prevented the prohibition. A 1954 Illinois (United States) court ruled that donor insemination constituted adultery, even in cases where the husband consented. Subsequent legislation and case law rebuked this decision, with the bulk of the states now statutorily acknowledging the use of donor sperm for legitimate family-building purposes.[2]

Reproduction, personal autonomy, and equal protection were all features of a United States Supreme Court ruling in 1972 that found unconstitutional a Massachusetts law restricting the sale and distribution of contraceptives solely to married persons and further extended the right to reproductive privacy (established in 1965, in *Griswold v. Connecticut*) to all persons.[3] The following year, *Roe v. Wade*[4] established a woman's privacy right to her own 'bodily integrity' and held that the unborn are not persons ("...persuades us that the word 'person,' as used in the Fourteenth Amendment, does not include the unborn..."), thereby extending women's rights to a legal abortion.

In the meantime, infertility was emerging as a growing health problem. Prospective parents began examining diverse options in their quest to build families. As a consequence, the first reported surrogate mother contract was arranged in 1976. And, in a long-sought medical breakthrough, Louise Brown, the first in vitro fertilization (IVF) baby, was born in England in 1978, followed in 1981 by a successful attempt in the United States. The world's first donor oocyte baby was born in Australia in 1984, followed by the birth of a child from frozen oocytes in 1986, also in Australia. The 'Baby M' case in New Jersey allowed a surrogate to enjoy parental rights to her genetic child (although the father and intended mother were awarded custody).[5]

Controversy seemed to multiply exponentially with the new developments in the science of assisted reproductive technology (ART). In response to this debate and to the unregulated practice of infertility treatment, the Human Fertilization and Embryology Authority (HFEA) was created in the United Kingdom in 1991, as a licensing authority in the regulation of reproductive treatments.[6] It continues to monitor these practices and revise policies and legislation in response to medical advances, opinions from the public sector, professional feedback, and decisions from its members.

With the need to involve others in the reproductive effort (e.g., medical providers and gamete donors), disagreements often evolve between reproductive partners and disagreeing parties increasingly turned to the courts for help in resolving their disputes. In 1991, a Canadian woman, who contracted HIV from donated sperm, won her lawsuit. In the mid-1990s, a Virginia

fertility doctor, Cecil Jacobson, was sentenced to five years in prison on various counts of fraud, for using his own sperm, without disclosure to his patients, to father somewhere between a dozen and seventy-five children with his fertility clients. He had claimed the sperm was from anonymous donors. This behavior, compounded by other fraudulent practices in the treatments he administered, also caused his medical license to be revoked. The American Society of Reproductive Medicine (ASRM) responded to this case by instituting practice guidelines against clinic personnel serving as gamete donors.[7] In 1992, the *Davis v. Davis* case was litigated in Tennessee. The court held that frozen embryos were, while deserving of special respect, nonetheless property and that each of the parties who created them had a right to privacy that included the right to not reproduce.[8] In 1993, the California Supreme Court ruled that, in a gestational carrier case where a dispute arose between the intended parents and the gestational carrier, the intention of the genetic parents determined the parentage of the child.[9]

More court cases continued to emerge as result of ART. In 1996, twins conceived in the U.S. after their father's death were awarded the right to seek social security death benefits.[10] In 2000, the parents of donor-conceived child, who had developed a genetic kidney disease, challenged sperm donor anonymity. California Cryobank was ordered to reveal the identifying information.[11] An interesting case in France raised public ire, when the court declared that a child has a right not to be born. In this case, the physician did not diagnose a birth defect prior to the birth of the child. The French parliament overturned the decision.[2] Case law continues to develop in this constantly shifting area of the law.

While the majority of fertility treatments have been accomplished professionally and appropriately, others have generated heated debate and controversy. A sixty-two-year-old woman gave birth in 1994, giving rise to public debate about the artificial extension of the natural childbearing years. A scandal surfaced in 1997, involving unauthorized use of gametes by a group of reproductive endocrinologists at the University of California (at Irvine), to achieve pregnancies for their patients.[2]

Partly due to the commercial aspect of infertility treatments, and the high cost involved, the United States Congress passed the Fertility Clinic Success Rate and Certification Act, in 1992, requiring fertility clinics to publicly post their success rates.[12]

During the past decade, controversy has swirled around the field of biotechnology, as issues involving cloning, genetic selection, the Human Genome Project, preimplantation genetic diagnosis (PGD), and stem cell research are discussed and debated. Constantly emerging ethical, moral, and scientific challenges constitute the backdrop for patient treatment with assisted reproductive technologies. The informed infertility counselor approaches the professional relationship mindful of these issues that, directly or indirectly, confront patients seeking resolution of their infertility.

LITERATURE REVIEW

To practice effective infertility counseling is to be aware of the differences among cultures and religions, to be sensitive to those differences, and to assist the client in working through the infertility process within this framework. It is also crucial that the mental health professional understand the various regulatory frameworks surrounding treatment options. Obviously, patients are most benefited by knowing of treatment methods that are legally available to them where they live and seek care. (Although reproductive tourism seems to be an increasing trend, it is an option available only to the relatively select few with the means to fund what may be long-term travel.) The legal climate is affected by the same factors influencing medical ethics, and it must deal with practical application of its contents as well. Consequently, laws regarding infertility treatments and counseling are not consistent across countries and often not even within countries. Following is a brief review of pertinent laws in selected countries.

The United States

There is minimal federal oversight of assisted reproductive technologies in the United States. At the current time, there are two statutory federal laws that specifically have an impact on fertility practices in the states. The first imposes mandatory reporting requirements and was initiated in 1992.[13] The law requires all U.S. medical facilities performing ART to submit annual data regarding ART cycles and success rates to the Centers for Disease Control (CDC). In turn, the CDC publishes the success rates relative to each reporting clinic.

The second federal mandate is the Federal Food and Drug Administration (FDA) regulation governing the use of human tissue and by-products. On May 25, 2005, the FDA issued its Current Good Tissue Practice (CGTP) for Human Cells, Tissues, and Cellular and Tissue-Based Products (HCT/P).[14] This was the latest of three rules designed to prevent the transmission of communicable disease by human cells, tissues, and cellular and tissue-based products. The regulations impose restric-

tions and record-keeping requirements on businesses that recover, store, and otherwise handle human tissue. It also requires all such facilities to report any serious adverse reactions involving HCT/P and communicable disease. Its impact on fertility clinics is still being evaluated, but the time restrictions on testing of gamete donors, and the scope of the testing, have already caused many treatment centers to modify policies and procedures. As a consequence, ART participants are undergoing additional screening and the commissioning (i.e., intended) parents are paying more for the process.

At least one state, New Hampshire, mandates that a mental health professional provide services in certain cases involving assisted reproductive technology. The New Hampshire law requires a nonmedical evaluation of intended parents, by a social worker, pastoral counselor, psychologist or psychiatrist, in surrogacy arrangements, and further requires that the counselor provide a copy of the evaluation to the court that oversees the finalization of parental rights.[15] ASRM Mental Health Professional Group (MHPG) recommends psychological assessment of both recipients and donors in gamete donation procedures, as well as in those processes involving embryo donation.[16] Resolution of parental rights is handled on a state-by-state basis.

The United Kingdom

The United Kingdom's Human Fertilisation and Embryology Authority (HFEA), introduced in 1990 by authority of the Human Fertilisation and Embryology Act, regulates assisted reproduction in the United Kingdom. It requires that mental health counseling (psychosocial counseling) be offered to those patients requesting certain assisted conception techniques.[17] Consistent with guidelines developed internationally but independently, HFEA notes that the purpose of psychological intervention is to support patients during the decision-making process and throughout treatment, helping them to make adjustments in their lives attendant to those choices. Those considering oocyte or sperm donation, whether as a donor or a recipient, are required to have "a suitable opportunity to receive proper counseling on the implications of taking the proposed steps" and their consent would not be effective unless such counseling has been offered. Furthermore, all medical centers offering ARTs must provide access to a qualified infertility therapist (credentialing is available through the British Infertility Counseling Association and the British Fertility Society, but is not required[18]), although patients do not have to accept the offer of counseling to receive treatment. Added emphasis is placed on the need for such counseling when donor gametes are used.[19]

HFEA permits a broad range of ARTs, including donor gametes, embryo donation, and both traditional and gestational surrogacy. It prohibits cloning for reproductive purposes. All practices providing such services must be licensed by the HFEA. The Act is 'child-centered,' imposing restrictions on treatment unless the welfare of a potential child, and any other child who may be affected by the potential child's birth, has been considered. Key segments of the Act address parental rights. For instance, a sperm donor has no parental rights unless his sperm was used contrary to his consent and not taken in accordance with the Act's consent provisions. A woman who gives birth is considered the mother of any child, regardless of genetic connection, although a court order supersedes this presumption. Limited payment to donors is allowed, with a cap on compensation, but reimbursement for expenses is permitted as well.[6] In 1998, HFEA considered prohibiting new clinics from offering payment, but was ultimately persuaded to allow continuation of payment because it was convinced of the chilling effect of such action.[20] In its original form, the Act dictated that a man's sperm might be used after his death, but that he would not be the child's father. However, in response to *R v. Human Fertilization and Embryology Authority* ex parte *Blood*,[21] the government commissioned a review of this section, and upon its recommendation, the Human Fertilization and Embryology (Deceased Fathers) Bill was approved and HFEA was amended to include designation of deceased men as fathers in circumstances similar to the *Blood* case.[6]

The HFEA also maintains a record of licensed treatments and outcomes, while maintaining anonymity of donors who entered information prior to April 1, 2005 (subject to any court order to the contrary). After April 1, 2005, the Authority will provide identifying information to adult donor-conceived children upon request, but the Act prohibits any licensed practice from retrospective disclosure of a donor's identity.[6]

Canada

Canada is a federated government, that is, a shared governmental alliance of national and provincial/territorial governments that controls its ten provinces and three territories. Healthcare is a responsibility of the federal government that sets and administers standards for the health provisions system, under the auspices of the Canada Health Act of 1985.[22] At the current time, only the province of Ontario continues to fund IVF and only in limited circumstances. Donor insem-

ination is funded, and it is the most widely used ART procedure, although about half of Canada's approximately twenty-five clinics offer oocyte donation.[23] However, the Assisted Human Reproduction Act (AHR), passed on March 26, 2004, bans payment of fees and expenses to donors and surrogates, raising concerns that an already slim population of donors and surrogates will become increasingly sparser.[24] Section 6 of the AHR Act also prohibits anyone from paying a person to act as a surrogate. Furthermore, it proscribes payment for arranging, offering to arrange, or advertising to arrange the services of a surrogate. Additionally, the Act requires that counseling services be received by patients prior to any licensed practice accepting health information or accepting donor genetic material. (The Act defines donor as anyone supplying gametes for ART, thereby including people supplying reproductive tissue for their own use. Consequently, all ART participants must be given access to infertility counseling before entering these treatments.) As of May 2, 2005, Health Canada launched an initiative for a pilot project to explore strategies for altruistic donation of gametes and, on May 9, announced that Vancouver will headquarter the new Assisted Human Reproduction Agency of Canada, to be established in January 2006 to oversee assisted human reproduction activities.[25]

Anonymity of donors is currently maintained for the participants in the arrangements, although in defined circumstances, disclosure might be made to other physicians, regulatory bodies, and so on.[24]

Legal parentage issues fall within the purview of the provinces and territories, as opposed to within the federal government. Therefore, there is no uniform policy applicable to children born of third-party ART. Specifically, only Newfoundland, Quebec, and the Yukon have instituted laws defining parental rights in children born of these procedures.[26] In the absence of legislation, most intended parents, whether genetically related to the child or not, pursue an adoption of a surrogate-born child. Commonly, couples working with oocyte donors are advised to retain an attorney to draft an oocyte donation contract to, among other things, outline the parties' understanding of the parentage of any child.[23]

Australia

Australia is a federation, with some states regulating the practice of ART, but all legislatively defining the legal status of the child born through assisted conception with donor gametes. Subsequent to the first IVF birth in Australia, the government of Victoria began a review of IVF research and practice that culminated in the establishment of the Infertility (Medical Procedures) Act of

1984, the first legislation to regulate IVF and its associated human embryo research. The Commonwealth Family Law Act of 1975, and the various state acts, gave intended parents in donor situations parental rights, thereby terminating any rights the donor might have held.[27]

The states offer different versions of counseling imperatives, ranging from mandatory counseling, to the requirement that clinics offer counseling, to suggestions that it should be offered. Many of the states adhere to the ethical guidelines in the National Health and Medical Research Council, rather than promulgate their own legislation. The states also differ on the provision of information to children born of donor arrangements. The developing trend appears to follow the belief that people have a right to know their genetic progenitors, and at least two of the states now provide identifying information to children upon their attainment of a certain, specified age. One of the states stipulates that the child must have received appropriate counseling prior to the release of information.

Australian law does not provide for commercial surrogacy. Most jurisdictions prohibit surrogacy for money and hold any such contracts unenforceable. Furthermore, any paid solicitation of a surrogacy arrangement is illegal. Ambiguity in the laws may make it difficult to arrange an altruistic surrogacy,[28] but even when the arrangements are successful, there is no statutory provision specifying the status of the child, except for within the Australian Capital Territory. The Artificial Conception Act of 2000 requires that, among other things, the genetic and birth couples must have received assessment and counseling from a service other than that which is performing the IVF procedure. These requirements were set into place after a disastrous case in 1998. In *Re Evelyn*,[29] a traditional surrogate, having been inseminated with the sperm of the intended and genetic father, conceived. This was a private arrangement, with no screening, experienced medical management, or counseling. After Evelyn was born, the surrogate refused to relinquish the child. The Family Court returned Evelyn to her birth mother, limiting and specifying the type of contact the father might then have with his daughter.

Israel

Israel has a very active infertility treatment community, with the world's highest per capita concentration of IVF clinics.[30] Israel is structured as a parliamentary democracy, and judicial institutions of the various religious communities hold jurisdiction in matters involving personal liberties. Israel's population is about 80%

Jewish, with ever smaller segments of the population espousing Muslim, Christian, and Druze faiths. Here, in addition to the impact religion is generally seen to have on ethics, legislation and societal attitude, religious beliefs and tenets are fundamental to the development of laws. A Jewish couple's religious directive is to practice at least replacement fertility, that is, to replace themselves with a son and a daughter, but, in fact, many of the Israeli Jewish population go on to have larger families, especially the ultra-Orthodox, with a birth rate as high as 7–7.5%.[31] Islamic views are similar.

The Israeli National Insurance Law mandates healthcare coverage for all citizens, and coverage for ARTs is an important part of these benefits.[32] Treatment is guaranteed until the birth of two children occurs, but recently, restrictions on age and number of cycles have been applied (a woman must be no older than forty-five to use her own oocytes and no older than fifty-one for donor oocytes, and may not undergo more than six IVF cycles per year.[33]) The use of donor sperm is permitted, but is restricted to the use of sperm from single men and under full anonymity. Rabbinical permission may be necessary in some circumstances, but is not required or recommended. Counseling is not required.[34] Oocyte donation is also permitted, and a new law allows clinics to compensate the donors for harm, loss of time, risk, loss of income, or temporary loss of ability to work. Formerly, donors could only be women who were undergoing IVF for their own reproductive purposes, and who chose to donate extra (unused) oocytes. Under current legislation, first proposed in March, 2001, an unmarried Israeli woman may donate oocytes as long as no more than seven offspring are born from her donations and she undergoes no more than three oocyte retrievals. The oocytes must be inseminated with the sperm of the recipient's husband. While oocyte donation is allowed, it is practiced under strict anonymity. However, a national center safeguards donor information, for release only in dire circumstances and with the donor's permission. The center also provides information to donor-born children who wish to establish that they are not genetically related to a possible sexual partner.[35]

While embryo donation is not permitted,[35] the Surrogacy Arrangement Act of 1996 governs gestational surrogacy (also known as gestational carrier). A panel of experts must approve all such arrangements. The couple must be prepared to supply the panel with five required documents, including a psychological evaluation addressing the suitability of the parties, and a representation by a mental health professional that the intended parents have received appropriate counseling, including information about alternative means of achieving parenthood. The surrogate may be compensated for actual and reasonable expenses, including loss of time. Counseling for the surrogate's children is also included in the costs the commissioning couple pays.

As a result of a law passed on May 19, 2005, Israeli parents who have at least four children of the same sex may be allowed the use of PGD for gender selection to have a child of the opposite sex. Couples may apply to choose embryos according to their sex, but a seven-member committee composed of experts in law, medicine, ethics, religion, and psychology must approve the request. Prior PGD for gender selection in Israel had been allowed solely for the avoidance of genetic disease. The Health Ministry issued detailed guidelines for parents, and promised to only apply the new exception in cases of apparent, substantial harm to the mental health of the intended parents, or to the mental health of a planned child who is not of the sex desired by the parent.[36]

Family and procreation are central to the Jewish religion, so much so that a marriage may be dissolved if the couple is not able to have children. Judaism encourages ART as a means of fulfilling personal and religious duty.

The Israeli law provides for mandatory psychological evaluations of intended parents in oocyte donation, and also requires that psychological counseling be provided to surrogates/gestational carriers.

Latin America

Latin American nations share an ill-defined regulatory approach. Generally, ART is offered to married or committed couples, and, while gamete donation is allowed, there is no provision for embryo donation. In contrast, though, Costa Rica severely restricts assisted reproduction through constitutional amendment, allowing only homologous insemination. Other countries labor under informal guidelines or regulations with no enforcement capabilities. Critical and precedent-setting decisions are left to the individual practitioners, who essentially operate within a system that has no set limits and in which they make decisions on a case-by-case basis. Compounding the difficulty is the marked influence of the Roman Catholic Church, with its well-known opposition to virtually all forms of ART. Unfortunately, although the practice of ART would likely benefit from well-reasoned and appropriate regulation, providers and consumers seem hesitant to approach the question for fear of over-reaching and restrictive intervention, and the not unreasonable concern that the services they are seeking to protect will be prohibited all together.[37] However, a consortium of Latin American representatives, meeting in Chile in 1996, drafted a consensus paper on ethical and legal aspects of ARTs. The

group reached a confluence of thought on the following issues: ART is provided to infertile heterosexual couples; every cryopreservation program must in some way be associated with an embryo donation program; embryo freezing is acceptable; and the only acceptable research on embryos is that which will not result in harm to the embryos, as the right to life possessed by the embryo takes precedence.[38] These policies seem reflective of the heavy Roman Catholic influence in this region, especially with regard to the status of the embryo. The Church adds even more restrictions: ART that separates procreation from sexual intercourse is unacceptable; donor gametes are not permitted; and any use of the embryo other than for conception is banned.[39]

Interestingly, the consensus policies were ostensibly developed to reflect the cultural background and have been disseminated to legislators, healthcare providers, and patients as directives. However, statistics reveal that despite the prohibitions, 7,000 cycles of IVF, with 351 transfers of embryos created with donor oocyte, were completed in fifty-nine centers throughout Latin America.[37]

At least one commentator is concerned that such morally rigid policies may result in psychological dissonance for patients. The only option for using supernumerary embryos is donation, and if the couple does not agree to this option, then they may only attempt fertilization for a number of embryos they reasonably anticipate they will implant. This amounts to little choice at all, if the couple is trying to maximize their chance for a pregnancy. So, they are forced to donate whatever embryos they do not use themselves. Furthermore, should the couple not achieve a pregnancy, the troubling thoughts of what happened to the excess embryos must surely be disturbing. Additionally, the prevailing terminology for what amounts to embryo donation is 'antenatal adoption,' which, at minimum, conveys the idea of an orphan child in need of care.[37]

The Latin American Federation of Fertility and Sterility Societies (FLASEF) provides a degree of private oversight. The mental health corollary to the Society is the newly formed GLASMI, along with a Latin American section of the MHPG. The latter group has established counseling guidelines, and these, along with a specific section of the FLASEF practice guidelines, recommend, but do not require, counseling for ART participants.[40]

THEORETICAL FRAMEWORK

Professional competency provides the basic theoretical approach of infertility counseling in the context of the law. Competency involves a cluster of skills, abilities, habits, character traits, and knowledge a person must have to perform a specific job well. An individual performs effectively within the professional construct when he or she possesses the skills, abilities, and knowledge that constitute competence. Accordingly, while one might not lose knowledge, a skill, or an ability, he or she could still lose a competence, if the requirements of good practice change. Competency is based upon knowledge, training, and standards that a profession has identified to perform a job effectively.

Professional societies relative to the mental health professional's specialty have guidelines regarding qualifications and standards of practice that set the foundation for professional competency. The MHPG of the ASRM was the first infertility counseling organization to establish competency guidelines in 1995. The guidelines[41] recommend that the minimum qualifications for infertility counselors include

- a graduate degree in a mental health profession;
- a license to practice;
- training in the medical and psychological aspects of infertility;
- a minimum of one year of experience;
- regular attendance at certified continuing education programs.[42]

In 2001, the Psychology Special Interest Group (PSIG) of the European Society for Human Reproduction and Embryology (ESHRE) established similar guidelines for competency in infertility counseling. The *Guidelines for Counselling in Infertility* provide an overview of the counselor's role.[43] They begin by addressing fundamental issues in counseling, the definition of counseling, who should provide counseling services, and who are the likely recipients of these services. Sections that follow discuss the integration of counseling and patient-centered care into the medical care scenario; situations giving rise to the need for counseling; third-party reproduction and the special concerns of gamete donation, surrogacy for gay couples, and single people. Lastly, the guidelines address ancillary methods to supplement the counseling sessions, such as written surveys, telephone counseling, support groups, and the mediated group session.

While these guidelines fall short of law, they provide assistance in the development of a framework of professional standards, competency, and possibly future credentialing for infertility counselors. Professional standards of licensing and credentialing currently exist for many mental health professions worldwide. As an example, this discussion will focus on professional practice standards in the United States. While similar guidelines apply in other countries and will be reviewed, defining every country's or province's approach is beyond the scope of this chapter. However, much of this information is universal and applicable in the professional practice of infertility counseling. It is the responsibility of the infertility counselor in his or her own place of practice to know the professional requirements of licensing, credentialing, and standards specific to his or her profession. The counseling professional should also be familiar with local and national laws and regulations regarding the specific profession and infertility counseling in general.

In the United States, psychologists, counselors, therapists, and social workers are credentialed separately, usually under separate legislative titles. Each state has a licensing entity, established by statute, that specifies licensing and certification requirements, and enumerates prohibited actions, as well as penalties, including suspension and revocation of license, for violations of the code. Standards of practice and ethical guidelines are typically promulgated by professional associations, and in some countries, are the basis for licensure, as in Canada and the United Kingdom. Once adopted by the organization, they become, at least arguably, the legal standards against which practitioners in each category may be judged. Of interest here are the American Psychological Association's (APA) *Ethical Principles of Psychologists and Code of Conduct*, the National Association of Social Workers (NASW) *Code of Ethics*, and the National Board for Certified Counselors (NBCC) *Code of Ethics*. Also pertinent may be: the American Association for Marriage and Family Therapy (AAMFT), *Code of Ethics*; The American Psychiatric Association (The APA), Ethics Primer of the APA, *Opinions of the Ethics Committee on the Principles of Medical Ethics with Annotations Especially Applicable to Psychiatry*; and the American Psychiatric Nurses' Association (APNA), *Scope and Standards of Psychiatric and Mental Health Nursing*.[44]

The APA sets out the aspired principles of beneficence and nonmalfeasance (assist and do no harm), fidelity and responsibility, integrity, justice, and respect for people's rights and dignities. Similarly, the NASW Code references service, social justice, dignity and worth of the person, importance of human relationships, and competence. The Certified Counselor's Code describes the relationship between the professional counselor and patient, as well as delineates business practice for its certificates. All detail the specific behavior of its members within the helping relationship. In the event of a legal controversy, the ethics codes will be invoked to establish the appropriateness of a practitioner's behavior. Unfortunately, none of the codes indicate which of its sections is most important, or should be first considered when analyzing a dilemma. Although helpful in furthering the ideals of the profession, they may not lend themselves to application in a particular clinical situation, or promote the greater good of the community. Because of this inherent weakness, it is reasonable to suggest that they should be read and understood in conjunction with relevant legal precepts: duty to practice with reasonable competence, obligation to seek informed consent, responsibility to identify the primary client, and the charge to treat clients equitably and with 'due process.'[44] For example, the APA Ethics Code states, "If psychologists' ethical responsibilities conflict with law, regulations or other governing legal authority, psychologists make known their commitment to the Ethics Code and take steps to resolve the conflict. If the conflict is irresolvable via such means, psychologists may adhere to the requirements of the law, regulations, or other governing legal authority."[44]

Other countries have differing policies for regulation of mental health professionals. Generally, psychiatrists and psychologists are regulated separately from other mental health professionals, and systems for regulating social workers and other types of counselors are not uniform. For instance, statutory registration systems function in some Canadian provinces, and in Japan, Hong Kong, Israel, Germany, France, South Africa, and The Netherlands. England, Wales, and Scotland regulate the training of social workers. In contrast, Australia allows social workers to self-regulate, based on an agreement between the profession, educators, and employers. An interesting deviation from this is the system practiced in Scandinavia and Finland, which allows self-regulation in conjunction with industrial union representation. The majority of registration systems operate in tandem with a competency evaluation and a disciplinary procedure, and registration is defined by statute.[45]

In the United Kingdom, credentialing of infertility counselors is available through the British Infertility Counselling Association (BICA) and the British Fertility Society (BFS), but is not required.[46] The Infertility Counselling Award is a recently developed joint project of BICA and the BFS. Counselors in the reproductive and assisted conception field may earn this professional designation by completing workshops and other training seminars and by demonstrating the expected competency in professional conduct. The award is recognized by HFEA as a qualifying tool for infertility counselors. Additionally, participants receive credit toward professional development for reaccreditations by the British Association for Counselling and Psychotherapy Professionals and the United Kingdom Council for Psychotherapy. There are plans to develop stages of BICA/BFS accreditation reflecting higher levels of skills in practice. Founded in 1988, the BICA remains the only

professional association for infertility counselors in the United Kingdom.

HFEA, in 1991, recommended that the minimum qualifications required for a counselor be a certificate of qualification of Social Work; an equivalent qualification recognized by the Central Council of Education and Training in Social Work; or an accreditation by the British Association of Counselling or Chartered Psychologist status.[6]

Canada's governmental system allows for some degree of separate regulatory authority among its ten provinces and three territories, so regulations pertaining to mental health professionals may vary. For instance, Ontario's healthcare professionals are governed by the Regulated Health Professionals Act, which allows for nonstatutory, self-regulated mental health professionals for those counselors who are not overseen by legislated regulation, such as psychologists and psychiatrists. These mental health professionals are subject to certification through a private agency or organization, provided they meet that organization's professional requirements and conditions. One such organization is the Canadian Counselling Association, a national organization inviting membership from all parts of the country. Its standards of practice apply to professional behavior for the Canadian mental health professional.[47] During a Spring 2004 workshop that reviewed Canada's Assisted Human Reproduction Act and its impact on infertility counseling,[48] a group of Canadian infertility counselors formed the Canadian Infertility Counsellor's Association which subsequently became a special interest group of the Canadian Fertility and Andrology Society (CFAS) in 2005. However, it has not yet formally adopted standards or provided ethics information.

Australia requires that working psychologists comply with registration requirements of the State and Territory Psychologists Registration Boards. Generally, all states or territories require completion of a four-year course of undergraduate study in psychology, and two full-time, additional years of postgraduate work or supervised fieldwork as a probationary/conditional registered psychologist.[49] Social workers, are expected to comply with the ethical requirements of state regulatory bodies, such as the South Australian Council on Reproductive Technology (established as a function of the Reproductive Act of 1998).[50]

Australian and New Zealand infertility counselors joined efforts to establish the Australian and New Zealand Infertility Counsellor's Association in 1988. Members include infertility counselors, social workers, and psychologists. The organization has adopted practice guidelines for professional infertility counselors, as well as a Code of Ethics.[51] In 2005 this organization became a special interest group of the Fertility Society of Australia (FSA) (see Chapter 31).

CLINICAL ISSUES

This section examines issues facing infertility counselors regarding their professional legal duties. The discussion includes the duty to practice with reasonable competence; the obligation to provide information for securing an informed consent; responsibility to identify the client; equal protection and the right to refuse treatment to a patient; confidentiality and privacy; and lawsuits avoidance.

Duty to Practice with Reasonable Competence

Understanding the meaning of 'practicing with reasonable competence' requires a review of the relevant state or country's licensing criteria. However, the statutes tend to broadly define what the practice is, not usually how to go about competent practice. Furthermore, the laws vary from country to country and from state to state within a given country, at which point common law (court decisions rendered over time and in response to controversy) must be examined for guidance. Practitioners are expected to exhibit the skill and care that a prudent practitioner within that specialty, and operating under substantially similar circumstances, would demonstrate. Several cases help to underscore this standard: In *Figueiredo-Torres v. Nichols*,[52] the Maryland Court of Appeals noted that a psychologist had a duty of care to his clients to practice within the relevant standard of care, meaning, "...that degree of care and skill which is expected of a reasonably competent practitioner in the same class ... acting in the same or similar circumstances."[53] The courts cloak social workers with the same responsibilities, as noted in *Heinmiller v. Department of Health*, attaching a duty to act in a professional manner and to practice with reasonable skill and safety.[54] Other factors, such as proper licensure, certification, research and review in the field of expertise, and appropriate documentation of patient files all lend weight to the reasonably competent practice of mental health providers. Additional factors, among others, might include engaging in conduct reasonably anticipated to help the client; appropriate professional conduct; avoidance of harmful conduct to the client or to other members of society; practice within statutory guidelines and within ethical standards; and honoring policies and procedures of the employing facility.[55] Although counselors' credentials and background may well be different from that of psychologists, psychi-

atrists, marriage and family therapists and/or social workers, courts have been willing to impose very similar standards of practice on this broad group.[56] Failure to uphold professional competency standards has civil and sometimes criminal implications, the severity dependent on whether the violations were simply negligent, reckless or intentional, and whether statutory regulations were violated.

Holding oneself out as an infertility counselor implies appropriate training and experience. At this basic level, formal education must be completed for licensure. Beyond that, attendance at seminars, classes and other continuing education programs, membership in a related professional association, such as the MHPG of ASRM, or the PSIG of ESHRE, as well as seeking mentorship and/or supervision will help establish the necessary credentials for the practitioner. Willingness to conduct treatment may be interpreted as holding oneself out as competent. Failure to possess such competency is a potential cause of action, as recognized by the Supreme Court of New Hampshire in *Hungerford v. Jones*.[57] There, a social worker, whose only 'expertise' in the treatment of patients with repressed memories was a single lecture on the topic, provided counseling to a patient using techniques to uncover such memories. This led the patient to believe that her father had abused her, when this was later shown not to be the case. The court permitted the patient's father to sue the therapist.

Equally important to the concept of competent practice is the responsibility to be informed of the law. Laws and regulations, and resultant standard of practice, vary widely among states, provinces and countries. Infertility counselors practicing in areas with ART friendly laws, or at least those with an absence of prohibitions, may expect to see travelers from areas that restrict certain treatments, such as gamete donation or surrogacy. In some cases, these patients may face penalties, as in Michigan, where state law imposes both civil and criminal penalties on participants and intermediaries in surrogacy arrangements.[58] Intended parents may also be prohibited from establishing parental rights to any child born through third-party collaboration. Just as importantly, cultural tolerance may be a significant factor in the patients' acceptance of certain treatments and in the development of beliefs about openness, secrecy, and shame, as well as in their adjustment to the child and comfort in establishing themselves as a family when they return home.

Reproductive tourism is now responsible for a small but steadily increasing segment of the fertility patient population. While there is continuing debate on the ethics and repercussions of this phenomenon,[59] it remains uncontested that potentially oppositional laws will impact these peripatetic patients. A recent example is a Japanese couple, both of whom were over the age of fifty, who sought assistance from a gestational carrier and an oocyte donor in the United States. The Japanese Justice Ministry requires that every birth to a mother over the age of fifty be confirmed with 'details.' Following the investigation, the children resulting from ART were not recognized by the Japanese government as the children of the couple, and were not awarded a certificate of family membership. The court indicated it denied the request because the intended mother did not give birth, nor were her oocytes used in the conception of the child, and ruled that the American birth certificate was inapplicable because the case should have been considered under the laws of Japan. The court opined that the case could be resolved by adoption. Gestational surrogacy is not illegal in Japan, but a Health, Welfare and Labor Ministry panel has recommended that it be prohibited by statute.[60]

While the mental health professional may not be expected to know the law applicable to any given area, he or she should advise the client that legal problems may arise from participation in these procedures and insist that the patient seek legal counsel before consenting to treatment. To the extent that the treatment requested is lawful in the place where it is administered, there is currently no specific legal prohibition to treating the visitor. However, the infertility counselor may be at some legal risk if the concern about potential legal problems is not raised with the client. If the client proceeds with treatment, even in the face of likely unfavorable or hostile reception at home, the infertility counselor should document both the client's acknowledgement of potential or certain legal difficulty and the counselor's attempts to discuss the emotional implications of this situation.

Obligation to Provide Information for Securing an Informed Consent

Part of the infertility counselor's responsibility is to educate the client about potential material risks and benefits of counseling, and inform the client about the nature of any evaluation the therapist will perform. In this context, 'material' means, "if a reasonably prudent person in the position of the patient or his representative would attach significance to it in deciding whether or not to submit to the proposed treatment."[61] It is also crucial that the client understand the nature of the relationship, especially in facilities that employ their own counselors. Generally, the elements of informed consent are diagnosis; description of the proposed treatment; possible benefits of the treatment; potential risks, including the possibility that some risks

may, as yet, be unknown; and alternatives to treatment, including no treatment. ASRM practice guidelines reference psychological screening and potential psychological issues as matters to discuss when obtaining an informed consent.[62] The doctrine of informed consent has been extended to behavioral science professionals by the courts[63] and adherence to it is stipulated in the ethic codes of the APA (Ethical Standard 4.02), NASW (Ethical Standard 1.03), and the NBCC (Section B8). Included in the construct of consent are the concepts of 'voluntaries' and 'capacity.' Reasonably complete disclosure of facts surrounding treatment or evaluation allows the client to give a voluntary consent. Capacity is the ability to fully join in a rational discussion about risks and benefits of a proposed treatment, and, based on that discussion, arrive at a reasoned decision.[64]

Responsibility to Identify the Client

A legal concept that deserves strict attention, particularly by those who work with participants in third-party reproduction, is the duty to identify the primary patient. This does not mean that one person from among the group of gamete donors, the gestational carrier, the carrier's husband, and intended parents has to be the sole primary client. Rather, the responsibility is identification of the party to whom a duty is owed. In the case of complex third-party reproduction, it is likely that *each* of the parties involved is a primary client, with perhaps competing interests, but to whom professional duties are, nonetheless, owed. The potential for conflict of interest is apparent, and care must be taken to secure consent to treat all parties, to ask each to waive a claim as to conflict of interest, where appropriate, and to refer to other, qualified practitioners, if conflict issues arise. As part of competent practice, and integral to the concepts of informed consent, all participants must be informed of the therapist's relationship with the other parties, and be given the opportunity to seek separate counseling. Also, if the provider is an employee of the medical practice, especially if the practice will ultimately decide the suitability of the candidates for treatment, that fact must be relayed to the clients. Clear and direct explanations of what information will be shared and with whom is critical to the clients' informed consideration of whether to proceed. The discussion should be carefully documented.

Equal Protection and the Right to Refuse Treatment to a Patient

As part of the infertility treatment team, the counselor is often entrusted with screening and evaluating participants in the various treatments. Several issues are raised by this responsibility. The most obvious is the inherent potential conflict of interest. The mental health professional, if an employee of the practice (or an employee of an independent donor or surrogate recruiting agency), may be subject to pressure, however subtle, to approve candidates. Considerable funds are expended in the recruitment of, for instance, oocyte donors. One study found that of 315 inquiries to a donor advertisement, only thirty-eight potential candidates eventually entered the donor pool. Cost analysis showed the ultimate cost to recruit one donor was approximately $1,869.[65] Every candidate who is declined represents a cost to the practice, the recipients, or the agency. The universal application of regular, customary, and approved guidelines in the evaluation and ultimate acceptance or rejection of donors will serve to protect the counselor from disgruntled applicants and questioning referral sources. Ideally, the referring practice will have known in advance what standards the infertility counselor will use in his or her evaluation and recommendations.

The American constitutional notion of equal protection may not, at first blush, appear to be applicable to practice in the private sector. However, many of the principles found in the fair employment acts, as well as in civil rights and antidiscrimination laws, flow from the liberties established in the Fifth and Fourteenth Amendments. Much of the discussion on this topic stems from restriction on personal liberties, a question not typically encountered by mental health professionals working in the ARTs, with perhaps one exception: when a decision is made to withhold treatment based on concerns about the patient's parenting ability. It begs the question: Does a person have the right to any treatment that is medically appropriate? If a provider refuses treatment to a patient, is that provider then at legal risk?[44] The answer is multilayered. Law pertinent to this area developed as a response to civil rights violations, spawning the Civil Rights Act of 1964.[66] Later, the Rehabilitation Act of 1973[67] codified penalties for discriminating on the basis of disability.

The Americans with Disabilities Act, a statutory compendium thoroughly addressing prejudices and discrimination against the disabled, was enacted in 1990. While based on its previously mentioned predecessors, it is a more complete attempt to correct disparities in public and private accommodations. According to the ADA, disability is "... a physical or mental impairment that substantially limits one or more of the major life activities of the individual...."[68] The ADA established certain rights for those in the class considered 'disabled,' but it is not an affirmative action statute. Instead, its mission is to guarantee equality of opportunity, independent living (where possible), and financial self-sufficiency for people who are disabled. Doctors' offices, clinics, and other providers of care are addressed in Title III, *Prohibition of Discrimination by Public Accommodations*.[68] The law does not require that each provider treat every patient who seeks treatment, but, rather, that a provider may not refuse care to a patient in a protected class on the basis of that person's disability.[68] Should a practitioner decline to recommend a patient for treatment based on a disability, then clear justification must be demonstrated: The statute provides that if a direct threat of risk to self or others can be shown, then the discrimination may be excused. To establish such a direct threat defense, certain strict and specific requirements must be met.[69] Accordingly, the practitioner must conduct a reasonable, individualized assessment based on current medical knowledge or best information available. Relying on this objective evidence, the provider must then determine that a risk is present, what that risk is, how long the risk will exist, how severe the risk or threat is, and the probability of the risk actually causing harm. Finally, the practitioner must consider whether reasonable modifications, policies, practices, or procedures would make treatment for the individual possible, by mitigating the risks.[68]

As an alternative, the provider might argue that refusal to treat is not based on the disability, but on other factors. The ASRM Ethics Committee Report on *Child-rearing Ability and the Provision of Fertility Services* addresses this kind of situation.[70] The Ethics Committee concluded that fertility providers may decline to treat a patient on "well-substantiated" conclusions that the potential parent will not or cannot safely care for a child. The committee went on to recommend that practices develop clear, written exclusion policies, based on parenting abilities. In so doing, it suggested a team approach to such decisions and indicated that the disabled should not be denied treatment except when they fall within the narrowly defined parameters outlined within the recommendations. The policies should be applicable to all patients. Caution should be exercised so that the counselor's personal feelings or his or her particular social and cultural mores do not influence the decision not to treat. Practitioners must realize that constitutional rights to family privacy, that is, the right to raise children as the parent sees fit, are well established.[71] In at least one case, the court determined that a social worker for the Department of Child Protective Services could be sued for violating a child's rights by separating him from his family. In this case, the social worker was allegedly involved in a conspiracy to remove children from a home because the extended family did not agree with the children's parents' religious beliefs and practices.

Although allegations of child abuse were made, and the social worker claimed the directive she issued to remove the children was based on those claims, the court found that the removal of the children was likely not the result of those claims. The court noted that, "Specifically, a reasonable person would have known that it was unconstitutional to use the government's power to cause, or conspire to cause, the unjustified removal of a six-year-old child from his parents in order to destroy the family, based simply on the family's religious beliefs."[72]

As an integral part of the team approach to treatment, the mental health professional provides crucial input in assessing concerns about a patient. Evaluations may reveal undiagnosed psychiatric illness or potentially serious psychosocial contraindications. In performing these evaluations, the therapist should review and consider the following:

- Professional society practice guidelines (e.g., ASRM, ESHRE, MHPG, APA, NASW, etc.)
- State/country licensing regulations
- Pertinent case law
- Documented medical/psychiatric/criminal/social history of the patient
- Internal policies and procedures of the practice
- Possible referral to an ethics committee, in-house counsel or the Institutional Review Board (IRB), or governing/licensing commission, for example, The Human Fertilization and Embryology Authority (UK) or the Assisted Reproduction Authority (Canada), as applicable.

Confidentiality

The professional infertility counselor has a duty to maintain confidentially as to client matters. This goes to the heart of the therapist–client relationship, and this obligation is imposed worldwide by professional guidelines, ethics standards, legislation, and case law.[73] An exception to this duty is the client who the therapist determines, or should determine, represents a serious danger to himself or to reasonably identifiable others, in which case, the therapist must make a reasonable effort to notify both the intended victim and the police.[74]

Privacy in the United States: Health Insurance Portability and Accountability Act (HIPAA)

On April 14, 2003, the United States Government initiated the implementation of HIPAA, the first-ever federal privacy standards for individual health information.[75] These new standards, developed by the Department of Health and Human Services, allow patients greater control over their private health information

(PHI) and provide easier and more complete access to their medical records. HIPAA was designed to facilitate and enable electronic transactions of medical information while strictly safeguarding the private nature of health data. Although not all health care entities are covered in its final regulation, most physicians and other healthcare providers must comply with the Act. The regulations cover medical records and other individually identifiable health information, whether paper, digital, or other electronic or oral communication. The privacy rules are inclusive of the following:

- *Access to medical records* – patients have the right to review and obtain a copy of their records (in almost all situations), and request corrections if they see mistakes. The records should be provided within thirty days. The requesting party may be charged for the service of copying and forwarding the records.
- *Notice regarding use of PHI* – practitioners must provide patients with notice about how their information might be used. Usually, the patients must provide acknowledgment of such notification.
- *Limitation on use of PHI* – For purposes of healthcare, PHI may be shared by providers on an as needed basis. A separate, specific release must be provided if the PHI is to be shared with any entity not providing care to the patient.
- *Marketing prohibition* – A specific consent to the use of PHI for marketing is required before such information may be released. The privacy rule does not prohibit doctors and other providers from communicating freely with patients about their treatments and alternatives, as these are not within the intended use of the term 'marketing.'
- *Confidential communications* – Reasonable steps must be taken to ensure that confidential communications between doctor and patient remain private.

The HIPAA privacy rule is intended to establish a balance between patients' privacy rights and appropriate disclosure of PHI as needed for treatment and other pertinent purposes. Unfortunately, largely due to misconceptions and concerns about inadvertent violations, it has often been applied with an overreaching hand. For instance, HIPAA does not require that each provider obtain a signed authorization before discussing patient care or treatment with another healthcare practitioner. It also does not require that providers eliminate all 'incidental disclosures.' In fact, HIPAA was modified in August 2002 to accommodate reasonable policies regarding things like patient sign-in sheets, nursing unit posting boards, and so on. Similarly, the law does not eliminate contact between healthcare providers and the families and friends of patients. Unless the patient objects, a provider may share information about the patient with family, friends, or whomever else the patient designates. Additionally, a provider may share that information, even when the patient is incapacitated, if he believes that doing so is in the patient's best interest.[76]

In the infertility counseling practice, all clients should sign HIPAA-compliant authorizations for release of information, and must indicate they are aware of the persons or entities with whom their information would be shared (see Appendix 8). In the professional relationship, the client (or designated proxy) is the only person who may elect to waive the confidentiality privilege.

Privacy in Healthcare Elsewhere

The United Kingdom regulates privacy in healthcare through common law, Article 8 of the European Convention on Human Rights, incorporated into United Kingdom law by the Human Rights Act of 1998 and the Data Protection Act of 1998.[77] The Data Protection Act is the most encompassing legislative instrument governing the disclosure of health information, especifically with regard to mental health professionals in Statutory Instrument 2001 No. 3968, Private and Voluntary Health Care. It imposes strict duties of confidentiality on healthcare professionals, and allows for civil suit if an individual believes that the Act has been violated.

Canada enacted the Personal Information Protection and Electronic Documents Act (PIPEDA) in 2004.[78] This law encompasses all collections, uses, and disclosures of personal information in the course of commercial activity. The law governs healthcare providers in the private sector who are engaged in commercial activity, unless governed by provincially enacted substantially similar legislation. The essential elements of PIPEDA include necessity of consent from an individual whose information is disclosed, disclosure to the individual of the purposes for the consent, as well as the scope of the information, what protections are afforded for the information, and the need for additional and sometimes specific consent for secondary uses. Furthermore, any requesting or disclosing organizations must provide a means for an individual to dispute the organization's compliance with the Act.

The Australian Federal Privacy Act and Privacy Amendment was enacted in 1988 and applies to confidential health communication throughout all of the country. As of December 21, 2001, the private-sector amendments to the Privacy Act 1988 became operative.[79] The new provisions provide for ten National Privacy Principles found in Schedule 3 of the Act, which apply to health service providers. Recently, in a ruling by the Queensland District Court that allowed for a successful claim in tort for breach of privacy, a district court judge found that the right to privacy exists outside of statute and regulation. However, the ruling is limited to the district and to facts substantially similar to those in the case.[80]

Avoiding Lawsuits

Lawsuits involving infertility counseling seem to derive from general legal issues rather than from those specifically relating to infertility. Accordingly, caveats regarding legally safe practice are derived from general practice pointers.

1. The therapist should avoid extreme self-disclosure to patients. Before raising personal experiences, the counselor should consider whether an experience is shared for the benefit of the patient or the therapist, and whether the revelation is appropriate for a particular patient with whom the disclosure is shared. More than 70% of therapists report using self-disclosure as a therapeutic device,[81] but careful assessment of the situation and the client is key to its safe application. This comment is especially pertinent for infertility counselors who have had their own personal experience with infertility.

2. Diagnosis should be accurate per ICD-9 and/or DSM-IV and consistent with treatment, in order to provide appropriate care and maintain truthful billing practices. In the United States, managed care gatekeepers and strident guidelines for authorization of payment have led to a reported increase in insurance fraud cases involving mental health practices.[82] An illustrative example is the therapist who provides a diagnosis that she knows will be covered by an insurance plan, but provides a different and more accurate description for treatment records. However, "the law does not recognize or permit the therapist to have one diagnosis for treatment purposes and one diagnosis for billing or insurance purposes."[83]

3. Generally speaking, mental health professionals are expected to follow the 'medical model' in their treatment practices. Stemming from this are the requirements of informed consent, documentation, adequate procurement and review of client history, confidentiality and privacy, standards of care, and so on. While the individual infertility counselor may not believe the medical model is applicable to his or her practice, it is quite certain that this is the standard against which the practice would be held. Perhaps this is even more relevant in the infertility milieu, as the counselor is working within a medical practice, as a member of an interdisciplinary team and/or as a consultant to a medical practice.

Practitioners should take care to follow the guidelines inherent in the medical model.

4. Engaging in a sexual relationship with any client, whether a current client or one with whom the professional relationship has terminated, is never legally or ethically acceptable. Such behavior is a violation of ethical codes worldwide and is illegal in some places. There is no 'true love' exception. Engaging in such a relationship is tantamount to rejecting continued practice of one's career.

5. Over the course of the past decade, a number of heretofore unidentified 'syndromes' have appeared in the counseling literature or have been summoned as defenses in litigation. These are conditions that have not been recognized by any authority and are not defined in the ICD-9 and/or the DSM-IV.[84] One of the most controversial of such syndromes is that of recovered memory, ultimately, in many cases, found to be *false* memory. Also included would be therapies or therapeutic techniques that have no basis in evidentiary medicine. Careful, standardized testing to establish efficacy should be required and reviewed by the mental health professional before attempting any treatment with a client. Otherwise, the mental health professional may be subject to liability if the patient does not improve, worsens, or forgoes another treatment that is likely to be helpful, in favor of a rogue technique.

6. The infertility counselor should be guided by institutional policies, guidelines and standards of practice within his or her own professional associations, and pertinent state/provincial/national governing laws. Deviation from any of these may open the counselor to liability, if a client suffers harm and alleges that the harm is due to the counselor's lack of adherence to these standards. For example, if the infertility counselor evaluates third-party collaborators for participation in donor or gestational carrier cycles, the institutional acceptance/rejection criteria must be applied. Additionally, the mental health professional would be expected to adhere to the practice guidelines established by ASRM, ESHRE or other applicable professional association, as well as to general guidelines pertaining to his or her own professional standing. This would include administration of any recommended standardized testing. Failure to follow these guidelines could result in two diverse but equally undesirable outcomes. On the one hand, the rejected candidate might allege that she was turned down for some prohibited reason, for example, a physical disability, religion, or race. On the other hand, a candidate who is accepted may later regret her decision, and allege that she should never have been accepted, and that her acceptance caused her emotional trauma. Acceptance or rejection is easier to defend if institu-

tional and professional policies and guidelines are followed, and there is documentation to show this. That said, all professionals in this area practice with a degree of uncertainty.

Because ART is a developing medical, legal, and social process, even with a careful and methodical approach, problems may still arise. A suit filed several years ago is illustrative: A potential gestational carrier applied to a program that employed a staff psychologist. The candidate underwent the usual and customary clinical interview and psychological testing, and, in accordance with the parameters established by the program and general guidelines in this area, was accepted. A pregnancy occurred, the child was born and subsequent to this, the carrier claimed to have severe psychological trauma. She sued the fertility center and the psychologist, claiming that she should not have been allowed to be a carrier, based on her emotional state, and the psychologist should have detected the underlying psychopathology. In this particular case, the infertility counselor had the MMPI-2 scored at a reputable outsourced scoring company, and the candidate was found to be acceptable under its scoring paradigm. However, the plaintiff's attorney submitted the test for scoring by another company, which supplied a different interpretation. Ultimately, the case settled, leaving unresolved the question of whether the mental health professional would have been found responsible.[85] Nevertheless, the lawsuit illustrates the risk of practice in this area, as well as the necessity of strictly following guidelines and protocol.

THERAPEUTIC INTERVENTIONS

In the United States, legal commentators may rely on a constitutional basis for analysis of legal trends. Procreative liberty or reproductive freedom is a principle rather firmly entrenched in American society, based on the national view of personal privacy. Procreative liberty is a derivative right, based on the doctrine of personal autonomy and freedom from governmental interference in private matters.[86] The nation's courts traditionally view the right to beget children with favor, acknowledging it as a basic right of the individual, and one not to be burdened by governmental interference.[87] The Supreme Court has recognized that an individual's right to reproduce is a major life activity.[69] However, the right to assistance in building a family, and the extension of specific constitutional protection to assisted reproduction, has not been established. At least one legal authority has theorized that no distinction should be drawn between coital and noncoital reproduction. Inability to procreate through sexual intercourse is not reflective of parenting abilities, nor does it diminish the person's wish to have children. A natural extension of these principles would be granting the same protection to noncoital reproduction as is extended to sexual procreation.[86] The Court has also endorsed the right of the individual to make decisions about whether or not to have children, remarking that persons may make decisions independent of governmental interference [in such matters] "involving the most intimate and personal choices a person may make in a lifetime, choices central to personal dignity and autonomy, [and they] are central to the liberty protected by the Fourteenth Amendment."[88] Following this logic, third-party reproductive collaborators have that same freedom in their participatory choices.

While matters of personal freedom are generally addressed by the Constitution, specific matters of parentage and child custody are left to the individual states. There is no uniformly applied law pertaining to determination of parental rights, so laws vary from state to state.

Other countries may analyze reproductive choices and access them in different ways, such as using, perhaps, a more child-centered approach. Still others focus on cultural forces and religious tradition. This section will review reproductive law and the issue of consent as an aspect of therapeutic intervention.

Reproductive Law

The following is a brief review of reproductive law regarding donor sperm, donor oocytes, embryo donation and disposition, lost or misappropriated embryos, surrogates and gestational carriers, and posthumous reproduction.

Donor Sperm

In approximately two-thirds of the United States, parental rights in cases of sperm donation are determined by statute.[1] Current law codifies the rights of the intended father, but may not explicitly terminate rights of the donor. Additionally, a number of the statutes qualify the circumstances in which the law may apply. For instance, a state law may require that a qualified medical practitioner perform the insemination. Another statute may require specific consent (usually written) of the mother to the 'artificial insemination,' while in others, her consent is implied.

[1] Alabama, Alaska, Arizona, Arkansas, California, Colorado, Connecticut, Florida, Georgia, Idaho, Illinois, Kansas, Louisiana, Maryland, Massachusetts, Michigan, Minnesota, Missouri, Montana, Nevada, New Hampshire New Jersey, New Mexico, New York, North Carolina, North Dakota, Ohio, Oklahoma, Oregon, Tennessee, Texas, Virginia, Washington, Wisconsin, Wyoming.

Issues arising in this area might include: children wishing to locate their genetic fathers, the need for medical information about donors, or inadvertent consanguinity and financial responsibility of donors to children born of their donation. Attempts have been made to address some of these issues. For instance, ASRM suggests that limitations on the number of pregnancies a donor produces should be imposed, based on population density in the area where donated sperm is used.[89] However, others of these issues, while being discussed and debated, have yet to be formally addressed in guidelines.

Parental rights and responsibilities in sperm donation were considered by an Illinois court, when the legal father (i.e., married to the biological mother) of a child born through donor insemination argued that because he had no biological connection to the child, he was not responsible for child support. The court found that since no adoption had occurred, the man could not be considered the father.[90] Subsequent American court decisions have taken an opposite course, finding that a man's consent was sufficient to attach the responsibilities of fatherhood, even in states with no statute regarding paternity in donor insemination cases.[91]

Demands for parental rights, including visitation, have arisen in the course of known sperm donor arrangements. A New York appellate court determined that a known sperm donor, despite agreements to the contrary, should be afforded paternal rights to the child.[92] In other jurisdictions, there appears to be little consistency to the rulings, although generally the courts rely on statute, where available, intention of the parties (within statutory framework), and best interest of the child.[93] In the case of *Re Patrick*, an Australian court held that a known sperm donor, who provided sperm to a lesbian couple, was entitled to continuing contact with the child, as the court determined that such visitation was in the best interest of the child. The court, however, also held that the donor was not a 'parent' under Australia's pertinent laws. This case had a tragic turn: The biological mother of the child, after psychiatric treatment to assist her in dealing with emotional issues, including the visitation schedule, killed herself and the child.[94] (No information was available as to whether this woman and the other parties had pretreatment counseling.)

Men whose intent was to donate sperm have also been found responsible for child support. A Victorian (Australia) man had intercourse with a lesbian, with the intention of donating his sperm to her so that she could conceive a child. The Australian court noted that if the child had been conceived through artificial insemination and not coitus, or if an adoption had occurred, then financial liability for supporting the child would not have resulted. The Justice specifically noted that one parent could not waive the child's right to support from the other (see Chapter 17).[95]

Donor Oocyte

Anonymous, recruited donor oocyte arrangements have become more widely accepted, although many aspects of donation remain controversial. Approximately 80% of U.S. clinics offering IVF also offer oocyte donation, and quote a success rate of about double that of traditional IVF (when using the oocytes of the infertile woman).[96] As of 2003, 10.5% of all American IVF cycles report the use of donor oocytes in transferred embryos.[97] In addition to recruited donors, family members and other women known to the recipient participate as donors in treatment cycles. The ASRM Ethics Committee examined this practice and determined that, in many cases, these types of known gamete donation (and surrogacy) arrangements may be appropriate, but also may come with their own set of ethical problems, including consanguinity, confusion regarding parentage, and coercion of parties to participate.[98]

As previously noted, counseling and/or evaluation are recommended by ASRM in its published guidelines on gamete donation.[16] Donor oocyte procedures are permitted in the U.K., France, Australia, Japan and Israel, among other countries, but the process is regulated to a much greater degree than in the United States.

Currently, fewer than ten states in the United States have oocyte donation laws. In jurisdictions without statutory resolution of parental rights, there is no absolute assurance that the intended mother would be considered the legal mother. Most often, there is not controversy generated by these arrangements, so there is very little case law. Rather, problems develop from collateral issues, and one of the first disputes involving an oocyte donor did not involve a claim by the donor.[99] The situation arose when a couple divorced after their twins, conceived through donor oocyte, were born. The father sought sole custody of the children, basing his argument on his genetic connection to them. The court noted that the parents had entered into the donor agreement, both intending to be parents, and the father had no superior claim to the girls. Recently, a Texas appeals court reached the same conclusion under similar circumstances.[100] A California court of appeals ruled that a woman who gave her oocytes to her lesbian partner, who, with donated sperm, conceived and gave birth to a child, was not a parent. The court reviewed the pre-birth intentions of the parties, as reflected in the standard 'oocyte-donor' consent forms used by the medical facility, and noted that no further action was taken

to establish the maternity of the oocyte provider.[101] However, on appeal to California's Supreme Court, the ruling was reversed, the court holding that, ". . . when partners in a lesbian relationship decide to produce children (by one partner providing her ova for IVF, with resultant embryos implanted into the other partner), both the woman who provides her ova and her partner who bears the children are the children's parents."[102] In a recent development, an Ohio appeals court ruled that an oocyte donor has parental rights to triplets born to a gestational carrier. The court ordered a new custody hearing in Ohio for the boys, who are now almost two years old. The carrier removed the children from the hospital following their birth because the genetic father and his fiancée, according to the carrier, did not exhibit sufficient interest in the children.[103] This ruling challenges a prior Pennsylvania court's decision that the gestational carrier of the boys was entitled to primary custody. This matter continues to be litigated.

Oocyte and sperm donation have not enjoyed the same mainstream approval as that surrounding child adoption. It is no surprise, then, that recipients may struggle with shame, ambivalence, and other issues when considering whether or not to tell their child of his or her origins. ASRM encourages recipient parents to share information about their child's genetic origins with their offspring, and in support of this have issued these suggestions: Before the donation, all participants should agree as to how much information may be released; sperm banks and fertility centers should maintain genetic and medical records on donors; all parties should receive counseling about disclosure; and clinics should expect inquiries from ART children and should consider developing a written policy (see Chapter 18).[104]

Embryo Donation and Disposition

Depending on the country, excess embryos may be stored for a period of time (although in the United Kingdom storage time is statutorily limited[6]), donated for research, destroyed (although this option is illegal in some places and restricted in many others by private policy), used by the intended parents for procreation, or donated to others for transfer and gestation, with the intention that the recipients become the parents.

Early case law on the subject of embryo disposition determined that the genetic progenitors of extracorporeal embryos owned those embryos.[105] However, the case involved individuals using their own gametes for the creation of the embryos and the case was silent as to what should happen if donor gametes were used. Later disputes involved the assignation of rights to cryopreserved embryos when the progenitors parted ways, as in divorce. Although the cases have varied in the details and the basis for the court opinions may often be divergent, the consistent trend is the courts' refusal to force parenthood upon a protesting party.[106] Even in cases where the parties had clearly stated their intentions to allow the other to use the embryos, the courts have found that the party trying to *avoid* procreation had a greater interest than that of the person *seeking* reproduction. While a cryopreservation informed consent document may be given probative weight by a court, it is, properly, not viewed as a contract between the parties and may not be controlling in a dispute. However, in at least one case, the court ruled inapposite to this principle. In this Massachusetts case, the clinic had transferred frozen embryos to the estranged wife of Richard Gladu, allegedly without his knowledge or consent. The court held the clinic liable for breach of contract, relying on the cryopreservation informed consent document and characterizing it as a contract. This was decided at a trial level and, therefore, is not binding precedent.[107] The court in *Litowitz*[106] also used a contract analysis of the informed consent document, but in reference to the rights of the parties as between themselves (not in Litowitz's rights as against the clinic).

In some countries, another option for persons with stored frozen embryos is donation to another person or couple. A small number of states in the United States have laws pertaining to donation for reproductive purposes, and in those states, the donors' rights are terminated upon the donation. There is, however, little consistency in the way subsequent parentage is established, what documentation is necessary, and in other procedural matters.[108] Three additional states regulate the disposal of embryos,[2] and current federal law restricts embryonic research.[109] If gamete donors contribute to the creation of an embryo, it adds a new level of scrutiny. While sperm donors are generally releasing rights to a sperm bank, oocyte donors almost always donate their oocytes to a specific couple, presumably with the intention that the couple will use any resultant embryos only. The donor should provide written acknowledgment of and agreement to subsequent donation, if that is her intention.[110] Once again, a written agreement is critical, and should detail how parental rights will be established, any issues regarding future contact, and any financial agreements. Although there should be no payment for the embryos, in places where it is permissible, the recipients may pay embryo storage costs.[3] It is also common for the recipients to pay

for any additional medical, genetic, and psychological screening.

In the United States, there has been some dispute as to whether the giving of embryos should be termed 'donation' or 'adoption.' While discussion of the controversy is beyond the scope of this chapter, current trends and existing law appear to support the term 'donation', because, despite their potential for becoming persons, without the intervening medical manipulation and gestation and birth, they are not considered juridical persons with the exception of Louisiana, which bestows juridical personhood on the embryo.[111]

Mental health practitioners should also be aware of embryo research laws in their states and countries. At least in the United States, many of these were enacted in response to abortion legislation, and have not met constitutional challenges.[112]

Again, there are no laws in the United States requiring psychological evaluation or counseling for any of the parties involved in embryo donation. The issues seem to be more complex than in gamete donation and would appear to warrant increased involvement of the counselor. ASRM guidelines[16] suggest, in part, that embryo donors receive counseling about the potential psychological issues, discuss dispositional choices (prior to cryopreservation), and that they be assessed for appropriateness, including standardized psychological testing, and be excluded if deemed inappropriate. Similarly, recipients should receive counseling about the implications of participating, impact on any relationship with the donors, and should also be assessed for appropriateness, in accordance with the guidelines. There are at least two embryo donation agencies that require a home study prior to recommending clients for receipt of a donated embryo.

In the United Kingdom, HFEA requires that any person undergoing treatment involving IVF and/or donor gametes (including donor embryos) be given the opportunity to receive counseling. The Act further requires that the counselors meet the qualifications defined within the Act. The counseling must be differentiated from information given to secure an informed consent.[6] The Assisted Human Reproduction Act of Canada requires counseling prior to the acceptance of a donated embryo (see Chapter 20).[24]

Lost or Misappropriated Embryos

Medical practices likely face liability for losing, mishandling, or misappropriating embryos. A number of cases have arisen over misuse, or unauthorized donation, of

---

[2] Louisiana, New Mexico, and Minnesota.
[3] California, Connecticut, Delaware, DC, Georgia, Florida, Illinois, Louisiana, Maine, Michigan, Minnesota, Nevada, New Mexico,

North Dakota, Pennsylvania, Rhode Island, Texas, Virginia, West Virginia, and Wisconsin all have laws which may interfere with payments in an embryo donation arrangement.

oocytes and embryos.[113] In at least one state, criminal penalties now exist for the unauthorized use of gametes or embryos.[114] In a recent case, a clinic unintentionally implanted embryos from two different couples into one of the genetic mothers, a Caucasian woman. The embryo that was not from her oocytes was from an African American couple. The first woman became pregnant with twins. The clinic revealed the mix-up, and both couples sued. After protracted litigation, the matter was finally settled for an undisclosed amount of money. The parentage issues were settled, after a heated trial, in favor of the genetic parents.[115] A similar case arose in England, where a clinic inseminated the oocytes from a Caucasian woman with the sperm of an African man, who was not her partner and not the intended father of the child.[116] The High Court named the biological father as the legal father of the black twins but ruled that the twins were to stay with the white couple.[117] And, in a case originating in The Netherlands, a Caucasian woman underwent insemination with her husband, who was white. But, because the lab instruments had been inadequately cleaned, they also contained sperm from a black man. She became pregnant with twins, one of whom was white and the other black. Although the biological father was notified, he did not express an interest in the child and both boys remain with the gestating mother and the rearing father.[118]

Notwithstanding the above, establishment of parental rights may be difficult or nearly impossible in cases where a patient received the wrong embryos or gametes. In one case, a California clinic mistakenly transferred a number of the embryos from a married couple (Mr. and Mrs. D, who used donor oocyte) to another patient, Ms. S., who intended to use both donor oocyte and sperm from unknown donors. After both women gave birth, the clinic revealed the mistake and Mr. and Mrs. D sought contact with Ms. S's son, the couple's intended child and Mr. D's biological son. Ms. S. refused to relinquish custody of the boy, and was found to be the 'mother,' because Mrs. D had no biological connection to the child. In so ruling, the court refused to apply the principles expounded in *Johnson v. Calvert*[9] and *In Re Marriage of Buzzanca*,[119] and distinguished the case on the grounds of intent, noting, [if we were to] "…invoke the concept of intended mother here, which party would qualify? Both and neither: (Ms. S) intended to be the mother of the child created from an embryo implanted in her uterus that day at the clinic – but not that embryo…(Mrs. D) intended to be the mother of the child created from this very embryo – but not at that time, and she did not intend for another woman to bear the child."[120]

Surrogates and Gestational Carriers

Traditional surrogacy has long been a medical possibility. In this process, the gestational mother is inseminated with the sperm of the intended father. Standard practice is a written agreement that the child will be placed with the father, and if married, his wife, after the birth. Some number of surrogates achieve their pregnancies by 'home-insemination,' but, as performed by a medical professional after appropriate screening and documentation, it is a safer procedure, both from the medical and legal perspective (a number of statutes defining legal paternity in donor sperm situations stipulate that the procedure be performed by a medical professional).

Gestational carrier arrangements differ in that the woman carrying the pregnancy is genetically unrelated to the baby, and the intended parents may have used their own gametes or those of donors in the conception of the child. Because the legal assumption and the medical fact have traditionally been that the woman who gives birth is the mother, this shift in the paradigm represents a major challenge to the determination of parenthood.

Fewer than two dozen of states in the United States have statutes governing surrogacy. Of those, a handful prohibits it outright,[4] while other states regulate the practice.[5] In the remaining, there is no legislation that encourages, prohibits, or regulates surrogacy, but case law may have developed. In the absence of legislation or case law affording protection, and even if those safeguards are provided, it is customary for the parties to enter into a written agreement. Generally, the courts approach traditional surrogacy with greater caution because of the birth mother's genetic connections to the child, and these arrangements have often been termed 'unenforceable' or even 'illegal' by some courts.[121] In any event, in most situations involving traditional surrogacy, an adoption is required to finalize the parental rights of the intended mother.

Gestational surrogacy issues were litigated early on in *Johnson v. Calvert*.[9] The commissioning couple used their own gametes for IVF, and the resultant embryos were transferred to the carrier, who, despite contractual agreement, changed her mind about the placement during the pregnancy. The court held that the genetic ties between the intended parents and the child were controlling, and noted that it also recognized the intent of the parties as a factor.

But, as seen in the *Buzzanca* case (where the child was a result of both oocyte and sperm donation and

---

[4] Arizona, Michigan, New York, Utah and Washington.
[5] Florida, New Hampshire and Virginia.

was born to a gestational carrier),[119] the courts may not rely on the genetic connection, but rather on the intentions of the parties at the time of the arrangement.

Only a handful of the state surrogacy statutes address mental health counseling and screening.[122] However, the standard of care informally developed by practitioners in this area demands that each of the parties have the opportunity to receive counseling prior to participation, and that, at minimum, the surrogate to have an evaluation. The MHPG is currently developing practices guidelines for evaluation of surrogates (see Chapter 21 and Appendix 7).

The first reported case of gestational surrogacy in England was that of a young woman, Ms. Cotton, who agreed to carry a pregnancy for a couple and accepted installment payments for this service. Public controversy arose when it was discovered that Ms. Cotton was paid £15,000 by a London newspaper for her story. After the birth, the commissioning couple adopted the child.[123]

Posthumous Reproduction

The more obvious type of posthumous procreation involves the disposition of frozen gametes or embryos after the death of one or both partners. Unless there are specific instructions to the contrary, the survivor or heir should have the legal right to make dispositional decisions.[124] Although these are difficult emotional issues, the ethical debate may be mitigated if the decedent has given instructions as to what should occur in the event of death. More problematic is a man dying unexpectedly, without leaving permission to procure his sperm posthumously for use in procreation. While not common, there have been a number of cases involving a decedent's loved one (almost always, the wife) requesting sperm retrieval immediately following death, with decision making as to its use deferred to a later date. A study conducted in 1997 found eighty-two requests for post-mortem sperm retrieval at forty ART centers, over the fifteen-year period from 1980–1995.[125] It is medically possible to obtain viable sperm for approximately twenty-four hours following death, and retrieval and storage of the sperm may offer the widow and family some measure of comfort. However, even if the couple was actively trying to have a baby during the decedent's lifetime, consent to conceive and raise a child is very different than consent to conceive a child who would be raised without the presence of his or her genetic father. The ASRM has indicated that practitioners need not honor requests to obtain sperm from dead individuals, without the prior consent or known wishes of the person.[126] It urges a case-by-case analysis of each circumstance, including the consideration of any

state law.[127] There is no dispositive case in the United States addressing the use of sperm retrieved in this fashion.

A British court decided that sperm retrieved from a man in a coma who later died could not be used for the purpose of conceiving a child. In this case, the husband had not given his consent to the storage or use of his gametes. The court suggested to the widow, though, that the insemination might occur in another country, and ordered that the sperm be released to her (in Belgium).[128] In Japan, a 2004 high court ruling recognized a boy as his dead father's legitimate offspring. In this case, the child was born after his deceased father's frozen sperm and his mother's oocyte created an embryo through an IVF procedure. The court indicated that it would require the same set of facts to rule similarly in future cases: natural blood-parental relationship between child and father and the father had given his consent to such a pregnancy. The court went on to say that it was immaterial whether the father was dead or alive.[129] The trend in the U.S. courts has been to approve survivor benefits for children conceived after the death of the father.[130]

Informed Consent

Informed consent is an essential element of the ART process. Because it does not involve interventional procedures, informed consent for sperm donation is almost solely focused on the psychological issues, although counseling and evaluation are not widely required. Federal, state, and local regulations might also apply because the tissue is stored in facilities subject to licensing and regulation. In New York, for instance, such consent must be in compliance with the requirements of the state's sperm bank regulations.[131] However, informed consent for oocyte donors is not so simple. Because of the invasive nature of the donation, as well as the potential emotional repercussions, a truly informed consent is essential to maintain the integrity of the process. While a number of commentators have expressed concern that this strict standard is not uniformly applied, inroads are being made with regard to consent procedures. ASRM has issued practice guidelines that offer detailed specifics for inclusion in informed consent for ART.[132] ASRM recommends, consistent with standards in other areas of medicine, that all consents be in writing and signed with appropriate witnesses. Particular to ART procedures is the requirement that the clinic report data regarding ART cycles, which is mandated by federal law. Patients must be told of this requirement and the possibility that they may be asked for follow-up information. Patients should be informed that their identity may be held in confidence by the CDC, or they may opt that their identifying statistics be omitted.[12]

FUTURE IMPLICATIONS

In this constantly evolving field, law and medicine have become inextricably and inexorably entwined. Lacking a central, standardized system of regulation in the U.S., the law has developed on a case-by-case basis, resulting in great variation in statutory and case law. The American experience mirrors that of many nations, with a few notable exceptions, such as the United Kingdom and Canada. Professionals working in this field find few easy answers about how to best protect the integrity of the ART arrangements and preserve their own professional standards. Careful attention to professional guidelines, observance of pertinent regulations and rules, and adherence to professional standards of care will assist the practitioner in the competent performance of counseling. Ignorance of the law is no excuse.

SUMMARY

■ Reproductive law continues to evolve in this area.
■ The mental health professional should follow professional standards of practice, become familiar with the applicable law, and document carefully.
■ Mental health professionals must comply with all applicable licensing standards and should comply with additional, available credentialing and continuing education.
■ In areas where there is no legislative directive or established case law, the intentions of the parties in reproductive controversies seem to be the best predictor of how courts might rule.
■ A global perspective is essential, particularly in light of burgeoning reproductive travel and the learning potential reflected in shared experience.

REFERENCES

1. *Skinner v. Oklahoma*, 316 U.S. 535, 541 (1942).
2. http://www.pbs.org/bloodlines/timeline/text timeline.html. Retrieved from the website 09/25/05.
3. *Eisenstadt v. Baird*, 405 US 438 (1972).
4. 410 US 113, 93 S.Ct. 705, 35 L.Ed.2d 147 (1973).
5. 217 NJSuper.Ct. 313 (NJSuper. Ct. 1987).
6. Human Fertilisation and Embryology Act, 1990, and *seq.*
7. *St. Paul Fire and Marine Insurance Co. v. Cecil B. Jacobson, Jr. Reproductive Genetics Center Ltd.*; *United States v. Jacobson*, No. 92-5406, slip op. (4th Cir. Sept. 3, 1993) (unpublished), *cert. denied*, 62 U.S.L.W. 3717, 3722 (U.S. May 2, 1994).
8. *Davis v. Davis*, 842 S.W.2d 588, 597 (Tenn. 1992).
9. *Johnson v. Calvert*, 5 Cal.4th 84 (1993).
10. *Woodward v. Commissioner of Social Security*, 435 Mass. 536 760 N. E. 2nd 257 (Mass. 202) (1996).
11. *Diane L. Johnson et al., v. California Cryobank Ind., et al.*, 80 Cal. App. 4th 1050; 2000.
12. The Fertility Clinic Success Rate and Certification Act of 1992 (Pub. L. 102-493, 42 U.S.C. 263a-1 et seq.);.
13. Fertility Clinic Success Rate and Certification Act of 1992 [FCSRCA], Section 2 [a] of P.L. 102-493 [42 U.S.C. 263 (a) -1].
14. Federal Register: 66 FR 5447, January 19, 2001; 66 FR 29786, May 25, 2004; and 69 FR 68612, November 24, 2004.
15. New Hampshire Code, *Revised Statutes Annotated*, Title XII, Public Safety & Welfare, §168-B:18.
16. American Society for Reproductive Medicine. Guidelines for gamete and embryo donation: A practice committee report: *Fertil Steril* 2002; 77:S11–S13.
17. Human Fertilisation and Embryology Authority (HFEA) *Code of Practice*, 2nd ed. London HFEA, 1995; 31–2.
18. www.bica.net/CPD/Accreditation, Retrieved from the website on May 10, 2005.
19. Braude P, Muhammed S. Assisted conception and the law in the United Kingdom. *BMJ* 2003; 327:978–81.
20. Blyth E, The United Kingdom: Evolution of a statutory regulatory approach. In: E Blyth, R Landau, eds. *Third-Party Assisted Conception Across Cultures: Cultural, Legal and Ethical Perspectives*. London: Jessica Kingsley Pub., 2004; 226–45.
21. *R v Human Fertilisation and Embryology Authority ex parte Diane Blood* [1997], 2 All ER 687.
22. Canada Health Act (1985) R.S.C. 1985, c. C-6.
23. Haase J. Canada. The long road to regulation. In: E Blyth, R Landau, eds. *Third-Party Assisted Conception Across Cultures: Cultural, Legal and Ethical Perspectives*. London: Jessica Kingsley Pub., 2004; 55–72.
24. Assisted Human Reproduction Act, Bill c-13, *An Act respecting assisted human reproduction and related research*, S.C. 2004, c.2.
25. http://www.hc-sc.gc.ca/english/media/releases/2005/2005_37.htm, retrieved from the website on May 12, 2005.
26. Newfoundland Welfare of the Child Act Part II; 1990; Quebec Civil Code, 2002, Sections 538–542; and, Yukon Children's Act, Part 1, 1992.
27. Status of Children (Amendment) Act 1984 (Victoria); Family Relationships Amendment Act 1984 (South Australia); Artificial Conception Act 1984 (New South Wales); and amendment in 1985 to the Status of Children Act 1974 (Tasmania); Artificial Conception Act 1985 (Queensland); and, Artificial Conception Act 196 (Western Australia).
28. South Australia-Reproductive Technology Act 1988; Queensland-Surrogate Parenthood Act 1988; Western Australia-Human Reproductive Technology Act 1991; Australian Capital Territory-Substitute Parent Agreement Act 1994; Tasmania-Surrogate Contracts Act 1994; Victoria-Infertility Treatment Act 1995.
29. *Re Evelyn*, 1998 FLC 92-807.
30. Landau R. Israel: Every person has the right to have children. In: E Blyth, R Landau, eds, *Third-Party*

Assisted Conception Across Cultures: Cultural, Legal and Ethical Perspectives, London: Jessica Kingsley Pub., 2004.

31. Trabman T. Demography. The Jewish Agency for Israel, Department for Jewish Zionist Education. http://www.haaretz.com/hasen/ spages1478066.html. Retrieved from the website on November 18, 2005.

32. National Health Insurance Law. *Book of Laws* 1469, 156 [Hebrew]: 1994.

33. Ministry of Health. *The People's Health Regulations*: [Assisted Human Reproduction-Amendments]. Jerusalem: Ministry of Health [in Hebrew]: 1999a.

34. Paz G, *Do You Want a Child? A Manual for Couples Planning Pregnancy*. Tel Aviv: Hakipod Hakachol Ltd., 1998 [in Hebrew].

35. Siegel-Itzkovic L. Israel to allow women to donate their ova, http://www.bmj.com, 4/7/01, and Ministry of Health (2001b) *Public-Professional Committee for the Examination of Egg Donations* and (2001c) Women Who Are Not Undergoing Fertility Treatments Will Also Be Allowed to Donate Eggs. Jerusalem: Ministry of Health [in Hebrew].

36. Horsey K. Israel allows "social sex selection," http://ivf.net. Retrieved from the website 6/3/05.

37. Luna F. Assisted reproductive technology in Latin America: Some ethical and sociocultural issues. In: E Vayena, P Rowe, D Griffin, eds, *Current Practices and Controversies in Assisted Reproduction: Report of a meeting on "Medical, Ethical and Social Aspects of Assisted Reproduction,"* 9/17 9/21, 2001, World Health Organization, Geneva, Switzerland, 2002.

38. Red Latino Americana de Reproduccion Asistida. *Sonsenso Latinoamericano en aspectos etico-legales relativos a las tecenicas de reproduccion assistido*. Reflaca, Chile, 1996.

39. Zegers-Hochshild F. Cultural expectations from IVF and reproductive genetics in Latin America. *Hum Reprod Update*, 1999; 5:21–5.

40. American Society for Reproductive Medicine, *Mental Health Professional Group Winter Newsletter* 2004. Birmingham, AL.

41. American Society for Reproductive Medicine. *Qualification Guidelines for Infertility Counselors*. American Society for Reproductive Medicine and Mental Health Professional Group, 1995.

42. Burns LH, Covington SN. *Infertility Counseling: A Comprehensive Handbook for Clinicians*. New York: Parthenon Publishing Group, 1999; 529.

43. Boivin J, Appleton TC, Baetens P, et al. Guidelines for counselling in infertility: Outline version. *Hum Reprod* 2001; 16:1301–4.

44. American Psychological Association. *Ethical Principles of Psychologists and Code of Ethics*. Washington, DC 2002; 1996 & Supp. 1999; National Board for Certified Counselors, Inc. and Affiliates, www.nbcc.org/ethics, Greensboro, North Carolina. Retrieved from the website June 23, 2005; American Association of Marriage and Family Therapists. Ethics Committee, *Code of Ethics*, Revised, Alexandria, Virginia (2001); The Principles of Medical Ethics with Annotations Especially Applicable to Psychiatry, American Medical Association, Council of Ethical and Judicial Affairs, Code of Medical Ethics, Washington, D.C. (2001, includes 2003 amendments); American Psychiatric Nurses' Association, *Scope and Standards of Psychiatric and Mental Health Nursing*, Arlington, Virginia (2001).

45. New Zealand Ministry of Social Development, Discussion Paper on Registration of Social Workers (2000). Retrieved from the website on September 15, 2005. www.msd.govt.nz/documents/publications/csre/reg_socwork_discpaper.pdf.

46. British Infertility Counseling Association. *Infertility Counselling for Practising Counsellors*. Sheffield S1 4GE, http://www.bica.net/. Retrieved from the website on September 15, 2005.

47. Canadian Counseling Association, Ottawa, Ontario. http://www.ccacc.ca/SOP.htm. Retrieved from the website on September 15, 2005.

48. Health Canada, Assisted Human Reproduction Implementation Office (2004), Infertility counselling workshop report, http://www.hc-sc.gc.ca/hl-vs/alt formats/hpb-dgps/pdf/reprod/counselling_e.pdf. Retrieved from the website, September 10, 2005.

49. ACT Health: *Health in the Australian Capital Territory, About Us-Psychologists*, http://health.act.gov.au/c/health?a=da&did=10033491. Retrieved from the website September 15, 2005.

50. South Australian Department of Human Resources, South Australian Council on Reproductive Technology, as established under provisions of the Reproductive Technology Act of 1998 (amended July, 2000). http://www.dh.sa.gov.au/reproductive-technology/sacrt.asp. Retrieved from the website on September 14, 2005 .

51. ANZICA, http://www.ANZICAorg/ethics.html. Retrieved from the website on September 14, 2005.

52. *Figueiredo v. Nichols*, 321 Md. 642, 584 A.2d 69 (1991).

53. *Shilkret v. Annapolis Emergency Hosp.*, 276 Md. 187, 349 A.2d 245, 23 (1975).

54. *Heinmiller v. Department of Health*, 127 Wash. 2d 595, 903 P.2d 433 (1995).

55. Israel A. *Applied Law in the Behavioral Health Professions: A Textbook for Social Workers, Counselors, and Psychologists*. New York: Peter Lang Publishing, Inc., 2002.

56. *F.G. v. McDonell*, 150 N.J. 550, 696 A.2d 697 (1997).

57. *Hingerford v. Jones*, 722 A.2d 478 (1998).

58. MCLS §722.851–861.

59. Spar D. *The Baby Business: Elite Eggs, Designer Genes, and the Thriving Commerce of Conception*. Boston, MA: Harvard Business School Press, 2005.

60. The Japan Times. Court rejects attempt to register babies from U.S surrogate mother. 2004. http://search.japatimes.co.jp/print/news/nn08-2004/nn-20040815a2htm. Retrieved from the website September 3, 2005.

61. *Backlund v. University of Washington*, 137 Wn.2d 651, 664, 975 P2d 950 (1999).

62. American Society of Reproductive Medicine. Practice Committee Guidelines: Elements to be considered in obtaining informed consent for ART. *Fertil Steril* 2004; 82(Supp. 1):S202.

63. *Laskowitz v. Ciba Vision Corp.*, 632 N.Y.S.845, 215 A.D.2d 25 (App.Div.1995) (Dicta).

64. *Bee v. Greaves*, 744 F.2d 1387 (10th Cir. 1984).

65. Gorrill M, Johnson L, Patton P, Burry K. Oocyte donor screening: The selection process and cost analysis. *Fertil Steril* 2001; 75(2):400–4.

66. Civil Rights Act of 1964, Pub. l. 88–352.

67. Rehabilitation Act of 1973, Pub.L. 93–112, Vol. 29 §791.

68. Americans with Disabilities Act, Pub. L. 101–336, U.S.C. Title 42 §12101 *et seq.*, at §12102(2)(A).

69. Swain M. *The ART Practice and Refusing Treatment to a Patient Requesting Service*, Opinion Article in ASRM Mental Health Professional Group Newsletter, Spring, 2005 (portions appear throughout this section, by permission of ASRM); *Bragdon v. Abbott*, 524 U.S. 624, 649–650 (1998).

70. Ethics Committee of the American Society for Reproductive Medicine. Child-rearing and the provision of fertility services. *Fertil Steril* 2004; 82:S1.

71. *Brokaw v. Mercer County*, 235 F. 3d 1000 (7th Cir. 2000), *Santosky v. Kramer*, 455 U.S. 745, 753 (1982).

72. *Brokaw v. Mercer County*, 235. F.3d 1000 (nth Cir. 12/19/2000.

73. *Eckhardt v. Charter Hosp.*, 124 N.M. 549, 953 P. 2d 722 (Ct. App.1997); *Jaffee v. Redmond*, 518 U.S, 1, 116 S.Ct. 1923, 135 L.Ed. 2d 337 (1996).

74. *Tarasoff v. Regents of the Univ.Cal.*, 17 Cal. 3d 425, 551 P,2d 334, 131 Cal. Rptr. 14 (1976).

75. Pub.L. 104-191.

76. Summary of the HIPAA Privacy Rule, www.hhs.gov/ocr/hipaa/guidelines/sharinsfortpo.pdf, www.hhs.gov/ocr/privacysummary.pdf.

77. *Confidentiality: RNC Guidance for Occupational Health Nurses*. Royal College of Nursing (2003). http://www.rcn.org.u/publications/ pdf/confidentiality.pdf. Retrieved from the website September 11, 2005; Data Protection Act 1998 (UK) c. 69(l)(i).

78. Personal Information and Electronic Documents Act 2000 (Canada) c.5.

79. Privacy Act of 1988 cht. (1988) amended 2001, Australia.

80. *Grosse v. Purvis* (2003).ODC 151, Dist. Ct. Brisbane, Qld.

81. Pope KS, Tabachnick BG, Keith-Spiegel P. Ethics of Practice: The beliefs and behaviors of psychologists as therapists. In: *AAMFT Ethics Casebook*, 175. *A National Survey of the Ethical Practices and Attitudes of Marriage and Family Therapists* 1998; 42:993–1006.

82. Sparrow MK. *License to Steal: Why Fraud Plagues America's Healthcare System*. Boulder, CO: Westview Press, 1998.

83. Caudill OB. Twelve pitfalls for psychotherapists. *Family Therapy News*, Oct/Nov. 2000; 17–20.

84. *Diagnostic and Statistical Manual of Mental Disorders*, Fourth Edition (DSM-IV), American Psychiatric Publishing, Arlington, Virginia; National Center for Health Statistics, *International Classification of Diseases*, Tenth Revision, Clinical Modification, (ICD-9), 1999.

85. Personal correspondence with a party to the case, on September 13, 2005. Names withheld by request. Case filed in 1995.

86. Robertson JA. *Children of Choice*. Princeton, NJ: Princeton University Press, 1994.

87. *Skinner v. Oklahoma*, 316 U.S 535, 541 (1942); *Meyer v. Nebraska, 262 U.S. 390, 393 (1923); Cleveland Bd. Of Ed. v.*

LaFleur, 414 U.S. 632, 639–40, (1973); *Eisenstadt v. Baird*, 405 U.S. 438, 453 (1972).

88. *Planned Parenthood of SE PA v. Casey*, 505 U.S. 833, 851 (1992).

89. American Society for Reproductive Medicine. Practice Committee Guidelines for Sperm Donation. *Fertil Steril* 2004; 82:S11.

90. *Doornbos v. Doornbos*, 112 Ill. App. 2d 473, 139 N.E. 844 (1956).

91. *Anonymous v. Anonymous*, 41 Misc. 2d 886, 246 N.Y.S.2d 1835 (Sup. Ct., Suffolk Co.1964).

92. *Thomas v. Rubin*, 209 A.D. 2d 298, 619 N.Y.S.2d 356 (1st Dep't. 1994).

93. *In re Guardianship of I. H.* 2003 Me.130, 834 A.2d 922, 2003 ME 130 (Me. 11/04/2003); *People v. Shreve*, 756 N.E.2d 422 (2001); *In the Matter of the Parentage of J.M.K. and D.R.K.*, 89 P.3d 309, Wa.Ct. of App. (May 4, 2004); *Ferguson v. McKiernan*, No. 1430 MDA 2003 (Pa. Super.Ct., 7/22/04), *In re Sullivan*, No. 14-04-00514-CV (Tex.App.Dist.14 02/24/2005).

94. McConvil J, Mills E. *Re Patrick* and the rights and responsibilities of sperm donor fathers in Australian family law. *QUT Law Justice* 2003; 3:2.

95. *The Australian* (2003). www.theaustralain.com.au. Retrieved from the website September 1, 2005.

96. Wright et al., *Assisted Reproductive Technology Surveillance-United States*, 2000, CDC/MMWR Surveillance summaries, August 29, 2003/52; 1–16.

97. Blyth E. The United States of America: Regulation, technology, and the marketplace. In: E Blyth, R Landau, eds, *Third-Party Assisted Conception Across Cultures: Cultural, Legal and Ethical Perspectives*. London: Jessica Kingsley Pub., 2004; 246–65.

98. Ethics Committee of the American Society for Reproductive Medicine. Family members as gamete donors and surrogates. *Fertil Steril* 2003; 80:5.

99. *McDonald v. McDonald*, 196 A.D.2d 7, 608 N.Y.S.2d 477 (2d Dep't. 1994).

100. *In re C.K.G.*, No. M2003–01320-COA-R3-JV (Tenn.App. 06/22/2004).

101. *K.M. v. E.G.*, 118 Cal.App4th 477, 13 Cal.Rptr.3d 136, (Cal. App.1st Dist.2004). Petition for review granted by Supreme Court of California, 97 P.3d 72, Cal.Rptr.3d 667 (September 1, 2004).

102. *K.M. v E.G.*, Ct.App.1/5 A101754, S125643, 8/22/05.

103. *Rice v. Flynn*, 2005-Ohio-467 (Ohio App.Dist.9, 09/07/05).

104. Ethics Committee of the American Society for Reproductive Medicine. Informing Offspring of their Conception by Donor Gamete. *Fertil Steril* 2004; 81:3, S27.

105. *York v. Jones*, 717 F. Supp. 421 (E.D. Va. 1989).

106. *Davis v Davis*, 842 S.W.2d 588 (Tenn. 1992), *Kass v. Kass,*, 91 N.Y.2d 554, 673 N.Y.S.2d 350 (1998), *A.Z. v. B.Z.*, 431 Mass. 150, 725 N.E.2d 1051 (2000), *J.B. v. M.B.* No. A-9-00 (8/14/01), *Litowitz v. Litowitz*, 146 Wash.2d 514, 48 P.3d 261, 2002.

107. *Gladu v. Boston* IVF, 32 M.L.W. 1195 (2/9/04).

108. Crockin S. Law, Language and Liability: Defining Issues, Determining Outcomes? Proceedings of ART and Embryo Law: Practice, Policy, Regulation and Ethics, Serono Symposia International, Cambridge, MA, November, 2004.

109. Pub. L. No. 104-99, 110 Stat. 26 (1996), as amended, Consolidated Appropriations Resolution, 2003, Pub. L. No. 108–7, 117 Stat. 11 (2003).

110. Crockin S. *Embryo Law: Legal Aspects of Embryo Status and Disposition*. 2001; CME Presentation, Serono Symposia.

111. La. Rev. Stat. Ann. § 9:123, § 9:126 (West 1991).

112. *Lifches v. Hartigan*, 735 F.Supp.1361, aff'd without opinion, sub nom. *Scholberg v. Lifchez*, 914 F.2d.

113. Franz L. UCSD Announces Funding of Fertility Program Review (University of California at Irvine press release, January 30, 1996); *Moore v. UCI*, et. al; *Clay v. UCI*, et. al., (Orange Cty. Sup.Ct.) CA#s 752293–752294.

114. Cal.Bus. and Prof. Code § 2260(a) (West 1997).

115. *Fasano v. Nash*, 723 N.Y.S.2d 181 (App. Div. 2001), *Perry-Rogers v. Obasaju*, 723 N.Y.S.2d 28 (App. Div. 2001), *Perry-Rogers v. Fasano*, 276 A.D.2d 67; 715 N.Y.S.2d 19 (2000).

116. *Leeds Teaching Hospitals NHS v A*[2003], EWHC 259 (QB)[2003]1FLR.

117. Court rules on father of IVF mix-up twins. BBC News (health section) 2003 Feb 26 www.news.bbc.co.uk. Retrieved from website August 15, 2005.

118. Stuart W. Child with two fathers: The unbelievable story of a hospital's mistake 1999. In: V Cotrell, ed, Kind van twee vaders: de ongeloofijke gevolgen van een ziekenhuisfout (Arbeiderspers).

119. *In re Marriage of Bazzanca*, 61 Cal.App.4th 1410, 72 Cal.Rptr.2d 280 (Cal.App. Dist.4 03/10/1998).

120. *Robert B. v. Susan B.*, 109 Cal.App.4th 1109, 135 Cal.Rptr.2d 785, fn7 (Cal.App. Dist.6 06/13/2003).

121. *In re Baby M*, 537 A.2d 1227 (NJ 1988); *In re Marriage of Moschetta*, 30 Cal.Rptr.2d 893, 25 Cal. App. 4th 1218(1994).

122. New Hampshire Title XII, Cap. 68-B:18; Virginia Code 20–160, for example.

123. Surrogacy: *some facts*. 2005. http://www.BBC.co.uk. Retrieved from the website 09/28/05.

124. *Hecht v. Superior Court of County of Los Angeles*, 50 Cal.App.4th 1289, 59 Cal.Rptr.2d 222 (Cal.App. Dist2 11/13/1996).

125. Kerr SM, et al. Post-mortem sperm procurement *J Urol* 1997; 167:2154–6.

126. Ethics Commmittee of the American Society for Reproductive Medicine. Posthumous Reproduction, *Fertil Steril* 2004; 82: S.1 (currently under revision).

127. N.Y. Public Health Law §§ 4300–4309.

128. Aston J, Howard S. Widow Has No Legal Right to Family. Press Association Newsfile, Oct. 3, 1996.

129. www.medicalnewstoday.com. Retrieved from the website on June 2, 2005.

130. *Woodward v. Comm'r of Social Security*, 435 Mass. 536 (1996), *In re Estate of Kolacy*, 332 N.J. Super. 593, 753 A.2d 1257 (N.J. Super.Ct.Ch.Div. 2000); *Gillett-Netting v. Barnhart*, 231 F.Supp. 2d 961 (D.Ariz.2002).

131. N.Y.C.R.R. §52–8.7.

132. Practice committee of the American Society for Reproductive Medicine. A Committee Opinion. *Fertil Steril* 1998.

31 Global Perspectives on Infertility Counseling

JEAN M. HAASE AND ERIC BLYTH

The world only exists in your eyes – your conception of it. You can make it as big or as small as you want to.
– F. Scott Fitzgerald, 1945

Since the 1980s, infertility counseling has gained increasing recognition in a number of countries, with considerable growth occurring in the past ten years. This has coincided with the expansion of reproductive technologies, particularly in the developed world. Globally, the provision of infertility counseling is now supported by many medical societies, governments and consumer organizations, and a new International Infertility Counseling Organization (IICO).

A number of key factors have had an impact on the development of infertility counseling. First, government legislation and regulation in some countries and jurisdictions addresses specific requirements for counseling provision. Legislation in the United Kingdom,[1] the state of Victoria in Australia,[2] and recently, Canada[3] were preceded by influential advisory reports that recommended the provision of counseling services in fertility clinics.[4–6] Second, there has been a growth in the number of professional infertility counseling associations that have been established at national (e.g. United Kingdom, Japan, Germany, Switzerland) and pan-national (e.g., Europe, Australia and New Zealand, United States/Latin America) levels. These have been influential in various ways, such as the provision of professional education and collegial support, and contributions to practice standards and policy development. A third factor is the opportunity for professional development through conference participation, training opportunities, and communication through the use of the internet and world wide web. Many infertility counselors have expressed a sense of professional isolation in the past, but the establishment of IICO and the first global symposium for counselors held in 2004[7] are important milestones, suggesting that there is considerable interest in expanding collaboration between professionals. These combined developments seem likely to ensure the continued growth worldwide of infertility counseling as a recognized profession.

While cross-cultural issues in infertility counseling are the focus of Chapter 4, this chapter addresses:

- the emergence of infertility counseling as a specialized activity in assisted conception;
- the development and influence of infertility counseling associations;
- the impact of legislation and professional guidelines;
- clinical and theoretical issues related to infertility counseling;
- future implications for the international development of infertility counseling.

HISTORICAL OVERVIEW

The development of infertility counseling at a global level can be traced, in large part, through a review of how mental health professionals have organized and formed professional associations facilitating academic and clinical collaboration with medical professionals working in the field of infertility. This section provides an overview of the chronological development of these associations, noting any relevant legislative or regulatory counseling requirements to date.[1]

USA – Mental Health Professional Group (affiliated with ASRM)

What is now the MHPG had its origins as an informal network of counselors who met at the 1985 meeting

---

[1] Although we are aware of individuals offering infertility counseling in many countries not cited here (and space precludes a detailed discussion of infertility counseling in each country), we know of no other infertility counseling organizations, at this point in time.

of the American Fertility Society [later becoming the American Society for Reproductive Medicine (ASRM)]. By 1987, the group was formally established as the Psychological Aspects of Infertility Special Interest Group of AFS, as a multidisciplinary group committed to the study and treatment of the emotional components of reproductive health. Membership grew and the group was promoted to professional group status within ASRM, becoming the Psychological Special Interest Group (PSIG) in 1995. It is now known as the Mental Health Professional Group (MHPG). Membership is open to all active members of ASRM – regardless of professional discipline – and in 2005, membership was 343 individuals.

In the United States, there is no national or state policy or regulation related to assisted conception, and consequently there is no *requirement* for fertility clinics to either provide or recommend counseling. Although the ASRM has various guidelines recommending that counseling services be available in programs offering assisted conception procedures,[8–15] adherence to these recommendations is voluntary on the part of clinics. Currently, infertility counseling appears to be provided within the United States in one of three ways. The infertility counselor may be an employee of the clinic; an independent mental health professional who has a contract with a clinic to provide specific services (e.g., for evaluations of donors/donor recipients); or an independent mental health professional in private practice, with no formal or informal affiliation with a clinic.

Current MHPG goals are to:

■ promote greater awareness of the psychosocial dimensions of reproductive health issues and treatment;
■ educate ASRM members and the general public about the emotional aspects of infertility and the need for support services in conjunction with medical care;
■ encourage research into the psychosocial aspects of reproductive health;
■ provide materials that enable practitioners to better meet clients' needs for information, support, and comprehensive care.

An Executive Committee governs the MHPG, and several standing committees have been established to undertake projects that allow the MHPG to fulfill its goals:

■ *Scientific Development Committee* (reviews recent relevant scientific information and encourages scientific study and research among members);

■ *Abstract Committee* (reviews and selects research projects that are submitted for oral or poster presentation at the ASRM Annual Meeting);
■ *Membership Committee* (encourages health and mental health professionals in reproductive health to join the MHPG); and
■ *Education Committee* (promotes further learning and educational growth among members).

In addition to the Standing Committees, the MHPG supports a number of *ad hoc* Task Forces whose aim is to gather specific information and data and make recommendations regarding guidelines and policies relevant to client care and professional responsibility. These currently include:

■ International Infertility Counseling Task Force
■ Accreditation of Infertility Counselors Task Force
■ Psychological Assessment of Egg Donors Task Force
■ Embryo Donation Task Force
■ Children of the ARTs Task Force
■ Internet Task Force
■ Egg Donor Recruitment Programs Task Force
■ Mentoring and Training Task Force
■ Regulatory Issues Task Force
■ Oocyte Donors Follow-up Task Force
■ Latin American Task Force

As a component of the ASRM, the Chair of MHPG communicates directly with the President and Executive Director of ASRM. MHPG members have gained representation on essential committees within ASRM such as ASRM's Ethics Committee, the Society for Assisted Reproductive Technology (SART), and ASRM Patient Education Committee. In addition, consumer advocacy groups and other mental health professional associations have recognized the role of mental health professionals in the treatment, education, and research of psychosocial issues in reproductive health.

Key activities undertaken by MHPG include:

■ helping to develop ASRM guidelines for fertility counselors and other professionals in reproductive health[8–15] and MHPG qualification guidelines for mental health professionals in reproductive health;[16]
■ developing ASRM patient education information[17] about the psychological aspects of infertility, and resources for finding infertility counselors;
■ participating in multidisciplinary seminars and symposia, and presenting abstracts, papers, poster sessions, and roundtables at ASRM annual meetings;
■ organizing annual postgraduate courses nationally and regionally;

■ encouraging research in reproductive health psychology including collaboration with other MHPG members, among members, or on various topics decided on by MHPG membership or the executive committee;

■ publishing a bibliography of articles addressing psychological aspects of infertility including a bibliography on books for children – that are available online at the ASRM website;[18]

■ publishing a triennial members' newsletter that is accessible online for members;

■ instituting an internet listserve consultation and discussion service for members, to facilitate professional collaboration and discussion, and information sharing;

■ introducing a mentoring program at annual ASRM meetings in which senior members of MHPG arrange one-on-one meetings with conference attendees to discuss clinical, ethical, and research issues of mutual interest; a program to offer year-round program telephone/email mentoring to newer members is being established; and

■ working to establish an infertility counseling credentialing system.

United Kingdom: British Infertility Counselling Association (BICA)

Infertility counseling is mandated in the United Kingdom under the Human Fertilisation and Embryology Act 1990.[1] Prospective donors of gametes and embryos and people considering licensed treatments (i.e., treatments involving an embryo created outside the human body and treatments involving donated gametes or embryos) under the Act, must be offered a 'suitable opportunity' to receive 'proper' counseling. The Act does not define proper, and while infertility counseling has been able to develop in the United Kingdom because of its statutory basis, there remain considerable variations in the provision of counseling made available by fertility clinics across the country. This has occurred despite elaboration of counseling standards in the *Code of Practice* published by the statutory regulatory body, the Human Fertilisation and Embryology Authority (HFEA).[19]

BICA was founded in 1988 as an independent association and is a registered charity that "aims to encourage and facilitate its members to provide the highest standards of counselling support to people affected by fertility issues." BICA draws its membership, currently at 175, from a wide professional field, including social workers, psychologists, nurses, and others, and represents most of those offering counseling services at licensed fertility clinics.

Since its inception, BICA has assumed an increasingly active role in the development of assisted conception services in the United Kingdom. It is in regular communication with the Department of Health, the HFEA, and the multidisciplinary British Fertility Society (BFS), and has participated in policy consultations undertaken by the government, the HFEA, and the U.K. Parliament. BICA members (although acting in a personal capacity rather than representing BICA) serve on the Executive Committee of the BFS, as inspectors for the HFEA, and a founder member of BICA is currently a member of the HFEA. BICA is also represented on a multidisciplinary body originally set up under the auspices of the British Association of Social Workers, the Project Group on Assisted Reproduction (PROGAR), which comprises representatives from social services, children's services, adoption services, and donor-conceived families. BICA has engaged in an extensive program of member information and support through a *Practice Guide* series and publication of the *Journal of Fertility Counselling* three times annually. Further professional development for members is provided through national and regional meetings, conferences, and study days. Information for members and the public is available through an information officer and a website that also provides access to a nationwide infertility counselor referral system.

In collaboration with the BFS, BICA has developed a voluntary accreditation process for infertility counselors, the Infertility Counselling Award, which has university recognition. The award is based on a portfolio documentation of academic credentials, knowledge base, and supervised clinical experience. A two-tiered award program is now under consideration to increase the number of counselors undertaking the award.

Australia and New Zealand Infertility Counselling Association – ANZICA

Infertility counseling in Australia and New Zealand evolved during the 1980s, and the inaugural meeting of ANZICA took place in Canberra in 1989. ANZICA was formed to:

■ represent the particular interests of infertility counselors;

■ promote recognition and understanding of counseling and the counseling process in the context of infertility;

■ promote training of counselors in the area of infertility;

■ undertake research leading to an understanding of the counseling needs of people with fertility problems and improve the effectiveness of counseling services;

■ provide professional development for members;

■ maintain a regular newsletter;

■ be a consultative group on issues pertaining to infertility;

■ actively cooperate with organizations with similar aims and objectives.

Since inauguration, membership of ANZICA – which is restricted to licensed social workers, psychologists, and psychiatrists – has grown to approximately 100, of whom about three-quarters are employed in clinics. ANZICA members sit on the National Ethics Advisory Board of the National Medical and Research Council of Australia, the Reproductive Technology Accreditation Council (RTAC), Fertility Society of Australia (FSA), and various other organizations; and an ANZICA member has served as President of FSA. Clinic accreditation by RTAC – a peer-accreditation body – is well respected, and several state and national authorities will only license (and provide federal funding for patients treated at) RTAC accredited clinics. Under RTAC guidelines:

■ all counselors hired by clinics must be members of ANZICA;

■ prospective donors and recipients and their partners must undergo counseling for a minimum of two sessions; and

■ counselors must be present during accreditation visits.

Assisted conception is regulated variably across Australia and New Zealand, thus impacting differentially on practice and, concomitantly, the provision of infertility counseling services. Legislation is in force in the states of Victoria,[2] South Australia,[20] Western Australia,[21] and in New Zealand[22] and is about to be implemented in the state of New South Wales in Australia.[23] Victoria was the first Australian state to afford a donor-conceived person the legal right to learn the identity of his or her donor, and has established both statutory and voluntary donor registers,[24] as well as regulations for 'donor linking' counseling[25] (counseling that is available when a donor-conceived person formally requests his or her donor's identity). In 1995, Victoria became the first jurisdiction in the world to mandate counseling for *all* infertility patients and/or donors. In 2004, Western Australia's legislation was amended to give a donor-conceived person the legal right to learn the identity of his or her donor.

Donor conception has been one of the main issues addressed at ANZICA professional development sessions, but other topics include access to treatment, the best interests of children conceived following assisted conception, and psychosocial research and practice standards. ANZICA's annual meeting is held in conjunction with the FSA yearly conference, and ANZICA publishes a newsletter. The ANZICA website provides a communications network not only for members, many of whom work in geographical and professional isolation, but also for developing links internationally. Initially, it was considered important for ANZICA to be independent of, but closely linked with, FSA to enable counseling to establish a clear professional identity. Recently, however, ANZICA has become a special interest group of FSA in order to facilitate increased integration.

Psychology and Counselling Special Interest Group of the European Society for Human Reproduction and Embryology (ESHRE)

The Psychology and Counselling Special Interest Group of the European Society for Human Reproduction and Embryology (ESHRE) was founded in 1993. Membership of the group is open to any member of ESHRE. As ESHRE is an international, multiprofessional society, members come from a variety of countries and professions. As of 2005, the P&C Special Interest Group had a membership of 190.

The group's purpose is to address the psychosocial issues and needs of clients and professionals working in infertility by:

■ promoting awareness about the significance and importance of psychosocial issues;

■ facilitating the study and discussion of psychosocial aspects of reproductive health;

■ conducting research into the psychosocial aspects of reproductive health;

■ educating professionals about psychosocial issues that may affect the individual and/or couple facing reproductive health problems;

■ fostering cooperation and multidisciplinary collaboration among professionals working in different disciplines; and

■ cooperating with other societies having similar goals.

Members of the group conduct research on the psychosocial aspects of

■ specific reproductive conditions;

■ medical treatments;

■ family-building options;

■ child-free living;

■ stress and its effect on biological functioning;

the development of children conceived following assisted conception; and

family processes in families using assisted conception procedures.

The group promotes the psychosocial aspects of reproductive health in a number of ways:

arranging precongress courses at ESHRE annual meetings;

arranging symposia;

authoring ESHRE's *Counselling Guidelines*;[26]

undertaking an international initiative for the development of the Fertility Quality of Life (FertiQoL) measure; and

promoting the establishment of the International Infertility Counselors Organization (IICO).

Germany – Beratungsnetzwerk Kinderwunsch Deutschland e.V. (BKiD)

Interest in the psychosocial aspects of infertility developed in Germany during the late 1980s, gaining momentum during the 1990s. Between 1989 and 2000, a number of universities collaborated in federal research projects devoted to psychosocial issues in infertility. One group carried out research on developing a concept for infertility counseling, publishing in 2004 the first, and only, book on infertility counseling in German, *Couple Counseling and Therapy for Infertility*.[27]

There is no legislation regarding assisted conception in Germany, although this is anticipated. While medical guidelines for assisted conception recommend the provision of counseling prior to treatment, doctors usually see themselves as providing this because the German term used for 'counseling' in the guidelines is vague. Furthermore, the guidelines do not specify the criteria regarding the qualifications of counselors.

There are currently more than ninety certified infertility counselors in Germany whose main professional backgrounds are in social work, psychology, and medicine. Most counselors offer individual and couple counseling, and some offer group work. Few infertility counselors are employed by fertility clinics or work within the reimbursement system of the German health insurance program. Instead, the majority work in private practice or in counseling institutions funded either by the state or by churches, where counseling services are provided free (increasingly less likely for financial pressure), for a nominal fee, or at market rates.

BKiD was founded in June 2000 and was formally organized as a charitable organization in 2002. In 2001,

it developed guidelines for accreditation of infertility counselors. In order to be accredited, a person must

have completed a professional training in a psychosocial discipline;

have completed a training in counseling/therapy;

have a minimum two years counseling/therapy experience and have carried out infertility counseling for a minimum of one year;

have ongoing and evidence-based basic knowledge of the psychosocial implications of infertility;

undergo further training and supervision.

BKiD organizes two annual meetings, which include training for new members and continuing education training events on various topics related to infertility counseling. It has been proactive in raising awareness about psychosocial aspects of infertility, has established a website, and developed a brochure that is distributed to fertility clinics. As of 2005, BKiD had ninety-eight members. While the organization aims to attract counselors nationwide to improve access to high-quality counseling, there are several areas in Germany (especially in the former East Germany) where there are a number of clinics providing infertility treatment, but few or no infertility counselors. Closer collaboration with clinics is essential to make counseling available more easily for those in treatment, and to increase medical professionals' awareness of psychosocial issues.

International Infertility Counseling Organisation (IICO)

Infertility counselors have been communicating informally with each other for years. At the International Federation of Fertility Societies' meeting in 2002, held in Melbourne, ANZICA organized a postgraduate course that included the attendance of many international infertility counselors. This set the stage for the formation of what subsequently became IICO through discussions and meetings involving leaders from several national associations. An initial organizational meeting took place at the annual meeting of ESHRE in Madrid in 2003, and further progress was made at a second meeting held during the annual meeting of ASRM/MHPG in San Antonio in October 2003. IFFS also gave approval for IICO to organize a postgraduate course at the IFFS 2004 meeting to take place in Montreal. The 2004 IFFS meeting therefore became IICO's official launch with a postgraduate course, "Global Perspectives in Infertility Counseling," and IICO's inaugural business meeting. Fifty-nine counselors from fourteen different countries attended the postgraduate course.[7] In Montreal, the

IFFS executive board voted in favor of IICO becoming a liaison group of IFFS. IICO's declared objectives are:

■ to promote a comprehensive and ethical approach to the care of people affected by or involved with infertility;
■ to define quality standards of communicative and counseling interventions within the context of infertility care;
■ to encourage and support international cooperation and education among mental health professionals working in reproductive health and cooperation with other specialized societies in the field of infertility;
■ to establish global professional standards and practice guidelines for the provision of psychological care regarding reproductive issues and to develop curricula and training programs for mental health professionals;
■ to organize international meetings and congresses on subjects of infertility counseling at regular intervals in conjunction with (but not exclusive to) the tri-annual meeting of IFFS and meetings of other relevant societies; and
■ to promote the study of the ethical and psychosocial aspects of reproductive health.

At the inaugural business meeting, much of the discussion centered on developing the IICO constitution, work that was progressed subsequently through email contact between the constituent organisations (ANZICA, ASRM/MHPG, BICA, Bkid, ESHRE/PCSIG, FertiForum, GLASMI, and JAPCRM) and the 2004 meetings of ESHRE (Berlin) and ASRM (Philadelphia). IICO has developed by-laws, a logo, and website that will facilitate effective member communications between members; provide information on professional and patient education materials and resources as well as professional meetings and educational opportunities; and an internet listserve facilitating consultation, discussion, and information sharing. As a new, and obviously diverse, international organization, much remains 'under construction' including the plans for IICO's second international postgraduate course.

Japan Association of Psychological Counseling for Reproductive Health (JAPCRM)

IVF has been provided in Japan since the 1980s, and donor insemination for much longer. Currently, nearly 600 institutions are registered to provide IVF in Japan, although there is no law regulating services. More than twenty Japanese scientific societies and associations issue their own qualifications for practicing in psychotherapy or professional counseling, the most widely recognized qualification being that of Certified Clinical Psychologist (CCP), which demands a master's degree in clinical psychology and a minimum of one year clinical experience. Fewer than 20 of the 13,000 CCPs in Japan currently work in reproductive health. Furthermore, many Japanese doctors and nurses believe that infertility counseling is their job, not that of mental health professionals, although few have the additional training in counseling that physicians in countries like Switzerland, Austria, and Germany do.

During the mid-1990s, some infertility specialists realized that infertility counseling should be provided by properly qualified professional counselors, and employed psychologists in their clinics. During the 1990s, this first generation of infertility counselors developed their expertise and exchanged their views and experiences with other professions in reproductive health. In September 2003, the Japan Association of Psychological Counseling for Reproductive Medicine (JAPCRM) was established. The founding members include CCPs, other mental health professionals, gynecologists, and medical staff working in reproductive health. There is no strict requirement for membership, and as of 2005, there were about 120 members – about half nurses, twenty mental health professionals, and forty gynecologists.

The primary aim of JAPCRM is to provide infertile couples[2] with professional counseling services. JAPCRM holds annual meetings, promotes education, training, research, and publications, and collaborates with other academic and medical associations. In 2005, the organization launched a one-year training course that will provide a specialist qualification in infertility counseling. JAPCRM is an independent organization committed to the autonomy of infertility counselors from other professionals in reproductive health. In addition, it provides assistance to consumer support organizations and conducts research, most recently on treatment outcomes.

Switzerland – Association of Infertility Counselling ("FertiForum")

Under Swiss legislation,[28] infertility clinics must offer psychological assistance to clients before, during, and after all forms of medically assisted procreation, without defining the credentials of those who would and should provide such assistance. Very few fertility clinics employ designated infertility counselors, so referrals for counseling are made to a range of external mental

---

[2] In some countries, heterosexual couples only may access assisted conception services, either because of legislation or, in its absence, customary practice.

health professionals including psychologists, family planning counselors, social workers, nurses, and physicians – the latter are mainly psychiatrists and specially trained gynecologists with special training in mental health counseling. With the exception of a limited number of stimulation cycles, assisted conception treatment is generally not covered by health insurance in Switzerland. Therefore, access to services, including access to adequate psychosocial support, is often limited by or affected by personal financial resources.

The decision to establish FertiForum was taken in 2004 as a direct consequence of proposals to create the IICO. Each fertility clinic in Switzerland was contacted to identity those professionals who were providing infertility counseling. As a result, a dozen interested counselors met on four occasions in 2004 and 2005, and another twenty people expressed interest in the association. Currently, it is proposed that FertiForum will be established under the auspices of the Swiss Society for Reproductive Health (SSRM) to ensure access to a wider number of professionals engaged in assisted conception in Switzerland, and that one of the founders of FertiForum will be appointed to the committee of SSRM to promote the new organization. Key activities to date have been the development of a constitution, informing interested parties and potential members of the existence of FertiForum, and identifying priorities in relation to practice, research, and training. The goals of FertiForum are:

■ providing support for infertility counselors at local, national, and international, levels;
■ promoting awareness of the role of counseling in reproductive health;
■ establishing common criteria for training infertility counselors;
■ encouraging postgraduate training;
■ participating in the development of government policies that are related to infertility counseling;
■ promoting communication between different associations concerned with infertility;
■ promoting research to develop understanding of the psychosocial needs of those experiencing infertility and improve the efficiency of counseling practice;
■ providing information about infertility and counseling;
■ informing members of the association's activities; and
■ collaborating with other associations promoting similar goals.

Currently the key issues facing the organization are to define its place and role within SSRM and – given that three languages (French, German, and Italian) are spoken in different parts of Switzerland – to develop communications with people in different parts of the country.

Latin America – Grupo Latinoamericano de Interes en Salud Mental en Infertilidad (GLASMI)

Assisted conception services have been available in Latin America since the late 1970s, although it was not until the early 1990s that some clinics began to acknowledge the importance of psychosocial intervention and the role of counselors in reproductive health. Subsequently, more counselors began to participate as staff members in infertility clinics. The majority of mental health professionals offering counseling are qualified to master's or doctoral level in psychology, psychiatry, or marriage and family therapy. It is less common to find social workers and psychiatric nurses working as infertility counselors in Latin America. Although fertility clinics have offered courses on the psychosocial, medical and legal dimensions of infertility, there has been insufficient availability of relevant information and training in most Latin American countries. Consequently, many mental health professionals from Latin America have become members of the MHPG of the ASRM and have used the MHPG's continuing education program to help enhance their knowledge base, theoretical understanding, and clinical skills. In 1998, MHPG established a Latin American Task Force to offer networking opportunities and a cross-cultural interchange of knowledge, research, and experiences between Latin American members and other members of the MHPG.

Following proposals to launch the IICO, a decision was taken to launch a designated Latin American infertility counseling group. In 2004, GLASMI was established as an interest group of the Latin American Federacion Latinoamericana de Sociedades de Esterilidad y Fertilidad (FLASEF). The goals of GLASMI are to:

■ encourage multidisciplinary work and collaboration in reproductive health;
■ provide a forum for exchange of ideas, experiences, and research results for professionals involved in reproductive health;
■ be a source of educational reference and support in psychosocial aspects for professionals involved in reproductive health;
■ encourage continued education about psychosocial aspects of infertility through courses, symposia, and workshops;
■ encourage training of mental health professionals in infertility counseling;

■ develop guidelines for assessment and counseling in infertility;

■ promote the importance of research in psychosocial aspects of infertility, counseling in infertility, and the impact of assisted conception procedures on clients, offspring, and families;

■ develop educational material for clients and professionals working in reproductive health;

■ establish a network for communication and support between Latin American professionals interested in mental health in infertility; and

■ establish a close relationship with the IICO and the ASRM MHPG Latin American Task Force.

As a fledgling organization with a small, but growing, membership and facing a historical tendency to marginalize the importance of infertility counseling, GLASMI faces a number of challenges – many similar to those faced by the organizations mentioned earlier. These challenges include establishing communications with mental health professionals and patient groups over a vast geographical area; promoting awareness about the contribution of infertility counseling to reproductive healthcare; and establishing new and significant ways of collaborating with and contributing to FLASEF.

Canadian Infertility Counselling Association (CICA)

Given the recent passage of Canadian legislation that mandates counseling for most participants in assisted conception, Health Canada sponsored a consultation workshop on infertility counseling in May 2004. Twenty-two Canadian infertility counselors attended, together with seven counselors from five other countries. The primary goals of the workshop were to: discuss the impact of the Assisted Human Reproduction Act on infertility counseling in Canada; to promote dialogue about infertility counseling services in Canada; and to discuss the development of a regulatory framework for infertility counseling in support of the Assisted Human Reproduction Act.[29] Although a regional network of infertility counselors had been meeting for several years in Toronto, this was the first national meeting of Canadian infertility counselors. At the end of the two-day workshop, Canadian counselors decided to establish the Canadian Infertility Counseling Association (CICA), which remains in the preliminary stages of development. Early in 2006, CICA became a special interest group of the Canadian Fertility and Andrology Society (CFAS), to be known as Counselling Special Interest Group (CSIG). The regu-

lations about mandatory counseling under the Assisted Human Reproduction Act are still being developed, with consultations planned among Health Canada, counselors, consumer groups, and other stakeholders.

THEORETICAL FRAMEWORKS

Although counselors have identified many common interests and concerns at a global level, their clinical roles and theoretical perspectives are characterized by wide variations. While understandably influenced by international differences and cultural issues, other factors affecting theoretical approaches to infertility counseling include the:

■ academic discipline and clinical training/background of counselors;

■ requirements of legislation, regulations, professional policies, and codes of practice;

■ practice standards developed by infertility counseling associations.

Academic and clinical training, scope of practice, codes of ethics, and professional values have a significant influence on the ways in which various mental health professions provide infertility counseling. For example, some favor a nondirective approach of traditional, client-centered psychotherapies, while others favor the addition of a certain degree of guidance, advice, and even assessment or evaluation. Many counselors (for theoretical or practical purposes) have adopted a perspective somewhere between these two, respecting client self-determination but focusing on the provision of education, support, advocacy, and liaison with the medical team. For some counselors with an interest in social policy development, the regulation of assisted conception has provided a unique opportunity for consultation, analysis, and advocacy regarding the broader societal aspects of assisted conception, such as rights of access by donor-conceived people to genetic origins information, and access to assisted conception services by minority groups such as single women and lesbian couples. Others have focused on the more personal and psychological impact of infertility, contributing clinical expertise and knowledge to the development of practice guidelines, research, and training for other professionals.

As might be expected, a wide range of therapeutic skills are used by infertility counselors, and it is virtually impossible to identify specific theories or techniques that are universally favored. Mind–body approaches have become respected in North America by a number of professionals, and are based on cognitive-behavioral theories of stress management.[30,31] However, family systems theory, grief and loss perspectives, crisis intervention, group counseling, feminist oriented, emotionally focused, psychodynamic, psychoanalytic, marital and sex therapies, brief solution-focused, strategic, and self-psychology approaches are all found within the varied practice domains of infertility counselors.[32] Preferred frameworks may be influenced by the professional background of the counselor, selected on the basis of specific client needs, or chosen for a combination of reasons.

In many countries, certain mental health professions are regulated by legislation and licensing requirements (e.g., psychiatry, psychology, social work, and genetics counseling), while others are self-regulated (e.g., marital and family counseling). This has implications for professionals' use of title, scope of practice, areas of expertise, need for continuing professional accreditation, and public accountability through complaints and discipline procedures. Some professional organizations, such as ANZICA, restrict membership to licensed, regulated professions. These standards are upheld in both the Victoria legislation and through the requirements of RTAC accreditation (see earlier discussion). However, other counseling organizations such as BICA, ESHRE's Psychology and Counselling Special Interest Group, BKiD, and MPHG have less restrictive membership criteria. In the United Kingdom, the HFEA's *Code of Practice* states that it 'expects' counselors to be members of a regulated profession, although this is not a mandatory requirement.[33] Canadian regulations about the credentials and training of counselors have not yet been drafted, although it is proposed by the government that consultation about such matters will take into account the views of counselors, and draw upon existing standards in other countries.[29]

One of the most debated issues among counselors themselves is whether infertility counseling should include an assessment component to evaluate the suitability of individuals for assisted conception services, and if such an assessment essentially places the counselor in the role of 'gatekeeper.' Opponents of the assessment role claim that it can undermine the therapeutic relationship with clients; create tensions; inhibit open discussion; focus on personal deficits rather than strengths; and reinforce the impression that the counselor's role is to screen them for their suitability as parents. It is argued that infertility counseling should more appropriately focus on the provision of information and support; an exploration of the implications of treatment, especially in relation to the use of donor gametes and embryos, or surrogacy; preparation for the treatment process; therapeutic work to deal with stress,

anxiety, grief, and failed cycles; and information about alternative resources such as adoption.

However, advocates of assessment as part of the counseling process, point to the benefits of identifying risk factors that have implications for coping with treatment (e.g., depression, stress, anxiety, and marital discord); helping to determine whether expectations and understanding of the treatment process are accurate; or, finally, if the client is mentally or emotionally capable of providing informed consent. The ability to identify such factors potentially enhances the therapeutic aspect of the counseling role, allows for the interaction with clients to be focused on improvement of their emotional well-being, reduction of stress levels, development of better coping strategies, and avoidance of potential harm to the client and/or any prospective children. In this respect, assessment may have less to do with 'gatekeeping' and more to do with improving the overall quality and experience of care for individuals and couples. However, if the counselor's role does involve gatekeeping, then this needs to be clearly communicated to the clients at the outset.[34]

Counselors who consider clinical assessment is integral to their role often work as part of a multidisciplinary team, contributing to discussions about client eligibility rather than making independent judgments. The view that decisions about acceptability are more appropriately made by the team as a whole is supported by a recent ASRM Ethics Committee recommendation that they be based on a group assessment or review which "might involve evaluation by a mental health worker and consideration by psychological or other consultants."[13] Similarly, the United Kingdom's HFEA advises that: "In deciding whether to provide treatment, treatment centres are expected to take into account views from the staff who have had involvement with the prospective patients."[35] The Code also provides some guidance regarding the grounds on which refusal might be considered and on how to manage the refusal of treatment.[36]

Assessment may often, although not always, use psychometric testing, and this is another issue that has stirred some debate among counselors. It has been noted that the advantages of using standardized assessment tools include the prevention of counselor or team biases; the ability to identify individuals with psychological risk factors; and the potential to protect against litigation.[37] However, the use of testing should never be considered a substitute for a face-to-face clinical interview, although it is often considered beneficial in supplementing, confirming, or refuting information gathered in the interview.[38] The use of testing may be more related to the specific discipline of the counselor than any explicit requirement or policy. In many places, such testing must be conducted by a licensed professional, in most cases a counselor with a psychology background. The ASRM guidelines for psychological assessment of gamete donors and recipients recommend that there be psychological assessment and counseling,[11] with the guidelines for embryo donation making explicit reference to the use of *psychological testing* "to document and validate in a standardized, objective manner the information gathered from the clinical interview," including "an objective personality test and other self-report measures to assess potential instability or psychopathology."[12] The use of psychological testing to screen participants in third-party conception and surrogacy is most prevalent in the United States, but is much less in evidence in countries such as Australia, New Zealand and the United Kingdom, where other professions that do not conduct standardized psychometric testing (i.e., social work, clinical counseling, and marital and family therapy) are more prominent, and where more exclusive emphasis is placed on the provision of psychosocial and implications counseling, including education, preparation for parenthood, and emotional support.

In some places, the issue of assessment is tied to the welfare of children conceived from assisted conception procedures, and is required as a matter of government policy. Legislation that includes a child welfare requirement is currently in force in three Australian states (South Australia,[20] Victoria,[2] Western Australia[21]), Canada,[3] the United Kingdom,[1] and New Zealand,[22] and in proposed legislation in New South Wales.[23] As an example, U.K. legislation requires that the welfare of the child be taken into account before providing assisted conception services, although the HFEA does not indicate that counselors be responsible for these decisions other than their potential role as members of the multidisciplinary team (see earlier discussion). Concerns about welfare of the child assessments in the United Kingdom prompted a review by the HFEA[39] while a committee of lawmakers has called for the complete overhaul of the welfare of the child provisions.[40]

CLINICAL ISSUES

Despite major differences in attitudes toward counseling and in how counseling is provided, the recent inaugural symposium of international infertility counselors addressed a number of common clinical concerns.[7] These included disclosure issues in third-party assisted conception; access to counseling and to assisted con-

ception services; counselor training; professional and academic credentials; and reproductive tourism.

Disclosure Issues in Third-Party Conception

The issue of disclosure is undeniably affected by cultural norms and values related to how infertility is perceived at a personal and social level; dominant religious beliefs; perceptions of genetic versus social relationships in families; the influence of parties providing third-party conception services; and the social and legal recognition of third-party conception. Questions of whether donor-conceived children should be informed about their genetic origins, and if it is appropriate for counselors to adopt a specific stance with regard to disclosure, are matters of considerable debate among counselors everywhere. In many parts of the world there are strong cultural, social, religious, and legal pressures to maintain secrecy in third-party assisted conception,[7,41] while there has been a suggestion that in countries where legislation permits donor-conceived people to learn the identity of their donor, counseling should be focused toward disclosure.[42]

Elsewhere, there is evidence of apparently contradictory developments. In some countries, an increasing number of parents have told – or are intending to tell – their children about their conception,[43,44] although even in countries where donor-conceived people have the legal right to know the identity of their donors, research suggests that a substantial proportion of parents still indicate that they do not intend to inform their children.[44]

In terms of the clinical roles for counselors, BICA has noted that they are increasingly likely to be called upon to offer support in regard to the long-term implications of third-party conception, helping families to deal with the actual telling process, and with late or unplanned disclosure.[45] Indeed, given a general global reduction in the use of donor procedures, counselors' involvement in third-party assisted conception procedures might increasingly become focused on postconception issues.

The complex relationships and dynamics that are often present in families created by third-party conception highlight the need for the availability of counseling services *after* the birth of children, and where there is any potential for linkages between offspring and their donors. Counselors in Australia and New Zealand are increasingly becoming involved in this role, helping to develop clinic policies or using existing counseling regulations for donor–offspring linking, such as those developed by the state of Victoria.[24] The Western Australia Reproductive Technology Council publishes a list of accredited infertility counselors, with particular indication of those "qualified to assist with child-related telling issues associated with donor conception."[46] These are strong indicators that third-party assisted conception counseling is emerging as a recognized and valued area of expertise, addressing the needs of parties at all stages of the process, including relationships within the resulting families.

Access to Counseling

Many experienced infertility counselors acknowledge that it has been a struggle to raise the profile of psychosocial issues within the predominantly medical and scientific domains of reproductive technologies. Even where the number of infertility counselors has increased significantly, such as the United States, the United Kingdom, and Australia, there are still many factors that have an impact on access, such as geographic isolation and financial barriers. It is also apparent that the vast majority of infertility counselors are female, raising the potential issue of gender barriers for male clients. In general, infertility consumer groups support wider access to counseling services to be more available, and for more emphasis on the ethical and psychosocial implications of infertility. The collaborative links that many consumer groups have established with counselors may extend to positions on consumer group boards and advisory committees, or to counselors leading support groups sponsored by consumer organizations. There is also growing use of the internet and telephone to access counseling and 'coaching,' although this is a relatively new development that might have legal and ethical implications for some counselors.

Even in countries with legislation, there can be wide variations between clinics regarding accessibility, standards, and provision of counseling services, not to mention 'interpretation' of the legislation to fit the specific clinic or caregiver's personal biases about infertility counseling or counseling in general. There are also mixed opinions among counselors themselves about the appropriateness of mandated counseling, with some believing that it compromises client self-determination and motivation. Countries such as Canada face some challenges in the mandatory provision of counseling for all participants in assisted conception because the number of experienced infertility counselors is currently very small and the geographic size of the country so large.

One implication of the counselor shortage is 'counseling' and 'advice giving' by other healthcare professionals who are not qualified mental health professions. This is an issue that would appear to cross international and cultural boundaries.

Counselor Training

Neither legislation mandating counseling, nor guidelines recommending it, are sufficient without a strategy to train more counselors and to establish practice standards. Currently, there are limited opportunities for specific infertility counselor training beyond basic training and qualification in a mental health profession. Geographic and financial barriers often confront those wishing to attend conferences, courses, and workshops or obtain supervision or mentoring. Furthermore, evaluating and comparing counseling credentials from so many disciplines, and so many countries, presents major challenges. Professional counseling organizations are, however, working on addressing some of these issues. BICA has developed a university accredited 'counseling award' (see above discussion), holds 'study days' for its members twice annually, and publishes counseling practice guides.[47] ANZICA also provides workshops for members, and MHPG has a well-established annual postgraduate program held in conjunction with ASRM meetings, a mentoring program, and is in the early stages of establishing a credentialing process (see earlier discussion). Other counseling associations, such as BKiD in Germany and those in Japan and Switzerland, have also begun to address the need for professional development and training (see earlier discussion). The establishment of IICO is a further indication of the potential for future collaborative learning initiatives among counselors.

Professional and Academic Credentials

Just as there is no single practice standard or model of infertility counseling, there is little agreement as to the specific academic credentials, training, and experience that are appropriate for the title of 'accredited infertility counselor.' The issue may be addressed in legislation (cf. Victoria) but is more often expressed through recommended guidelines and standards. For example, RTAC accredits only those clinics having ANZICA members as counselors, and in turn, ANZICA requires members to be licensed psychologists, social workers, or psychiatrists. In the United States, MHPG has published *Qualification Guidelines for Mental Health Professionals in Reproductive Health* (see Appendix 1), which suggests a combination of academic credentials (master's or doctoral degree in a mental health profession); license to practice; training in the medical and psychological aspects of infertility; a minimum of one year infertility counseling experience, preferably under supervision from an experienced infertility counselor; and a commitment to ongoing professional development.[16] As already noted, legislation in the

United Kingdom indicates a preference for counseling professionals to be licensed, but this is not required, nor does BICA have restrictions on membership. Similarly, counseling organizations in Switzerland, Japan, and Latin America have not developed specific criteria for membership credentials, although BKiD in Germany requires that there have been professional training in a psychosocial area. See Appendix 2 for a comparison of standards and guidelines for infertility counselors.

Reproductive Tourism

It is recognized that increasingly, people are crossing international and geographic boundaries to seek assisted conception services, while others – as potential gamete providers or surrogates – may do so following enticement by a 'contracting' couple or offers of financial reward or other benefits. This phenomenon has become widely known as 'reproductive tourism.' Reasons for doing so include specific procedures not being available within the country of origin or the existence of restrictions concerning eligibility.[48] The United States is a popular destination due to the wide range of services available and relatively unrestricted access, as are Eastern European countries because of limited regulation and cheaper labor. Furthermore, the tourists may be infertile clients seeking a specific medical treatment (e.g., IVF) or may be potential gamete donors or surrogates enticed by a contracting couple or offers of financial reward or other benefits. Reproductive tourism presents a dilemma for counselors, especially if clients are proposing to engage in activities that are illegal in their home country. While counselors will need to ensure that they operate within the law in their own country, the emerging international links should be developed to offer appropriate client care and, in particular, to try to ensure protection of the interests of any children that may subsequently be born.

FUTURE IMPLICATIONS

Formal infertility counseling organizations exist in very few countries and, even where they do, infertility counseling as a discrete specialty is largely undeveloped. In many parts of the world, in particular in countries outside Western Europe, North America, and Oceania, the rapid expansion of assisted conception services has not been accompanied by developments in counseling provision. As we have noted above, this is compounded by the development of reproductive tourism, often involving the very countries where both counseling and regulatory safeguards may be lacking. These present evident challenges to the international community.

From a global perspective, the initial priority for infertility counseling is to establish an effective communications network that is not reliant for its success on face-to-face contact. While annual and triennial international meetings such as ESHRE, ASRM, and IFFS are invaluable forums for such gatherings, the limited ability of counselors to attend these on a regular basis means that they cannot provide the sole or even the principal mode of communication. Inevitably, an effective global network will be centered on electronic communications. As we have indicated in this chapter, there are many issues that will exercise counselors in respect of their specific role, methods of working, and relationships with consumers and fellow reproductive health professionals. It is unlikely – even undesirable – that such collaboration will result in a homogenized global model of infertility counseling. Rather, it is our hope – as members of this network – that what we have in common will provide a sound basis for solidarity, and that where we differ will provide a basis for challenging and engaging debate.

SUMMARY

■ Recent years have been marked by considerable achievements in the development of infertility counseling, although there remains very limited access and availability in some countries.

■ Legislation and/or regulation play an important role in supporting counseling provision in many countries. Counselors have often contributed to such legislative and policy development.

■ Infertility counseling organizations continue to play a pivotal role in facilitating communication and collaboration between counselors, and helping to establish standards and training.

■ Clinical practice issues affecting counselors are often similar from country to country, but the contexts of practice such as policies, regulations, and overall recognition of counseling may be quite different.

■ Most counselors welcome opportunities for professional contact at meetings and conferences. There are also opportunities for global contact through electronic communication such as the internet.

■ Establishing common international standards for infertility counseling is likely to present significant challenges, partly due to the diversity of mental health disciplines involved.

ACKNOWLEDGMENTS

We gratefully acknowledge the assistance of a number of colleagues who have provided information about infertility counseling organizations in different parts of the world: Linda D. Applegarth, Jacky Boivin, Andrea Braverman, Joelle Darwiche, Joann Paley Galst, Tetsuya Goto, Anne Graham, Elizabeth Grill, Shiro Hirayama, Jim Monach, Peggy Orlin, Corrine Palatchi, Bill Petok, Sheila Pike, Jan Elman Stout, and Petra Thorn. Any errors or omissions are our responsibility.

REFERENCES

1. Human Fertilisation and Embryology Act 1990, United Kingdom.
2. Infertility Treatment Act 1995, Victoria.
3. Assisted Human Reproduction Act 2004, Canada.
4. Department of Health and Social Security. *Report of the Committee of Inquiry into Human Fertilisation and Embryology (The Warnock Report)*. London: HMSO, 1984.
5. Royal Commission on New Reproductive and Genetic Technologies. *Proceed with Care*. Ottawa: Minister of Government Services, 1993.
6. Waller L. *Report on Donor Gametes in IVF*. Melbourne: Committee to Consider the Social, Ethical and Legal Issues Arising from In Vitro Fertilisation, 1983.
7. International Infertility Counselors Organization (IICO). *Global Perspectives on Infertility Counseling*. Postgraduate Program. Montreal, Canada, May 23, 2004.
8. American Society for Reproductive Medicine. Guidelines for sperm donation. *Fertil Steril* 2004; 82:S9–12.
9. American Society for Reproductive Medicine. Guidelines for oocyte donation. *Fertil Steril* 2004; 82(Suppl 1): S13–14.
10. American Society for Reproductive Medicine. Guidelines for cryopreserved embryo donation. *Fertil Steril* 2004; 82: S16–17.
11. American Society for Reproductive Medicine. Psychological assessment of gamete donors and recipients. *Fertil Steril* 2004; 82:S18–19.
12. American Society for Reproductive Medicine. Psychological guidelines for embryo donation. *Fertil Steril* 2004; 82: S20–21.
13. American Society for Reproductive Medicine Ethics Committee. Child-rearing ability and the provision of fertility services. *Fertil Steril* 2004; 82:S211.
14. American Society for Reproductive Medicine Ethics Committee. Informing offspring of their conception by gamete donation. *Fertil Steril* 2004; 82:S212–216.
15. American Society for Reproductive Medicine. Family members as gamete donors and surrogates. *Fertil Steril* 2004; 82:S217–222.
16. Mental Health Professional Group of the American Society for Reproductive Medicine (1995). Qualification Guidelines for Mental Health Professionals in Reproductive Medicine. Appendix I. In: LH Burn, SN Covington, eds, *Infertility Counseling: A Comprehensive Handbook for Clinicians*. New York: Parthenon, 1999.
17. The Psychological Component of Infertility: Frequently asked questions (also available in Spanish) on ASRM website. http://www.asrm.org/Professionals/PG-SIG-Affiliated Soc/MHPG/mhpgfaqs.html.
18. Gordon E, Speyer E. (2005) Children's Bibliography. http://www.asrm.org/Professionals/PG-SIG-Affiliated Soc/MHPG/MHPG Childrens Bibliography.pdf.
19. Human Fertilisation and Embryology Authority. *Code of Practice* (6th ed.). London: Human Fertilisation and Embryology Authority, 2004.
20. Reproductive Technology Act, 1988, South Australia.
21. Human Reproductive Technology Act, 1991, Western Australia.
22. Human Assisted Reproductive Technology Act 2004, New Zealand.
23. Assisted Reproductive Technology Bill, 2003, New South Wales.
24. The "1984 Central Register," established under the Infertility [Medical Procedures] Act 1984; the "1995 Central Register," established under the Infertility Treatment Act 1995, and the "Donor Treatment Procedure Information Register" (known as the 'Voluntary Register'), established under the Infertility Treatment Act 1995.
25. Infertility Treatment Authority. *Conditions for Approval – Donor Linking: Application by Counsellors*. Melbourne: November, 2001.
26. ESHRE Guidelines for counselling in infertility. Grimbergen, Belgium: ESHRE, 2001. http://www.eshre.com/file.asp?filetype=doc/04/005/003/psyguidelines.pdf.
27. Stammer H, Verres R, Wischmann T. Paarberatung und – therapie bei unerfülltem Kinderwunsch [Couple counseling and therapy for infertility]. Göttingen: Hogrefe, 2004.
28. Loi Fédérale sur la Procreation Médicalement Assistée, 1998.
29. Infertility Counseling Workshop Report, May 28–29, 2004. Available on request from Health Canada: http://www.hc-sc.gc.ca/hl-vs/reprod/index_e.html.
30. Domar AH, Kelly AL. *Conquering Infertility: Dr. Alice Domar's Mind–Body Guide to Enhancing Fertility and Coping with Infertility*. New York: Penguin, 2002.
31. Hunt J, Monach JH. Beyond the bereavement model: The significance of depression for infertility counselling. *Hum Reprod* 1997; 12:188–94.
32. Burns LH, Covington SN, eds. *Infertility Counseling: A Comprehensive Handbook for Clinicians*. New York: Parthenon, 1999.
33. Human Fertilisation and Embryology Authority (2004) op cit. para 1.9.
34. Gordon EG, Barrow RG. Legal and ethical aspects of infertility counseling. In: LH Burns, SN Covington, eds, *Infertility Counseling: A Comprehensive Handbook for Clinicians*. New York: Parthenon, 1999; 491–512.
35. HFEA 2004, op cit. para 3.21.
36. HFEA 2004, op cit. para 3.22–3.24.
37. Burns LH. Use of standardized psychological testing in infertility counseling. *Special Topics in Infertility Counseling: An Emphasis on Therapeutic Interventions*. Presented at the 32nd annual meeting of the American Society for Reproductive Medicine Postgraduate Program, Toronto, September 25–26, 1999.
38. Klock S. Psychosocial evaluation of the infertile patient. In: LH Burns, SN Covington, eds, *Infertility Counseling: A Comprehensive Handbook for Clinicians*. New York: Parthenon, 1999; 49–63.
39. Human Fertilisation and Embryology Authority. Tomorrow's Children – Review of the HFEA's guidance on Welfare of the Child. London: Human Fertilisation and Embryology Authority, 2005. http://www.hfea.gov.uk/AboutHFEA/HFEAPolicy/TomorrowsChildren-ReviewoftheHFEAsguidanceonWelfareoftheChild.

40. House of Commons Science and Technology Committee. Human Reproductive Technologies and the Law, Fifth Report of Session 2004–05. Vol I, 2005. http://www.publications.parliament.uk/pa/ cm200405/cmselect/cmsctech/7/7i.pdf.
41. Blyth E, R Landau, eds. *Third Party Assisted Conception Across Cultures: Social, Legal and Ethical Perspectives*. London: Jessica Kingsley, 2004.
42. Gottlieb C, Lalos O, Lindblad F. Disclosure of donor insemination to the child: The impact of Swedish legislation on couples' attitudes. *Hum Reprod* 2000; 15:2052–6.
43. Golombok S, Jadva V, Lycett E, et al. Families created by gamete donation: Follow-up at age 2. *Hum Reprod* 2004; 1:286–93.
44. Brewaeys A, de Bruyn JK, Louwe LA, et al. Anonymous or identity-registered sperm donors? A study of Dutch recipients' choices. *Hum Reprod* 2005; 20:820–4.
45. British Infertility Counselling Association. *'Opening the Record': Planning the Provision of Counselling to People applying for Information from the HFEA Register*. Report of the HFEA Register Counselling Project Steering Group. Sheffield: British Infertility Counselling Association, 2003. http://www.bica.net/.
46. Western Australia Reproductive Technology Council. *Infertility Counselling: The role of approved counsellors under the Human Reproductive Technology Act 1991(WA), 2004*. http://www.rtc.org.au/counsellors/index.html.
47. British Infertility Counselling Association. *Implications counselling for people considering donor-assisted conception*. Sheffield: British Infertility Counselling Association, 2004.
48. Blyth E, Farrand A. Reproductive tourism – a price worth paying for reproductive autonomy? *Critical Social Policy* 2005; 25:91–114.

APPENDIX 1

Qualification Guidelines for Mental Health Professionals in Reproductive Medicine*

These guidelines were developed by the Mental Health Professional Group of the American Society for Reproductive Medicine to help determine the qualifications and training for mental health professionals working in reproductive medicine. Mental health professionals are playing an increasingly important role in reproductive medicine due to technological advances and recognition of the complex psychosocial issues faced by infertility patients. As a result, there is a growing need for the skills and services of trained infertility counselors to assist patients and staff. Infertility counseling includes psychological assessment, psychotherapeutic intervention, and psychoeducational support of individuals and couples who are experiencing fertility problems. A qualified infertility counselor should be able to provide the following services:

- psychological assessment and screening
- diagnosis and treatment of mental disorders
- psychometric testing (psychologist)
- decision-making counseling
- couple and family therapy
- grief counseling
- supportive counseling
- education/information counseling
- support group counseling
- referral/resource counseling
- staff consultation
- crisis intervention
- sexual counseling
- psychotherapy

The following guidelines suggest minimum qualifications and training of mental health professionals providing infertility counseling and psychological services. The mental health professional should have

1. Graduate Degree in a Mental Health Profession
A master's or doctorate degree from an accredited program in the field of psychiatry, psychology, social work, psychiatric nursing, or marriage and family therapy. Curriculum and training should include psychopathology; personality theory; life cycle and family

---

*These guidelines serve as an example. Other guidelines for infertility counseling services are available through the European Society of Human Reproduction and Embryology at www.eshre.com or Human Fertilization and Embryology Authority at www.hfea.gov.uk.

development; family systems theory; bereavement and loss theory; crisis intervention; psychotherapeutic interventions; individual, marital, and group therapy; and a supervised clinical practicum or internship in counseling.

2. License to Practice

A license (or registration/certification, where applicable) to practice in the mental health field in which the professional holds a graduate degree and as required by the state in which the individual practices.

3. Training in the Medical and Psychological Aspects of Infertility

Training in the medical aspects of infertility indicating knowledge of

1. basic reproductive physiology;
2. testing, diagnosis, and treatment of reproductive problems;
3. etiology of male and female infertility;
4. assisted reproductive technologies.

Training in the psychology of infertility indicating knowledge of

1. marital and family issues associated with infertility, and the impact on sexual functioning;
2. approaches to the psychology of infertility including psychological assessment, bereavement/loss, crisis intervention, post-traumatic stress, and typical/atypical responses;
3. family-building alternatives including adoption, third-party reproduction, child-free lifestyle;
4. psychological and couple treatments;
5. the legal and ethical issues of infertility treatments.

4. Clinical Experience

The mental health professional should have a minimum of one year clinical experience providing infertility counseling, preferably under the supervision of or in consultation with a qualified and experienced infertility counselor.

5. Continuing Education

Continuing education helps ensure continued growth in knowledge and skills. Regular attendance at courses offered by the American Society for Reproductive Medicine or other professional organizations and educational institutions is recommended to provide continuing education in both the medical and psychological issues in reproductive health care.

Prepared by the Committee on Infertility Counseling Guidelines:
Sharon N. Covington, MSW, Chair
Linda D. Applegarth, EdD, Vice-Chair
Linda Hammer Burns, PhD, Vice-Chair
Suzan A Aydinel, PhD
Paul R Feldman, MD
Judith Parkes, MSW, RN
Deidra T Rausch, MSN, RNC
September 1995

APPENDIX 2

International Comparison of Standards/Guidelines for Infertility Counselors

JEAN M. HAASE AND ERIC BLYTH

APPENDIX 2. Comparison of standards/guidelines for infertility counselors

Country or jurisdiction	Legislation or guidelines	Degree required or recommended	License to practice	Disciplines providing counseling	Professional counseling association	Training/professional development offered
United Kingdom	Legislation	Required: diploma level or above in counseling, psychology, social work	Regulations recommend membership in regulated profession	Psychology Social work Counseling	BICA [British Infertility Counseling Association]	Courses through BICA www.bica.net
Australia/ New Zealand	Legislation varies but accreditation guidelines apply to all	Required: Bachelor, Masters, or Doctorate	Required membership in ANZICA	Psychology Social work MD	ANZICA/FAS [Australia/New Zealand Infertility Counseling Association of Fertility Society of Australia]	Courses through ANZICA, FAS; and government (donor linking counselor training) www.fas.org
United States of America	Guidelines ARSM and MHPG	Recommended: graduate level degree	Required to practice in every state	Psychology Social work Marriage/family therapy Nurses (psychiatric) MD (psychiatrist)	MHPG/ASRM [Mental Health Professional Group of American Society of Reproductive Medicine]	Annual courses at ASRM www.asrm.org
Germany	Guidelines BKid	Recommended: training in psychosocial discipline and training in counseling or therapy	MD	Psychology Social work Counseling MD (psychiatry, ob/gyn with counseling credentialing)	BKiD [Beratungsnetzwerk Kinderwunsch Deutschland]	Courses through BKiD www.bkid.de

(continued)

APPENDIX 2 *(continued)*

Country or jurisdiction	Legislation or guidelines	Degree required or recommended	License to practice	Disciplines providing counseling	Professional counseling association	Training/professional development offered
Latin America	GLASMI Guidelines	Recommended: graduate level degree	Varies between countries	Psychology MD (psychiatry)	GLASMI/FLASEF [Grupo Latinamericana de interes en salud mental en infertili-dad/Federacion Latinamericana de sociedades de Esterilidad y Fertilidad]	Courses through FLASEF, ASRM, ESHRE
Japan	JAPCRM Developing guidelines	Recommended: Masters or doctorate degree	Psychologists	Psychologists Nurses MD (psychiatry)	JAPCRM [Japan Association of Psychological Counseling for Reproductive Medicine]	Courses offered through JAPCRM
Europe	ESHRE Guidelines	Recommended: graduate level degree	Varies among countries	Psychology Social work Counseling Nurses MD (psychiatry, ob/gyn special counseling credentialing)	PSIG/ESHRE [Psychosocial special interest group of European Society of Human Reproduction and Embryology]	Annual courses at ESHRE www.eshre.com
Switzerland	Legislation	Recommended: graduate level degree	Psychologists, MD (psychiatry, ob/gyn special counseling credentialing)	Psychology Social work Family planning Counselors MD	FertiForum Special Interest Group of Swiss Society of Reproductive Medicine (SGRM)	Members attend Swiss Society of Reproductive Medicine, ESHRE www.sgrm.org
Canada	Legislation	Recommended: graduate level degree	MD	Psychology Social work Marriage/family Therapy Nurses MD (psychiatry)	CSIG/CFAS [Counseling Special/Canadian Fertility and Andrology Society]	Members attend CFAS, ASRM, ESHRE, ANZICA, BICA www.cfas.ca/csig
Spain	Guidelines in development	Recommended: graduate level degree	Required in every state	Psychology Social work	Grupo de Interes de Psicologia SEF	Courses through SEF www.sefertilidad.es

Comprehensive Psychosocial History for Infertility (CPHI)

This is not a psychometric test. Instead, it is a comprehensive psychological and social history of infertility designed to be used by a mental health or medical professional. It should provide the clinician with a global impression of the patient's history, stressors, functioning, and current psychosocial status relevant to infertility. Although the history provides guidelines for potentially disruptive responses, there are some areas that are red flags and indications for referral for more complete psychological evaluation and intervention. They include (1) use or consideration of a donor/surrogate program, (2) prior psychiatric illness, (3) change in current mental status and/or exacerbation of prior psychiatric symptoms, (4) history of pregnancy loss, (5) history of cancer, (6) history of rape, (7) ambisexual patterns, and (8) current problems with substance abuse.

I. Reproductive History

A. Infertility
1. Current infertility: primary or secondary
2. History of past infertility

B. Pregnancy
1. Living children (stepchildren, adopted, donor offspring, placed for adoption)
2. Therapeutic abortion(s)
3. Spontaneous abortion(s)
4. Other perinatal loss: SIDS, death of child
5. High-risk pregnancy

C. History of genetic/chromosomal abnormalities
1. Cancer of the reproductive tract and/or chemotherapy
2. DES exposure
3. Congenital abnormalities of the reproductive tract
4. Family history of genetic disorders

II. Mental Status

A. Psychiatric history
1. Hospitalization for psychiatric illness
2. Psychiatric treatment
3. Treatment with psychotropic medication
4. Substance abuse

Reproduced from Burns LH, Greenfeld DA, for the Mental Health Professional Group. *CPHI: Comprehensive Psychosocial History for Infertility*. Birmingham, AL: American Society for Reproductive Medicine, 1990.

B. Current mental status
1. Symptoms of depression
2. Symptoms of anxiety/panic attacks
3. Symptoms of obsession
4. Current use of psychotropic medications
5. Current problem with substance abuse/addiction

C. Change in mental status

D. Exacerbation of prior psychiatric symptoms

III. Sexual History

A. Frequency and response

B. Function/dysfunction

C. Religious or cultural influence on sexual patterns or procreation beliefs

D. Sexual history
1. Function/dysfunction
2. Sexually transmitted disease
3. Prior sperm donor/surrogate mother/consideration of use of donor gametes
4. Homosexual or ambisexual patterns
5. History of rape or incest

E. Changes in any sexual patterns secondary to infertility or medical treatment

IV. Relationship Status

A. Marital
1. History of marriages/divorces
2. History of marital discord/therapy
3. Extramarital relationships
4. Current satisfaction/dissatisfaction
5. Ambivalence about medical treatment and reproductive technologies

B. Familial
1. History of dysfunctional family of origin
2. Recent deaths or births in family
3. History of numerous familial losses

C. Social
1. Available support system
2. Career disruptions or pressures
3. History of or current legal problems
4. Criminal conduct

APPENDIX 4

Psychological Fertility-Related Questionnaires

JACKY BOIVIN

NEGATIVE AFFECT, DISTRESS AND STRAIN ABOUT INFERTILITY

Multidimensional

Infertility Questionnaire

- self-image, guilt/blame, sexuality
- negative feelings and thoughts about infertility
- middle-class American women in treatment

Bernstein J, Potts N, Mattox J. Assessment of psychological dysfunction associated with infertility. *J Obstet Gynaecol Neonatal Nurs (supplement)*, 1985; suppl:63–65.

Infertility Reaction Scale

- need for parenthood, social and work efficiency and social pressure to have a child
- middle-class American couples about to begin IVF

Collins A, Freeman EW, Boxer AS, Tureck R. Perceptions of infertility and treatment stress in females as compared to males entering in vitro fertilization treatment. *Fertil Steril* 1992; 57:350–56.

Fertility Problem Inventory

- social, sexual, relationship, need for parenthood, rejection of child-free living
- level of psychological strain or stress in each area of concern
- middle-class Canadian men and women attending fertility clinic

Newton CR, Sherrard W, Glavac I. The Fertility Problem Inventory: Measuring perceived infertility stress. *Fertil Steril* 1999; 72:54–62.

Infertility Cognitions Questionnaire

- helplessness and acceptance in regards to the fertility problem
- Dutch women about to begin first IVF cycle

Verhaak CM, Smeenk JMJ, Evers AWM, van Minnen A, Kremer JAM, Kraaimaat FW. Predicting emotional response to unsuccessful fertility treatment: A prospective study. *J Behav Med* 2005; 28:181–90.

Unidimensional

Fertility Problem Stress Inventory

- infertility stress
- American middle-class couples referred to study by infertility specialist

Abbey A, Andrews FM, Halman LJ. Gender's role in responses to infertility. *Psychol Women Quarterly* 1991; 15:295–316.

Infertility Feelings Questionnaire

* negative feelings in relation to infertility
* infertility patients

Stanton A, Tennen H, Affleck G, Mendola R. Cognitive appraisal and adjustment to infertility. *Women and Health* 1991; 17:1–15.

Infertility Distress Scale

* assesses self-reported stress, appraisals of infertility and cognitive involvement in infertility
* German, male infertility patients attending andrology clinic for the first time

Pook M, Rohrle B, Krause W. Individual prognosis for changes in sperm quality on the basis of perceived stress. *Psychother Psychosom* 1999; 68:95–101.

MOTIVATIONS, THOUGHTS AND FEELINGS ABOUT BECOMING A PARENT AND PARENTHOOD

Wikman Reproduction Scale

* motivation and conflict about parenthood
* presumed fertile medical personnel

Wikman M, Gustavsson L, Jacobsson L. von Schoultz B. Development of a psychometric instrument for the assessment of reproductive profile in men and women. *J Psychosom Obstet Gynaecol* 1990; 11:37–45.

Child Project Questionnaire

* endorsement of family life-events and of motivational and/or sexual factors which were theorized to predict fertility
* presumed fertile French couples, no previous children

Stoleru S, Teglas JP, Fermanian J, Spira A. Psychological factors in the etiology of infertility: A prospective cohort study. *Human Reprod* 1993; 8:1039–1046.

Fertility Adjustment Scale

* need for parenthood
* British men and women attending a fertility clinic

Glover L, Hunter M, Richards JM, Katz M, Abel PD. Development of the Fertility Adjustment Scale. *Fertil Steril* 1999; 72:623–28.

Irrational Parenthood Thoughts Scale

* irrational cognitions concerning the need to have children to have a happy life
* Dutch couples attending IVF clinic

Fekkes M, Buitendijk SE, Verrips GHW, Braat DDM, Brewaeys AMA, Dofing JG, Kortman M, Leerentveld RA, Macklon NS. Health-related quality of life in relation to gender and age in couples planning IVF treatment. *Human Reprod* 2003; 18:1536–43.

TREATMENT-SPECIFIC

Daily Record-Keeping Sheet

* negative (depression, anxiety, uncertainty), positive affect and coping during treatment
* middle-class Canadian couples undergoing a first IVF cycle

Boivin J, Takefman JE. Stress levels across stages of in vitro fertilization in subsequently pregnant and nonpregnant women. *Fertil Steril* 1995; 64:802–10.

Psychological Evaluation Test after ART

- negative reactions to specific aspects of ART
- Brazilian men and women with at least one past ART cycle

Franco JG, Baruffi RLR, Mauri AL, Petersen CG, Felipe V, Garbellini E. Psychological evaluation test after the use of assisted reproduction techniques. *J Assisted Reprod Genetics* 2002; 19:274–78.

Concerns About Reproductive Technologies

- level of concern about different aspects of ART technologies: procedural (e.g., side effects and anaesthetics), treatment failure, disruption to work and financial considerations
- white Caucasian, professional American women

Klonoff-Cohen H, Natarajan L. The concerns during assisted reproductive technologies (CART) scale and pregnancy outcomes. *Fertil Steril* 2004; 82:982–88.

COPING

Coping Scale for Infertile Couples

- assesses the use of coping strategies from four categories (e.g., increasing space and sharing the burden)
- Chinese infertile couples attending fertility clinic

Lee TY, Sun GH, Chao SC, Chen CC. Development of the coping scale for infertile couples. *Arch Androl* 2000; 45:149–54.

QUALITY-OF-LIFE

FertiQoL

- assesses impact of fertility problems in eight domains: affective, psychological, physical, spiritual, partner relationship, social network, occupation and need for psycho-educational help
- developed on an international sample and will be available in eight languages

(**For FertiQoL contact:** boivin@cardiff.ac.uk)

Polycystic Ovary Syndrome Quality-of-life

- assesses quality of life in five domains relevant to people with PCOS: emotions, body hair, weight, infertility and menstrual problems.
- North American women with PCOS

Cronin L, Guyatt G, Griffith L, Wong E, Azziz R, Futterweit W, Cook D, Dunaif A. Development of a health-related quality-of-life questionnaire (PCOSQ) for women with polycystic ovary syndrome (PCOS). *J Clin Endo Metabol* 1998; 83:1976–87.

Endometriosis Health Profile-30

- assesses symptomatology in five domains: pain; control and powerlessness; emotional well-being; social support; and self-image
- British women symptomatic for endometriosis and British women contacting a support group for endometriosis

Jones G, Kennedy S, Barnard A, Wong J, Jenkinson C. Development of an endometriosis quality-of-life instrument: The Endometriosis Health Profile-30. *Obstet Gynecol* 2001; 98:258–264.

Quality-of-Life in Infertile Men

- assesses functioning in four domains: desire for a child, sexual relationship, gender identity, psychological well-being
- German male patients attending andrology and urology clinics

Schanz S, Baeckert-Sifeddbine IT, Braeunlich C, Collins SE, Batra A, Gebert S, Hautzinger M, Fierlbeck G. A new quality-of-life measure for men experiencing involuntary childlessness. *Human Reprod* 2005; 20:2858–65.

Recommended Guidelines for the Screening and Counseling of Oocyte Donors*

Anonymous Oocyte Donor

I. Clinical interview: psychosocial history based on a semi-structured interview

A. Comprehensive Psychosocial History for Infertility (CPHI) (see Appendix 2)

B. If the CPHI is not used, then target these essential elements:
   1. Family history (with or without genogram) – investigate history through grand-parents and offspring
   2. Assessment of stability (e.g., job history and relationships)
   3. Motivation to donate
   4. Current life stressors and coping skills
   5. Difficult or traumatic reproductive history
   6. Interpersonal relationships
   7. Sexual history (including sexual abuse)
   8. History of major psychiatric disorders, including personality disorders
   9. Alcohol, drug use, and/or dependence in donor and family of origin (current and past)
   10. Legal history (lawsuits, misdemeanors and felonies)
   11. History of abuse or neglect (sexual and physical)
   12. Educational background

C. Determination of motivation to participate (psychological, financial and physical)

D. Ability to comprehend and assimilate information provided

E. Education about treatment for donor and recipient (and respective partners, if applicable)
   1. Purpose
   2. Description of procedures
   3. Success and failure rates
   4. Potential health risks and complications
   5. Reasons why treatment would be discontinued
   6. Financial issues
   7. Time commitment
   8. Potential psychological risks

---

*These guidelines serve as an example. Other guidelines for infertility counseling services are available through the European Society of Human Reproduction and Embryology at www.eshre.com or Human Fertilization and Embryology Authority at www.hfea.gov.uk.

Developed by the Mental Health Professional Group Ovum Donor Task Force of the American Society for Reproductive Medicine, 1994.

F. Counseling: pre- and post-treatment and during treatment
   1. Potential impact on relationships (e.g., marital, sexual, work, social, family)
   2. Potential impact on relationship between donor and recipient (known donors)
   3. Implications
      a. What if treatment is not successful
      b. What if pregnancy is not successful
      c. What if pregnancy is terminated or selectively reduced
      d. What if donor changes her mind
      e. What if the child has a physical problem

G. Counseling on recipient-specific issues
   1. Impact of the failure of treatment
      a. Emotional issues associated with infertility, including feeling out of control or failure
      b. Terminating treatment
      c. Grieving process
      d. Developing alternatives (e.g., child-free living or adoption)
   2. Impact of success of treatment
      a. Feelings during pregnancy
      b. Transition to parenthood
      c. Privacy versus openness with the child
      d. Potential impact of multiple pregnancy
      e. Parenting at an older age (if applicable)
      f. Family relationships

H. Information and consents
   1. Provide a reasonable time interval between giving of information, assessment, and consent
   2. Specifically state risks involved
   3. Specifically state who has parental rights and responsibilities
   4. State and designate financial responsibilities
   5. Require maintenance of medical records of all participants and applicable state law
   6. Delineate specific responsibilities of each participant
   7. Provide for anonymity of all parties to the best of the clinician's ability

II. Psychological testing

A. Structured personality tests (examples listed below)
   1. Minnesota Multiphasic Personality Inventory-2
   2. California Personality Inventory
   3. Personality Assessment Inventory

B. Self-report measures (examples listed below)
   1. Marital Satisfaction Inventory
   2. Dyadic Adjustment Scale
   3. Life Events Checklist
   4. Beck Depression or Anxiety Inventory
   5. Sentence Completion
   6. Pennsylvania Reproductive Associate Infertility Survey (PRAIS)
   7. Brief Symptom Inventory

III. Known oocyte donors

For known donors, the protocol of the interview and psychological testing is the same, although psychological testing is optional in some known-donor programs. The clinical interview should include the recipient and her husband/partner and the donor and her husband/partner. The interview should also include a group meeting in which all parties come together for discussion, summary, and recommendations. The interview should include the following elements that are not included in the anonymous donor interview.

A. **Additional content areas for known donor interview**
1. Assessment for the presence of coercion (financial or emotional)
2. Information from both the donor and recipient regarding their interpersonal relationship
3. In sister-to-sister donation: parents' role
4. Issues of disclosure or privacy
5. Interactions among all three or four parties
6. Dysfunctional family history
7. Plans for future relationships
8. Information regarding intentions of all four parties regarding custody arrangements in the event of the death of the recipients
9. Issues regarding cryopreservation and future disposition of the frozen embryos
10. Prenatal testing and selective reduction
11. Donor's role and relationship with future child(ren)
12. Impact on donor if treatment is unsuccessful
13. Estimation of number of cycles in which donor is willing to participate

IV. Criteria for acceptance or rejection of oocyte donors

The following indicators can be used to decide on a case-by-case basis who is suitable as an oocyte donor. While the following list is not exhaustive and each program may over time add to or delete from this list, it is offered as a preliminary guide. The caveat is to err on the side of caution to protect all parties.

A. **Positive indicators**
1. Absence of significant psychopathology
2. Absence of unusual life stressors
3. Use of adaptive coping skills
4. Ability to provide informed consent
5. Supportive and stable interpersonal and/or marital relationships
6. Economic stability
7. Psychological testing within normal limits
8. Employment stability

B. **Negative indicators**
1. Significant DSM-IV axis I or II disorder (including psychological standardized testing which is two standard deviations above the mean)
2. Positive family history for heritable psychiatric disorder (e.g., schizophrenia, bipolar disorders)
3. Two or more first degree relatives with substance dependence
4. Current use of psychoactive medications
5. Family history of sexual or physical abuse with no professional treatment for the donor
6. Chaotic lifestyle
7. Significant current stress
8. Marital instability
9. Impaired cognitive functioning or mental incompetence
10. History of legal difficulties

If the potential donor is in a crisis, appropriate psychological help should be provided. Objection to donation by the husband or partner of the donor should be grounds at least for a deferment of treatment.

APPENDIX 6

Psychological Guidelines for Embryo Donation*

These recommendations should be understood as general guidelines for addressing the many complex moral, ethical, and psychosocial issues that embryo donors, recipients, and potential offspring may confront as we move forward with this family-building option. Providing thorough information and adequate time for decision making will increase the likelihood for establishing well-adjusted families.

I. Donors

1. Prior to signing an informed consent document, all potential donor couples should be educated about all aspects of their medical treatments and the relevant psychological and ethical issues inherent in donating embryos. These issues should be addressed during the clinical interview and are included in recommendations for the interview.

2. It is recommended that there should be a discussion of embryo disposition options at the time of cryopreservation. After couples have concluded their own reproductive attempts, they should again be apprised of embryo-disposition options, including donation.

3. Psychological assessment is strongly recommended to ascertain appropriateness of potential donors, including determining psychopathology. This assessment should include a clinical interview and psychological testing. The timing of this assessment should occur after couples have concluded their own reproductive attempts and have clearly indicated their desire to donate embryos (including signing informed consent), and their embryos are medically appropriate for donation.

4. The clinical interview should include a psychosocial history of both partners that addresses educational background; current life stressors; difficult or traumatic reproductive history; interpersonal relationships; sexual history; history of major psychiatric and personality disorders; legal problems; history of abuse or neglect; substance abuse; and family history (at least first-degree relatives) of major psychiatric and personality disorders; substance abuse; physical or sexual abuse; and legal problems.

5. The clinical interview should also address the unknown potential psychological impact and/or risks, assessment for presence of coercion (financial and/or

---

*These guidelines serve as an example. Other guidelines for infertility counseling services are available through the European Society of Human Reproduction and Embryology at www.eshre.com or Human Fertilization and Embryology Authority at www.hfea.gov.uk.

Developed by the Mental Health Professional Group of the American Society for Reproductive Medicine Task Force on Embryo Donation, 1996.

emotional), emotional attachment to embryos, disclosure or nondisclosure of the donors' involvement, amount and type of information to be exchanged, if any, between donors and recipients.

6. Psychological testing is recommended to document and validate in a standardized, objective manner the information gathered from the clinical interview and should include an objective personality test and other self-report measures to assess potential instability or psychopathology.

7. Positive indicators for embryo donors include: absence of significant psychopathology; absence of current or significant history of substance abuse/addiction; absence of unusual life stressors; use of adaptive coping skills; ability to provide true informed consent; supportive and stable marital relationship; economic stability; employment stability; lack of coercion; and psychological testing within normal limits.

8. Negative indicators for embryo donors include: presence of significant psychopathology; positive family history for heritable genetic and psychiatric disorders; substance abuse/addiction; two or more first-degree relatives with substance abuse; family history of sexual or physical abuse with no professional treatment; chaotic lifestyle; significant current life stress; marital instability; impaired cognitive functioning or mental incompetence; history of legal difficulties, high-risk sexual practices, and objection by either partner.

9. A minimum three-month waiting period is recommended between the time a couple signs the consent form to donate embryos and the actual donation to a recipient couple.

10. Employees of the infertility program or physician should be excluded from embryo donation within their own program.

11. Donors should not be compensated for their donated embryos.

12. Donors should be a least twenty-one years of age.

II. Recipients

1. Recipients of donor embryos should receive counseling about the potential psychosocial implications of this parenting option prior to signing an informed consent document.

2. Counseling should address the impact of success of treatment, such as the feelings during pregnancy; positive and negative aspects of disclosure and nondisclosure with offspring; potential impact of multiple pregnancy; transition to parenthood (if applicable); parenting at an older age (if applicable); and nongenetic parenting issues.

3. The impact of treatment failure should also be addressed, including treatment termination, the grieving process, and developing alternatives for the future.

4. Related issues such as the potential impact of the relationship between known donors and recipients and potential offspring should be addressed when relevant.

5. Psychological assessment is strongly recommended to assess appropriateness of potential recipients (not to assess parenting abilities). This assessment would attempt to rule out significant psychiatric illness, current substance abuse/addiction, and ability to cope with the stress of assisted reproductive technologies.

Psychological Guidelines for Evaluation and Counseling of Gestational Carriers and Intended Parents*

I. Application Criteria for Carriers

A. Minimum age 21
B. High school diploma or GED
C. Prior deliveries and experience parenting a child
D. Free of major medical problems
E. Lifestyle that would not interfere with prenatal care and management

II. Written Informed Consent for the Psychological Evaluation of Carrier or Intended Parent

A. Elements of the evaluation: purpose, clinical interview and psychometric tests administered
B. The credentials of the evaluator
C. Release of information to carriers, medical/psychological team and intended parents
D. Storage of records and documentation
E. Limitations of confidentiality

III. Pre-Patient Counseling of Carrier

One purpose of the pre-patient counseling for a Gestational Carrier is to provide the Carrier with a clear understanding of the potential psychological issues and risks associated with the process. It is suggested that the Carrier's partner attend the clinical interview and education.

Limitations of an Evaluation

A. Screening does not predict human behavior and the possibility of psychological harm.
B. There are no long-term prospective studies about psychological risks.

Preparation for Medical Protocol

A. It is recommended that the following aspects of the medical protocol be discussed: schedule demands, risks of canceled cycle, risk of unsuccessful cycle, risk of the

*These guidelines serve as an example. Other guidelines for infertility counselling services are available through the European Society of Human Reproduction And Embryology at www.eshre.com or Human Fertilization and Embryology Authority at www.hfea.gov.uk.

Prepared by the Gestational Carrier Task Force, Mental Health Professional Group of the American Society of Reproductive Medicine, Co-chairs Carol Wolf, MFCC and Ellie Schwartzman, PhD, 2000.

multiple pregnancy, possibility of selective reduction, prenatal testing, and elective termination.

Carriers always have the right to refuse any of these treatments and should inform the Intended Parents and treatment team of their opinions prior to entering into a contract with Intended Parents. There should be congruency between the Intended Parents and the Gestational Carrier on the above-listed issues.

Involvement of the Evaluator, Intended Parents, and Attorneys

A. The mental health professional should define his or her role in his or her relationship with the Carrier:
   1. Carrier's right to request a referral for outside counseling.
B. The Carrier should have an opportunity to explore the psychological issues of the pregnancy and the risks of emotional stress. These issues include
   1. Managing the relationship with the Intended Parents
   2. Coping appropriately with the pregnancy
   3. Risks of attaching to the baby and risk to the Carrier's children
   4. Impact on Carrier's marriage
   5. Impact on Carrier's employment
   6. The balance between the Carrier's right to privacy and the Intended Parents' right to information about their baby
C. The relationship between the Gestational Carrier and Intended Parents
   1. A group meeting should be encouraged with the mental health professional.
   2. If the Carrier and the Intended Parents are being matched by a third party, the procedure for accepting or rejecting a match should be clearly stated. The Carrier and the Intended Parents should understand that they always have the right to refuse a match.
D. Every Gestational Carrier and set of Intended Parents should have a legal contract.
   1. The Carrier and Intended Parents should have separate legal counsel.
   2. A contract should clearly define the financial obligations.

IV. Psychological Testing for Carrier

It is recommended that more than one test be administered; a minimum of one objective instrument and one self-report or projective instrument. Suggested instruments:

A. Measure of psychopathology (e.g., MMPI-2, PAI)
B. Projective screen (e.g., RISB, Sentence Completion for Marriage, TAT)
C. Measure of current stressors (Life Events Checklist, SCL 90 R)

V. Clinical Interview of Carrier

A. Social history, including family of origin
B. Occupational and financial history
C. Sexual and reproductive history
D. History of substance use, eating disorders, and physical or sexual abuse
E. Psychiatric history
F. Religious beliefs that may influence behavior
G. Maturity, judgment, assertiveness, and decision making skills
H. Personality style and coping skills
I. Capacity for empathy
J. Current life stressors and anticipated changes within the next two years
K. Previous Carrier experience or application to another facility
L. Motivation to become a Carrier
M. Support of significant other
N. Social network
O. Desire for more children of her own

P. Anticipated impact of Carrier experience upon her children and significant other
Q. Anticipated type and duration of relationship with Intended Parents
R. Ability to separate from and relinquish the child
S. Anticipated feelings toward the child
T. Feelings about multiple pregnancy, bed rest, hospitalization, pregnancy loss
U. Feelings about sexual abstinence
V. Feelings and decisions about termination of pregnancy, selective reduction, amniocentesis, and chorionic villi sampling
W. Agreement with the financial compensation arrangement
X. Reactions to the possibility of becoming infertile as a result of this process

VI. Suggested Rejection Criteria

A. Cognitive or emotional inability to comply or to understand
B. Evidence of financial or emotional coercion
C. Failure to evidence altruistic commitment to become a Carrier
D. Psychological testing not within normal limits
E. Unresolved or untreated addiction, child abuse, sexual abuse, physical abuse, depression, eating disorders, or traumatic pregnancy, labor and/or delivery
F. History of major depression, bipolar disorder, psychosis, or diagnosis of a personality disorder
G. Insufficient emotional support from partner/spouse or support system
H. Current marital or relationship instability
I. Excessively stressful family demands, without a sufficient social support system
J. Chaotic lifestyle
K. Inability to maintain respectful and caring relationship with Intended Parents
L. Evidence of emotional inability to separate from/surrender the baby at birth
M. History of conflict with authority
N. Inability to perceive and understand the perspective of others
O. Motivation to use compensation to solve own infertility
P. Unresolved issues with a previous abortion

VII. Repeat, Known, or Childless Carriers

Repeat Carriers

It is recommended that a woman be a Carrier no more than three times in her lifetime. If a Carrier is considering a second or third gestational arrangement, the following additional issues should be explored, for example, motivation, goals not achieved, unresolved feelings about prior pregnancies; potential physical risks; and risks to her children and marriage.

Additional Issues with Carriers Acquainted with or Related to Intended Parents

A. Issues of conflict in the historical relationship, including methods of coping with conflict and loss, should be explored. In addition, unique issues should be explored regarding amount of contact, privacy issues, and potential for negative impact on relationship.

Childless Carriers

A. As a general rule, childless women are not considered as Carrier candidates. Applicants should have given birth and parented a child.

VIII. The Carrier's Family Members

A. Husband or Partner evaluation should include: Level of support, motivation, maturity and judgment, desired relationship with Intended Parents, risks of a multiple pregnancy, impact of pregnancy on relationship and children, and community reaction.

B. Evaluation of the Carrier experience on her children.

C. Evaluation of impact and reactions of the extended family.

IX. Counseling of Carrier

1. Individual counseling should be available as desired or needed by the Carrier. If group counseling is not possible, phone counseling sessions are recommended as a minimum.

X. Compensation of Carrier

A fee for the Carrier may be provided to compensate her and her family for time, energy, and risks. The fee should be reasonable but not coercive.

XI. Psychological Evaluation of Intended Parents

An evaluation is recommended to ensure that the couple is capable of maintaining a warm and respectful relationship with a Carrier. Determining the Intended Parents' ability to parent is *not* the purpose of this evaluation.

A. A clinical interview, including the couple's history of infertility and methods of coping, and all of the elements in the Carrier's interview.

B. Psychological testing (optional and in the discretion of the evaluator)

XII. Pre-Patient Counseling of Intended Parents

A session specifically to help prepare the couple for this relationship may include discussion of the following issues:

A. Desired relationship with the Carrier and expectations

B. Meeting the emotional and physical needs of the carrier and her family

C. Understanding the "my body/your baby" issues

D. Rights of the Carrier to refuse medical interventions such as amniocentesis, chorionic villi sampling, selective reduction, and abortion

E. Number of embryos to be transferred and number of cycles planned

F. Carrier's desires regarding number of cycles, medical interventions, and a multiple pregnancy

G. Multiple pregnancy and associated risks

H. Selective reduction and psychological concerns

I. Therapeutic abortion in the event of an abnormal fetus

J. Carrier's behavior during pregnancy and how to handle conflicts that may arise (e.g., eating habits, prescription drugs, and alcohol)

K. Intention to disclose to offspring

L. Disclosure to family members and friends

M. Future relationship with Carrier and Carrier's family

N. Need for Carrier and her children to interact with baby after birth

O. Disposition of extra embryos

P. Feelings about the carrier's pregnancy

Q. Need for separate legal consultation and a written contract

R. Potential guilt reaction of Carrier at failed attempts or if problem occurs

S. Explanation of medical procedures

XIII. Matching of Carrier and Intended Parents

The success of a Carrier arrangement is largely contingent on the compatibility among all involved parties. Thorough evaluation and subsequent recommendation of a Carrier candidate does not guarantee a positive outcome. Compatibility of personality styles may be a significant factor in whether these relationships provide a meaningful and satisfying experience. A Carrier should be allowed to choose the Intended Parents with whom she will work. Both the Carrier and the Intended Parents should have the right to refuse a match. A group session is recommended, with a mental health professional and all parties, including the Carrier's partner, prior to a final commitment to the arrangement.

XIV. Counseling of Intended Parents

Counseling should be available to the Intended Parents throughout the arrangement. It should be recommended in the event a Carrier has any difficulties, or if misunderstandings occur.

Release of Information Example

This document is only to be construed as an example. Local standards and practice may vary and practitioner is cautioned to seek qualified legal advice before adapting any form for his or her own use.

AUTHORIZATION TO DISCLOSE PROTECTED HEALTH INFORMATION

Patient name: _____

Date of Birth: _____ Social Security No: _____

Address: _____

I hereby authorize _____ to disclose the above-named individual's health information as described below.

The type and amount of information to be disclosed is any and all psychological testing, evaluations, clinical interview materials, reports, summaries of therapy and therapeutic treatment and/or recommendations.

_____

I understand that this information may include information about my mental health status.

This information may be disclosed to and used by the following person or organization:

_____

_____

The disclosure and use is for the following purpose: _____

I understand I have a right to revoke this authorization at any time, and that if I chose to do so, I must revoke in writing and present it to the health information management department or the provider of services. I understand that the revocation will not apply to my insurance company when the law provides my insurer with the right to contest a claim under my policy. Unless otherwise revoked, this authorization will expire one year from the signature date.

I understand that authorizing the disclosure of this health information is voluntary. I may refuse to sign this authorization but such refusal may affect my ability to participate in certain treatments or programs.

By signing this authorization, I understand that any disclosure of information carries with it the potential for an unauthorized redisclosure and the information may not be protected by federal privacy rules. I further understand I may request a copy of this signed authorization. A photostatic copy of this authorization shall serve in its stead.

_____   _____
Witness   Signature of Individual or Legal Representative

Date: _____   Relationship of Representative: _____

                                                 Date: _____

Informed Consent

Pre-Psychological Counseling and/or Evaluation Example

This document is only to be construed as an example. Local standards and practice may vary and the practitioner is cautioned to seek qualified legal advice before adapting any form for his or her own use.

I/we,_____, hereby acknowledge that I/we have requested psychological services from *(mental health professional's name), (professional designation).* Such services may include (please initial all appropriate choices):

❑ Counseling regarding infertility and/or psychological implications of fertility treatments.
❑ Psychological evaluation regarding suitability to participate in one or all of the following:
    ❑ IVF or other assisted reproductive treatment using my own gametes and not involving a third-party collaborator
    ❑ Egg donation
        ❑ Recipient   ❑ Donor
    ❑ Sperm donation
        ❑ Recipient   ❑ Donor
    ❑ Gestational surrogacy/carrier
        ❑ Intended parent   ❑ Surrogate/carrier
    ❑ Traditional surrogacy (surrogate's own egg used in conception)
        ❑ Intended parent   ❑ Surrogate
    ❑ PGD
    ❑ Other_____

I/we understand that not every potential participant for third-party procedures will be accepted for treatment. As necessary, I/we hereby authorize _____(MHP)_____ to discuss the results of testing and clinical interviews with members of the fertility treatment team, and understand that the results of said tests will be used to assess my ability to participate. I/we hereby release _____(MHP)_____ from any liability in the event that I am not accepted for treatment.

I/we understand that there are potential psychological risks posed by counseling and evaluation. These may include risks that are presently unknown or unidentified. I/we also understand that any psychological and emotional risks may vary widely among individuals, so it is impossible to accurately state the likelihood of my/our personal risk and I/we cannot expect any mental health professional (MHP) to state with certainty whether or not I/we may suffer any psychological consequences of counseling and evaluation. Further, should I/we accept treatment, I/we understand that there are psychological risks associated with fertility treatments, and these may include risks that are presently unknown or unidentified. Fully understanding the above, I/we voluntarily agree to proceed with counseling and/or evaluation.

I/we, as a participant(s), specifically waive the right to claim any conflict of interest on the part of the MHP, which may arise since Intended Parents may pay the third-party participant's fees. Further, I/we understand that the MHP may counsel and/or evaluate other proposed participants involved in my/our treatment. I/we understand that the MHP has a professional responsibility to each client, individually and regardless of the interests of other participants who might be involved. I/we acknowledge and agree that the MHP may give certain advice to one client, or make certain recommendations about a client, which may negatively impact the ultimate success of any proposed treatment for me/us or other participants. I/we specifically release the MHP (and his/her employees, agents and assignees) from liability, and release and hold harmless said MHP to the extent that his/her actions are reasonably within standards of professional practice. None of the above may be construed, however, as a waiver of my right to pursue a negligence or malpractice claim.

_____   _____
Signature of Participant   Signature of MHP

_____
Signature of Participant

_____
Date

(to be signed in conjunction with HIPAA release)

Informed Consent: Proceeding with Fertility Treatments

Post-MHP Consultation/Evaluation Example

This document is only to be construed as an example. Local standards and practice may vary and the practitioner is cautioned to seek qualified legal advice before adapting any form for his or her own use.

I/we,_____, hereby acknowledge that I/we requested and participated in psychological services from _ *(mental health professional's name)*, *(professional designation)*. Such services included (please initial all appropriate choices):

❑ Counseling regarding infertility and/or psychological implications of fertility treatments.
❑ Psychological evaluation regarding suitability to participate in one or all of the following:
    ❑ IVF or other assisted reproductive treatment using my own gametes and not involving a third-party collaborator
    ❑ Egg donation
        ❑ Recipient   ❑ Donor
    ❑ Sperm donation
        ❑ Recipient   ❑ Donor
    ❑ Gestational surrogacy/carrier
        ❑ Intended parent   ❑ Surrogate/carrier
    ❑ Traditional surrogacy
        ❑ Intended parent   ❑ Surrogate
    ❑ PGD
    ❑ Other_____

During the course of consultation with the mental health professional noted above, we discussed, among others that may not be listed here, the following matters (please initial where applicable):

    ❑ Future contact with donor/recipient/surrogate
    ❑ Anonymity
    ❑ Third-party contact with child, including likelihood this may never happen
    ❑ Curiosity about other party(ies)
    ❑ Feelings of loss of control
    ❑ Feelings toward child
    ❑ Dealing with the unknown
    ❑ General attitude toward infertility
    ❑ Feelings about and effect on spouse/significant other
    ❑ Financial concerns
    ❑ Success of treatment
    ❑ Dealing with family, friends, co-workers
    ❑ Other:_____

I/we have considered all of the above in my/our decision to participate in the proposed assisted reproductive technology treatment. Based on my/our discussions with the above-named mental health professional (MHP), the psychological risks and benefits of participation in the treatments and procedures. Further, I/we understand there may be risks that are presently unknown or unidentified. I/we also understand that any psychological and emotional risks may vary widely among individuals, so it is impossible to accurately state the likelihood of my/our personal harm and I/we cannot expect any mental health professional to state with certainty whether or not I/we may suffer any psychological consequences of treatment. I/we hereby release _____ (MHP) _____ (and his/her agents, employees and assignees) from any liability in the event that I/we suffer psychological or emotional harm from participation in the contemplated behavior, to the extent that his/her actions are reasonably within standards of professional practice. None of the above may be construed, however, as a waiver of my/our right to pursue a negligence or malpractice claim.

Fully understanding the above, I/we freely and voluntarily agree to proceed with treatment. No person has coerced or forced me to consent to any treatment or evaluation.

_____   _____

Signature of Participant   Signature of MHP

_____

Signature of Participant

_____

Date

Embryo Donor Consents

Consent of Couple to Donate Frozen Embryos Example

This document is only to be construed as an example. Local standards and practice may vary and the practitioner is cautioned to seek qualified legal advice before adapting any form for his or her own use.

We wish to donate our frozen embryos (oocyte, provided by the undersigned female donor, that has been fertilized in the laboratory by a sperm provided by the undersigned male donor, and permitted to divide) to a recipient couple who have been unable to achieve or sustain a pregnancy.

We understand that in order to participate in this program we will first undergo a screening process (includes a detailed medical and genetic history, a full physical exam, with blood tests and cultures), an interview with a mental health professional who may administer a standardized personality test (MMPI-2), and an interview with a genetic counselor. We further understand that the costs of the above-described screening will be covered by the program. Upon satisfactory completion of all exams, the frozen embryos from our previous IVF cycle will be released for donation. Upon identification of recipients and their preparation for embryo transfer, the embryos will be allowed to thaw. Embryos that survive the thaw and continue to grow, if any, will be transferred to the uterus of the recipient woman. The disposition of any nonviable or remaining (thawed or frozen) embryos will be decided solely by the recipient couple. Their options include designation as medical waste or for medical research, donation to another couple or individual, implantation into a gestational carrier for the original recipient, if it is deemed medically necessary, or indefinite storage.

We understand that this process is intended to be anonymous, that is, it is intended that any identifying information obtained during this program will remain confidential and will be disclosed only with our permission. The recipients of our embryos will only have access to non-identifying information about our physical characteristics and medical history. We understand and agree that the couple(s) will receive part of the application we completed, a report by the mental health professional, and medical information that we have provided to the genetic counselor. Likewise, we understand that we will not have access to identifying information concerning the recipient of our embryos or will we be informed whether a pregnancy results. It is impossible for anyone to predict whether rule, regulation, or law will allow or require recipients or potential offspring to receive additional information in the future, or whether any such rule, regulation, or law, will be retroactively applicable.

We understand and agree that the donation of embryos is intended to be anonymous and that no entry will be made in our record as to the disposition of any embryos. Furthermore, there will be no entry on the record of any recipient as to the source of the donated embryos. We understand that it is necessary for the physician to keep certain medical records as part of hospital records as to the source and disposition of donated embryos. This information and any other information that would directly or indirectly identify us will not be disclosed or released to any person or entity, except upon our written consent, with the exception of release to authorized employees of the Department of Health, or as required by law or court of competent jurisdiction.

We understand that it is impossible to know with any degree of certainty or specificity the psychological implications of my/our participation as an embryo donor(s) in the Embryo Donation Program. We assume all psychological risks.

We understand and agree that we may receive no money or anything of value in exchange for our agreement to donate our embryos, and no one has offered any such payment to us. However, we understand that the Program may pay for any required medical and/or psychological testing/counseling, without which we may not participate in the embryo donation program.

We have discussed feelings and thoughts related to embryo donation with the mental health professional so that we can make a responsible and informed decision. A number of areas of potential difficulty were discussed, including (1) anonymity of the donation process, (2) curiosity regarding the potential child or children, (3) break in connectedness and continuity traditionally experienced in a genetic parent-child relationship, and (4) possible feelings and questions that may arise in the future. We also discussed feelings and concerns regarding the fact that our child(ren) may have fully genetic siblings who are being parented by someone else.

We acknowledge that, in accordance with current understanding and good practice, the program mental health professional has informed us of the potential psychological risks involved in embryo donation. We acknowledge that we are voluntary participants in the program and that neither the mental health professional nor anyone else in the program has acted in a coercive manner or pressured us to participate in any way.

WE FULLY UNDERSTAND AND AGREE THAT WE WAIVE ANY RIGHT TO AND RELINQUISH ANY CLAIM TO THE DONATED EMBRYOS and TO ANY RESULTANT PREGNANCY, OR OFFSPRING. WE AGREE THAT THE RECIPIENT(S) WILL REGARD THE DONATED EMBRYOS OR OFFSPRING THEREFROM AS THEIR OWN. WE UNDERSTAND THAT WE MAY NOT CLAIM ANY RESPONSIBILITY OR PARENTING RIGHTS FOR OR OBLIGATIONS TO THOSE CHILDREN. WE UNDERSTAND THAT THE RECIPIENT COUPLE IS FULLY RESPONSIBLE FOR ALL OFFSPRING, REGARDLESS OF THE OUTCOME OF THE PREGNANCY, UNTIL THE CHILD REACHES THE AGE OF CONSENT.

We understand that standardized test data as well as other non-identifying information may be used for future research and publication, and we authorize such use of our data. We also understand that we may be contacted in the future for additional information. Our participation is fully voluntary, to the extent that all information remains confidential and data are coded, and, as embryo donors, we are not identified in any published data.

We understand that we may request a copy of this consent form for our records.

We acknowledge that we have been given an opportunity to undergo medical and psychological counseling, which has been met to our satisfaction.

With full understanding of all of the above, we affirm that our signatures indicate we have read the information provided and have voluntarily decided to participate and comply with the program described above.

Signature of Female Partner   Date

Signature of Witness   Date

Signature of Male Partner   Date

Signature of Witness   Date

Embryo Recipients' Consents

Consent to Receive Thawed Donated Embryos Example

This document is only to be construed as an example. Local standards and practice may vary and the practitioner is cautioned to seek qualified legal advice before adapting any form for his or her own use.

We have asked the reproductive medicine clinic [specific name] for treatment using donor embryos. It is our intention to undergo this treatment in hopes of becoming pregnant from the donor embryos. We understand that there are several steps involved in this procedure. The undersigned female recipient will receive medication to mature the endometrium in preparation for an embryo transfer. During this time period, the female recipient will undergo blood testing and ultrasound to determine the response to the medication. When the physicians determine the endometrial lining is ready, the embryos, which have been donated to us, will be thawed. Embryos that survive the thaw will be transferred to the female recipient's uterus via a catheter placed through the cervix into the uterine cavity. We understand that each of these steps carries some risk, including, but not limited to those detailed in the following paragraphs.

Endometrial Preparation

We understand that a variety of medications are used for endometrial preparation including leuprolide acetate (Lupron), transdermal estradiol patches (Climara), and progesterone. We understand that some of these medications are given by intra-muscular or subcutaneous injections and may cause bruising and discomfort at the injection site. Lupron may result in fatigue, muscle and joint pain, or transient menopausal-like symptoms (headaches, hot flashes, mood swings, sweats, and insomnia, etc). Climara may result in headache, nausea, weight gain, breast tenderness, or irritation of the skin.

Monitoring Protocol

We understand that while receiving the medications described above, the female recipient will be closely monitored by the embryo donation team. This monitoring will include frequent blood drawing, which carries the risk of mild discomfort and bruising at the puncture site. We understand that transvaginal ultrasound examinations will be performed as necessary. There may be some discomfort with this procedure although there is no known medical risk associated with its use. The female recipient may also be asked to collect urine samples for further hormone analysis. We understand that if monitoring suggests a low probability of successful maturation of the endometrial lining, the cycle may be canceled. We also understand that some or all of the embryos may not survive the thawing process.

We understand that research supports the use of small doses of corticoids and antibiotics to protect the embryos from possible invasion of blood cells and bacteria following the transfer into the uterus. We understand that the female recipient will receive corticosteriods in the form of methylprednisolone and antibiotics in the form of tetracycline or a similar antibiotic prior to transfer of the embryos.

The following side effects, although extremely rare, may occur after treatment with corticosteriods:

- Treatment may mask signs of infection; new infections may appear during corticosteriod use; there may be an inability to localize an infection, if one occurs.
- Blood pressure elevation, salt and water retention, and increased excretion of potassium and calcium may occur. These medications in high doses have been reported to cause mood swings, insomnia, depression, and psychotic manifestations, muscle weakness, impaired wound healing, increased sweating, headache, vertigo, allergic reaction, loss of muscle mass, osteoporosis, and abdominal distention.

The use of tetracycline may result in the following dose-related side effects:

- Nausea, vomiting, diarrhea, loss of appetite, rash
- Vaginal yeast infection
- Sensitivity to the sun
- Although rare, hypersensitivity reactions resulting in shock, blood diseases including reduced platelets or fractured red blood cells that can result in anemia or bleeding.

Embryo Transfer

When appropriate, thawed donated embryos will be transferred into the uterine cavity via a catheter passed through the cervix. We understand that this may cause some cramping, discomfort, and possibly a small amount of bleeding. Infection is a possible result of the catheter insertion and may require antibiotic treatment. We understand that there is no guarantee that any of the embryos transferred will result in pregnancy.

We understand that transferring multiple embryos and, less commonly, even a single embryo, places us at risk for multiple gestation (more than one baby), and the risk correlates directly with the number of embryos transferred. There are obstetrical risks of multiple gestation including pre-term labor and delivery of premature infants who require intensive care and could have long term complications associated with pre-maturity. It is the policy of the reproductive medicine clinic to limit the number of embryos transferred to maximize the chance of pregnancy while reducing the high order multiple rate when possible.

Post-Transfer Management

In an attempt to increase the chance of successful implantation, post-transfer management will include intra-muscular progesterone injections and transdermal estrogen patches. The progesterone and estrogen are continued, in most cases, for approximately ten to twelve weeks. We understand that during this period the female recipient will be asked to have hormonal evaluations performed as instructed by the program.

If pregnancy should result from this procedure, the pregnancy will be monitored by frequent hormone blood tests. We understand that the female recipient might suffer a miscarriage or an ectopic (tubal) pregnancy, or any of the other complications that might occur during any pregnancy. There is no current consensus as to whether the likelihood of certain birth defects or other abnormalities may be increased in children conceived with IVF technologies, as opposed to non-IVF conceived children. We understand that the program cannot guarantee the normality or health of any infant who results from this procedure. Alternative options (if any) have been explained to us by the IVF team. These include procedures that are not performed here, and other non-medical options such as adoption or non-treatment.

In the event the pregnancy progresses to sixteen weeks, depending upon the female donor age and/or if intra-cytoplasmic sperm injection was utilized in the fertilization of the embryos, amniocentesis, for determination of chromosome status of the fetus, may be advisable. If any serious abnormalities are discovered prior to birth, we understand that we should then discuss the various alternatives including elective termination of the pregnancy, with our obstetrician. We will assume full responsibility for any decision or action required should a fetal abnormality be detected, and understand that no guarantee as to the health of any pregnancy or child has been promised or given.

We understand that we will be responsible for all costs incurred in the procedure, including, but not limited to, the cost of medications, hormonal monitoring, thawing and transferring the embryo, and the cost for screening embryo donors.

Thawed embryos that show arrested growth may also result from this process. These nonviable embryos will be discarded as medical waste unless otherwise specified by us. As an alternative, we may elect to permit Institutional Review Board (IRB) approved research of these nonviable embryos. The IRB serves to protect the human rights of individuals who participate in clinical research. Separate IRB approved research consents will be attached if we elect this option.

We understand that it is impossible, at this time, to estimate the possibility of success. We understand that all of the information and data resulting from this procedure will remain confidential. This information will not be disclosed or released to any person or entity except to authorized employees of the Department of Health or as permitted or required by law, rule, or regulation.

We understand that, we will not have access to identifying information concerning the donors of our embryos or will we be informed whether a pregnancy results. It is impossible for anyone to predict whether rule, regulation, or law will allow or require donors or potential offspring to receive additional information in the future, or whether any such rule, regulation, or law, will be retroactively applicable.

It is not possible to state with any degree of certainty or specificity the psychological implications of participation as recipients of anonymously donated embryos in the Embryo Donation Program at_____.

We consulted with a mental health professional during which the psychosocial issues surrounding embryo donation and the possible implications for our family were discussed. Our thoughts and feelings regarding building my family by embryo donation have been addressed so that we can make an informed and responsible choice.

The areas of potential difficulty that were discussed included (1) disclosure to the child and possible curiosity of the child regarding his or her genetic heritage; (2) potential implications of non-disclosure to the child; (3) discontinuity of traditional biologic and genetic connectedness in the parent–child relationship; (4) the real possibility that my child will have full genetic siblings who are being parented by other parents; and (5) questions and feelings that might arise in the future either within the child, myself, or my partner. As with any child, temperament, personality style, intelligence, and physical characteristics cannot be known or accurately predicted.

We acknowledge that, in accordance with current understanding and good practice, the program mental health professional has informed us of the potential psychological risks involved in embryo donation. We acknowledge that we are voluntary participants in the program and that neither the mental health professional nor anyone else in the program has acted in a coercive manner or pressured us to participate in any way.

We agree that any psychological information deemed relevant to our participation in embryo donation may be shared with the medical staff, and hereby specifically authorize this disclosure of information.

We understand that standardized test data as well as other non-identifying information may be used for future research and publication, and we authorize such use of our data. We also understand that we may be contacted in the future for additional information. Our participation is fully voluntary, to the extent that all information remains confidential and data are coded, and, as embryo donor recipients, we are not identified in any published data.

In accordance with government regulation, we understand the Medical Center's policy in the event physical injury occurs. If, as a result of our participation, we experience physical injury from known or unknown risks of the procedure as described, hospitalization, if necessary, will be available. No monetary compensation is available and we will be responsible for the cost of such medical treatment, directly or through medical insurance and/or other forms of medical coverage.

After carefully considering the alternatives, the risks, the benefits and likelihood of success of the proposed treatment, we have decided to proceed with embryo donation, and our signature hereon indicates that we have listened to and read the information provided, had the opportunity to ask questions of our doctor, had our questions answered, and are giving our fully informed consent to proceed.

_____   _____
Signature of Patient Recipient   Date

_____   _____
Witness   Date

_____   _____
Signature of Recipient Partner   Date

_____   _____
Witness   Date

Resources

OVERVIEW

Professional Organizations – Medical

American Society for Reproductive Medicine (ASRM)
www.asrm.org

European Society of Human Reproduction
and Embryology (ESHRE)
www.eshre.com

International Federation of Fertility Societies (IFFS)
www.iffs-reproduction.org

World Health Organization (WHO)
www.who.int

Human Fertilization and Embryology Authority
(HFEA)
www.hfea.gov.uk

Professional Organizations – Psychological

ASRM Mental Health Professional Group
http://www.asrm.org/Professionals/PG-SIG-
Affiliated_Soc/MHPG/ index.html

ESHRE Mental Health Group
www.eshre.com/emc.asp?pageId=368

Australia and New Zealand Infertility Counselling
Association – ANZICA
www.anzica.org

British Infertility Counselling Association (BICA)
www.bica.net

Germany – Beratungsnetzwerk Kinderwunsch
Deutschland e.V. (BKiD)
www.bkid.de

International Society of Psychosomatic Obstetrics and
Gyneacology
http://www.ispog.org

Patient Organizations

Resolve, The National Infertility Association
www.resolve.org

The American Fertility Association
www.theafa.org

Canada: Infertility Network
http://www.infertilitynetwork.org

POF International Support group
www.pofsupport.org

The Endometriosis Association
www.endometriosisassn.org

The Polycystic Ovarian Syndrome Association
www.pcosupport.org

International Council on Infertility Information
Dissemination (INCIID)
http://www.inciid.org

The Fertility Awareness and Natural Family Planning
Service UK
http://www.fertilityuk.org

Medical

Society of Assisted Reproductive Technology (SART) –
patient information
http://www.sart.org/

ASRM Patient Fact Sheet *is a series produced under
the direction of the ASRM Patient Education Committee
and the Publications Committee. These fact sheets may
be printed and distributed to patients to enhance patient
education.*
http://www.asrm.org/Patients/FactSheets/fact.html

World Health Organization – "Medical, Ethical and Social Aspects of Assisted Reproduction"
http://www.who.int/reproductive-health/infertility/index.htm

Disorders associated with infertility:
http://www.nichd.nih.gov/womenshealth/infertility.cfm

The Impact of Environmental Factors, Body Weight and Exercise on Fertility:
http://www.resolve.org/main/national/preview/publication/pdf/The%20Impact%20of%20Environmental%20Factors,%20Body%20Weight%20and%20Exercise%20on%20 Fertility.pdf

Med Help *provides patient medical information*:
www.medhelp.org

Bio News *provides news, information, and comment in assisted reproduction and genetics*
www.bionews.org.uk

U.S. National Institutes of Health
www.nih.gov

Cross-Cultural

Guidelines on multicultural education, training, research, practice, and organizational change for psychologists.
www.apa.org

TREATMENT MODALITIES

Behavioral Medicine

Mind-Body Medicine Institute at Harvard University
www.mbmi.org

Association for the Advancement of Behavioral Therapy
AABT
www.aabt.org

Complementary and Alternative Medicine

National Center for Complementary and Alternative Medicine, NIH
http://nccam.nih.gov/

Public Broadcasting Service (PBS)
http://thenewmedicine.org

Sexual Counseling

Sexuality Special Interest Group (SSIG) of ASRM
www.asrm.org

American Association of Sex Educators, Counselors, and Therapist AASECT
www.aasect.org

Female Sexual Dysfunction Online *from Baylor College of Medicine provides clinicians and researchers with edu-*

cational materials, including the contributions that relationship factors and psychosocial issues make to these disorders:
SiteInfo@FemaleSexualDysfunctionOnline.org

MEDICAL COUNSELING ISSUES

Medically Complicating

Fertile HOPE *offers resource information, support services, and at times financial grants for cancer survivors dealing with reproductive issues:*
http://www.fertilehope.org

Premature Ovarian Failure information:
http://pof.nichd.nih.gov

DES at website – Center for Disease Control
www.cdc.gov/des

DES Action
www.desaction.org

DES Cancer Network
www.descancer.org

Turner's Syndrome
www.turner-syndrome-us.org

Genetic Counseling

Alliance of Genetic Support Groups
www.geneticalliance.org

CDC Genomics and Disease Prevention *provides lectures, slices, audio, video and downloads including Importance of Race, Ethnicity, and Genetics in Biomedical Research and Clinical Practice:*
www.cdc.gov/genomics/info/presentations.htm

American Board of Genetic Counselors
www.abgc.net

Genetic Counseling Special Interest Group (GCSIG) of ASRM
www.asrm.org

Genetic Interest Group
www.gig.org.uk

Human Genetics Commission
www.hgc.gov.uk

Preimplantation Genetic Diagnosis International Society
www.pgdis.org

Pregnancy Loss

March of Dimes – pregnancy and newborn loss
http://www.marchofdimes.com/pnhec/572_4009.asp

Request to put a "stop" on baby mailings is:
www.meadjohnson.com or 1-800-BABY123

Share Pregnancy and Infant Loss and Support Office
http://www.nationalshareoffice.com/index.shtml

Miscarriage Support Auckland, Inc.
http://www.miscarriagesupport.org.nz/what_mis.html

Center for Loss in Multiple Births (CLIMB)
www.climb-support.org

Angels Forever – a parental support network for
multiple loss
www.angels4ever.com

SIDS Alliance
http://www.sidsalliance.org

Pregnancy Termination Support
www.aheartbreakingchoice.com

ASRM Recurrent Pregnancy Loss Fact Sheet
http://www.asrm.org/Patients/FactSheets/
recurrent_preg_loss.pdf

Medline at National Institutes of Health
http://www.nlm.nih.gov/medlineplus/
pregnancyloss.html

THIRD-PARTY REPRODUCTION

Donor Recipients and Offspring

Donor Conception Network (England)
http://www.dcnetwork.org

Donor Conception Support Group (Australia)
http://www.dcsg.org.au

Information Donogene Insemination (Germany)
http://www.spendersamenkinder.de

Embryo Donation

See www.resolve.org for additional information regarding embryo donation patient and professional resources, and a directory listing of member clinics of the Society of Assisted Reproductive Technology (www.sart.org) in the United States that provide embryo donation services.

Snowflakes
www.nightlight.org/snowflakeslanding.asp

Embryos Alive
www.embryosalive.com

National Embryo Donation Center
www.embryodonation.org

Surrogacy

The American Surrogacy Center, Inc. offers a website with information regarding surrogacy.
www.surrogacy.com

COTS (Childlessness Overcome through Surrogacy) –
an organization from the UK providing information regarding surrogacy and IVF.
http://www.surrogacy.org.uk/

Surrogate Parenting Services
www.surrogateparenting.com

OPTS (The Organization for Parents through
Surrogacy)
http://www.opts.com/

ALTERNATIVE FAMILY BUILDING

Adoption

Joint Council on International Children's Services
www.jcics.org

National Adoption Information Clearinghouse
www.naic.acf.hhs.gov

Evan B. Donaldson Adoption Institute
www.adoptioninstitute.org

Rainbow Kids – international adoption newsletter
www.rainbowkids.com

Families with Children from China
www.FWCC.org

Families for Russian and Ukrainian Adoptions
www.FRUA.org

National Adoption Center
www.adopt.org

www.adopting.org *(includes link to EurAdopt, an association of adoption organizations in 12 western European countries, as well as worldwide links)*

The Center for Adoption Support and Education
www.adoptionsupport.org

Department for Education and Skills (England)
www.dfes.gov.uk/adoption

Australian Society of Intercountry Aid for Children
www.asaic.org

Australians Caring for Children
www.accau.org

General Adoption Information (U.S.)

www.Adoption.com

General Adoption Information (U.K.)

www.adoption.org.uk
www.adoptionuk.org

Adoption Groups and Discussion Boards

www.adoptionboards.com

Childfree

Global Infertility and Childlessness
World Health Organization – Infertility
http://www.who.int/reproductive-health/infertility/
report_content.htm

No Kidding! *Non-profit social club/resource with local, national and international chapters based in Canada*
http://www.nokidding.net

Kidding Aside – The British Childfree Association
http://www.kiddingaside.net

Internet Mailing List
http://groups/yahoo.com/group/CF_and_like_kids/

POST-INFERTILITY COUNSELING ISSUES

Pregnancy

Depression After Delivery
www.depressionafterdelivery.com or (800) 944–4773

Postpartum Support International
www.postpartum.net/ or (631) 422–2255

Marce Society – Professional organization on postpartum depression
www.marcesociety.com

Triplet Connection
http://www.tripletconnection.org

The Center for Study of Multiple Births
www.multiplebirth.com

Resource for Parenatal Complications and Loss
www.aplacetoremember.com

Parenting

Advice for New Parents *provides resources for parents of infants, babies and toddlers*:
www.babycenter.com/

Family.Com *columnists who dispense advice on every topic*:
www.family.com/

ParentsPlace.Com *parenting advice on the net*:
www.parentsplace.com/

PositiveParenting.Com *offers on-line parenting classes and links to other good parenting sites*:
www.positiveparenting.com/

Fatherhood

Father's World *is an on-line community for men who want to learn more about fatherhood*:
www.fathersworld.com

Fatherwork *web site to encourage good fathering*:
www.fatherwork.byu.edu

Gay Parenting

Family Pride Coalition *advances the well-being of lesbian, gay, bisexual, and transgendered parents and their families*:
www.familypride.org

Alternative Family Magazine *provides information for gay parents*:
www.altfammag@aol.com

Colage (Children of Lesbians and Gays Everywhere) *support network for children of gay and bisexual parents*:
www.colage.org/

Rainbow Families *is a midwest organization for gay and lesbian parents and their children*:
www.rainbowfamilies.org

Children

Talking to Children about Donor Conception:
http://www.theafa.org/faqs/afa_
talktoovumdonorchildren.html

Bibliography on Children's Books:
http://www.asrm.org/Professionals/PG-SIG-Affiliated_
Soc/MHPG/MHPG_Childrens_Bibliography.pdf

www.mybeginnings.org

www.thewaywardstork.com

www.xyandme.com

INFERTILITY COUNSELING IN PRACTICE

Ethics

ASRM Ethics Committee Reports
http://www.asrm.org/Media/Ethics/ethicsmain.html

President's Council on Bioethics
www.bioethics.gov

International Bioethics Committee
www.unesco.org/shs/bioethics

European Group on Ethics in Science and New Developments
http://europa.eu.int/comm/europea_group_ethics/
index_en.htm

Glossary*

Abdominal Pregnancy. A pregnancy that has implanted on structures in the abdomen other than the uterus, fallopian tubes, or ovaries. It usually implants on tissue in the abdomen known as the omentum.

Acquired Immunodeficiency Syndrome (AIDS). A disease caused by the Human Immunodeficiency Virus (HIV) that impairs the body's immune system and leads to severe infections and eventually death.

Acrosome. A membrane-bound portion of the end of the sperm head that contains enzymes necessary to penetrate the egg's outer covering (zona pellucida).

ACTH. See adrenocorticotropic hormone.

Addison's Disease. Failure of the adrenal glands resulting in a deficiency in the secretion of adrenocortical hormones.

Adenoma. A benign (non-cancerous) growth of cells that usually does not invade adjacent tissue. A pituitary adenoma can disrupt ovulation and menstruation.

Adenomyosis. A benign (non-cancerous) invasion of endometrial tissue into the muscular wall (myometrium) of the uterus; can be associated with painful or heavy menses.

Adhesions. Bands of fibrous scar tissue that may bind the pelvic organs and/or loops of bowel together. Adhesions can result from previous infections, endometriosis, or surgeries.

Adoptive Parents. Parents who have children by adoption.

Adrenal Glands. Glands located above each kidney that secrete hormones, such as cortisol, aldosterone,

adrenaline, and androgens, that help the body withstand stress and regulate metabolism. Altered function of these glands can disrupt menstruation.

Adrenal Hyperplasia. An abnormal or unusual increase in the production of androgens by the adrenal glands. This disorder is the result of a genetic problem.

Adrenocorticotropic Hormone (ACTH). A pituitary hormone that stimulates the adrenal gland to produce androgens and cortisol.

Agency Adoption. An adoption that takes place through an established institution, either public or private, that exists for the purpose of facilitating adoptions.

Amenorrhea. The absence of menstrual periods.

American Society for Reproductive Medicine (ASRM). A nonprofit, professional medical organization of more than 8,000 health care specialists interested in reproductive medicine. Contact info: American Society for Reproductive Medicine, 1209 Montgomery Highway, Birmingham, AL 35216; (205) 978–5000; asrm@asrm.org; www.asrm.org.

Amniocentesis. A procedure in which a small amount of amniotic fluid is removed through a needle from the fetal sac at about 16 weeks into a pregnancy. The fluid is studied for chromosomal abnormalities that may affect fetal development.

Amnion. Thin membrane that expands to enclose a developing fetus. This membrane (sac) holds the amniotic fluid that protects the developing fetus.

Anabolic Steroid. A synthetic androgen-like hormone sometimes used to increase muscle size.

Androgens. Hormones produced by the testes, ovaries, and adrenal glands responsible for encouraging masculine characteristics. Often referred to as "male"

*Used with permission, American Society of Reproductive Medicine, Birmingham, AL, 2005.

hormones. Androgens are produced in males and females, but males have much higher levels.

Androstenedione. An androgenic hormone naturally made by the ovaries, testes, and adrenal glands. The body turns it into testosterone. Androstenedione sold as a "natural" supplement is made from plant chemicals and is not regulated by the FDA. It is often marketed as an athletic performance and muscle enhancer, but its safety and effectiveness are controversial.

Anemia. A reduction in the number of red blood cells, which carry oxygen in the body. Anemia is characterized by weakness or listlessness.

Anovulation. Absent ovulation.

Antibodies. Proteins that are produced by the body to attack and destroy foreign substances, such as bacteria and viruses. Antibodies are an important part of the body's immune system.

Anticardiolipin Antibodies. A type of a group of antiphospholipid antibodies that may be associated with miscarriage.

Antiphospholipid Antibodies. See anticardiolipin antibodies.

Antisperm Antibodies. Immune or protective proteins (immunoglobulins) that attack and destroy the sperm because they recognize it as a foreign substance. Antisperm antibodies may be present in the male in blood or sperm or in the female in blood or cervical mucus.

Appendicitis. A condition where the appendix (a tubular structure attached to the colon) becomes infected and inflamed and can be associated with the formation of adhesions in the proximity of the fallopian tube.

Arcuate Uterus. A birth defect in which the uterine cavity is slightly indented at the central upper portion.

ART (Assisted Reproductive Technology). Procedures performed in a laboratory or physician office that facilitate pregnancy. Examples of ART include in vitro fertilization (IVF) and gamete intrafallopian fertilization (GIFT).

Assay. A medical term meaning "test."

Assisted Hatching (AH). A procedure in which the zona pellucida (outer covering) of the embryo is partially opened, usually by application of an acid, to facilitate embryo implantation and pregnancy.

Assisted Reproductive Technology (ART). All treatments that include laboratory handling of eggs, sperm, and/or embryos. Some examples of ART are in vitro fertilization (IVF), gamete intrafallopian transfer (GIFT),

pronuclear stage tubal transfer (PROST), tubal embryo transfer (TET), and zygote intrafallopian transfer (ZIFT).

Asymmetric. Not symmetrical. Each side is not equal.

Atherosclerosis. A condition that results from the collection of fatty substances in the inner layer of the arteries. It is a common cause of arterial blockage.

Atresia. The natural process by which eggs age and degenerate.

Autoimmune. A condition in which the body's immune system attacks its own tissues, falsely recognizing them as foreign.

Azoospermia. The complete absence of sperm in semen.

Basal Body Temperature (BBT). The body temperature at rest. The temperature is taken orally each morning immediately upon awakening and recorded on a BBT chart. The readings are studied to help identify ovulation, which usually occurs at approximately the same time as the rise in BBT.

Bicornuate Uterus. A birth defect in which the external contour of the uterus and the contour of the uterine cavity appear to be heart-shaped with a central indentation. This condition may result in premature labor or abnormal positioning of the fetus in the uterus.

Biochemical Pregnancy. A pregnancy that is detected by the presence of pregnancy hormone (human chorionic gonadotropin – hCG) in the blood, but no fetus is visible on ultrasound and the woman has a menstrual period.

Biological Child. The child produced by the union of the sperm and the egg of the birth parents.

Biological Parents. The parents who supply the egg and sperm that produce a child.

Biopsy. The removal of a small tissue sample for microscopic examination. The term "biopsy" also refers to the tissue removed during the procedure.

Birth Control Pills. Also known as oral contraceptives. The pills contain a mixture of synthetic estrogen and progestin. Proper usage prevents pregnancy by suppressing ovulation and decreasing the ovarian secretion of hormones, including androgens.

Bladder. A bag-like structure located in the lower abdomen that holds urine flowing from the kidneys.

Blastocyst. An embryo that has formed a fluid-filled cavity, and the cells begin to form the early placenta and embryo, usually 5 days after ovulation or egg retrieval.

Bone Densitometry. A radiological procedure used to measure the density of bone.

Bone Density. The amount of bone material in a given volume of bone.

Bromocriptine (Parlodel®). A drug used to suppress the production of prolactin by the pituitary gland.

Carcinoma. The medical term for cancer.

Centers for Disease Control and Prevention. Federal agency for protecting the health and safety of people at home and abroad, providing credible information to enhance health decisions, and promoting health through strong partnerships.

Cerclage. Placement of a non-absorbable suture around an incompetent (weak) cervical opening in an attempt to keep it closed and thus prevent miscarriage. Also know as a cervical stitch.

Cerebral palsy. A disorder causing damage to one or more specific areas of the brain usually occurring during fetal development; before, during or shortly after birth; or infancy. Cerebral palsy is characterized by an inability to fully control motor function, particularly muscle control and coordination. Other problems that may arise are difficulties in feeding, bladder and bowel control, problems with breathing, skin disorders and learning disabilities.

Cervical Agenesis. An undeveloped or absent cervix that obstructs the opening of the uterus.

Cervical Canal. The passageway leading from the vagina into the uterus.

Cervical Mucus. The substance in the cervix through which sperm must swim in order to enter the uterus.

Cervix. The narrow, lower part of the uterus that opens into the vagina. The cervical canal runs through the cervix and connects the vagina with the uterine cavity. The cervix produces mucus through which sperm must swim before entering the uterine cavity and then the fallopian tubes.

Cesarean Section. Removal of a fetus through an incision in the mother's abdomen rather than by vaginal delivery.

Chemical Pregnancy. See biochemical pregnancy.

Chemotherapy. The treatment of diseases with chemicals that have a toxic effect on the disease-causing process and may be acutely harmful to the individual.

Chlamydia. A sexually transmitted bacteria that causes pelvic infections and subsequent damage to the fallopian tubes.

Chorionic Villus Sampling (CVS). A procedure in which a small sample of cells is taken from the placenta early in a pregnancy for chromosomal testing.

Chromosomes. Rod-shaped structures located in the nucleus of a cell that contain hereditary (genetic) material. Humans have 23 pairs of chromosomes (46 total). Two of the 46 are the sex chromosomes, which are the X and Y chromosomes. Normally, females have two X chromosomes and males have one X and one Y chromosome.

Cleavage. The cell division of a fertilized egg.

Clinical Pregnancy. A pregnancy confirmed by an increasing level of human chorionic gonadotropin (hCG) and the presence of a gestational sac detected by ultrasound.

Clomid®. See clomiphene citrate.

Clomiphene Citrate. An oral anti-estrogenic drug used to induce ovulation in the female. It is also sometimes used to increase testosterone levels in the infertile male, which may, in turn, improve sperm production. The trade names are Clomid® and Serophene®.

Clomiphine Citrate Challenge Test (CCCT). A test of ovarian reserve in which serum FSH is checked on days 3 and 10 of the menstrual cycle and clomiphene citrate is taken on days 5 through 9.

Closed Adoption. An adoption in which no information is exchanged between the birth parents and the adoptive parents.

Coagulator. An instrument used to cauterize bleeding points or to "burn" away patches of endometriosis.

Collagen. The main protein of the white fibers of connective tissue, cartilage, and bone.

Computerized Tomography (CT scan). An x-ray imaging technique that creates a three-dimensional image of internal organs.

Congenital. A physical abnormality that is present at birth. The defect(s) may be due to an inherited problem, such as abnormal chromosomes or genes, or due to an influence occurring during pregnancy.

Contraindication. A medical situation that a particular medication or treatment should not be used because of possible risks and/or side effects.

Controlled Superovulation. The administration of ovulation drugs that stimulate the ovaries to produce multiple eggs: also called superovulation, enhanced follicular recruitment, controlled ovarian hyperstimulation, or controlled ovarian stimulation.

Cornu. The area in the uterus where the fallopian tube opens into the uterine cavity.

Corpus Luteum. Literally, a "yellow body." A mass of yellow tissue formed in the ovary from a mature follicle that has collapsed after releasing its egg at ovulation. The corpus luteum secretes estrogen and large quantities of progesterone, a hormone that prepares the lining of the uterus (endometrium) to support a pregnancy.

Cortisol. A hormone produced by the adrenal glands, which are located on top of the kidneys in the area of the back near the waistline. Cortisol is responsible for maintaining the body's energy supply, blood sugar, and control of the body's reaction to stress.

Cryopreservation. Freezing at a very low temperature, such as in liquid nitrogen (-196 °C), to keep embryos viable so as to store them for future transfer into a uterus or to keep sperm viable.

Croypreserved. Frozen.

Danazol. An androgen-like drug used to treat endometriosis. Danazol blocks ovulation and suppresses estrogen levels. The brand name is Danocrine®.

Degenerate. A condition of breakdown or decay, such as when a fibroid outgrows its blood supply, begins to deteriorate, and changes in size.

Dehydroepiandrosterone (DHEA). A hormone naturally made by the adrenal glands. The body turns it into other hormones such as estrogen and testosterone. DHEA sold as a "natural" supplement is made from plant chemicals and is not regulated by the FDA. It is often marketed as an anti-aging medication, but its safety and effectiveness are controversial.

DES. A synthetic hormone given in part during pregnancy to prevent miscarriage. Children from pregnancies treated with DES can have abnormalities of the reproductive system, including an increased risk of ectopic pregnancy.

Dexamethasone (Decadron®). A synthetic drug, similar to cortisone or cortisol, often used to treat an overactive adrenal gland.

Diabetes Mellitus. A condition due to a lack of insulin or lack of response to insulin, resulting in blood glucose (sugar) levels that are too high.

Diagnostic Hysteroscopy. The insertion of a long, thin, lighted telescope-like instrument, called a hysteroscope, through the vagina, cervix, and into the uterus in order to look inside the uterine cavity.

Diagnostic Laparoscopy. The insertion of a long, thin, lighted telescope-like instrument, called a laparoscope, through the navel into the abdomen in order to look at the internal pelvic organs, such as the uterus, ovaries, and fallopian tubes.

Diazoxide. A medication that is used to lower blood pressure. The brand name is Proglycem™.

Didelphic Uterus. A complete double uterus and double cervix. It is often also associated with a partial or complete double vagina.

Dilantin™. An anti-seizure medication. The generic name is phenytoin.

Dilation and Curettage (D&C). An outpatient surgical procedure during which the cervix is dilated and the tissue contents of the uterus are emptied. The tissue is often used for microscopic examination.

Dilator. Instrument(s) used to enlarge a small opening, such as the cervix.

Disorders of Descent. Birth defects in the female reproductive system that result when the mullerian ducts and the upper part of the urogenital sinus do not properly join.

Disorders of Fusion. Birth defects in the female reproductive system that result from the failure of the two mullerian ducts to join together.

Distal Tubal Blockage. Blockage at the end of the fallopian tube farthest away (distal) from where it joins the uterus and near where it meets the ovary.

Diuretic. A medication or drug that increases the loss of water from the body in the form of urine.

Dizygotic. Di-two; zygote-fertilized egg. Two separate eggs fertilized by separate sperm in a single pregnancy. Fraternal twins.

Domestic Adoption. An adoption of a child from the same country of citizenship as the adoptive parents.

Dominant Follicle. The largest follicle among developing follicles in the ovary.

Donor. A woman who provides eggs, a man who provides sperm, or a couple who provide embryos for a recipient man, woman, or couple.

Donor Eggs. The eggs taken from the ovaries of a fertile woman and donated to an infertile woman to be used in an assisted reproductive technology procedure using IVF or GIFT. Also see Egg Donation.

Donor Embryo. Embryos produced from the sperm and egg of one couple and donated to an infertile woman or couple.

Donor Embryo Transfer. The transfer of an embryo donated by one couple into the uterus of an infertile woman.

Donor Insemination (DI). The process of placing sperm from a donor (a man who is not a woman's sexual partner) into a woman's reproductive tract for the purpose of producing a pregnancy. The resulting child will be biologically related to the woman but not to her partner.

Donor Sperm. The sperm donated by a fertile man who is not the recipient's partner.

Down Syndrome. A genetic disorder caused by the presence of an extra chromosome 21 and characterized by mental retardation, abnormal facial features, and medical problems such as heart defects.

Dysfunctional Uterine Bleeding (DUB). Abnormal uterine bleeding with no evidence of mechanical or structural cause. The cause of DUB is deficient or excessive production of estrogen and/or progesterone.

Dyspareunia. Pain with intercourse; sometimes a symptom of endometriosis.

Early Menopause. Cessation of menstrual periods due to failure of the ovaries before age 40. The average age of menopause in the United States is 52. Also see Premature Ovarian Failure.

Ectopic (Extrauterine) Pregnancy. A pregnancy in the fallopian tube or elsewhere outside the lining of the uterus.

Efferent Ducts. Tubular structures that conduct sperm from the seminiferous tubules in the testis to the epididymis.

Egg (ooycte). The female sex cell (ovum) produced by the ovary, which, when fertilized by a male's sperm, produces an embryo.

Egg Retrieval (harvest). The procedure in which eggs (oocytes) are obtained by inserting a needle into the ovarian follicle and removing the fluid and the egg by suction. Also called oocyte aspiration or follicle aspiration.

Ejaculation. The expulsion of semen (sperm and glandular fluid) from the urethra at the time of male orgasm. Semen is also referred to as the "ejaculate."

Ejaculatory Duct. A duct formed by the joining of the seminal vesicles with the vas deferens.

Electroejaculation (EEJ). Procedure to cause ejaculation of sperm, performed by electrical stimulation of tissue in the region of the prostate.

Electrosurgical Instrument. A surgical instrument using electric current to burn, incise (cut), and eliminate unwanted tissue.

Embryo. An organism in the early stages of development, arising after the union of sperm and egg (fertilization).

Embryo Culture. Growth of an embryo in a laboratory (culture) dish.

Embryo Transfer. Placement of an embryo into the uterus through the vagina and cervix or, in the case of zygote intrafallopian transfer (ZIFT) or tubal embryo transfer (TET), into the fallopian tube.

Endocrinologist. A physician who specializes in endocrinology, which is the medical specialty concerned with hormonal secretions and their actions.

Endometrial Ablation. A hysteroscopic procedure used to remove portions of the endometrium (uterine lining); sometimes used to treat abnormal uterine bleeding.

Endometrial Biopsy. Removal of small pieces of tissue from the endometrium (lining of the uterus) for microscopic examination. The results may indicate whether or not the endometrium is at the appropriate stage for successful implantation of a fertilized egg (embryo) and/or if it is inflamed or diseased.

Endometrial Polyp. Benign (non-cancerous) tissue mass in the endometrial (uterine) lining which can lead to excessive uterine bleeding and cramping.

Endometriomas. Blood-filled cysts that can occur when endometrial tissue develops in the ovary.

Endometriosis. A condition where endometrial-like tissue (the tissue that lines the uterus) develops outside of the uterine cavity in abnormal locations such as the ovaries, fallopian tubes, and abdominal cavity. This tissue can grow with hormonal stimulation and cause pain, inflammation, and scar tissue. It may also be associated with infertility.

Endometritis. An inflammation of the endometrial lining caused by bacterial invasion.

Endometrium. The lining of the uterus that is shed each month with the menstrual period. As the monthly cycle progresses, the endometrium thickens and thus provides a nourishing site for the implantation of a fertilized egg (embryo).

Epididymis. A tightly coiled system of tiny tubing where sperm collect after leaving the testis. Sperm continue to mature as they are pushed through the epididymis, which covers the top and back sides of each testis.

Estradiol. The predominant estrogen (hormone) produced by the follicular cells of the ovary.

Estrogen. A class of female sex hormones produced by the ovaries that are responsible for the development of female sex characteristics. Estrogens are largely responsible for stimulating the uterine lining to thicken during the first half of the menstrual cycle in preparation for ovulation and possible pregnancy. They are also important for healthy bones and overall health. A small amount of these hormones is also produced in the male when testosterone is converted to estrogen. Estradiol is the main estrogen. Estradiol and estrone are the main two estrogens in ovulating women. Ninety-five percent of all estradiol is produced by the developing follicle.

Estrogen Therapy. The term commonly used to indicate the administration of exogenous estrogens to post-menopausal women and those who have had their ovaries removed.

Fallopian Tubes. A pair of tubes attached to the uterus, one on each side, providing the path by which the egg travels from the ovary to the uterus and in which the egg can be fertilized by the sperm.

Familial Hyperlipidemia. The presence of abnormally high amounts of fat cells (lipids) in the circulating blood. Familial means affecting several members of the same family.

Fecundity. Probability of conception occurring in a given period of time, usually one month.

Fertilization. The fusion of sperm and egg.

Fetus. An unborn child.

Fibroids. Benign (non-cancerous) tumors of the uterine muscle wall that can cause abnormal uterine bleeding. Also see Leiomyomas or Myomas.

Fimbriae. The flared end (fingers) of the fallopian tube that sweeps over the surface of the ovary and helps to direct the egg into the tube.

Finasteride. An antiandrogen medication that blocks the conversion of testosterone to its more active metabolite, dihydrotestosterone. May be prescribed to reduce hair loss associated with male pattern baldness and for enlarged prostate in men. Brand names are Propecia® and Proscar®.

Flutamide. Flutamide is an antiandrogen medication that blocks androgen receptors, preventing the actions of androgens. Flutamide is used in the treatment of prostate cancer, and as off-label, it has been used to treat excess hair in women. The brand name is Eulexin®.

Foley Catheter. A catheter usually used to drain urine and retained in the bladder by a balloon inflated with air or liquid. The balloon of the catheter may be placed in the uterus to prevent scar tissue formation following uterine surgery.

Folic acid. A B-complex vitamin present in many supplements that is important for fetal development.

Follicle, hair. A tubular sheath that surrounds the lower part of the hair shaft, supplies the growing hair with nourishment, and gives life to new hairs.

Follicle, ovarian. A fluid-filled sac located just beneath the surface of the ovary, containing an egg (oocyte) and cells that produce hormones. The sac increases in size and volume during the first half of the menstrual cycle and at ovulation, the follicle matures and ruptures, releasing the egg. As the follicle matures, it can be visualized by ultrasound.

Follicle-Stimulating Hormone (FSH). The pituitary hormone responsible for stimulating the growth of the cells that form the follicle that surrounds the egg. In women, FSH is the pituitary hormone responsible for stimulating follicular cells in the ovary to grow, stimulating egg development and the production of the female hormone estrogen. In the male, FSH is the pituitary hormone that travels through the bloodstream to the testes and helps stimulate them to manufacture sperm. In addition, FSH is the hormone in injectable ovulation drugs that promotes growth of the follicles, and which also may be used to promote spermatogenesis in hypogonadal men.

Follicular Phase. The first half of the menstrual cycle (beginning on day one of bleeding) during which the dominant follicle grows, matures, and secretes large amounts of estrogen.

Frank Technique. A technique to elongate and enlarge a vaginal pouch by using a series of increasingly larger dilators.

Fructose. In men, a sugar made in the seminal vesicles that normally appears in the semen. The presence or absence of fructose in the semen may indicate the location of a blockage in the duct system.

Galactorrhea. A small amount of breast milk production by a woman who is not nursing; caused by elevated levels of the pituitary hormone prolactin.

Gamete Intrafallopian Transfer (GIFT). An assisted reproductive technology that involves surgically removing eggs from a woman's ovary, combining them with sperm, and immediately injecting the eggs/sperm mixture into the fallopian tube. Fertilization then hopefully takes place inside the fallopian tube. One disadvantage of GIFT is the inability to know whether or not fertilization took place if the woman does not become pregnant.

Gametes. Germ cells referring to either sperm and/or eggs.

Genes. Structures located on chromosomes that contain "blueprints" for inherited characteristics.

Genetic. Referring to inherited conditions, usually due to the genes located on the chromosomes.

Genitourinary Tract. Refering to the organs of the reproductive and urinary tracts.

Gestation. Pregnancy.

Gestational Carrier. A woman who carries a pregnancy for another couple. The pregnancy is derived from the egg and sperm of persons not related to the carrier. Although the carrier carries the pregnancy to term, she has neither a genetic relationship nor rearing rights or responsibilities to the resulting child.

Gestational Diabetes. Elevated blood sugar levels in the mother while she is pregnant. During pregnancy, the placenta normally produces hormones that antagonize insulin. With a multiple pregnancy, more of these hormones are produced and lead to a rise in the mother's blood sugar.

Gestational Sac. The fluid-filled sac surrounding an embryo that develops within the uterine cavity. Ultrasound can detect the sac in the uterus at a very early stage of pregnancy.

GnRH Agonists. Synthetic hormones similar to the naturally occurring gonadotropin-releasing hormones (GnRH) secreted by the hypothalamus. GnRH agonists, when given in short pulses, stimulate FSH and LH production by the pituitary gland. However, when given in more prolonged doses, they decrease FSH and LH production by the pituitary, which in turn decrease ovarian hormone production. Brand names include Lupron®, Synarel®, and Zolodex®.

GnRH Analog. A long-acting synthetic hormone similar to the naturally occurring gonadotropin-releasing hormone produced by the hypothalamus. There are two types of GnRH analogs: GnRH agonists and GnRH antagonists. Both types will suppress the secretion of FSH and LH from the pituitary gland.

GnRH antagonists. Synthetic hormones similar to the naturally occurring gonadotropin releasing hormone that have an immediate suppressive effect on the pituitary gland. GnRH antagonists are used to prevent premature ovulation.

Gonadotropin-Releasing Hormone (GnRH). The natural hormone secreted by the hypothalamus that prompts the pituitary gland to release follicle stimulating hormone (FSH) and luteinizing hormone (LH) into the bloodstream. This in turn stimulates the ovaries to produce estrogen, progesterone, and to ovulate. Factrel® and Lutrepulse® are brand names.

Gonadotropins. Follicle stimulating hormone (FSH) and luteinizing hormone (LH). FSH and LH may be purified or synthetically produced to be used as ovulatory drugs. hMG (human menopausal gonadotropin – Pergonal®, Humegon™, Repronex™, Menopur™); hFSH (human follicle stimulating hormone – Metrodin®, Fertinex™, Bravelle™); rFSH (recombinant follicle stimulating hormone – Gonal F™, Follistim™); and hCG (human chorionic gonadotropin – Profasi®, APL®, Pregnyl®, Novarel™, Ovidrel®.

Gonorrhea. A sexually transmitted disease caused by the gonococcus bacterium that can cause pelvic infections, scar tissue, and tubal damage in the female. In the male, gonorrhea can cause obstructions in the ducts that transport sperm.

HAIR-AN Syndrome (Hyperandrogenism, Insulin Resistance, Acanthosis Nigricans). A genetic disorder associated with very high circulating levels of insulin and androgens.

Hair Follicle. A tubular sheath that surrounds the lower part of the hair shaft and supplies the growing hair with nourishment.

Hair Shaft. The part of the hair that is visible above the skin.

HDL Cholesterol. The "good" type of cholesterol that is composed of a high proportion of protein and is associated with a decreased chance of developing heart disease.

Hematomas. Localized collections of blood that seep from the blood vessels into tissue, like a very large bruise.

Hemivagina. One side of a double vagina.

Hemophilia. An inherited blood defect found almost exclusively in males. It is characterized by delayed blood clotting and bleeding problems.

Hemorrhoids. A painful swelling of a vein in the anal region often accompanied by bleeding.

Heparin. A blood-thinning medication given by injection.

Hepatitis B and C. Viruses that may be sexually transmitted, or transmitted by contact with blood and other bodily fluids, that can cause infection of the liver leading to jaundice and liver failure.

Hirsutism. The growth of long, coarse hair on the face, chest, upper arms, and upper legs of women in a pattern similar to that of men. Hirsutism may be due to ethnic background or to excess levels of androgens.

Home Study. Part of the adoptive process, either public or private, in which an adoption worker examines the home environment where the adoptive child will be placed.

Hormone. A substance secreted from organs of the body, such as the pituitary gland, adrenal gland, or ovaries, which is carried by a bodily fluid such as blood to other organs or tissues where it exerts a specific action.

Hormone Therapy. The term commonly associated with the use of synthetic hormonal medications to substitute for the natural hormones that are lost due to menopause.

Hot Flash. Also called vasomotor flush. A sudden brief flushing and sensation of heat caused by dilation of skin capillaries. Hot flashes are associated with menopausal hormonal imbalances.

Human chorionic gonadotropin (hCG). A hormone produced by the placental tissue. Its detection is the basis of most pregnancy tests. Also refers to the medication used during ovulation induction to cause ovulation and the final stages of egg maturation. The U.S. trade names are A.P.L.®, Pregnyl®, and Profasi®.

Human Immunodeficiency Virus (HIV). A retrovirus that causes acquired immune deficiency syndrome (AIDS), a disease that destroys the body's ability to protect itself from infection and disease. It is transmitted by the exchange of bodily fluids or blood transfusions.

Human Menopausal Gonadotropins (hMG). A fertility drug containing follicle stimulating hormone (FSH) and luteinizing hormone (LH). It is derived from the urine of postmenopausal women. hMG is used to stimulate the growth of multiple follicles. Examples of trade names are Pergonal®, Humegon™, Repronex™, Menopur™.

Humegon™. Brand name of human menopausal gonadotropins (hMG): see human menopausal gonadotropins (hMG).

Huntington's Disease. An inherited disorder of the central nervous system that develops in adulthood and may cause irregular, spasmodic, involuntary movements of the limbs or facial muscles.

Husband Insemination (HI). A procedure in which sperm from a woman's partner is placed into her reproductive tract for the purpose of increasing the chance of pregnancy.

Hydrosalpinx. A blocked, dilated, fluid-filled fallopian tube.

Hymen. The remnant of the hymenal membrane which normally partially covers the entrance to the vagina. If the hymenal membrane does not resorb, it will be "imperforated" and can result in blood accumulation above the membrane when menstruation begins.

Hymenal Membrane. A thin layer of tissue that covers the end of the vagina in the developing fetus.

Hyperandrogenism. A condition in which women have elevated levels of androgens (male hormones).

Hyperplasia. The excessive formation of normal cells within tissue or organs.

Hyperthyroidism. An abnormal increase in the amount of thyroid hormone produced by the thyroid gland.

Hypospadias. A congenital abnormality of the penis in which the urethra opens on the underside of the penis rather than at the tip. This condition may prevent the semen from being deposited into the female reproductive tract during intercourse.

Hypothalamic Disorders. Disorders that occur in the hypothalamus, which is the thumb-sized area at the base of the brain that secretes hormones to regulate the pituitary gland.

Hypothalamus. A thumb-sized area in the base of the brain that controls many body functions, regulates the pituitary gland, and releases gonadotropin releasing hormone (GnRH).

Hysterectomy. The surgical removal of the uterus. Hysterectomy may be performed through an abdominal incision (laparotomy), through the vagina (vaginal hysterectomy), or through laparoscopy-assisted vaginal hysterectomy (LAVH). Sometimes the ovaries and fallopian tubes are also removed.

Hysterosalpingogram (HSG). An x-ray procedure in which a special media (a dye-like solution) is injected through the cervix into the uterine cavity to illustrate the inner shape of the uterus and degree of openness (patency) of the fallopian tubes.

Hysteroscope. A thin, lighted, telescope-like instrument that is inserted through the vagina and cervix into the uterine cavity to allow viewing of the inside of the uterus.

Hysteroscopic Metroplasty. Surgical repair of a uterine defect using a hysteroscope and other surgical instruments.

Hysteroscopy. A procedure in which a long, thin, lighted telescope-like instrument, (hysteroscope), is inserted through the cervix and into the uterus to examine the inside of the uterine cavity. Hysteroscopy can be used to both diagnose and surgically treat uterine conditions.

Identified Adoption. Also known as agency-assisted adoption. An adoption where the prospective adoptive parents locate a child or birth parents and use the services of an agency to assist with and finalize the adoption.

Idiopathic. Unexplained.

Immune System. The body system that is responsible for protecting against foreign substances such as viruses and bacteria.

Immunoglobulins. Proteins in the body that act like antibodies; they attack foreign substances such as viruses and bacteria and are important components in the body's immune system.

Immunologic Factors. Antibodies or allergic responses that may cause certain types of infertility.

Imperforate Hymen. A birth defect in which the hymenal membrane does not break down before birth and therefore obstructs the vagina.

Implantation. The process whereby an embryo embeds in the uterine lining to obtain nutrition and oxygen. Sometimes an embryo will implant in areas other than the uterus, such as in a fallopian tube. This is known as an ectopic pregnancy.

Implants (of endometriosis). Patches of endometrial tissue (tissue that lines the uterus) growing outside of the uterus in abnormal locations such as the abdominal cavity or ovaries.

Impotence. The inability of a male to achieve or maintain an erection.

Incompetent Cervix. A cervix (the narrow, lower end of the uterus) that is incapable of staying closed and holding a pregnancy without surgical correction.

Independent or Private Adoption. An adoption that takes place outside an agency. It is usually facilitated by a lawyer, minister, and/or physician who serves as an intermediary between the birth parents and the adoptive parents.

Infertility. Infertility is the result of a disease (an interruption, cessation, or disorder of body functions, systems, or organs) of the male or female reproductive tract that prevents the conception of a child or the ability to carry a pregnancy to delivery. The duration of unprotected intercourse with failure to conceive should be about 12 months before an infertility evaluation is undertaken, unless medical history, age, or physical findings dictate earlier evaluation and treatment.

Infertility Workup. A series of tests performed to determine the cause(s) of infertility.

Inhibin. A substance produced by granulosa cells in the ovaries in females and the testes in males. It signals the pituitary gland to slow down the release of follicle stimulating hormone (FSH).

Insemination. Placement of sperm into the uterus or cervix for producing a pregnancy, or adding sperm to eggs in IVF procedures.

International Adoption. Adoption of a child from a country other than that of the adoptive parents.

Interracial Adoption. Adoption of a child of a race other than that of the adoptive parents.

Interstitial Cells. Cells in the interstitium of the testes; see Leydig cells.

Interstitium. The area in the testes outside the seminiferous tubules that contains Leydig cells and other interstitial cells.

Intracervical Insemination (ICI). Placement of semen via a syringe directly into the cervical canal.

Intracytoplasmic Sperm Injection (ICSI). A micromanipulation technique used in conjunction with IVF that involves injecting a sperm directly into an egg to facilitate fertilization. The fertilized egg is then transferred to the uterus.

Intramural Fibroids. Fibroids located in the muscular wall of the uterus.

Intrauterine Device (IUD). A contraceptive device placed within the uterus; also sometimes used to prevent scar tissue formation following uterine surgery.

Intrauterine Insemination (IUI). The process whereby sperm are injected directly into the uterine cavity to bypass the cervix and place the sperm closer to the egg. The sperm are usually washed first to remove chemicals that can irritate the uterine lining and to increase sperm motility and concentration.

Intrauterine Pregnancy. An embryo that has implanted appropriately on the wall of the uterus.

Intrauterine Synechiae. Adhesions (scar tissue) within the uterus.

Intravenous Pyelogram (IVP). An x-ray of the urinary system.

In Vitro Fertilization (IVF). A method of assisted reproduction that involves combining an egg with sperm in a laboratory dish. If the egg fertilizes and begins cell division, the resulting embryo is transferred into the woman's uterus where it will hopefully implant in the uterine lining and further develop. IVF bypasses the fallopian tubes and is usually the treatment choice for women who have badly damaged or absent tubes.

IVF Culture Medium. A special fluid into which sperm, eggs, and embryos are placed outside the human body.

Karyotype. A blood or tissue test that analyzes a person's chromosomes.

Laparoscope. A thin, lighted, telescope-like viewing instrument that is usually inserted through the navel into the abdomen to visually inspect the contents of the pelvic and abdominal cavities. The laparoscope can be used as both a diagnostic and operative instrument.

Laparoscopy. A surgical procedure that allows viewing of the internal pelvic organs. During the procedure, a long, narrow fiber-optic instrument, called a laparoscope, is inserted through an incision in or below the woman's navel. Other incisions may also be made through which additional instruments can be inserted to facilitate diagnosis and treatment of pelvic disease.

Laparotomy. Major abdominal surgery performed through an incision in the abdominal wall, usually a "bikini" or "up and down" cut.

LDL Cholesterol. A type of cholesterol that is composed of a moderate proportion of protein with fat. High levels are associated with an increased probability of developing heart disease.

Leiomyomas. Benign (non-cancerous) tumors of the uterine muscle wall that can cause abnormal uterine bleeding. Also called fibroids or myomas.

Leiomyosarcoma. A malignant tumor arising from smooth muscle tissue such as the uterus.

Leydig Cells. The interstitial cells in the testes that produce the male hormone testosterone.

LH Surge. The rapid rise and secretion of luteinizing hormone (LH) that the pituitary gland releases in the middle of the menstrual cycle to trigger ovulation.

Libido. Sexual drive and desire.

Lipid. A fat or fat-like substance. Elevated lipids are associated with an increased risk of cardiovascular disease.

Lipoprotein. A compound containing lipids and proteins.

Liquefaction. The process by which semen turns from a jelly-like consistency to liquid.

Lumen. The interior passageway of a tubular structure; its central cavity.

Lupron®. Brand name of leuprolide acetate, a GnRH analog.

Lupus Anticoagulant. See anticardiolipin antibodies.

Luteal Phase. The second half of the menstrual cycle after ovulation when the corpus luteum secretes large amounts of progesterone. This progesterone is important in preparing the endometrium to receive an embryo for implantation.

Luteal Phase Defect. A shorter than normal luteal phase or one with a progesterone deficit. A condition present when the lining of the uterus (endometrium) does not mature properly in response to progesterone secretion by the ovaries after ovulation. A luteal phase defect can result in early pregnancy loss.

Luteinizing Hormone (LH). In women, the pituitary hormone that triggers ovulation and stimulates the corpus luteum of the ovary to secrete progesterone and estrogen during the second half of the menstrual cycle. In the male, LH is the pituitary hormone that stimulates the testes to produce the male hormone testosterone.

Lutrepulse®. Brand name of gonadotropin releasing hormone (GnRH) given intravenously at regular intervals.

Magnetic Resonance Imaging (MRI). A diagnostic procedure that absorbs energy from specific high-frequency radio waves. The picture produced by measurement of these waves can be used to form precise images of internal organs without the use of x-ray techniques.

Male Factor. Infertility caused by a problem in the male reproductive tract, for example, inability of ejaculate or insufficient number of sperm.

Mammogram. An x-ray examination of the breasts.

McIndoe Procedure. A surgical procedure in which a skin graft is used to create a vagina.

Menarche. The age that an adolescent experiences her first menstrual period. The average age of menarche is approximately 12.8 years of age in the United States.

Menometrorrhagia. Heavy or irregular bleeding during and between menstrual periods.

Menopause. Natural cessation of ovarian function and menstruation. Menopause can occur between the ages of 42 and 56 but usually occurs around the age of 51, when the ovaries stop producing eggs and estrogen levels decline.

Menorrhagia. Regular but heavy menstrual bleeding which is excessive in either amount (greater than 80 cc – approximately five tablespoons) or duration (greater than seven days).

Menstruation. The normal, cyclic shedding of the endometrial lining (lining of the uterus), which appears as a bloody discharge from the uterus.

Methotrexate. A medication that hastens re-absorption of tissue in a woman with an ectopic pregnancy.

Metrorrhagia. Irregular bleeding from the uterus between normal menstrual periods.

Microepididymal Sperm Aspiration (MESA). Outpatient microsurgical procedure used to collect sperm in men with blockage of the male reproductive ducts such as prior vasectomy or absence of the vas deferens. Used in IVF-ICSI procedures.

Microinsemination. The IVF laboratory process whereby a small number of sperm are concentrated and placed close to the eggs to maximize the chance of fertilization.

Micromanipulation. The IVF laboratory process whereby the egg or embryo is held with special instruments and surgically altered by procedures . Micromanipulation techniques to facilitate fertilization include injection of a single sperm into an egg (intracytoplasmic sperm injection), injection of sperm under the membrane surrounding the egg (subzonal injection), and drilling a small hole in the membrane to allow the sperm easier access to the egg (partial zona dissection). The two most common embryo micromanipulation procedures are assisted hatching, a procedure in which the zona pellucida (outer covering) of the embryo is partially disrupted, usually by injection of acid, to facilitate embryo implantation and pregnancy, and embryo biopsy, in which one or more cells are removed from the embryo for the purposes of prenatal diagnosis.

Microsurgery. A type of surgery that uses magnification, meticulous technique, and fine suture material to get precise surgical results. Microsurgery is important for certain types of tubal surgery in the female, as well as for vasectomy reversal in the male.

Minoxidil. A medication used to lower blood pressure that was also found to promote hair growth. Loniten® and Rogaine® are brand names.

Miscarriage. The naturally occurring expulsion of a nonviable fetus and placenta from the uterus; also known as spontaneous abortion or pregnancy loss.

Mittelschmerz. A pain in the lower abdomen that is associated with ovulation.

Monozygotic. From "Mono" – one and "zygotic" – fertilized egg. One egg fertilized by a single sperm that divides into two embryos. Monozygotic twins are also called identical twins.

Morphology. The form, structure, and shape of sperm. Using World Health Organization criterial for normal, at least 30% of the sperm in a semen sample should have oval heads and slightly curving tails.

Motile. Moving.

Motility. The percentage of all moving sperm in a semen sample. Normally 50 percent or more are moving rapidly.

Mullerian Anomalies. Congenital abnormalities (birth defects) of the female reproductive organs that are derived from the mullerian ducts.

Mullerian Duct System. A pair of ducts parallel to the vertebrae in embryonic life. They develop into the female reproductive tract (fallopian tubes, uterus, cervix, and upper vagina).

Mullerian Dysgenesis. A birth defect in which the internal female reproductive organs do not develop completely, generally leading to the absence (agenesis) of the uterus, cervix, and upper part of the vagina. Also known as the Rokitansky Syndrome.

Multifetal Pregnancy Reduction. Also known as selective reduction. A procedure to reduce the number of fetuses in the uterus. This procedure is sometimes performed on women who are pregnant with multiple fetuses who are at an increased risk of late miscarriage or premature labor. These risks increase with the number of fetuses.

Myasthenia Gravis. A disorder of neuromuscular function characterized by extreme muscular weakness and fatigue. It may affect any muscle of the body, but especially those of the eye, face, lips, tongue, throat, and neck.

Mycoplasma. A class of bacteria that lack cell walls and may adversely affect the reproductive system.

Myomas. Benign (non-cancerous) tumors of the uterine muscle wall that can cause abnormal uterine bleeding and miscarriage. Also see Fibroids or Leiomyomas.

Myomectomy. The surgical removal of myomas (fibroids) from the uterus.

Myometrium. The muscular wall of the uterus.

Nodules. Knot-like growths of endometriosis.

Non-classic Adrenal Hyperplasia (NCAH). An inherited disorder in which the adrenal glands do not produce enough of the hormone cortisol and overproduce androgens. Elevation of the hormone 17a-hydroxyprogesterone is characteristic of NCAH. NCAH is a genetic disorder most commonly seen in certain ethnic groups including Ashkenazi Jews, Eskimos, and French-Canadians.

Oligomenorrhea. Light or infrequent uterine bleeding occurring at intervals of greater than 35 days.

Oligo-ovulatory. Infrequent ovulation.

Oocyte. Medical term for egg, the female gamete. Also called ovum.

Open Adoption. An adoption in which information is exchanged between birth parents and adoptive parents.

Operative Hysteroscopy. Surgery, such as removal of adhesions or tumors, performed inside the uterus using a hysteroscope.

Operative Laparoscopy. Surgery, such as removal of adhesions or endometriosis, performed inside the abdomen with a laparoscope and other long, slender instruments. The surgeon can sometimes cut and remove scar tissue and open closed fallopian tubes during this procedure.

Oral Contraceptive. Also known as birth control pills. The pills contain a mixture of synthetic estrogen and progestin. Proper usage prevents pregnancy by suppressing ovulation and decreasing the ovarian secretion of hormones, including androgens.

Osteoporosis. A condition characterized by loss of bone mass, decreased bone density, and enlargement of bone spaces resulting in bone fragility. Osteoporosis results from disturbances of gastrointestinal absorption, nutrition, mineral metabolism, and low estrogen levels in women and often occurs with menopause.

Ova (plural of ovum). Eggs.

Ovarian Cysts. Fluid-filled cysts on the ovaries.

Ovarian Drilling. A laparoscopic procedure, using laser or electrocautery, to destroy the androgen-producing tissue in the ovaries. This procedure is usually a last resort for ovulation induction in PCOS patients who have not responded to hormonal treatments.

Ovarian Hyperstimulation Syndrome. A condition that may result from ovulation induction characterized by enlargement of the ovaries, fluid retention, and weight gain.

Ovarian Reserve. Refers to a woman's fertility potential in the absence of any problems in the reproductive tract (fallopian tubes, uterus, and vagina). It mainly depends on the number and quality of eggs in the ovaries and how well the ovarian follicles are responding to the hormonal signals from the brain. Diminished ovarian reserve is associated with depletion in the number of eggs and worsening of oocyte quality.

Ovarian Stimulation. See Ovulation induction.

Ovulation. The release of a mature egg from its developing follicle in the outer layer of the ovary. This usually occurs approximately 14 days before the next menstrual period (the 14th day of a 28-day cycle).

Ovulation Detection Kit. These commercially available kits use paper dip sticks that show changes in the levels of luteinizing hormone (LH) in the urine. Once the LH surge has occurred, ovulation usually takes place within 12 to 44 hours. Urine testing usually begins two days prior to the expected day of ovulation. Also called ovulation prediction kit.

Ovulation Induction. Originally used to refer to the administration of ovulation drugs to achieve follicle development and ovulation in women who were anovulatory. It also refers to the administration of ovulation drugs that stimulate the ovaries to produce multiple mature follicles. Sometimes called enhanced follicular recruitment or controlled ovarian hyperstimulation.

Parathyroid. Any of four small kidney shaped glands that lie in pairs near the thyroid gland and secrete parathyroid hormone, which is necessary for calcium and phosphorous metabolism.

Partial Salpingectomy. An operation where the section of a fallopian tube containing an ectopic pregnancy is removed. This procedure attempts to preserve most of the tube for future fertility.

PCOD. See polycystic ovarian syndrome.

Percutaneous Epididymal Sperm Aspiration (PESA). A sperm aspiration procedure in which a needle is inserted into the epididymis (gland that carries sperm from testicle to vas deferens) to retrieve sperm for use in an IVF procedure.

Pergonal®. Brand name of the first commercially marketed human menopausal gonadotropins (hMG): see human menopausal gonadotropins (hMG).

Perimenopausal Transition. The end of a woman's reproductive years when the ovaries lose their ability to secrete estrogen and progesterone in a regular fashion.

Perimenopause. The years that immediately precede cessation of menstrual periods (menopause); usually about five years before menopause.

Perinatologist. A maternal-fetal medicine specialist.

Peritoneum. The smooth transparent membrane that lines the abdominal and pelvic cavities.

Pituitary Adenoma. Benign (non-cancerous) tumors of the pituitary gland that are often associated with excessive prolactin production.

Pituitary Gland. A small hormone-producing gland just beneath the hypothalamus in the brain that controls the ovaries, thyroid, and adrenal glands, and also produces growth hormone. Ovarian function is controlled through the secretion of follicle stimulating hormone (FSH) and luteinizing hormone (LH). Disorders of this gland may lead to irregular or absent ovulation in the female and abnormal or absent sperm production in the male.

Placenta. A disk-shaped vascular organ attached to the wall of the uterus and to the fetus by the umbilical cord. It provides nourishment to the fetus.

Platelets. Circulating blood components that aid in blood clotting and prevention of bleeding.

Pneumonia. Lung inflammation.

Polycystic Ovarian Disease (PCOD). See polycystic ovarian syndrome.

Polycystic Ovarian Syndrome (PCOS). A condition associated with chronic anovulation and overproduction of androgens (male hormones), in which the ovaries contain many small cystic follicles. Symptoms may include irregular menstrual periods, obesity, excessive growth of body hair in a male-like pattern (hirsutism), and infertility. Also called Stein-Leventhal Syndrome.

Polymenorrhea. Uterine bleeding occurring at regular intervals of fewer than 21 days.

Polyps. A general term that describes any mass of tissue that bulges or projects outward or upward from the normal surface level.

Postcoital Test (PCT). The microscopic analysis of a cervical mucus sample, usually collected within 18 hours after intercourse. This test determines the quality of cervical mucus and the ability of sperm to enter and penetrate the mucus. Also called the Sims-Huhner test.

Postmenopausal. A term used to refer to the time after menopause.

Prednisone. A synthetic cortisone-like steroid medication sometimes prescribed to treat immune disorders or an overactive adrenal gland.

Preeclampsia. A disorder occurring during pregnancy that affects both the mother and the fetus. Preeclampsia is characterized by high blood pressure, swelling, and protein found in the urine. This disorder, also known as toxemia, can restrict the flow of blood to the placenta.

Preimplantation genetic diagnosis (PGD). A test performed by an embryologist in which one or two cells are removed from an embryo and then tested for genetic abnormalities, chromosomal abnormalities, or genetic sex. PGD is performed in conjunction with IVF.

Premature Ovarian Failure. Cessation of menstrual periods due to failure of the ovaries before age 40. Also see Early Menopause.

Primary Dysmenorrhea. Lower abdominal pain associated with menstrual periods that decrease with age.

Primary Infertility. Infertility in those who have never had children.

Private Adoption. An adoption that takes place outside an agency. It is usually facilitated by a lawyer, minister, or physician who serves as an intermediary between the potential birth parents and the adoptive parents.

Progestational Agents. Medications that mimic the effect of progesterone. Also called progestogens.

Progesterone. A female hormone secreted by the corpus luteum after ovulation during the second half of the menstrual cycle (luteal phase). It prepares the lining of the uterus (endometrium) for implantation of a fertilized egg and also allows for complete shedding of the endometrium at the time of menstruation. In the event of pregnancy, the progesterone level remains stable beginning a week or so after conception.

Progestin. A synthetic hormone that has an action similar to progesterone. Synonymous with progestational hormones.

Progestogen. Progesterone or any progestin. Analogous to progestational agent.

Prolactin. A hormone secreted by the pituitary gland into the bloodstream for the purpose of maintaining milk production during lactation. When secreted in excessive amounts, it may lead to irregular or absent menstrual periods and may produce a milk-like discharge from the breasts.

Pronuclear Stage. Also called zygote. A one cell embryo, an early stage of fertilization, in which the sperm has penetrated the egg but before cell division has begun. The nucleus of the sperm and the nucleus of the egg (2-pronuclei) are visible under a microscope. Each pronucleus contains 23 chromosomes. The egg and sperm pronuclei later fuse together, which sets the stage for the first cell division.

Pronuclear Stage Transfer (PROST). See zygote intrafallopian transfer (ZIFT).

Pronuclei. The nucleus of a male or female gamete (egg or sperm) seen in the one cell embryo (zygote).

Prostaglandins. A group of acids found throughout the body, especially in semen, that stimulate smooth muscle tissue and affect blood pressure, metabolism, body temperature, and other body processes. In women, prostaglandins are hormone-like chemicals produced in large amounts by endometrial cells. They stimulate the uterine muscles to contract and are largely responsible for menstrual cramps.

Prostate Gland. The gland located below the bladder in males where the ejaculatory ducts, the two vas deferens, and the urethra join. It contributes fluid to the ejaculate.

Proximal Tubal Blockage. Tubal blockage that occurs near where the fallopian tubes join the uterus.

Pseudo-menopause. A hormonal state created by taking medication that mimics the symptoms of menopause and characterized by low estrogen levels similar to those found at menopause.

Pubic Region. The region at the base of the abdomen above the external genitalia and covered in part with hair.

Pubis. The bony region at the base of the abdomen.

Radiation Therapy. Treatment with high-energy rays to kill or damage cancer cells. External radiation therapy uses a machine to aim high-energy rays at the cancer growth. Internal radiation therapy is the placement of radioactive material inside the body as close as possible to the cancer.

Recipient. A person who receives donated eggs, sperm, or embryos.

Rectum. The lowest segment of the intestines attached to the anus.

Recurrent Miscarriage. Consecutive pregnancy loss (two or three) before 20 weeks gestation. The fetus usually weighs less than one pound.

RESOLVE. A national support group for people with infertility. RESOLVE's mailing address is 7910 Woodmont Ave, Suite 1350, Bethesda, MD 20814. 301-654-8585. www.resolve.org

Respiratory Distress Syndrome (RDS). A lung disease that effects premature infants and causes increasing difficulty in breathing.

Retrograde Ejaculation. A condition that causes the ejaculate to be released backward into the bladder at male climax.

Reversible Menopause. A temporary hormonal state created by taking GnRH analogs in which estrogen levels fall to menopause levels, ovulation does not occur, the endometrium does not grow, and menstruation does not occur.

Rheumatoid Arthritis. A chronic autoimmune disease of the joints characterized by inflammation and deterioration of the bones.

Rh sensitized. A condition whereby an Rh-negative woman has been immunized (sensitized) to the Rh-factor through previous exposure to this antigen. An Rh-positive fetus may suffer significant intrauterine and immediate post-delivery consequences that can lead to significant handicaps and/or death.

Rubella. A viral infection also known as German measles and characterized by general redness and swollen glands. Infection during pregnancy can cause severe congenital abnormalities (birth defects) in the fetus.

Sacrum. The last lumbar vertebra of the spinal column; the base of the spine.

Salpingectomy. An operation where one or both of the fallopian tubes are removed.

Salpingitis Isthmica Nodosa (SIN). A thickening or nodular appearance of the interior walls of the fallopian tubes.

Salpingo-oophorectomy. Removal of the fallopian tube and ovary together.

Salpingostomy. A surgical procedure where the wall of the fallopian tube is opened and the ectopic pregnancy is removed. The tubal incision heals spontaneously.

SART Registry. An ongoing collection of results from participating assisted reproductive technology clinics developed and maintained by the Society for Assisted Reproductive Technology (SART), a society affiliated with the American Society for Reproductive Medicine (ASRM).

Scrotum. The pouch of skin and other tissues that contain the testes in the male.

Secondary Dysmenorrhea. Lower abdominal pain associated with menstrual periods that begins later in a woman's reproductive lifespan. It may be due to an abnormal condition such as endometriosis or infection.

Secondary Infertility. Infertility in those who have previously been fertile.

Semen. The fluid in which sperm are located that comes out of the urethra when a man ejaculates.

Semen Analysis. The microscopic examination of semen (the male ejaculate) to determine its volume, the number of sperm (sperm count), their shapes (morphology), and their ability to move (motility) in addition to other parameters.

Semen Viscosity. The thickness of semen. Semen is ejaculated as a liquid, then becomes jelly-like and then turns to liquid again.

Semen Volume. The amount of semen. The normal amount of semen per ejaculate is two to five milliliters (approximately one teaspoon).

Seminal Plasma. The fluid in which the sperm is ejaculated. Seminal plasma makes up most of the fluid volume of semen.

Seminal Vesicles. Two oblong glands behind the bladder that join each vas deferens and empty into the urethra. They contribute about 90 percent of the fluid volume of semen.

Seminiferous Tubules. The tiny tubes in the testes where sperm cells grow and mature.

Septate Uterus. A congenital abnormality (birth defect) in which the uterus has a normally appearing outer surface, but has a central wall of fibrous tissue (septum) within the uterine cavity.

Septum. See uterine septum.

Serophene®. See clomiphene citrate.

Serotonin. A neurochemical that affects mood and appetite.

Sexually Transmitted Infection (STI). An infection, such as chlamydia or gonorrhea, that is transmitted by sexual activity. In the female, some STIs can cause pelvic infections and lead to infertility by damaging the fallopian tubes and increasing the risk of ectopic pregnancy. In the male, STIs can cause blockage of the ductal system that transports sperm.

Singleton. Offspring (child) born singly.

Skin Graft. A piece of skin that is taken from one area and grafted to another area.

Society for Assisted Reproductive Technology (SART). A society affiliated with the American Society for Reproductive Medicine (ASRM) and comprised of representatives from assisted reproductive technology programs that have demonstrated their ability to perform IVF and other assisted reproductive technologies.

Sonogram. An image produced by ultrasound, which uses high-frequency sound waves to form a picture of internal organs on a monitor screen.

Sonohysterography. A technique that involves injecting fluid into the uterus and fallopian tubes and using ultrasound to observe the image of these structures on a monitor screen. Also called saline infusion sonography.

Special needs adoption. Adoption of a child who has special health or emotional needs.

Speculum. A device inserted into the vagina to allow visualization of the cervix.

Sperm. The male reproductive cells that fertilize a woman's egg. The sperm head carries genetic material (chromosomes), the midpiece produces energy for movement, and the long, thin tail wiggles to propel the sperm.

Sperm Aspiration. A technique that uses a very fine needle to remove (aspirate) sperm from the testes or from the tubes leading from the testes. This technique may be recommended for a male who has no sperm in his ejaculate.

Sperm Antibody Test. A test in which the blood, semen, or cervical mucus is examined to detect antibodies to sperm. Antibodies can contribute to infertility in men or women.

Sperm Autoimmunity. An allergy to sperm that may be present in a man against his own sperm. This can lead to abnormalities of sperm function and infertility.

Sperm Capacitation. A laboratory process to increase the ability of sperm to penetrate and fertilize an egg.

Sperm Count. The number of sperm per milliliter of semen. A normal count is usually 20 million or more per milliliter.

Sperm Morphology. The shape of individual sperm as seen under a microscope. At least 30 percent of the sperm in a routine semen analysis should have oval heads and slightly curving tails.

Sperm Motility. The percentage of all moving sperm in a semen sample. Normally 50 percent or more are moving rapidly.

Sperm Penetration Assay. A test to help evaluate the fertilizing ability of a man's sperm. A semen sample is incubated with specially treated hamster eggs to determine if the sperm can penetrate them.

Sperm Preparation. A procedure to remove seminal fluid from sperm cells.

Sperm Washing. A procedure to remove seminal fluid from sperm cells before intrauterine insemination or other assisted reproductive technologies.

Spina Bifida. A birth defect of the spinal column. Spina bifida is the failure of the spine to close properly during development.

Spironolactone (Aldactone®). A synthetic steroid hormone that directly blocks the effect of androgens on the skin. It initially was used as a diuretic or water pill to increase urine output and treat hypertension.

Spontaneous Ovulation. Naturally occurring ovulation.

Stein-Leventhal Syndrome. See polycystic ovarian syndrome.

Steroids. Hormones that are derived from cholesterol. Categories of steroids include sex steroids (estrogens, androgens, and progestogens), glucocorticoids (hormones that closely resemble cortisol), and mineralcorticoids (hormones related to aldosterone and involved in fluid and electrolyte control). Man-made steroids closely resemble cortisol, a hormone naturally produced by the adrenal glands. Steroids decrease inflammation, reduce immune system activity, and are used to treat a variety of inflammatory diseases and conditions.

Strassman Procedure. A major abdominal surgery in which a bicornuate uterus is reconstructed to form a more normal uterus.

Submucous Fibroids. Fibroids that are found underneath the uterine lining within the uterine cavity.

Subserous Fibroids. Fibroids that are located beneath the outer covering of the uterus.

Superovulation. The administration of fertility medications in a manner intended to achieve development and ovulation of multiple ovarian follicles. Superovulation is often combined with intrauterine insemination as an infertility treatment (see controlled superovulation).

Superovulation with Timed Intrauterine Insemination. A procedure to facilitate fertilization. The woman is given ovulation inducing drugs that cause her ovaries to produce multiple eggs. When the eggs are ready to be released, the woman is inseminated with her partner's sperm or donated sperm.

Suprapubic Punctures. Incisions made directly above the pubis.

Surrogacy. An arrangement in which a woman is inseminated with the sperm of a man who is not her partner in order to conceive and carry a child to be reared by the biologic (genetic) father and his partner. The surrogate is genetically related to the child. The biologic father and his partner usually must adopt the child after its birth.

Surrogate. A woman who carries a pregnancy intended for another family.

Suture. Thread used to close an incision made during surgery. It is generally absorbable or self-dissolving.

Symmetric. Able to divide into equal similar sides.

Synarel®. Brand name of a GnRH analog.

Systemic Lupus Erythematosus. A disorder where antibodies are produced against an individual's own tissues, which can result in damage to many body systems or tissues.

Tay-Sachs Disease. A fatal heredity disorder characterized by mental retardation and paralysis. This condition is most common in offspring from Jewish couples of eastern European descent.

Terminal Hair. The long, coarse, thick hairs that normally grow in the scalp, pubic, and armpit areas of men and women, and the face, chest, abdomen, upper arms and upper thighs of men.

Testes. The two male reproductive glands located in the scrotum that produce testosterone and sperm.

Testicular Sperm Extraction (TESE). Operative removal of testicular tissue in an attempt to collect living sperm for use in an IVF-ICSI procedure.

Testosterone. In men, the primary male hormone produced by the testes which is responsible for the development of sperm, male physical characteristics, and sex drive. Testosterone is also produced in small quantities by the ovaries in women.

Thrombophlebitis. An inflamed vein caused by a blood clot.

Thyroid Gland. A large, two-lobed, endocrine gland located in front of and on either side of the trachea (windpipe) in the neck that secretes the hormone thyroxin, which maintains normal body growth and metabolism.

Thyroid Hormone. A hormone produced by the thyroid gland that regulates growth and metabolism.

Tocolytic Agents. Medications that may slow or stop premature labor.

Toxemia. See Preeclampsia.

Transcervical Cannulation. An x-ray technique for opening a fallopian tube that is blocked proximally (at the junction of the uterus) using a narrow, flexible tube inserted through the vagina into the tube; can also be used for GIFT or ZIFT. Also known as selective salpingography or retrograde hysterosalpingography.

Transvaginal Ultrasound Aspiration. An ultrasound guided technique for egg retrieval whereby a long, thin needle is passed through the vagina into the ovarian follicle and suction is applied to accomplish retrieval. Also known as ultrasound-guided egg aspiration and transvaginal egg retrieval.

Transverse Vaginal Septum. A birth defect in the form of a thick ridge across the vagina. The blockage can be either complete or partial.

Trocar. An instrument used to make an incision in the abdominal wall through which the laparoscope is placed for diagnostic or operative laparoscopy.

Tubal Embryo Transfer (TET). A process where an early stage embryo is transferred to the fallopian tube.

Tubal Ligation. A surgical procedure where the fallopian tubes are clamped, clipped, or cut to prevent pregnancy.

Tubal (ectopic) Pregnancy. A fertilized egg that implants within the fallopian tube rather than the uterine cavity. Under these conditions, the tube can rupture and bleed. Tubal pregnancies can be fatal if they are not identified and treated early.

Turner Syndrome. A condition in which the female has only one X chromosome instead of two and is associated with short stature, failure to undergo normal sexual development, and other physical abnormalities.

Ulcer. A lesion (sore) on the surface of the skin or on a mucous surface, usually inflamed. As an occasional side effect of methotrexate therapy, temporary ulcers may form in the mouth.

Ultrasound. Also called a sonogram. A picture of internal organs produced by high frequency sound waves viewed as an image on a video screen; used to monitor growth of ovarian follicles, retrieve eggs, and evaluate a pregnancy. Ultrasound can be performed either abdominally or vaginally.

Ultrasound-Guided Egg Aspiration (retrieval). A technique in which an ultrasound-guided needle is passed into the ovary, and an egg is removed by suction. Usually the needle is passed through the vagina. Also known as transvaginal ultrasound aspiration. See Egg Retrieval.

Unicornuate Uterus. A congenital abnormality (birth defect) in which only one-half of the uterus is formed from either the left or right side of the mullerian duct system. The other side of the Mullerian system fails to develop into the other half of the uterus. Also called hemiuterus.

Ureters. Tubes connecting each kidney to the bladder, often abnormal in females with mullerian duct defects or males with an absent vas deferens.

Urethra. In men, the tube leading from the bladder that carries urine and semen out of the body. In women, the tube leading from the bladder that carries urine out of the body.

Urinary Retention. The inability to spontaneously empty the bladder.

Urogenital Sinus. A tube-like organ in the fetus where the bladder, part of the vagina, and the rectum begin to develop in the female. In the male, the urogenital sinus develops into the bladder, urethra, and rectum.

Uterine Fibroids. Abnormal masses of smooth muscle tissue (non-cancerous tumors) that grow within the uterine wall. Also called fibroids, myomas, or leiomyomas.

Uterine Fundus. The large upper end of the uterus.

Uterine Remnant. The remains of an abnormally developed portion of the uterus.

Uterine Septum. A band of fibrous tissue present from birth that forms a wall extending from the top of the uterine cavity. A septum may increase the risk of miscarriage and other pregnancy complications.

Uterosacral Ligaments. Ligaments that attach the lowest part of the uterus and the cervix to the sacrum.

Uterus (womb). The hollow, muscular organ in the pelvis where an embryo implants and grows during pregnancy.

Vagina. The genital canal in the female that leads from the vulva (external genitalia) to the cervix and uterus.

Vaginal Hysterectomy. Removal of the uterus through the vagina.

Vaginal Suppository. A solid but meltable cone of medicated material inserted into the vagina.

Vaginoplasty. Surgical creation of a vagina.

Varicocele. A varicose or dilated vein within the scrotum that can cause infertility in some men.

Vascular. Relating to blood vessels.

Vascular Thrombosis. A blood clot in a blood vessel.

Vas deferens. The two muscular tubes that carry sperm from the epididymis to the urethra.

Vasoepididymostomy. A surgical procedure to connect the vas deferens to the epididymis in order to bypass an obstruction in the epididymis, sometimes used for vasectomy reversal.

Vasovasostomy. A surgical procedure to reconnect the severed ends of the vas deferens. Often called "vasectomy reversal."

Vellus Hair. The soft, fine, usually short hairs that appear on the face, chest, and back of women, giving the impression of "hairless" skin.

Venous Thrombosis. A blood clot in a vein.

Viable Intrauterine Pregnancy. An embryo that has implanted appropriately in the wall of the uterus and appears to be growing well.

Vulva. Outer lips of the vagina.

Zona Pellucida. The egg's outer layer that a sperm must penetrate to fertilize the egg.

Zygote. A fertilized egg before cell division (cleavage) begins. See Pronuclear Stage Embryo.

Zygote Intrafallopian Transfer (ZIFT). An assisted reproductive technology procedure in which an egg is fertilized in the laboratory and the zygote is transferred to the fallopian tube at the pronuclear stage (after fertilization but before cell division) takes place. The eggs are retrieved and fertilized on one day and the embryo is transferred the following day.

Author Index

Subject Index

AAMFT. *See* American Association of Marriage and Family Therapy
ACMG. *See* American College of Medical Genetics
ACOG. *See* American College of Obstetricians and Gynecologists
acupuncture, 202–203
  electroacupuncture, 202
  β endorphin levels after, 202–209
  GnRH normalization from, 202
  IVF and, 202
  male infertility and, 203, 211
  ovulation and, 202
  pregnancy and, 202–203
ADA. *See* Americans with Disabilities Act
Adjustment Disorder, 99, 103
adolescence, as parenthood stage, 472
adopted children. *See* children, adopted
adoption, 15, 33, 406–407
  See also adoption agencies; complex adoption theory; domestic adoption; independent adoption; international adoption; transracial adoption
  aboriginal, in Australia, 388
  Adoption and Safe Families Act, 396
  attachment and loss theory and, 393
  birth parent relationships, 402–403
  in China, 388
  complex adoption theory, 11, 395
  DI v., 306–307, 314
  domestic, 389, 395–397
  embryo v. ED, 358
  enforced Native-American, in United States, 388
  EuroAdopt program, 400
  family systems theory and, 394–395
  as family-building, 8, 9, 10, 12, 403–405
  fears about, 401
  grief therapy during, 405
  home studies for, 400–401
  identity formation and, 393–394
  after infertility, 387

  infertility counseling and, 390, 401–402, 407
  information disclosure as part of, 391
  information sources about, 405–406
  intercountry, 389
  international, 388, 389, 391–393, 398–399
  Islam and, 74
  migration's influence on, 388
  parent education of, 395–401
  prenatal, 526
  Protection of Children and Co-Operation in Respect of Intercountry Adoption, 389, 398
  psychological issues as part of, 401
  psychosocial adjustment to, 390–391
  as relationship realignment, 387
  in Romania, 388
  social stigma of, 388, 389
  social transitions towards, 407
  transnational policies for, 388
  transracial, 392–393, 399–400
adoption agencies
  domestic, 395–397
  Welcome Home, 388
Adoption and Safe Families Act, 396
adrenal hormones, 241
advanced maternal age, 270–271, 450, 466–467
  American Society for Reproductive Medicine on, 513
  Canadian Fertility and Andrology Society on, 513
  Down syndrome from, 271
  European Society of Human Reproduction and Embryology on, 513
  infertility counseling for, 513–514
  OD and, 332–333, 513
  post-infertility pregnancy during, 450–451
  pregnancy risks for, 450
  prenatal testing for, 451
advocacy organizations. *See* organizations, advocacy

affective disorders, 98–99, 103
  Adjustment Disorder, 99, 103
  bipolar disorders, 99
  depression, 98–99
  pathological grief, 98
Africa. *See also* Egypt; Mozambique; Nigeria
  childlessness in, 415
  DI in, 306
  female circumcision in, 214, 413
  female sexual expression in, 214–215
  fertility rites in, female, 3, 74
  male infertility in, 40, 413
  reproduction in, social importance of, 413
  sub-Saharan, female infertility in, 42, 71
age
  advanced maternal, 270–271, 466–467
  ART and, as factor for, 173
  childlessness and, for females, 415
  female infertility and, 50–51
  fertility and, for males, 271
  infertility treatment withdrawal and, 430
  male infertility and, 47
  miscarriages and, 300
  OD and, 332–333
  parental, surrogacy and, 385
  preconception counseling and, 270–271
  pregnancy rates by, Spain,
  pregnancy rates by, United States, 50
  semen analysis and, 246
AHR. *See* Assisted Human Reproduction Act
AHRA. *See* Assisted Human Reproduction Agency
alarm reactions, 170
alcohol/drug usage, 190–191
  male reproductive hormones and, 191
  sperm production after, 188
Alcoholics Anonymous, 49
alexithymia, from male infertility, 40
allocentrism, 69

counseling, couples (*cont.*)
  social support outside of, 89
  spoiled identity in, 152
  stage theories and, 144
  welfare of the child as goal of, 147
counseling, genetic, 13, 261–262, 264,
  265–267. *See also* counseling,
  preconception; counselors, genetic
  ART and, 268, 269
  biopsychosocial medicine approach
    to, 264
  client-centered, 263
  collaborative treatment approach to,
    264
  communication approach to, 263
  family pedigree assessment for, 262
  family systems theory and, 264
  gender responses to, 266
  Internet resources for, 594
  non-directive, 263
  preconception, 269–272
  psychological aspects of, 265, 269
  psychotherapy v., 263
  reproductive, 272–277
  requirements for, 261
counseling, grief, 137
counseling, group, 15, 156
  altruism as part of, 160
  Beck Depression Inventory in, 159
  behaviorally oriented, 103
  catharsis in, 160
  CBT in, 158, 164–165, 168
  cognitive restructuring from, 157
  collective therapy as, 157
  confidentiality as part of, 162
  coping strategies and, 164
  curative factors of, 159
  decision-making as part of, 164
  diagnostic conditions and, 157–158
  emotive-interactional, 165
  encounter groups and, 157
  gender differences within, 163–164
  grief therapies under, 163
  history of, 156–157
  imitative behaviors within, 160
  for infertility, 405
  Internet groups, 166
  interpersonal learning from, 160
  loss of control in, 163
  for medical staff, 166
  membership in, 162
  pregnancy during, 159, 164
  psycho-educational, 165
  social cohesion within, 160
  socialization development in, 160,
    164
  stages of, 162–163
  structure of, 161–162
  support groups v., 161
  technology-mediated, 166
  themes within, 163
  Transcendental Meditation as, 157
  treatment teams in, 164
  universality of, 160
  weight loss under, 158

counseling, infertility, 2, 5, 55, 493, 527.
  See also Collaborative Reproductive
  Healthcare Model; counseling,
  couples; counseling, group;
  counseling, multicultural;
  counselors, infertility; psychological
  evaluations
  abnormality issues as part of, 252–253
  access to, 554
  adoption as part of, 390, 401–402, 407
  for advanced maternal age, 513–514
  American Society for Reproductive
    Medicine guidelines, 527
  for ART, 129, 486
  ART's influence on, 494
  behavioral medicines in, 15
  Boulder model for, 120
  after breast cancer, 251
  British Infertility Counseling
    Association guidelines, 505
  Canadian regulation of, 528
  for cancer, 54–59
  children's welfare as factor in, 553
  clinical issues within, 126
  cognitive-behavioral treatments for,
    15
  Collaborative Reproductive
    Healthcare Model for, 495–497
  common factors within, 121
  compassion fatigue v. burnout in,
    498
  competency in, 14
  complementary and alternative
    medical approaches to, 15
  coping strategies as part of, 119
  counter-transference in, 253–254, 497
  for couples, 15, 23, 26
  CPHI, 88, 125, 178, 563
  crisis intervention therapy in, 15
  cultural resistance to, 75
  culturally-sensitive, 12
  denial of treatment, 405
  for DI, 310–312
  after diabetes diagnosis, 251
  for endometriosis, 52
  ethics literature for, 511
  European Society of Human
    Reproduction and Embryology
    guidelines, 24
  family therapies in, 15
  fear as factor in, 405
  for gamete donations, 341
  for gay males, 506, 514
  genetic counseling as part of, 13
  goals of, 13, 119
  grief and, 15
  gynecologists as part of, 23
  history of, 129, 493–494
  after HIV diagnosis, 251
  hostility in, 180–181
  Human Fertilization and Embryo
    Authority guidelines, 15
  after hypertension diagnosis, 251
  implication/decision-making
    therapies as part of, 15

independent clinical practice for,
  499–500
for individuals, 15
Infertility Counseling Award, 505,
  528
initial visits for, 24, 25
integrationist approach to, 121
International Infertility Counseling
  Organization, 14
intervention-focused, 120–121
legislation for, 5
with limited life expectancy, 252
literature about, 494
medical examinations as part of, 25
medical issues for, 12–13, 252
medical organizations and, 5
medical staff collaboration with, 498
mind-body programs for, 120
models for, 11, 12
mortality issues as part of, 252
multicultural, 63, 65, 66, 67, 77–78
multi-modal approach to, 123
National Association of Social
  Workers guidelines, 527
for OD, 333
patient collaboration as part of,
  497–498
PGD during, 22, 35
for physicians, 436, 441
for post-infertility pregnancy, 16, 17,
  451–452, 454–455
post-treatment, 435, 441
practice issues for, 13–14
with pre-existing illnesses, 513
pregnancy loss and, 13
psychodynamic therapy in, 15,
  133–134
psycho-education in, 181–183
in psychological consequences theory,
  7
Psychological Special Interest Group
  guidelines, 322
psychometric testing as part of,
  552–553
psychosocial assessment during, 14
psychotherapy v., 132–133
RCTs and, 120, 123
relaxation training as part of, 119
religion as factor in, 78
reproductive health psychology as,
  169
sexual counseling as part of, 15, 119,
  230
for S/GCs, 449
shame and, 405
S-P model for, 120, 122–123
standards of care for, 505–506
strategic/solution-focused brief
  therapies in, 15
stratification of services, 2, 8, 18,
  215
study parameters for, 118
tasks as part of, 501, 502
teams for, 23–24
testicular cancer and, 48, 249

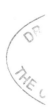